Y0-AQL-064

Surgical Nutrition

Surgical Nutrition

Edited by

Josef E. Fischer, M.D.
Chairman and Christian R. Holmes Professor, Department of Surgery, University of Cincinnati College of Medicine; Surgeon-in-Chief, University Hospital, Christian R. Holmes Hospital, and Children's Hospital Medical Center, Cincinnati, Ohio

Little, Brown and Company, Boston, Toronto

First Edition

Library of Congress Catalog Card No. 82-82687

ISBN 0-316-28371-1

Printed in the United States of America

MV

Contents

Contributing Authors

Ronald M. Abel, M.D.
Associate Professor of Surgery, College of Medicine and Dentistry of New Jersey—New Jersey Medical School; Director, Nutritional Support Service and Associate Director, Department of Thoracic and Cardiovascular Surgery, Newark Beth Israel Medical Center, Newark
Chapter 20

J. Wesley Alexander, M.D., Sc.D.
Professor of Surgery, University of Cincinnati College of Medicine; Director, Transplantation Division, University of Cincinnati Medical Center; Director of Research, Shriners Burns Institute, Cincinnati Unit, Cincinnati, Ohio
Chapter 16

Louis H. Aulick, Ph.D.
Clinical Adjunct Assistant Professor of Surgery, Uniformed Services University of the Health Sciences, Bethesda, Maryland; Research Physiologist, Surgical Study Branch, U.S. Army Institute of Surgical Research, Brooke Army Medical Center, Fort Sam Houston, Texas
Chapter 3

Richard A. Becker, M.D.
Assistant Professor of Medicine, The University of Texas Medical School at San Antonio, San Antonio; Consulting Physician, University of Health Sciences Center at San Antonio, San Antonio, and Institute of Surgical Research-Burn Unit, Brooke Army Medical Center, Fort Sam Houston, Texas
Chapter 3

W. Fraser Bremner, M.D., Ph.D.
Associate Professor of Medicine, Internal Medicine, Cardiology Division, University of Cincinnati College of Medicine; Attending Physician, University Hospital, Cincinnati, Ohio
Chapter 7

Murray F. Brennan, M.D., F.A.C.S.
Professor of Surgery, Cornell University Medical College; Attending Surgeon and Chief, Gastric and Mixed Tumor Service, Memorial Sloan-Kettering Cancer Center, New York
Chapter 14

Bruno Cianciaruso, M.D.
Assistant, Division of Nephrology, Second Faculty of Medicine, University of Naples; Assistant, Nuovo Policlinico, Second Faculty of Medicine and Surgery, University of Naples, Naples, Italy
Chapter 18

Edward M. Copeland III, M.D.
Professor and Chairman, Department of Surgery, University of Florida College of Medicine, Gainesville
Chapter 15

John M. Daly, M.D.
Associate Professor of Surgery, Cornell University Medical College; Associate Attending Surgeon, Memorial Sloan-Kettering Cancer Center, New York
Chapter 15

Stanley J. Dudrick, M.D., F.A.C.S.
Professor of Surgery, The University of Texas Medical School at Houston; Director, Nutritional Support Services, Saint Luke's Episcopal Hospital, Houston
Chapter 15

Robert J. Fairfull-Smith, M.B., F.R.C.S.(C)
Assistant Professor of Surgery, University of Ottawa Faculty of Medicine; Director, Nutrition and Metabolism Laboratory, Ottawa General Hospital, Ottawa, Ontario, Canada
Chapter 23

Josef E. Fischer, M.D.
Chairman and Christian R. Holmes Professor, Department of Surgery, University of Cincinnati College of Medicine; Surgeon-in-Chief, University Hospital, Christian R. Holmes Hospital, and Children's Hospital Medical Center, Cincinnati, Ohio
Chapters 17, 22

Joel B. Freeman, M.D., C.M., F.R.C.S.(C), F.A.C.S.
Associate Professor of Surgery, University of Ottawa Faculty of Medicine; Chief, Division of General Surgery, Ottawa General Hospital, Ottawa, Ontario, Canada
Chapter 23

Herbert R. Freund, M.D.
Associate Professor of Surgery, Hebrew University-Hadassah Medical School; Chief Physician, Department of Surgery and Director, Nutritional Support Unit, Hadassah University Medical Center, Jerusalem, Israel
Chapter 22

Zvi Gimmon, M.D.
Senior Lecturer in Surgery, Hebrew University-Hadassah Medical School; Chief Physician, Department of Surgery A, Hadassah University Medical Center, Jerusalem, Israel
Chapter 8

J. Thomas Goodgame, Jr., M.D.
Associate Surgeon, Morton F. Plant Hospital, Clearwater, Florida
Chapter 26

Khursheed N. Jeejeebhoy, M.B., B.S., Ph.D., F.R.C.P.(C)
Professor of Medicine, University of Toronto Faculty of Medicine; Senior Physician, Department of Medicine, Toronto General Hospital, Toronto, Ontario, Canada
Chapter 21

Bengt Jeppsson, M.D., Ph.D.
Associate Professor of Surgery, University of Lund, Lund, Sweden; formerly Clinical and Research Fellow, Nutritional Support Service, University Hospital, Cincinnati, Ohio
Chapter 8

Ronald G. Kay, M.B., F.R.C.S. (Eng.), F.R.A.C.S.
Associate Professor of Surgery, University of Auckland School of Medicine; Consulting Surgeon, Auckland Hospital, Auckland, New Zealand
Chapter 9

John M. Kinney, M.D.
Professor of Surgery, Columbia University College of Physicians and Surgeons; Attending Surgeon, The Presbyterian Hospital, New York
Chapter 4

Grant S. Knight, Ph.D.
Biochemist, Department of Surgery, University of Auckland School of Medicine, Auckland, New Zealand
Chapter 9

Joel D. Kopple, M.D.
Professor of Medicine and Public Health, UCLA School of Medicine (University of California, Los Angeles), Los Angeles; Chief, Division of Nephrology and Hypertension, Harbor-UCLA Medical Center, Torrance
Chapter 18

Kenneth A. Kudsk, M.D.
Resident in Surgery, The Ohio State University College of Medicine and Ohio State University Hospital, Columbus; formerly Fellow in Trauma and Burn Research, University of California, San Francisco, School of Medicine and San Francisco General Hospital, San Francisco
Chapter 12

Stanley M. Levenson, M.D.
Professor of Surgery, Albert Einstein College of Medicine of Yeshiva University; Attending Surgeon and Director, Surgical ICU-Burn Unit, Jacobi Hospital-Bronx Municipal Hospital Center, Bronx, New York
Chapter 13

Sheldon Margen, M.D.
Professor of Public Health, Public Health and Nutrition Program, School of Public Health, University of California, Berkeley, Berkeley, California
Chapter 11

Errol B. Marliss, M.D., F.R.C.P.(C)
Director, McGill Nutrition and Food Science Center, McGill University Faculty of Medicine; Staff Physician, Department of Medicine, Royal Victoria Hospital, Montreal, Quebec, Canada
Chapter 21

Laura E. Matarese, M.S., R.D.
Nutritional Support Dietitian, Nutritional Support Service, University Hospital, Cincinnati, Ohio
Chapter 24

Roger J. May, M.D.
Instructor in Medicine, Harvard Medical School; Assistant in Medicine, Massachusetts General Hospital, Boston
Chapter 19

Francis D. Moore, M.D.
Moseley Professor of Surgery Emeritus, Harvard Medical School; Surgeon-in-Chief Emeritus, Peter Bent Brigham Hospital and Brigham and Women's Hospital, Boston
Chapter 10

Hamish N. Munro
Director, USDA Human Nutrition Research Center on Aging, Tufts University, Boston
Chapter 5

Craig A. Nachbauer, M.D.
Clinical Fellow, Nutritional Support Service, Department of Surgery, University Hospital, Cincinnati, Ohio
Chapter 17

Barbara J. Nath, M.D.
Clinical Instructor in Medicine, Harvard Medical School, Clinical Assistant in Medicine, Massachusetts General Hospital, Boston
Chapter 19

David M. Ota, M.D.
Assistant Professor of Surgery, The University of Texas Medical School at Houston; Assistant Surgeon, University of Texas System Cancer Center, M. D. Anderson Hospital and Tumor Institute, Houston
Chapter 15

Martin B. Popp, M.D.
Assistant Professor of Surgery, University of Cincinnati College of Medicine; Assistant Chief, Surgical Service, Cincinnati Veterans Administration Medical Center, Cincinnati, Ohio
Chapter 14

Harry Rudney, Ph.D.
Professor and Director, Department of Biological Chemistry, University of Cincinnati College of Medicine, Cincinnati, Ohio
Chapter 6

John A. Ryan, Jr., M.D.
Clinical Assistant Professor of Surgery, University of Washington School of Medicine; Surgeon, The Mason Clinic, Seattle
Chapter 25

Robert H. Schapiro, M.D.
Associate Clinical Professor of Medicine, Harvard Medical School; Physician, Gastrointestinal Unit, Massachusetts General Hospital, Boston
Chapter 19

Eli Seifter, Ph.D.
Professor of Surgery and Biochemistry, Albert Einstein College of Medicine of Yeshiva University, Bronx, New York
Chapter 13

George F. Sheldon, M.D.
Professor of Surgery, University of California, San Francisco, School of Medicine; Attending Surgeon and Chief, Trauma and Hyperalimentation Services, San Francisco General Hospital, San Francisco
Chapter 12

Harry M. Shizgal, M.D.
Professor of Surgery, McGill University Faculty of Medicine; Associate Surgeon, Royal Victoria Hospital, Montreal, Quebec, Canada
Chapter 1

David B. A. Silk, M.D., M.R.C.P.
Director, Department of Gastroenterology and Nutrition, Central Middlesex Hospital, London, England
Chapter 2

J. Dwight Stinnett, Ph.D.
Associate Professor of Research Surgery, University of Cincinnati College of Medicine, Cincinnati, Ohio
Chapter 16

Jane L. H. C. Third, M.D., M.R.C.P.(UK)
Assistant Professor of Medicine, University of Cincinnati College of Medicine; Director, Coronary Primary Prevention Trial and Associate Director, Lipid Clinic, University Hospital, Cincinnati, Ohio
Chapter 7

Katrin Valgeirsdóttir
Department of Food and Nutrition, Massachusetts Institute of Technology, Cambridge
Chapter 5

John W. Vester, M.D.
Professor of Medicine and Clinical Biochemistry and Assistant Dean, CONMED and AHEC, University of Cincinnati College of Medicine; Attending Physician and Director of Research, Good Samaritan Hospital, Cincinnati, Ohio
Chapter 6

Douglas W. Wilmore, M.D.
Associate Professor of Surgery, Harvard Medical School; Associate in Surgery, Nutrition Support Service, Brigham and Women's Hospital, Boston
Chapter 3

Preface

This volume is an attempt to characterize the relatively new field of nutritional support in its current developmental phase. Since the demonstration by Dudrick, Rhoads, and coworkers of the feasibility of total parenteral nutrition using primarily glucose-protein hydrolysate mixtures administered into a central vein, the field of nutritional support has grown rapidly. The phase when the technique was popularized, roughly between 1968 and 1976 or 1977, manifested almost unabashed and probably, in retrospect, appropriate enthusiasm for what was justifiably seen as a new, important, and therapeutically lifesaving technique. Acclaim was uncritical, and excesses, as with any new form of therapy, were common. Popularization substituted for careful scientific investigation and application of this powerful technique.

In a previous volume, *Total Parenteral Nutrition,* my coauthors and I attempted to summarize the knowledge as it existed until 1975. The emphasis in that volume was on the characterization of the field and its uses, and a rough appreciation of what the indications and complications were, but in general the book was a practical guide to a new and important therapeutic tool. Since that time, a necessary period of retrenchment, evaluation, and contemplation has taken place in the field of nutritional support. In the best sense, this period has consisted of an attempt to place the field of nutritional support on a more firm scientific basis by the somewhat overdue application of new research techniques and technology to the clinical and laboratory area. Thus, unabashed enthusiasm has been replaced by a more careful and balanced appreciation for such things as energy requirements, the question of caloric source, trace metals, and, above all, a concern for the requirement for the demonstration of efficacy.

To a certain extent, this current volume reflects the alteration in the field of nutritional support. It is entitled *Surgical Nutrition* because I am, in fact, a practicing surgeon and because, although the contributions of others to this field have been notable, it has been and largely remains an area of interest to surgeons since their patients are, by and large, the ones in most critical need of nutritional support. This is not to say that physicians would not benefit from a more critical and aggressive appraisal of their patients' nutritional needs, nor does it deny the need for the more widespread teaching of nutritional requirements in medical school curricula, which still remains woefully lacking. Rather, it acknowledges that other disciplines have been somewhat less prone to adopt nutritional support as an essential part of their armamentarium.

This volume also reflects changing interests in the field of nutritional support. Growing appreciation for the importance of the preclinical sciences toward progress in clinical areas is reflected in the first several sections, including chapters on protein, carbohydrate, fat, vitamin, and trace metal metabolism, as well as other areas that are important, such as body composition, hormone and energy interchange, fluid and electrolytes, and methods of evaluation of efficacy. The growing appreciation that the enteral route may offer significant advantages, not the least of which may be in the immunologic area, is reflected in the inclusion of several chapters on enteral techniques emphasizing both the theoretical and practical applications of the enteral approach in normal and disease states. The preponderance of discussion of the importance of caloric source, be it glucose or fat, and the multiple references in this regard represent not careless editing, as the casual reader might suppose, but rather the growing importance of this debate within the area of nutritional support. To my count, there are no less than five individual statements of the proper ratios of calorie distribution between glucose and fat. All five differ in perspective and indicate both the depths of division and the breadth of interest in this particular topic. Other topics that may overlap are also included because of my feeling that open discussion and widespread debate of controversial points is not only necessary but desirable, and because in a field that is so immature, there must be free discussion rather than dogmatically held points of view.

Once again, I have been privileged to work with the members of the staff at Little, Brown. Many of them are friends in addition to collaborators, including Fred Belliveau, Vice President and General Manager of the Medical Division, and Lin Richter Paterson, Editor-in-Chief. Cynthia Baron has been invaluable in her position as Associate Book Editor for the volume. I would also like to acknowledge the friendship, collaboration, and inspiration of the many colleagues with whom I have had the privilege of working over the past decade or so, including Ronald Abel, John Ryan, Herbert Freund, Alfonso Aguirre, Bengt Jeppsson, Robert Bower, Kenneth Kern, Howard James, and Bill Chance, to name but a few. Rita Colley, Jean Wilson, and Vickie Duty are excellent representatives of our nursing staff, and Laura Matarese, our Dietitian, is represented in this volume. It has been my good fortune, over my professional career, to have been blessed with an excellent office staff, including Catherine Sullivan, Pat Walk, Kay Powell, Tricia Robertson, Shirley Davis, Marty Ridder, and Barbara Daria, all of whom have contributed to this volume.

Finally, and most importantly, one must not forget one's family, whose forbearance, support, and love make possible the tasks that are accomplished. *Surgical Nutrition* in every way belongs not only to my wife, Karen, but to my children, Erich and Alexandra, as well, who shoulder the burden of the inevitable intrusion upon our family life, yet manage to keep our relationship intact.

J. E. F.

General Considerations

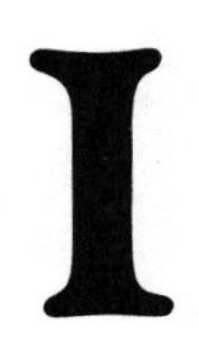

Body Composition

Harry M. Shizgal

1

LEAN BODY MASS AND BODY FAT

Total body mass, or body weight (BWt), is composed of two major components: body fat and the lean body mass (LBM). The lean body mass was originally defined by densitometric measurements based on underwater weighing procedures. This methodology was based on the concept that the lean body mass was that component of body composition with a density of 1.100, whereas the neutral body fat had a density of 0.900 [1]. Thus, Behnke et al. [2], employing the diving tank of Bethesda, determined the LBM by measuring total body water (TBW) and specific gravity (*d*).

$$\%\text{LBM} = 100 - \frac{213.66}{d} - 77.49\frac{(\text{TBW})}{\text{BWt}} - 137.4$$

The lean body mass, as defined by densitometry, was originally regarded as containing between 2 and 10 percent essential lipids. Thus, conceptually there was a small difference between the lean body mass, as defined by densitometry, and the "fat-free body." The measurement of specific gravity by underwater weighing is difficult to perform, especially in the clinical setting. Currently, lean body mass is commonly determined by measuring total body water (TBW) and using the relationship

$$\text{LBM} = \frac{\text{TBW}}{0.73}$$

This relationship is based on the observations of Pace and Rathburn [8] that the water content of the fat-free body is 73 percent. The lean body mass, as defined by this relationship, is equivalent to the fat-free mass. Thus, body fat (BF) can be determined as follows:

$$\text{BF} = \text{BWt} - \text{LBM}$$

The calculations of body fat and lean body mass from the measurement of TBW are based on the assumption that the water content of the fat-free mass is constant. The hydration of the fat-free mass is fairly constant in a healthy homogeneous population, but varies considerably with illness. The water content of the fat-free body has been estimated to vary from a maximum of 85 percent with severe anasarca to a minimum of

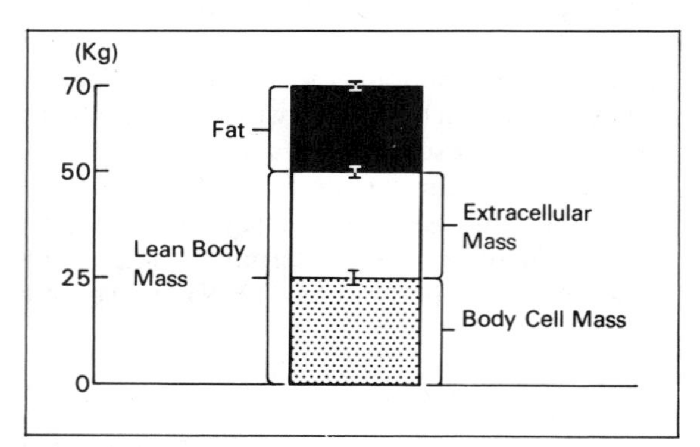

Figure 1-1. *The mean (± SEM) body composition of 25 normal volunteers. Body weight is the sum of body fat and the lean body mass, which in turn is subdivided into two compartments: the extracellular mass and the body cell mass.*

67 percent with marked dehydration. The Pace-Rathburn formula thus results in a first approximation of body fat and lean body mass.

Moore et al. [7] developed a nomogram to calculate the hydration of the fat-free body and thus improve the precision of the body fat and lean body mass determination. The ratio of intracellular water volume to total body water (ICW/TBW) and the ratio of observed to expected extracellular water (ECW) are the indices that are used to determine the hydration of the fat-free body. Although this nomogram was described by Moore et al., they have seldom used it to calculate either body fat or LBM, but have instead employed the Pace-Rathburn formula.

In a healthy and homogeneous population, a relationship exists between the lean body mass and metabolic indexes such as oxygen consumption, carbon dioxide production, caloric requirement, and work performance. However, such a relationship does not exist with heterogeneous populations or in the presence of pathologic states. This is because the lean body mass is anatomically and metabolically heterogeneous, being composed of both the body cell mass and the extracellular mass (Figure 1-1). The latter represents the extracellular supporting component of body composition and is composed of such composition elements as the skeleton, cartilage, fascia, tendons, plasma volume, extracellular fluids, and pathologic water accumulations. These components of the body are not metabolically active, do not consume oxygen, and do not perform work. Rather, they are largely concerned with transport and support.

BODY CELL MASS

The body cell mass is the metabolically active, energy-exchanging mass of the body. The body cell mass was defined by Moore et al. [7] "as that component of body composition containing the oxygen-exchanging, potassium-rich, glucose-oxidizing, work-performing tissue." It is therefore that component of body composition that can serve as a reference for the metabolic activity of the body as measured by oxygen consumption, carbon dioxide production, caloric requirement, and work performance. The body cell mass is the sum of all the cellular elements of the body and thus includes the cellular components of both skeletal and smooth muscle, the viscera (liver, kidneys, lungs, gastrointestinal tract), and the central nervous system. Also included are the cells of tissues with a sparse cellular population such as bone, cartilage, tendon, and adipose tissue. In the normal healthy individual, the skeletal muscle cell mass has been estimated to comprise 60 percent of the total cell mass, whereas the visceral cell mass accounts for 20 percent. The remaining 20 percent is made up by the red cell mass and the cells in the peripheral connective tissues such as bone, cartilage, tendon, adipose, and so forth [6].

A direct measure of the body cell mass is currently unavailable. However, the size of the body cell mass can be estimated by a variety of indirect measurements. The approach most commonly employed is the measurement of total body potassium. Potassium is the most abundant intracellular cation, with over 98 percent of total body potassium located within the intracellular compartment. Furthermore, the intracellular potassium concentration varies within a narrow range. As a result, total body potassium is linearly related to the size of the body cell mass [7]. In addition, total body potassium is linearly related to both the intracellular water volume [7] and to total body nitrogen [3]. The ratio of potassium to nitrogen is fairly constant in all tissues in both normal and pathologic states [13, 14]. Kinney et al. have also demonstrated a relationship between body potassium and resting metabolic expenditure [4]. Considerable data therefore exist supporting the use of body potassium to estimate the size of the body cell mass.

Total exchangeable potassium (K_e), as measured by isotope dilution with an isotope of potassium, is equivalent to total body potassium. Several studies have reported differences between K_e and total body potassium. However, in each instance these differences were extremely small, statistically insignificant, and less than the measurement errors of the techniques employed. The most precise and accurate measurement of K_e is obtained by isotope dilution using a radioactive isotope of potassium. However, the radioactive isotopes of potassium that are currently available are relatively unstable and decay rapidly. The half-life of ^{42}K is 12.5 hours. As a result, 86.6 percent of the available ^{42}K decays in the initial 36 hours. By three days only 1.7 percent remains. This short half-life is not a problem if the K_e measurement can be planned to coincide with the delivery of the isotope. However, with clinical studies, this is often difficult because the availability of patients is usually unpredictable.

To overcome the difficulties and expense associated with the use of the rapidly decaying radioactive isotopes of potassium, a technique for the indirect measurement of K_e was developed. This technique is based on the fact that in all tissues, except for bone, the ratio of the sodium plus potassium content divided by the water content is a constant and is equal to the ratio of the sum of exchangeable sodium (Na_e) plus K_e divided by TBW, i.e.,

$$\frac{Na_e + K_e}{TBW} = \frac{Na + K}{H_2O} = R$$

Thus,

$$K_e = R \times TBW - Na_e$$

Total body water and Na_e are easily measured by standard isotope dilution using tritiated water and ^{22}Na, respectively. The constant, R, is determined by measuring the sodium, potassium, and water content of a sample of whole blood. The validity of this measurement was experimentally verified both in the experimental animal and in a group of patients [12]. The indirect measurement of K_e was identical to the measurement obtained simultaneously by either carcass analysis or by ^{42}K dilution.

Total body potassium also can be measured by means of a whole body counter. The whole body counter measures the total mass of ^{40}K, a naturally occurring radioactive isotope of potassium which comprises 0.012 percent of all naturally occurring potassium. The whole body counter is an expensive installation. In addition, its calibration remains a difficult problem, since the ^{40}K count detected by the whole body counter is a function of both total body potassium and the geometric configuration of the subject. The geometric configuration of the individual determines the degree of self-absorption of the emitted gamma rays and thus the percentage of emitted ^{40}K gamma rays detected. In the majority of installations, the body counter is calibrated by injecting ^{42}K into a group of volunteers and measuring ^{42}K with the whole body counter. Potassium-42 is used, as it emits a gamma ray with an energy similar to the gamma emitted by ^{40}K. The counting efficiency (i.e., counts detected/counts injected) is correlated with weight and/or height. The resultant regression is then used to determine the counting efficiency arising from the geometry of the individual and thus correct the ^{40}K count. The error introduced by the use of this regression may be considerable, especially since the background count is usually large relative to the ^{40}K count. With some total body counters the background count may also be a function of body weight. Thus, although the reproducibility of the whole body potassium determination is usually excellent, the accuracy is often poor because of the low ^{40}K count, the large background count, and the difficulty associated with determining the ^{40}K counting efficiency. The low ^{40}K counts also necessitate long counting times, which may pose a problem with ill patients.

The body cell mass (BCM) can be calculated from K_e based on the assumption that the average potassium to nitrogen ratio in tissue is 3 mEq/gm. Thus,

$$\text{Total body nitrogen} = \frac{K_e}{3} \text{ (gm)}$$

$$\text{Total body protein} = \frac{6.25}{3} K_e \text{ (gm)}$$

$$\text{Body cell mass} = \frac{4 \times 6.25}{3} K_e = 8.33\ K_e \text{ (gm)}$$

Because the BCM is related to K_e by a simple constant, the calculation of the BCM results in an approximation of its absolute size, but does not yield additional compositional information.

The body cell mass can also be calculated from the intracellular water volume (ICW), by assuming that the average water content of the body cell mass is 70 percent, i.e.,

$$\text{BCM} = \frac{\text{ICW}}{0.70}$$

This approach is much less accurate, since ICW cannot be measured directly, but is calculated as the difference between TBW and the extracellular water volume (ECW). The accuracy of ICW determination is therefore dependent on the errors associated with both the TBW and ECW measurements. The accuracy of the TBW measurement is excellent, since the TBW space is well defined anatomically and is measured by a tracer, usually tritiated water, which does not "leak" out of the TBW space. The equilibrated concentration of the tracer is used to calculate the TBW volume. In contrast, the majority of the tracers used to measure the ECW space leak out of the ECW at varying rates. The volume is therefore calculated from the kinetics of the disappearance curve, as defined by the slope and the intercept. The ECW volumes obtained with the larger and less diffusible tracers, such as mannitol and insulin, are smaller than those obtained with the ions, such as sodium, bromide, and sulfate. The ECW volume is in part, therefore, a function of the distribution volume of the tracer used. Since the ECW is not well defined anatomically, biologic validation of an ECW measurement is impossible. The inaccuracies of the ICW measurement, therefore, result from the difficulties associated with the ECW determination and not from the TBW measurement. As a result, the ICW is seldom used to calculate the body cell mass.

The body cell mass can also be calculated from total body nitrogen (TBN) from

$$\text{BCM} = \text{TBN} \times 6.25 \times 4$$

Because body nitrogen does not exist in well-defined "pools," TBN cannot be measured by isotope dilution. However, neutron activation analysis has been used to measure TBN. This involves the irradiation of the subject with neutrons from either a cyclotron or from a plutonium source [3, 5]. When any material is irradiated with neutrons, nuclear changes result, with the production of gamma rays specific for the substance that captured the neutron. In the case of nitrogen a 10.83 Mev gamma ray is produced. By using large sodium iodine crystal detectors, a measure of TBN can be obtained. In one study involving 190 measurements in 65 patients, an excellent correlation was obtained between TBN and K_e [3].

EXTRACELLULAR MASS

The extracellular mass (ECM) is that component of the fat-free mass which exists outside the cells and is composed of both fluids and solids. The fluid component of the extracellular mass consists of plasma, and interstitial and transcellu-

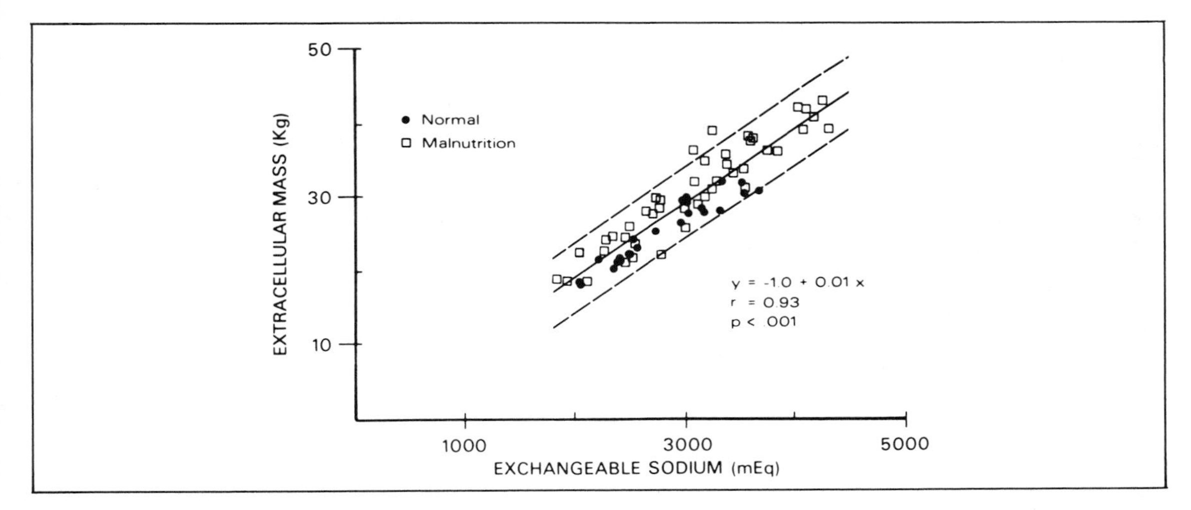

Figure 1-2. *The extracellular mass is plotted as a function of the total exchangeable sodium, in 25 normal volunteers and 50 patients with malnutrition. The regression and 95 percent confidence limits for the sample are included.*

lar water. Transcellular water is extracellular water that is secreted into a well-defined space by the surrounding cells, often against an electrochemical gradient. Examples are fluid within the lumen of the gastrointestinal tract and cerebral, spinal, and joint space fluids. The solid component of the extracellular mass includes collagen, elastin, dermis, tendon, fascia, and the skeleton. Of the extracellular solids, the largest by weight is the skeleton. The principal function of the extracellular mass is support and transport.

Sodium is the principal extracellular cation, the majority of total body sodium being restricted to the extracellular space. However, a large fraction of total body sodium is tightly incorporated into the skeleton and does not exchange with the isotopes of sodium. Total body sodium therefore is not equivalent to total exchangeable sodium (Na_e). Nevertheless, total exchangeable sodium is an excellent measure of the fluid component of the extracellular tissues. The extracellular water volume, which also is used to assess the size of the extracellular mass, can be measured directly by using a tracer that is principally restricted to the extracellular space. Neither exchangeable sodium nor extracellular water is an estimate of the solid component of the extracellular mass. However, the total extracellular mass, i.e., the sum of the solid and the fluid components, can be calculated from the difference between the lean body mass and the body cell mass, i.e.,

$$ECM = LBM - BCM$$

This relationship was used to determine the extracellular mass in 25 normal volunteers and in 50 patients with malnutrition. An excellent correlation exists between the ECM and Na_e (Figure 1-2). A similar regression analysis was performed for each group, i.e., for the 25 normal volunteers ($Y = 0.5 + 0.01X$; $r = 0.96$) and for the 50 malnourished patients ($Y = 0.2 + 0.01X$; $r = 0.94$). The two regression curves were not significantly different. These data therefore indicate that the difference between LBM and BCM results in a determination of the ECM that is accurate and independent of both the Na_e and ECW measurements.

MEASUREMENT OF BODY COMPOSITION

Multiple isotope dilution is the method usually employed to quantify body composition. The method employed in our laboratory involves the simultaneous intravenous injection of four radioactive isotopes: 10 μCi of iodine-labeled human serum albumin (RISA), 50 μCi of ^{51}Cr-tagged autologous red cells, 8 μCi of ^{22}Na, and 500 μCi of tritiated water [11]. The total radiation dose to the patient is 230 millirems, which is one-fourth to one-fifth the radiation associated with a barium meal examination.

The red cell mass (RBC) is determined from the equilibrated whole blood concentration of ^{51}Cr-tagged red cells. The plasma volume (PV) and extracellular water volume are determined by plotting the logarithm of plasma concentration of RISA and ^{22}Na, respectively, against time, as the independent variable, between 60 and 110 minutes. The volumes are determined by the reverse extrapolation of the respective straight lines, obtained by least square fitting. Total exchangeable sodium is determined from the equilibrated plasma ^{22}Na specific activity at 24 hours. Total body water is determined from the equilibrated plasma tritium concentration. Corrections are made, when appropriate, for plasma water concentration, the Donnan equilibrium, and the urinary excretion of isotope. Total exchangeable potassium is calculated from

$$K_e = TBW \times R - Na_e$$

where R is equal to the sum of the sodium and potassium content of a sample of whole blood, divided by its water content. The remaining parameters of body composition are calculated as indicated in Table 1-1.

Multiple isotope dilution was also employed by Moore et al. [7] to carry out their classic studies on body composition. However, the isotopes they injected were slightly different. Potassium-42 was used to measure total exchangeable potassium. The bromide distribution volume was determined as a measure of the extracellular water volume, whereas ^{24}Na was employed to measure total exchangeable sodium. Chromium-51-tagged red cells, RISA, and tritiated water were injected to measure red cell mass, plasma volume, and total body water, respectively.

Table 1-1. *Body Composition Measurement*

Parameter	Determination
RBC	Equilibrated ^{51}Cr-tagged cell distribution volume
PV	Early RISA distribution volume
TBW	Equilibrated tritiated water distribution volume
ECW	Early ^{22}Na distribution volume
Na_e	24-hour ^{22}Na specific activity
BV	$BV = PV + RBC$
ICW	$ICW = TBW - ECW$
K_e	$K_e = R \times TBW - Na_e$
BCM	$BCM = 0.0833\ K_e$
LBM	$LBM = TBW/0.73$
ECM	$ECM = LBM - BCM$
BF	$BF = BWt - LBM$

NORMAL BODY COMPOSITION

Body composition data obtained in two groups of normal volunteers are tabulated in Table 1-2. The first set of data was obtained in our laboratory in 25 normal volunteers consisting of 15 males and 10 females. The second set consists of similar data, published by Moore et al. [7], obtained in 34 normal volunteers, with an equal number of males and females. In both series, as expected, the body weight of the males exceeded that of the females, owing principally to a larger lean body mass. In the females, body fat accounted for approximately one-third of the body weight; in the males, approximately one-fourth of body weight was due to body fat. In both sexes, the body cell mass and the extracellular mass were equal in size.

To correct for body size, the various components of body composition are expressed as a function of total body water. Total body water is a better measure of body size than is body weight, as it is linearly related to a lean body mass. Thus, K_e/TBW and ICW/TBW are both measures of the body cell mass, whereas Na_e/TBW and ECW/TBW are similarly related to the extracellular mass. Body composition expressed as a function of TBW becomes inde-

Table 1-2. *Normal Body Composition*

	Author's Series			Moore et al.[a]		
	Males	Females	Total	Males	Females	Total
n	15	10	25	17	17	34
Weight (kg)	76.4 ± 3.0	61.5 ± 2.6[b]	70.4 ± 2.5	70.7 ± 2.8	61.2 ± 2.2[b]	65.9 ± 1.9
Fat (kg)	20.2 ± 1.9	19.8 ± 2.1	20.1 ± 1.4	19.8 ± 1.6	22.7 ± 1.7	21.3 ± 1.2
Lean body mass (kg)	56.2 ± 1.8	41.7 ± 1.5[b]	50.4 ± 1.9	50.8 ± 1.8	38.5 ± 0.9[b]	44.7 ± 1.5
Body cell mass (kg)	27.4 ± 1.3	20.5 ± 1.0[b]	24.6 ± 1.1	26.3 ± 1.2	18.7 ± 0.6[b]	22.4 ± 0.9
Extracellular mass (kg)	28.8 ± 0.7	21.2 ± 0.7[b]	25.8 ± 0.9	24.9 ± 1.0	19.8 ± 0.4[b]	22.4 ± 0.7
K_e/TBW(mEq/L)	79.6 ± 1.3	80.6 ± 1.7	80.0 ± 1.0	84.0 ± 1.8	79.6 ± 1.0[b]	81.8 ± 1.1
Na_e/TBW(mEq/L)	77.2 ± 1.1	77.9 ± 1.7	77.5 ± 0.9	77.5 ± 2.0	80.8 ± 1.0	79.2 ± 1.1
Na_e/K_e	0.97 ± .03	0.98 ± .04	0.98 ± .02	0.94 ± .04	1.02 ± .02	0.98 ± .02
ICW/TBW(%)	58.6 ± 1.2	55.8 ± 1.9	57.5 ± 1.1	54.2 ± 1.1	52.1 ± 0.6	53.1 ± 0.6[c]
ECW/TBW(%)	41.4 ± 1.2	44.2 ± 1.9	42.5 ± 1.1	45.8 ± 1.1	47.9 ± 0.6	46.9 ± 0.6[c]

[a] From F. D. Moore et al. *The Body Cell Mass and Its Supporting Environment.* Philadelphia: Saunders, 1963.
[b] Significant difference ($p < .05$) between males and females by impaired Student's t-test.
[c] Significant difference ($p < .05$) between the two groups by impaired Student's t-test.

pendent of the amount of the body fat. It also permits the comparison of individuals and groups of individuals with different body size. The body composition of the males and females are therefore similar when expressed as a function of total body water (Table 1-2). In addition, body composition is similar in the two normal groups, except for the ECW and ICW. The small differences are probably related to the different ions used to measure the ECW: ^{22}Na in our group; ^{82}Br by Moore et al. [7].

From the data obtained in the normal volunteers, Moore et al. derived a series of relationships that can be used to calculate normal body composition, based on age, sex, and body weight (Table 1-3). In our group of 25 normal volunteers, the various components of body composition were compared to the values predicted by these relationships. An excellent correlation was obtained between the measured and predicted values as illustrated for K_e in Figure 1-3. The resultant regression line approximated the line of identity. A similar comparison between the measured K_e and the predicted K_e was performed in 50 patients with an abnormal body composition (Figure 1-4). The resultant correlation was poor, with a large difference between the regression line and the line of identity. The data demonstrate that the equations developed by Moore (Table 1-3) are useful in predicting normal body composition, but are of little value in an individual with abnormal body composition. In a similar fashion, TBW has been used to calculate the various components of body composition. This approach is based on the observation that, in a group of normal individuals, a close correlation exists between TBW and the various body compositional components. In the normal individual, the body cell mass accounts for 50 percent of the lean body mass. In the presence of abnormal body composition, this relationship between the body cell mass and TBW ceases to exist. As a result, TBW accurately predicts the size of the body cell mass in the normal individual, but not when the body composition is abnormal.

EFFECT OF CATABOLIC STRESS

Surgery in normal man invariably results in a short catabolic period, the intensity and dura-

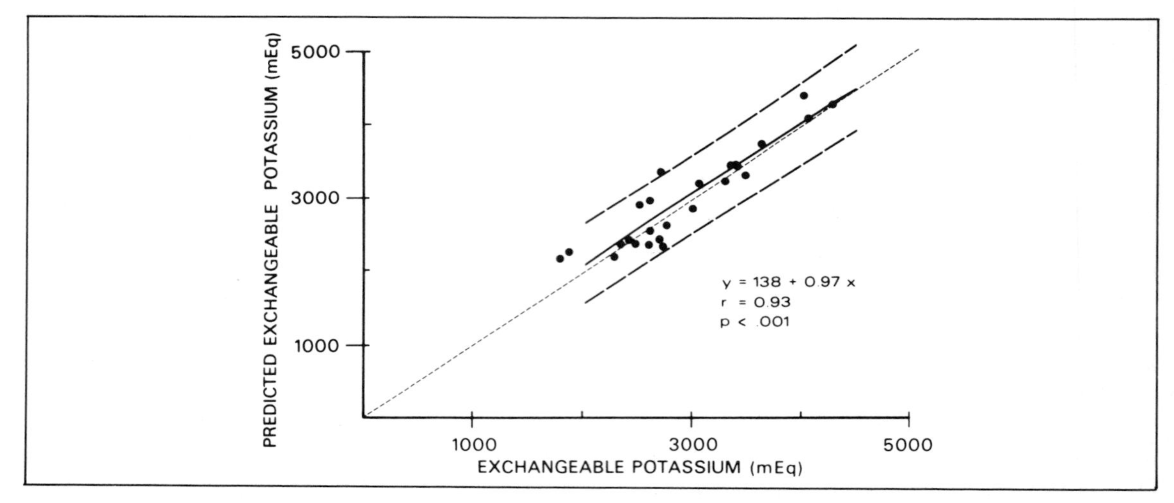

Figure 1-3. *In 25 normal volunteers the total exchangeable potassium, predicted by the relationship in Table 1-3, is plotted against the measured exchangeable potassium. The resultant regression is highly significant and approximates the line of identity. The 95 percent confidence limit for the sample is included.*

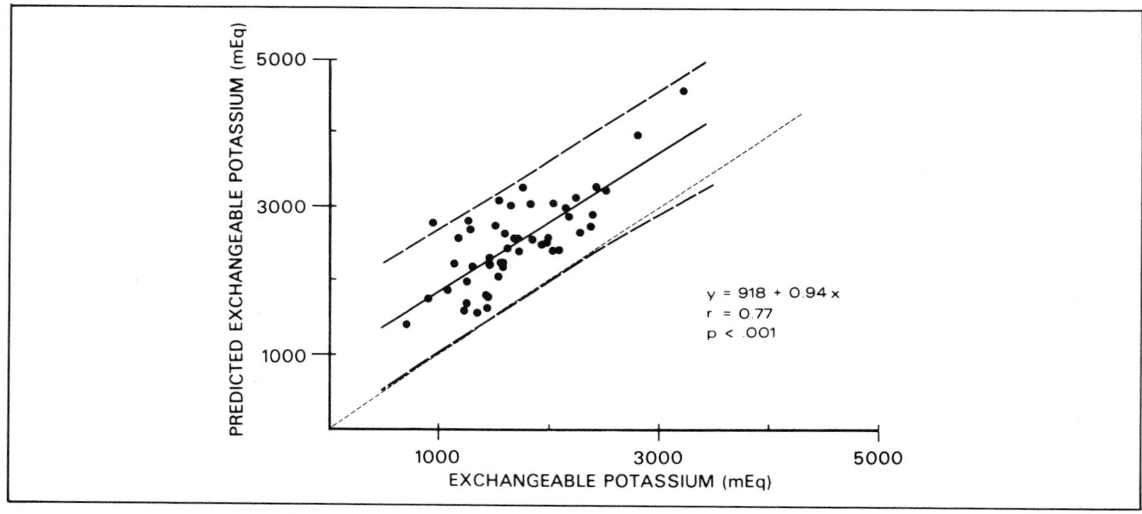

Figure 1-4. *In 50 patients with an abnormal body composition ($Na_e/K_e > 1.22$) the exchangeable potassium, predicted by the relationship in Table 1-3, is plotted against the measured exchangeable potassium. The resultant regression is significantly different from the line of identity. The 95 percent confidence limits for the sample are included.*

Table 1-3. *Prediction of Normal Body Composition*

$$TBW = 0.7945\,(BWt) - 0.0024\,(BWt)^2 - 0.0015\,(age)\,(BWt) \quad \text{(males)}$$
$$TBW = 0.6981\,(BWt) - 0.0026\,(BWt)^2 - 0.0012\,(age)\,(BWt) \quad \text{(females)}$$
$$ICW = 0.623\,(TBW) - 0.0016\,(age)\,(TBW) \quad \text{(males)}$$
$$ICW = 0.553\,(TBW) - 0.0007\,(age)\,(TBW) \quad \text{(females)}$$
$$FAT = BWt - TBW/0.732$$
$$ECW = TBW - ICW$$
$$K_e = 150\,(ICW) + 4\,(ECW)$$
$$Na_e = 163.2\,(TBW) - K_e - 69$$
$$RBC = 52.96\,(TBW) - 158$$
$$BV = \frac{RBC}{0.380} \quad \text{(males)}$$
$$BV = \frac{RBC}{0.348} \quad \text{(females)}$$
$$PV = BV - RBC$$

Source: F. D. Moore et al. *The Body Cell Mass and Its Supporting Environment.* Philadelphia: Saunders, 1963.

tion of which is directly related to the severity of the surgical trauma. The short but intense postoperative catabolic phase is characterized by weight loss, negative potassium, and nitrogen balance with positive salt and water balance, suggesting a postoperative decrease in the body cell mass accompanied by an expansion of the extracellular mass. These postoperative changes were confirmed in a group of 19 patients undergoing an elective surgical procedure [11]. The majority of the patients underwent either a gastrectomy or colon resection. Preoperatively, body composition was normal (Figure 1-5). However, by the fifth postoperative day the body cell mass had decreased by 14 percent from 23.5 ± 1.5 kg to 19.9 ± 1.4 kg ($p < .05$) and was accompanied by the concomitant expansion of the extracellular mass from 24.9 ± 0.9 to 27.3 ± 0.9 kg ($p < .05$). There were similar significant changes in the K_e/TBW and Na_e/TBW (Figure 1-5). Because the decrease in the body cell mass was accompanied by an increase in the extracellular mass the Na_e/K_e ratio increased significantly from a normal mean of 1.04 ± 0.08 to 1.29 ± 0.11 ($p < .05$) (Figure 1-5).

Similar compositional changes were recorded in 75 patients with chronic catabolic stress and/or starvation. The majority of these patients had experienced a surgical complication and were referred for total parenteral nutrition (TPN). Their body composition, which was determined prior to the onset of TPN, is compared to that of 25 normal volunteers (Figure 1-6). Their mean body weight was 58.9 ± 1.8 kg as compared to a mean weight of 70.4 ± 2.5 kg in the normal group, a 16 percent difference. This difference in body weight did not reflect the 41 percent difference in the body cell mass, because of the concomitant expansion of the extracellular mass. Their mean body cell mass was 14.7 ± 0.6 kg compared to 24.7 ± 1.1 kg in the normal group, whereas the extracellular mass was 31.9 ± 0.9 kg and 25.6 ± 0.9 kg in the two groups, respectively. These differences are reflected by the K_e/TBW and Na_e/TBW, which are plotted in Figure 1-6. Again, because the contracted body cell mass was accompanied by an expansion of the extracellular mass, there was an abnormal elevation in the Na_e/K_e ratio ($p < .001$).

Na_e/K_e RATIO

The Na_e/K_e ratio is a measure of the extracellular mass expressed as a function of the body cell

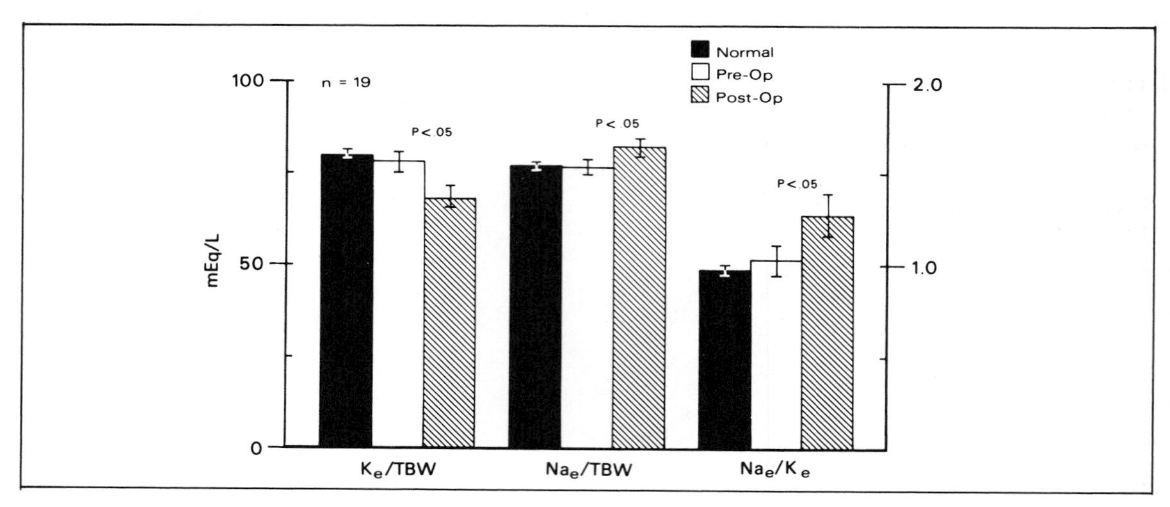

Figure 1-5. *The body composition in 19 normal individuals prior to and on the fifth day following a major surgical procedure. The data obtained in 25 normal volunteers are included (solid histograms).*

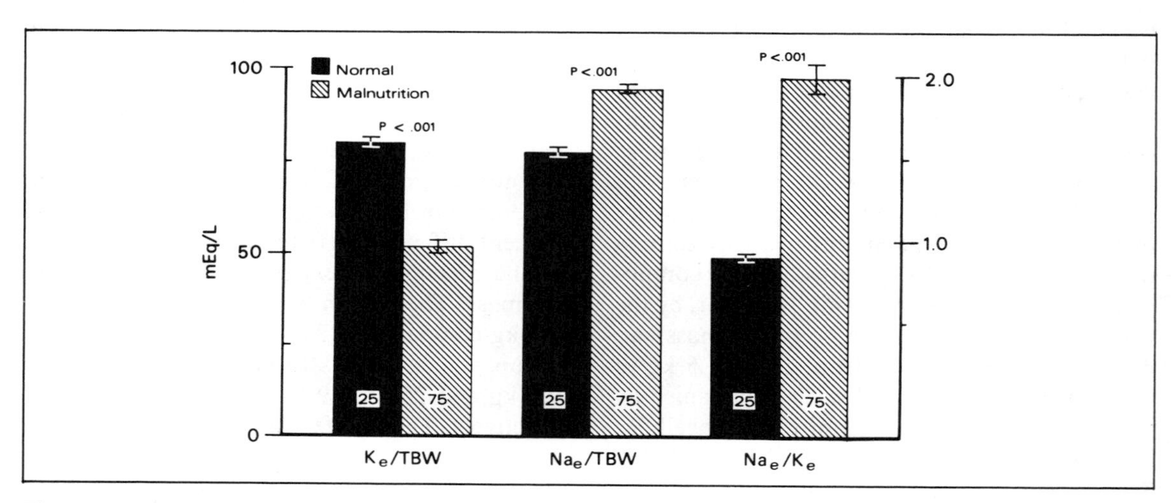

Figure 1-6. *The body composition of 75 patients subjected to prolonged catabolic stress or starvation or both is compared to the body composition of 25 normal volunteers.*

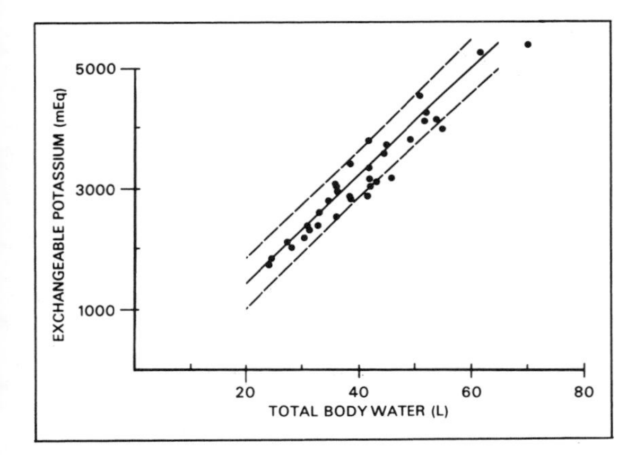

Figure 1-7. *Total exchangeable potassium plotted as a function of total body water in the 34 of 100 consecutive studies with $Na_e/K_e < 1.22$. The normal range is indicated by the regression and 95 percent confidence limits of the sample, obtained in 25 normal volunteers.*

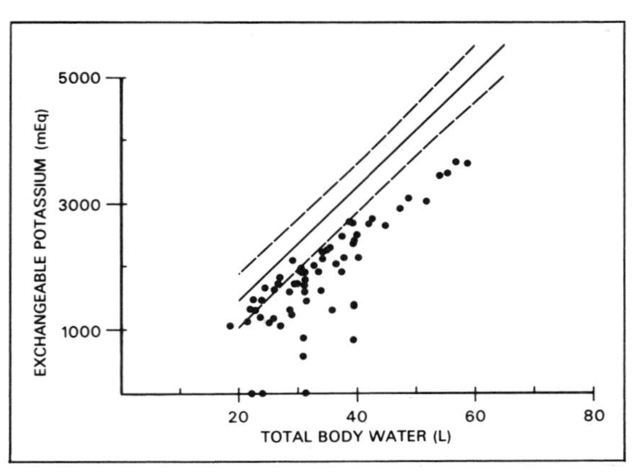

Figure 1-8. *Total exchangeable potassium plotted as a function of total body water in 66 of the 100 consecutive studies with $Na_e/K_e > 1.22$. The normal range is indicated by the regression and 95 percent confidence limits of the sample, obtained in 25 normal volunteers.*

mass. This ratio is normally close to unity with a small variance. In 25 normal volunteers, the mean Na_e/K_e was 0.98 ± 0.02, with an upper 95 percent confidence limit of 1.22.

With malnutrition, the decrease in the body cell mass is almost always accompanied by an expansion of the extracellular mass, and therefore an increase in the Na_e/K_e ratio. The Na_e/K_e was abnormally elevated in the patients who developed an abnormal body composition as a result of a chronic catabolic stress or starvation or both (Figure 1-6). Similarly, the decrease in body cell mass following a major operation was accompanied by an abnormal elevation in the Na_e/K_e (see Figure 1-5). In our personal experience, the Na_e/K_e ratio has proved to be a sensitive index of nutritional status. The validity of the Na_e/K_e ratio as a measure of nutritional status was confirmed by the following analysis of data obtained in 100 consecutive body composition studies performed on a variety of patients. The latter included both normal and malnourished patients receiving TPN, and several morbidly obese patients, before and at varying time intervals following surgery performed for weight reduction. This entire group of 100 patients were divided into a malnourished and a normal group on the basis of the Na_e/K_e ratio. The presence of malnutrition was defined by an Na_e/K_e ratio that exceeded 1.22. On this basis, 66 patients were considered to be malnourished; the remaining 34 patients were normal. For both groups, K_e, a measure of the body cell mass, was plotted against TBW. The normal range is defined by the regression and 95 percent confidence limits, calculated from the data obtained in normal volunteers. In the 34 patients with a normal ratio, the points were uniformly distributed about the regression line (Figure 1-7). In addition, the regression of K_e on TBW for these patients was not significantly different from the regression obtained in the normal volunteers. However, in the malnourished group, all of the K_e values were below the normal regression line, and the majority were below the lower 95 percent confidence limits (Figure 1-8). These data, obtained in 100 consecutive studies, indicate that the Na_e/K_e ratio accurately predicted the individuals with a normal body cell mass and those with a depleted body cell mass.

Table 1-4. *Effect of TPN on Body Composition*

		Normal Initial Body Composition		Preexisting Malnutrition	
	Normal	Pre-TPN	Post-TPN	Pre-TPN	Post-TPN
Weight (kg)	70.4 ± 2.5	59.7 ± 1.7	60.9 ± 1.6	56.1 ± 2.0	57.1 ± 2.0
Fat (kg)	20.2 ± 1.4	13.6 ± 1.2	14.7 ± 1.2	10.4 ± 1.1	11.7 ± 1.1[a]
Lean body mass (kg)	50.3 ± 1.9	46.2 ± 1.2	46.2 ± 1.1	45.7 ± 1.4	45.4 ± 1.2
Body cell mass (kg)	24.7 ± 1.1	21.4 ± 0.6	21.0 ± 0.6	15.8 ± 0.6	16.6 ± 0.5[a]
Extracellular mass (kg)	25.6 ± 0.9	24.8 ± 0.7	25.2 ± 0.7	29.9 ± 1.0	28.8 ± 1.1
K_e/TBW (mEq/L)	80.0 ± 1.0	76.1 ± 0.9	74.5 ± 1.3	57.0 ± 1.3[b]	61.1 ± 1.6[a,b]
Na_e/TBW (mEq/L)	77.5 ± 0.9	77.0 ± 0.7	77.6 ± 1.1	93.6 ± 1.3[b]	90.1 ± 1.6[a,b]
Na_e/K_e	0.98 ± .02	1.02 ± .02	1.07 ± .03	1.73 ± 0.08[b]	1.57 ± 0.07[a,b]
Number	25	55		52	
cal/kg/day		48.8 ± 1.4		48.8 ± 1.9	
Gm protein/kg/day		1.26 ± .04		1.23 ± .05	
Days on TPN		14.6 ± 0.4		14.6 ± 0.2	

[a]Significantly different ($p < .05$) from pre-TPN measurement by paired Student's t-test.
[b]Significantly different ($p < .05$) from normal by an analysis of variance and Scheffe's test (only K_e/TBW, Na_e/TBW and Na_e/K_e tested).

EFFECT OF TPN ON BODY COMPOSITION

The effect of TPN on body composition was evaluated in 79 patients receiving a solution containing 25 percent dextrose and 2.5 percent Crystalline Amino Acids (Travasol, Baxter Laboratories, Canada) [9]. To evaluate the efficacy of TPN, body composition studies were performed at the onset of TPN and at 2-week intervals. A total of 179 body composition studies were performed to evaluate 107 periods of TPN, of 14.6 ± 0.2 days duration. The efficacy of TPN was assessed by determining the change in the body cell mass. However, in the absence of malnutrition, the body cell mass should not increase, regardless of the calories and protein infused. In a normal individual, the excessive administration of calories and protein results in an increase in body fat without any change in the size of the body cell mass. As a result, the data were divided into two groups according to the presence or absence of malnutrition at the onset of each period of TPN. Malnutrition was defined by an Na_e/K_e greater than 1.22. In patients with an abnormally elevated ratio (Table 1-4, Figure 1-9), the pre-TPN body composition was characteristic of malnutrition, with a contracted body cell mass and an expanded extracellular mass. The administration of TPN at 48.8 ± 1.9 cal/kg/day for 14.6 ± 0.2 days resulted in a 5.1 percent increase in the body cell mass from 15.8 ± 0.6 to 16.6 ± 0.5 kg ($p < .05$). This was accompanied by a 3.7 percent contraction of the extracellular mass from 29.9 ± 1.0 to 28.8 ± 1.1 kg. In addition the Na_e/K_e ratio decreased from 1.73 ± 0.08 to 1.57 ± 0.07.*

In the patients with a normal ratio at the onset of TPN, body cell mass did not increase during the course of TPN (Table 1-4, Figure 1-10).

**Editor's Note:* The failure to observe gain in lean body mass, although alluded to by others, may be due in this case to a comparatively low nitrogen dose and a relatively high calorie: nitrogen ratio. It is not clear what would have resulted if a higher dose of nitrogen had been administered.

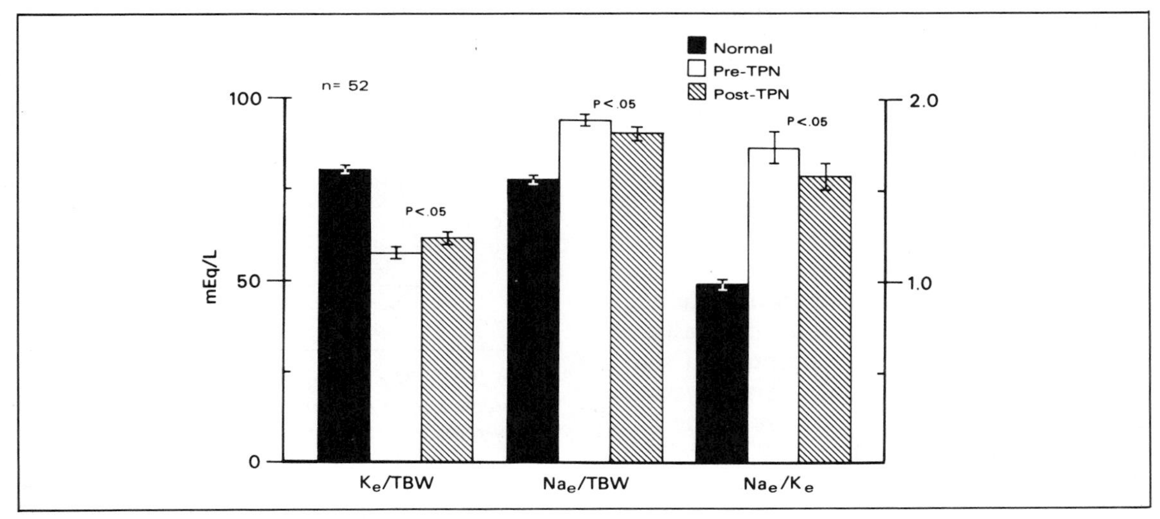

Figure 1-9. *The change in body composition resulting from 14.6 ± 0.2 days of TPN in patients with preexisting malnutrition as defined by an $Na_e/K_e > 1.22$. The pre-TPN data are significantly ($p < .05$) different from that obtained in 25 normal volunteers (solid histograms).*

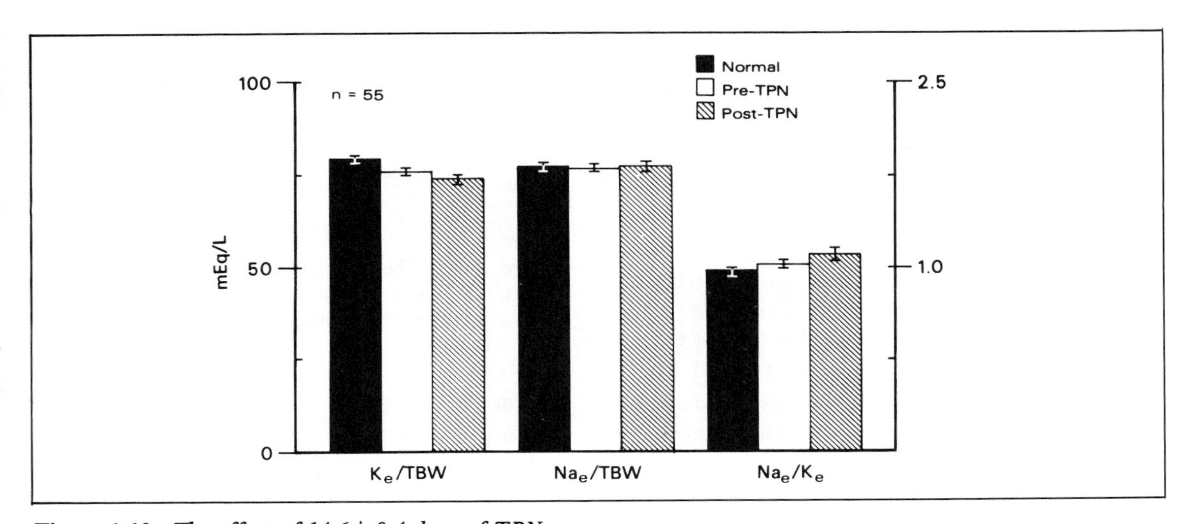

Figure 1-10. *The effect of 14.6 ± 0.4 days of TPN on the body composition of patients without preexisting malnutrition as defined by an $Na_e/K_e < 1.22$. The pre-TPN data are not significantly different from that obtained in 25 normal volunteers (solid histograms).*

Their body composition was normal when TPN was started and remained normal after 14.6 ± 0.4 days of TPN. These data thus provide additional support for the use of Na_e/K_e to assess nutritional status, as the ratio accurately predicted the presence of malnutrition. In addition, the data demonstrate that the body cell mass will increase in response to adequate TPN only in the presence of a depleted body cell mass, i.e., in the presence of preexisting malnutrition. In addition, multiple linear regression demonstrated that, in the presence of malnutrition, a statistically significant relationship exists between the repletion rate of the body cell mass and both the cal/kg/day infused and the Na_e/K_e ratio [9]. In the absence of malnutrition, i.e., in the normal individual, the BCM remained unchanged, with adequate or even excessive nutritional support. An accurate knowledge of an individual's nutritional status is therefore essential when assessing the efficacy of nutritional support, regardless of the methodology employed in performing this assessment. Thus, adequate nutritional support in the presence of preexisting malnutrition should result in positive nitrogen balance. However, in the normal individual, positive nitrogen balance will not be achieved, regardless of the caloric and protein intake.

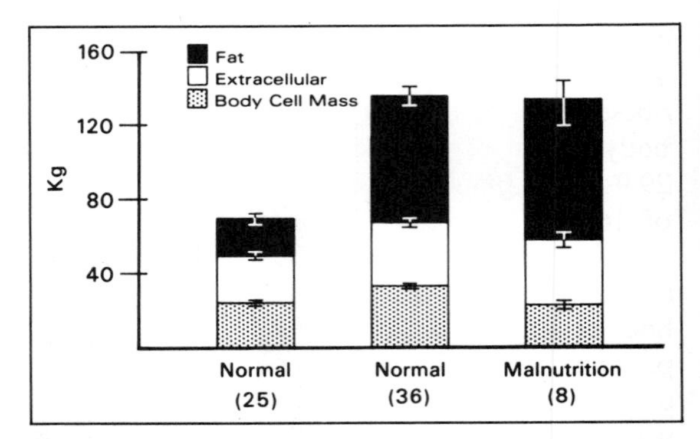

Figure 1-11. *The body composition of 25 normal volunteers and of 42 morbidly obese patients prior to weight-reducing surgery. Eight of the 42 morbidly obese patients were malnourished as defined by an $Na_e/K_e > 1.22$. (From H. M. Shizgal, Protein malnutrition following intestinal bypass for morbid obesity.* Surgery *86:60, 1979.)*

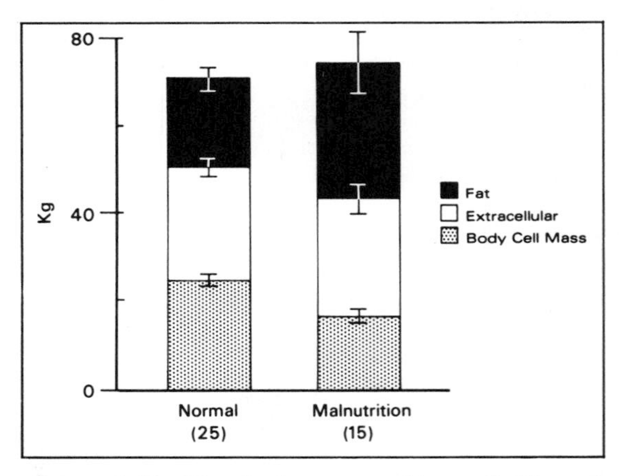

Figure 1-12. *The body composition of 15 malnourished obese patients compared to the body composition of 25 normal volunteers.*

OBESITY

Obesity is usually characterized by a relatively normal lean body mass covered by an excessive mantle of body fat. Body composition measurements performed in 42 morbidly obese patients just prior to jejunoileal bypass for weight reduction illustrate this point (Figure 1-11) [10]. These data also demonstrate that the obese individual can develop malnutrition in spite of an excessive amount of fat. In 8 of these morbidly obese patients, the body cell mass was abnormally decreased in size, while both extracellular mass and Na_e/K_e were abnormally increased. Their mean Na_e/K_e was 1.34 ± 0.03, indicating mild malnutrition. In the remaining 36 morbidly obese patients, the composition of lean body mass was normal. In this group, body fat accounted for 50 percent of their mean body weight of 136.9 ± 4.8 kg. Their lean body mass was 68.5 ± 2.3 kg, which was 36 percent greater than that of the 25 normal volunteers. Their body cell mass and extracellular mass were essentially equal in size, with a mean Na_e/K_e of 0.93 ± 0.02.

An intense catabolic stress can result in severe malnutrition that, because of excessive body fat, can be difficult to detect in the obese individual. This is demonstrated in the data collected in 15 obese individuals (Figure 1-12). Their mean body weight of 73.9 ± 6.9 kg was composed of 29.9 ± 4.8 kg of body fat, with a body cell mass of 16.2 ± 1.3 kg and an extracellular mass of 27.9 ± 1.5 kg. The 25 normal volunteers with a comparable body weight of 70.4 ± 0.5 kg had a body cell mass of 24.7 ± 1.1 kg. In these 15 obese patients, the mean Na_e/K_e was 1.56 ± 0.11, indicating moderate malnutrition. However, this was not suspected clinically because of their normal body weight and because their excessive body fat obscured the presence of muscle wasting.

REFERENCES

1. Behnke, A. R. Physiologic studies pertaining to deep sea diving and aviation, especially in relation to the fat content and composition of the body. *Harvey Lect.* 37:198, 1941.
2. Behnke, A. R., Guttentag, O. E., and Brodsky, C. Quantification of body weight and configuration from anthropometric measurements. *Hum. Biol.* 31:213, 1959.
3. Harvey, T. C., et al. Measurement of whole body nitrogen by neutron activation analysis. *Lancet* 2:359, 1973.
4. Kinney, J. M., Lester, J., and Moore, F. D. Relationship of energy expenditure to total exchangeable potassium. *Ann. N.Y. Acad. Sci.* 110:711, 1963.
5. Mernagh, J. R., Harrison, J. E., and McNeil, K. G. In vivo determination of nitrogen use Pu-Be sources. *Phys. Med. Biol.* 22:831, 1977.
6. Moore, F. D., and Brennan, M. F. Surgical Injury: Body Composition, Protein Metabolism and Neuroendocrinology. In the Committee on Pre- and Postoperative Care, American College of Surgeons (Eds.), *Manual of Surgical Nutrition.* Philadelphia: Saunders, 1975.
7. Moore, F. D., et al. *The Body Cell Mass and Its Supporting Environment.* Philadelphia: Saunders, 1963.
8. Pace, H., and Rathburn, E. N. Studies in body composition: III. The body water and chemically combined nitrogen content in relation to fat content. *J. Biol. Chem.* 158:685, 1945.
9. Shizgal, H. M. Protein requirements with total parenteral nutrition. *Surg. Forum* 24:60, 1978.
10. Shizgal, H. M., Forse, R. A., Spanier, A. H., and MacLean, L. D. Protein malnutrition following intestinal bypass for morbid obesity. *Surgery* 86:60, 1979.
11. Shizgal, H. M., Milne, C. A., and Spanier, H. A. The effect of nitrogen-sparing intravenously administered fluids on postoperative body composition. *Surgery* 85:496, 1979.
12. Shizgal, H. M., Spanier, A. H., Humes, J., and Wood, C. D. The indirect measurement of total exchangeable potassium. *Am. J. Physiol.* 233: F253, 1977.
13. Talso, P. J., Spafford, M. S., and Blaw, M. The metabolism of water and electrolytes in congestive heart failure: I. The electrolyte and water content of normal skeletal muscle. *J. Lab. Clin. Med.* 41:280, 1953.
14. Talso, P. J., Spafford, M. S., and Blaw, M. The metabolism of water and electrolytes in congestive heart failure: II. The distribution of water and electrolytes in skeletal muscle in edematous patients with congestive heart failure before and after treatment. *J. Lab. Clin. Med.* 41:405, 1953.

Intestinal Absorption of Nutrients

David B. A. Silk

2

Several recent studies have shown that there is a high prevalence of nutritional deficiencies in hospital inpatients with general medical and surgical disorders [47, 54, 55, 177, 220]. These deficiencies have been attributed to a failure to recognize the nutritional needs of patients and to the lack of emphasis given to nutrition in the medical curriculum [59].

The nutritional status of patients can be improved or maintained in a number of ways. The most physiologic and cheapest way is by maintaining or increasing normal food intake. In many patients this is often not possible, as for example when anorexia is a prominent symptom or when gastrointestinal cancer is a cause of a mechanical obstruction. Alternative choices of nutritional support usually lie between parenteral and enteral nutrition.

Enteral nutrition is defined as the administration of liquid nutritional products orally, or via a nasogastric feeding tube, or via feeding gastrostomies and jejunostomies. Although a number of factors have contributed to the interest currently being generated in this field, experiences of parenteral nutrition may have contributed more than most. The realization that parenteral nutrition is costly, requires considerable backup facilities, and is not without severe side effects has led to more critical appraisals being made of its indications. This, in turn, has led to the realization that many patients who previously might have received parenteral nutrition can be maintained perfectly well on enteral feeding. Other factors involved have been the development of narrow-bore nasogastric feeding tubes [24, 99, 380] that produce less discomfort and the possibility of longer-term use, the administration of liquid diets via gravity infusion [24, 99, 328, 380], and the recent availability of a number of proprietary, low-residue enteric feeds [328].

Despite the aforementioned advances, a number of problems in the field of enteral nutrition remain unsolved. The most important relates to the basic composition of enteric feeds. The composition of the energy and nitrogen constituents of the proprietary enteric feeds now available in the United Kingdom is extremely variable. For example, the nitrogen sources are composed of whole protein (e.g., Clinifeed), oligopeptides (Flexical), or of free amino acids (Vivonex). The carbohydrates that constitute part or most of the energy source are partial enzymic hydrolysates of starch, consisting of glucose polymers of varying mean chain lengths with greater or lesser proportions of free glucose. Some of the diets contain substantial proportions of unhydrolyzed triglycerides (e.g., Clinifeed); others contain medium chain triglycerides (Triosorbon) or only trace amounts of the essential fatty acid, linoleic acid (Vivonex).

The variability in diet composition is unlikely to have an adverse effect on the overall intestinal assimilation of nutrients in patients with normal gastrointestinal function because of the significant digestive and absorptive reserves of the human intestine. In contrast, when absorption is limited by reduced rates of luminal hydrolysis and/or intestinal transport—as in patients with short bowel syndrome, gastrointestinal fistulas, Crohn's disease, or severe pancreatic insufficiency—it becomes much more important that the composition of the energy and nitrogen constituents of enteric feeds be based on the formulations from which *maximal* absorption normally occurs. The optimal composition of the carbohydrate, nitrogen, and fat components of enteric feeds can only be determined once the processes involved in overall intestinal assimilation have been fully elucidated. The aim of this chapter is, therefore, to review some of the information that is available about the physiology of nutrient absorption.

DIGESTION AND ABSORPTION OF DIETARY CARBOHYDRATES

In the western hemisphere an adult ingests more than 300 gm of carbohydrate daily, which provides at least 50 percent of total caloric intake [187]. As Table 2-1 shows, most is in the form of starch and sucrose. Starch, the major food polysaccharide, consists of 85 percent amylopectin and 15 percent amylose. Amylose is composed of straight chains of glucose molecules, linked through α 1-4 glycosidic bands, whereas amylopectin, in addition to chains of α-linked glucose molecules, also has α 1-6 glycosidic linkages between glucose molecules in adjacent chains forming bridges.

Table 2-1. *Average Daily Carbohydrate Intake for an Adult Human Subject*

Saccharides	Intake (gm)	Percentage of Total
Polysaccharides		
Starch	200	64
Glycogen	1	0.5
Disaccharides		
Sucrose	80	26
Lactose	20	6.5
Monosaccharide		
Fructose	10	3

Site of Carbohydrate Assimilation

Using simple intestinal sampling techniques, most workers have agreed that dietary carbohydrate is predominantly absorbed in the proximal jejunum [50, 153]. More recently, using the multiple indicator dilution method [201, 202, 218], Johansson has confirmed these findings, showing that 75 percent of the sugar content of a composite liquid test meal was absorbed during transit in the proximal 70 cm of the intestine [200].

Luminal Digestion

The luminal hydrolysis of starch is catalyzed by two α amylases secreted by the pancreas and salivary glands. These enzymes have a pH optimum of approximately 7.0 [250], which corresponds to the luminal pH of the duodenum and proximal jejunum [252]. It is probable that in the lumen of the small intestine, pancreatic α amylase plays the predominant role [94, 130]. Both enzymes are capable of cleaving only the α 1-4 glycoside linkages of starch, and the products of luminal digestion of amylose are maltotriose and maltose. In the digestion of amylopectin, the α 1-6 linkages at the points of branching and the adjacent 1-4 linkages are resistant to the action of α amylases [43], and thus oligo 1-6 glucosides comprising four or more glucose units are formed (α-limit dextrins).

Thus, the final end-stage products of luminal digestion of starch are α-limit dextrins, maltotriose, and maltose. Neither α amylase is capable of hydrolyzing sucrose or lactose.

For many years it was presumed that the final stage of the digestion of carbohydrates to their constituent sugars takes place within the small bowel lumen by the action of enzymes of the succus entericus. This view was upheld despite the fact that various earlier authors had pointed out that carbohydrases occurred in far greater concentrations in the intestinal mucosa than in the succus entericus [61, 292, 302]. It was only at a much later stage, when the point was reemphasized that the luminal carbohydrase concentration was so low that they would be unable to account for the observed speed of hydrolysis and absorption of disaccharides [94], that the importance of mucosal digestion of dietary carbohydrate was recognized. Two more papers have now confirmed that there is *some* luminal carbohydrase activity in the bulk phase of the gut lumen [119, 147]. These studies are of interest because they both show that the intravenous injection of secretin and cholecystokinin causes a marked and highly significant release of solubilized oligosaccharidase activity in the gut lumen. The functional significance of this hormonally mediated enzyme release is unknown, but the phenomenon is certainly in keeping with the observation that the turnover rate of brush border disaccharidases is higher than the turnover rate of the epithelial cells themselves [199].

Membrane Digestion

In man, all the evidence points to the fact that dietary carbohydrate is translocated across the microvillus membrane of the intestinal mucosal cell predominantly in the form of monosaccharides. The final stages of the digestion of sucrose, lactose, maltose, maltotriose, and α-limit dextrins, as already mentioned, are cellular processes from which monosaccharides are formed. Small quantities of the disaccharide trehalose (α 1:1 glucose-glucose), which is present in mushrooms, may also require hydrolysis, and deficiency of its specific hydrolytic enzyme has been described [41]. The oligosaccharidases responsible for hydrolyzing these sugars have now been localized to the microvillus membrane fraction of human intestinal mucosa [231, 317, 370]. Confusion has arisen regarding the nomenclature and classification of these oligosaccharides, not least of all because the cross-reacting substrate specificity of these enzymes, even when highly purified, is not absolute [210].

α 1-4 Glucosidase (Maltase)

According to the technique of separation and the sensitivity of the chemical assay used, as many as five human intestinal enzymes capable of hydrolyzing maltose have been characterized [26, 33, 210, 231, 322]. All exhibit a pH optimum of around 6.0, which corresponds to the pH of the microclimates adjacent to the microvillus membrane [229]. One of the most functionally significant α 1-4 glucosidases is the enzyme isolated in a highly purified form from the brush border fraction of human intestinal mucosa by Kelly and Alpers [210]. This enzyme sequentially splits single glucose molecules from the nonreducing end of α 1-4 linked glucose chains. The enzyme is capable of hydrolyzing malto-oligosaccharides of chain length 2 to 9 glucose molecules and has a higher affinity for those of longer chain length (9 glucose units, Km 1.1 mM; maltose Km 3.8 mM).

Sucrose α-Glucohydrolase (Sucrase-Isomaltase)

The α 1-2 linkage of sucrose and the α 1-6 linkages of the α-limit dextrins are cleaved by sucrase isomaltase, which has recently been isolated from human intestinal mucosa and purified to homogeneity [74]. The enzyme is a hybrid molecule that can be split into two subunits, one of which exhibits absolute substrate specificity for sucrose and the other for the α 1-6 linkage of α-limit dextrins. The α-limit dextrins are thus hydrolyzed to glucose by the concerted action of sucrase-isomaltase and the oligosaccharidase with maltase specificity, predominantly glucamylase.

β-Galactosidases

Recent investigations have shown that the human intestinal mucosa contains three distinct β-galactosidases [25, 31, 32, 155]. One of these has a high substrate specificity for lactose and has been localized to the brush border fraction of human small intestinal mucosa. In addition, there is an acid β-galactosidase, which is localized to the lysomal fraction, and a hetero-β-galactosidase, which is localized to the soluble fraction of the cell.

Absorption of Carbohydrates in the Human

As mentioned previously, the digestion of carbohydrates has two phases, a luminal phase involving pancreatic α amylase and a membrane phase involving intestinal oligosaccharidases. As a result, dietary starch, sucrose, and lactose are hydrolyzed to monosaccharides of which 80 percent are glucose, 15 percent fructose, and 5 percent galactose [187].

There is still a great deal of speculation about the spatial and functional interrelationships between membrane saccharide hydrolysis and the transport processes that facilitate the absorption of monosaccharide hydrolysis products [85–89, 151, 187, 250, 286]. Not surprisingly, there is a disagreement about which model accords best with the currently available experimental data. At the outset, therefore, it seems advantageous to highlight some important observations about which there is general agreement.

First, with the possible exception of lactose [251], the results of steady-state perfusion experiments in the human have shown that over a wide range of solute concentrations, absorption of monosaccharide from the other disaccharides, sucrose and maltose, occurs at least as rapidly as from equivalent equimolar concentrations of constituent free monosaccharides [79, 125, 154, 251, 313]. Peripheral venous blood glucose increments are also at least as great after feeding of maltose and glucose [230, 241], as were portal venous blood glucose increments observed after duodenal instillations of maltose and glucose [106]. All these findings strongly suggest that in man, over the range of concentration of maltose and sucrose studied, disaccharide hydrolysis is not a rate-limiting step in absorption.

Second, a consistent feature of the human perfusion experiments with disaccharides has been the detection of monosaccharides in the intestinal contents aspirated from the distal end of the perfused segment [79, 125, 154, 251, 313]. This feature indicates release of disaccharide hydrolysis products into free solution during the process of absorption and, as all investigators have agreed, implies that at least components of infused disaccharide must be hydrolyzed at or on the luminal surface of the mucosal cell. In fact, these in vivo physiologic observations are in complete accord with what is currently known about the mode of integration of oligosaccharidases into the microvillus membrane. Thus, the amphipathic nature of these hydrolases has been demonstrated [234], and by comparisons of the molecular properties of enzymes released by treatments with papain and the neutral detergent Triton X-100 [228], it has been shown that the hydrophobic part of the enzyme molecules, which exhibited no hydrolase activity, are intercolated directly into the bilipid layer membrane [235], and the catalytic site on the hydrophobic part of the glycoprotein molecule is oriented outward from the surfaces of the membrane toward the lumen of the intestine [234].

It follows, therefore, that during the human digestive absorptive process of α-limit dextrins, maltotriose, maltose, sucrose, and lactose, there is at least *partial* dissociation between membrane hydrolysis and monosaccharide transport. Whether all or only a portion of monosaccharides liberated by membrane hydrolysis diffuse into free solution and require separate capture by specific transport mechanisms remains largely a matter of conjecture.

Transport of Freely Liberated Monosaccharides

Glucose

Results of in vitro experiments show that active glucose absorption is likely to depend on a gradient of sodium ion across the brush border membrane of intestinal epithelial cells [85, 88, 145]. The pattern of absorption observed during repeated in vivo perfusion studies, in which saturation of transport is reached at increasing glucose concentrations, has supported the existence in humans of a carrier-mediated mechanism for glucose absorption [184, 259]. The anticipated sodium dependency of glucose absorption could not be confirmed in two early human perfusion studies [284, 312], presumably owing to the bidirectional flux of sodium in vivo [128], which would allow considerable concentrations of sodium to build up in the microvillus microclimates despite low sodium concentrations in the bulk phase of the gut lumen. More recently, however, Fordtran and his colleagues have demonstrated, by replacing Na^+ in their perfusion systems with Mg^{2+} instead of mannitol, that 50 percent of the carrier-mediated absorption of glucose in vivo may be Na^+-dependent [42]. These results are, therefore, reminiscent of those of Debnam and Levin, who have also suggested that 50 percent of glucose absorption occurred by the Na^+-dependent electrogenic carrier-mediated mechanism [103].

Galactose

Until quite recently, most of the available in vivo and in vitro data indicated that galactose shares the glucose transport system.

Holdsworth had noted previously, in vivo in the human, inhibition of galactose uptake by glucose but not vice versa [183]. McMichael [249] has subsequently confirmed this result in rats in vivo and, in a study of the effects of various dietary manipulations on the Km and PD max of the electrogenic component of monosaccharide transport in vivo in the rat, Levin and his colleagues have also found support for the existence of multiple forms of sugar carriers [104]. If more than one functionally significant carrier-mediated transport system exists for glucose and galactose in human small intestine, however, they are likely to have to be controlled by the same gene, because in the congenital glucose-galactose malabsorption syndrome, neither sugar can be transported against a concentration gradient [120, 318, 378].

Fructose

In contrast to glucose and galactose, fructose absorption in the human appeared to be linearly related to concentration [183, 184] and not inhibited by glucose. At face value, these data suggested that fructose was absorbed by simple diffusion. However, in a separate series of experiments in humans, fructose was found to be absorbed much faster than two closely related monosaccharides, sorbose and mannose, which are known quite definitely to be absorbed passively [185]. It thus seems likely that in the human there must be a carrier mechanism for fructose, probably one with a very high Km. The recent in vitro studies of Gracey et al. [148] and the in vivo animal studies of Harries and coworkers [256] suggest that this carrier may also function by utilizing a transmembrane sodium gradient.

In different mammalian species, fructose is converted to glucose to a varying extent during intestinal absorption [149]. Human intestinal tissue also contains enzymes that are capable of metabolizing fructose [282], but fructose does not appear to be exposed to them during absorption in vivo; no significant fructose metabolism was observed in experiments where portal venous blood was sampled directly, or when peripheral venous blood levels were measured during jejunal infusion of fructose in patients whose liver had been bypassed by a portacaval anastomosis [183].

POSTULATED RELATIONSHIPS BETWEEN MUCOSAL HYDROLYSIS AND TRANSPORT OF SUGARS

Any proposed model for the membrane hydrolysis and subsequent transport of monosaccharide in humans has to account for the fact that monosaccharide transport from a disaccharide can occur as rapidly [154, 241, 251] or even faster than when the free form is presented to the mucosa for absorption [79, 125, 230, 313]. In addition, the model would have to account for the extremely efficient recapture of monosaccharide released following saccharide hydrolysis, for little of the monosaccharides diffuse back into the lumen of the bowel, especially when the concentration of disaccharides is low [94, 154, 251].

The original two-layer hypothesis proposed by Crane [85] remains one of the most attractive. In brief, it suggested that hydrolysis takes place on the surface or just within the membrane of the cell and that the monosaccharide transport mechanism is situated in a deeper layer of the cell wall. It was mentioned previously that recent topologic studies have indicated that the catalytic sites of microvillus membrane hydrolases are associated with the lipophobic moiety of the enzyme, which is that part located on the luminal side of bilipid layer membrane [228, 234, 235]. In view of this, there is no longer any need to invoke an intramembrane site of hydrolysis so that the monosaccharide transport mechanism (situated within or at the immediate surface of the membrane) and the hydrolysis site will be spatially separated. Hydrolysis of disaccharides will result in the setting up of a high local concentration of monosaccharide adjacent to the transport sites, which in the context of the human experimental studies might permit as rapid or even faster uptake of monosaccharide from the disaccharides than from free monosaccharide diffusing more randomly from the bulk phase of the gut lumen.

An alternative hypothesis of Hamilton and McMichael [160] is based more on the anatomy of the microvilli and an effect of the glycocolyx on diffusion. These workers envisaged that both the saccharidases and the transport mechanisms are scattered at random, like a mosaic, over the whole surface of the microvilli, and that once hydrolysis has taken place, the released monosaccharides are then free to move at random within the intermicrovillus space. They proposed that the intermicrovillus space, which is extremely long compared with its width, acts as a backwater so that released monosaccharides will have a greater chance of being absorbed by the transport mechanism before escaping into the gut lumen. Although this hypothesis can explain equal absorption rates from mono- and disaccharides, it is difficult to envisage how it can easily explain the faster rates of monosaccharide absorption from disaccharides [79, 125, 230, 313].

Most recently, Crane and his colleagues have proposed that the saccharidases of the brush border membrane act as true vectorial enzymes, thereby transferring their monosaccharide products directly across the membrane quite independently of the glucose or fructose transport carrier, hydrolase-related transport [89, 233, 300, 301]. Based on a series of experiments, hydrolase-related transport is purported not to require Na^+ and the glucose released is purported not to appear to mix with the pool of luminal glucose before crossing the membrane into the cell [233, 300, 301]. In addition, hydrolase-related transport is not the same as the efficient recapture mechanism described by others [286]. If hydrolase-related transport were to be shown to be biologically significant in the human, many, if not all, of the human experimental data could be explained. Unfortunately, as yet there is no evidence that there is any biologic significance of this hypothesis [89]. In the most recent in vivo perfusion study, addition of maltose to a

222 mM solution of glucose did not result in a significant increase in net uptake of glucose [313], and the possibility that hydrolase-related transport functions as a bypass mechanism for the deficit of carrier-mediated transport of free hexoses in congenital glucose-galactose malabsorption was not confirmed, as absorption of glucose from sucrose [193] and maltose [123] was negligible in two patients with the syndrome during intestinal perfusion in vivo.

Clinical Application

Most proprietary enteric foods contain at least some glucose as the energy source, which renders them hypertonic. Although it is still unclear whether hypertonicity forms the basis of the diarrhea that so often occurs following institution of enteric feeding [328], the apparent kinetic advantage transferred by maltose on glucose transport [79, 125, 230, 313] does suggest that there could be advantages to replacing the free glucose component of these diets with maltose. This is particularly so when the absorptive capacity of the intestine is reduced, for example, in patients with diffuse small bowel, Crohn's disease, or severe adult celiac disease or following small intestinal resection, as the aim of enteric feeding regimes in these cases should be to achieve maximum absorption at the lowest osmotic cost. At present, no information is available about the in vivo handling of higher glucose polymers by the human small intestine. It would be of interest, though, to determine whether partial enzymic hydrolysis of starch confers a kinetic advantage on glucose absorption, in which case the carbohydrate energy source of enteric foods could be further rationalized to ensure maximum glucose uptake, still keeping fluid and electrolyte secretion to the minimum.

DIGESTION AND ABSORPTION OF DIETARY PROTEIN

Although it has become clear that brush border hydrolysis and consequent utilization of the monosaccharide transport system is the predominant method of absorption of the luminal products of carbohydrate digestion in man, it now appears certain that two major mechanisms are involved in the absorption of the luminal products of protein digestion: on the one hand, transport of liberated free amino acid by group-specific active amino acid transport systems, and on the other hand, uptake of unhydrolyzed peptides by mechanisms independent of the specific amino acid entry mechanisms [12, 97, 169, 238, 240, 326].

Exogenous Protein

Dietary protein is derived from animal and vegetable sources and makes up 11 to 14 percent of the average caloric intake. In western diets this amounts to about 70 to 100 gm of protein per day.

Endogenous Protein

Proteins derived from endogenous sources, such as gastric, biliary, pancreatic, and intestinal secretions, consisting of secretory glycoproteins and digestive enzymes as well as protein derived from desquamated cells, also enter the intestinal lumen. The results of the animal studies of Nasset and coworkers indicate that the endogenous intestinal pool of protein is considerably larger than the exogenous pool [266, 268]. Nasset considered that the endogenous protein acted as a homeostatic device to prevent wide fluctuations in the amino acid mixture available for absorption [265], and in some early studies, the magnitude of the endogenous intestinal pool of protein was thought to be one of the reasons the pattern of appearance of amino acids in peripheral plasma was unrelated to the amino acid composition of material ingested [137, 382].

In the human, however, all the data point to the fact that this endogenous pool is much smaller. Using a simple intubation technique, Nixon and Mawer estimated that, at most, 8 gm of endogenous protein was secreted in response to oral ingestion of 30 gm of protein [276, 277], and using their multiple indicator dilution technique, Johansson found that, on the average, 3 gm of endogenous protein was secreted into the proximal small intestine in response to ingestion of 8 gm of protein [200]. Adibi and Mercer [16] have confirmed that exogenous protein is the principal source of increased free amino acids and peptides in intraluminal contents. In addition, unlike the aforementioned studies, recent studies in man show that the pattern of appearance of amino acids in peripheral plasma correlates well with the amino acid composition of the ingested materials [16, 236].

Site of Protein Assimilation

Most available data indicate that the bulk of undigested protein is absorbed in the proximal jejunum [50, 200, 276, 277, 329]. Two studies suggest, however, that some ingested protein and its luminal hydrolysis products reach the ileum [16, 68] and, as judged by the protein content of ileostomy effluent [143], protein assimilation may not be completed in the small intestine. The site of endogenous protein assimilation in the human has not been fully characterized. Recent animal experiments indicate the colon as the major site [93].

Luminal Protein Digestion

The initial step in protein digestion is the gastric phase: dietary protein is denatured at acid pH by the action of several pepsins with varying substrate specificities [353, 363, 373]. Negligible amounts of amino acids are released, and large polypeptides enter the duodenum, where they are further hydrolyzed by pancreatic, proteolytic enzymes. The functional significance in vivo of the gastric phase of digestion is normally thought to be minimal [50, 98]. In certain circumstances, however, it may play an important role in the assimilation of dietary protein. For example, recent studies indicate that in an animal model of massive pancreatic exocrine deficiency, intestinal absorption of exogenous protein is increased markedly by prior incubation with acid or pepsin [93].

The intraluminal digestion of proteins by pancreatic proteolytic enzymes has been reviewed in some detail by Gray and Cooper [152], and the zymogen enzyme exopeptidases by Keller [209]. Each of the proteolytic pancreatic enzymes is secreted as an inactive precursor. Trypsinogen is then activated by contact with enterokinase, an enzyme that has been isolated in a highly purified form from the brush border membrane fraction of human intestinal mucosa by a number of investigators [150, 174, 225, 279, 316]. Trypsin then hydrolyzes bonds in the other zymogens to form the active enzymes [209].

In addition to pancreatic, proteolytic enzymes, recent studies indicate the presence of solubilized intestinal brush border and cytoplasmic intestinal mucosal amino oligopeptidases in intestinal contents [205, 222, 333, 336, 338, 341]. As is the case with the succus entericus with respect to sugar digestion, the luminal peptidases of the jejunum are unlikely to be functionally significant [336]. In the ileum, the activity of these enzymes was considerably higher [333, 336], so that at this location a significant proportion of luminal peptides produced as a result of the action of pancreatic endo- and exopeptidases may be further hydrolyzed by luminal amino oligopeptidase released from the mucosa.

The products of luminal proteolysis are free amino acids and small peptides having a chain length of two to six amino acid residues [16, 64, 276, 277]. Analysis of postprandial intestinal contents aspirated from human jejunum reveals that only approximately one-third of the total amino acid content exists in the free form [16]. The nature of the oligopeptides in terms of distribution of chain length frequency and amino acid composition has not yet been characterized.

Free Amino Acid Transport

As with glucose transport, results of in vitro experiments have shown that active amino acid transport is dependent on a gradient of sodium ion across the brush border membrane of intestinal epithelial cells [320]. The absorptive patterns of free amino acids have been studied in some detail in humans using various in vivo steady-state perfusion techniques. In these experiments, saturation of transport was reached with increasing solute concentration compatible with the existence in the human of carrier-mediated mechanisms for amino acid transport [9, 10, 14, 15, 127, 171, 314]. Different free amino acids have markedly different affinities for free amino acid carrier systems. This is found to be so because the rates of absorption of individual free amino acids varied considerably when in vivo perfusion studies were performed using equimolar mixtures of different acids [9, 14, 15].

The sodium dependency of active free amino acid transport has not been confirmed in vivo in the human [10, 331]. Again, this is probably because of an artifact of the perfusion technique, and even in the presence of low sodium concentrations in the perfusion solutions, there is probably sufficient sodium entering the lumen from the gut wall to provide the necessary minimal sodium for interaction with the carrier.

The results of competition studies in animals have highlighted the likely existence of three major group-specific active transport systems [237, 242]:

1. Monoamino monocarboxylic (neutral amino acids).
2. Dibasic amino acids and cystine.
3. Dicarboxylic (acidic) amino acids.

It should be borne in mind that the subject is complicated by species differences, and by the fact that certain amino acids may be transported by more than one mechanism, e.g., glycine, proline, and hydroxyproline.

In vitro and in vivo studies of amino acid transport in patients with cystinuria and Hartnup disease have firmly established the existence of mechanisms 1 and 2 in man.

Hartnup Disease

Hartnup disease is a rare autosomal recessive disease named after the surname of the first affected family [35]. In this condition, the basic abnormality is a reduced efficiency of transport of neutral amino acids by the proximal renal tubular cells of the kidney [258]. Although earlier workers have considered that the kidneys alone were affected in this disorder, Milne and his coworkers considered that a more generalized defect could occur. To test this hypothesis, they have, over the years, investigated neutral amino acid transport from the intestines of these patients. In 1960, they reported that fecal excretion of tryptophan and tryptophan metabolites was increased in three patients with Hartnup disease after these patients had been fed tryptophan orally [258], and subsequently the results of oral tolerance tests [27, 28] confirmed the presence of a severe intestinal transport defect for histidine, phenylalanine, and tryptophan.

Cystinuria

Cystinuria is a related autosomal recessive disorder. The basic defect in this condition is a reduced efficiency of transport of the dibasic amino acids and cystine by the proximal tubular cells of the kidney [108]. In 1954 Dent and his coworkers demonstrated that blood levels of cystine were low in patients with homozygous cystinuria after the oral administration of 5 gm of cystine [107, 110]. Milne and his coworkers later showed that after oral administration of 20 gm lysine or 10 gm ornithine, the lysine, ornithine, and arginine levels in the feces of patients with cystinuria were elevated, as were the levels of cadavarin and putresin, the diamines of lysine and ornithine [257]. Following publication of these results, which strongly suggested that in homozygous cystinuria, an intestinal transport defect existed for the dibasic amino acids and cystine, two groups of workers in America independently demonstrated in vitro that there was a defect of carrier-mediated transport of the dibasic amino acids and cystine by jejunal mucosa obtained from patients with cystinuria [246, 355]. Later, in vivo absorption studies in cystinuria carried out by Milne's group and our own produced some conflicting results. Using a perfusion technique, impaired absorption of lysine, arginine, and cystine in homozygous cystinuria was confirmed [172, 339, 340]. However, when high doses of lysine and arginine were administered orally, convincing evidence of an intestinal transport defect could be demonstrated only for arginine [29, 171] and not for lysine [29, 171] or ornithine [171].

Thus, in cystinuria, in vitro and in vivo experimental data indicate that only at low concentrations (i.e., below the Km for lysine transport) does a defect exist throughout the small intestine for free lysine. At all concentrations thus far tested, however, there appears to be an intestinal transport defect for free arginine and cystine in cystinuria.

Other Amino Acid Transport Defects

There have also been a few reports of defective intestinal transport of individual amino acids, such as methionine [116, 189] and proline [146], but there is as yet insufficient evidence to establish the existence of more than one carrier system for an individual amino acid in human small intestine.

Finally, in view of the evidence that will be presented favoring the existence of carrier peptide transport systems in humans, it must be stressed that the nutritional significance of information obtained from studies of the absorption of mixtures of free amino acids is questionable. Thus, in vivo perfusion studies in the human have shown that the pattern of uptake of individual amino acids from partial enzymic hydrolysates of protein, whose amino acid and peptide composition closely simulates that of postprandial luminal contents [16, 64, 276, 277], is quite different from that of uptake from equivalent free amino acid mixtures [122, 330, 335]. The reason for the difference is the existence of peptide transport systems, to be discussed.

INTESTINAL HANDLING OF PEPTIDES

Historical Aspects

Nineteenth century physiologists believed that dietary protein was absorbed in the form of polypeptides [139, 302, 368], a view that seemed to be confirmed when Nolf [278] and Messerli [253] showed that peptones produced by tryptic hydrolysis of protein disappeared from the lumen of the small intestine more rapidly than equivalent amounts of free amino acids. When Cohnheim demonstrated in 1901 [71] that intestinal juice was capable of hydrolyzing peptones to amino acids, some early workers suggested that protein must be hydrolyzed to amino acids before absorption takes place. This hypothesis began to gain ground when all known free amino acids were detected in intestinal contents obtained during protein absorption in vivo [2, 72, 73], and when studies in vivo showed that hydrolysates of protein (consisting of amino acids) disappeared rapidly from the lumen of the small intestine [4, 62]. Furthermore, many of the investigators at the time speculated that free acids passed into the portal circulation during protein absorption as the nonprotein nitrogen values in peripheral and portal plasma increased during absorption of amino acids [7, 131, 364], protein hydrolysates, and whole protein [3, 191]. When only amino acids were isolated from the portal circulation during protein absorption [5], the idea that protein was completely hydrolyzed to amino acids within the intestinal lumen before absorption took place became the classic view of protein absorption [367]. This view was held despite later observations that intraluminal peptidase activity was insufficient to account for the absorption of peptone in the form of free amino acids [61].

The concept was questioned by a number of workers who claimed that peptides entered the portal venous circulation during protein absorption [162, 207, 216]. The quantitative significance of their findings was unknown, and later studies, using improved techniques, failed to detect an increase in peptide-bound amino acid levels in portal plasma during protein absorption [65, 66, 109, 111]. The final vindication of the classic view of protein absorption appeared to be provided by the demonstration, using ion exchange chromatography, that only free amino acids appeared in peripheral plasma after protein was administered to human subjects [343].

In 1954, Fisher strongly criticized the classic view of protein absorption [126]. He pointed out that it had previously been shown that upward of 200 hours were required for the liberation of 90 percent of the amino acids from different proteins subjected to successive action of pepsin, trypsin, and erepsin [117, 138] and made the following statement:

> Even on the most generous assumption, the time course of liberation of amino acids is too slow to fit with the view that protein must be digested to amino acids before they are absorbed [126].

He suggested that the idea of absorption of protein in the form of peptides deserved serious consideration [126]. His postulate did not, however, totally distinguish brush border peptide hydrolysis from absorption of unhydrolyzed peptides.

Mucosal Transport of Peptides

Initial experiments in vitro with dipeptides showed that small quantities of intact glycylglycine and glycyl-L-leucine crossed the intestinal wall [20]. Similar observations were made when glycyl-glycine was studied in vitro [374, 375] and in vivo [271] by other workers. Newey and Smyth [272] demonstrated that dipeptides could be taken up intact by intestinal mucosa and concluded [273] that the products of protein digestion could be transported into the mucosal cell in the form of oligopeptides as well as amino acids. The concept of intact peptide uptake as a second mode of protein absorption, although not disputed, was not thought to be quantitatively significant, as it seemed much more likely that absorption of peptides, analogous to disaccharides, would involve brush border hydrolysis with subsequent absorption of the released amino acids by amino acid transport systems.

The modern era of our knowledge of peptide absorption has stemmed from the results of oral load experiments carried out in the human by Matthews and his colleagues [83]. They found out that a given quantity of glycine was absorbed faster when administered orally as the dipeptide and tripeptide than when administered in the free form. It was concluded that the glycine peptides were probably transported into the mucosal cell in the unhydrolyzed form because if brush border hydrolysis of the peptides had preceded uptake of transport of liberated amino acids, then at best the net rates of glycine transport from the free and peptide forms of glycine would have been the same. In the light of recent in vivo perfusion data showing more rapid transport of glucose from maltose [79, 125, 313], their data were perhaps somewhat overinterpreted. Nonetheless their conclusions provided a powerful stimulus for further research in this area, which has subsequently provided unequivocal evidence for the existence in man of peptide transport systems that are distant from those used by free amino acids.

Evidence for Intact Transport of Dipeptides in Humans

Of all the experimental data available favoring dipeptide transport in human intestine, still the most persuasive is that derived from experiments performed in patients with Hartnup disease and cystinuria. The intestinal transport defect for neutral amino acids in Hartnup disease and dibasic amino acids in cystinuria has already been discussed. Despite these transport defects, the affected amino acids were shown to be absorbed normally or near normally when presented to the mucosa in the form of homologous or mixed dipeptides [27, 28, 30, 172, 269, 339]. To illustrate this, Figures 2-1 and 2-2 show results of perfusion experiments carried out in patients with cystinuria [339]. No significant absorption of L-arginine occurred when the jejunum of cystinuric patients was perfused with free L-arginine, whereas in contrast, absorption of L-arginine in these patients was normal when the test solution contained the dipeptide L-arginyl L-leucine.

If any of the dipeptides administered to these patients had been hydrolyzed to substantial degrees in the bulk phase of the gut lumen, or by brush border peptidases before transport of released amino acid by specific active transport processes, then absorption of the affected amino acids would not have occurred. This was clearly not the case in these experiments.

Additional evidence supporting the existence of intact dipeptide transport in human small intestine has included the following. First, the competition between free amino acids for mucosal uptake is avoided or much reduced when solutions of dipeptides, instead of corresponding free amino acid mixtures, are instilled into the gut lumen [11, 170, 338]. Such observations could not be explained if complete luminal or membrane hydrolysis occurred before transport of free amino acids. Similar observations, but on a wider scale, have been observed in animal studies [238].

Second, in all the human dipeptide perfusions in vivo, faster rates of uptake of at least one of the constituent residues has been observed from dipeptide than from corresponding free amino acid solutions [11, 77, 78, 170, 338]. As mentioned previously, this line of evidence is open to criticism because the same phenomenon has been observed in three perfusion studies with disaccharides [79, 125, 313], which are thought to be hydrolyzed at the brush border and not to be transported intact. Nonetheless, unlike the sugar experiments, the kinetic advantage conferred by dipeptides on amino acid transport has been a consistent finding and of much greater magnitude, and has been observed during perfusion of dipeptide substrates known to have a low affinity for human brush border peptidases [215].

Third, acidic pH abolishes the hydrolysis of dipeptides by brush border peptidases [167, 213, 215]. However, when the intraluminal pH was made highly acidic (pH less than 3), there was only a 40 percent reduction in uptake of two glycine-containing dipeptides [129]. Thus, dipeptide transport was observed even under conditions likely to completely inhibit brush border peptidase activity. The latter study is open to some criticism because of the uncertainty of what effect acidifying the bulk luminal phase has on unstirred layer pH.

Finally, glycyl-glycine has been detected in peripheral plasma samples during intestinal perfusion in vivo [11], an observation that has been quoted as evidence of intact intestinal absorption [12]. Since high concentrations of dipeptide were perfused in the aforementioned experiment, it does not necessarily follow that the peptide gained access to the circulation via specific transport process across the microvillus membrane. In other studies, however, carnosine, anserine, and hydroxyproline peptides have also been detected in the peripheral circulation during oral feeding experiments in the human [193, 288, 296, 297]. The qualitative significance is far from clear at present.

Characteristics of Dipeptide Transport in Humans

Matthews and coworkers have shown in vitro that intestinal transport of glycyl-sarcosine and carnosine occurs via a carrier-mediated sodium-dependent process [7, 239]. Doubt has subsequently been thrown upon the sodium dependency of peptide transport, because Rubino et al. have shown appreciable influx into rabbit ileal mucosa in vitro after sodium replacement [309]. Cheeseman and Parsons have reported that transport of glycyl-leucine by the small intes-

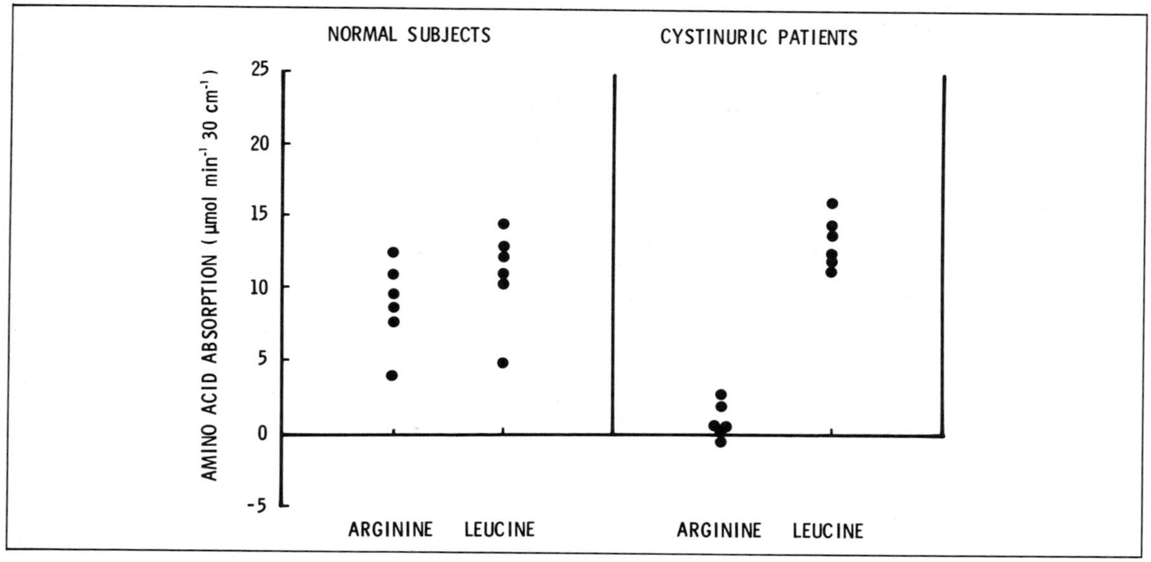

Figure 2-1. *Jejunal absorption of* L*-arginine and* L*-leucine during intestinal perfusion with solutions containing* L*-arginine (1 mM) +* L*-leucine (1 mM). Results of studies carried out in six normal subjects and six cystinuric patients. (From D. B. A. Silk, D. Perrett, and M. L. Clark, Jejunal and ileal absorption of dibasic amino acids and an arginine-containing dipeptide in cystinuria.* Gastroenterology *68:1426, 1975.)*

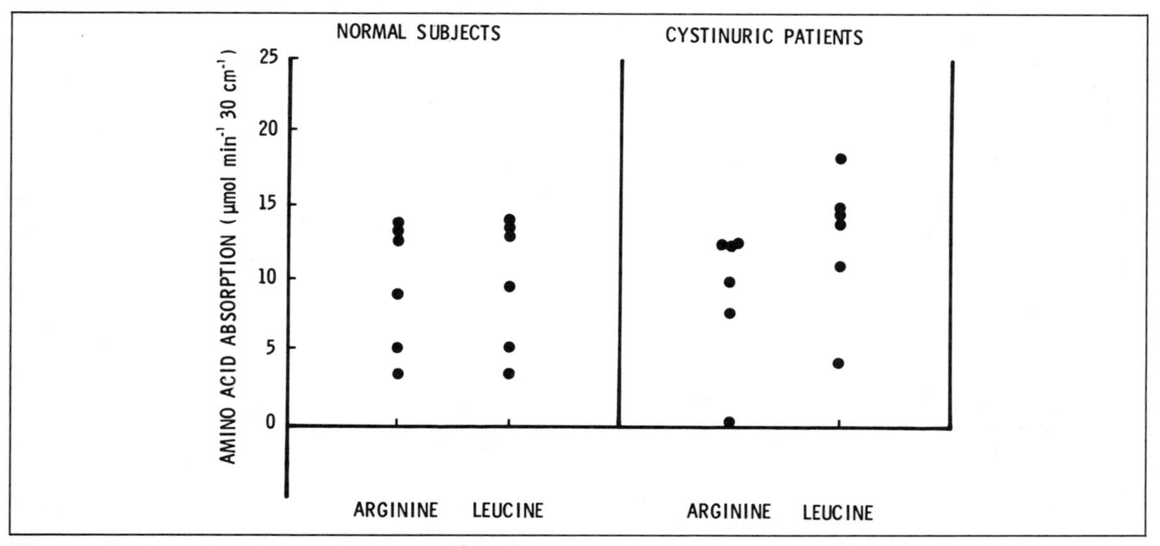

Figure 2-2. *Jejunal perfusion of amino acid residues of* L*-arginyl-*L*-leucine during the perfusions with a solution containing* L*-arginyl-*L*-leucine (1 mM). Results of studies carried out in six normal subjects and six cystinuric patients. (From D. B. A. Silk, D. Perrett, and M. L. Clark, Jejunal and ileal absorption of dibasic amino acids and an arginine-containing dipeptide in cystinuria.* Gastroenterology *68:1426, 1975.)*

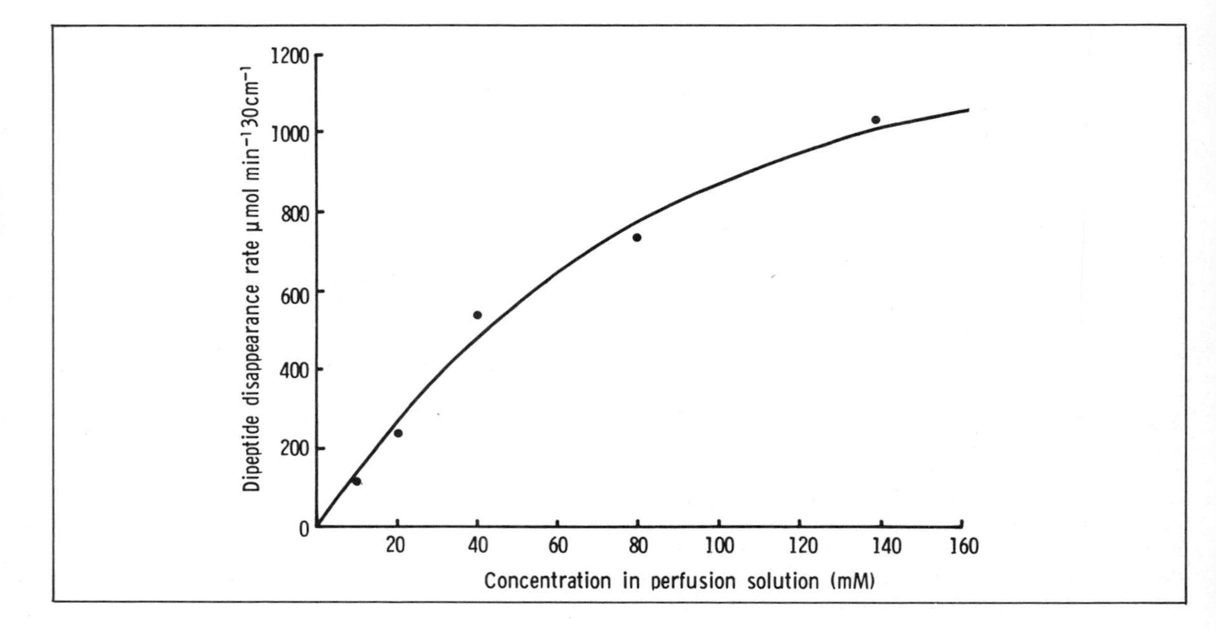

Figure 2-3. *Dipeptide disappearance rates during perfusion of 30-cm segments of human jejunum with test solutions containing glycyl-L-alanine. Each point is the mean of studies on at least four individual volunteers.*

tine of *Rana pipiers* in vivo was unaffected by replacement of intralumen sodium by potassium, whereas transport of glycine and leucine from the equivalent mixture of free amino acids was inhibited [63].

In the human, saturation of transport of three dipeptides has been reached during perfusion in vivo of increasing solute concentrations [11, 327], and this is illustrated in Figure 2-3 for the dipeptide glycyl-L-alanine (Gly-Ala). Competitive inhibition between two dipeptides has been observed [18], and this confirms the existence of a carrier-mediated dipeptide transport mechanism in human small intestine. The sodium dependency of this transport process has not yet been investigated.

Free amino acids have not been shown to alter substantially the absorption rates of either glycyl-glycine or glycyl-leucine in vivo, and this fact suggests that the carrier-mediated transport system for dipeptides in human small intestine is not shared by free amino acids [18].

The question whether more than one carrier-mediated transport system exists for dipeptides in the small intestine of animals or humans has not yet been fully resolved [238]. Based on the use of glycyl-glycine as an inhibitor dipeptide, Fairclough and colleagues have published evidence suggesting that there is more than one operative dipeptide transport system in human small intestine in vivo [124]. However, Das and Radhakrishnan have studied the inhibitory effects of a wide range of dipeptides on the intestinal uptake of glycyl-leucine by human intestine in vitro and have reached the alternative conclusion that there is a single dipeptide transport system with an extremely broad specificity [96, 299].

Appearance of Free Amino Acids in Lumen During Dipeptide Perfusion

A consistent finding during in vivo dipeptide perfusion experiments in human small intestine is the difference of free amino acids in intestinal contents aspirated from the distal end of the perfusion segment [11, 18, 77, 78, 170, 172, 338, 339, 341, 342]. The rate of appearance of free amino acids during perfusion of different dipeptides varies [11, 338], and substantially faster rates of appearance have been observed during ileal compared to jejunal dipeptide perfusion [11, 342].

Intraluminal peptidase activity is insufficient to account for the appearance of more than a small proportion of the released free amino acids [11, 338], which implies that, analogous to disaccharide transport, a close relationship exists between the mucosal transport and hydrolysis of dipeptides. According to numerous animal studies, two distinct groups of mucosal peptidases are located within the cytoplasmic compartment of the cell and at the brush border of the cell [115, 140, 168, 206, 211, 213, 214, 280, 281, 289, 304, 379]. Although not so complete, results of human studies indicate a similar subcellular distribution [211, 212, 215, 274, 275]. It follows, therefore, that the appearance of free amino acids during dipeptide perfusion is likely to be due either to hydrolysis of proportions of dipeptide by brush border enzymes before transport has occurred or hydrolysis of dipeptide by cytoplasmic peptidases after absorption, a process that would need to be followed by efflux of released free amino acids back out of the cell, across the unstirred water layer, into the bulk phase of the gut lumen. For two reasons the first explanation seems more probable.

First, the differential rates of appearance of free amino acids during perfusion of glycylalanine and alanyl-glycine [338] correlate with the differential specific activities of brush border peptidase against the two dipeptides [215]. Second, the appearance rates of hydrolytic products is greater during tripeptide than dipeptide perfusion [19, 341], and human mucosal brush border peptidases have a higher specific activity against tripeptides than against dipeptides [215, 274, 275]. To date there is no available experimental evidence to favor the second explanation.

Postulated Relationships Between Mucosal Hydrolysis and Transport of Dipeptides

Four hypothetical models for intestinal mucosal uptake of amino acids from dipeptides in human small intestine in vivo are depicted in Figures 2-4 through 2-6.

Scheme A, as depicted in Figure 2-4, proposes that all dipeptide presented to the mucosa for absorption is hydrolyzed by brush border peptidases, followed by absorption of the liberated amino acids by group-specific free amino acid transport mechanisms. While adequately explaining the appearance of free amino acids during in vivo perfusion, this scheme is not in keeping with the observations of normal uptake of dipeptides in patients with cystinuria and Hartnup disease, who have complete intestinal transport defects for free amino acids. Nor can it explain the avoidance of competition for mucosal uptake between dipeptide-bound amino acids.

Scheme B, as depicted in Figure 2-5, proposes that all dipeptide presented to the mucosa for

Figure 2-4. *Hypothetical model for intestinal mucosal uptake of amino acids from dipeptides. Complete hydrolysis of dipeptide by peptidase located on the luminal surface of the microvillus membrane (M-V-M). The liberated amino acids are transferred from the enzyme directly to the specific carrier-systems utilized by amino acids presented in the free form (Carrier F-A.A.).*

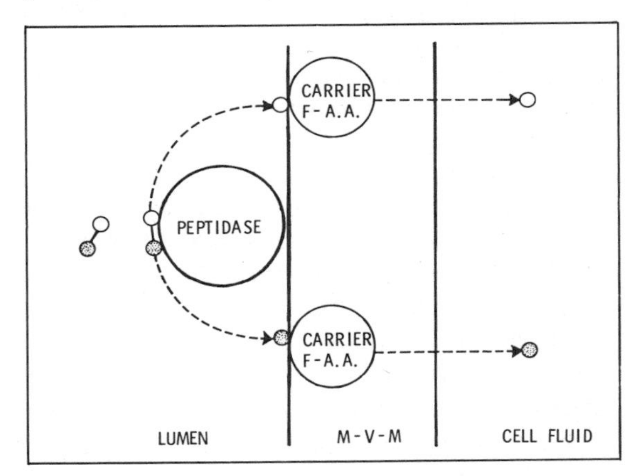

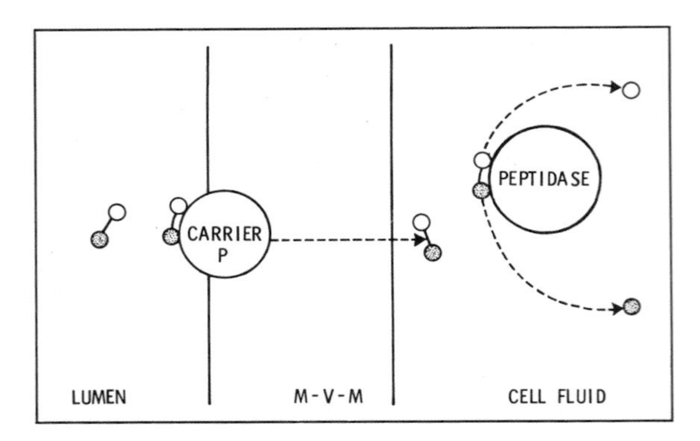

Figure 2-5. *Hypothetical model for intestinal mucosal uptake of amino acids from dipeptides. Transmembrane transfer of dipeptides using specific dipeptide carrier-system (Carrier P) located on the luminal surface of the microvillus membrane (M-V-M). Hydrolysis of intact peptide catalyzed by intracellular peptidase enzymes.*

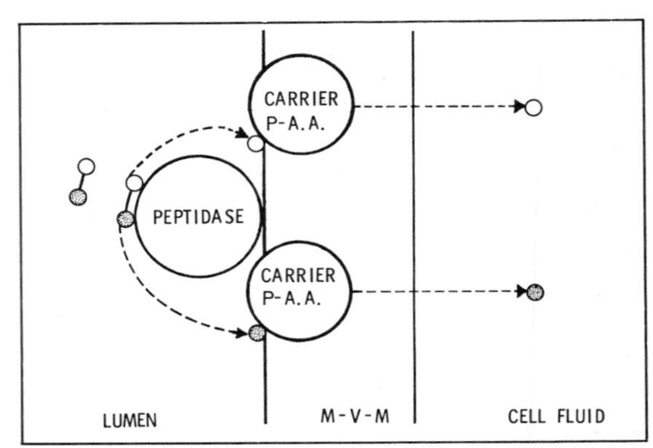

Figure 2-6. *Hypothetical model for intestinal mucosal uptake of amino acids from dipeptides. Complete hydrolysis of dipeptides by peptidases located on the luminal border of the microvillus membrane (M-V-M). The liberated amino acids are transferred from the enzyme directly to the carrier-systems (Carrier P-A.A.). The carrier-systems (Carrier-P-A.A.) are only accessible to amino acids liberated by peptidases on the luminal border of the M-V-M, and are separate from the carrier-systems (Carrier F-A.A.) utilized by amino acids presented in the free form (see Figure 2-4).*

absorption is transported intact and hydrolyzed by cytoplasmic peptidases. The specific activity of cytoplasmic peptidases is high [115, 140, 168, 206, 211, 213, 280, 281, 289], and the rapid hydrolysis of dipeptides can be expected to result in the formation of a concentration gradient for free amino acids between the cytoplasmic compartment of the cell and the microcirculation down which they would then diffuse. Such a scheme would be in keeping with the evidence supporting transport of intact dipeptide, as already discussed, but would not explain the back diffusion of free amino acids into the gut lumen during dipeptide perfusion.

Considering all the available experimental data as a whole, there are certain features that would obviously be compatible with schemes A and B. We have suggested, therefore [325–327], that neither of the two schemes should be mutually exclusive and that a dual hypothesis is applicable. Thus, those dipeptides with a high affinity for brush border peptidases would be predominantly handled according to scheme A, whereas greater proportions of those with a low affinity for brush border peptidases (e.g., proline-containing dipeptides) would be handled according to scheme B.

Although there is as yet little experimental evidence supporting it, consideration should be given to a further model, scheme C, as depicted in Figure 2-6, which proposes that brush border membrane hydrolysis of a dipeptide is followed by uptake of amino acids by carrier mechanisms only available to amino acids liberated by the action of these enzymes. It is essentially analogous to the concept of hydrolase-related transport proposed by Crane and colleagues for sugar transport [89, 233, 300, 301]. Its application to dipeptide transport has one theoretical drawback, however, because in contrast to disaccharides, hydrolysis of at least some dipeptides by brush border peptidases is likely to be a rate-limiting step in absorption [12, 215, 274, 275, 337].

Tripeptide Absorption in Humans

Absorption of three tripeptides has been investigated in humans [19, 83, 341]. During the in vivo intestinal perfusion studies [19, 341], the rate of amino acid uptake has been shown to be significantly greater from tripeptide than from corresponding free amino acid solutions. Whether this is indicative of intact transport of tripeptide or of constituent dipeptide released following brush border hydrolysis is not entirely clear. In all these experiments, constituent-free and dipeptide-bound amino acids were released into the lumen during tripeptide perfusion, and as with dipeptides, the relative rates of appearance of hydrolysis products varied according to the chemical structure of tripeptide perfused. Subfractionation studies using human intestine reveal approximately equal distributions of tripeptidase activity between brush border and soluble fractions [273, 274]. It seems reasonable, then, to conclude that substantial proportions of at least two of the infused tripeptides, alanylglycyl-glycine and trileucine, were hydrolyzed at the brush border prior to uptake of constituent dipeptide and amino acid by a peptide and a free amino acid transport mechanism, respectively. As with dipeptides, a dual mechanism for the intestinal handling of tripeptides may be proposed, as the available data indicate that substantially greater proportions of triglycine were absorbed intact. Again the quantitative importance of the brush border hydrolysis versus intact transport mechanisms is likely to be dictated by the affinity of the tripeptide substrate for the brush border peptidases.

As yet there is no evidence to confirm animal findings that intact uptake of tripeptides occurs via the system utilized by dipeptides [6, 8] and, moreover, it is not clear yet whether uptake of intact tripeptide in human intestine in vivo occurs via an energy-dependent carrier-mediated process [8].

Tetrapeptide Transport in Humans

The absorption of only one tetrapeptide, tetraglycine, has been studied in human intestine in vivo [17]. No evidence of intact absorption was found, and hydrolysis of the peptide at the brush border appears to be the rate-limiting step in absorption.

The results in animals are more conflicting, for evidence has been presented in one in vivo study to suggest that significant components of L-leucyl-triglycine may be absorbed intact and subsequently hydrolyzed by cytoplasmic peptide hydrolases [67]. However, in vitro work performed by Matthews and coworkers indicated that tetrapeptides are not absorbed intact, but are hydrolyzed to tri- and dipeptides by brush border peptide hydrolases prior to uptake [58].

Nutritional Significance of Oligopeptide Transport in Humans

The studies carried out in Hartnup disease and cystinuria have emphasized the nutritional importance of oligopeptide transport in these two conditions. As there are 400 possible dipeptides and 8,000 possible tripeptides, it would clearly be impossible to assess the overall nutritional importance of peptide absorption by studying the characteristics of absorption of each in turn.

A number of recent perfusion studies, however, do support a concept that mucosal uptake of peptides has an important, or possibly a major, role to play in protein absorption.

Total absorption of α amino nitrogen has been shown to be consistently greater during perfusion of solutions containing partial enzymic hydrolysates of protein (consisting mainly of peptides of chain length two to six amino acid residues) than protein perfusion of the corresponding free amino acid mixtures of identical amino acid composition [330, 335]. In addition, there was less variation in the extent to which individual amino acids were absorbed from the peptide solutions compared to absorption from the amino acid solutions. Figure 2-7 summarizes the results of one such perfusion study performed in vivo with a partial enzymic hydrolysate of lactalbumin [122], and it can be seen that the alteration in pattern of absorption of amino acids from the peptide solution was largely due to the fact that those amino acids, which were

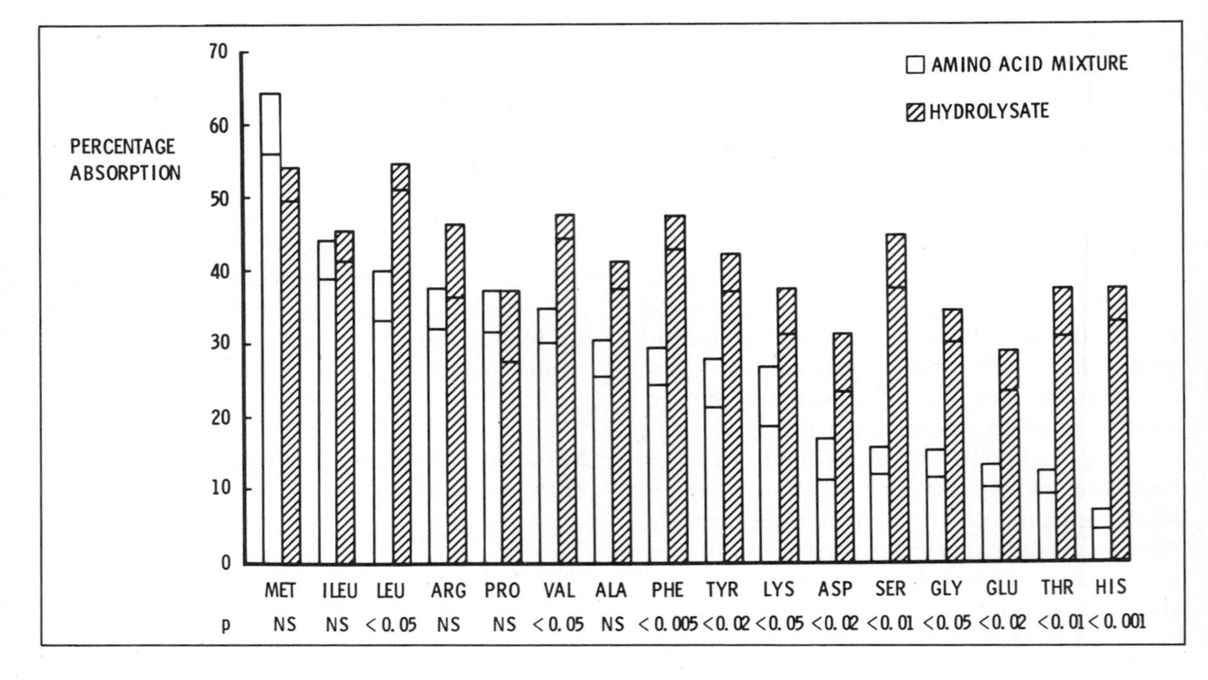

Figure 2-7. *Absorption of amino acids from an amino acid mixture simulating lactalbumin and a partial enzymic hydrolysate of lactalbumin. The total height of each column represents the mean value (n = 6) and the transverse line across each column shows one standard error. The significance of the difference between absorption from the amino acid mixture and the partial enzymic hydrolysate is given below each pair of columns. Open columns = amino acid mixture; shaded columns = partial enzymic hydrolysate of lactalbumin; NS = not significant.*

absorbed poorly from the free amino acid mixture, were absorbed to a greater extent from the peptide solution.

The possible importance of this and evening out of amino acid absorption rates conferred by the peptide component of the hydrolysate on the pattern of amino acid transport in relation to protein synthesis has been discussed in detail [287].

Clinical studies have shown that the kinetic advantage conferred by peptides on rates of amino acid transport is maintained even when the absorptive function of intestinal mucosa is reduced, as for example in untreated adult celiac disease [13, 334]. Moreover, there is experimental evidence from animal studies suggesting that long-term protein restriction causes a decrease in absorption of free amino acids but not peptides.

Conceivably, therefore, there could be advantages in administering oligopeptide mixtures (i.e., partial enzymic hydrolysates of protein) rather than free amino acid mixtures orally to patients with severe, long-standing protein-calorie malnutrition caused by disorders of intestinal mucosal function.

ABSORPTION OF LIPIDS

Triglycerides, cholesterol, and the fat-soluble vitamins A, D, and K constitute the major dietary lipids. Daily adult intake of triglyceride varies from 60 to 80 gm with an intake of cholesterol of 0.5 to 1 gm per day. Triglycerides are triesters of glycerol. Most contain fatty acids with 16 to 18 carbon atoms (long-chain triglycerides) and are highly insoluble in water. Some contain fatty acids with 8 to 12 carbon atoms (medium-chain triglycerides, MCT) and are more soluble. The processes involved in the digestion and absorption of lipids are complex, and involve a chemical event, the hydrolysis of ester lipids by lipases and esterases, and a physical event, the micellar solubilization of lipolytic products, which increases the diffusive flux through the unstirred water layer by a factor of 100 to 200 [182].

Intraluminal Digestion

Dietary lipid is emulsified in the stomach by mechanical means, and a coarse emulsion passes into the duodenum, where mixing with bile and pancreatic juice occurs. Although it was noted as long ago as 1957 that lipolysis of fed triglyceride occurred in the human stomach [50], it was not clear whether this lipolysis was an effect of regurgitated intestinal content or was attributable to a gastric lipase. A specific lipase was later isolated from gastric contents [70], and this lipase is currently thought to be secreted by glands in or near the pharynx. Thus it has been renamed pharyngeal lipase [161]. The action of this enzyme is not enhanced by bile salts, and its major effect is to hydrolyze triglyceride to diglyceride and fatty acid. The liberated fatty acids probably facilitate the further emulsification of triglycerides in the stomach and upper duodenum.

Intraluminal Lipolysis

The emulsified lipids undergo lipolysis in the lumen of the duodenum and upper jejunum, thus providing more polar lipid for further emulsification and eventual micellar solubilization. The enzyme responsible for lipolysis is pancreatic lipase, whose secretion is controlled by the hormon cholecystokinin-pancreozymin (CCK-PZ), which in turn is released from specific jejunal cells of the APUD series [293] in response to food ingestion. Lipase acts at the substrate water interface of the emulsion droplets, and Benzonana and Desnuelle [40] have shown that the

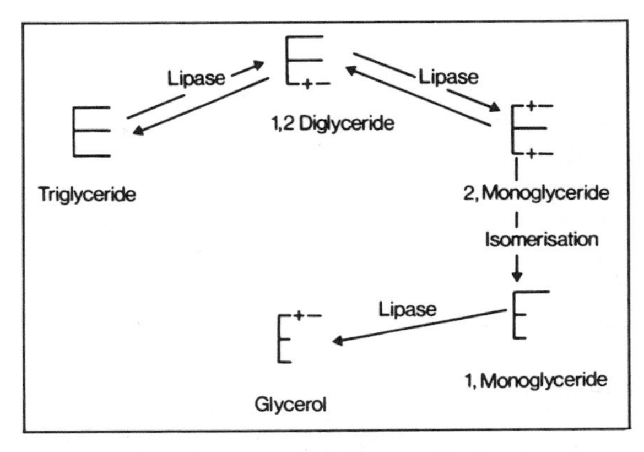

Figure 2-8. *Hydrolysis of triglycerides by pancreatic lipase.*

rate of lipid hydrolysis is proportional to the interfacial area of emulsion droplets, because increasing the concentration of triglyceride substrate had little effect on the rate of hydrolysis until the solution was saturated and an emulsion had been formed.

Pancreatic lipase hydrolyzes the one and three ester bonds of the triglyceride molecule, thereby producing free fatty acids and a 2-monoglyceride. Some further hydrolysis of the 2-monoglyceride occurs, but only after isomerization of the fatty acid to the one position (Figure 2-8) has taken place. The effect of luminal bile acids on the lipase-catalyzed hydrolysis of insoluble triglyceride has, in the past, mostly been described as an activation. However, recent results of experiments with purified or pure lipase show that bile salts inhibit lipase activity at concentrations in the critical micellar concentration range [49, 365]. Bile salts are presumed to exert their inhibiting effect by preventing binding of the enzyme to its substrate [48]. This inhibitory effect of bile acids is now thought to be prevented by the action of colipase, a polypeptide secreted in human pancreatic juice [261], which forms a lipase-colipase complex.

A further distinct lipase has been partially purified from homogenates of small intestinal mucosa. The physiologic importance of this enzyme has not yet been defined.

Cholesterol

All the evidence points to the fact that the hydrolysis of cholesteryl esters is important for cholesterol absorption [324], and the esterified cholesterol, which enters the small intestinal lumen, is hydrolyzed by pancreatic cholesteryl esterase. The activity of the enzyme is greatly increased by the presence of bile acids [243]. Indeed trihydroxy bile salts have been considered to act as cofactors [195]. According to the results published by Erlanson [121], the specificity for trihydroxy bile acids is not absolute, and a similar stimulating effect can be achieved by dihydroxy bile acids, albeit at higher concentrations.

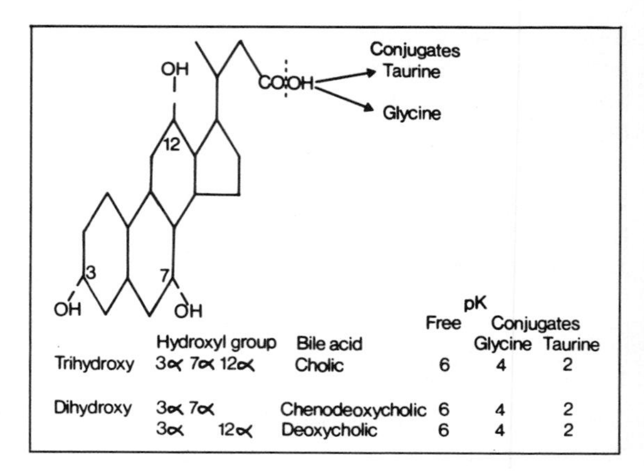

Figure 2-9. *Chemical structure of bile acids and effects of conjugation on their dissociation constants (i.e., pK).*

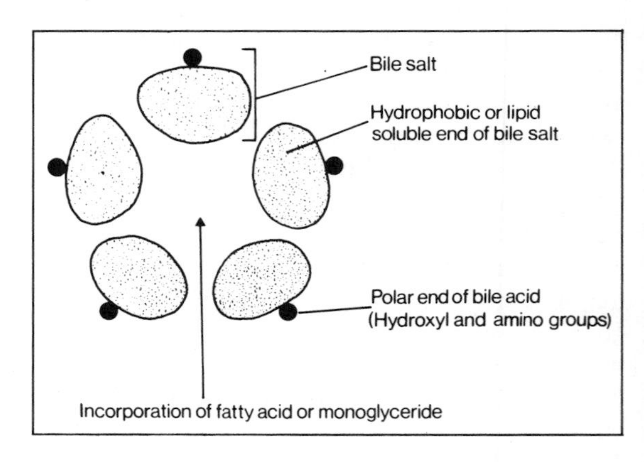

Figure 2-10. *Schematic representation of mixed bile salt micelle.*

Micellar Solubilization

The products of luminal lipid hydrolysis—free cholesterol, monoglycerides, and fatty acids—are poorly soluble in the water milieu of the gut lumen and, as such, diffuse very slowly across the unstirred water layer, the limiting barrier between the bulk water phase of the lumen and the surface of the mucosal cells. Efficient absorption requires that these products be solubilized to allow more rapid movement to absorptive sites. Solubilization is mediated by bile acids, the end products of hepatic cholesterol metabolism. Bile salts are secreted in bile as peptide conjugates of glycine and taurine; as such, they are readily soluble in jejunal contents (pH 6 to 7), since at this pH they are heavily ionized (Figure 2-9). Above a certain concentration, the critical micellar concentration (CMC), bile salts form molecular aggregates known as pure bile salt micelles. Each molecule is oriented in such a way that the hydrophilic polar hydroxyl and amino groups face outward, and the nonpolar end faces inward. The lipid-soluble fatty acids, monoglycerides, and phospholipids (derivatives of glycerol present in bile and the diet), are incorporated into the hydrophobic core of the aggregate (mixed micelle, Figure 2-10). Owing to the fact that these molecular aggregates have an outer rim of polar water-soluble hydroxyl and amino groups, they are able to diffuse easily across the unstirred water layer. In this way the products of lipolysis, packaged in the core of the micelle, reach the surface of the intestinal microvilli and, by virtue of their lipid solubility, are able to traverse the lipid membrane and enter the mucosal cells.

Mechanisms Involved in the Intestinal Uptake

Intestinal uptake may be considered to be a two-step process—diffusional transport across the

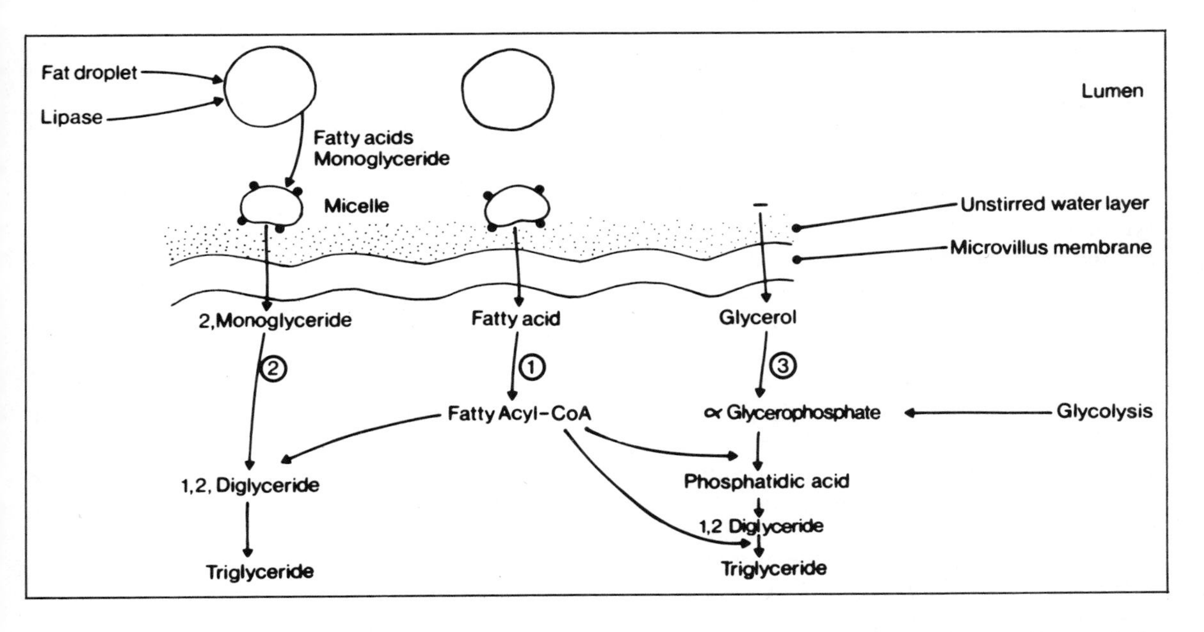

Figure 2-11. *Pathways for mucosal resynthesis of triglyceride.*

unstirred water layer up to the absorptive cell membrane, followed by penetration of the cell membrane [343]. Diffusion across the unstirred layer is a major determinant of lipid uptake. All the available evidence points to the fact that the rate of uptake is determined by the amount of solubilized lipid present (i.e., in micelles), and a linear relationship has consistently been formed between fatty acid uptake and amount of fatty acid in the micellar phase [181, 219].

The actual mucosal uptake of fatty acid and monoglyceride appears to be a passive process, and penetration of the cell membrane is probably a monomolecular process, consisting of partition of lipid molecules from the aqueous side of the interface into the cell membrane, followed by diffusion through the structural lipid membrane and then partition into aqueous cytoplasm [343].

Intracellular Metabolism of Absorbed Lipids

Most short- and medium-chain fatty acids (12 carbon atoms or less) pass through the mucosal cell and enter the portal plasma. Long-chain fatty acids, monoglycerides, and cholesterol are re-esterified and transported via the lymphatics to the systemic circulation.

The biosynthesis of triglyceride occurs in the endoplasmic reticulum [53, 305, 315] of mucosal cells in the tip of the villus, either by the monoglyceride pathway (reaction 2, Figure 2-11) or the glycerol-3-phosphate pathway (reaction 3, Figure 2-11) [52]. The first stage in the esterification process via either pathway is the acylation of fatty acids to their CoA derivatives by fatty acid thiokinase, which has been localized to the microsomal fraction of intestinal mucosal homogenates.

Although there is some controversy as to the relative importance of the monoglyceride and glycerol-3-phosphate pathways, many workers in this field hold the view that the synthesis of triglycerides occurs mainly via the monoglyceride pathway. Indeed evidence has been presented suggesting the existence of a control mechanism that favors the monoglyceride pathway, for monoglycerides actually decrease the incorporation of glycerol-3-phosphate into phosphatidic acid [203].

For many years it has been generally held that fatty acid uptake is rate-limiting for triglyceride synthesis in the intestinal mucosal cell. More recently, however, the availability of triglyceride has been shown to influence the activity of various enzymes associated with triglyceride biosynthesis [306, 352], and the addition of increased levels of triglyceride to the diet has been shown to be associated with an increase in the activity of the monoglyceride transacylase and increased absorptive capacity for triglycerides to the more distal portions of small intestine [203]. Similarly, when animals were placed on a fat-free diet, a decrease in the activity of this enzyme was observed [294, 295]. In the essential fatty acid-deficient rat, the incorporation of fatty acid into triglyceride was reduced, and the microsomal esterifying enzyme activities were lowered.

It seems, therefore, that the pathways involved in the mucosal triglyceride biosynthesis may be substrate-induced. Whether this is of functional significance in the clinical setting is at present unclear. It should be borne in mind, however, that the fat content of a number of proprietary enteric feeds consists only of essential fatty acids, so that the possibility exists that return to normal fat intake may be associated with temporary fat malabsorption because of reduced activities of the enzymes involved in mucosal triglyceride synthesis.

Lipid Transport out of the Cell

Once the triglyceride droplet has been formed within the smooth endoplasmic reticulum, it is subjected to a series of additions of specific apoproteins, phospholipid, and carbohydrate. These provide a polar coating, so that the spatial orientation of the chylomicron particle is analogous to the micelle, with the hydropic lipid in the core [383]. The chemical composition of the final lymph chylomicron is shown in Table 2-2 [144]. Although quantitatively small (one percent), the importance of specific chylomicron apoproteins is underscored by the disease abetalipoproteinemia, in which the apparent inability to synthesize one of the chylomicron apoproteins, apo B, is associated with a severe impairment of intestinal lipoprotein formation [221]. Impaired protein synthesis in human calorie malnutrition also appears to interfere with intestinal lipoprotein formation [354].

Table 2-2. *Characteristics of Rat Intestinal Lymph Chylomicrons*

Chemical Composition	%
Triglyceride	84
Phospholipid	13
Cholesterol	2
Protein	1
Density	< 1.006

The events that occur during chylomicron formation and the secretion of chylomicrons into the intercellular space have been viewed directly at the ultrastructural level in a unique series of electron micrograph studies [333]. The triglyceride droplets appear to be channeled through the endoplasmic reticulum to the Golgi zone. Within the Golgi, the lipid droplets assume the exact size and configuration of chylomicrons, and these are transported within Golgi residues to the lateral cell membrane, where their exocytosis occurs. Exocytosis occurs as a result of direct fusing of Golgi vesicles with the lateral cell membrane and furthermore, it is now evident that secretion of chylomicrons occurs by the bulk discharge of many chylomicrons from each vesicle. From the intercellular space the chylomicrons enter the lamina propria and thence the lymphatics via gaps in adjoining endothelial cells.

ABSORPTION OF THE FAT-SOLUBLE VITAMINS

Vitamins A, D, E, and K are relatively large nonpolar molecules and are dependent on micellar solubilization for absorption [44, 136, 164]. The major steps involved in the absorption of fat-

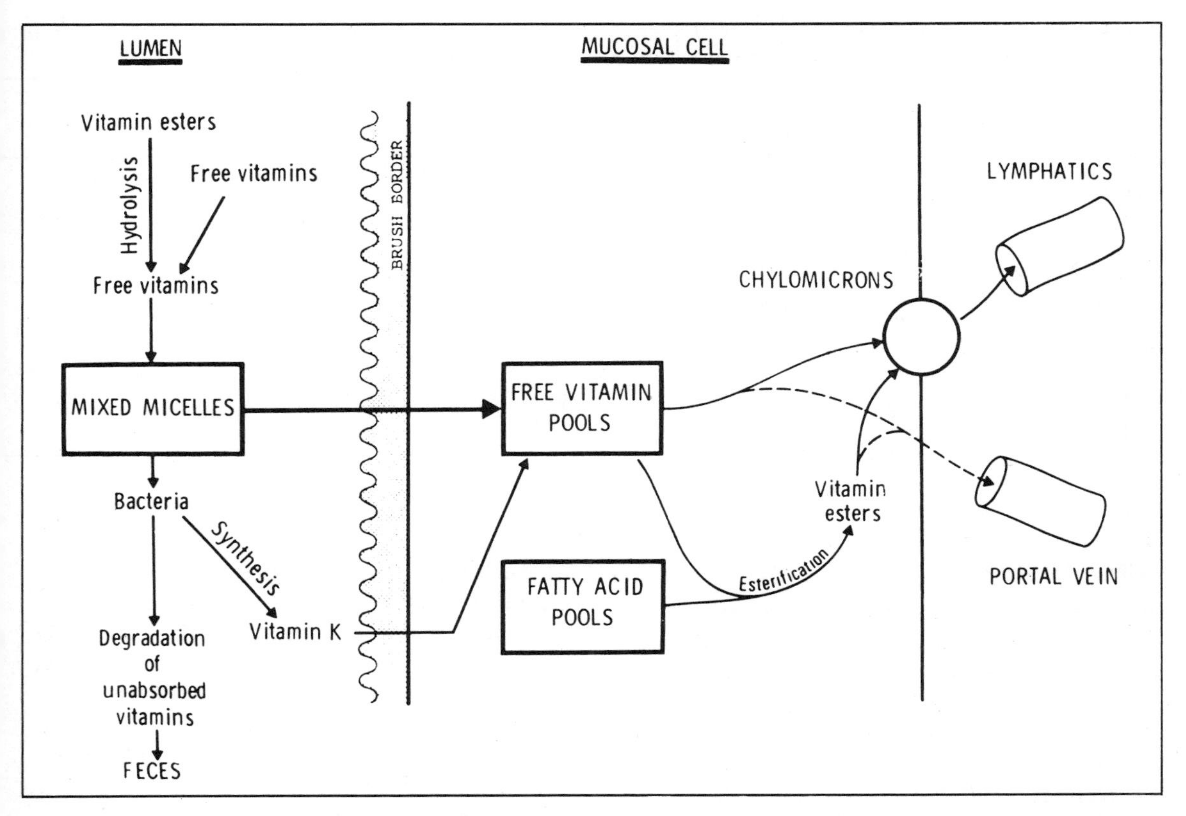

Figure 2-12. *The major steps of fat-soluble vitamin absorption.*

soluble vitamins are summarized in Figure 2-12. The fat-soluble vitamins are relatively large non-polar molecules, and the solubilizing properties of bile are of major importance for their absorption. Vitamin A esters are hydrolyzed by pancreatic retinyl hydrolase, and this reaction is an obligatory step to cellular uptake [69]. Hydrolysis of the other fat-soluble vitamins may also be an important absorptive step, but this has not yet been clearly established.

At present it is not clear how fat-soluble vitamins are translocated across the cell membrane. After gaining entrance to the mucosal cell, the fat-soluble vitamins become associated with chylomicrons and are transported from the mucosal cells mainly via the lymphatics, where they appear in the chylomicron fraction [44, 46, 163]. During transport from gut lumen to lymph, vitamin K and unesterified vitamin E remain chemically unaltered, whereas most of vitamin A and 3 to 28 percent of vitamin D are re-esterified, probably within the mucosal cell [36, 45, 141, 142, 323]. Absorption of all fat-soluble vitamins occurs predominantly via the lymphatic channels, but some absorption can occur via the portal vein for vitamins A and E [84, 163].

In addition to mucosal esterification, other metabolic events can occur in the mucosal cell. Vitamin A (retinol) can be oxidized to vitamin A aldehyde (retinal) and then to retinoic acid [142]. Retinoic acid is absorbed predominantly via the portal vein, and its formation from vitamin A may be an important compensatory mechanism whereby adequate absorption of vitamin A can be maintained when lymphatic transport is impaired.

Table 2-3. *Approximate Mean Quantities of Water, Sodium, Chloride and Potassium Handled by the Gut in 24 Hours in Normal Subjects and in Patients with Established Ileostomy*

	Water (ml)	Sodium (mEq)	Chloride (mEq)	Potassium (mEq)
Input				
Diet	1500	150	150	80
Gut secretions	7500	1000	750	40
Total	9000	1150	900	120
Output				
Ileostomy	450	60	45	4
Feces	150	5	3	12

FLUID AND ELECTROLYTE ABSORPTION

In the course of an average 24 hours, the human intestine handles large quantities of water and electrolytes [345] (Table 2-3). The bulk of the input into the upper small intestine comes from the various gastrointestinal secretions, and compared to this large input, fecal output of fluid and electrolytes is small. The figures in Table 2-3 do not in any way reflect the total absorptive capacity of the human intestine, however, and the studies of Love et al. [227] indicate that the daily absorptive capacity of the adult gut may, under certain conditions, be as high as 15 to 20 liters of water and 1,500 to 3,000 mM Na^+.

Table 2-3 indicates that the small intestine is the major site of fluid and electrolyte absorption; for example, net uptake of fluid is 9 liters, whereas ileostomy output is in the order of 450 ml. It should be remembered, however, that the ileal mucosa of established ileostomies undergoes a morphologic as well as functional adaptation with respect to fluid and electrolyte handling [357], and the intubation studies of Phillips and Giller [290] suggest that normal colonic inflows are two to three times as high as those observed in established ileostomy effluent.

The jejunum and ileum differ markedly with respect to their handling of fluid and electrolytes. Intubation studies in which intestinal contents have been sampled from different locations of the human small intestine following oral ingestion of liquid test meals containing a nonabsorbable marker, suggest that the bulk of the absorption of fluid and water-soluble digestive products occurs in the proximal 100 cm of the small intestine [50, 329]. In the normal situation, therefore, the ileum and colon are probably only concerned with the final conservation of fluid and electrolytes.

Role of Stomach and Duodenum

Negligible absorption of water and electrolytes takes place from the stomach, and gastric contents may remain nonisotonic for prolonged periods [133]. However, the duodenum is freely permeable to the net and bidirectional movements of fluids and electrolytes. Nonisotonic gastric contents rapidly come into osmotic equilibrium when they enter the duodenum [133], and by the time the upper jejunum is reached, gastric contents and added gastrointestinal secretions have been rendered isotonic. Moreover, the aqueous phase of the upper jejunal contents is in approximate ionic equilibration with plasma and consists largely of Na^+ and Cl^-, and the total contribution of nonelectrolyte to the tonicity of postprandial jejunal contents is less than 50 mOsm/L, irrespective of the nature of the meal [133].

Based on the original animal studies of Hindle and Code [178], it has been generally assumed that osmotic equilibration is achieved in the duodenum by a simple combination of bulk water movement in response to osmotic gradients and net movement of diffusable ions (Na^+ and Cl^-) in response to local concentration gradients. Earlier work by Nasset and colleagues, however, had implied that humoral factors could be involved [264], for instillation of food contents into proximal intestinal segments resulted in a net secretion of fluid and electrolytes into isolated distal segments [267]. A group of South African workers have now confirmed this in the human, by showing that duodenal infusion of simulated gastric meal contents elicited a net secretion of fluid and electrolytes into more distal isolated jejunal segments [381]. To date, the hormones responsible for eliciting this response and their modes of action have not been identified.

JEJUNAL ABSORPTION

Water and Electrolytes

The jejunum absorbs large quantities of water, Na^+, and Cl^- in the few hours after every meal from a luminal solution consisting largely of isotonic saline. Human perfusion studies indicate, however, that negligible absorption of water, Na^+, and Cl^- takes place from isotonic saline [332, 346, 371]. Net absorption of water, Na^+, and Cl^- can be promoted by the addition to the lumen of small concentrations of glucose [232, 346]. Maximum rates of water and electrolyte absorption take place from isotonic solutions containing approximately 56 mM glucose (Figure 2-13). A similar effect is shown by galactose [344], whereas fructose is relatively ineffective [179, 344].

At first sight, the physiologic significance of these findings may be questioned because only small amounts of monosaccharide accumulate in the lumen of the small intestine during the intestinal assimilation of carbohydrate. They diffuse back across the unstirred water layer following hydrolysis of disaccharide, α-limit dextrins, and maltrotriose by brush border-associated oligosaccharidases. However, additional human jejunal perfusion studies have shown that similar amounts of water and electrolytes are absorbed when equimolar amounts of glucose are presented to the mucosa in the forms of free glucose, maltose, and α 1-4, α 1-6, linked glucose polymers [204, 251]. These findings therefore confirm that the absorption of the products of carbohydrate digestion are important in securing concomitant absorption of fluid and electrolyte from the jejunum.

Recently, the effects of the products of luminal protein digestion, amino acid and oligopeptides, on net fluid and electrolyte absorption from the human jejunum have also been studied. The neutral amino acid, leucine, stimulates the jejunal absorption of water and Na^+ [10]. Two recent perfusion studies have shown that the dipeptide glycyl-L-alanine (Gly-Ala), as well as an equimolar mixture of its constituent amino acids, glycine (Gly) and L-alanine (Ala), also promote fluid and electrolyte absorption [173, 332]. Moreover, as Figure 2-14 shows, increasing the concentrations of free amino acids and dipeptide in the perfusion solutions resulted in a graded increase in water absorption, the pattern of which closely resembles the effects of glucose depicted in Figure 2-13. Not all amino acids stimulate jejunal water and electrolyte absorption, however, and as Figure 2-15 shows, the dibasic amino acids, L-lysine and L-arginine, actually promote a net jejunal secretion of fluid and electrolytes [165, 173]. These contrasting effects of free amino acids on jejunal water and electrolyte absorption may be one of the reasons why not all partial enzymic protein hydrolysates have a net stimulating effect on water absorption [166]. Thus, a partial pancreatic hydrolysate of lactalbumin, in which nearly 80 percent of the αNH_2 nitrogen existed in the form of small peptides and 20 percent as free amino acids, promoted net absorption of water, Na^+, and Cl^-, whereas a partial pancreatic hydrolysate of fish protein had no such effect, and in-

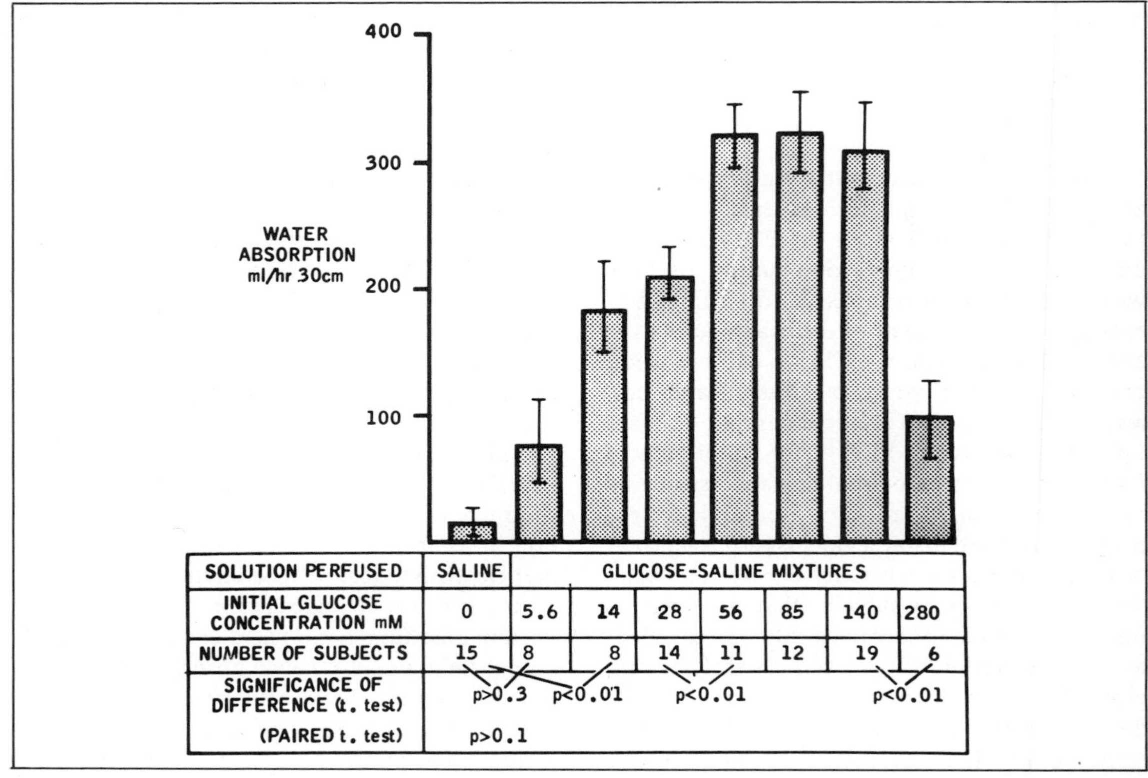
400
300
200
100
WATER
ABSORPTION
ml/hr 30cm
SOLUTION PERFUSED
SALINE
GLUCOSE-SALINE MIXTURES
INITIAL GLUCOSE CONCENTRATION mM
0
5.6
14
28
56
85
140
280
NUMBER OF SUBJECTS
15
8
8
14
11
12
19
6
SIGNIFICANCE OF DIFFERENCE (t. test)
p>0.3
p<0.01
p<0.01
p<0.01
(PAIRED t. test)
p>0.1

2-13

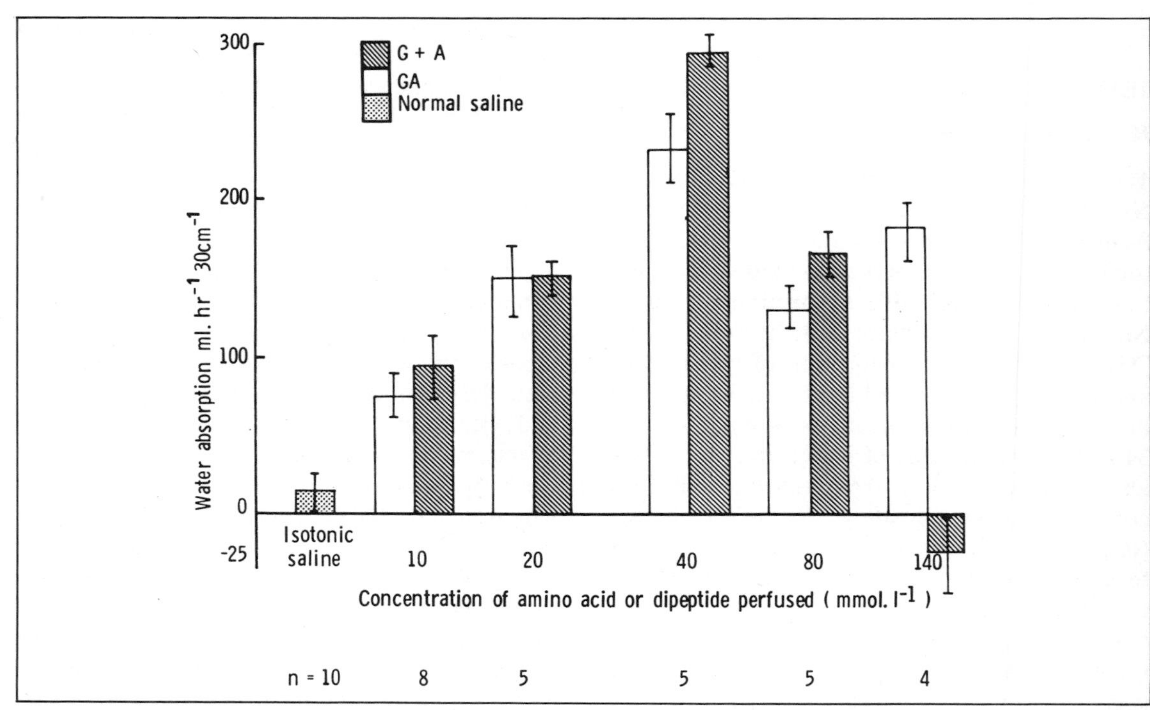
G + A
GA
Normal saline
300
200
100
0
-25
Water absorption ml. hr^{-1} 30cm^{-1}
Isotonic saline
10
20
40
80
140
Concentration of amino acid or dipeptide perfused (mmol. l^{-1})
n = 10
8
5
5
5
4

2-14

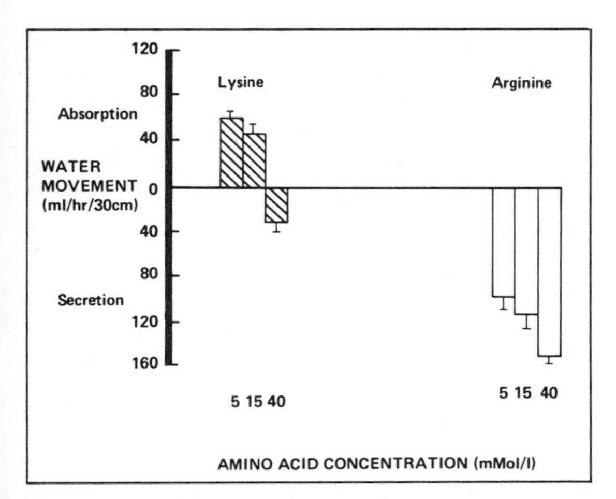

Figure 2-15. *Mean water movement (= 1 S.E.M.) from isotonic amino acid-saline mixtures perfused at 20 ml/min through 30-cm segments of upper jejunum in healthy adults. Absorption of water above the horizontal axis, secretion of water below the horizontal axis.*

deed in some of the subjects studied, net secretion occurred. Overall though, there certainly seems to be a link between the absorption mechanisms for water and Na^+, on the one hand, and the glucose-galactose, amino acid, and peptide transport systems on the other.

Mechanisms Involved in Jejunal Fluid and Electrolyte Transport

Studies with glucose have indicated that jejunal water transport occurs as a direct consequence of net solute transport, and that net solute and water transport occur in isotonic proportions [344]. The mechanisms whereby glucose interacts with electrolytes to produce an isotonic absorbate remain controversial. One hypothesis for which much supportive evidence has been furnished supposes that glucose and Na^+ combine with a common membrane carrier that facilitates the entry of both into the mucosal cell [86]. Basolateral membrane-associated Na^+-K^+ ATPase [298] then actively pumps Na^+ out of the cell into the lateral intercellular space, thereby generating a local osmotic gradient down which water flows. Cl^- ions accompany the Na^+ ions and the resultant isotonic solution in the lateral intercellular space is then driven toward the capillary lumen by local hydrostatic gradients. This hypothesis is based on the original Curran model [91], the various compartments of which have now been defined anatomically [113, 358]. Direct supportive evidence for this hypothesis has now been provided by Naftaline and coworkers [157], who have used a microprobe technique to directly measure Na^+, K^+, and Cl^- concentration profiles in rabbit ileal epithelial cells and their lateral intercellular spaces.

Fordtran and colleagues have proferred an alternative view [132–135], whereby glucose provides a drive for the bulk flow of water across the jejunal mucosa and Na^+ and Cl^- are absorbed as a consequence of this by a process of solvent drag. The "solvent drag" hypothesis has been based largely on observations showing that the magnitude and direction of net Na^+ movement could be influenced by manipulating the direction and bulk flow of water by alteration of luminal tonicity [135]. It has to be borne in mind, however, that hypertonic solutions have been shown to damage intestinal mucosa [208]. Moreover, it would seem to be difficult to account quantitatively for the observed rates of Na^+ and water absorption from the various isotonic glucose-saline mixtures studied by Sladen and colleagues [345, 346] on the basis of Fordtran's estimates of the permeability properties of human jejunum [135].

Figure 2-13. *Mean water absorption rates (= 1 S.E.M.) from isotonic saline and isotonic glucose-saline mixture perfused at 20 ml/min through 30-cm segments of upper jejunum in healthy adults.*

Figure 2-14. *Mean water absorption rates (= 1 S.E.M.) from isotonic saline and isotonic free amino acid-saline mixture (G + A) and dipeptide-saline mixtures (GA) perfused at 15 ml/min through 30-cm segments of upper jejunum in healthy adults.*

Although an absolute Na^+ dependency for free amino acid transport has not been shown in the human [331], it is probable that free amino acids interact with electrolytes in the same way as glucose to produce an isotonic absorbate. The mechanisms involved in the promotion of fluid and electrolyte absorption by oligosaccharides and oligopeptides are also thought to involve an initial reaction between solute and Na^+ at the carrier level. On the basis of the original work with glucose and amino acids, it was assumed that the absorbate would be isotonic [332, 346]. Recent studies, however, have shown this not to be the case, as the absorbates are slightly hypertonic [125]. In retrospect, this is not surprising, for the brush border hydrolysis of saccharides and peptides results in the release of free glucose and amino acids in at least 2:1 proportion, making the fluid in close proximity to the surface enzymes hypertonic. The finding that the rise in osmolality of gut contents during oligosaccharide and oligopeptide assimilation is a small one is due to the fact that the site of hydrolysis is in close proximity to the transport carrier, and that the unstirred water layer limits the back diffusion of liberated hydrolytic products into the bulk phase of the gut lumen.

Jejunal Bicarbonate Absorption

Bile and pancreatic juice are alkaline, bicarbonate-rich fluids. Although HCO_3^- serves to neutralize gastric acid, an equilibrium concentration of approximately 6 mEq/L has been found in human jejunal perfusion studies [291]. HCO_3^- can be absorbed against electrical and chemical gradients [361], which suggests that there is an active transport system in the jejunal mucosa for HCO_3^-. It is not clear, however, whether there is a Na^+-linked transport of anion across the mucosa or whether it is a consequence of an H^+–Na^+ exchange system with subsequent conversion of HCO_3^- to CO_2 and water. Certainly experiments have shown that the presence of HCO_3^- in the gut lumen promotes net absorption of Na^+ as well as water [134, 347], so that the outpouring of HCO_3^- into the jejunal lumen, followed by its rapid absorption, coupled to that of Na^+ and water, provides yet another mechanism whereby large quantities of fluid and electrolytes are conserved in the jejunum during digestion of a meal.

Clinical Implications

Although a number of chemically defined elemental diets are now being used in clinical practice, diarrhea frequently occurs and often limits their use [328]. It is popularly held that onset of this complication is related to the high osmolality of these preparations. The diets are hypertonic by virtue of their free amino acid and/or varying glucose content, and in the light of our current understanding of the mechanisms involved in the duodenal and jejunal handling of water and electrolytes, it seems reasonable that the respective monomeric nitrogen and carbohydrate components should be replaced by oligopeptides and oligosaccharides. Not only would less duodenal fluid and electrolyte secretion be required to achieve luminal isotonicity, but the terminal stages in digestion and the Na^+ monomer-linked interactions providing drive to water absorption would all take place on the mucosal side of the unstirred water layer.

Ileal and Colonic Absorption

The absorption of fluid and electrolytes remaining in the ileum and colon is not promoted either by the luminal products of carbohydrate and protein digestion or by HCO_3^-. In contrast to absorption in the jejunum, Na^+ is absorbed against a concentration gradient by an active transport process in both the ileum and the colon [112, 134] (Figure 2-17). Cl^- is absorbed from even lower concentrations than Na^+ and, in general, is absorbed more rapidly than Na^+ from identical luminal concentrations (Figure 2-16). Cl^- cannot, therefore, simply be absorbed as the accompanying anion for Na^+. The most likely mechanism to explain the discrepancies between

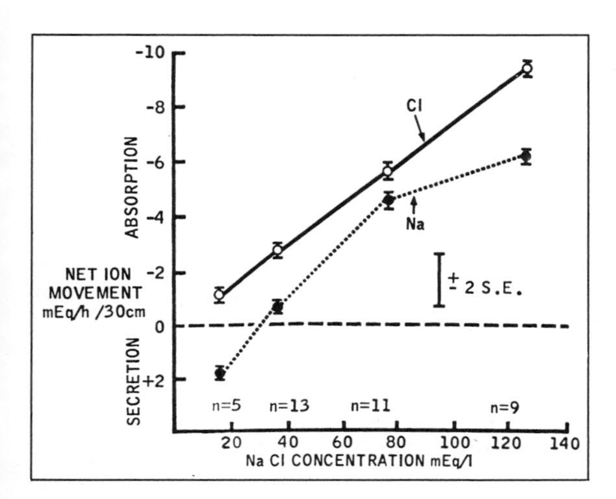

Figure 2-16. *Effect of luminal sodium chloride concentrations on sodium and chloride absorption from the normal human ileum. The number of studies at each concentration is indicated. In these studies, solutions made isotonic with mannitol were perfused through 30-cm ileal segments in healthy adults at approximately 10 ml/min. (After J. S. Fordtran et al. Permeability characteristics of the human small intestine.* J. Clin. Invest. *44:1935, 1965.) Very similar results in human colon are reported by Devroede and Phillips [112].*

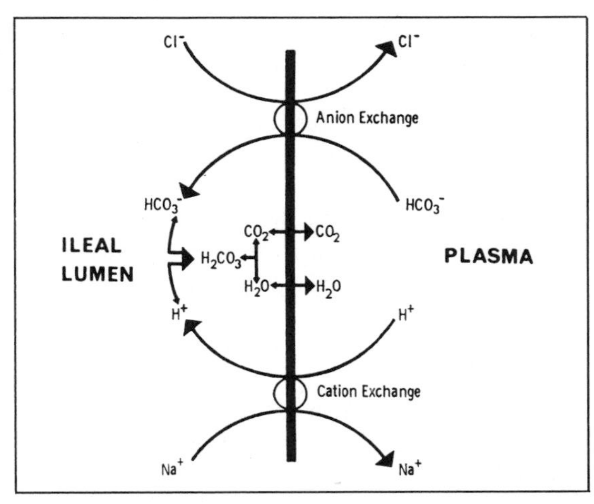

Figure 2-17. *Postulated double ion-exchange model proposed by Turnberg et al. to explain their observations on human ileal transport. (From L. A. Turnberg et al. Interrelationships of chloride, bicarbonate, sodium and hydrogen transport in the human ileum.* J. Clin. Invest. *49:557, 1970.)*

Na^+ and Cl^- movement is that Cl^- is partly exchanged for HCO_3^-. Experimental support for this hypothesis about the ileum comes from the evidence of Turnberg et al. [362], who showed that in the absence of luminal Cl^-, HCO_3^- does not enter the ileal lumen and the luminal contents become acid. These workers have postulated a double ion-exchange model to explain their observations in human ileal transport (Figure 2-17), in which Na^+ is absorbed in exchange for H^+, and Cl^- is absorbed in exchange for HCO_3^- anion. Although such a mechanism would not apparently promote net water absorption, since there would be no net disappearance of solute from the lumen, it is suggested that the combination of H^+ and HCO_3^- in the lumen results in the loss of osmotically active solute molecules, with consequent bulk flow of water out of the lumen [362].

Similar paired ion exchanges probably do not take place in the colon, and it seems more likely that active electrogenic rather than cation exchange is the major mechanism responsible for colonic Na^+. HCO_3^- clearly moves against an electrochemical gradient in the colon. As in the ileum, HCO_3^- secretion by the colon is dependent on the presence of Cl^- in the lumen [51, 112], again suggesting that an anion exchange mechanism is operational at this site.

Hormonal Content of Intestinal Water and Electrolyte Transport

Considerable effort has been directed toward investigation of the effects of various hormones on intestinal fluid and electrolyte transport. Glucagon, secretin, pentagastrin, cholecystokinin (CCK), gastric inhibitory polypeptide (GIP), and vasoactive intestinal polypeptide (VIP) have all been the subject of study. It is difficult to be sure that their described effects are meaningful in terms of physiology, and many of their actions may represent more pharmacologic phenomena. The experimental data may nevertheless be of clinical relevance in respect to the fluid diarrhea associated with pancreatic islet cell adenomas as well as that associated with enteric feeding.

Glucagon at an infusion dose of 0.6 and 1.2 μg/kg/hr significantly decreased water, Na^+, and Cl^- absorption to zero in the normal human jejunum [176]. Secretin has been shown to significantly reduce absorption, as well as to cause a secretion of water, Na^+, and Cl^- in the human jejunum [175, 264]. Likewise, CCK has been found to result in a net secretion of fluid and electrolytes [244, 262]. In the latter study, unidirectional movements determined with ^{22}Na revealed that CCK caused a reduction in lumen-to-plasma movement without significant change in plasma-to-lumen fluxes. VIP [260], GIP [34], prostaglandin E [90], and thyrocalcitonin [156]—the four hormones that have all been implicated as the etiologic agents responsible for the diarrhea in the Verner-Morrison syndrome—have all been variously shown to cause a secretion of fluid and electrolytes in the mammalian small intestine [260].

ABSORPTION OF HEMATINICS

Iron Absorption

The total amount of iron in the body of a healthy adult is maintained between 3 and 4 gm by the absorption of iron. The principal factors that regulate absorption are:

1. Those acting in the lumen of the gastrointestinal tract which determine the availability of iron for mucosal uptake.
2. Intra-epithelial mechanisms controlling uptake of iron across the mucosa.
3. Changes within the body which signal iron requirements to the intestinal cells [56].

INTRALUMINAL FACTORS AFFECTING IRON ABSORPTION

In both organic and inorganic compounds, iron commonly exists in one of the two oxidation forms, ferrous (Fe^{2+}) and ferric (Fe^{3+}) iron. The fate of ionizable iron released from food in the gut lumen is largely determined by its chemical reactions [196]. Ferric ions undergo increasing polymerization forming colloidal gels as the pH rises toward neutrality and finally form a precipitate of ferric hydroxide. Ferrous ions do not undergo such marked polymerization, and their solubility is greater than ferric ions at any given pH, which accounts, at least in part, for their greater availability. The unpolymerized ions of both species found at the low pH of gastric contents are chemically reactive, and when the gastric contents pass into the jejunum and neutralization occurs they combine with available ligands to form complexes. Iron binding in this situation may result in the formation of soluble or insoluble complexes, and the absorption will therefore be dictated by the proportion of ingested iron that is presented to the mucosa in the form of soluble complexes. Ascorbid acid [75], succinic acid [376], mannitol, sorbitol [226], and some amino acids [217, 236] all form stable and soluble complexes with iron, preventing its precipitation and thereby promoting absorption. Substances that inhibit iron absorption are in general constituents of food and pharmaceuticals. Thus, vegetable foodstuffs are rich in phytates and phosphates, which form insoluble salts with iron, and cholestyramine, an ion exchange resin, which strongly binds inorganic and hemoglobin iron [356].

Gastric Juice. It is now generally accepted that gastric acid enhances the absorption of iron, and that this is due to the fact that acid secretion ensures that iron released as a result of peptic digestion of food remains in a chemically reactive form which can produce soluble complexes [56]. A good deal of controversy has arisen recently as to the possible role of a factor or factors in gastric juice (other than acid) in the overall regulation of iron absorption. Initially, Deller and coworkers suggested that a high-molecular-weight glycoprotein capable of chelating iron (gastroferrin) probably formed part of the control mechanism regulating the extent of iron absorption [102]. This conclusion was largely based on their own findings, showing an absence of gastroferrin in hemochromatosis [101, 105]. This observation was later challenged, and most recently Bella and Kim have shown that no single molecular entity is responsible for the binding of iron in the gastric juice [37] and that a variety of mucins and other macromolecular substances all have rather similar iron-binding capacities. It seems probable, therefore, that under normal circumstances, most of the ionizable iron released from the food in the stomach either binds to the mucopolysaccharides in gastric secretions to form high-molecular-weight complexes or becomes unavailable on neutralization. This would explain why only 5 to 10 percent of the 10- to 15-mg daily iron intake is absorbed. However, as mentioned, the presence of low-molecular-weight chelating agents, such as ascorbic acid, in the diet will lead to the formation of soluble complexes, thereby facilitating the absorption of iron.

Pancreatic and Biliary Secretions. The role of exocrine pancreatic secretions in iron absorption in humans is controversial [100, 263]. On the one hand, evidence has been presented to suggest that iron absorption is reduced by orally administered pancreatic extracts [57]; on the other hand, the action of pancreatic proteolytic enzymes results in the release of free amino acids and peptides, which would be expected to facilitate iron absorption by removing ionizable iron from the high-molecular-weight mucopolysaccharide complexes and forming low-molecular-weight complexes.

Although bicarbonate is known to promote the formation of macromolecular iron complexes when free iron is present, no consistent effect of bicarbonate on iron absorption has been found experimentally [38].

Animal experiments have suggested that bile may facilitate iron absorption [75]. The original suggestion that this was due to its ascorbic acid content [75] has not been confirmed [197]. The possible beneficial effect of bile on iron absorption seems more likely to be due to its content of free amino acids [285].

Intestinal Mucosal Absorption of Iron

The whole small intestine has the capacity to absorb iron. Absorption is efficient in the duodenum and proximal jejunum, and these are the likely sites of absorption in the normal situation. Uptake of ionic iron by the human intestine has been shown to occur via an energy-dependent carrier-mediated process [82]. For a number of years, it has generally been accepted that the transported iron is then transferred to the serosal surface by intracellular iron-binding protein carriers. Recently, however, Munro and coworkers have been unable to identify these so-called "carrier" proteins and conclude that they probably represented partially digested mucosal cell constituents [223]. Their experimental data are more in keeping with a view that ionic iron is chelated with amino acids and in equilibrium with part of the ferritin iron pool, and in those forms is transported to the serosal surface for transfer to unsaturated, or partially saturated, transferrin molecules present in the adjacent plasma and interstitial fluid.

In one of the most recent studies in this field, Hopkins and Peters [190] have established that mitochondria are actively involved at an early stage in the intestinal transport of ferric ion. The significance of this finding is unclear; an intriguing possibility, which requires confirmation, is that ionic iron undergoes a valency change in this organelle.

Regulation of Mucosal Iron Absorption. Regulation of iron absorption at the mucosal level is thought to be achieved by independent control of the number of iron receptors (carriers) on the brush border and serosal membrane, as well as by alterations in the form and reactivity of plasma transferrin, which removes the iron from the serosal surface [223]. Kinetic studies using human intestinal tissue confirm that the increased absorption in iron deficiency is likely to be due to an increase in the number of normally functioning carriers in the brush border [82]. Except in primary idiopathic hemochromatosis [81], iron overload is associated with a reduction in iron absorption. This, in turn, is largely due to a decrease in iron transfer across the serosal, and not the mucosal, surface of the cell [223].

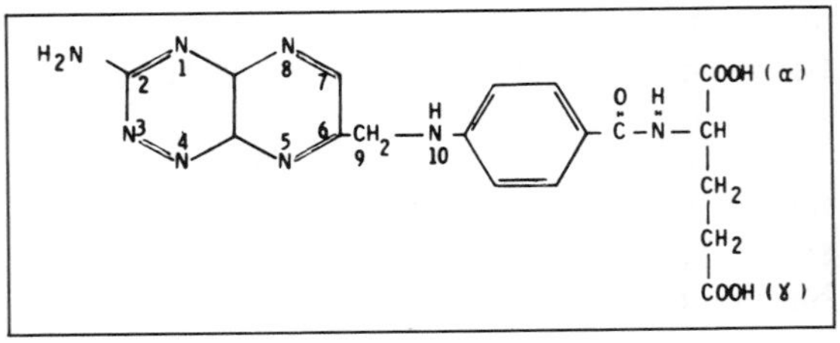

Figure 2-18. *Formula for folic acid (pteroylglutamic acid). Dietary folates may contain: (1) additional hydrogen atoms at positions 7 and 8 (dihydrofolate) or 5, 6, 7, and 8 (tetrahydrofolate); (2) a formyl group at N5 or N10 or a methyl group at N5; (3) additional glutamate moieties attached to the gamma-carboxyl group of the glutamate moiety.*

FOLATE ABSORPTION

Folate deficiency is probably the most common clinical vitamin deficiency and often occurs as a complication of gastrointestinal disease or of therapy with certain drugs, and in patients receiving parenteral or enteral nutrition if folate supplements are not given.

Chemistry of the Folates

Folic acid, or pteroylglutamic acid, is the parent substance of a large group of related compounds called folates. The structure of pteroylglutamic acid and its principal plant pteroylglutamyl conjugate is shown in Figure 2-18. All folate compounds have the same basic molecular structure consisting of three parts: pteridine, para-aminobenzoate (these two together forming the pteroyl group), and L-glutamic acid. More than 80 percent of dietary folate occurs in the form of conjugates of pteroylglutamic acid bearing multiple glutamyl units bound in γ peptide linkages. The principal polyglutamate in plants is pteroylheptaglutamic acid. The γ-linked glutamyl peptide chain is resistant to hydrolysis by the usual pancreatic proteolytic and intestinal mucosal amino oligopeptidase enzymes, but is cleaved by a group of specific enzymes properly known as pteroylpolyglutamyl hydrolases, and in the ensuing text as folate conjugases.

Intestinal Absorption of Polyglutamates in Humans

Available experimental evidence suggests that following oral administration of polyglutamates, only di- and monoglutamyl folate forms appear in the portal circulation [198], and only monoglutamyl folate in peripheral blood [60, 307]. This suggests that hydrolysis of the polyglutamate forms occurs either before absorption takes place in the gut lumen or at the surface of the mucosal cell or following absorption within the cytoplasmic compartment of the absorptive cell.

Jägerstad and colleagues [198] have investigated the activity of folate conjugase in gastric and pancreatic juice. Enzyme activity was found in both biologic fluids, albeit in low amounts. Nevertheless, the authors concluded that sufficient activity was present to hydrolyze the 500 μg or so of the conjugated polyglutamates assimilated each day. Recently, however, human perfusion studies have questioned the functional significance of intraluminal folate conjugase activity [80, 159]. Halstead and coworkers have perfused heptaglutamylfolate into segments of normal human jejunum [159] and have demonstrated the appearance in intestinal aspirates of mono- and triglutamyl folates at concentrations that could not be accounted for by the amount of luminal folate conjugase activity detected in intestinal aspirates. The foregoing studies therefore have suggested that the intestinal mucosal cell itself is the major site of polyglutamate hydrolysis, a conclusion that would be in keeping with the concepts of Rosenberg, who has recently purified folate conjugase from mucosal homogenates obtained from chicken intestine [307, 311].

Initial subcellular fractionation studies indicated that the bulk of folate conjugase activity resides in the intracellular compartment of the mucosal cell [180]. It therefore seemed likely that polyglutamates are absorbed intact by the mucosal cell and subsequently hydrolyzed by intracellular folate conjugases to mono- and diglutamyl folate forms. Halstead and coworkers have considered this to be an unlikely sequence of events on the basis that it would be hard to explain the mechanisms involved in the uptake process of the large (MW 1,215), negatively charged polyglutamate molecules. Consequently, the same group of workers pursued their subcellular fractionation studies, and have now shown that there are two distinctive human intestinal mucosal folate conjugases, one with a pH optimum of 4.5, localized to the intracellular compartment of the cell, and one with a pH optimum of 7.5, localized to the brush border fraction of mucosal homogenates [303].

In the light of their work, a plausible scheme for the intestinal assimilation of dietary folates can be proposed. Hydrolysis of pteroylheptaglutamate ($PteGlu_7$) by brush border folate conjugases to mono-($PteGlu_1$) and di-($PteGlu_2$) glutamyl folates is rapid. $PteGlu_1$ and $PteGlu_2$ are the likely forms in which the dietary folates are absorbed. Under appropriate conditions, a substantial amount of absorbed $PteGlu_1$ is reduced and methylated within the mucosal cell to appear in the portal circulation as 5-methyltetrahydrofolate ($CH_3H_4PteGlu_1$). It is not clear at present whether $PteGlu_1$ and $PteGlu_2$ are absorbed by passive diffusion or via specific carrier-mediated transport systems.

ABSORPTION OF VITAMIN B_{12}

Until recently it has generally been accepted that vitamin B_{12} is bound to intrinsic factor (IF) in the acid environment of the stomach and that the IF-vitamin B_{12} complex remains intact until some time after it becomes bound to specific receptors located in the ileum. The suggestion that this model could be an oversimplification of the mechanisms involved in the intestinal assimilation of vitamin B_{12} was prompted by clinical observations that patients with pancreatic insufficiency, who secrete IF normally, malabsorb crystalline vitamin B_{12} [245, 248, 358, 365], and that this could be completely corrected with oral pancreatic extract [245, 366]. A number of investigations have now isolated a protein with a rapid mobility on electrophoresis (R-protein) from gastric juice, saliva, and bile. It binds vitamin B_{12} [21, 22], and it has been subsequently suggested that R-protein could act as an endogenous inhibitor of vitamin B_{12} absorption [283, 369]. Allen and colleagues have now shown that orally administered vitamin B_{12} is bound by R-protein in the stomach at acid pH and remains bound at the nearly neutral pH of the small intestine until the R-protein moiety is degraded by the synergistic action of trypsin and chymotrypsin together possibly with elastase [23].

It therefore seems likely that IF-vitamin B_{12} binding occurs in the small intestine and not in the stomach, and only after vitamin B_{12} is released from the R-protein–vitamin B_{12} complex by the action of pancreatic proteases.

ABSORPTION OF WATER-SOLUBLE VITAMINS

Ascorbic acid, niacin, riboflavin, thiamine, pyridoxine, folic acid, and vitamin B_{12} are the water-soluble vitamins essential to man. Absorption of folic acid and vitamin B_{12} have been discussed. Compared to other water-soluble nutrients, less is known about the characteristics of the transport processes responsible for mediating the absorption of the nonhematinic water-soluble vitamins. The absorption of riboflavin is thought to occur via passive diffusion [348], and the mechanisms operative for niacin have not yet been defined.

Until recently there has been disagreement about the mechanisms involved in thiamine absorption. It now appears, however, that there is a dual system: at very low concentrations, there exists a saturable active sodium-dependent process, while at concentrations above 2 μm, transport occurs largely by passive diffusion [192]. Available evidence indicates that absorption of pyridoxine occurs by a nonsaturable nonenergy-dependent passive diffusional process [254, 360]. In the most recent experiments, however, relatively high concentrations of the vitamin (0.2 to 1 mM) were studied [255], and it remains to be determined whether absorption occurs via a carrier-mediated process at lower concentrations. The vitamin is phosphorylated during absorption [254, 360], a reaction catalyzed by pyridoxal kinase [247]. Phosphorylation is saturable, and it appears that this reaction may have the net effect of delaying exit of the vitamin from the intestine without affecting the rate of uptake of pyridoxine from the lumen [255].

Uptake of ascorbic acid by human intestinal mucosa has been shown to occur via a sodium-dependent active transport mechanism [350]. Although studies have been restricted to ileal tissue, the absorptive characteristics are similar to those observed in the guinea pig [351]. In this mammal, absorption occurs throughout the length of the small intestine with the highest activity in the ileum, so it seems probable that a similar profile exists throughout the length of the human small intestine.

REFERENCES

1. Abderhalden, E., Gigon, A., and London, E. S. Das verhalten von d-alanin im organismus des hundes unter verschiedenen bedingungen. *Hoppe Seylers Z. Physiol. Chem.* 53:113, 1907.
2. Abderhalden, E., and Lampe, A. Weiterer beitrag zur frage nach der vertretbarkeit von eiweiss resp. eines vollwertigen aminosauregemiseches durch gelatine und ammonsalze. *Hoppe Seylers Z. Physiol. Chem.* 80:160, 1912.
3. Abderhalden, E., and Lampe, A. E. Weiterer beitrag zur kenntnis des schicksals von in den magendarmkanal eingefuhrten einzelnen aminosauren, aminosauregemischen, peptonen und proteinen. *Hoppe Seylers Z. Physiol. Chem.* 81:473, 1912.
4. Abderhalden, E., and London, E. S. Weiterer beitrag zur frage nach dem ab- und aufban der proteine im tierischen organismus. *Hoppe Seylers Z. Physiol. Chem.* 65:251, 1910.
5. Abel, J. J., Rowntree, L. G., and Turner, B. B. On the removal of diffusible substances from the circulating blood of living animals by dialysis: II. Some constituents of the blood. *J. Pharmacol. Exp. Ther.* 5:611, 1913–1914.
6. Addison, J. M., et al. A common mechanism for transport of di and tripeptides by hamster jejunum in vitro. *Clin. Sci. Mol. Med.* 49:313, 1975.
7. Addison, J. M., Burston, D., and Matthews, D. M. Evidence for active transport of the dipeptide glycyl sarcosine by hamster jejunum in vitro. *Clin. Sci.* 43:907, 1972.
8. Addison, J. M., et al. Evidence for active transport of tripeptides by hamster jejunum in vitro. *Clin. Sci. Mol. Med.* 49:305, 1974.
9. Adibi, S. A. The influence of molecular structure of neutral amino acids on their absorptive kinetics in the jejunum and ileum of human intestine in vivo. *Gastroenterology* 56:903, 1969.
10. Adibi, S. A. Leucine absorption rate and net movements of sodium and water in human jejunum. *J. Appl. Physiol.* 28:753, 1970.
11. Adibi, S. A. Intestinal transport of dipeptides in man: Relative importance of hydrolysis and intact absorption. *J. Clin. Invest.* 50:2266, 1971.
12. Adibi, S. A. Intestinal phase of protein assimilation in man. *Am. J. Clin. Nutr.* 29:205, 1976.
13. Adibi, S. A., Fogel, M. R., and Agrawal, R. M. Comparison of free amino acid and dipeptide absorption in the jejunum of sprue patients. *Gastroenterology* 67:586, 1974.
14. Adibi, S. A., and Gray, S. J. Intestinal absorption of essential amino acids in man. *Gastroenterology* 52:837, 1967.
15. Adibi, S. A., Gray, S. J., and Menden, E. The kinetics of amino acid absorption and alteration of plasma composition of free amino acids after intestinal perfusion of amino acid mixtures. *Am. J. Clin. Nutr.* 20:24, 1967.
16. Adibi, S. A., and Mercer, D. W. Protein digestion in human intestine as reflected in luminal, mucosal and plasma amino acid concentrations after meals. *J. Clin. Invest.* 52:1586, 1973.
17. Adibi, S. A., and Morse, E. L. The number of glycine residues which limits intact absorption of glycine oligopeptides in human jejunum. *J. Clin. Invest.* 60:1008, 1977.
18. Adibi, S. A., and Soleimanpour, M. R. Functional characterization of dipeptide transport system in human jejunum. *J. Clin. Invest.* 53:1368, 1974.

19. Adibi, S. A., et al. Evidence for two different modes of tripeptide disappearance in human intestine, uptake by peptide carrier systems and hydrolysis by peptide hydrolases. *J. Clin. Invest.* 56:1355, 1975.
20. Agar, W. T., Hird, F. J. R., and Sidhu, G. S. The uptake of amino acid by the intestine. *Biochim. Biophys. Acta* 14:80, 1954.
21. Allen, R. H. Human vitamin B_{12} transport proteins. *Prog. Hematol.* 9:57, 1975.
22. Allen, R. H., and Mehlman, C. S. Isolation of gastric vitamin B_{12}-binding proteins using affinity chromatography: II. Purification and properties of hog intrinsic factor and hog nonintrinsic factor. *J. Biol. Chem.* 248:3670, 1973.
23. Allen, R. H., et al. Effect of proteolytic enzymes on the binding of cobalamin to R protein and intrinsic factor. *J. Clin. Invest.* 61:47, 1978.
24. Allison, S. P., et al. Practical aspects of nutritional support. *Res. Clin. Forums* 1:49, 1979.
25. Alpers, D. H. Separation and isolation of rat and human intestinal β-galactosidases. *J. Biol. Chem.* 244:1238, 1969.
26. Alpers, D. H., and Isselbacher, K. J. Disaccharidase deficiency. *Adv. Metab. Disord.* 4:75, 1970.
27. Asatoor, A. M., et al. Intestinal absorption of carnosine and its constituent amino acids in man. *Gut* 11:250, 1970.
28. Asatoor, A. M., et al. Intestinal absorption of two dipeptides in Hartnup disease. *Gut* 11:380, 1970.
29. Asatoor, A. M., et al. Intestinal absorption of oligopeptides in cystinuria. *Clin. Sci.* 41:23, 1971.
30. Asatoor, A. M., Harrison, D. D. W., Milne, M. D., and Prosser, D. I. Intestinal absorption of an arginine-containing peptide in cystinuria. *Gut* 13:95, 1972.
31. Asp, N. G. Human small intestinal β-galactosidases. Separation and characterization of three forms of an acid β-galactosidase. *Biochem. J.* 121:299, 1971.
32. Asp, N. G., and Dahlqvist, A. Human small intestinal β-galactosidase: Specific assay of three different enzymes. *Anal. Biochem.* 47:527, 1972.
33. Auricchio, S., Semenja, G., and Rubino, A. Multiplicity of human intestinal disaccharidases: II. Characterization of the individual maltases. *Biochim. Biophys. Acta* 96:498, 1965.
34. Barbezat, G. O., and Grossman, M. I. Intestinal secretion: Stimulation by peptides. *Science* 174:442, 1971.
35. Baron, D. N., et al. Hereditary pellagra-like skin rash with temporary cerebellar ataxia, constant renal amino aciduria and other bizarre biochemical features. *Lancet* 2:421, 1956.
36. Bell, N. H. Comparison of intestinal absorption and esterification of 4-C^{14} Vitamin D_3 and 4-C^{14} cholesterol in the rat. *Proc. Soc. Exp. Biol.* 123:529, 1966.
37. Bella, A., and Kim, Y. S. Iron binding of gastric mucins. *Biochim. Biophys. Acta* 304:580, 1973.
38. Benjamin, B. I., Cortell, S., and Conrad, M. E. Bicarbonate-induced iron complexes and iron absorption: One effect of pancreatic secretions. *Gastroenterology* 53:389, 1967.
39. Bennet Clark, S., et al. Fat absorption in essential fatty acid deficiency: A model experimental approach to studies of the mechanism of fat malabsorption of unknown etiology. *J. Lipid Res.* 14:581, 1973.
40. Benzonana, G., and Desnuelle, P. Etude cinetinique de l'action de la lipase pancreatique sur les triglycerides en emulsion. Essai d'une enzymologue en milieu heterogene. *Biochim. Biophys. Acta* 105:121, 1965.
41. Bergoz, R. Trehalose malabsorption causing intolerance to mushrooms. *Gastroenterology* 60:909, 1971.
42. Biederdorf, F. A., Morawski, S., and Fordtran, J. S. Effect of sodium, mannitol and magnesium on glucose, galactose, 3-0-methylglucose, and fructose absorption in the human ileum. *Gastroenterology* 68:58, 1975.
43. Bines, J., and Whelan, W. J. The mechanism of carbohydrase action. *Biochem. J.* 76:253, 1960.
44. Blomstrand, R., and Forsgren, L. Intestinal absorption and esterification of vitamin D_3-1,2,^3H in man. *Acta Chem. Scand.* 21:1662, 1967.
45. Blomstrand, R., and Forsgren, L. Vitamin K_1-^3H in man. Its intestinal absorption and transport in the thoracic duct lymph. *Int. J. Vitam. Nutr. Res.* 38:45, 1968.
46. Blomstrand, R., and Werner, B. Studies on the intestinal absorption of radioactive B-carotene and vitamin A in man. *Scand. J. Clin. Lab. Invest.* 19:339, 1967.
47. Bollet, A. J., and Owens, S. Evaluation of nutritional status of selected hospitalized patients. *Am. J. Clin. Nutr.* 26:931, 1973.
48. Borgström, B. On the interactions between pancreatic lipase and co-lipase and the substrate and the importance of bile salts. *J. Lipid Res.* 16:411, 1975.
49. Borgström, B., and Erlanson. Pancreatic lipase and co-lipase. Interactions and effects of bile salts and other detergents. *Eur. J. Biochem.* 37:60, 1973.
50. Borgström, B., et al. Studies of intestinal digestion and absorption in the human. *J. Clin. Invest.* 36:1521, 1957.

51. Bown, R. L., et al. A study of water and electrolyte transport by the excluded human colon. *Clin. Sci.* 43:891, 1972.
52. Brindley, D. N. The Intracellular Phase of Fat Absorption. In Smyth (Ed.), *Intestinal Absorption.* New York: Plenum, 1974. Pp. 621–672.
53. Brindley, D. N., and Hübscher, G. The intracellular distribution of the enzymes catalyzing the biosynthesis of glycerides in the intestinal mucosa. *Biochim. Biophys. Acta* 106:495, 1965.
54. Bristian, B. R., Blackburn, G. L., Hallowell, E., and Heddle, R. Protein status of general surgical patients. *J.A.M.A.* 230:858, 1974.
55. Bristian, B. R., Blackburn, G. L., Vitale, J., Cochrane, D., and Naylor, J. Prevalence of malnutrition in general medical patients. *J.A.M.A.* 235:1567, 1976.
56. Brozović, B. Absorption of Iron. In I. McColl and G. E. G. Sladen (Eds.), *Intestinal Absorption in Man.* London: Academic, 1975. P. 263.
57. Brozović, B., et al. Iron absorption in normal and d, 1-ethionine treated rats before and after the administration of pancreatin. *Gut* 7:531, 1966.
58. Burston, D., Taylor, E., and Matthews, D. M. Intestinal handling of two tetrapeptides by rodent small intestine in vitro. *Biochim. Biophys. Acta* 553:175, 1979.
59. Butterworth, C. E. The skeleton in the hospital closet. *Nutr. Today* 9:4, 1974.
60. Butterworth, C. E. Nutritional support for hospitalized patients: How do we cope? How should we cope? *J. Am. Diet. Assoc.* 75:227, 1979.
61. Cajori, F. A. The enzyme activity of dog's intestinal juice and its relation to intestinal digestion. *Am. J. Physiol.* 104:659, 1933.
62. Cathcart, E. P., and Leathes, J. B. On the absorption of proteins from the intestine. *J. Physiol.* 33:462, 1905–1906.
63. Cheeseman, C. I., and Parsons, D. S. Intestinal absorption of peptides. Peptide uptake by small intestine of rana pipiens. *Biochim. Biophys. Acta* 373:523, 1974.
64. Chen, M. L., Rogers, Q. R., and Harper, A. G. Observations on protein digestion in vivo: IV. Further observations on the gastrointestinal contents of rats fed different dietary proteins. *J. Nutr.* 76:253, 1962.
65. Christensen, H. N. Conjugated amino acids in portal plasma of dogs after protein feeding. *Biochem. J.* 44:333, 1949.
66. Christensen, H. N., et al. The conjugated non-protein, amino acids of plasma: V. A study of the significance of peptidemia. *J. Clin. Invest.* 26: 853, 1947.
67. Chung, Y. C., Silk, D. B. A., and Kim, Y. S. Intestinal transport of a tetrapeptide, L-leucylglycylglycylglycine, in rat small intestine, in vivo. *Clin. Sci. Mol. Med.* 94:454, 1979.
68. Chung, Y. C., et al. Protein digestion and absorption in human small intestine. *Gastroenterology* 76:1415, 1979.
69. Clark, M. L., and Harries, J. T. Absorption of Lipids. In I. McColl and G. E. G. Sladen (Eds.), *Intestinal Absorption in Man.* London: Academic, 1975. P. 187.
70. Cohen, M., Morgan, R. G. H., and Hofmann, A. F. Lipolytic activity of human gastric and duodenal juice against medium and long chain triglycerides. *Gastroenterology* 60:1, 1974.
71. Cohnheim, O. Die Umwandlung des eiweiss durch die darmwand. *Hoppe Seylers Z. Physiol. Chem.* 33:451, 1901.
72. Cohnheim, O. Zur frage der eiweissresorption: III. *Hoppe Seylers Z. Physiol. Chem.* 76:293, 1912.
73. Cohnheim, O. Die wirkung vollstandig abgebauter nahrung auf den verdauungskanal. *Hoppe Seylers Z. Physiol. Chem.* 84:419, 1913.
74. Conklin, K. A., Yamashiro, K. M., and Gray, G. M. Human intestinal sucrose-isomaltase: Identification of free sucrase and isomaltase and cleavage of the hybrid into active distinct subunits. *J. Biol. Chem.* 250:5735, 1975.
75. Conrad, M. E., and Schade, S. G. Ascorbic acid chelates in iron absorption: A role for hydrochloride acid and bile. *Gastroenterology* 55:35, 1968.
76. Cook, G. C. Absorption products of D-fructose in man. *Clin. Sci.* 37:675, 1969.
77. Cook, G. C. Comparison of intestinal absorption rates of glycine and glycylglycine in man and the effect of glucose in the perfusing fluid. *Clin. Sci.* 43:443, 1972.
78. Cook, G. C. Independent jejunal mechanisms for glycine and glycylglycine transfer in man in vivo. *Br. J. Nutr.* 30:13, 1973.
79. Cook, G. C. Comparison of absorption rates of glucose and maltose in man in vivo. *Clin. Sci.* 44:425, 1973.
80. Corcino, J. J., Reisenauer, A. M., and Halstead, C. H. Jejunal perfusion of simple and conjugated folates in tropical sprue. *J. Clin. Invest.* 58:298, 1976.
81. Cox, T. M., and Peters, T. J. In vitro: Uptake of iron by human duodenal biopsies. *Gut* 18:A961, 1977.
82. Cox, T. M., and Peters, T. J. Duodenal iron uptake in vitro: Studies in iron overloaded subjects. *Gut* 19:A973, 1978.
83. Craft, I. L., et al. Absorption and malabsorp-

tion of glycine and glycine peptides in man. *Gut* 9:425, 1968.
84. Crain, F. D., Lotspeich, F. J., and Krause, R. F. Biosynthesis of retinoic acid by intestinal enzymes of the rat. *J. Lipid Res.* 8:249, 1967.
85. Crane, R. K. Hypothesis for mechanisms of intestinal active transport of sugars. *Fed. Proc.* 21:891, 1962.
86. Crane, R. K. Na^+-dependent transport in the intestine and other animal tissues. *Fed. Proc.* 24:1000, 1965.
87. Crane, R. K. Structural and Functional Organization of an Epithelial Cell Brush Border. In K. B. Warren (Ed.), *Symposia of the International Society for Cell Biology*. New York: Academic, 1966. Vol. 5, pp. 71–102.
88. Crane, R. K. Absorption of Sugars. In C. F. Code (Ed.), *Handbook of Physiology*. Washington, DC: American Physiological Society, 1968. Vol. 3, p. 1323.
89. Crane, R. K. Digestion and Absorption: Water Soluble Organics. In R. K. Crane (Ed.), *MTP International Review of Physiology, Gastrointestinal Physiology II*. Baltimore: University Park Press, 1977. Vol. 12, pp. 325–365.
90. Cummings, J. H., et al. Effect of intravenous prostaglandin $F_{2\alpha}$ on small intestinal function in man. *Nature* 243:169, 1973.
91. Curran, P. F. Na, Cl and water transport by rat ileum in vitro. *J. Gen. Physiol.* 43:1137, 1960.
92. Curtis, K. J., Gaines, H. D., and Kim, Y. S. Protein digestion and absorption in rats with pancreatic duct occlusion. *Gastroenterology* 74: 1271, 1978.
93. Curtis, K. J., et al. Protein absorption and digestion in the rat. *J. Physiol.* 274:409, 1978.
94. Dahlqvist, A., and Borgström, B. Digestion and absorption of disaccharides in man. *Biochem. J.* 81:411, 1961.
95. Dahlqvist, A., and Thomson, D. L. The digestion and absorption of sucrose by the intact rat. *J. Physiol.* 167:193, 1963.
96. Das, M., and Radhakrishnan, A. N. Studies on a wide-spectrum intestinal dipeptide uptake system in the monkey and in the human. *Biochem. J.* 146:133, 1975.
97. Das, M., and Radhakrishnan, A. N. Role of peptidases and peptide transport in the intestinal absorption of proteins. *World Rev. Nutr. Diet* 24:58, 1976.
98. Davenport, H. W. Intestinal Digestion and Absorption of Protein. In *Physiology of the Digestive Tract* (3rd ed.). Chicago: Year Book, 1971. Pp. 191–196.
99. Davenport, P. J. Nutritional support in severe burns. *Res. Clin. Forums* 1:80, 1979.
100. Davis, A. E., and Biggs, J. D. The pancreas and iron absorption: Current views. *Am. J. Dig. Dis.* 12:293, 1967.
101. Davis, P. S., Luke, C. G., and Deller, D. J. Reduction of gastric iron-binding protein in haemochromatosis. A previously unrecognized metabolic defect. *Lancet* 2:1431, 1966.
102. Davis, P. S., Luke, C. G., and Deller, D. J. Gastric iron binding protein in iron chelation by gastric juice. *Nature (London)* 214:1126, 1967.
103. Debnam, E. S., and Levin, R. J. An experimental method of identifying and quantifying the active transfer electrogenic component from the diffusional component during sugar absorption measured in vivo. *J. Physiol.* 246:181, 1975.
104. Debnam, E. S., and Levin, R. J. Influence of specific dietary sugars on the jejunal mechanisms for glucose, galactose and methylglucoside absorption: Evidence of multiple sugar carriers. *Gut* 17:92, 1976.
105. Deller, D. J., et al. Gastric iron binding substance (gastroferrin) in a family with haemochromatosis. *Aust. Ann. Med.* 18:36, 1969.
106. Dencker, H., et al. Absorption of maltose as measured by portal vein catheterization. *Scand. J. Gastroenterol.* 7:707, 1972.
107. Dent, C. E., Heathcote, J. G., and Joran, G. E. The pathogenesis of cystinuria: I. Chromatographic and biological studies of the metabolism of sulphur containing amino acids. *J. Clin. Invest.* 33:1210, 1954.
108. Dent, C. E., and Rose, G. A. Amino acid metabolism in cystinuria. *Q. J. Med.* 20:205, 1951.
109. Dent, C. E., and Schilling, J. A. Studies on the absorption of proteins: The amino acid pattern in portal blood. *Biochem. J.* 44:318, 1949.
110. Dent, C. E., Senior, B., and Walshe, J. M. The pathogenesis of cystinuria: II. Polarographic studies of the metabolism of sulphur containing amino acids. *J. Clin. Invest.* 33:1216, 1954.
111. Denton, A. E., and Elvehjem, C. A. Availability of amino acids in vivo. *J. Biol. Chem.* 206:449, 1954.
112. Devroede, G. J., and Phillips, S. F. Conservation of sodium, chloride and water by the human colon. *Gastroenterology* 56:101, 1969.
113. Diamond, J. M., and Tormey, J. McD. Studies on the structural basis of water transport across epithelial membranes. *Fed. Proc.* 25ii:1458, 1966.
114. Donhoffer, S. Uber die elektive resorption der zucher. *Arch. Exp. Pathol. Pharmakol.* 177:689, 1935.
115. Donlon, J., and Fottrell, P. F. Studies on substrate specificities and subcellular location of

multiple forms of peptide hydrolases in guinea pig intestinal mucosa. *Comp. Biochem. Physiol. (B)* 41:181, 1972.
116. Drummond, K. N., et al. The blue diaper syndrome; familial hypercalcemia with nephrocalcinosis and indicanuria. *Am. J. Med.* 37:928, 1964.
117. Dunn, M. S., and Lewis, H. B. A comparative study of the hydrolysis of casein and deaminized casein by proteolytic enzymes. *J. Biol. Chem.* 49:343, 1921.
118. Dunne, W. T., Cooke, W. T., and Allan, W. Enzymatic and morphometric evidence for Crohn's disease as a diffuse lesion of the gastrointestinal tract. *Gut* 18:290, 1977.
119. Dyck, W. P., et al. Hormonal stimulation of intestinal disaccharidase release in the dog. *Gastroenterology* 66:533, 1974.
120. Elsas, L. J., et al. Renal and intestinal hexose transport in familial glucose-galactose malabsorption. *J. Clin. Invest.* 49:576, 1970.
121. Erlanson, C. Purification, properties and substrate specificity of a carboxyl esterase in pancreatic juice. *Scand. J. Gastroenterol.* 10:401, 1975.
122. Fairclough, P. D. Jejunal absorption of water and electrolytes in man: the effects of amino acids, peptides and saccharides. University of London M.D. thesis, 1978.
123. Fairclough, P. D., Clark, M. L., Dawson, A. M., Silk, D. B. A., Millar, P., and Harries, J. T. Absorption of glucose and maltose in a patient with glucose-galactose malabsorption. *Pediatr. Res.* 12:1112, 1978.
124. Fairclough, P. D., Silk, D. B. A., Clark, M. L., Matthews, D. M., Marrs, T. C., Burston, D., and Clegg, K. M. Effect of glycyl glycine on absorption from human jejunum of an amino acid mixture simulating casein and a partial enzymic hydrolysate of casein containing small peptides. *Clin. Sci. Mol. Med.* 53:27, 1977.
125. Fairclough, P. D., Silk, D. B. A., Webb, J. P. W., Clark, M. L., and Dawson, A. M. A reappraisal of "osmotic evidence" for intact peptide transport. *Clin. Sci. Mol. Med.* 53:241, 1977.
126. Fisher, R. B. *Protein Metabolism.* London: Methuen, 1954.
127. Fleshler, B., Butt, J. H., and Wismar, J. D. Absorption of glycine and L-alanine by the human jejunum. *J. Clin. Invest.* 45:1433, 1966.
128. Fleshler, B., and Nelson, R. A. Sodium dependency of L-alanine absorption in canine Thiry-Vella loops. *Gut* 11:240, 1970.
129. Fogel, M. R., and Adibi, S. A. Assessment of the role of brush border peptidases in luminal disappearance of dipeptides in man. *J. Lab. Clin. Med.* 84:327, 1974.
130. Fogel, M. R., and Gray, G. M. Carbohydrate digestion and absorption. *Gastroenterology* 58:96, 1970.
131. Folin, O., and Denis, W. Protein metabolism from the standpoint of blood and tissue analysis. *J. Biol. Chem.* 11:87, 1912.
132. Fordtran, J. S. Speculations on the pathogenesis of diarrhea. *Fed. Proc.* 26:1405, 1967.
133. Fordtran, J. S., and Locklear, J. W. Ionic constituents and osmolality of gastric and small-intestinal fluids after eating. *Am. J. Dig. Dis.* 11:503, 1966.
134. Fordtran, J. S., Rector, F. C., Jr., and Carter, N. W. The mechanisms of sodium absorption in the human small intestine. *J. Clin. Invest.* 47:884, 1968.
135. Fordtran, J. S., et al. Permeability characteristics of the human small intestine. *J. Clin. Invest.* 44:1935, 1965.
136. Forsgren, L. Studies on the intestinal absorption of labelled fat-soluble vitamins (A, D, E and K) via the thoracic-duct lymph in the absence of bile in man. *Acta Chir. Scand. (Suppl.)* 399:1, 1969.
137. Frame, E. J. The levels of individual free amino acids in the plasma of normal man at various intervals after a high protein diet. *J. Clin. Invest.* 37:1710, 1958.
138. Frankel, E. M. A comparative study of the behavior of purified proteins towards proteolytic enzymes. *J. Biol. Chem.* 26:31, 1896.
139. Freidlander. Ueber die resorption gelosser eiweissstoffe im dunndarm. *Z. Biol.* 33, 264.
140. Fujita, M., Parsons, D. S., and Wojnarowska, F. Oligopeptidases of brush border membranes of rat small intestinal mucosal cells. *J. Physiol.* 227:377, 1972.
141. Gallo-Torres, H. E. Intestinal absorption and lymphatic transport of d, 1-3,$4^{-3}H_2$-α-tocopheryl nicotinate in the rat. *Int. J. Vitamin. Nutr. Res.* 40:505, 1970.
142. Ganguly, J. Absorption of vitamin A. *Am. J. Clin. Nutr.* 22:923, 1969.
143. Gibson, J. A., Sladen, G. E., and Dawson, A. M. Protein absorption and ammonia production: The effects of dietary protein and removal of the colon. *Br. J. Nutr.* 35:61, 1976.
144. Glickman, R. M. Chylomicron Formation by the Intestine. In K. Rommel and H. Goebell (Eds.), *Lipid Absorption: Biochemical and Clinical Aspects.* Lancaster: MTP Press, 1976. P. 99.
145. Goldner, A. M., Schultz, S. G., and Curran, P. F. Sodium and sugar fluxes across the mucosal

border of rabbit ileum. *J. Gen. Physiol.* 53:362, 1969.

146. Goodman, S. I., McIntyre, C. A., and O'Brian, D. Impaired intestinal absorption of proline in a patient with familial aminoaciduria. *J. Pediatr.* 71:246, 1967.
147. Götze, H., et al. Hormone-elicited enzyme release by the small intestinal wall. *Gut* 13:471, 1972.
148. Gracey, M., Burke, V., and Oshin, A. Intestinal transport of fructose. *Biochim. Biophys. Acta* 266:397, 1972.
149. Gracey, M., Burke, V., and Oshin, A. Transport of Fructose by the Intestine. In W. L. Burland and P. D. Samuel (Eds.), *Transport Across the Intestine.* London: Churchill Livingstone, 1972. Pp. 99–104.
150. Grant, D. A. W., and Hermon-Taylor, J. The purification of human enterokinase by affinity chromatography and immunoadsorption: Some observations on its molecular characterization and comparisons with the pig enzyme. *Biochem. J.* 155:243, 1976.
151. Gray, G. M. Progress in gastroenterology: Carbohydrate digestion and absorption. *Gastroenterology* 58:96, 1970.
152. Gray, G. M., and Cooper, H. L. Protein digestion and absorption. *Gastroenterology* 61:535, 1971.
153. Gray, G. M., and Ingelfinger, F. J. Intestinal absorption of sucrose in man: The site of hydrolysis and absorption. *J. Clin. Invest.* 44: 390, 1965.
154. Gray, G. M., and Ingelfinger, F. J. Intestinal absorption of sucrose in man: Interrelation of hydrolysis and monosaccharide product absorption. *J. Clin. Invest.* 45:1433, 1966.
155. Gray, G. M., and Santiago, N. A. Intestinal B-galactosidases: I. Separation and characterization of three enzymes in normal human intestine. *J. Clin. Invest.* 48:716, 1969.
156. Gray, T. K., Bieberdorf, F. A., and Fordtran, J. S. Thyrocalcitonin and the jejunal absorption of calcium, water and electrolytes in normal subjects. *J. Clin. Invest.* 52:3084, 1973.
157. Gupta, B. L., Hall, T. A., Naftaline, R. J. Microprobe measurement of Na, K and Cl concentration profiles in epithelial cells and intercellular spaces of rabbit ileum. *Nature* 272:70, 1978.
158. Hallberg, L., Sölvell, L., and Zederfeldt, B. Iron absorption after partial gastrectomy: A comparative study on the absorption from ferrous sulfate and hemoglobin. *Acta Med. Scand.* 179:Suppl. 445:269, 1966.
159. Halstead, C. H., Baugh, C. M., and Butterworth, C. E. Jejunal perfusion of simple and conjugated folate in man. *Gastroenterology* 68:261, 1975.
160. Hamilton, J. D., and McMichael, H. B. Role of the microvillus in the absorption of disaccharides. *Lancet* 2:154, 1968.
161. Hamosh, M., et al. Pharyngeal lipase and digestion of dietary triglyceride in man. *J. Clin. Invest.* 55:908, 1975.
162. Hannaert, L., and Wodon, R. Contribution a l'etude de l'hemo clasie digestive. *C. R. Soc. Biol. (Paris)* 88:636, 1923.
163. Harries, J. T. Absorption of vitamin E in children. University of London M.D. thesis, 1971.
164. Harries, J. T., and Muller, D. P. R. Absorption of vitamin E in children with biliary obstruction. *Gut* 12:579–584, 1971.
165. Hegarty, J. E., et al. Jejunal water and electrolyte secretion induced by L-arginine in man. *Gut* 22:108, 1981.
166. Hegarty, J. E., Fairclough, P. D., Silk, D. B. A., Clark, M. L., and Dawson, A. M. Are peptides best? *Gut* 20:A438, 1979.
167. Heizer, W. D., and Laster, L. Peptide hydrolase activities of the mucosa of the human small intestine. *J. Clin. Invest.* 48:210, 1969.
168. Heizer, W. D., Kerley, R. L., and Isselbacher, K. J. Intestinal peptide hydrolases: Differences between brush border and cytoplastic enzymes. *Biochim. Biophys. Acta* 264:450, 1972.
169. Hellier, M. D., and Holdsworth, C. D. Digestion and Absorption of Proteins. In I. McColl and G. E. Sladen (Eds.), *Intestinal Absorption in Man.* London: Academic, 1975.
170. Hellier, M. D., Holdsworth, C. D., McColl, I., and Perrett, D. Dipeptide absorption in man. *Gut* 13:143, 1972.
171. Hellier, M. D., Holdsworth, C. D., and Perrett, D. Dibasic amino acid absorption in man. *Gastroenterology* 65:613, 1973.
172. Hellier, M. D., Holdsworth, C. D., Perrett, D., and Thirumalai, C. Intestinal dipeptide transport in normal and cystinuric subjects. *Clin. Sci.* 43:659, 1972.
173. Hellier, M. D., Thirumalai, C., and Holdsworth, C. D. The effect of amino acids and dipeptides on sodium and water absorption in man. *Gut* 14:41, 1973.
174. Hermon-Taylor, J., et al. Immunofluorescent localization of enterokinase in human small intestine. *Gut* 18:259, 1977.
175. Hicks, T., and Turnberg, L. A. The influence of secretin on ion transport in the human jejunum. *Gut* 14:485, 1973.
176. Hicks, T., and Turnberg, L. A. Influence of

glucagon on the human jejunum. *Gastroenterology* 67:1114, 1974.
177. Hill, G. L., et al. Malnutrition in surgical patients. An unrecognized problem. *Lancet* 1:689, 1977.
178. Hindle, W., and Code, C. F. Some differences between duodenal and ileal sorption. *Am. J. Physiol.* 203:215, 1962.
179. Holdsworth, C. D., and Dawson, A. M. The absorption of monosaccharides in man. *Clin. Sci.* 27:371, 1964.
180. Hoffbrand, A. V., and Peters, T. J. The subcellular distribution of radio-labelled iron during intestinal absorption in guinea pig enterocytes with special reference to the mitochondrial localization of the iron. *Clin. Sci.* 56:179, 1979.
181. Hoffman, N. E. The relationship between uptake in vitro of oleic acid and micellar solubilization. *Biochim. Biophys. Acta* 196:193, 1970.
182. Hofmann, A. F. Fat Digestion: The Interaction of Lipid Digestion Products with Micellar Bile Acid Solutions. In K. Rommel and H. Goebell (Eds.), *Lipid Absorption: Biochemical and Clinical Aspects.* Lancaster: MTP Press, 1976. P. 3.
183. Holdsworth, C. D. The absorption of monosaccharides in man. University of Leeds M.D. thesis, 1964.
184. Holdsworth, C. D., and Dawson, A. M. The absorption of monosaccharides in man. *Clin. Sci.* 27:371, 1964.
185. Holdsworth, C. D., and Dawson, A. M. Absorption of fructose in man. *Proc. Soc. Exp. Biol. Med.* 118:142, 1965.
186. Holdsworth, C. D., Hulme-Moir, I., and Thirumalai, C. Effect of posture on glucose intolerance after gastric surgery. *Br. Med. J.* 4:198, 1972.
187. Holmes, R. Carbohydrate digestion and absorption. *J. Clin. Pathol.* 5:Suppl. 24:10, 1971.
188. Holmes, R. The intestinal brush border. *Gut* 12:668, 1971.
189. Hooft, C. J., et al. Methionine malabsorption in a mentally defective child. *Lancet* 2:20, 1964.
190. Hopkins, J. M. P., and Peters, T. J. Subcellular distribution of radio-labelled iron during intestinal absorption in guinea pig enterocytes with special reference to the mitochondrial localization of the iron. *Clin. Sci.* 56:179, 1979.
191. Howell, W. H. Note upon the presence of amino acids in the blood and lymph as determined by the β-naphthalinsulphochloride reaction. *Am. J. Physiol.* 17:273, 1906.
192. Hoyumpa, A. M., Middleton, H. M., Wilson, M. D., and Schenker, S. Thiamine transport across the rat intestine: I. Normal characteristics. *Gastroenterology* 68:1218, 1975.
193. Hueckel, H. J., and Rogers, Q. R. Urinary excretion of hydroxyproline-containing peptides in man, rat, hamster, dog, and monkey after feeding gelatin. *Comp. Biochem. Physiol.* 32:7, 1970.
194. Hughes, W. S., and Senior, J. R. The glucose-galactose malabsorption syndrome in a 23-year-old woman. *Gastroenterology* 68:142, 1975.
195. Hyun, J., et al. Purification and properties of pancreatic juice cholesterol esterase. *J. Biol. Chem.* 244:1937, 1969.
196. Jacobs, A. Iron absorption. *J. Clin. Pathol.* (Suppl.) (Roy. Coll. Pathol.) 24:55, 1971.
197. Jacobs, A., and Miles, P. M. The formation of iron complexes with bile and bile constituents. *Gut* 11:732, 1970.
198. Jägerstad, M., Dencker, H., and Westesson, A. K. The hydrolysis and absorption of conjugated folates in man. *Scand. J. Gastroenterol.* 11:283, 1976.
199. James, W. P. T., et al. The turnover of disaccharidases and brush border proteins in rat intestine. *Biochim. Biophys. Acta* 230:194, 1971.
200. Johansson, C. Characteristics of the absorption pattern of sugar, fat and protein from composite meals in man: A quantitative study. *Scand. J. Gastroenterol.* 10:33, 1975.
201. Johansson, C., Ekelund, K., Kulsdom, N., Larsson, I., and Lagerlöf, H. O. Calculation of gastric evacuation in an in vitro model. *Scand. J. Gastroenterol.* 7:391, 1972.
202. Johansson, C., Lagerlöf, H. O., Ekelund, K., Kulsdom, N., Larsson, I., and Nylind, B. Determination of gastric secretion and evacuation, biliary and pancreatic secretion, intestinal absorption, intestinal transit time and flow of water in man. *Scand. J. Gastroenterol.* 7:489, 1972.
203. Johnston, J. M. Triglyceride biosynthesis in the intestinal mucosa. In K. Rommel and H. Goebell (Eds.), *Lipid Absorption: Biochemical and Clinical Aspects.* Lancaster: MTP Press, 1976. P. 85.
204. Jones, B. J. M., et al. Comparison of oligosaccharide and free glucose absorption from a normal human jejunum. *Gut* 21:A905, 1980.
205. Josefsson, L., and Lindberg, T. Intestinal dipeptidases: IX. Studies on dipeptidases of human intestinal mucosa. *Acta Chem. Scand.* 21:1965, 1967.
206. Josefsson, L., Sjöström, H., and Noren, O. Intracellular hydrolysis of peptides. *Ciba Found. Symp. 50 (New Series):*199, 1977.
207. Kalmykoff, M. P. Abbau im darm und aufbau in der leber bei eiweissresorption. *Arch. Gen. Physiol.* 205:493, 1924.
208. Kameda, H., et al. Functional and histological

injury to intestinal mucosa produced by hypertonicity. *Am. J. Physiol.* 214:1090, 1968.
209. Keller, P. J. Pancreatic Proteolytic Enzymes. In C. F. Code (Ed.), *Handbook of Physiology.* Washington, DC: American Physiological Society, 1968. Vol. 5, Pp. 2605–2628.
210. Kelly, J. J., and Alpers, D. H. Properties of human intestinal gluco-amylase. *Biochim. Biophys. Acta* 315:113, 1973.
211. Kim, Y. S. Intestinal mucosal hydrolysis of proteins and peptides. *Ciba Found. Symp. 50 (New Series):* 159, 1977.
212. Kim, Y. S., Birtwhistle, W., and Kim, Y. W. Peptide hydrolysases in the brush border and soluble fraction of small intestinal mucosa of rat and man. *J. Clin. Invest.* 51:1419, 1972.
213. Kim, Y. S., and Brophy, E. J. Rat intestinal brush border peptidases. 1. Solubilization, purification and physio-chemical properties of two different forms of the enzyme. *J. Biol. Chem.* 251:3199, 1976.
214. Kim, Y. S., Brophy, E. J., and Nicholson, J. A. Rat intestinal brush border peptidases. 2. Enzymic properties, immunochemistry and interactions with lectins of two different forms of the enzyme. *J. Biol. Chem.* 251:3206, 1976.
215. Kim, Y. S., Kim, Y. W., and Sleisenger, M. H. Studies on the properties of peptide hydrolases in the brush border and soluble fractions of small intestinal mucosa of rat and man. *Biochim. Biophys. Acta* 370:283, 1974.
216. Kotschneff, N. Weitere untersuchungen uber das verhalten verschiedener eiweissabbauprodukte im intermidiargebiet nach versuchen an angiostromierten hunden. *Pfluegers Arch.* 218: 635, 1928.
217. Kroe, D. J., et al. Interrelation of amino acids and pH on intestinal iron absorption. *Am. J. Physiol.* 211:414, 1966.
218. Lagerlöf, H. O., Ekelund, K., and Johansson, C. A mathematical analysis of jejunal indicator concentrations used to calculate jejunal flow and mean transit time. *Scand. J. Gastroenterol.* 7: 379, 1972.
219. Lee, K. Y., Hoffman, N. E., and Simmonds, W. J. The effect of partition of fatty acid between oil and micelles on its uptake by everted intestinal sacs. *Biochim. Biophys. Acta* 249:548, 1971.
220. Leevy, C. M., et al. Incidence and significance of hypovitaminemia in a randomly selected municipal hospital population. *Am. J. Clin. Nutr.* 17:259, 1965.
221. Levy, R. E., Frederickson, D. S., and Lester, L. The lipoproteins and lipid transport in abetalipoproteinemia. *J. Clin. Invest.* 45:531, 1966.
222. Lindberg, T., Noren, O., and Sjöström, H. Peptidases of the Intestinal Mucosa. In D. M. Matthews and J. W. Payne (Eds.), *Peptide Transport in Protein Malnutrition.* New York: American Elsevier, 1975. Pp. 204–242.
223. Linder, M. C., et al. Ferritin and intestinal iron absorption: Pancreatic enzyme and free iron. *Am. J. Physiol.* 228:196, 1975.
224. Lis, M. T., Crampton, R. F., and Matthews, D. M. Effects of dietary changes on intestinal absorption of L-methionine and L-methionyl-L-methionine in the rat. *Br. J. Nutr.* 27:159, 1972.
225. Lobley, R. W., Moss, S., and Holmes, R. Brush border localization of human enterokinase. *Gut* 14:817, 1973.
226. Loria, A., Medal, S. L., and Elizonodo, J. Effect of sorbitol on iron absorption in man. *Am. J. Clin. Nutr.* 10:124, 1962.
227. Love, A. H. G., Mitchell, T. G., and Phillips, R. A. Water and sodium absorption in the human intestine. *J. Physiol. (London)* 195:133, 1968.
228. Louvard, D., et al. Topological studies on the hydrolases bound to the intestinal brush border membranes: 1. Solubilization by papain and Triton X-100. *Biochim. Biophys. Acta* 375:236, 1975.
229. Lucas, M. L., et al. Further investigations with pH microelectrodes into the jejunal microclimate in rat and man. *Gut* 16:844, 1975.
230. MacDonald, I., and Turner, L. J. Serum-fructose levels after sucrose or its constituent monosaccharides. *Lancet* 1:841, 1968.
231. Maestracci, D., et al. Enzymes of the human intestinal brush border membrane, identification after gel electrophoretic separation. *Biochim. Biophys. Acta* 383:147, 1975.
232. Malawer, S. J., et al. Interrelationships between jejunal absorption of sodium, glucose and water in man. *J. Clin. Invest.* 44:1072, 1965.
233. Malathi, P., et al. Studies on transport of glucose from disaccharides by hamster small intestine in vitro: 1. Evidence for a disaccharidase related transport system. *Biochim. Biophys. Acta* 307:613, 1973.
234. Maroux, S. Intestinal brush border peptides. *Ciba Found. Symp. 50 (New Series):*191, 1976.
235. Maroux, S., and Louvard, D. On the hydrophobic part of aminopeptidase and maltases which bind the enzyme to the intestinal brush border membrane. *Biochim. Biophys. Acta* 419:189, 1976.
236. Marrs, T. C., et al. Changes in plasma amino acid concentrations in man after ingestion of an amino acid mixture simulating casein, and a

tryptic hydrolysate of casein. *Br. J. Nutr.* 34: 259, 1975.
237. Matthews, D. M. Protein absorption. *J. Clin. Pathol.* 5:Suppl. 24:29, 1971.
238. Matthews, D. M. Intestinal absorption of peptides. *Phys. Rev.* 55:537, 1975.
239. Matthews, D. M., Addison, J. M., and Burston, D. Evidence for active transport of the dipeptide carnosine (β-alanyl-L-histidine) by hamster jejunum in vitro. *Clin. Sci. Mol. Med.* 46:693, 1974.
240. Matthews, D. M., and Adibi, S. A. Peptide absorption. *Gastroenterology* 71:151, 1976.
241. Matthews, D. M., Craft, I. L., and Crampton, R. F. Intestinal absorption of saccharides and peptides. *Lancet* 2:49, 1968.
242. Matthews, D. M., and Laster, L. Absorption of protein digestion products: A review. *Gut* 6:441, 1965.
243. Mattson, F. H., and Volpenheim, R. A. Carboxylic ester hydrolases of rat pancreatic juice. *J. Lipid Res.* 7:536, 1966.
244. Matuchansky, C., Huet, P. M., Mary, J. Y., Rambaud, J. C., and Bernier, J. J. Effects of cholecystokinin and metoclopramide on jejunal movements of water and electrolytes and on transit time of luminal fluid in man. *Eur. J. Clin. Invest.* 2:169, 1972.
245. Matuchansky, C., Rambaud, J. C., Modigliani, R., and Bernier, J. J. Vitamin B_{12} malabsorption in chronic pancreatitis. (Letter) *Gastroenterology* 67:406, 1974.
246. McCarthy, C. F., et al. Defective uptake of basic amino acids and L-cystine by intestinal mucosa of patients with cystinuria. *J. Clin. Invest.* 43:1518, 1964.
247. McCormick, D. B., Gregory, M. E., and Snell, G. E. Pyridoxal phosphokinases: 1. Assay, distribution, purification and properties. *J. Biol. Chem.* 236:2076, 1961.
248. McIntyre, P. A., et al. Pathogenesis and treatment of macrocytic anemia: Information obtained with radioactive vitamin B_{12}. *Arch. Intern. Med.* 98:541, 1956.
249. McMichael, H. B. A second intestinal glucose carrier. *Gut* 14:428, 1973.
250. McMichael, H. B. Absorption of Carbohydrates. In I. McColl and G. E. Sladen (Eds.), *Intestinal Absorption in Man.* London: Academic, 1975. Pp. 99–141.
251. McMichael, H. B., Webb, J., and Dawson, A. M. The absorption of maltose and lactose in man. *Clin. Sci.* 33:135, 1967.
252. Meldrum, S. J., et al. PH profile of gut as measured by a radiotelemetry capsule. *Br. J. Med.* 2:104, 1972.
253. Messerli, H. Ueber die resorptions geschwindigkeit der eiweisse und ihrer abbauprodukteim dunndarm. *Biochem. Z.* 54:446, 1913.
254. Middleton, H. M. Uptake of pyridoxine hydrochloride by the rat jejunal mucosa in vitro. *J. Nutr.* 107:126, 1977.
255. Middleton, H. M. In vivo absorption and phosphorylation of pyridoxine HCl in rat jejunum. *Gastroenterology* 76:43, 1979.
256. Milla, P. J., et al. Fructose absorption and the effects of other monosaccharides on its absorption in the rat jejunum in vivo. *Gut* 18:425, 1977.
257. Milne, M. D., Asatoor, A. M., Edwards, K. D. G., and Loughridge, L. W. The intestinal absorption defect in cystinuria. *Gut* 2:323, 1961.
258. Milne, M. D., Crawford, M. A., Girao, C. B., and Loughridge, L. W. The metabolic disorder in Hartnup disease. *Q. J. Med.* 29:407, 1960.
259. Modigliani, R., and Bernier, J. J. Absorption of glucose, sodium and water by the human jejunum studied by intestinal perfusion with a proximal occluding balloon and at variable flow rates. *Gut* 12:184, 1971.
260. Modlin, I. M., Bloom, S. R., and Mitchell, S. J. Experimental evidence for vasoactive intestinal peptide as the cause of the watery diarrhea syndrome. *Gastroenterology* 75:1051, 1978.
261. Morgan, R. G. H., and Hoffman, N. E. The interaction of lipase, lipase co-factor and bile salts in triglyceride hydrolysis. *Biochim. Biophys. Acta* 248:143, 1971.
262. Moritz, M., et al. Effect of secretin and cholecystokinin on the transport of electrolyte and water in human jejunum. *Gastroenterology* 64:76, 1973.
263. Murray, M. J., and Stein, N. Does the pancreas influence iron absorption? A critical review of information to date. *Gastroenterology* 51:694, 1966.
264. Nasset, E. S. Enterocrinin, a hormone which excites the glands of the small intestine. *Am. J. Physiol.* 121:481, 1938.
265. Nasset, E. S. The role of the digestive tract in protein metabolism. *Am. J. Dig. Dis.* 9:175, 1964.
266. Nasset, E. S., and Ju, J. S. Mixture of endogenous and exogenous protein in the alimentary tract. *J. Nutr.* 74:461, 1961.
267. Nasset, E. S., Pierce, H. B., and Murlin, J. R. Proof of a humoral control of intestinal secretion. *Am. J. Physiol.* 111:145, 1935.
268. Nasset, E. S., Schwartz, P., and Weiss, H. V.

The digestion of proteins in vivo. *J. Nutr.* 56:83, 1955.
269. Nawab, F., and Asatoor, A. M. Studies of intestinal absorption of amino acids and a dipeptide in a case of Hartnup disease. *Gut* 11:373, 1970.
270. Neal, G. Disaccharidase deficiencies. *J. Clin. Pathol.* 5:Suppl. 24:22, 1971.
271. Newey, H., and Smyth, D. H. The intestinal absorption of some dipeptides. *J. Physiol.* 145:48, 1959.
272. Newey, H., and Smyth, D. H. Intracellular hydrolysis of dipeptides during intestinal absorption. *J. Physiol.* 152:367, 1960.
273. Newey, H., and Smyth, D. H. Cellular mechanisms in intestinal transfer of amino acids. *J. Physiol.* 164:527, 1962.
274. Nicholson, J. A., and Peters, T. J. Subcellular distribution of di and tripeptidase activity in human jejunum. *Clin. Sci. Mol. Med.* 52:168, 1977.
275. Nicholson, J. A., and Peters, T. J. Subcellular distribution of di, tri, tetra and penta-peptidase in human jejunum. *Gut* 18:A960, 1977.
276. Nixon, S. E., and Mawer, G. E. The digestion and absorption of proteins in man: 1. The site of absorption. *Br. J. Nutr.* 24:227, 1970.
277. Nixon, S. E., and Mawer, G. E. The digestion and absorption of protein in man: 2. The form in which digested protein is absorbed. *Br. J. Nutr.* 24:241, 1970.
278. Nolf, P. Les albumoses et peptones sont-elles absorbees par l'epithelium intestinal? *J. Physiol. Pathol. Genet.* 9:925, 1907.
279. Nordström, C., and Dahlqvist, A. Localization of human enterokinase. *Lancet* 1:933, 1972.
280. Noren, O., Dabelsteen, E., Sjöström, H., and Josefsson, L. Histological localization of two dipeptidases in the pig small intestine and liver, using immunofluorescence. *Gastroenterology* 72:87, 1977.
281. Noren, O., Sjöström, H., Svensson, B., Jeppesen, L., Staun, M., and Josefsson, L. Intestinal brush border peptidases. *Ciba Found. Symp. 50 (New Series)*:177, 1977.
282. Öckerman, P. A., and Lundborg, H. Conversion of fructose to glucose by human jejunum: Absence of galactose-to-glucose conversion. *Biochim. Biophys. Acta* 105:34, 1965.
283. Okuda, K., Kitazaki, T., and Takamatsu, M. Inactivation of vitamin B_{12} by a binder in rat intestine and the role of intrinsic factor. *Digestion* 4:35, 1971.
284. Olsen, W. A., and Ingelfinger, F. J. The role of sodium in intestinal glucose absorption in man. *J. Clin. Invest.* 47:1133, 1968.
285. Owens, C. W. J., and Albuguergue, Z. P. Changes in rat bile amino acid concentrations following exposure to oral tetracycline, phenobarbitone and paracetamol. *Clin. Sci. Mol. Med.* 52:70, 1977.
286. Parsons, D. S., and Pritchard, J. S. Hydrolysis of disaccharides during absorption by the perfused small intestine of amphibia. *Nature (London)* 208:1097, 1965.
287. Payne, J. W., and Matthews, D. M. Peptides in the Nutrition of Microorganisms and Peptides in Relation to Animal Nutrition. In D. M. Matthews and J. W. Payne (Eds.), *Peptide Transport in Protein Nutrition.* Amsterdam: Associated Scientific, 1975., Pp. 1–60.
288. Perry, T. L., et al. Carnosinemia: A new metabolic disorder associated with neurologic disease and mental defect. *N. Engl. J. Med.* 277:1219, 1967.
289. Peters, T. J. The subcellular localization of di and tripeptide hydrolase activity in guinea pig small intestine. *Biochem. J.* 120:195, 1970.
290. Phillips, S. F., and Giller, J. The contribution of the colon to electrolyte and water conservation in man. *J. Lab. Clin. Med.* 81:733, 1973.
291. Phillips, S. F., and Summerskill, W. H. J. Water and electrolyte transport during maintenance of isotonicity in human jejunum and ileum. *J. Lab. Clin. Med.* 70:686, 1967.
292. Plimmer, R. H. A. On the presence of lactase in the intestines of animals and on the adaptation of the intestine to lactose. *J. Physiol.* 35:20, 1907.
293. Polak, J. M., Pearse, A. G. E., Bloom, S. R., Buchan, A. M. J., Rayford, P. L., and Thompson, J. C. Identification of cholecystokinin secreting cells. *Lancet* 2:1016, 1975.
294. Polheim, D., and Johnston, J. M. The activity of monoglyceride transacylase in response to various diets. In preparation, 1975.
295. Powell, G. K., and McElveen, M. A. Effect of prolonged fasting on fatty acid re-esterification in rat intestinal mucosa. *Biochim. Biophys. Acta* 369:8, 1974.
296. Prockop, D., and Sjoerdsma, A. Significance of urinary hydroxyproline in man. *J. Clin. Invest.* 40:843, 1961.
297. Prockop, D. J., Keiser, H. R., and Sjoerdsma, A. Gastrointestinal absorption and renal excretion of hydroxyproline peptides. *Lancet* 2:527, 1962.
298. Quigley, J. P., and Gotterer, G. S. Distribution of (Na^+K^+) stimulate. ATPase activity in rat intestinal mucosa. *Biochim. Biophys. Acta* 173: 456, 1969.

299. Radhakrishnan, A. N. Intestinal dipeptidases and dipeptide transport in the monkey and man. *Ciba Found. Symp. 50 (New Series)*:37, 1977.
300. Ramaswamy, K., Malathi, P., and Crane, R. K. Demonstration of hydrolase-related glucose transport in brush border membrane residues prepared from guinea pig small intestine. *Biochem. Biophys. Res. Commun.* 68:162, 1976.
301. Ramaswamy, K., et al. Studies on the transport of glucose from disaccharides by hamster small intestine *in vitro*: II. Characteristics of the disaccharidase-related transport system. *Biochim. Biophys. Acta* 345:39, 1974.
302. Reid, E. W. On intestinal absorption, especially on the absorption of serum, peptone and glucose. *Philo. Trans. R. Soc. Lond. (Biol.)* 192:211, 1900.
303. Reisenauer, A. M., Krumdieck, C. L., and Halstead, C. H. Human jejunal brush border folate conjugase. *Gastroenterology* 72:1118, 1977.
304. Rhodes, J. B., Eicholz, A., and Crane, R. K. Studies on the organization of the brush border intestinal epithelial cells: 4. Amino peptidase activity in microvillus membranes of hamster intestinal brush borders. *Biochim. Biophys. Acta* 135:959, 1967.
305. Robins, S. J., et al. Localization of fatty acid re-esterification in the brush border region of intestinal absorptive cells. *Biochim. Biophys. Acta* 233:550, 1971.
306. Rodgers, J. B., Jr., and Bochenek, W. Localization of lipid re-esterifying enzymes of the rat small intestine. Effects of jejunal removal on ileal enzyme activities. *Biochim. Biophys. Acta* 202:426, 1970.
307. Rosenberg, I. H. Folate absorption and malabsorption. *N. Engl. J. Med.* 293:1303, 1975.
308. Rosenzweig, N. S. The Influence of Dietary Carbohydrates on Intestinal Disaccharidase Activity in Man. In B. Borgström, A. Dahlqvist, and L. Hambraens (Eds.), *Intestinal Enzyme Deficiencies and Their Nutritional Implications.* Symposium of the Swedish Nutrition Foundation, Stockholm 51:52, 1973.
309. Rubino, A., Field, M., and Shwachman, H. Intestinal transport of amino acid residues of dipeptides: 1. Influx of the glycine residue of glycyl-L-proline across mucosal border. *J. Biol. Chem.* 246:3542, 1971.
310. Sabesin, S. M. Ultrasound Aspects of the Intracellular Assembly. Transport and Exocytosis of Chylomicrons by Rat Intestinal Absorptive Cells. In K. Rommell and H. Goebell (Eds.), *Lipid Absorption: Biochemical and Clinical Aspects.* Lancaster: MTP Press, 1976. P. 113.
311. Saini, P. K., and Rosenberg, I. H. Isolation of pteroyl-γ-oligoglutamyl endo peptidase from chicken intestine with the aid of affinity chromatography. *J. Biol. Chem.* 249:5131, 1974.
312. Saltzman, D. A., Rector, F. C., and Fordtran, J. S. The role of intraluminal sodium in glucose absorption in vivo. *J. Clin. Invest.* 51:876, 1972.
313. Sandle, G. I., Lobley, R. W., and Holmes, R. Effect of maltose on the absorption of glucose in the jejunum in man. *Gut* 18:A944, 1977.
314. Schedl, H. P., et al. Absorption of L-methionine from human small intestine. *J. Clin. Invest.* 47:417, 1968.
315. Schiller, C. M., David, J. S. K., and Johnston, J. M. The subcellular distribution of triglyceride synthetase in the intestinal mucosa. *Biochim. Biophys. Acta* 210:489, 1970.
316. Schmitz, J., Preiser, H., Maestracci, D., Crane, R. K. Troesch, V., and Hadorn, B. Subcellular localization of enterokinase in human small intestine. *Biochim. Biophys. Acta* 343:435, 1974.
317. Schmitz, J., Preiser, H., Maestracci, D., Ghosh, B. K., Cerda, J. J., and Crane, R. K. Purification of the human intestinal brush border membrane. *Biochim. Biophys. Acta* 323:98, 1973.
318. Schneider, A. J., Kinter, W. B., and Stirling, C. E. Glucose-galactose malabsorption: Report of a case with autoradiographic studies of a mucosal biopsy. *N. Engl. J. Med.* 274:305, 1966.
319. Schultz, F. M., and Johnston, J. M. The synthesis of higher glycerides via the monoglyceride pathway in hamster adipose tissue. *J. Lipid Res.* 12:132, 1971.
320. Schultz, S. G., and Curran, P. F. Coupled transport of sodium and organic solutes. *Physiol. Rev.* 50:637, 1970.
321. Schütz, H. B., and Reizenstein, P. Radio vitamin B_{12} as a dilution indicator in gastrointestinal research. *Am. J. Dig. Dis.* 8:904, 1963.
322. Semenza, G., Auricchio, S., and Rubino, A. Multiplicity of human intestinal disaccharidases: 1. Chromatographic separation of maltases and of two lactoses. *Biochim. Biophys. Acta* 96:487, 1965.
323. Shearer, M. J., Barkhan, P., and Webster, G. R. Absorption and excretion of an oral dose of tritiated vitamin K_1 in man. *Br. J. Hematol.* 18:297, 1970.
324. Shiratori, T., and Goodman, D. S. Complete hydrolysis of dietary cholesterol esters during intestinal absorption. *Biochim. Biophys. Acta* 106:625, 1965.
325. Silk, D. B. A. The absorption of peptides in man. University of London M.D. thesis, 1974.

326. Silk, D. B. A. Peptide absorption in man. *Gut* 15:494, 1974.
327. Silk, D. B. A. Amino acid and peptide absorption in man. *Ciba Found. Symp. 50 (New Series)*: 15, 1977.
328. Silk, D. B. A. Clinical nutrition in hospitals: 2. Enteral nutrition. *Hospital Update* 4:543, 1978.
329. Silk, D. B. A., Chung, Y. C., Berger, K. L., Conley, M., Beigler, M., Sleisenger, M. H., Spiller, G. A., and Kim, Y. S. Comparison of oral feeding of peptide and amino acid meals to normal human subjects. *Gut* 20:291, 1979.
330. Silk, D. B. A., Clark, M. L., Marrs, T. C., Addison, J. M., Burston, D., Matthews, D. M., and Clegg, K. M. Jejunal absorption of an amino acid mixture simulating casein and an enzymic hydrolysate of casein prepared for oral administration to normal adults. *Br. J. Nutr.* 33:95, 1975.
331. Silk, D. B. A., and Dawson, A. M. Intestinal Absorption of Carbohydrate and Protein in Man. In R. K. Crane (Ed.), *International Review of Physiology (III. Gastrointestinal Physiology).* Baltimore: University Park Press, 1979. P. 151.
332. Silk, D. B. A., Fairclough, P. D., Park, N. J., Lane, A. E., Webb, J. P. W., Clark, M. L., and Dawson, A. M. A study of relations between the absorption of amino acids, dipeptides, water and electrolytes in the normal human jejunum. *Clin. Sci. Mol. Med.* 49:401, 1975.
333. Silk, D. B. A., and Kim, Y. S. A study of intraluminal peptide hydrolase activity in the rat. *Clin. Sci. Mol. Med.* 49:523, 1975.
334. Silk, D. B. A., Kumar, P. J., Perrett, D., Clark, M. L., and Dawson, A. M. Amino acid absorption in patients with coeliac disease and dermatitis herpetiformis. *Gut* 15:1, 1974.
335. Silk, D. B. A., Marrs, T. C., Addison, J. M., Burston, D., Clark, M. L., and Matthews, D. M. Absorption of amino acids from an amino acid mixture simulating casein and a tryptic hydrolysate of casein in man. *Clin. Sci. Mol. Med.* 45: 715, 1973.
336. Silk, D. B. A., Nicholson, J. A., and Kim, Y. S. Hydrolysis of peptides within the lumen of small intestine. *Am. J. Physiol.* 231:1323, 1976.
337. Silk, D. B. A., Nicholson, J. A., and Kim, Y. S. Relationships between mucosal hydrolysis and transport of two phenylalanine dipeptides. *Gut* 17:870, 1976.
338. Silk, D. B. A., Perrett, D., and Clark, M. L. Intestinal transport of two dipeptides containing the same two neutral amino acids in man. *Clin. Sci. Mol. Med.* 45:291, 1973.
339. Silk, D. B. A., Perrett, D., and Clark, M. L. Jejunal and ileal absorption of dibasic amino acids and an arginine-containing dipeptide in cystinuria. *Gastroenterology* 68:1426, 1975.
340. Silk, D. B. A., Perrett, D., Stephens, A. D., Clark, M. L., and Scowan, E. F. Intestinal absorption of cystine and cysteine in normal human subjects and patients with cystinuria. *Clin. Sci. Mol. Med.* 47:393, 1974.
341. Silk, D. B. A., Perrett, D., Webb, J. P. W., and Clark, M. L. Absorption of two tripeptides by the human small intestine: A study using a perfusion technique. *Clin. Sci. Mol. Med.* 46:393, 1974.
342. Silk, D. B. A., Webb, J. P. W., Lane, A. E., Clark, M. L., and Dawson, A. M. Functional differentiation of human jejunum and ileum: A comparison of the handling of glucose, peptides and amino acids. *Gut* 15:444, 1974.
343. Simmonds, W. J. Uptake of Fatty Acid and Monoglyceride. In K. Rommel and H. Goebell (Eds.), *Lipid Absorption: Biochemical and Chemical Aspects.* Lancaster: MTP Press, 1976. P. 51.
344. Sladen, G. E. A study of the intestinal absorption of fluid and electrolytes in man. University of Oxford M.D. thesis, 1970. Pp. 130, 141.
345. Sladen, G. E. Absorption of Fluid and Electrolytes in Health and Disease. In I. McColl and G. E. Sladen (Eds.), *Intestinal Absorption in Man.* London: Academic, 1975. P. 51.
346. Sladen, G. E., and Dawson, A. M. Interrelationships between the absorption of glucose, sodium and water by the normal human jejunum. *Clin. Sci.* 36:119, 1969.
347. Sladen, G. E., and Dawson, A. M. Effect of bicarbonate on sodium absorption by the human jejunum. *Nature (London)* 218:267, 1970.
348. Spencer, R. P. S., and Zamcheck, N. Intestinal absorption of riboflavin by rat and hamster. *Gastroenterology* 40:794, 1961.
349. Stein, W. H., and Moore, S. The free amino acids of human blood plasma. *J. Biol. Chem.* 211:915, 1954.
350. Stevenson, N. R. Active transport of L-ascorbic acid in the human ileum. *Gastroenterology* 67: 952, 1974.
351. Stevenson, N. R., and Brush, M. K. Existence and characteristic of Na^+-dependent active transport of ascorbic acid in guinea pig. *Am. J. Clin. Nutr.* 22:318, 1969.
352. Tandom, R., Edwards, R. H., and Rodgers, J. B. Effects of bile diversion on the lipid re-esterifying capacity of the rat small bowel. *Gastroenterology* 63:990, 1972.
353. Taylor, W. H. Biochemistry of Pepsins. In C. F. Code (Ed.), *Handbook of Physiology.* Wash-

ington, DC: American Physiological Society, 1968. Vol. 5, pp. 2567–2588.
354. Theron, J. J., Wittmann, W., and Prinslove, J. G. The fine structure of the jejunum in kwashiorkor. *Exp. Mol. Path.* 14:184, 1971.
355. Thier, S. O., et al. Cystinuria: Defective intestinal transport of dibasic amino acids and cystine. *J. Clin. Invest.* 44:442, 1965.
356. Thomas, F. B., McCullough, F. S., and Greenberger, N. J. Inhibition of the intestinal absorption of inorganic and hemoglobin iron by cholestyramine. *J. Lab. Clin. Med.* 78:70, 1971.
357. Tilson, M. D., and Wright, H. K. Adaptation of functioning and bypassed segments of ileum during compensatory hypertrophy of the gut. *Surgery* 67:687, 1970.
358. Tomasini, J. T., and Dobbins, W. O., III. Intestinal mucosal morphology during water and electrolyte absorption. A light and electron microscopic study. *Am. J. Dig. Dis.* 15:226, 1970.
359. Toskes, B., et al. Vitamin B_{12} absorption in chronic pancreatic insufficiency. Studies suggesting the presence of a pancreatic "intrinsic factor." *N. Engl. J. Med.* 248:627, 1971.
360. Tsuji, T., Yamada, R., and Nose, Y. Intestinal absorption of vitamin B_6: 1. Pyridoxal uptake by rat intestinal tissue. *J. Nutr. Sci. Vitaminol. (Tokyo)* 19:401, 1973.
361. Turnberg, L. A., Bieberdorf, F. A., Morawski, S. G., and Fordtran, J. S. Interrelationships of chloride, bicarbonate, sodium and hydrogen transport in the human ileum. *J. Clin. Invest.* 49:557, 1970.
362. Turnberg, L. A., Fordtran, J. S., Carter, N. W., and Rector, F. C., Jr. Mechanism of bicarbonate absorption and its relationship to sodium transport in the human jejunum. *J. Clin. Invest.* 49: 548, 1970.
363. Turner, M. D. Pepsinogens and pepsins. *Gut* 9:134, 1968.
364. Van Slyke, D. D., and Meyer, G. M. The amino acid nitrogen of the blood: Preliminary experiments on protein assimilation. *J. Biol. Chem.* 12:399, 1912.
365. Vandermeers, A., et al. On human pancreatic triacylglycerol lipase isolation and some properties. *Biochim. Biophys. Acta* 370:257, 1974.
366. Veeger, W., et al. Effects of sodium bicarbonate and pancreatin on the absorption of vitamin B_{12} and fat in pancreatic insufficiency. *N. Engl. J. Med.* 267:1341, 1962.
367. Verzar, F., and MacDougall, E. J. *Absorption from the Intestine.* London: Longmans, 1936.
368. Voit, C., and Bauer, J. Ueber die aufsaugung im dick-und dunndarme. *Z. Biol.* 5:536, 1869.
369. Von der Lippe, G., Anderson, K., and Schjonsby, H. Pancreatic extract and the intestinal uptake of vitamin B_{12}: III. Stimulatory effect in the presence of a non-intrinsic factor vitamin B_{12} binder. *Scand. J. Gastroenterol.* 12:183, 1977.
370. Welsh, J. D., et al. An enriched microvillus membrane preparation from frozen specimens of human small intestine. *Gastroenterology* 62: 572, 1972.
371. Whalen, G. E., Harris, J. A., Geenen, J. E., and Soergel, K. H. Sodium and water absorption from the human small intestine. The accuracy of the perfusion method. *Gastroenterology* 51: 975, 1966.
372. Whalen, G. E., Wu, W. C., Ganeshappa, K. P., Wall, M. J., Kalkhoff, R. K., and Soergel, K. H. The effect of endogenous glucagon on human small bowel function. *Gastroenterology* 64:822, 1973.
373. Whitecross, D. P., et al. The pepsinogens of human gastric mucosa. *Gut* 14:850, 1973.
374. Wiggans, D. S., and Johnston, J. M. Absorptive patterns of peptides through the isolated rat intestine. *Fed. Proc.* 17:335, 1958.
375. Wiggans, D. S., and Johnston, J. M. The absorption of peptides. *Biochim. Biophys. Acta* 32:69, 1959.
376. Will, G., and Boddy, K. Influence of succinic acid on absorption of iron studied by whole-body monitoring. *Am. J. Clin. Nutr.* 23:779, 1970.
377. Wilson, F. A., and Dietschy, J. M. The intestinal unstirred layer: Its surface area and effect of active transport kinetics. *Biochim. Biophys. Acta* 363:112, 1974.
378. Wimberely, P. D., and Harries, J. T. Congenital glucose-galactose malabsorption. *Proc. R. Soc. Med.* 67:755, 1974.
379. Wojnarowska, F., and Gray, G. M. Intestinal surface peptide hydrolases: Identification and characterization of three enzymes from rat brush border. *Biochim. Biophys. Acta* 403:147, 1975.
380. Woolfson, A. M. J., et al. Prolonged nasogastric tube feeding in critically ill and surgical patients. *Postgrad. Med. J.* 52:678, 1976.
381. Wright, J. P., Barbezat, G. O., and Clain, J. E. Jejunal secretion in response to a duodenal mixed nutrient perfusion. *Gastroenterology* 76:94, 1979.
382. Yearick, E. S., and Nadeau, R. G. Serum amino acid response to isocaloric test meals. *Am. J. Clin. Nutr.* 20:338, 1967.
383. Zilversmit, D. W. The composition and structure of lymph chylomicrons in dog, rat and man. *J. Clin. Invest.* 44:1610, 1965.

Hormones and the Control of Metabolism

Douglas W. Wilmore
Louis H. Aulick
Richard A. Becker

3

Claude Bernard first suggested that the composition of the fluid bathing the body cells is controlled, and proposed that the constancy of the *milieu intérieur* allows the organism a degree of functional freedom from the external environment. Since that time, it has become apparent that such internal stability is attained by very intricate systems of control; this overall regulatory function is coordinated between the endocrine system and the autonomic nervous system. Starling proposed the name hormone (from the Greek root *hormaein,* meaning to excite, arouse, or set in motion) to describe chemical agents that are released from one group of cells, travel by the bloodstream, and affect other cell populations. Huxley placed less emphasis on the mode of travel of these substances and suggested that the prime role of hormones is to transfer information from one set of cells to another, to evoke a response beneficial for the cell population as a whole. In this discussion, hormonal control is considered in the context of Huxley's definition, and the regulatory function of both the endocrine system and autonomic nervous system will be presented. Although there are many physiologic alterations that initiate these control mechanisms in patients during critical illness, homeostatic adjustment to alterations of salt, water, and mineral metabolism and regulation of blood volume will not be considered. However, blood flow is often altered in patients with surgical problems, and this perturbed circulation may affect substrate utilization and energy metabolism. Therefore, interaction occurs between tissue perfusion and metabolism, and the effect of the circulation on regional metabolism in surgical patients will be discussed.

LEVELS OF METABOLIC CONTROL

Cellular Control Mechanisms

Although a wide variety of intricate and interacting metabolic control mechanisms exist in the body, the regulating systems that are present in complex, highly specialized, multicellular populations have evolved from control systems that are operative in simple unicellular organisms. Single cells have elegant control processes, and these systems serve important and vital functions in maintaining cellular integrity and basal metabolic functions. The most widely used cellular control mechanisms operate by simple stoichiometry—that is, when substrates accumulate, the reaction removing them proceeds more rapidly, if the responsible enzymes are not saturated. Conversely, if a substrate diminishes, reactions become slower to maintain substrate concentration.

Stoichiometric control is particularly applicable to the regulation of intracellular metabolism by the nucleotides, primarily, the adenine nucleotides. The intracellular concentration of ADP regulates oxygen consumption and, hence, cellular energy utilization [34]. ADP is generated from ATP, a compound that stores energy to be used for cellular work and synthetic processes. As soon as the ADP appears, it promotes biochemical oxidation, which generates energy and converts ADP back to ATP, thus removing ADP from the reaction (Figure 3-1). As ADP is reduced, oxidative metabolism slows and returns to basal, while cells maintain a constant *high-energy phosphate balance*. Similar systems utilize NAD-NADH and coenzymes to control cellular metabolism. All of these mechanisms operate because the quantity of the regulator substance (the nucleotide or coenzyme) is small compared to the mass of substrate passing through the metabolic reaction [89]. As the regulator (the nucleotide or coenzyme) is converted back to its initial state, the reaction slows or stops.

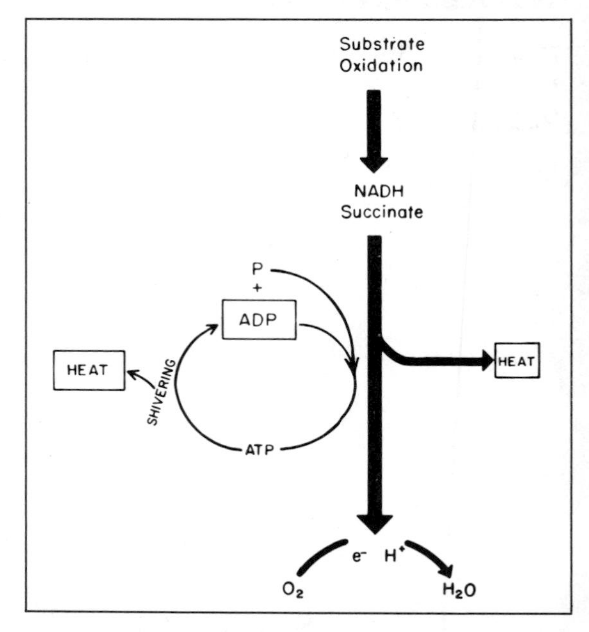

Figure 3-1. *When respiration and phosphorylation in the mitochondria are "coupled" or linked together, the production of high-energy bond compounds (ATP) is directly related to the rate of oxidation. However, the rate with which substrate is oxidized depends on the quantity of ADP and P available; i.e., respiratory control is determined by the availability of these substances. In this example, shivering converts skeletal muscle ATP to ADP+ P, which then increases substrate oxidation and heat production. When the shivering stops, ATP accumulates, ADP and P diminish, and the reaction rate slows.*

Cellular control may also occur at the membrane level, either at the cell or mitochondrial membrane [34]. With an isolated heart preparation, Neely demonstrated that transport of glucose remains the rate-limiting step for its utilization [96]. Membrane transport across the cell wall remained the limiting factor even during increased external work; impaired glucose transport resulted in a decline in intracellular energy levels. Transport of many metabolites across the mitochondrial membrane appears to be carrier-dependent and may serve as a control point for metabolic processes. For example, with skeletal muscle stimulation, carbohydrate uptake increases, but the quantity of pyruvate generated in the cytosol may exceed mechanisms for mitochondrial membrane transport and Kreb's cycle oxidation [89]. Hence, pyruvate is converted to lactate in the cytosol, which is released back into the bloodstream. Thus, intracellular partitioning provides an important directional component in the control of cellular energy metabolism and a portion of this control is expressed through the regulation of mitochondrial membrane transport.

An additional mechanism of cellular metabolic control is the regulation of enzyme concentrations, which govern, in part, enzyme-catalyzed reactions. The concentration of enzymes in the cell varies widely in response to environmental changes, and mechanisms have evolved for increasing or decreasing the rate of synthesis and/or degradation of these specific protein molecules. In addition, some enzymes may be converted from an active to an inactive form. In functional terms, all these mechanisms preserve metabolic efficiency: enzyme molecules are synthesized or activated during times of need, and concentration and/or activity is suppressed when substrate deficiency occurs.

Substrate Control

It has already been noted that a change in the external environment of a cell can induce a variety of alterations in cellular metabolic control. The most common adjustments occur in response to *substrate availability*. For example, as blood glucose is elevated, concentration gradients across cell membranes increase, glucose flux into the cell is augmented, and cystolic concentrations of glucose are elevated. Because of the mass action effect created by this substrate, increased flow of glucose through the metabolic pathways occurs, and soon more intermediary metabolites (lactate) will accumulate or glycogen will be formed. With prolonged glucose loading, which occurs with high dietary carbohydrate intake, specific enzymatic machinery adapts to accommodate this increased substrate load. Other substances that commonly exert profound effects on metabolism are glycerol, lactate, and the gluconeogenic amino acids. Increased concentrations of these substances augment hepatic gluconeogenesis.

In contrast to the mass action effect of excess substrate, which stimulates reaction rates, a biochemical product may be produced that inhibits other metabolic events. The formation of acetoacetate and β-hydroxybutyrate during starvation are examples of this *end product inhibition.* Ketone bodies serve as negative feedback signals to a variety of tissues signaling them to decrease glucose utilization or minimize protein breakdown, and these compounds are essential substrates that minimize skeletal muscle proteolysis during prolonged starvation [29]. Competitive inhibition may also occur between glucose and fatty acid oxidation; when fatty acid levels in the blood are raised, glucose utilization is depressed, and when glucose is elevated, fat oxidation decreases. These findings led Randle to propose the glucose-fatty acid cycle, which suggests that the rates of utilization of these substances are related to their concentrations in blood; the substance that achieves the highest concentration relative to the other inhibits entry and oxidation of the other substrate [103].

Hormonal and Autonomic Nervous System Regulation

The endocrine and autonomic nervous systems provide yet another dimension to the control of the body's metabolic machinery. The transmitting materials (hormones or neurotransmitters) occur in three general biochemical forms: steroids, polypeptides, and amines. These substances are liberated from the endocrine cell or nerve ending following stimulation by an afferent signal. The hormone is released into the bloodstream while other neurotransmitters (norepinephrine and acetylcholine) travel only a few microns across a synaptic cleft.

Chemical transmitters excite specific cells that are genetically programmed to respond to the biochemical messenger. This preselection is implemented through a system of specialized receptors, which bind the transmitter substance rapidly and with sufficient affinity to detect the molecule at extremely low concentrations (physiologic effects of circulating hormones occur at blood concentrations of 10^{-7} to 10^{-12} M) [55]. The transmitter-receptor complex combines to form a signal, which is then transduced (or amplified) within the cell to initiate a specific biologic response. Receptors may be on the cell membrane, as is the case of the receptors for polypeptide hormones and amines, or they may be housed within the cell, which is the site of

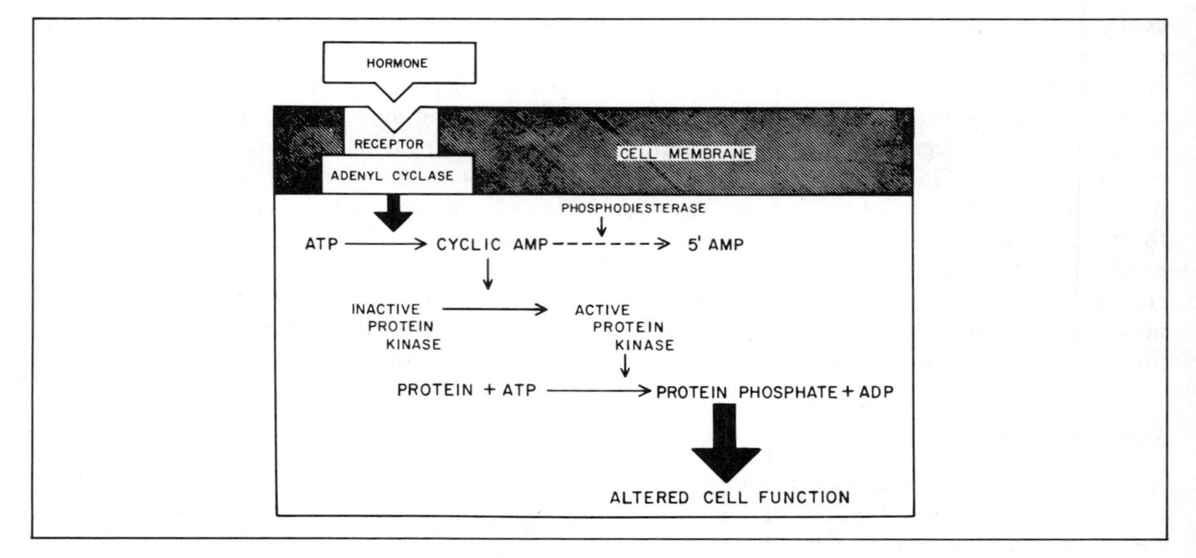

Figure 3-2. *The role of cyclic AMP as a "second messenger" in the actions of many hormones.*

action for most steroids [105]. The cellular location of the receptor determines, in part, the time between hormonal release and biologic response (the polypeptides evoke rapid action, whereas the steroid response is more prolonged) and also influences the half-life of the transmitter material (peptides have a short half-life; steroids have a longer half-life).

Once stimulated, the cellular receptor complex evokes a response. In the case of the peptide hormones, however, this action leads to a rise in concentration of another substance, cyclic AMP, which is thought to serve as the second or "intracellular" messenger [106]. Peptide hormones regulate the concentration of a membrane-bound enzyme, adenylcyclase, which catalyzes the conversion of ATP to cyclic AMP, thus causing a rise in concentration of cyclic AMP within the cell (Figure 3-2). The increase in cellular concentration of cyclic AMP activates protein kinases, a class of enzymes that catalyze phosphorylation of proteins, eventually inducing changes in cell function. Other hormones initiate responses more directly, but all the biologic transmitters act to: (1) enhance or inhibit the activity of differentiated cells; (2) increase the number of responsive cells by inducing differentiation of precursor cells or stimulating mitosis of active cells; or (3) stimulate both functions. An example of this latter function occurs when adrenocorticotropin (ACTH) is released at sustained levels; it not only stimulates steroid hormone production from the adrenal cortex, but also causes hypertrophy and hyperplasia of the gland.

Hormones and the autonomic nervous system maintain exacting and finite regulation of body substrate and energy metabolism, and these intricate and coordinated functions are maintained, in part, by an elaborate number of feedback signals. A simple closed-loop, negative-feedback system may regulate serum concentration of a substance (for example, the control of blood glucose by insulin) without involving higher centers (the hypothalamus or pituitary). More elaborate systems monitor hormone concentration and regulate hormonal output to maintain a precise blood concentration (i.e., cortisol regulation). In other systems, several levels of feedback control exist (both the hypothalamus and pituitary receive feedback signals from thyroid hormones). Through all of these sensitive feedback processes, a precise amount of hormone is elaborated to achieve the appropriate response.

In spite of these elaborate control systems, the target tissue response to a hormone may be inadequate. Recent advances in endocrine research have suggested that a hormone's effect on the target cell is determined by the concentration and affinity of the receptor and by many steps in metabolism beyond the receptor. Exposure of receptor-bearing cells to high concentrations of hormone causes (often within hours) a decrease in the number of receptors per cell [55]. The decrease in receptor concentration is referred to as "down regulation," which has been described following cellular exposure to high concentrations of insulin, glucagon, thyroid hormones, and growth hormone. The role of receptor concentration and affinity during critical illness, with aging, or during chronic debilitating disease is unknown.

Another stabilizing effect in the integration of hormonal and autonomic nervous system control is the interaction that occurs between the individual hormones. For every hormonal action, there may be a subsequent hormonal reaction; elaboration of one hormone will cause adjustments and alterations in the secretion of other hormones. A discussion of direct effects of a single hormone on metabolism aids conceptualization and understanding of a control process. However, this type of presentation is an extreme simplification of a complex and interacting biologic control process.

Circulation and Metabolic Control

No discussion of metabolic control is complete without emphasizing the interdependence of circulation and metabolism. Although the metabolic needs of the body primarily determine blood flow requirements, all metabolically induced hemodynamic changes must be balanced against thermoregulatory and pressure and/or volume demands on the circulation. During stress (physiologic or pathologic), the cardiovascular system is often faced with conflicting demands; the resultant compensatory adjustments may limit perfusion and alter local metabolism of different regional beds.

Most tissues have two levels of vascular control [109]. *Extrinsic* vasomotor control is that regulation effected through the vasomotor center in the medulla oblongata and mediated via autonomic nerves and circulating neurohormones. *Intrinsic* or *local control* occurs within a specific organ or tissue, whereas vasomotor adjustments develop with changes in the immediate environment and are independent of autonomic nerves or systemically released circulatory mediators [70]. In some tissues, where basal flow commonly exceeds local metabolic requirements (i.e., skin, kidney, and gastrointestinal tract), extrinsic vasomotor control predominates. Blood flow to the heart, brain, and active skeletal muscle, on the other hand, is principally determined by local, metabolic factors. The basic functional difference between these two levels of vasomotor control is that one (the extrinsic form) involves a higher center, which integrates multiple afferent stimuli and coordinates a generalized, vasomotor outflow to the entire organism, whereas the other (the local controller) is sensitive *only* to the immediate metabolic changes of that one particular tissue.

Because of the dual nature of vasomotor control, the ultimate level of perfusion for any particular organ results from the interaction between local and systemic signals. There are many situations during stress in which total body circulatory requirements compete with regional blood flow. For example, during hypotension associated with sepsis, the metabolic demands of the liver may be increased, but these local drives for increased hepatic perfusion are overridden by baroreceptive vasoconstrictor signals, which maintain or reduce visceral blood flow to restore blood pressure. If normal pressure cannot be reestablished, the liver remains relatively vasoconstricted and hepatic metabolism becomes *flow-limited.* In other words, increased liver function can continue only as long as the imbalance between local flow and metabolism can be met by increased extraction of oxygen and the necessary fuels from the blood; once maximal levels of extraction develop, liver function is impaired. Thus, during altered hemodynamic states that occur in surgical patients during shock, injury, sepsis, cardiac failure, and fluid and electrolyte imbalance, the impact of circulation on metabolism of the patient must be considered.

AFFERENT SIGNALS THAT INITIATE METABOLIC RESPONSES

Simple Starvation

The signals that initiate the response to starvation are: (1) lack of metabolic substrate, and (2) end product inhibition signaled by ketone bodies. With fasting, concentrations of key circulating substrates are altered: blood glucose falls, free fatty acids and ketone bodies rise, and levels of total serum amino acids gradually fall. These alterations in plasma concentrations generally reflect the decrease in glucose as a primary fuel, and the relative increase in fat oxidation as the body's major energy source. Insulin appears to play a central role in man's adaptation to fasting [29]. As glucose concentration is reduced, insulin falls and fatty acid mobilization and utilization are favored at high rates of oxidation. Increased concentrations of fatty acids compete with glucose for entry into muscle cells and therefore act as potent peripheral glucose antagonists [103]. Within several days of starvation, fatty acids are partially oxidized in the liver to form acetoacetate, acetone, or β-hydroxybutyrate, or "ketone bodies." The parent body of ketones, acetoacetyl CoA, is a normal intermediate of lipogenesis and fatty acid degradation, and fatty acid oxidation appears unimpaired to the level at which acetyl CoA is formed. For acetyl CoA to be utilized in the citric acid cycle, it must combine with oxaloacetate, which is an end product of carbohydrate breakdown, arising from the conversion of pyruvate to oxaloacetate (Figure 3-3). However, with glucose availability limited by starvation, the citric acid cycle is rate-limited by the diminished amount of oxaloacetate present. Hence, fatty acid breakdown is shunted by way of CoA into ketone-body formation. During starvation, ketones are a main source of body fuel, and either directly or indirectly provide the signal to muscle cells to minimize amino acid release, which aids protein conservation during long-term caloric deprivation. In addition, utilization of ketone bodies by the central nervous system further spares glucose utilization and dampens

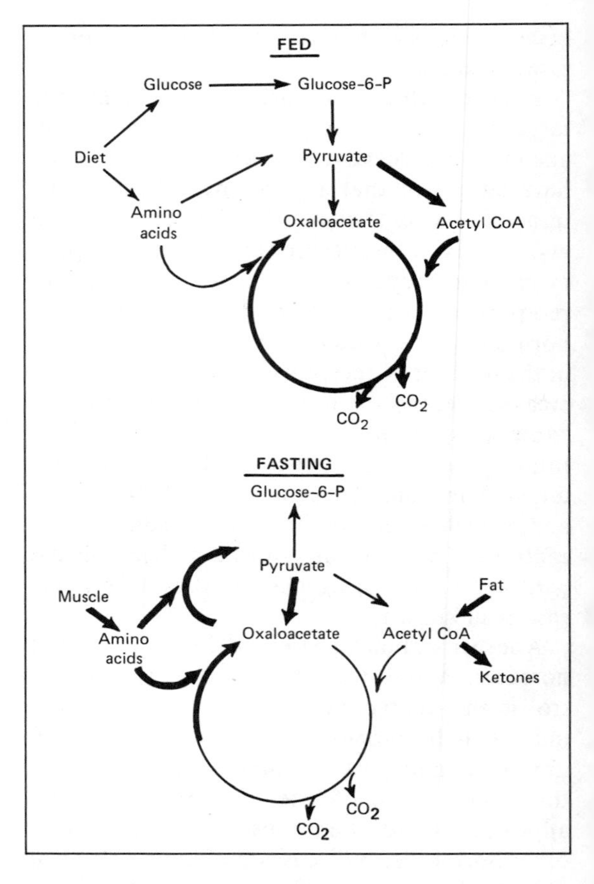

Figure 3-3. *The flow of substrate during the fed and fasting state. During fasting the movement of pyruvate into the Kreb's cycle is limited because of the endocrine environment (low insulin, elevated glucagon), which induces enzymes favoring conversion of 3-carbon intermediates to glucose.*

CNS function and sympathetic outflow during long-term fasts.

With the initial fall in insulin, amino acid release from skeletal muscle is increased [102], and the gluconeogenic amino acids are converted to new glucose in the liver [52]. In the first several days of fasting, catecholamine excretion rate may increase [92], probably in response to the initial fall in blood glucose. The increased irritability and palpitations that frequently occur on the second to third day of fasting may be clinical manifestations of increased adrenergic discharge. The initial catecholamine discharge may accelerate release of free fatty acid and amino acids, although lack of central autonomic regulation does not appear to alter the initial adaptive response to starvation [24]. Catecholamine levels then fall and remain low throughout the remainder of the fast [21]. Glucagon rises with fasting and the insulin/glucagon ratio is low, favoring hepatic gluconeogenesis [1]. Other hormones, such as ACTH and growth hormone, are altered, but are of minor importance in the overall adaptation.

Injury

In contrast to the substrate lack that initiates metabolic alterations following starvation, the responses to injury result in a series of centrally controlled events that mobilize an apparent excess of body substrate. The metabolic alterations to injury result from a series of integrated neurohormonal signals that, for the most part, originate in the central nervous system. The magnitude of these signals depends primarily on the extent of stress, related to the mass of tissue damage, although tissue responses to these signals may be modulated by the age and sex of the patient, physiologic reserve (i.e., stress capacity), nutritional status, and underlying disease processes.

The causative factors and afferent stimuli that evoke the stress response in the injured patient appear specific and are related in time following the initial insult. Cuthbertson described the posttraumatic events and labeled the first part of the response to injury as the "ebb" phase, which occurs immediately and is characterized by a general depression of the body's physiologic function [38]. Following successful resuscitation and restoration of blood volume, cardiopulmonary function increases, heat production and body temperature rise, and substrate is mobilized from peripheral tissues. This elevation in physiologic activity characterizes the "flow" phase of injury, which describes metabolic and hemodynamic alterations associated with tissue repair and patient recovery.

During the "ebb" phase of injury, three general types of stimuli signal the central nervous system to initiate homeostatic adjustment:

1. *Fluid loss* from the vascular compartment results in stimulation of volume and pressure receptors, initiating a series of CNS-mediated cardiovascular adjustments. Cardiac output falls, peripheral resistance increases, and blood is redistributed to vital organs to maintain function. With progressive volume loss into the area of injury, the resulting hypoperfusion reduces tissue oxygenation and causes disturbances in the acid-base equilibrium. Chemoreceptor stimulation thus serves as additional afferent input to both vasomotor and respiratory centers during hypovolemia. Because loss of fluid volume following injury is closely related to the extent of tissue damage, these specific mechanisms allow a quantitative response to occur following trauma (i.e., the response is directly proportional to the size of the injury).

2. *Afferent sensory nerve fibers* provide the most direct and quickest route for signals to arrive at the central nervous system following stress. It has frequently been suggested that pain may serve as the initial afferent signal following injury, and a variety of studies suggest that the afferent nervous signals from the injured area are essential for the stimulation of the pituitary-adrenal axis. The adrenocortical response to injury was not observed in animals after section of the peripheral nerves to the area of injury, tran-

section of the spinal cord above the injury, or section through the medulla oblongata [79]. A similar pattern of response to denervation before injury has been described in man. Both growth hormone (GH) and ACTH levels in the serum rise within one hour following incision in patients receiving general anesthesia and undergoing cholecystectomy or inguinal herniorrhaphy. However, this hormonal response did not occur in patients undergoing herniorrhaphy who received spinal anesthesia [97], nor did the usual rise in serum cortisol occur in patients undergoing abdominal procedures when epidural blockade was utilized in conjunction with the general anesthetic [23, 27]. Studies of the pituitary-adrenal axis following operation in paraplegic patients demonstrate a markedly diminished cortisol response when the operation is performed in a denervated area [77]. Nervous afferents also appear to stimulate the elaboration of antidiuretic hormone following trauma [122]. In addition, a number of factors that accompany the "stress" of critical illness—restraint, immobilization, environmental disturbances—most likely alter nervous afferent impulses and affect the response to injury.

3. *Circulating substances* may directly or indirectly stimulate the central nervous system and set in motion the injury response. Alterations in serum electrolytes, release of cell breakdown products [71], changes in the amino acid pattern, and release of endogenous pyrogens, all originating from or a direct result of the wound, may initiate homeostatic adjustments that develop during the early phase of injury.

With initial nonfatal injuries, the "ebb" phase evolves into the "flow" phase response, which is characterized by hypermetabolism and the increased loss of nitrogen and other intracellular constituents from the body. During the "flow" phase, the increased vascular permeability resolves, and blood volume and composition of other fluid compartments stabilize. Hypovolemia or abnormalities in acid-base composition of the blood are not signals that explain the alterations that occur during this hypermetabolic phase of injury.

To determine the role of afferent nervous signals from the area of injury during the "flow" phase, a variety of clinical studies have been conducted in injured patients. First, a patient with traumatic spinal cord transection and burns of the lower extremities has been studied: hypermetabolism and the associated metabolic responses occurred despite denervation of a major portion of the wound [119]. In three burn patients, a topical anesthetic was applied to the wound to achieve anesthesia and to ensure that afferent nervous stimulation from pain receptors was blocked in the injured area. No alteration in metabolic rate or body temperature occurred following the application of the topical anesthetic for up to six hours, although most patients were rendered pain-free and slept throughout the study. Finally, a spinal anesthetic was placed and maintained in a patient with multiple long bone fractures and 33 percent total body surface burns over the lower extremities. No significant effect on metabolic rate or core temperature was detected following denervation of the injured area. Therefore, there is little evidence from these studies that sensory nerves play a major role in the afferent limb of this stress response.

At one time, it was thought that the increased evaporative water loss that occurs from the damaged surface of burn patients stimulated cold receptors, causing a rise in metabolic heat production. Subsequent studies have demonstrated that the hypermetabolism following thermal injury is temperature-sensitive, but not temperature-dependent [135]. Although heat production can be minimized by treating burn patients in a warm ambient environment, the marked elevation in metabolic rate does not return to normal with external heating [6].

Although nervous afferent stimulation may not be responsible for the "flow" phase response, pain following treatment and patient manipulation will increase metabolism above the already elevated level that occurs following injury. However, when burn patients were studied in ambient conditions of comfort and allowed to sleep with or without analgesics, the hypermetabolic response was not abated but maintained at levels 50 to 80 percent above normal. Patient care should be oriented to minimize all painful stimuli: judicious use of analgesics and tranquilizers may be necessary in the treatment of critically ill patients.

Because of the inability to identify specific nervous afferent stimuli as the initiators and propagators of the "flow" phase injury response, a search for a circulating afferent signal has begun. In one study, heparinized blood was collected from burn patients and normals in pyrogen-free syringes [130]. A micro-aliquot of each sample was injected through indwelling chronic cannulae in rabbits, placed by standard stereotactic technique so that the distal tip lay in the preoptic area of the hypothalamus. Injection of normal serum from 6 control subjects in the rabbits resulted in no more than a 0.1°C rise in rectal temperature. Hypothalamic injection of serum from 9 of the 13 patients elicited a febrile response (0.63 to 0.93°C over 2 hours). Limulus lysate assay for endotoxin was negative in all these samples. After heat treatment of the serum, the febrile response was attenuated, suggesting that endogenous pyrogens (the product of the body's cells participating in the inflammatory reaction) mediated this response.

Prostaglandins are known to affect hypothalamic function, and increased concentrations of these substances are found in lymph-draining areas of injury and in exudate from burn wounds [4]. To evaluate these substances as possible "wound hormones," arterial and venous concentrations of PGA, E, and F were determined, using specific antibody assay techniques [130]. Twenty-one patients were studied and blood was drawn specifically from the femoral vein in 15 of these subjects with burned lower extremities to determine the contribution of injured tissue to the prostaglandin level. However, arterial and venous concentrations of prostaglandins A, E, and F were similar to those observed in normals: patients with and without leg burns showed similar concentrations of these substances in the femoral vein when studied between the third to thirty-first day postinjury. Although these products of tissue injury may have profound local metabolic and circulatory effects in the wound, it does not appear that these substances exert a major systemic metabolic effect.

Infection

It is well known that the injection of pus or exudate from infected tissue into a test animal will stimulate a systemic response. A constant feature of many early bacterial studies was that microorganisms secreted a substance into the culture media which was regularly pyrogenic in animals and would often invoke a leukocytic response. At the turn of the nineteenth century, it was realized that bacteria produced pyrogenic factors in addition to the exotoxins that were secreted by the microorganisms into the culture media. This new toxin was described as being tightly anchored to, if not a part of, the cell wall; this substance was called endotoxin and was later biochemically characterized as a lipopolysaccharide [18].

In spite of the identification of pyrogenic substances associated with microorganisms, a recurrent concept appeared in the medical literature that products of the host's own cells served as a signal to stimulate fever and the response to infection. In 1948, Bennett and Beeson developed techniques to exclude endotoxin from their test system, and reported that a fever-inducing substance could be extracted from rabbit granulocytes [17]. Further studies revealed that the leukocytic substance was regularly pyrogenic, whereas similar extracts from a wide variety of tissues carried no fever-inducing effect. In addition, the host pyrogen (called "endogenous pyrogen") differed in many respects from the pyrogen of microbial origin [5].

A number of investigators have contributed to our knowledge of endogenous pyrogen, with most of the experimental work performed in animals. Tissue pyrogen does not exist in storage form in host's cells, but is synthesized shortly before being liberated into the bloodstream. Activation occurs following a variety of stimuli which include exogenous pyrogens (endotoxin), viruses, bacteria, antigen-antibody complexes, and specific steroids. These stimulators cause a variety of cells to synthesize and then liberate the pyrogen. Granulocytes were once thought to be the only cell type with the capacity to elaborate endogenous pyrogen, but later it was established that monocytes and macrophages—all cells capable of phagocytosis—also serve as pyrogenic sources [43]. When stimulated, these cells produced and released a heat-labile protein of 100,000 to 200,000 molecular weight, which produced a prompt monophasic fever spike.

Partial species cross-reactivity to this substance has been observed, but tolerance in the animal does not develop after repeated injection. In contrast, an animal becomes unresponsive or tolerant after repeated injections of "endotoxin" (exogenous pyrogen). The fever response to injection of endogenous pyrogen into the central nervous system is much greater than the response to a comparable intravenous dose. Although the presence and activity of tissue pyrogen have been demonstrated in man, repeated attempts to assay circulating pyrogen during high fevers have been unsuccessful, hampering definition of the specific role of tissue pyrogen in human infection and injury.

More recently, other properties have been attributed to endogenously produced pyrogens. One such substance is referred to as leukocyte endogenous mediator (LEM), which is closely related to (or may be the same as) endogenous pyrogen but has effects other than the induction of fever [126]. When injected into normal rats, LEM has specific and direct effects on the liver to promote hepatic uptake of plasma zinc and iron, increase plasma copper (elevate ceruloplasmin), and stimulate hepatic uptake of plasma amino acids, which are utilized in the synthesis of acute-phase proteins. LEM may also decrease insulin levels and stimulate glucagon release. Thus, the inflammatory cells involved in phagocytosis appear to regulate (either through direct organ effects or indirectly through the central nervous system) body redistribution of trace elements and nitrogen and stimulate acute-phase globulin synthesis to participate in the host defense mechanisms (Figure 3-4).

CENTRAL NERVOUS SYSTEM ADJUSTMENTS FOLLOWING STRESS

The brain receives a variety of signals that a "stress" has occurred and integrates this afferent input. Although the sympathetic nervous system is not essential to the adaptation to starvation, the central nervous system is essential to the hypermetabolic response to injury: patients with "brain death" and associated soft tissue injury failed to mount a "flow" phase response [119]. Similarly, in severely burned patients, morphine anesthesia, which markedly reduced hypothalamic function, resulted in a prompt decrease in hypermetabolism, rectal temperature, and cardiac output. In contrast, however, quadriplegic patients with high spinal cord transections that totally interrupted sympathetic efferent activity failed to generate a febrile response to infection, but were able to increase the leukocyte count and blood glucose concentration during sepsis (Figure 3-5). Moreover, when low-molecular-weight extracts from granulation tissue were injected (both intravenously and subcutaneously) into normal animals fibroblast proliferation and collagen biosynthesis were observed [83]. These findings suggest that several circulating mediators with direct and specific cellular effects may exist and initiate catabolic responses. However, in all patients with intact central nervous systems, a variety of adjustments are observed within the hypothalamus and pituitary gland; these alterations in neurohumoral control appear to be specific compensatory adjustments to stress. These alterations in central nervous system control have an impact on thermoregulation, substrate mobilization, and intra-organ energy transfer.

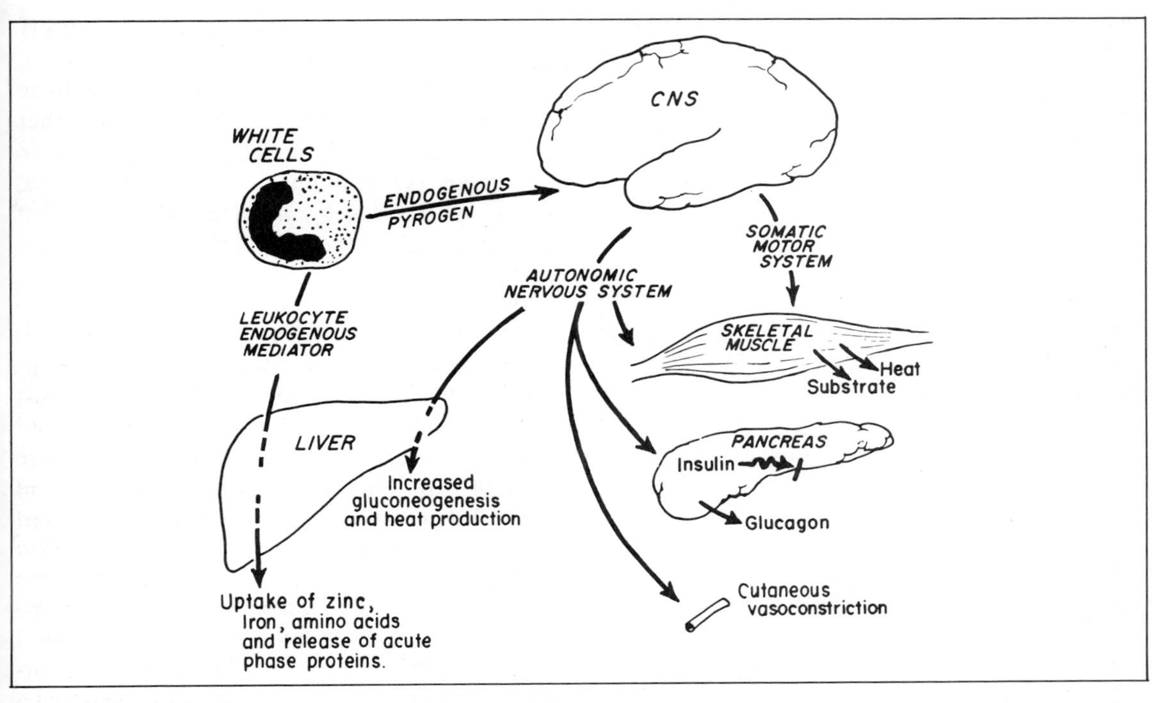

Figure 3-4. *Messenger substances liberated by cells involved in the inflammatory reaction influence a variety of physiologic responses by altering hypothalamic "setpoint" or by acting directly on the liver or other tissues to affect metabolism.*

The most prominent clinical expression of the hypothalamic alterations are the marked adjustments in thermoregulation that occur following infection and severe injury. At any ambient temperature studied, core and mean skin temperature are above those observed in normal individuals [44, 135]. When allowed to adjust ambient temperature, these febrile patients select a warmer environment than normals to achieve comfort, in spite of the fact that the patients have elevated core and mean skin temperatures [137]. The ambient temperature selected is generally related to the extent of injury or severity of infection. Administration of a variety of pharmacologic agents known to affect temperature "setpoint" in man has not generally reduced the hypermetabolism and hyperpyrexia that occur following injury. In contrast, the injury response in a burn rat model is consistently reduced by the administration of prostaglandin blocking agents, possibly through their central effects on the thermoregulatory mechanism [73].

Other alterations in normal hypothalamic neuroendocrine regulation are observed in starved individuals and in critically ill surgical patients, and these adjustments will be discussed with the function of the individual hormones.

THE HORMONES

Glucocorticoid Response

In normal man, metabolism is finely regulated between anabolic and catabolic processes. These events are primarily under hormonal control; insulin acts as the principal anabolic agent while glucocorticoids, glucagon, and catecholamines serve to integrate catabolic responses [129]. With stress and hypothalamic stimulation, increased pituitary secretion of adrenal cortico-

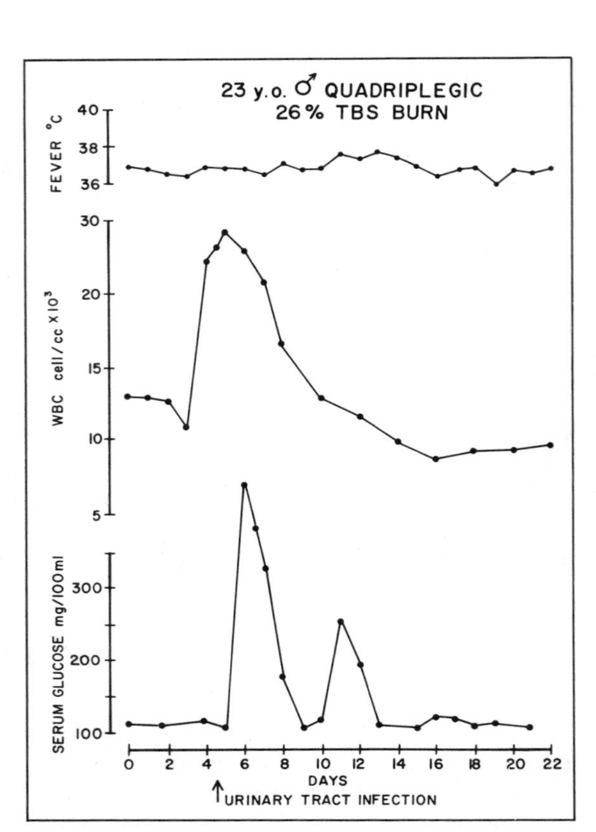

Figure 3-5. *The presence of circulating mediators associated with infection is demonstrated by the leukocytosis and hyperglycemia observed in this C4-5 quadriplegic (without sympathetic outflow) when he developed a urinary tract infection. In spite of his inability to elaborate catecholamines and generate a febrile response, a variety of metabolic events occurred (for example, acute phase protein concentrations were also markedly altered), suggesting that the circulating messengers liberated as a consequence of the infection exerted a direct effect on other tissues.*

tropic hormone (ACTH) occurs, causing liberation of glucocorticoids from the adrenal cortex. The hypothalamic centers that stimulate ACTH release are under three types of control [20]. Dur-

inversely with the concentrations of corticosteroids in the plasma, and plasma concentrations are thought to provide a feedback signal to maintain adrenal control. Similarly, administration of exogenous corticoids suppresses ACTH release, resulting in adrenal cortical atrophy.

It is clear, however, that the major physiologic cause for liberation of ACTH is stress, either psychologic or physiologic. With exposure to unfamiliar surroundings or with emotional stress, ACTH level may rise, indicating that higher centers in the brain influence the glucocorticoid response. Direct stimulation of a peripheral afferent nerve or exposure of an animal to intense stimuli of sound and light will also produce increased adrenocortical activity [56].

In 1950, Gordon demonstrated that the discharge of adrenal ascorbic acid (a marker used to assay corticosteroid secretion) after fracture or mild scald burn was minimal in normal and adrenal-demedullated rats if the traumatized limb was denervated [67]. However, denervation had no effect on discharge of adrenal ascorbic acid after a more severe scald burn. Hume studied eosinophil counts in peripheral blood as an assay for release of ACTH and adrenal cortical stimulation after injury in dogs. He noted a diminished or absent response to injury of a denervated extremity and concluded that afferent nerve impulses from the injured area were essential to initiate adrenocorticotropic hormone secretion after trauma [78]. Other afferent pathways were not excluded after severe trauma.

In a series of classic studies, Hume and Egdahl measured adrenal venous 17-hydroxycorticosteroids in experimental animals and demonstrated that adrenocorticoid secretion was not elicited after trauma to a denervated hind limb [79]. The adrenocortical response to injury was not observed following operative transection of the afferent pathway between the injury and the hypothalamus. Results of other studies demonstrated that post-traumatic elevation of ACTH and adrenocorticoids could be abolished in animals subjected to standard operative trauma with previously placed electrical lesions in the anterior medial eminence, or after hypophysectomy [77]. Removing the cortex of the brain did not ablate the ACTH response to injury. Results of similar studies revealed that the initial response of epinephrine and norepinephrine was dependent on nervous signals from the injured area, but the catecholamine response in dogs could be dissociated from the increased corticosteroid secretion and diminished by using Nembutal anesthesia [78]. As previously reported, a similar pattern of responses to denervation before injury has been described in humans [23, 27, 97].

With marked hypothalamic stimulation, primarily from afferent nerves, the initial blood concentrations of corticoids are elevated and return slowly to normal levels after the acute phase response. Measurements of cortisol turnover during severe infection indicate that the adrenal cortisol secretion may increase up to 2 to 5 times normal and return to baseline levels during convalescence [15]. Elevated cortisol concentrations are also associated with periods of cardiovascular instability and hypotension, and incresed serum concentrations may also occur during hepatic dysfunction when deconjugation processes are impaired. During stable, prolonged, infectious or traumatic illness, the serum cortisol remains in the high-normal range, but this stable state usually maintains normal circadian rhythm.

The effects of steroids can be classified into two general categories: (1) those concerned with organic metabolism (metabolism of fat, carbohydrate, and protein; inflammation; wound healing; and myocardial metabolism), and (2) those affecting mineral metabolism. The primary metabolic effects of steroids are to produce substrate flux and metabolism of body fuels. Glucocorticoids provide specific signals, which augment hepatic gluconeogenesis by stimulating enzymes that direct conversion of 3-carbon fragments into synthesis of new glucose [48]. Glucocorticoids augment other hormonal signals, which call for the production of new glucose, and increased gluconeogenesis occurs when corticosteroids are administered in conjunction with glucagon and catecholamines [48, 58]. In addition, glucocorticoids promote storage of carbohydrate as glycogen, but this could occur because of increased glucose synthesis. Adrenalectomized animals demonstrate reduction of urinary nitrogen, blood glucose, and liver glycogen, and these concentrations are restored to normal with steroid administration [86].

The stable adrenalectomized animal cannot mobilize amino acids from skeletal muscle. However, there is no impairment in utilization of free amino acids provided in the diet or by intravenous administration. As long as the animal is fed, it can maintain carbohydrate stores and continue protein biosynthesis; when forced to depend on its own protein stores for carbohydrate precursors or for hepatic protein synthesis, the adrenalectomized animal cannot meet this demand [20]. This effect is reversed by glucocorticoid administration. However, accelerated myofibrilar protein breakdown in skeletal muscle occurs in experimental animals only when plasma levels of corticosteroids exceed normal concentrations [120]. If these data are applicable to critically ill patients, then corticosteroid-mediated breakdown of muscle protein would only be associated with more severe injury and infection, which elevate serum cortisol concentration. Although glucocorticoids facilitate amino acid mobilization from the periphery, protein biosynthesis is favored in the liver, resulting in the overall transfer of protein from the carcass to visceral organs.

Although the precise effect of cortisol on lipid metabolism is not completely clear, steroids are known to increase body fat. Adrenal insufficiency is associated with decreased triglyceride and cholesterol synthesis in humans. Glucocorticoids augment lipolysis and catecholamine-stimulated glycogen oxidation in skeletal muscle. The overall effect on body composition following glucocorticoid administration is the erosion of lean body mass while body fat is maintained or increased. Extracellular water is also increased.

Although the specific catabolic effects of corticoids are well known, their role in the metabolic response to infection and injury appears to promote events in concert with other hormones.

Glucocorticoids are participatory in their catabolic function (some say permissive), and adrenal ablation studies demonstrate that catabolic responses still occur in adrenalectomized, stressed animals receiving a maintenance dose of cortisol [73]. Moreover, administering large doses of glucocorticoids to fed [16] or fasting control subjects [99] failed to increase urinary urea excretion or accelerate total body nitrogen loss. Thus, cortisol participates with other hormones to facilitate gluconeogenesis and mobilize 3-carbon glucose precursors. It is not *the* catabolic *hormone per se,* but acts with other hormonal stimuli to promote the transfer of substrate from carcass to viscera.

Glucagon

It has long been known that a hyperglycemic factor could be extracted from the pancreas, and almost 50 years have elapsed since glucagon was discovered as the hyperglycemic component of partially purified insulin. The measurement of glucagon in plasma has been considerably more difficult than that of insulin, primarily because similar circulating materials arise from the gastrointestinal tract. The gut substances had a heavier molecular weight, but demonstrated immunologic properties similar to glucagon. Since the 1960s, however, specific antibodies to pancreatic glucagon have been developed, and this advance, coupled with the definition and synthesis of the hormone molecule, has led to a virtual plethora of data concerning the importance of glucagon in normal physiology and disease.

Glucagon is a polypeptide with a molecular weight of 3,485, containing 29 amino acid residues. It is produced exclusively by the α-2 cells of the islets of Langerhans in the pancreas. In general, the biologic role of glucagon is to act in concert with insulin to ensure a steady supply of substrate from the liver under a wide range of physiologic conditions [124]. While insulin has been referred to as the hormone of energy storage, glucagon has been viewed as the (a) hormone of energy release [124]. Glucagon is suppressed following ingestion of a meal containing carbohydrate and rises during starvation [1]. Glucagon is elevated in traumatized [85, 132] and infected patients [108] and then returns to normal with resolution of the disease process [132].

Glucagon is stimulated by hypoglycemia, specific amino acids, other 3-carbon glucose intermediates, and the sympathetic nervous system. Glucagon, which is released into the portal venous system, signals the liver to release glucose during states of body glucose need, and hypoglycemia is a major signal for glucagon release. Glucagon also participates in the regulation of gluconeogenesis, and its release is stimulated by amino acids, particularly the gluconeogenic amino acids that are converted in the liver to new glucose [107]. Amino acids also stimulate insulin elaboration: essential amino acids have the greatest insulinogenic potential (signaling for synthesis and storage of protein), whereas nonessential amino acids have the most marked glucagon-stimulating effect (favoring conversion to glucose and/or transamination). Alanine administration has been utilized as a standard provocative stimulus for glucagon response, which has been measured in a variety of disease states. In addition to amino acids, other 3-carbon precursors, such as lactic acid, stimulate glucagon elaboration. As insulin-producing cells monitor and normalize blood glucose concentration in the extracellular compartment, glucagon-producing cells sense alterations in the concentration of 3-carbon fragments and act to normalize these levels, primarily by promoting conversion of these substances to glucose. Finally, glucagon elaboration is also under the influence of the autonomic nervous system, mediated by way of the beta adrenergic receptor system [80]. The close relationship between glucagon and catecholamines in severely injured patients suggests that post-traumatic adrenergic activity may mediate the post-traumatic hyperglycemia that occurs with injury.

Glucagon signals the liver through the cyclic AMP second messenger system [106] to make new glucose from hepatic glycogen stores or from gluconeogenic 3-carbon precursors [48, 106]. Unger and Orci have demonstrated that every hyperglycemic state except exogenous glucose administration is associated with hyperglucagonemia [125]; the hyperglycemia of insulin-dependent diabetes mellitus is improved with glucagon suppression [104]. Maintenance of basal levels of blood glucose in normal man may also depend on a basal quantity of glucagon elaboration; suppression of basal glucagon blood concentrations lowers fasting glucose levels significantly [3]. In addition to its hyperglycemic effect, glucagon may augment ketosis and lipolysis, a reaction that does not occur in the presence of insulin [84].

Although pharmacologic infusions of the hormone may result in significant peripheral effects [110], marked catabolic events have not been observed under physiologic conditions. For example, glucagon infused in quantities that achieve levels observed in the posttraumatic state, does not have peripheral effects, but rather acts centrally on the liver to promote gluconeogenesis [54]. Glucagon exerts its primary effect on the hepatocyte, which is in keeping with the anatomic connection between the pancreas and liver via the portal venous system.

Unger has proposed that the insulin/glucagon (I/G) ratio be utilized in a quantitative and qualitative sense to describe hepatic glucose balance in fed and fasting man and in diabetic patients [123]. Anabolism and protein conservation occur when insulin is increased relative to glucagon ($I/G > 5$), a hormonal environment that favors energy storage, limits gluconeogenesis, increases protein biosynthesis, and decreases urea nitrogen excretion. Starvation in normal man, diabetes, or infusion of glucagon into fasting man increases glucagon relative to insulin ($I/G < 3$), and this hormonal milieu is associated with increased glycogenolysis, gluconeogenesis, and ureagenesis at the expense of protein biosynthesis.

In summary, glucagon levels are elevated in critically ill patients, even in the face of glucose administration and hyperglycemia [132]. The close relationship between glucagon and catecholamines in severely injured and infected patients suggests that increased adrenergic activity may mediate the hyperglycemia that occurs after critical illness. The return of glucagon to normal coincides with healing of the wound, when urine catecholamines fall to normal levels. Therefore, in stressed patients, the autonomic nervous system may direct the pancreatic islet cell elaboration of glucagon (and insulin)—that is, adjust setpoints for the hormonal response of the endocrine pancreas. Glucagon, in turn, controls the disposition of key body-fuel substrates. Glucagon exerts its effect primarily on the liver, augmenting or amplifying catecholamine-directed, cyclic-AMP-mediated hepatic gluconeogenesis. Glucagon does not contribute to the efflux of amino acids from skeletal muscle. Pancreatectomized patients can generate appropriate metabolic response to stress. Glucagon does not appear to be the "primary" stress hormone, but is augmentative in its actions, which appear to be primarily on the liver.

Insulin

The peptide hormone insulin is synthesized in the beta pancreatic cell as a single-chain precursor, proinsulin. This molecule is then broken and forms the active protein hormone, which contains two peptide chains joined by two disulfide bridges of cystine. About 200 units of insulin are stored in the granules of the beta cell of the pancreas; only 40 to 60 units are required daily. The insulin stores in the pancreas decrease with age and vary with the quantity of carbohydrate in the diet. Pancreatic insulin content markedly decreases with starvation.

Insulin is released from the beta cells into the portal venous blood, exposing the liver to high insulin concentrations. Normal metabolism and replication of the hepatocyte may be dependent on the high portal concentrations of insulin [115]. Studies of endogenously secreted and exogenously administered labeled insulin indicate that approximately 50 percent of the insulin in the portal system is degraded by the liver during a single passage through the portal system [111]. The remaining insulin that passes through the liver exerts its effect on peripheral tissue; the concentration of insulin measured in peripheral blood is a reflection of the quantity of insulin that is not degraded in the liver. In some patients with liver disease, hepatic extraction of insulin may be diminished, and an increased quantity of insulin may reach the periphery when compared to normals. In functional terms, this may be reflected in decreased serum concentrations of the branched-chain amino acids leucine, isoleucine, and valine, essential amino acids that pass through the liver and have their transport into skeletal muscle augmented by insulin. Serum concentration of these amino acids reflects the insulin effect on peripheral tissue; branched-chain amino acid concentrations are elevated in the diabetic and decrease following insulin administration. In the patient with cirrhosis, insulin may bypass the liver, and peripheral tissue may receive too much insulin, which accounts for the low concentrations of branched-chain amino acids observed in patients with liver disease [95]. In contrast, dietary carbohydrate restriction leads to accumulation of plasma branched-chain amino acids after protein feeding, and this may result from alterations in insulin elaboration [61].

Studies of labeled insulin demonstrate that the hormone molecule is removed from the blood stream quite rapidly and the half-life appears to be less than 10 minutes [121]. Thus, insulin is most effective if administered either subcutaneously or intramuscularly, or if given in a constant intravenous infusion, utilizing a syringe pump, rather than by periodic intravenous injections of regular insulin. Insulin release occurs following glucose administration, and similar sugars exert comparable effects. The amount of insulin released is related quantitatively to the level of glucose in the blood. Nonmetabolized congeners of glucose (such as 2-deoxy-D-glucose) inhibit insulin secretion, suggesting that insulin release is regulated by the metabolism of glucose in the beta pancreatic cell. Insulin release is also stimulated by amino acids and products of lipid metabolism, long-chain free fatty acids, and possibly ketone bodies. Thus, the elevated blood concentrations of the body's fuels determine the secretion rate of insulin.

It is well known that insulin response to an oral load of glucose is much greater than the response following a comparable intravenous dose of glucose. The differences in insulin responses have been attributed to hormonal factors in the upper duodenum (secretin and possibly pancreozymin), which act to prepare the beta pancreatic cell for, or sensitize it to, the intraluminal glucose. Other hormones affect insulin secretion, usually by altering insulin sensitivity to glucose, or by increasing the insulin response to a provocative stimulus. Glucagon and ACTH directly stimulate insulin elaboration.

The interaction between the autonomic nervous system and the endocrine pancreas is fundamental to the regulation of substrate storage or mobilization following stress. Catecholamines serve as a setpoint controller for insulin release, and the increased sympathetic nervous system activity appears to be responsible for the insulin suppression and glucose intolerance observed during operation, volume depletion, mild or severe infection, and burn shock [100]. The insulin inhibitory effect of the sympathetic nervous system is mediated by alpha receptors, whereas adrenergic beta receptor stimulation augments insulin elaboration [80]. During periods of marked sympathetic nervous system discharge, such as shock, myocardial infarction, or systemic infection, the alpha receptor effects appear to dominate, resulting in glucose intolerance. However, hypermetabolism secondary to increased adrenergic activity is characterized by increased heat production (a beta adrenergic effect), and increased mass flow of glucose from the liver to the peripheral tissue is related to the increased heat production and insulin secretion that occur. Beta adrenergic receptors may augment insulin elaboration during the "flow" phase of injury [134].

Insulin is essential to glucose homeostasis: pancreatectomized man requires insulin for survival [30]. Insulin facilitates glucose entry into many tissues, increasing the flow of glucose along all pathways concerned with intracellular glucose metabolism. Thus, insulinized muscle increases formation of glycogen, lactic acid, and CO_2, and fat cells increase conversion of glucose to triglycerides in the presence of insulin. Glucose enters the liver and brain much more readily than it enters muscle in the absence of insulin. In the liver, insulin induces key hepatic enzymes that favor storage of glycogen, suppresses hepatic enzymes concerned with glycolysis and gluconeogenesis, and reduces hepatic glucose production, an effect that is explained by the action of insulin on intracellular enzymes and is not dependent on increased hepatic membrane transport of glucose by insulin. Insulin lowers blood glucose by promoting membrane transport of glucose by peripheral tissue and inhibiting hepatic glucose release; insulin also facilitates intracellular storage and/or metabolism of glucose.

Lipogenesis decreases in insulin-deprived man, and in the presence of lipolytic stimuli (such as catecholamines), the rate of triglyceride breakdown is greatly accelerated when insulin concentrations are low. The mobilized free fatty acids may be converted in the liver to ketone bodies. During the glucose-deprived state, the rate of ketone production may exceed peripheral uptake, resulting in "ketosis"; significant quantities of ketones are found in blood and urine. Administration of carbohydrate and insulin reverses ketosis, promotes lipogenesis, and reduces the mobilization of free fatty acids and glycerol from the fat mass. The triglyceride stores are so sensitive to insulin that lypolysis is inhibited by insulin alone in the absence of glucose. Insulin with dietary carbohydrate facilitates lipogenesis by aiding generation of acetyl CoA from carbohydrate (a precursor of fatty acids), by providing alpha-glycerol phosphate for esterification of fatty acids to form triglycerides, and by generation of NADPH, which is necessary for a key step in fat synthesis [89]. The net result of the antilipolytic, lipid-synthetic, glycerologenic actions of insulin is to convert energy ingested as carbohydrate to a storage form as lipid.

When the insulin concentration falls or insulin is absent, the efflux of amino acid from skeletal muscle increases. Insulinization of the skeletal muscle reverses this effect by augmenting the transport of amino acids in the muscle cell [101], favoring protein synthesis. The increased amino acid transport, which occurs primarily in muscle, appears independent of the enhanced intracellular protein synthesis that is stimulated by insulin. In microsomes prepared from diabetic livers, amino acid incorporation is impaired and can be restored to normal by insulin.

Insulin is a critical hormone for the storage of carbohydrates and fat, and synthesis of new protein. It is a potent anabolic hormone that can counteract the negative nitrogen balance and catabolism of severe injury and infection when administered with large quantities of glucose and potassium [76]. Further studies have demonstrated that this impact on nitrogen conservation in catabolic patients is primarily the effect of insulin and not the result of the calories per se [139]. The marked protein-sparing effect of high-carbohydrate diets (whether administered by enteral or parenteral routes) is the result of stimulation of endogenous insulin or may occur because exogenous insulin is administered with the nutrient. In critically ill patients, high-carbohydrate feedings (with or without exogenous insulin) elevate serum insulin levels, but have minimal effects on reducing glucagon concentrations. However, in terms of the bihormonal endocrine environment, the I/G ratio increases with carbohydrate feedings, favoring protein biosynthesis and fuel storage. Similar effects on the endocrine environment or protein conservation are not observed in stressed patients when fat is substituted isocalorically for carbohydrate calories [87, 139]; protein breakdown is not effected because insulin is not stimulated, and other biochemical mechanisms (i.e., starvation adaptation and ketone formation) that usually occur during fat feedings are suppressed by the stressed state [128].

In contrast to critically ill patients following injury and/or infection, patients who are simply starved without additional stresses, have a metabolic state characterized by substrate depletion—hormonal concentrations are easily modulated by the exogenous fuel source. A high-fat meal in normals or in starved patients lowers the I/G ratio [94], but positive nitrogen balance usually occurs in this hormonal environment because of other compensatory biochemical adjustments that occur [82, 138]. When the stress of the illness is minimal, fat may be substituted for carbohydrate in the diet with no major deterioration in nitrogen balance [82, 138, 139]. During simple starvation, nutrient energy is the rate-limiting substance necessary for protein synthesis, and the hormonal environment is determined by the substrate administered. During stress states, catabolic hormone levels (glucagon, glucocorticoids, and catecholamines) are relatively fixed, and insulin is the primary anabolic signal necessary for protein conservation.

Growth Hormone (GH)

Growth hormone, a polypeptide hormone liberated from the anterior pituitary gland, has the unique role of promoting growth and improving nitrogen storage. Growth hormone secretion occurs following a wide variety of stressful situations, including hypoglycemia, exercise, hemorrhage, operation [97], thermal injury, infection, pyrogen administration [41], and starvation [90]. Some stimuli that promote growth hormone elaboration may be suppressed by hyperglycemia; others augment growth hormone elaboration in spite of the elevation of blood glucose (Table 3-1).

Amino acids are potent stimulating agents, and arginine infusion has been utilized to test the pituitary capacity to release growth hormone. Insulin hypoglycemia is also a strong provocative stimulus utilized to assess growth hormone elaboration. Basal growth hormone concentrations are elevated following injury or infection in spite of persistent hyperglycemia, which would suppress growth hormone elaboration in normal man. Moreover, the hormonal response to both insulin hypoglycemia and arginine infusion is decreased in injured man, demonstrating alterations in hypothalamic control that may occur following stress [137]. Morphine anesthesia will diminish or abolish the increase in growth hormone that occurs during operations [62]. Unlike other hormones, the basal level of growth hormone remains elevated into convalescence, presumably to promote anabolism. Also during convalescence, the growth hormone response to insulin hypoglycemia and arginine infusion returns to normal [137].

This single-chain polypeptide stimulates nucleic acid and protein synthesis in a wide variety of tissues and stimulates synthesis of chondroitin sulfate and collagen [40]. The dramatic effect of this highly potent anabolic hormone is demonstrated with growth hormone administration to an immature, deficient organism: prompt linear growth and weight gain result. Growth hormone promotes protein storage, increases fat mobilization and utilization, and resets the insulin response to glucose.

The precise role of growth hormone in starvation and stress states is not known at this time, although it is generally thought that this hormone does not exert major effects on the numerous metabolic adjustments which occur. Human growth hormone has been administered with sufficient calories and protein to maintain energy and nitrogen balance to severely injured patients and has preserved protoplasmic mass and improved nitrogen retention during the catabolic phase of injury [136]. The protein-sparing effects and enhanced recovery of the injured patients appeared to be dose-related, to require adequate nutrient loading, and to be mediated by alterations of carbohydrate metabolism in the presence of augmented insulin pro-

Table 3-1. *Normal Stimuli for Growth Hormone Secretion*

Suppressed by Glucose	Independent of Glucose
Basal resting	Pyrogen
Hypoglycemia	Major operations and injury
Rapid fall in blood glucose without hypoglycemia	Intravenous amino acids
Inhibition of intracellular glucose utilization	L-Dopa administration
Prolonged fasting	
Muscular exercise	

duction. In contrast, growth hormone has been administered to starved [51] or injured persons receiving an inadequate caloric intake and nitrogen sparing does not occur. Adequate calories appear necessary for expression of the anticatabolic effect of growth hormone.

Thyroid Hormones

The iodinated thyronine molecules (thyroxine, T_4, and triiodothyronine, T_3) which originate in the thyroid gland exert strong influences on metabolism and growth. The classification of thyroid hormone as an anabolic or catabolic hormone depends on the dose which is administered, as well as the metabolic state of the organism at the time of hormonal administration. The anabolic effects of the hormone are clearly seen in a newborn animal in which thyroidectomy results in a reduction of muscle mass, carcass protein, and protein content of the liver and kidneys. Small amounts of thyroid hormone allow normal growth and development to proceed. In contrast, administration of a large dose of thyroid to the adult results in a catabolic response, characterized by increased excretion of urinary nitrogen, hypermetabolism, and weight loss. However, thyroid hormone has specific anabolic effects on wounds to promote wound healing [12, 63].

Thyroid hormone stimulates protein synthesis; increased liver mitochondrial protein synthesis appears to be one of the early effects of administered thyroid hormone [127]. Thyroid hormone causes an increased incorporation of labeled RNA precursor into the muscle cell, increased production of messenger RNA, and increased formation of polysomes. Excess administration of T_4 causes loss of protein from muscle, but increases amino acid incorporation into liver protein. Continual administration reduces both the liver and the carcass protein stores. Cholesterol levels fall with thyroid administration, and this decrease is correlated closely with the rise in basal metabolic rate. The mechanism for the increase in oxygen consumption is not known, but thyroxine requires about 10 days before its peak effect on metabolic rate is seen, whereas triiodothyronine exerts its peak effect 24 to 36 hours after administration.

Thyroid hormone appears to interact closely with the sympathetic nervous system. Serum concentrations of these two calorigenic hormones move in a reciprocal manner: during hyperthyroidism catecholamines are low, and during hypothyroidism catecholamine levels rise above normal [35]. Moreover, some of the manifestations of clinical thyrotoxicosis resemble excessive adrenal medullary activity, and this clinical observation has been strengthened by the successful management of some manifestations of thyrotoxicosis with catechol receptor blocking agents. Recent work in cellular biology has suggested two possible mechanisms by which this thyroid-catechol interaction occurs [116]: (1) thyroid hormone increases β-adrenergic receptor sites on cardiac and skeletal muscle, and (2) thyroid hormone increases transduction of information between the β-adrenergic receptor and the intracellular cycle AMP.

A variety of intrinsic physiologic adjustments following illness or operation result in alterations of thyroid hormone concentrations in surgical patients. Glucocorticoids suppress thyroidal elaboration of T_4, although there appears to be a breakthrough of this inhibition after 5 to 7 days [98]. Following caloric deprivation [114], injury [13], and infection [28], protein-bound iodine levels and concentration of T_3 fall, whereas serum levels of reverse-T_3 rise. T_4 may decrease slightly or remain normal. Kinetic studies demonstrate that clearance of the thyroidal hormones may be altered during acute illness [33], and tissue analysis of autopsy material demonstrates a marked deficiency of intracellular T_3 resulting from impaired deiodination of T_4 and/or reduced T_3-binding protein [117]. As the T_3 level decreases during starvation, the effect of thyroid on the regulation of heat production and protein catabolism appears to decrease, as if to compensate for the diminished exogenous energy source [60]. The very rapid fall in serum T_3 concentrations with starvation can be reversed by feeding 800 calories as carbohydrate but not fat [114]. In addition, Danforth and associates have observed that serum T_3 levels vary directly (and reverse T_3 inversely) with the carbohydrate content of the diet [39], and low T_3 levels in critically ill patients have returned toward normal with high carbohydrate feedings. These data suggest that the deiodination process, which regulates T_4 conversion to T_3, may be related to or affected by the carbohydrate-insulin system.

Finally, the alterations that occur in thyroid hormone economy reflect concurrent adjustments in the hypothalamic pituitary axis. In spite of the low serum concentrations of active thyroid hormones, the pituitary elaboration of thyrotropin-releasing hormone (TRH) does not increase as it does during hypothyroidism [118] (Table 3-2). This suggests that associated adjustments have also occurred in the hypothalamus, which limit TRH release from the pituitary and ultimately control the output of thyroid hormone. TRH is also markedly inhibited during the administration of dopamine, a commonly used vasoactive agent administered to septic patients during cardiovascular instability. These alterations in thyroid hormone concentration appear at a time when concentrations of thyroid-binding proteins are also reduced. The interrelationships between free and bound hormone and the effects of these low serum concentrations on tissue metabolism in critically ill patients are not well understood, but preliminary observations suggest that T_3 hypothyroidism may exist during critical illness [14, 117]. It has been suggested that the decreased concentration of T_3 observed following acute illness is the result of phagocytic cells utilizing the iodine for bactericidal functions [42]. However, this hypothesis remains to be proved.

AUTONOMIC NERVOUS SYSTEM

A major portion of the body's metabolic processes are regulated by the autonomic nervous system. This system exerts *direct* effects on metabolism [75] through cell stimulation, enzyme induction, and hormonal adjustments, but also influences metabolism in an *indirect* manner by reflex changes in the circulatory system in order to maintain blood pressure, ensure the constancy of the internal chemical environment, and regulate body temperature. These involuntary control pathways of the vegetative nervous system maintain the internal environment by integrating respiration, circulation, digestion, and metabolism for the benefit of the whole organism.

The autonomic nervous system is generally separated into two components, the sympathetic and parasympathetic systems, which exert contrasting functions in regulating the internal environment. The sympathetic nervous system is not essential to life if the animal is maintained in a controlled environment [31]. However, during circumstances of stress, the sympathetic nervous system is essential to survival. The dramatic

Table 3-2. *Thyroid-Stimulating Hormone (TSH) Response to a Bolus Injection of Thyrotropin-Releasing Hormone (TRH 500 μg)*

	Basal Hormone Concentrations			Δ TSH Response To TRH
Patient Group	T_4 (μg/dl)	T_3 (ng/dl)	TSH (μIU/dl)	μIU/dl
Normal range	4.5–11.0	80–180	< 10	7–20
Hypothyroid	< 4.5	< 80, normal	> 10, normal	> 20
Starvation*	Low normal	Low normal	< 10	Normal or blunted
Trauma	3.2 ± 1	100 ± 32	3.6 ± 1	10.2 ± 1.5
Infection*	Low normal	Low to low normal	Normal	Normal
Trauma-infection receiving dopamine infusion	3.4 ± 0.5	72 ± 29	2.0 ± 2	1.6 ± 0.4

*Data based on K. K. Talwar, R. C. Sawhney, and G. K. Rastogi, *J. Clin. Endocrinol. Metab.* 44:398, 1977; R. A. Becker, D. W. Johnson, K. A. Woeber, and D. W. Wilmore, *Fed. Proc.* 35:216, 1976; and R. A. Becker, D. W. Wilmore, C. W. Goodwin, C. A. Zitzka, L. Wartofsky, K. D. Burman, A. D. Mason, Jr., and B. A. Pruitt, Jr., *J. Trauma* 20:713, 1980.

effect of sudden sympatho-adrenal discharge is observed when a normal animal is subjected to severe stress. The "fight-or-flight" syndrome is characterized by tachycardia, pupillary dilatation, pilo-erector activity of the skin, alterations in skin and muscle blood flow, and increased respiratory rate associated with bronchial dilatation. This physiologic response is accompanied by an outpouring of glucose and free fatty acids into the bloodstream and a release of hormones that signal for salt and water retention. This mass response is the result of the sympathetic nervous system and the adrenal medulla discharging as a unit. However, the sympathetic system is normally active at all times, making fine adjustments in the control of the internal environment from moment to moment.

The parasympathetic system is designed for discrete and localized control, not mass discharge. It is concerned with conservation, restoration, and storage of energy rather than with energy expenditure [19]. It slows heart rate, aids digestion and absorption of nutrients, and stimulates bladder emptying. Evidence indicates, however, that during stress there is discharge of both the sympathetic and parasympathetic nervous systems [50], but the effects of the sympatho-adrenal system dominate and contribute the major portion of the clinical signs observed in "stress" states. Although the function of the sympathetic nervous system in critically ill patients is the focus of this discussion, increased discharge of the parasympathetic nervous system also participates in the stress response.

The catecholamines, epinephrine and norepinephrine, are synthesized from the essential amino acid phenylalanine. Enzymatic conversion of phenylalanine to tyrosine occurs in the liver by a complex hydroxylation system. Tyrosine is transported by the blood stream to various sites for catecholamine biosynthesis. It is transported across the cell membrane in specialized tissues by a tyrosine concentrating mechanism and undergoes a series of intracellular migrations—mitochondria, cytoplasm, storage vesicle—in which specific enzymatic transformations occur, producing norepinephrine. The enzyme for conversion of norepinephrine to epinephrine is found in high concentrations in the adrenal medulla, but not in the sympathetic nerve endings.

The sympathetic neuron consists of a cell body, a long axon, and highly branched nerve terminals. The nerve terminals have swellings or varicosities that lie in close proximity to the effector cell, and it has been estimated that one neuron, with its highly branched nerve endings, may innervate some 25,000 effector cells [140]. Norepinephrine undergoes final biochemical processing and is stored as a nondiffusible complex of protein in the "granulated vesicles," which account for the varicosities of the nerve endings. With arrival of a nervous impulse, there is a change in ionic permeability of the membrane, permitting an influx of calcium. Although the effector mechanism is not known, norepinephrine and the other soluble compounds of the vesicle are discharged to the exterior of the nerve terminal. The released norepinephrine diffuses across the synaptic cleft between the nerve ending and the effector cell, where it interacts with specific adrenergic receptors [9].

Epinephrine is stored in the adrenal medulla and is released by sympathetic nerve stimulation. Epinephrine exerts its effects on distant target organs and, unlike norepinephrine, is carried to effector cells by the bloodstream. Dopamine is a specific intermediate compound for the synthesis of epinephrine and norepinephrine, but it also stimulates specific receptors in the central nervous system and may act as a transmitter in the peripheral autonomic nervous system.

The sympathetic nervous system is stimulated by a variety of signals including pain, anxiety, anesthesia, dehydration, blood loss, operations, infection, hypoglycemia, increased intracranial pressure, and alterations in tissue perfusion and metabolism that affect the chemical environment of the body. The hypothalamus receives these afferent signals and integrates this input into a meaningful response. This is accomplished by a variety of interactions in various hypothalamic nuclei, all of which are located close to, and interconnected by, numerous nervous pathways. These discrete areas of the brain regulate temperature, blood glucose and other fuels, appetite, thirst, blood pressure, and respiration. These nuclei are also connected to an area in the posterior hypothalamus through which all sympathetic nerve traffic flows (often referred to as the "sympathetic center" of the brain, but rather than a discrete control center, this area serves as a relay station); the hypothalamic nuclei are also intimately related to the pituitary gland via neurons and the pituitary portal system [49]. Many of the afferent mediators that stimulate the hypothalamus are known and can be duplicated experimentally. A response may also be evoked by electrically stimulating the discrete control area of the hypothalamus.

Central to hypothalamic control of metabolism is the function of the ventral medial and ventral lateral nuclei of the hypothalamus, which are important for regulation of food intake, substrate flow, and heat production. The first experimental evidence for this association was presented by Hetherington and Ranson [74], who reported that bilateral destruction of the ventromedial hypothalamus of the rat resulted in hyperphagia and massive obesity. Later, it was found that destructive lesions of the ventrolateral nucleus of the hypothalamus resulted in reduction or cessation of food intake. The ventromedial nucleus was labeled the satiety center and the ventrolateral area the feeding center. A variety of additional studies have demonstrated that these centers were intimately involved in the control of blood glucose [57, 59, 91], fatty acids [66], insulin, glucagon [59], and possibly other fuels and metabolic substrates.

There is, however, no recognized central nervous center for the control of metabolic rate, and it is thought that this function is determined by basal oxidative cell processes. (However, it has been suggested that the membrane transport of sodium and potassium may serve as a metabolic pacemaker of the body [46].) The basal metabolic rate is modified by the chronic elaboration of thyroid hormones and is affected by the acute release of catecholamines. Because the liver is the single most active metabolic organ in the body and reflects a major portion of the oxidative metabolism of the host, a close communication system exists between the hypothalamus and the liver [11]. Hepatic function is significantly altered by autonomic nervous system function. This is best demonstrated by the hepatic response to hypoglycemia; mobilization of glycogen stores can occur by release of epinephrine from the adrenal medulla [64], by enhanced glucagon secretion, or by release of norepinephrine from sympathetic nerve endings contiguous with hepatocytes. Administration of 2-deoxy-D-glucose blocks glucose oxidation and induces intracellular glucopenia, causing marked glycogenolysis and hyperglycemia. This response is not observed in patients with high spinal cord transections, an injury that interrupts central sympathetic nervous system outflow [25]. The response to intracellular glucopenia is present in adrenalectomized patients and occurs despite the absence of significant alterations in glucagon concentrations, suggesting that the sympathetic neurotransmitter norepinephrine released from hepatic sympathetic nerve endings is the mediator of this response [26]. This conclusion is in keeping with the demonstrations that hyperglycemia occurs following stimulation of the sympathetic nerves to the liver in both animals [47] and man [81], and that the liver is incapable of responding to hypoglycemia directly, but requires extrinsic stimulation [113].

Hyperglycemia occurs following the injection of epinephrine as a response to a complex series of interactions. First, there is a direct effect on the liver, increasing the conversion rate of glycogen to glucose and simultaneously directing conversion of 3-carbon precursors to glucose. Second, epinephrine acts directly on skeletal muscle, converting skeletal muscle glycogen to lactic acid, which is transported to the liver and converted to new glucose (Cori cycle) [10]. Beta receptors characteristically mediate this effect. Finally, epinephrine has a direct effect on the pancreas, suppressing the release of insulin that would normally occur in response to an elevated blood glucose level. Simultaneously, pancreatic glucagon is stimulated, augmenting the signal for hepatic glucose release.

Mobilization of free fatty acids occurs following sympathetic stimulation, a result of the direct action of catecholamines on fat cells. This effect is blocked by adrenergic blocking agents and nicotinic acid [32]. The lipolytic effect of catechols is potentiated by suppression of insulin release from the pancreatic beta cell; low insulin levels favor fat mobilization, whereas high insulin concentrations augment fat storage. Glucose administration to critically ill patients will stimulate endogenous insulin, limit fat mobilization, and allow oxidation of the infused carbohydrate. Thus, fat mobilization is regulated by an interaction of insulin and catecholamines, with insulin favoring fat storage and sympathetic activity stimulating mobilization.

Catecholamines are elevated following injury [65, 133], and adrenergic activity has been related to the extent of stress and to the oxygen consumption of the patient. Carefully controlled adrenergic blockade in patients with large surface area burns demonstrated a consistent decrease in metabolic rate with α- and β- or β-adrenergic blockade alone [133]. Administration of epinephrine and norepinephrine to normal man increases metabolic activity. Increased catecholamines (increased adrenergic activity) are the major calorigenic mediators responsible for the post-traumatic hypermetabolic response and this is related to, or the result of, their effect on the mobilization of body fuels.

Plasma epinephrine and norepinephrine have also been measured in patients following uneventful major surgical procedures and in similar individuals with severe postoperative infection [68]. The patients without complications had mean arterial plasma catecholamine levels near the upper limits of normal, whereas the catecholamine values were significantly elevated in the septic individuals. Norepinephrine was consistently greater than epinephrine. The increase in plasma catecholamines did not appear in response to circulatory reflexes, since it occurred when blood pressure was normal and there were no other clinical indices suggesting hypovolemia. In studies of bacteremic, normotensive, trauma patients, the normal relationship between urinary catecholamine excretion rate and oxygen consumption, which occurs in uncomplicated cases, appeared disturbed: high levels of catecholamines were present in these septic individuals, but oxidative processes were attenuated [133]. This suggests that severe sepsis with multiple organ system failure results in an inability of the body to respond appropriately to this calorigenic hormone. Because catecholamines are central to the metabolic and cardiovascular adjustments to infection, the nature of this response in critically ill, infected, traumatized, or postoperative patients, may limit appropriate homeostatic adjustments to these complications.

Finally, it should be noted that sympathetic outflow is influenced by nutritional state. Sympathetic activity is suppressed during fasting [21] and rises above normal with overfeeding [141]. This suggests that the sympathetic nervous system may play a role in the nutritionally induced thermogenesis that occurs with large caloric intakes.

EFFECT OF ALTERED CIRCULATION ON METABOLISM

Low-Flow States

With absolute hypovolemia (hemorrhagic shock), relative hypovolemia (low-flow septic shock), or central pump failure (heart failure, myocardial infarction, cardiac tamponade), hormonal elaboration occurs in response to tissue ischemia, and the extent of the response correlates closely with the severity of the hypoperfusion [93]. Marked stimulation of the sympathoadrenal system is associated with maximal output of ACTH and glucocorticoids. However, the tissue response pattern to these hormones is modified because of the blood flow limitations imposed on vital organs during anaerobic metabolism. Gluconeogenesis is stimulated, and the lactic acid generated as a result of the tissue anoxia is converted in part to new glucose. Oxygen consumption is reduced because of the limitations in blood flow [112]. Because turnover rates of substrates are depressed, increased serum concentrations of many substances appear in the bloodstream [36]. This substrate excess and the associated hormonal profile quickly return to normal with restoration of circulation.

With only minimal or moderate blood volume deficits, increased extraction of substrate may initially compensate for the reduction in organ flow. Thus, central pressure and chemoreceptive sympathetic drives adjust the circulation to maintain the internal milieu [109]. Blood flow to such critical organs as the liver and kidney will fall, but associated with the reduced blood flow are a widening of the arterial-venous oxygen gradient and an increased extraction ratio of metabolic substrates. With minimal alterations in blood volume, these adjustments may be made with no significant limitations in metabolism—as volume deficits increase, oxidative processes are limited and the patient progresses to the low-flow state.

Posttraumatic Hypermetabolic States

The increased cardiac output following successful resuscitation from major injury provides the additional flow necessary to maintain wound perfusion [8] and also to serve the increased metabolic demands of the visceral tissues [7, 131]. These circulatory adjustments are accompanied by marked elaboration of catecholamines, glucocorticoids, and glucagon, with or without insulin suppression. During this compensated circulatory state, no major limitations in blood flow appear to exist, and a full metabolic expression of all the hormones elaborated results in the characteristic hypermetabolic response associated with increased gluconeogenesis and skeletal muscle protein catabolism. However, this hyperdynamic circulatory state may be tenuous, making further circulatory adjust-

Table 3-3. *Summary of Stimulus-Response Patterns that Occur in Critically Ill Patients*

	Fed State	Starvation	Post-Traumatic Hyper-metabolic State	Low-Flow States	High-Flow Sepsis
Afferent limb	Increased substrate concentration	Decreased substrate concentration	Not known	Baro- and chemo-receptors	Pyrogens and other circulating factors
Central nervous system integration	Yes, but cephalic phase not required for responses	No	Yes	Yes	Yes, although circulating factors may exert direct effects
Efferent limb					
Circulating					
Insulin	+++	−−	0;++	0;−	++
Glucagon	−−	++	+++	+++	++
Glucocorticoids	0	0	++	+++	++
Epinephrine	0	−	++	+++	++
Nervous	0	0	+++	+++	++
Responses					
Substrate concentration					
Glucose	+++	−−	++	++	++
Lactate	+	−	0;+	+++	++
Free fatty acids	−−	++	0;+	+++	0;++
Ketones	0	++	0;+	0	0;+
Amino acids	+++	0;−	0;±	++	0;±
Substrate turnover					
Glucose	++	−−	++	0;±	++
Lactate	+	−	++	+++	++
Free fatty acids	−−	+++	+++	0;+	++
Ketones	0	+++	0	0	0
Amino acids	+++	−−	+++	0;+	++
Oxidative metabolism					
Total body VO_2	0;+	−	+++	−−	+
Splanchnic bed	+	−	++	−−	++
Renal	0	0;−	++	−−	0;++
Muscle	0	−	++	−−	0;+
Circulation					
Cardiac output	0	−	+++	−	++
Splanchnic	++	−	++	−−	++
Renal	0	0;−−	0;+	−−	++
Muscle	0;+	±	0	−−	0;+

0 = normal postabsorptive man; + = increase; − = decrease.

ments to sepsis or hypovolemia impossible without causing regional flow limitations and subsequent deleterious effects on metabolism and the function of many vital organs.

High-Flow Sepsis

The relationship between blood flow and metabolism in infected patients has attracted much research interest and speculation; the findings can only be briefly summarized in this chapter. The increased cardiac output provides flow through the area of infection [2, 37, 72], and the tissues involved in the inflammatory response appear to obtain their energy requirements through anaerobic means [37, 72]. Blood flow to the visceral organs also rises. The increased renal flow [88] is accompanied by a narrowing of the arterial-venous oxygen difference and appears to be mediated by circulating vasodilators, most probably pyrogens [22, 72]. Splanchnic blood flow also increases, but oxygen extraction is maintained at normal levels, suggesting that blood flow responds appropriately to the increased aerobic metabolic requirements [69]. If muscle blood flow is increased [45, 53], the elevation is only slight and, in general, rarely exceeds the upper limit of expected physiologic norms (2 to 4 ml per 100 gm muscle per minute) [109]. However, even a slight loss of arterial tone in the large mass of skeletal muscle may account for the loss of vascular resistance and the hypotension that are observed in septic patients. Regardless of the peripheral perfusion, however, increased release of skeletal muscle amino acids occurs during the septic state. Lactate release from skeletal muscle, when observed, may be an effect of impaired oxygen transport, the result of other mitochondrial dysfunctions or accelerated glycolysis. The expression of hormonal signals in well-oxygenated tissues is markedly altered, with the development of hypotension and low flow.

The alterations in metabolism that occur in critically ill patients are the result of afferent stimuli which usually, but not always, are integrated in the central nervous system (Table 3-3). Most of the metabolic alterations observed are appropriate responses to changes in substrate and hormone concentrations and activity of the sympathetic nervous system. However, circulating pyrogens and/or other wound factors may also stimulate metabolic changes by acting directly on specific tissues. The full expression of the efferent mediators of the metabolic responses occurs only if circulation is not limited and cellular metabolism is unimpaired. Metabolism in nonstressed patients is controlled primarily by exogenous substrates, and the hormonal pattern varies depending on the type and quantity of nutrients administered. In critically ill patients, however, the catabolic signals are relatively fixed and not greatly altered by food intake. Insulin is the primary anabolic hormone that can override these catabolic drives and stimulate tissue synthesis and nitrogen conservation. Following life-threatening disease, prompt and appropriate surgical care (e.g., débridement and closure of a wound, drainage of an abdominal abscess, support of the circulation, administration of appropriate antimicrobial therapy) is the most important therapy to diminish these catabolic signals and allow tissue synthesis to progress following balanced nutrient administration.

REFERENCES

1. Aguilar-Parada, E., Eisentraut, A. M., and Unger, R. H. Effects of starvation on plasma pancreatic glucagon in normal man. *Diabetes* 18:717, 1969.
2. Albrecht, M., and Clowes, G. H. A., Jr. The increase of circulating requirements in the presence of inflammation. *Surgery* 56:158, 1964.
3. Alford, F. P., Bloom, S. R., Nabarro, J. D. N., Hall, R., Besser, G. M., Coy, D. H., Kastin, A. J., and Schally, A. V. Glucagon control of fasting glucose in man. *Lancet* 2:974, 1974.
4. Arturson, G. Prostaglandins in human burn wound secretion. *Burns* 3:112, 1978.
5. Atkins, E., and Bodel, P. Fever. *N. Engl. J. Med.* 286:27, 1972.
6. Aulick, L. H., Hander, E. W., Wilmore, D. W., Mason, A. D., Jr., and Pruitt, B. A., Jr. The rela-

tive significance of thermal and metabolic demands on burn hypermetabolism. *J. Trauma* 19:559, 1979.
7. Aulick, L. H., Wilmore, D. W., Goodwin, C. W., and Becker, R. A. Increased visceral blood flow in burn patients. *Fed. Proc.* 38:902, 1979.
8. Aulick, L. H., Wilmore, D. W., Mason, A. D., Jr., and Pruitt, B. A., Jr. Influence of the burn wound on peripheral circulation in thermally injured patients. *Am. J. Physiol.* 233:H520, 1977.
9. Axelrod, J., and Weinshilboum, R. Catecholamines. *N. Engl. J. Med.* 287:237, 1972.
10. Baltzan, M. A., Andres, R., Cader, G., and Zierler, K. L. Effects of epinephrine on forearm blood flow and metabolism in man. *J. Clin. Invest.* 44:80, 1965.
11. Ban, T. The hypothalamus and liver metabolism. *Med. J. Osaka Univ.* 15:275, 1965.
12. Barklay, T. H. C., et al. The influence of metabolic stimulants in wound healing: The influence of thyroid and 2-4-Dinitrophenol. *Q. J. Exp. Physiol.* 32:309, 1943.
13. Becker, R. A., Johnson, D. W., Woeber, K. A., and Wilmore, D. W. Decreased serum triiodothyronine (T_3) levels following thermal injury. *Fed. Proc.* 35:216, 1976.
14. Becker, R. A., Wilmore, D. W., Goodwin, C. W., Zitzka, C. A., Wartofsky, L., Burman, K. D., Mason, A. D., Jr., and Pruitt, B. A., Jr. Free T_4, free T_3 and reverse-T_3 in critically ill, thermally injured patients. *J. Trauma* 20:713, 1980.
15. Beisel, W. R. Metabolic response to infection. *Annu. Rev. Med.* 26:9, 1975.
16. Beisel, W. R., Sawyer, W. D., Ryll, E. D., and Crozier, D. Metabolic effects of intracellular infections in man. *Ann. Intern. Med.* 78:744, 1967.
17. Bennett, I. L., Jr., and Beeson, P. B. Studies on the pathogenesis of liver; effect of injection of extracts and suspensions of uninfected rabbit tissues upon the body temperature of normal rabbits. *J. Exp. Med.* 98:477, 1953.
18. Berry, L. J. *Bacterial Toxins, Critical Reviews in Toxicology.* Cleveland: CRC Press, 1977. Vol. 5, p. 239.
19. Best, C. H., and Taylor, N. B. *The Physiological Basis of Medical Practice: A Test in Applied Physiology.* Baltimore: Williams & Wilkins, 1955. P. 1098.
20. Bondy, P. K. The Adrenal Cortex. In P. K. Bondy (Ed.), *Diseases of Metabolism.* Philadelphia: Saunders, 1969. P. 829.
21. Bourgeois, B., Schmidt, B. J., and Bourgeois, R. Some Aspects of Catecholamines in Undernutrition. In L. I. Gardner and P. Amacher (Eds.), *Endocrine Aspects of Malnutrition.* Santa Ynez, CA: The KROC Foundation, 1973. P. 163.
22. Bradley, S. E., Chasis, H., Goldring, W., and Smith, H. W. Hemodynamic alteration in normotensive and hypertensive subjects during the pyrogenic reaction. *J. Clin. Invest.* 24:749, 1945.
23. Brandt, M. R., Kehlet, H., Skovsted, L., and Hansen, J. M. Rapid decrease in plasma-triiodothyronine during surgery and epidural analgesia independent of afferent neurogenic stimuli and of cortisol. *Lancet* 2:1333, 1976.
24. Brodows, R. G., Campbell, R. G., Al-Aziz, A. J., and Pi-Sunyer, F. X. Lack of central autonomic regulation of substrate during early fasting in man. *Metabolism* 25:803, 1976.
25. Brodows, R. G., Pi-Sunyer, F. X., and Campbell, R. G. Neural control of the counter-regulatory events during glucopenia in man. *J. Clin. Invest.* 52:1841, 1973.
26. Brodows, R. G., Pi-Sunyer, F. X., and Campbell, R. G. Sympathetic control of hepatic glycogenolysis during glucopenia in man. *Metabolism* 24:617, 1975.
27. Bromage, P. R., Shibata, H. R., and Willoughby, H. W. Influence of prolonged epidural blockade on blood sugar and cortisol responses to operations upon the upper part of the abdomen and the thorax. *Surg. Gynecol. Obstet.* 132:1051, 1971.
28. Burger, A., Nicod, R., Suter, P., Vallotton, M. B., Vagenakis, A., and Braverman, L. Reduced active thyroid hormone levels in acute illness. *Lancet* 1:653, 1976.
29. Cahill, G. F., Jr. Starvation in man. *N. Engl. J. Med.* 282:668, 1970.
30. Cahill, G. F., Jr., Aoki, T. T., and Marliss, E. B. Insulin and Muscle Protein. In R. O. Greep and E. B. Astwood (Eds.), *Handbook of Physiology.* Washington, D.C.: Am. Physiol. Society, 1972. Section 7, vol. 1, p. 563.
31. Cannon, W. B. *The Wisdon of the Body.* New York: Norton, 1967. P. 177.
32. Carlson, L. A., Levi, L., and Oro, L. Plasma lipids and urinary excretion of catecholamines in man during experimentally induced emotional stress, and their modification by nicotinic acid. *J. Clin. Invest.* 47:1795, 1968.
33. Cavalieri, R. R., and Rapoport, B. Impaired peripheral conversion of thyroxine to triiodothyronine. *Annu. Rev. Med.* 28:57, 1977.
34. Chance, B., Estabrook, R. A., and Williamson, J. R. *Control of Energy Metabolism.* New York: Academic, 1965.
35. Christensen, N. J. Plasma noradrenaline and adrenaline in patients with thyrotoxicosis and

myxoedema. *Clin. Sci. Mol. Med.* 42:163, 1973.
36. Clowes, G. H. A., O'Donnell, T. F., Blackburn, G. L., and Maki, T. N. Energy Metabolism and Proteolysis in Traumatized and Septic Man. In G. G. A. Clowes, Jr. (Ed.), *Symposium on Response to Injury and Infection II. Surg. Clin. North Am.* 56:1169, 1976.
37. Cronenwett, J. L., and Lindenauer, S. M. Direct measurement of arteriovenous anastomotic blood flow in the septic canine hindlimb. *Surgery* 85:275, 1979.
38. Cuthbertson, D., and Tilstone, W. J. Metabolism during the postinjury period. *Adv. Clin. Chem.* 12:1, 1969.
39. Danforth, E., Jr., Tyzbir, E. D., Horton, E. S., Sims, E. A. H., Burger, A. D., Braverman, L. E., Vagenakis, A. G., and Ingbar, S. H. Reciprocal changes in serum triiodothyronine (T_3) and reverse (rT_3) triiodothyronine induced by altering carbohydrate content of the diet. *Clin. Res.* 24:271A, 1976.
40. Daughaday, W. H., and Parker, M. L. Human pituitary growth hormone. *Annu. Rev. Med.* 16:47, 1965.
41. Davidson, M. B., Maser, M., Killian, P., and Brawn, A. Metabolic and thermal responses to Piromen in man. *J. Clin. Endocrinol. Metab.* 32:179, 1971.
42. DeRubertis, F. R., and Kosch, P. C. Accelerated host metabolism of L-thyroxine during acute infection: Role of the leukocyte and peripheral leukocytosis. *J. Clin. Endocrinol. Metab.* 40:589, 1975.
43. Dinarello, C. A., and Wolfe, S. M. Pathogenesis of fever in man. *N. Engl. J. Med.* 298:607, 1978.
44. DuBoise, E. F. *Fever and the Regulation of Body Temperature.* Springfield, IL: Thomas, 1948.
45. Duff, J. H., Viidik, T., Marchuk, J. B., Holliday, R. L., Finley, R. J., Groves, A. C., and Woolf, L. I. Femoral arteriovenous amino acid differences in septic patients. *Surgery* 85:344, 1979.
46. Edelman, I. S. Thyroid thermogenesis. *N. Engl. J. Med.* 290:1303, 1974.
47. Edwards, A. V., and Silver, M. Comparison of the hyperglycaemic and glycogenolytic responses to catecholamines with those to stimulation of the hepatic sympathetic innervation in the dog. *J. Physiol.* 223:571, 1972.
48. Exton, J. H. Gluconeogenesis. *Metabolism* 21:945, 1972.
49. Ezrin, C., Louacs, K., and Horvath, E. A functional anatomy of the endocrine hypothalamus and hypothesis. *Med. Clin. North Am.* 67:229, 1978.
50. Feldman, J., and Gellborn, E. The influence of fever on the vago-insulin and sympathetico-adrenal system. *Endocrinology* 29:141, 1941.
51. Felig, P., Marliss, E. B., and Cahill, G. F., Jr. Metabolic response to human growth hormone during prolonged starvation. *J. Clin. Invest.* 50:411, 1971.
52. Felig, P., Owen, O. E., Wahren, J., and Cahill, G. F., Jr. Amino acid metabolism during prolonged starvation. *J. Clin. Invest.* 48:584, 1969.
53. Finley, R. J., Duff, J. H., Holliday, R. L., Jones, D., and Marchuk, J. B. Capillary muscle blood flow in human sepsis. *Surgery* 78:87, 1975.
54. Fitzpatrick, G. F., Meguid, M. M., Gitlitz, P., O'Connor, N. E., and Brennan, M. F. Effects of glucagon on 3-methylhistidine excretion: Muscle proteolysis or ureogenesis? *Surg. Forum* 26:46, 1975.
55. Flier, J. S., Kahn, C. R., and Roth, J. Receptors, antireceptor antibodies and mechanisms of insulin resistance. *N. Engl. J. Med.* 300:413, 1979.
56. Fortier, C., and Selye, H. Adenocorticotropic effect of stress after severance of the hypothalamo-hypophyseal pathways. *Am. J. Physiol.* 159:433, 1949.
57. Freinkel, N., Metzger, B. E., Harris, E., Robinson, S., and Mager, M. The hypothermia of hypoglycemia. *N. Engl. J. Med.* 287:841, 1972.
58. Friedmann, N., Exton, J. H., and Park, C. R. Interaction of adrenal steroids and glucagon on gluconeogenesis in perfused rat liver. *Biochem. Biophys. Res. Commun.* 29:113, 1967.
59. Frohman, L. A. The Hypothalamic and Metabolic Control. In H. L. Ioachim (Ed.), *Pathobiology Annual.* New York: Appleton-Century-Crofts, 1971. P. 353.
60. Gardner, D. F., Kaplan, M. M., Stanley, C. A., and Utiger, R. D. Effect of tri-iodothyronine replacement on the metabolic and pituitary responses to starvation. *N. Engl. J. Med.* 300:579, 1979.
61. Gelfand, R. A., Hendler, R. G., and Sherwin, R. S. Dietary carbohydrate and metabolism of ingested protein. *Lancet* 1:65, 1979.
62. George, J. M., Reier, C. E., Lanese, R. R., and Rower, J. M. Morphine anesthesia blocks cortisol and growth hormone response to surgical stress in humans. *J. Clin. Endocrinol. Metab.* 38:736, 1974.
63. Glickman, A. S., et al. Modification of late radiation injury with L-triiodothyronine. *Radiology* 73:178, 1959.
64. Goldfien, A., Moore, R., Zileli, S., Havens, L. L., Boling, L., and Thorn, G. W. Plasma epinephrine and norepinephrine levels during insulin-

induced hypoglycemia in man. *J. Clin. Endocrinol. Metab.* 21:296, 1961.

65. Goodall, M. C., Stone, C., and Haynes, B. W., Jr. Urinary output of adrenaline and noradrenaline in severe thermal burns. *Ann. Surg.* 145:479, 1957.
66. Goodner, C. J., Koerker, D. J., Werrback, J. H., Toivala, P., and Gale, C. C. Adrenergic regulation of lipolysis and insulin secretion in the fasted baboon. *Am. J. Physiol.* 224:534, 1973.
67. Gordon, M. L. An evaluation of afferent nervous impulses in the adrenal cortical response to trauma. *Endocrinology* 47:347, 1950.
68. Groves, A. C., Griffiths, J., Leung, F., and Meek, R. N. Plasma catecholamines in patients with serious postoperative infection. *Ann. Surg.* 178: 102, 1973.
69. Gump, F. E., Price, J. B., Jr., and Kinney, J. M. Whole body and splanchnic blood flow and oxygen consumption measurements in patients with intraperitoneal infection. *Ann. Surg.* 171:321, 1970.
70. Haddy, F. J., and Scott, J. B. Metabolically linked vasoactive chemicals in local regulation of blood flow. *Physiol. Rev.* 48:688, 1968.
71. Haist, R. E., and Hamilton, J. K. Reversibility of carbohydrate and other changes in rats shocked by a clamping technique. *J. Physiol.* 102:471, 1944.
72. Hermreck, A. S., and Thal, A. P. Mechanisms for the high circulatory requirements in sepsis and septic shock. *Ann. Surg.* 170:677, 1969.
73. Herndon, D., Wilmore, D. W., Mason, A. D., Jr., and Pruitt, B. A., Jr. Humoral mediators of nontemperature-dependent hypermetabolism in 50% burned adult rats. *Surg. Forum* 28:37, 1977.
74. Hetherington, A. W., and Ranson, S. W. Hypothalamic lesions and adiposity in the rat. *Anat. Rec.* 78:149, 1940.
75. Himms-Hagen, J. Effects of Catecholamines on Metabolism. In H. Blaschko and E. Muscholl (Eds.), *Catecholamines.* New York: Springer-Verlag, 1972. P. 363.
76. Hinton, P., Allison, S. P., Littlejohn, S., and Lloyd, J. Insulin and glucose to reduce catabolic response to injury in burn patients. *Lancet* 1:767, 1971.
77. Hume, D. M. The Endocrine and Metabolic Response to Injury. In S. I. Schwartz (Ed.), *Principles of Surgery.* New York: McGraw-Hill, 1969. P. 2.
78. Hume, D. M. The secretion of epinephrine, norepinephrine and corticosteroids in the adrenal venous blood of the dog following simple and repeated trauma. *Surg. Forum* 8:111, 1957.
79. Hume, D. M., and Egdahl, R. H. The importance of the brain in the endocrine response to injury. *Ann. Surg.* 150:697, 1959.
80. Iverson, J. Adrenergic receptors and the secretion of glucagon and insulin from the isolated, perfused canine pancreas. *J. Clin. Invest.* 52: 2102, 1973.
81. Jarhult, J., Falck, B., Ingemansson, S., and Nobin, A. The functional importance of sympathetic nerves to the liver and endocrine pancreas. *Ann. Surg.* 189:96, 1979.
82. Jeejeebhoy, K. N., Anderson, G. H., Nakhooda, A. F., Greenberg, G. R., Sanderson, I., and Marliss, E. B. Metabolic studies in total parenteral nutrition with lipid in man: Comparison with glucose. *J. Clin. Invest.* 57:125, 1976.
83. Lerman, M. I., Abakumoua, O. Y., Kucenko, N. G., and Kobrina, E. M. Stimulation of growth of connective tissue by low-molecular weight constituents from rapidly growing tissues. *Lancet* 1:1225, 1977.
84. Liljenquist, J. E., Bomboy, J. D., Lewis, S. B., Sinclair-Smith, B. C., Felts, P. W., Lacy, W. W., Crofford, O. B., and Liddle, G. W. Effects of glucagon on lipolysis and ketogenesis in normal and diabetic man. *J. Clin. Invest.* 53:190, 1974.
85. Lindsey, A., Santeusanio, F., Braaten, J., Faloona, G. R., and Unger, R. H. Pancreatic alpha-cell function in trauma. *J.A.M.A.* 227: 757, 1974.
86. Long, C. N. H., Katzin, B., and Fry, E. G. The adrenal cortex and carbohydrate metabolism. *Endocrinology* 26:309, 1940.
87. Long, J. M., Wilmore, D. W., Mason, A. D., Jr., and Pruitt, B. A., Jr. The effect of carbohydrate and fat intake on nitrogen excretion during total intravenous feedings. *Ann. Surg.* 185:417, 1977.
88. Lucas, C. E., Rector, F. E., Werner, M., and Rosenberg, I. K. Altered renal homeostasis with acute sepsis: Clinical significance. *Arch. Surg.* 106:444, 1973.
89. McGilvery, R. W. *Biochemistry: A Functional Approach.* Philadelphia: Saunders, 1970.
90. Martin, J. B. Neural regulation of growth hormone secretion. *N. Engl. J. Med.* 288:1384, 1973.
91. Mayer, J., and Marshall, N. B. Specificity of gold thioglucose for ventromedial hypothalamic lesions and hyperphagia. *Nature* 178:1399, 1956.
92. Misbin, R. I., Edgar, P. J., and Lockwood, D. H. Influence of adrenergic receptor stimulation on glucose metabolism during starvation in man: Effects on circulating levels of insulin, growth hormone and fatty acids. *Metabolism* 20:544, 1971.

93. Moore, F. D. La Maladie Post-operatoire: Is There Order in Variety? The Six Stimulus-Response Sequences. In G. G. A. Clowes, Jr. (Ed.), *Symposium on Response to Infection and Injury, I. Surg. Clin. North Am.* 56:803, 1976.
94. Muller, W. A., Faloona, G. R., and Unger, R. H. The influence of the antecedent diet upon glucagon and insulin secretion. *N. Engl. J. Med.* 285:1450, 1971.
95. Munro, H. N., Fernstrom, J. D., and Wurtman, R. J. Insulin, plasma amino acid imbalance, and hepatic coma. *Lancet* 1:722, 1975.
96. Neely, J. R., Denton, R. M., England, P. J., and Randle, P. J. The effects of increased heart work on the tricarboxylate cycle and its interactions with glycolysis in the perfused rat heart. *Biochem. J.* 128:147, 1972.
97. Newsome, H. H., and Rose, J. C. The response of human adrenocorticotrophic hormone and growth hormone to surgical stress. *J. Clin. Endocrinol. Metab.* 33:481, 1971.
98. Nicoloff, J. T., Fisher, D. A., and Appleman, M. D., Jr. The role of glucocorticoids in the regulation of thyroid function in man. *J. Clin. Invest.* 49:1922, 1970.
99. Owen, E. E., and Cahill, G. F., Jr. Metabolic effects of exogenous glucocorticoids in fasted man. *J. Clin. Invest.* 52:2596, 1973.
100. Porte, D., Jr., and Robertson, R. P. Control of insulin secretion by catecholamines, stress, and the sympathetic nervous system. *Fed. Proc.* 32:1792, 1973.
101. Pozefsky, T., Felig, P., Tobin, J. D., Saeldner, J. S., and Cahill, G. F. Amino acid balance across tissues of the forearm in postabsorptive man: Effects of insulin at two dose levels. *J. Clin. Invest.* 48:2273, 1969.
102. Pozefsky, T., Tancredi, R. G., Moxley, R. T., Dupre, J., and Tobin, J. D. Effects of brief starvation on muscle amino acid metabolism in nonobese man. *J. Clin. Invest.* 57:444, 1976.
103. Randle, P. J., Hales, C. N., Garland, P. B., and Newsholme, E. A. The glucose-fatty-acid cycle. Its role in insulin sensitivity and the metabolic disturbance of diabetes mellitus. *Lancet* 1:785, 1963.
104. Raskin, P., and Unger, R. H. Hyperglucagonemia and its suppression. Importance in the metabolic control of diabetes. *N. Engl. J. Med.* 299:433, 1978.
105. Rasmussen, H. Organization and Control of Endocrine Systems. In R. H. Williams (Ed.), *Textbook of Endocrinology.* Philadelphia: Saunders, 1974. P. 1.
106. Robison, G. A., Butcher, R. W., and Sutherland, E. W. *Cyclic AMP.* New York: Academic, 1971.
107. Rocha, D. M., Faloona, G. R., and Unger, R. H. Glucagon-stimulating activity of 20 amino acids in dogs. *J. Clin. Invest.* 51:2346, 1972.
108. Rocha, D. M., Santeusanio, F., Faloona, G. R., and Unger, R. H. Abnormal pancreatic alpha-cell function in bacterial infections. *N. Engl. J. Med.* 288:700, 1973.
109. Ruch, T. C., and Patton, H. D. *Physiology and Biophysics... Circulation, Respiration and Fluid Balance.* Philadelphia: Saunders, 1974.
110. Salter, J. M., Ezrin, C., Laidlaw, J. C., and Gornall, A. G. Metabolic effects of glucagon in human subjects. *Metabolism* 9:753, 1960.
111. Samols, E., and Ryder, J. A. Studies on tissue uptake of insulin in man using a differential immunoassay for endogenous and exogenous insulin. *J. Clin. Invest.* 40:2092, 1961.
112. Shoemaker, W. C., Elwyn, D. H., Levin, H., and Rosen, A. L. Use of nonparametric analysis of cardiorespiratory variables as early predictors of death and survival in postoperative patients. *J. Surg. Res.* 17:1, 1974.
113. Sokal, J. E., and Weintraub, B. Failure of the isolated liver to react to hypoglycemia. *Am. J. Physiol.* 210:63, 1966.
114. Spaulding, S. W., Chopra, I. J., Sherwin, R. S., and Lyall, S. S. Effect of caloric restriction and dietary composition in serum T_3 and reserve T_3 in man. *J. Clin. Endocrinol. Metab.* 42:197, 1976.
115. Starzl, T. E., Porter, K. A., and Putnam, C. W. Intraportal insulin protects from the liver injury of portacaval shunt in dogs. *Lancet* 2:1241, 1975.
116. Sterling, K. Thyroid hormone action at the cell level. *N. Engl. J. Med.* 300:173, 1979.
117. Sullivan, P. R. C., Bollinger, J. A., and Reichlin, S. Selective deficiency of tissue triiodothyronine: A proposed mechanism of elevated free thyroxine in the euthyroid sick. *J. Clin. Invest.* 52:83a, 1973.
118. Talwar, K. K., Sawhney, R. C., and Rastogi, G. K. Serum levels of thyrotropin, thyroid hormones and their response to thyrotropin releasing hormone in infective febrile illness. *J. Clin. Endocrinol. Metab.* 44:398, 1977.
119. Taylor, J. W., Hander, E. W., Skreen, R., and Wilmore, D. W. The effect of central nervous system narcosis on the sympathetic response to stress. *J. Surg. Res.* 20:313, 1976.
120. Tomas, F. M., Munro, H. N., and Young, V. R. Effect of glucocorticoid administration on the rate of muscle protein breakdown in vivo in rats,

as measured by urinary excretion of N$^{\tau}$-methylhistidine. *Biochem. J.* 178:139, 1979.
121. Tomasi, T., Sledz, D., Wales, J. K., and Recant, L. Insulin half-life in normal and diabetic subjects. *Proc. Soc. Exp. Biol.* 126:315, 1967.
122. Ukai, M., Moran, W. H., Jr., and Zimmerman, B. The role of visceral afferent pathways on vasopressin secretion and urinary excretory patterns during surgical stress. *Ann. Surg.* 168:16, 1968.
123. Unger, R. H. Glucagon and the insulin:glucagon ratio in diabetes and other catabolic illnesses. *Diabetes* 20:834, 1971.
124. Unger, R. H. Glucagon physiology and pathophysiology. *N. Engl. J. Med.* 285:443, 1971.
125. Unger, R. H., and Orci, L. The essential role of glucagon in the pathogenesis of diabetes mellitus. *Lancet* 1:14, 1975.
126. Wannemacher, R. W., Jr., DuPont, H. L., Pekarek, P. S., Powanda, M. C., Schwartz, A., Hornick, R. B., and Beisel, W. R. An indogenous mediator of depression of amino acids and trace metals in serum during typhoid fever. *J. Infect. Dis.* 126:77, 1972.
127. Werner, S. C., and Ingbar, S. H. *The Thyroid* (4th ed.). Hagerstown, MD: Harper & Row, 1978.
128. Wilmore, D. W. Energy Requirements for Maximum Nitrogen Retention. In H. G. Green, M. A. Holliday, and H. N. Munro (Eds.), *Proceedings of a Symposium on Amino Acids.* AMA, 1977. P. 47.
129. Wilmore, D. W. Hormonal responses and their effect on metabolism. *Surg. Clin. North Am.* 56:999, 1976.
130. Wilmore, D. W. Studies of the effect of variations of temperature and humidity on energy demands of the burned soldier in a controlled metabolic room. U.S. Army Institute of Surgical Research Annual Research Progress Report, 1 July 1975–30 June 1976.
131. Wilmore, D. W., and Aulick, L. H. Metabolic changes in burn patients. *Surg. Clin. North Am.* 58:1173, 1978.
132. Wilmore, D. W., Lindsey, C. A., Moylan, J. A., Faloona, G. R., Pruitt, B. A., Jr., and Unger, R. H. Hyperglucagonaemia after burns. *Lancet* 1:73, 1974.
133. Wilmore, D. W., Long, J. M., Mason, A. D., Jr., Skreen, R. W., and Pruitt, B. A., Jr. Catecholamines: Mediator of the hypermetabolic response to thermal injury. *Ann. Surg.* 180:653, 1974.
134. Wilmore, D. W., Mason, A. D., Jr., and Pruitt, B. A., Jr. Insulin response to glucose in hypermetabolic burn patients. *Ann. Surg.* 183:314, 1976.
135. Wilmore, D. W., Mason, A. D., Jr., Johnson, D. W., and Pruitt, B. A., Jr. Effect of ambient temperature on heat production and heat loss in burn patients. *J. Appl. Physiol.* 38:593, 1975.
136. Wilmore, D. W., Moylan, J. A., Jr., Bristow, B. F., Mason, A. D., Jr., and Pruitt, B. A., Jr. Anabolic effects of human growth hormone and high caloric feedings following thermal injury. *Surg. Gynecol. Obstet.* 138:875, 1974.
137. Wilmore, D. W., Orcutt, T. W., Mason, A. D., Jr., and Pruitt, B. A., Jr. Alterations in hypothalamic function following thermal injury. *J. Trauma* 15:697, 1975.
138. Wolfe, B. M., Culebras, J. M., Sim, A. J. W., Ball, M. R., and Moore, F. D. Substrate interaction intravenous feeding. *Ann. Surg.* 186:518, 1977.
139. Woolfson, A. M. J., Heatley, R. V., and Allison, S. P. Insulin to inhibit protein catabolism after injury. *N. Engl. J. Med.* 300:14, 1979.
140. Wurtman, R. J. Catecholamines. *N. Engl. J. Med.* 273:637, 1965.
141. Young, J. B., and Landsberg, L. Stimulation of the sympathetic nervous system during sucrose feeding. *Nature* 269:615, 1977.

Energy Metabolism

John M. Kinney

4

The most basic requirement for sustaining life is energy. The human energy surplus in obesity is a major public health problem of the affluent countries, while the energy shortage of starvation threatens many of the underdeveloped countries. Paradoxically, the most frequent and severe form of protein-calorie malnutrition, which is seen in technologically advanced countries, is found in the acutely ill patients who require hospitalization for their care. The nutritional deficits associated with the medical care of such patients involve not only reduced intake, but also the increased requirements related to their disease or injury. No other segment of clinical nutrition has been associated with less concern for achieving daily balance than in the need for energy. Several reasons may account for this:

1. The difficulties of estimating the total energy expenditure of individual ambulatory subjects.
2. The lack of suitable equipment for measuring the resting energy expenditure of an acutely ill patient.
3. The general attitude among clinicians that body energy stores can be depended on to meet any reasonable energy deficit without penalty (an idea undoubtedly reinforced by the relatively high incidence of excessive calorie intake among the adult population in the United States).

The agriculturists have long had a particular interest in energy balance, since an efficient conversion of food energy to animal products, such as meat, milk, and eggs, has an obvious economic advantage. Consequently, animal calorimetry has received more governmental support than human calorimetry. The recent oil crisis has raised the possibility of an industrial energy shortage. It is interesting that during the same decade there has been increased interest in the problems of energy balance in man, whether the energy excesses of obesity or the energy depletion related to starvation, disease, or injury.

CALORIMETRY: BIRTH AND EARLY DEVELOPMENT

The middle of the eighteenth century saw the birth of both direct and indirect calorimetry. At the beginning of that century, air was still considered to be a simple, single substance, and it was generally thought that all gases were simply different forms of atmospheric air, rather than different chemical entities. The growth of calorimetry depended on the recognition—from botanical, chemical, and physiologic evidence—of the composition and behavior of the constituents of atmospheric air. Joseph Priestley was honored by England's Royal Society in 1733 for his discovery that plants could restore the atmosphere in some manner, which only later was recognized as removing CO_2 and producing O_2. After many years spent in searching for chemicals such as potassium nitrate, which "could restore the atmosphere," he returned to experiments on what we now call photosynthesis [51]. In 1772, he prepared a specimen of air in which a mouse had been allowed to die; sprigs of mint were allowed to stand in this air for one week. At the end of this time, not only was the mint still healthy, but the air had been restored to the point at which a candle would burn or a mouse could live in it. Benjamin Franklin, who saw the experiment, concluded that the air had been improved by taking something from it and not by adding to it. It took Priestley more than twelve years to find out that both processes occurred, side by side.

A Scottish medical student, Joseph Black, was assigned the problem in 1752 of finding a less caustic solvent to dissolve bladder stones, which were a common clinical problem [106]. After four years of work, Black had become interested in the effervescence that occurred when bladder stones were exposed to certain chemicals and termed the gas that was released "fixed air"; this was later identified as CO_2. Because of this research, Black was appointed Chairman of Anatomy and soon after became Chairman of Medicine at the University of Glasgow.

Joseph Priestley, in England, and Carl Scheele, in Sweden, were independently engaged in research during the 1760s, which demonstrated that small animals kept in a closed space would die at approximately the same time that the flame of a burning candle, in the same space, would be extinguished. However, neither scientist was able to grasp the significance of this observation because of their belief in the phlogiston theory, which claimed that a "substance" was given out by burning which no one had been able to identify. In the period of 1774 to 1784, Lavoisier and coworkers conducted experiments on the composition of air and concluded that the combustion of a candle, or the respiration of an animal, involved the removal from the air of a gas which was termed "oxygene." During this time, it was shown that the combination of O_2 with various other chemical elements was fundamental to the understanding of the behavior of acids and alkalis [82]. Therefore, Lavoisier, together with the work of other natural philosophers of his time, established the foundation of modern chemistry and particularly of modern biochemistry.

It is of particular interest that as Priestley, Black, Scheele and Lavoisier began to recognize the biochemical role of O_2 consumption and CO_2 production in both combustion and respiration, they all extended their research into related subjects of heat production and changes in temperature. Joseph Black [17], while maintaining an active practice of medicine in Glasgow and later in Edinburgh, became interested in the change of heat content when ice changed to water and water changed to steam. This led him to identify the concept of latent heat in contrast to the temperature of a material, an insight that was essential to the development of calorimetry. He designed an ice-jacketed container in an effort to relate the CO_2 given off by combustion or respiration with the heat production, which was measured by the amount of ice melted to water. Lavoisier used this type of device in more precise experiments to relate O_2 consumption to a measured amount of heat output [84] (Figure 4-1). The observation that there was a fixed relationship between gas exchange and heat production caused Lavoisier and his associates to fashion a metal face-piece for the measurement of gas exchange in man. Lavoisier wrote the results of these preliminary human investigations in a letter he sent from Paris to Joseph Black in Edinburgh, dated November 19, 1790. He presented

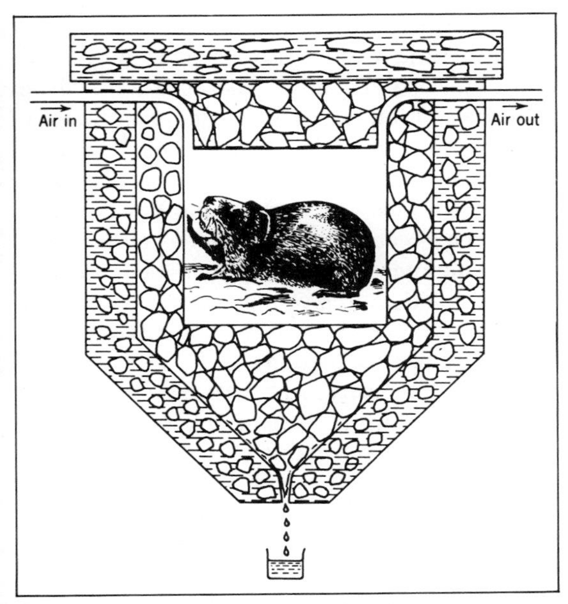

Figure 4-1. *A sketch of Lavoisier's calorimeter for the study of heat production in a guinea pig. The animal melts the ice to produce water. The weight of the ice measures the animal's heat production (80 kcal of heat will melt 1 kg of ice). The mixture of ice and water in the jacket prevents heat flow through the walls of the apparatus. (M. Kleiber,* Fire of Life: An Introduction to Animal Energetics. *Melbourne, FL: Krieger, 1975. P. 116.)*

results of the O_2 absorbed per hour by a man without food, with food, and during physical work; the data are in remarkable accord with measurements made over a century later [114]. We do not know the exact method employed by Lavoisier, but the form of his apparatus is illustrated by two watercolor drawings made by Madame Lavoisier. It is unfortunate that the details of his methodology were never published before his execution by the Paris commune, May 8, 1794.

The birth of both indirect and direct calorimetry in the second half of the eighteenth century was followed by rapid advances in organic chemistry and the emergence of nutrition as a science [104]. Liebig showed that it was not carbon and hydrogen that was burned in the body, but rather protein, carbohydrate, and fat [86]. Liebig's contribution stimulated the research of Voit and his students at Munich, thus establishing such concepts as the specific dynamic action of foodstuffs, nitrogen balance, and the apparent relationship of basal metabolism to surface area. Pettenkofer and Voit extended the previous animal studies of indirect calorimetry by building a respiration apparatus around a small room that was ventilated by a current of air [105]. This apparatus was used for detailed measurements of changes in body weight, together with continuous measurements of gas exchange and calculation of the total loss of carbon and nitrogen from the body during one day of starvation in man. Subsequent work showed that increased energy expenditure, associated with physical activity, did not increase protein metabolism. These studies also made it evident that the absorption of O_2 did not drive metabolism, but rather that the level of metabolism determined the amount of O_2 to be absorbed.

Rubner [111], a student of Voit's, built a special chamber for the study of both direct and indirect calorimetry in the dog. This led to confirmation of the agreement between direct and indirect calorimetry during a metabolic steady state. The specific dynamic action of foodstuffs was observed and named by Rubner. By 1900, the energy value of individual foods had been carefully determined and introductory efforts were under way to study the energy requirements of animals and man under different physical conditions.

Atwater followed his studies with Voit by enlisting the aid of a physicist, Rosa, to construct a large calorimeter of sufficient size to measure the heat given off by a man while living and exercising within the chamber [8]. This device allowed measurements of sufficient precision to compare direct and indirect calorimetry in active man. Three different individuals were studied over 40 days while receiving an ordinary mixed diet. These individuals averaged 2717 kcal per day by indirect calorimetry, and 2723 kcal by direct calorimetry, or an average difference per day of only 0.2 percent. The estimated energy values that

Rubner had assigned to protein, fat, and carbohydrate were shown to be in excellent agreement with feeding studies of normal subjects measured in the Atwater-Rosa chamber [9]. This pioneer calorimeter in the United States was followed by similar devices for the study of cattle and the founding of two particularly well-known laboratories for the study of calorimetry in man. One was the Nutrition Laboratory of the Carnegie Institute in Boston, under the direction of F. G. Benedict. The other was the calorimeter at the Russell Sage Institute of Pathology, at the Bellevue Hospital in New York City, under the direction of Graham Lusk. Much of the understanding of energy metabolism up to 1930 was presented in the classic volumes entitled *Elements of Nutrition,* by Lusk [88] and *Basal Metabolism in Health and Disease,* by DuBois [37].

CALORIMETRY: THE LAST FIFTY YEARS

The pioneering investigations of human calorimetry from 1890 to 1930 were followed by a quarter of a century characterized by the popularization of the basal metabolic rate (BMR) test for diagnosing and treating thyroid disease [40], while little interest was shown in the energy expenditure of other clinical conditions. The years since 1955 witnessed the replacement of the BMR test with more sophisticated chemical measurements for thyroid disease, and many hospitals have disposed of their facilities for measuring BMR. Thus, we are caring for both chronic and acute diseases by increasingly sophisticated methods of diagnosis and treatment, which are often based on an assumed level of energy expenditure that is never measured.

The principles of indirect calorimetry have recently been reviewed by Johnson [69], with careful attention to the assumptions and sources of error in application of the method. Clinical studies have emphasized that the pattern of breathing, and sometimes the values for gas exchange, may be altered by a tight-fitting mask or by a mouthpiece and noseclip [79]. A system has been designed, by Kinney and coworkers [75], in which a clear head canopy is ventilated by a continuous stream of air passed through piping in the wall to an analyzer in an adjacent room, where there is a continuous measurement of air flow, O_2 consumption, and CO_2 production. The only connection between the patient and the head canopy is a lightweight plastic neck seal, which allows the patient to breathe exactly as he would when lying quietly in bed. The ambient concentration of CO_2 in the canopy does not exceed 1 percent and, therefore, does not influence the level of minute ventilation.

A portable instrument has been developed commercially, which can be taken around the wards for measurement of O_2 consumption and CO_2 production under conditions of rest and also under some types of stress testing [100]. One of the most difficult circumstances under which to measure gas exchange is when patients are on mechanical ventilation. A Servo ventilator has recently been introduced with built-in equipment for the measurement of O_2 consumption and CO_2 production [34]. Therefore, it seems reasonable to expect that measurements of indirect calorimetry will be utilized in increasing numbers of clinical situations to provide reference values for ventilation and circulation, as well as useful information upon which to establish the amount of enteral or parenteral nutrition, which should be provided on a daily basis.

Since World War II, the development of direct calorimetry has largely been related to the perfection of a chamber whose walls employ the gradient layer principle, which provides an electrical signal associated with the passage of heat across the calorimeter wall. A precise instrument of this kind was built and used by Benzinger [14] for the study of human thermoregulation. Jequier and coworkers [68] are utilizing a chamber that employs the gradient-layer principle for direct calorimetry, while serving as a respiration chamber for indirect calorimetry. This experience led Jequier to note that due to limitations in size, gradient-layer calorimeters do not allow long-term studies of human energy balance. The principle of this construction imposes a limit on the size of the chamber, since the larger the wall area, the lower the rate of heat flow per unit surface and the weaker the resultant signal. Therefore, long-term studies on energy expenditure in man are easier to perform using large respiration chambers with the indirect calorimetric approach.

The new concepts involved in building space suits for the astronauts prompted Webb [125] to measure the heat removed from the human body within such a suit by measuring the heat added to water passing through a fine network of tubing that passed over the body beneath a heavy layer of insulation. A face shield was continuously ventilated with a stream of air, which was measured for gas exchange after passing the subject's face. The Webb suit therefore allowed an individual to move around and exercise while measurements were being made of both direct and indirect calorimetry. Excellent correspondence between direct and indirect calorimetry has been demonstrated for subjects at rest, but a curious deviation has been noted when subjects are studied continuously for approximately 2 days under conditions of varying food intake.

The measurement of heat loss by calorimetry is widely accepted, but this method is costly and complex, and the size of the measurement space is small. There are energy balance accounting methods in which indirect measurements of energy loss can be combined in various ways. Such methods are often referred to as "partitional calorimetry." Methods for partitional calorimetry were first described by Winslow, Gagge, and coworkers [127] in 1936. These workers demonstrated that heat loss by evaporation could be determined by the rate of weight loss, so that the loss of weight in grams per unit time multiplied by the heat of vaporization produces the rate of heat loss by evaporation. Similarly, they indicated that the heat loss by radiation is equal to a constant multiplied by the difference between the fourth powers of the absolute temperature of the skin and the environment and by the effective radiation surface area. Convective heat losses could be determined by measuring the effective air velocity and the difference between skin temperature and ambient air temperature. In the study of human thermoregulation, partitional calorimetry has the advantage of being able to deal with changing environmental conditions or with changes in metabolic rate more easily than can be done with direct calorimetry. An additional advantage of partitional calorimetry is that it makes experiments possible in large rooms that are not especially equipped, to allow the conduct of a study outdoors [121]. This is in contrast to direct calorimetry, in which measurements are made in spaces that must be kept as small as possible to retain sensitivity and rapidity of response.

METABOLIC BODY SIZE

The gross body weight per se has some direct significance to energy expenditure, to the extent that it determines the content of actively metabolizing cells. The major importance of using total body weight as a reference for energy expenditure has to do with body fatness. Many sedentary persons are excessively fat but not overweight, whereas the opposite condition, overweight without fat, is common among people doing heavy physical work. In addition to distinguishing between fat and muscle in the gross body weight, variations in the water content of the body must be considered. Adult subjects have been reported to vary in their daily body weight from 0.5 to 1.0 kg, or the equivalent of approximately 0.5 percent of the adult body weight. Most of the short term fluctuations of body weight can be explained by changes in the water content of the body. Such fluctuations, however, do not detract from the fact that, over periods of a week or more, food intake and energy expenditure are closely balanced and the body weight remains relatively constant.

Metabolic body size is a concept encountered in the literature relating to energy expenditure. Energy requirements must be adjusted for variation that results from differences in body size. The relation of energy expenditure to the body surface area was clearly expressed by Rubner in 1883 and became known as Rubner's surface law. Both Rubner and a French physiologist, Richet, showed that with animals of different size, the heat production was approximately the same per square meter of body surface, though it differed greatly per kilogram of body weight. DuBois [39] was interested in the surface law in relation to his calorimeter studies at the Russell Sage Institute and wrote the following:

> We can only apply the physical laws of cooling if we conceive of a world at a uniform temperature inhabited by warm-blooded animals with a uniform body temperature, with similar surface coverings living under similar physiologic conditions of nourishment. In such a world the loss of heat from each animal would be proportional to its surface area. The heat production must equal the heat loss. If it were smaller than the loss, the animal would cool to the temperature of the surrounding medium. If the heat production were greater than the loss, the animal would become warmer and warmer and finally burn up.

Investigators have shown that the blood volume, cross section of the aorta, and cross section of the trachea are all proportional to the body surface in warm-blooded animals as well as the vital capacity and other components or functions of the human body. Some of these may show this relationship because they are affected by the metabolism and need of the body for oxygen. Some one of these factors may be the determining cause of the level of the basal metabolism. Rubner, Magnus-Levy, and others demonstrated that the basal metabolism of man was more closely proportional to surface area than to any other standard [89]. They used, however, Meeh's formula—surface area = 12.312 times the cube root of the body weight squared—a relation that holds only for individuals of the same body shape. It became evident to workers at the Russell Sage Institute of Pathology in New York that their measurements of heat production were of greater accuracy than their calculation of each individual's body surface area by the Meeh formula. Therefore, Delafield DuBois undertook a more precise characterization of the surface area of five individuals by covering them with small paraffin blocks that were then laid out for measurement on photographic paper. The final surface area was related to height and weight by a linear formula, which proved to be surprisingly reliable.

Kleiber was particularly interested in the surface law and noted that the DuBois formula was probably the best method of estimating the "actual" surface area of man. In 1932, however, Kleiber [80] pointed out that the various refinements of surface area measurement did not help to clarify the underlying question of whether surface area was indeed a function of the metabolic rate. Theories advanced for the interpretation of the surface law of energy metabolism were classified and analyzed by Kleiber [81] according to six major contentions: The metabolic rate of animals must be in proportion to the body surface because of (1) the rate of heat transfer, (2) the flow of nutrients, (3) the relation of blood flow to the cross section of blood vessels, (4) the chemical composition of an animal as a function of body size, (5) the anatomic composition as a function of body size, and (6) an inherited metabolic requirement of tissue as related to body size. After criticizing all of these theories, Kleiber concludes, "In natural selection, those animals probably prove to be the fittest whose cells are adapted to a level of O_2 consumption at which the overall metabolic rate is suitable for the maintenance of a constant body temperature and commensurate with an efficient transport of O_2." Because the surface law is unreliable owing to poor definition and difficulties of measurement, Kleiber recommended that metabolic rate be expressed as a function of body weight. The laws of geometry indicate that the surface area of a sphere can be expressed in terms of the two-thirds power of the volume. However, the animal body is not a perfect sphere, and Kleiber recommended that the surface area be expressed in relation to the body weight to the three-fourths power as the basis for metabolic body size. There appears to be no advantage in using a power of body weight other than unity for comparing human studies, unless the heaviest individual in the group is more than 3 times heavier than the lightest individual. This covers a range of 40 to 120 kg for man. Thus, the greatest importance of using a power function of weight as the metabolic body size only becomes evident in comparative studies of energy metabolism in large and small species (Figure 4-2).

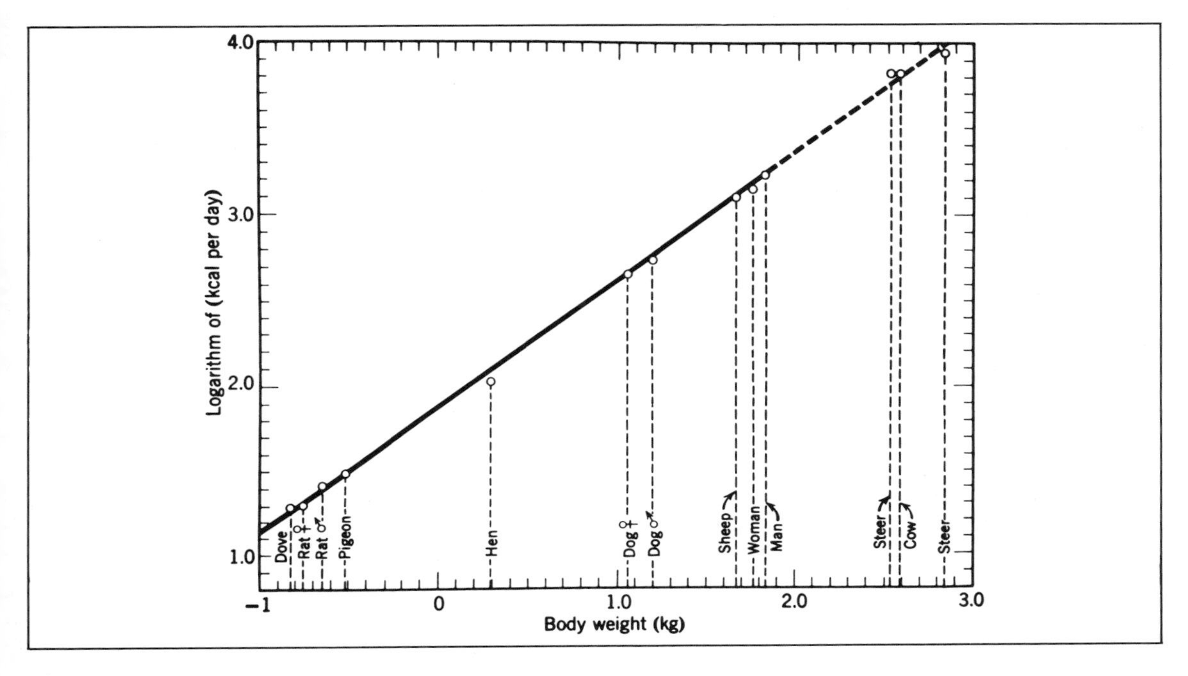

Figure 4-2. *The close correlation for ten groups of mammals between the logarithm of the fasting metabolic rate and the logarithm of body weight, supporting the use of a power of body weight to express metabolic rate. (M. Kleiber,* Fire of Life: An Introduction to Animal Energetics. *Melbourne, FL: Krieger, 1975. P. 203.)*

The traditional DuBois formula for calculating surface area has been reported to give an answer that is about 6.6 percent too low and has a coefficient of variation of 11 percent. Durnin [42] has emphasized that, in practice, body weight is as good a reference standard as the calculated surface area. Durnin and Passmore [43] suggest abandoning the "BMR" and substituting *resting metabolic rate.* They note that the 12- to 18-hour period of fasting is inconvenient for the subject, and if the measurement is made 2 to 4 hours after a light breakfast, as much information is gained by making the test less trying as is lost by abandoning the true fasting state. Children have a higher metabolic rate than adults, expressed in relation to either body weight or surface area. Garrow [54] notes that the use of surface area, because different species have a constant metabolic rate, cannot be taken seriously when within our own species there is roughly a halving of metabolic rate per square meter during our lifetime. The high metabolic rate of children is generally explained as representing the energy cost of growth. The metabolic rate of men is about 15 percent higher than that of women of the same body mass. The higher metabolic rate of men than women is explained by the greater lean body mass in men, or the greater fat mass in women.

Behnke [11] proposed that the body could be divided into two parts: the fat and the lean body mass. The latter was conceived of as the body with the least amount of fat compatible with health and was considered to include a minimum, but essential, amount of fat amounting to perhaps 2 percent of the lean body mass. Because it is difficult to know how much fat is really essential, recent investigations have redefined the lean body mass to represent the body devoid of all fat and consider the body fat to be the sum of lipid extractable substances in the body. Another approach [102] has been to measure the total amount of body water by isotope dilution and multiply by a factor from the average hydration of lean tissue, which would then be subtracted from the total body weight to indicate the amount of body fat.

Grande, Keys, and coworkers [57, 72] suggested in 1950 that much of the variation in reports of the normal basal metabolic rate could be eliminated when expressed in units of fat-free body, or active tissue mass. For persons of a given sex and age, the basal oxygen consumption is correlated to about the same extent with surface area as with fat-free body weight. The utility of fat-free body weight as a standard of reference becomes evident when persons of different sex and age are compared. For both males and females 20 to 60 years of age, a single value can be used to indicate the normal metabolic rate. The single value of 4.4 ml of oxygen per minute (or about 1.3 calorie per hour) per kilogram of fat-free body weight can be used instead of the customary tables and graphs, based on the artificial concept of surface area as the determinant of basal metabolism. The "active tissue mass" is similar to the "body cell mass" estimated by Moore and coworkers [92] from the isotope dilution measurements of total exchangeable potassium. The body cell mass may represent anything from one-third to two-thirds of the total body weight, but it accounts for essentially all the energy consumption and heat production. The highest values for this active tissue mass as a percentage of body weight will be found in lean muscular males who are dehydrated; the lowest values occur in sedentary women who are both fat and overhydrated.

The energy expenditure of all organs and tissues that are part of the active tissue mass of the body do not have equal rates of metabolism per unit of mass [58]. In man, the brain and liver together, representing about 4 percent of the normal body mass, account for over 40 percent of the total resting oxygen consumption, whereas the skeletal muscle, amounting to about 40 percent of the body weight, contributes only about 25 percent of the basal metabolism. These facts help to explain that early in starvation the basal metabolism falls far more rapidly than would be predicted from a consideration of the change in total body weight.

PARTITION OF ENERGY EXPENDITURE

The energy expenditure of adult subjects is usually divided into the resting metabolic rate and the amount associated with physical activity. The average sedentary adult tends to underestimate his resting energy expenditure and to overestimate the energy expenditure associated with exercise. Resting metabolic rate is usually taken to represent the basal metabolic rate plus whatever additional energy expenditure is associated with the intake of food. These categories of daily energy expenditure will be briefly discussed in this section as they relate to normal subjects; the energy expenditure of hospitalized patients will be considered in a subsequent section.

The term *basal metabolic rate,* or BMR, became popular when indirect calorimetry was introduced to investigate thyroid disease. The BMR is usually defined as the energy expenditure of an individual under standardized resting conditions, which means 10 to 18 hours after a meal and physically relaxed in a neutral thermal environment [38]. In practice, it is far more difficult to achieve the conditions for basal metabolism than it is to define them. Special transparent enclosures about the head have been designed to avoid the stimuli and discomfort of something tightly fastened to the upper airway [79]. The extensive work of DuBois [38] at the Bellevue Hospital, and Boothby and Sandiford [19] at the Mayo Clinic, established normal standards per square meter of surface area.

Specific dynamic action (SDA) is the increase in metabolic rate, which reaches a peak in 1 to 2 hours after a meal and slowly declines over the next 2 to 3 hours. Protein has usually been thought to have an SDA of 15 to 30 percent, whereas the comparable effect for carbohydrate or fat was 5 percent or less. Krebs [82] reported that the increased SDA of protein reflected energy losses associated with urea production, but experiments by Garrow and Hawes [54] could not demonstrate any relationship between the metabolic rate after a meal and the amount of urea produced. Glick and coworkers [56] have found that the brown adipose tissue of the rat increased in amount and O_2 uptake following a single low-protein, high-carbohydrate meal. These investigators suggest that dietary thermogenesis in the rat may be an extension of the SDAs of single meals. In addition, they propose that "the oxidation of substrate by brown fat may serve as a homeostatic mechanism by which a diet unbalanced in its macronutrient composition can become more balanced by selective oxidation of one or more macronutrients present in excess."

It is well known that severe exposure to either heat or cold will increase the metabolic rate. The thermic effect of food and cold exposure were previously considered to be independent. Buskirk and coworkers [23, 24] and Rochelle and Horvath [107] tested both stimuli separately and together and found no significant interaction. Previous controversy surrounding the subject of cold exposure and nonshivering thermogenesis tended to obscure some of the recent observations [61] which indicate close similarities with dietary thermogenesis.

Rothwell and Stock [110] have reviewed the similarities between brown adipose tissue from hyperphagic rats and that of cold-adapted rats; both had increased mitochondrial mass and respiratory enzyme activity as well as higher in vitro rates of mitochondrial respiration. This subject is discussed further under the influence of diet on energy expenditure.

People engaged in heavy work have been found to utilize approximately 800 kcal more than people in sedentary jobs. Passmore and Durnin [103] have observed that a rate of energy expenditure of 5 kcal per minute is approximately the upper limit of work that can be performed without an increasing accumulation of lactic acid, or a rise in body temperature. This exercise is equivalent to a daily walk of about 30 miles. Work at 5 kcal per minute for 8 hours corresponds to 2400 kcal expended at work. According to Garrow [55], if we allow 500 kcal for 8 hours in bed and about 1400 kcal for the 8 hours spent outside of work, the total energy expenditure for 24 hours is 4300 kcal. This has been considered the upper range of daily energy expenditure that could be maintained regularly in heavy industry.

The exact definition of energy requirements for a healthy diet remains uncertain because of marked variation in basal metabolic rate and mechanical work efficiency of individuals on high and low energy intakes, suggesting adaptation to low energy intakes. In developing countries, it is common to see individuals subsisting on an energy intake far below the recommended dietary allowance and yet leading an apparently healthy life. Does a low energy intake necessarily result in poor physical performance or can some adaptation result that permits productive physical activity at levels of energy intake much less than are usually recommended? Studies by Edmundson [46] of farmers in East Java indicated that the output of work was not affected by calorie intake. Farmers eating an intake of approximately 2389 kcal/day were studied in comparison to those receiving an average of 1535 kcal/day. The high intake group had a BMR that was almost twice that of the low energy intake group, and the high energy intake group expended significantly more energy in performing standard work tasks than the low energy intake group. The assessment of the daily energy balance is particularly difficult in field studies of energy balance because of difficulty in assessing the energy expenditure related to physical activity. Buskirk and coworkers [25] have recently discussed methodology for indirectly estimating physical activity. The amount of energy expended in exercise is much smaller in hospitalized patients than in normal ambulatory subjects, but is equally difficult to measure. Elwyn and Kinney [50] have suggested a unique method for determining total energy expenditure in the group of patients who are receiving their nutrition as hypertonic glucose and amino acids by vein.

CONTROL OF ENERGY INTAKE

The patient who receives his food intake by intravenous or enteral tube feeding has lost the ability to influence the composition and amount of his food intake. Therefore, it is important to consider the control of food intake that is normally present in the absence of artificial nutrient intake. The control of food intake has usually been thought of in terms of energy intake. Such control may be exerted by the nervous system, the gastrointestinal system, and metabolic factors, which may combine to stimulate the initiation of feeding, the termination of feeding, and/or the length of the interval between meals.

The neurologic role in the control of energy intake first received attention when Hetherington and Ranson [60] discovered that bilateral lesions in the ventromedial hypothalamus of rats caused excessive eating, which led to obesity. This effect has subsequently been observed in other rodents, cats, monkeys, and man. This type of brain damage results in rapid weight gain until a new increased level of weight is achieved, followed by a normal food intake and no further accumulation of body fat. Hyperphagia recurs if these obese animals are made to lose weight. About ten years after the discovery of the relationship between the ventromedial hypothalamus and food intake, Anand and Brobeck [1] discovered that lesions in the lateral hypothalamus produced rats that did not eat. This led to the "dual center" hypothesis for the neural control of feeding: that the ventromedial hypothalamic area inhibited feeding, while the lateral hypothalamic area increased feeding. This concept has come to appear as an oversimplification during the past decade, with reports that lesions and stimulations of the hypothalamus can affect many other forms of behavior in addition to feeding. However Bray and Gallager [20] described 8 patients with obesity related to hypothalamic injury and observed that hyperphagia was a characteristic in each case. Celesia and coworkers [31] report a case in which the onset of voracious eating led to obesity as a tumor invaded the ventromedial hypothalamus. Food is the primary stimulus for gastrointestinal function, but with a rapidly expanding list of neural and neuroendocrine relationships that also play a definite, but poorly defined, role in the control of feeding. Hunger sensations are complex and may, or may not, be associated with gastric hunger contractions. The gastric hunger contractions are primarily controlled by local and vagovagal reflexes. In summary, deficits of the body energy stores can give rise to a complex sensation called *hunger*. It is generally believed that the gastric hunger contractions play a less important role in the sensation of hunger than specific metabolic stimuli. However, it has been the common belief that the regulation of energy intake is controlled with considerable precision through mechanisms governing food intake. Janowitz and Hollander [66] maintained 3 dogs under standardized conditions and fed them once daily. These animals had a coefficient of variation of spontaneous food intake amounting to 12 percent, while the coefficient of variation of body weight was only 1 percent.

Carbohydrate and fat are the major sources of energy for cells and tissues. They represent the short-term energy sources that must cover energy needs until food intake occurs. Therefore, it has been suggested that some aspects of carbohydrate or fat metabolism may integrate cellular energy needs with energy expenditure.

Mayer and Bates [90] proposed a glucostatic hypothesis that linked the metabolism of glucose to feeding behavior. This hypothesis suggested that (1) glucose levels control feeding on a meal-to-meal basis; (2) the rate of glucose utilization by centers in the brain was the critical parameter by which glucose metabolism controlled food intake; and (3) food intake was inversely related to the rate of glucose utilization, so that increased glucose utilization would inhibit feeding and decreased utilization would stimulate feeding. Efforts to support this concept by measurement of cerebral arteriovenous glucose* differences in

***Editor's Note:* It should be pointed out that the amounts of amino acids given in the glucose group, 70 gm/24 hr, were less than those given to the group receiving no glucose, 90gm/24 hr. This accounts for the superior nitrogen balance in the group receiving no dextrose. It is generally accepted that 5% dextrose improves the retention of administered nitrogen, probably because less of the administered amino acid is utilized for energy.

man were reported to show little change before or after meals. However, local changes in glucose utilization could still occur, as suggested by the glucostatic hypothesis. Russek [113] has recently proposed that glucose metabolism may control food intake by way of the liver rather than the brain. He suggested that some relationship might exist between glycogenolysis in liver cells and their membrane potential. Thus, when the rate of glycogen breakdown is high during food deprivation, glucose flux across the liver cell membrane would increase, leading to depolarization of the cell membrane and activation of central neuromechanisms for feeding. This hypothesis is ingenious, but remains to be proved.

Kennedy [71] observed that the amount of depot fat in relation to body weight appears to be constant in most adult mammals that have completed growth and before the onset of old age. This correlation was interpreted to indicate that the amount of body fat reaches a threshold value in the adult beyond which there is inhibition of food intake. When body fat and body weight are both increased by the daily administration of insulin [63], or by excessive tube feeding [33], food intake is markedly decreased. When insulin treatment or tube feeding is stopped, the food intake remains partially inhibited until body fat and body weight have decreased to normal, whereupon normal feeding is resumed. Fat cell size has been suggested as the critical parameter of adipose tissue that correlates with inhibition of food intake [62]. It is not clear how enlarged fat cells could cause a reduction in food intake, but humoral factors, particularly hormone related to glucose and fatty acid metabolism, may play a central role.

It is a part of common knowledge that food intake is increased as a result of the environmental temperature, eating more in the cold and less in the heat. In conditions of the heat and cold stress, feeding may serve as a part of temperature regulation [21]. It is possible that the increased heat production that is the consequence of food intake is involved in the control of food intake, either to cause the termination of feeding or to regulate the frequency of meals. However, many physiologic events follow the ingestion of food, and the precise role of heat production as the result of food is difficult to separate from other factors associated with food intake.

INFLUENCE OF DIET ON ENERGY EXPENDITURE

Dietary surveys conducted over the years have shown reasonable agreement between estimates of energy intake and energy expenditure for groups of subjects. However, when energy balance has been examined carefully, particularly for one individual on a day to day basis, significant discrepancies have been observed between dietary intake, energy output, and changes in body weight. A well-known study by Edholm [45], in which dietary intake and energy expenditure were measured in soldiers who were continuously observed day and night, led to the following conclusions:

1. For a group of 10 or more subjects, intake and expenditure over a period of 5 to 7 days are in close agreement.
2. For an individual, on a single day, intake and expenditure are not related.
3. For an individual, over a period of 5 to 7 days, intake and expenditure are significantly related, but the scatter of results is considerable.
4. There is no significant relationship between body weight and food consumption.
5. After a period of calorie deficit, food intake exceeds energy expenditure, but over a period of 5 days the excess is not closely related to the size of the deficit.

Other studies have examined the influence on body weight of prolonged food intake in excess of measured energy expenditure. From observations such as these, Durnin and three other well-known British scientists [44] published their conclusions that the energy requirements of man are not known, nor is the balance of energy intake and energy expenditure understood for adult man. These authors challenged the conclusion that approximately two-thirds of the world's population is undernourished, offering the possibility that the 30 percent of the world's population who have an "adequate" intake are really eating too much, and that an unknown proportion of the remaining population may not be undernourished.

Energy balance in man may be defined as the balance between energy intake and total of energy stored by the body, plus energy produced as heat; intake must equal output, plus energy gain. In order to carry out such an energy balance study in man, one would have to measure O_2 consumption, CO_2 production, and N losses for periods of 24 to 48 hours. This would require the use of a large-chamber calorimeter in which normal activities could be carried out. A total balance for carbon and nitrogen would also be required to calculate changes in body energy stores. Garrow [55] has observed that most studies in man have been based on limited measurements of gas exchange throughout the waking day, with physical activity being estimated by assessing the energy cost of various types of activity and utilizing a diary system to estimate the daily energy cost of all activities. The laws of thermodynamics must be observed, and thus the total energy in the food consumed minus the energy output must equal the change in the energy content of the body. There is, however, no requirement to assume that different individuals, or even the same individual, at different times or under different conditions would utilize food energy with the same efficiency. The precision of measuring energy balance makes it difficult to account for the gain or loss of body fat stores over periods lasting one year or more. An excess of intake over expenditure of only 50 kcal per day can produce 6 or 7 gm of adipose tissue per day, which would represent 2 kg per year. Yet, an individual consuming 2500 kcal per day will have 50 kcal represent only 2 percent of the total intake. Considering the variability of food composition; the fact that different kinds of carbohydrate, fat, and protein do not have exactly the same potential energy; the difficulties in exact measurement of the amount of food eaten; and the limits of analytic methods, it becomes clear that the energy intake cannot be measured with high precision, and that actual precision represented in any given study is seldom known. The equally severe problems in measuring the energy expenditure have already been mentioned.

The route and the rate of food intake may influence the utilization of that food. Rats tube-fed varying proportions of their normal daily food intake, while being allowed free access to the stock diet, reduced their voluntary intake, so that the total daily energy intake was identical to that of the control animals [110]. However, all the animals receiving the tube feeding showed excessive weight gain, which was largely due to an increase in body fat, and all of this gained weight was lost when the tube feeding was discontinued.

Protein deficiency is associated with a wasteful utilization of energy intake. Miller and associates [91] found that young pigs fed a diet so low in protein that it did not allow growth consumed a large excess of calories which could not be accounted for in body tissue. Ashworth and associates [4] have observed that infants recovering from malnutrition take in an excessive number of calories. When the malnourished infants recover their normal size, the rate of growth and the calorie intake fall to normal levels.

Individual differences in the efficiency of utilizing dietary energy have long been appreciated in the field of animal husbandry. Yet nutritionists and clinicians are content to treat medical and surgical conditions on the basis of assumed energy expenditures, which are never measured. The original concept of specific dynamic action [111] needs to be considered in the light of current beliefs concerning the utilization of food energy. The energy and chemical bonds of food must be converted into free energy by the body, most frequently in the form of high-energy phosphate bonds, in order to be used for mechanical, synthetic, osmotic, or transport work. Hegsted [59], in an interesting discussion of this problem, notes that the maximum conversion of ATP from fat or carbohydrate approximates 38 or 40 percent, whereas the ATP realized from protein is only 32 to 34 percent. The recycling of pyruvate to glucose, hydrolyzing triglyceride with a subsequent re-esterification of the glycerol and fatty acid moieties, or maintaining the dynamic state of protein synthesis and breakdown, all have high costs of free energy, with a particularly high cost involved in protein synthesis. All of the energy released at rest when nutrients are metabolized to CO_2 and H_2O must eventually be dissipated as heat, unless stored by the tissues. However, the total metabolizable energy of food does not all pass through the form of free energy, as the unused fraction is immediately converted to heat. Heat energy cannot be transferred back to a biologically utilizable form of energy, since the body is not a heat engine. A decreased efficiency of conversion of food energy means that more energy must be provided in order to maintain a sufficient rate of free energy production as ATP. Since ATP cannot be stored to any extent, any rise in ATP utilization must be accompanied by a corresponding increase in ATP synthesis. This increased demand for nutrient conversion, whether derived from endogenous or exogenous sources, will bring about a rise in heat production. Energetic efficiency varies for different metabolic pathways, and thus the various factors determining the utilization of each pathway will influence the extent of heat production related to the ingestion of food.

The phenomenon of "waste heat" is influenced by many factors, some of which are not directly associated with food intake, and for this reason the term *thermogenic response* is a more general term and includes the specific dynamic action. For example, dinitrophenol uncouples oxidative phosphorylation and increases heat production, whereas thyroxine influences mitochondrial functions to increase heat production. Epinephrine and norepinephrine also increase heat production, but by a different mechanism. Thermogenesis is increased by certain nutrient deficiencies. Changing metabolic pathways also alter thermogenesis. Increasing the level of nutritional intake increases thermogenesis, as does a rapid growth rate.

Several hypotheses have been advanced which involve thermogenesis with the regulation of body fat content. Shapiro [117] has offered the hypothesis that fat accumulation and mobilization in adipose tissue is regulated by a so-called set point of adiposity. Shapiro relates the total metabolic activity of adipose tissue to the adipocyte cell surface area, which in turn is a function of both cell number and cell size, as well as the total mass of adipose tissue. Presumably, regulation of energy balance could be achieved by regulation of thermogenesis, for example, an increased thermic response to food when adipose tissue exceeds an individual set point, and a decreased thermogenesis when the amount of adipose tissue falls below the set point.

Stirling and Stock [120] have suggested that when alpha-glycerolphosphate levels are low due to a lack of carbohydrate precursors, or to an elevated enzyme activity, fatty acid oxidation is increased and re-esterification is decreased. This would result in thermogenesis owing to the fact that the step catalyzed by acyl CoA dehydrogenase has a low efficiency of ATP formation. Furthermore, fatty acids are well-known uncouplers of oxidative phosphorylation, and owing to a partial loss in respiratory control, there is a tendency toward an increased rate of oxidation. On the other hand, Ball [10] calculated that if adequate glucose or glycogen is present to furnish the alpha-glycerolphosphate for adipose tissue of the rat, cyclic lipolysis and subsequent re-esterification can proceed with concomitant heat loss, amounting to as much as 15 percent of the animal's resting metabolism. It is evident that thermogenesis can vary in amount dependent on which metabolic pathways are involved and on the availability of particular substrates, which ultimately depend on the nutrients ingested as well as the nutritional and metabolic status of the individual.

Trenkle [122] has reviewed the role of the endocrine system in partitioning nutrients among the tissues of the ruminant body. The energy metabolism of ruminants is complicated by the lack of absorption of glucose because of the fermentation of carbohydrates in the rumen. Increased secretion of glucagon after feeding may play a special role in stimulating hepatic gluconeogenesis from absorbed amino acids. During fasting, gluconeogenesis appears to be maintained by an increased secretion of glucocorticoids. Growth hormone causes a flow of carbon away from adipose tissue and the mammary gland, whereas insulin promotes the flow of carbon toward these tissues. Larger, leaner breeds of cattle tend to have more growth hormones and less insulin in the plasma, which favors increased and more prolonged growth of skeletal muscle rather than shifting energy to adipose tissue.

RELATION OF ENERGY INTAKE TO NITROGEN METABOLISM

A major objective of any nutritional program is to achieve a satisfactory nitrogen balance. It is generally accepted that the level of energy intake plays an important role in nitrogen metabolism and, in particular, the utilization of dietary nitrogen. This area has been the subject of several extensive reviews [29, 94, 96]. The subject has received recent attention because of new interest in determining (1) the appropriate energy intake to treat or prevent obesity while preserving body protein and (2) the appropriate energy intake for achieving the optimum nitrogen balance in acute catabolic states. Nitrogen equilibrium was traditionally considered to be impossible in the presence of a negative calorie balance. However, studies over the past decade have tended to question this conventional wisdom. It is commonly stated that dietary protein will be degraded for fuel purposes in the absence of an adequate calorie intake. However, Blackburn and associates [18] reported that the intravenous administration of a mixture of amino acid without any accompanying energy source had a more beneficial effect on the nitrogen balance of postoperative patients than the administration of these same amino acids along with a hypocaloric amount of glucose. This observation was followed by studies in normal subjects and in patients with varying degrees of injury and surgical infection. There is now general agreement that amino acids given alone can improve the negative nitrogen balance to a greater degree than hypocaloric dextrose given by peripheral vein. However, three groups have reported an improvement in nitrogen balance when glucose was added to the amino acid solution [47, 64, 128].

The proportion of the resting energy metabolism that is directly related to the maintenance of nitrogen equilibrium remains obscure. The endogenous urinary nitrogen excretion is somehow associated with the rate of resting energy metabolism, which in turn is a function of the body cell mass. Extensive animal studies [22] have suggested that most mammals demonstrate a value of approximately 2 mg of urinary nitrogen per basal kcal when receiving no nitrogen intake. However, the authorities who prepared the handbook on *Recommended Dietary Allowances* reviewed a group of experimental studies in man, which yielded an average of 1.35 mg of nitrogen per basal kcal. To this nitrogen loss may be added an average of 0.9 gm per day for fecal loss and 0.3 gm per day for cutaneous loss, producing, for a 70-kg man receiving no nitrogen intake, a ratio of nitrogen loss to energy expenditure of 3.7 gm per 1800 kcal. When the loss of efficiency in nitrogen utilization is taken into consideration, this value for the minimal nitrogen loss will be increased from 3.7 to approximately 5.2 gm per day on a minimal intake of high-quality protein.

Fatty acids from adipose tissue provide a large and ready source of 2-carbon energy, but cannot be used as a source of net production of glucose, glycogen, or carbohydrate intermediates in mammalian tissues. The glucogenic amino acids from either body protein or dietary sources represent the major gluconeogenic reserve of the body, along with the glycerol released from triglyceride breakdown. Therefore, in clinical conditions in which hypermetabolism and increased nitrogen excretion are associated with tissue catabolism, the increased urea synthesis and excretion are thought to represent accelerated gluconeogenesis and not simply the need to supply extra 2-carbon fragments for general fuel at the expense of body protein [78].

It has been emphasized by Munro [97] that variations in energy intake among normal individuals may contribute extensively to the apparent variability in minimal nitrogen intake required to achieve nitrogen equilibrium. Much of the variability may be due to the difficulty of finding a population of individuals whose normal energy intake exactly equals their energy expenditure. Consequently, deviations in intake, above or below the true energy needs of each individual, can be expected to contribute to the variability of any estimate of protein intake needed by normal individuals to achieve nitrogen balance.

A review of extensive metabolic studies in man led Calloway and Spector [29] to state:

> To the general principles set forth that on a fixed adequate protein intake, energy level is the deciding factor in N balance and that with a fixed adequate caloric intake, protein level is the determinant, may be added a corollary. That is, at each fixed inadequate protein intake there is an individual limiting energy level beyond which increasing calories without protein, or protein without calories, is without benefit.

The influence of energy intake on nitrogen metabolism has been demonstrated by Elwyn and coworkers [48] in a series of ten surgical patients receiving total parenteral nutrition in which the calorie intake was increased from 15 to 59 kcal per kg. This caused a retention of 1.7 gm of nitrogen per 1000 kcal, surprisingly similar to the relationship demonstrated by others in normal subjects.

The relation between nitrogen balance and energy metabolism is best considered when nitrogen balance is plotted against energy balance rather than energy intake, as this serves to differentiate the requirements to meet energy expenditure from the effects of energy intake on nitrogen balance. In the depleted patient, as in the normal adult, nitrogen balance can be increased by increasing either the nitrogen or the energy intake. However, the depleted subject differs from the normal in being able to achieve a positive nitrogen balance at a zero energy balance. This is usually not possible in normal adults, whose steady state behavior will reflect a zero nitrogen balance no matter how high the nitrogen intake, as long as a zero energy balance is present. If the energy balance is positive, nitrogen balance will be positive, and the slope of the line relating nitrogen and energy balance may increase somewhat with increasing nitrogen intake, but will always pass through the origin. The depleted patient in this respect seems to resemble a growing child, in that the protein tissues of the body can be increased without requiring a positive energy balance with the associated deposition of body fat. Thus, there is an important difference between achieving a positive nitrogen balance by increasing nitrogen intake vs increasing the energy intake. With the former, one increases the lean body mass without adding fat, but the latter requires a deposition of some body fat as well as lean tissue. This is an important consideration if the goal of nutritional therapy is to restore lean tissue and fat in approximately the proportion that has been lost. The effect of increasing energy intake on nitrogen balance is to deposit lean tissue and fat in a ratio of approximately 1 to 2. This is in contrast to weight loss due to starvation or acute catabolic states, in which the ratio of lean tissue to fat that is lost is between 2 to 1 and 4 to 1. Therefore, energy should be given in an amount that will meet energy expenditure and will provide, in addition, an appropriate rate of fat restoration, if that is desired. This is in contrast to the intake of nitrogen, which should be given to provide an appropriate rate of restoration of lean body mass, remembering that 1 gm of nitrogen is the equivalent of approximately 32 gm of lean body mass.

In addition to acting as a nonspecific energy source in the diet, carbohydrate exerts a specific protein-sparing action above and beyond that seen with the administration of fat. This is commonly thought to be related to the capacity of carbohydrate to stimulate the output of insulin. The administration of glucose and/or insulin to rats [95] has produced a decrease in urinary nitrogen and an increase in muscle protein, without benefiting the level of liver protein. Studies of 3-methylhistidine [124] indicate that carbohydrate administration causes both an increased synthesis and a reduced breakdown of muscle protein, which is typical of the action of insulin. These effects were not seen when fat was fed.

Long and coworkers [88] have reported that the administration of intravenous fat did not improve the nitrogen balance of severely burned patients when compared with isocaloric amounts of dietary carbohydrate. This difference in the response of nitrogen balance to the type of nonprotein energy source was noted by Shaffer and Coleman [116], who performed metabolic balance studies on patients with typhoid fever. Jeejeebhoy and coworkers [67] have reported that patients with moderate degrees of catabolism demonstrate a temporary increase in the protein-sparing effect of carbohydrate compared to fat, but that this advantage is less evident after the first week, and after ten days the two nonprotein calorie sources appear to be approximately equal in their protein-sparing effectiveness.

ENERGY INTAKE AND MUSCLE FATIGUE

Clinicians have known for many years that prolonged and complicated convalescence from a severe illness or injury is associated with weakness and easy fatigue, which persists well beyond the time when the patient has resumed regular meals and some degree of normal physical activity. The precise etiology of this prolonged weakness and easy fatigue has not been determined. However, it seems reasonable to suggest that the symptoms may be related to the breakdown of muscle constituents, which is a central part of the metabolic response in acute catabolic states. The extent to which these symptoms can be minimized by better attention to nutrition during the immediate period following illness or injury remains an important area for study. However, anyone interested in the nutrition of hospitalized patients should bear in mind the experimental work that has been done in normal man relating energy intake to muscle fatigue [16].

Christensen and Hanson [32] demonstrated in 1939 that work performance was significantly affected by dietary intake. With increasing intensity of work, the fraction of the energy supplied by carbohydrate was found to rise. After 3 to 7 days of a high-carbohydrate intake, the work time was 210 minutes compared with only 80 minutes after an equal time on an isocaloric fat diet. Protein does not seem to serve as a significant energy source during exercise. In fasting man, up to 50 percent of the energy utilized for physical activity may be supplied by the oxidation of free fatty acids. During short-term exercise, however, carbohydrate stores are an important factor in determining work performance [65]. Certain kinds of muscular exercise in fasting man have indicated that the major source of carbohydrate fuel is the muscle's own glycogen store. Bërgstrom and Hultman [15] have utilized a needle biopsy method to show a progressive decrease in muscle glycogen during muscular work. Fatigue ensues when glycogen becomes depleted. When glucose is infused continuously during muscular exercise, the decrease in glycogen consumption is reduced. Muscle glycogen concentration in man can be increased by giving a carbohydrate-rich diet, particularly if there has been a preceding period of carbohydrate depletion. The enhancement of glycogen stores is localized to the muscles that have worked and does not affect other muscle groups. This is in contrast to a diet of fat plus protein after exercise, which results in a slow and an incomplete restoration of glycogen. The aforementioned studies have been on relatively short periods of exercise; however, Bërgstrom has also demonstrated that diet affects the ability to perform prolonged exercise through its effect on glycogen stores. The administration of glucose may enable the previously exhausted subject to continue work during prolonged exercise. If exercise is prolonged, blood glucose may become an increasingly important substrate as glycogen stores are diminished.

The energy required for sustained exercise depends on two metabolic fuels: glucose and long-chain fatty acids. Glycogen reserves are limited, whereas fatty acid stores in adipose tissue are very large. Newsholme [98] has reviewed the interactions between these two fuels for the support of prolonged exercise. He presents evidence suggesting the metabolic limits to the rate of fatty acid utilization, so that sustained high level exercise requires the utilization of both fatty acids and glucose. The mechanism by which fatty acid oxidation reduces carbohydrate utilization in muscle plays an important part in ensuring that exercise can continue beyond the limits imposed by the level of glycogen storage. The availability of fatty acids for oxidation will allow the use of both fatty acids and glucose for a longer period of time. Since muscle fatigue occurs when glycogen stores are depleted, reduction in the rate of glucose utilization by the oxidation of fatty acids is obviously beneficial.

It is generally accepted that the increased urea nitrogen excretion with illness and injury is at the expense of muscle protein. The extent to which muscle protein may be lost before weakness and fatigue are evident is not clearly determined. Noltenius and Hartmann [99] studied the work performance of normal subjects during an 8-day fast. Work to exhaustion on a bicycle ergometer was essentially decreased to half the control value. The maximal strength of grip was not affected, but the fatigability was markedly increased. Benedict and coworkers [13], studying young, healthy males, found that weight loss during partial starvation reached 10 percent of normal body weight before loss of muscle function was measured. This is of interest since the majority of patients undergoing elective operation lose less than 10 percent of their normal body weight during convalescence, yet find that weakness and fatigue is commonly associated with the later stages of their recovery. Therefore, the extent of muscle protein breakdown may be only one of various factors contributing to these symptoms.

ENERGY EXPENDITURE IN OBESITY

For many years the problem of obesity has been simplified to the proposition that obese patients simply are the ones who consume energy in excess of their energy expenditure. A corollary assumption has been that energy intake is the major controlling factor in energy balance regulation and that a defective appetite control (i.e., hyperphagia) is the primary cause of obesity in man and experimental animals. However, a recent review by Rothwell and Stock [110] has summarized data showing that in man it is possible to observe a two- to threefold range of food intake in a population of subjects of the same age and weight, and that one can divide people who are apparently similar in other respects, into "large eaters" and "small eaters." The correlation between either body weight or body fat content and food intake has not been satisfactory [129]. A major difficulty in the study of human obesity remains the lack of precision with which daily energy intake and energy expenditure can be measured [54]. These difficulties make it easy for errors of 100 kcal per day, or more, to go unnoticed—errors that can easily result in obesity if continued over several years. It therefore seems naive to expect definitive information about the energy intake and energy expenditure of obese subjects when they are studied for only a few days.

Garrow [55] has reviewed most of the human overfeeding experiments to determine whether the resting metabolic rate was affected. In only five of ten studies did the authors conclude that energy expenditure was increased by overfeeding. It is possible that a large portion of the "excess energy" reported in some of these human studies might be due to methodologic error. However, it is difficult to assume sufficient error to explain the findings from the studies of Sims and coworkers [118, 119]. They persuaded lean volunteers to increase their food intake for several months to produce an average increase in body weight of 20 percent. The energy cost of maintaining this greater weight was 11.3 $MJ/m^2/day$

compared to a value of 7.5 before overfeeding and 5.4 in spontaneously obese subjects, indicating that overfeeding had resulted in a large increase in metabolic rate that was not accounted for in weight gain alone.

Rothwell and Stock [110] emphasize that over the past twenty years evidence has accumulated to indicate that energy expenditure is a major component in the regulation of energy balance and, in some situations, may be of greater importance than changes in food intake. Until recently, the contribution made by brown adipose tissue to the total metabolic rate was considered small even in nonshivering thermogenesis. This view has slowly changed to the idea that in the cold adapted rat, this small amount of tissue, which is less than 1 percent of body weight, can receive up to a third of the cardiac output and extract most of the oxygen supplied to it. These same investigators have shown that brown adipose tissue accounts for all of the increased thermogenic response to norepinephrine in hyperphagic cafeteria-fed rats.

Romsos [109] has discussed the efficiency of energy retention in genetically obese animals and in dietary-induced thermogenesis, emphasizing that these two conditions represent two extremes in efficiency of energy retention. The former deposits dietary energy with high efficiency; the latter deposits dietary energy with low efficiency. These differences in efficiency of energy retention must be associated at the cellular level with changes in the production or the utilization of high energy phosphate bonds. It has been speculated that the unique proton-conductance pathway of brown adipose tissue, which reduces the efficiency of ATP synthesis, is suppressed in the ob/ob mouse and accelerated in rats with dietary-induced thermogenesis. Romsos stresses the lack of data on the two largest components of energy expenditure in most tissues, namely Na^+, K^+-ATPase, and protein turnover, which is needed to understand the extreme difference in energy retention of these two conditions.

Many investigators are engaged in the search for mechanisms of thermogenesis that may be inhibited in the obese animal or man. There is increasing evidence that nonshivering thermogenesis occurs in man and perhaps could be associated with brown adipose tissue. Therefore, the control of dietary thermogenesis has become one of the central areas of investigation that may offer important insight into the development of obesity in man.

ENERGY EXPENDITURE DURING STARVATION

Numerous studies of protein-calorie malnutrition and experimental starvation have shown that dietary restriction causes a reduction in energy expenditure. From 1860 to 1910, various aspects of the metabolic response to starvation were studied by European investigators, first in the animal and then in adults who were professional fasters. One of the most complete studies of prolonged human starvation was conducted by Benedict and his associates at the Carnegie Institute of Nutrition in Boston in 1912 [12]. A normal, 40-year-old male was under continuous metabolic study for 31 days while receiving only distilled water. He spent his nights sleeping in a bed calorimeter; his days were occupied with respiration experiments, physical measurements, and psychologic tests. This period of fasting caused a weight reduction from 60.6 to 47.4 kg, or about 22 percent loss of body weight. The pattern of the weight loss showed a rapid fall during the first 10 days, followed by a relatively uniform loss of 320 gm per day. Perhaps the most striking feature of this experiment was the reduction of the basal metabolism. The average of direct and indirect measurements of calorimetry showed a starting basal metabolism of 1,432 calories per 24 hours, which dropped to 1,002 calories per day by the end of the third week and remained near this level for the last 10 days. Thus, by the twenty-first day of the fast the individual had reduced his heat production by 30 percent at a time when he had lost only 16.7 percent of his body weight. By the twenty-first day, this reduction in metabolism was associated with the cumulative loss of 200 gm of nitrogen. DuBois states, "It is evident that the fall in metabolism was caused not only by the decreased body and protoplasmic mass, but also by some specific and unknown factor which tends to protect the organism from the evil results of starvation" [37].

A monumental study of partial starvation in man was conducted by Keys and coworkers [73] during World War II at the University of Minnesota. These workers studied the effects of administering approximately 1,600 calories a day with low quality protein to a group of young, adult volunteers. Over a period of six months they lost approximately 24 percent of their body weight, and their basal energy expenditure decreased an average of 39 percent. These workers calculated that while the BMR decreased 39 percent per individual, the reduction amounted to 31 percent when calculated per square meter of body surface, and 19.5 percent when calculated per kilogram of body weight. At the end of the study, the rate of change of the BMR was close to 0, which indicated that the rate of change of the BMR roughly corresponded to the rate of weight loss. Eight of these individuals were placed in each of four groups, which received different amounts of food during the first 12 weeks of rehabilitation. These groups regained 35 to 70 percent of the decrease in BMR, which they had experienced during the period of partial starvation. The work output of the heart per minute was calculated to be reduced approximately 50 percent during partial starvation. This, and other, evidence was noted to support the idea that the metabolic rate is reduced more in starvation than would be expected from the reduction in body size. The intensity of the metabolism per unit of tissue mass is also reduced. Certain of the subjects in this study showed evidence of congestive heart failure during the early days of nutritional rehabilitation. This was interpreted as being the result of increasing the energy expenditure of the body faster than the depleted myocardium could regain its pumping capacity.

Plasma levels of thyroid hormones have been studied during dietary restriction, and serum thyroxine levels do not change. Those of reverse T_3 were first studied by Danforth and coworkers [35, 36], who showed that these levels fall during overeating. Leslie and coworkers [85] showed that rT_3 is initially high in patients with anorexia nervosa and that it falls within the normal range after a 25 percent gain in body weight. Serog and coworkers [115] studied the relationship between plasma and thyroid hormones and oxygen consumption in 14 healthy volunteers, who were given a restricted diet for two weeks, in which their average weight decreased from 63.46 to 59.00 kilograms, followed by two weeks on a diet that held their weight at that level. The oxygen consumption was reduced from an average of 140 to 103 ml per minute, and returned to 126 ml per minute during the weight-stabilizing diet. During the weight loss period, T_3 levels decreased from 150 to 105 ng/100 ml and rose to 125 ng/100 ml during the weight stabilization. The values for rT_3 rose sharply with weight loss and returned toward normal during the weight stabilization period. The authors suggest that one of the early steps in the process of adapting to a restricted energy intake is to alter the ratio of specific deiodination of T_4 to rT_3 versus T_3.

Cahill and Aoki [26] have emphasized that man is unique among the animals in the proportion of his basal metabolic expenditure that is devoted to the central nervous system. The overwhelming survival advantage given to man by his added intellect when compared to his animal competitors involves a metabolic price, i.e., the need to keep this critical tissue continuously supplied with appropriate fuel. A normal-sized individual may use one quarter of his total BMR for his brain, whereas in smaller individuals, particularly children, this proportion may be as high as 50 percent of the total resting energy utilization. Thus, the brain has two problems: its high energy need and its selective requirement for small water-soluble molecules as fuel. Owen, Felig, and Cahill [52, 101] have studied the various mechanisms by which the body adapts to starvation. Their investigations established that ketones could substitute for a substantial part of the glucose need of the brain during starvation; therefore, the metabolic response to starvation involves conservation of body tissues both by reduction in resting energy expenditure and by reduction in the demands of gluconeogenesis, with its associated depletion of muscle protein.

ENERGY EXPENDITURE OF HOSPITALIZED PATIENTS

The level of resting energy need of a hospitalized patient represents a balance between the decrease that normally occurs with tissue depletion from partial starvation and whatever increase may be present as the result of disease or injury. Among similar individuals with comparable basal metabolic rates, the amount of physical activity is usually the most important fact causing major variations in total energy expenditure. Hospitalized patients have a great reduction in the energy expenditure associated with physical activity [87]. Various activities from sitting beside the bed to slowly walking in the hospital corridors cause increases in energy expenditure from 25 to 250 percent above normal resting values. However, the short time involved with these limited physical activities means that the patient who moves between bed and chair will increase his daily energy expenditure only 5 to 10 percent, and the majority of ambulatory patients have total energy expenditures per day that are only 15 to 25 percent above their resting level of energy expenditure [76].

The conventional hospital diet approximates 2,100 calories per day, and the specific dynamic action associated with ingestion of a balanced meal is reported to be in the range of 8 to 10 percent of the caloric intake. Quantitative information is limited, but it appears that patients receiving total parenteral nutrition respond with a similar degree of specific dynamic action in the absence of extensive weight loss and tissue depletion.

Another factor influencing the energy expenditure of the hospitalized patient relates to body temperature. The pioneering work of DuBois and collaborators [41] examined the influence of fever on the BMR in a variety of medical conditions, including the administration of vaccines to produce fever for therapeutic purposes. When the results of all these studies were plotted together, each degree Centigrade of fever was associated with a 13 percent increase in energy expenditure (a 7.2 percent increase for each degree Fahrenheit) (Figure 4-3). Study of the original data

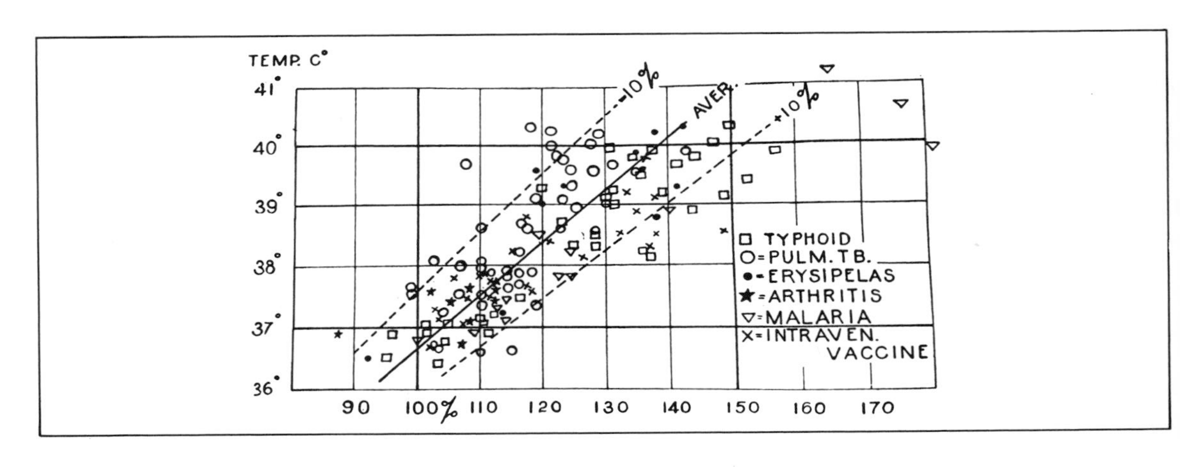

Figure 4-3. *The relation of basal metabolic rate to body temperature in six different types of clinical fever. (E. F. DuBois,* Basal Metabolism in Health and Disease. *Philadelphia: Lea & Febiger, 1924. P. 332.)*

reveals that patients with chronic pulmonary tuberculosis demonstrated fever with comparatively slight increase in energy expenditure and little or no "toxic destruction" of protein. At the other extreme were patients with acute typhoid fever who demonstrated much larger increases than average in energy expenditure for the degree of fever and had large increases in nitrogen excretion. DuBois writes of these patients: "On theoretical grounds we should give enough calories to cover the total expenditure of energy. If we wish to prevent all loss of body protein, we must give 50 to 100 percent more calories than the calculated heat production, but it is doubtful if this is necessary or advisable" [37].

Comparison of the resting metabolic expenditure with body temperature in postoperative patients was studied by Kinney and Roe [74]. In these patients, the 13 percent relationship reported by DuBois provided an approximate correlation for brief periods of low-grade fever. However, this was in distinct contrast to cases of major peritonitis and burns, in which the metabolic expenditure was increased well beyond the value predicted from the extent of the fever [108].

ENERGY EXPENDITURE IN SURGICAL CONDITIONS

Surgeons throughout history have tended to assume that the rate and extent of weight loss paralleled the magnitude of an injury or infection. A related assumption was that the energy expenditure was sufficiently high in surgical patients to account for the weight loss that was observed. The increase in energy expenditure during the first 10 days after injury was estimated to reach the range of 5,000 to 6,000 kcal per day, or 3 times the normal resting energy expenditure [3, 92]. It was even suggested that the large increases in energy expenditure with injury and infection exceeded the capacity of fat stores to meet these added demands and, therefore, the increased nitrogen loss represented the breakdown of amino acids from muscle protein to achieve more 2-carbon fuel.

When a noninvasive system was designed for prolonged measurements of gas exchange and nitrogen excretion in surgical patients [77], the extent of the increases in energy expenditure could be predicted for a given individual during the maximum catabolic period (Figure 4-4). Patients undergoing elective operation will not have their postoperative energy expenditure at rest vary from the preoperative values by more than 10 percent in the absence of any significant complications. Detailed studies with well-calibrated equipment may indicate increases of 5 to 8 percent during the first postoperative week; however, such changes are usually within the range of error of most measurement techniques. This is in contrast to the previously well-nourished patient who sustains multiple fractures, along with a variable amount of soft tissue injury. Such a patient commonly demonstrates an increase in resting energy expenditure of 10 to 25 percent, lasting over a period of 2 to 3 weeks following the injury. It is not uncommon for this period of mild hypermetabolism at rest to be followed by sufficient weight loss to cause the associated resting metabolism to decrease to 10 to 15 percent below normal. During the acute catabolic reaction associated with a major infection, such as peritonitis, the energy expenditure is commonly increased from 20 to 50 percent above normal levels. When the infection and the inflammatory response have subsided and body temperature has returned to normal, the patient will have lost a significant amount of body weight and will go through a period in which the resting energy expenditure may be decreased below normal. The only surgical condition associated with sustained levels of energy expenditure of 50 percent or more above normal levels is the major thermal burn, in which the energy expenditure commonly reaches 50 to 100 percent above predicted normal values (Figure 4-5). We have seen occasional situations in which the presence of unsuspected dead tissue has caused patients to have a resting energy expenditure elevated to the range of a major burn. Regardless of the stimulus to energy expenditure from injury or illness, the largest increases in

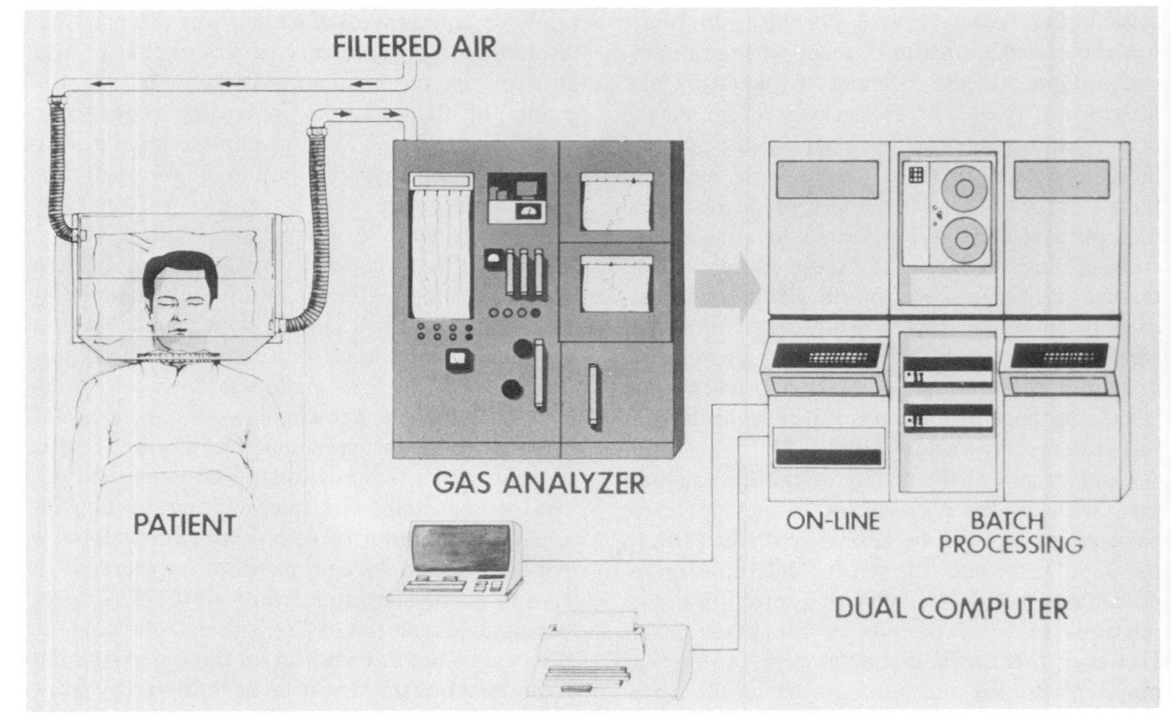

Figure 4-4. *A schematic representation of the noninvasive canopy-spirometer-computer system for prolonged measurements of gas exchange and the pattern of breathing without the artifacts of a mask or mouthpiece. (J. M. Kinney, The Application of Indirect Calorimetry to Clinical Studies. In J. M. Kinney (Ed.),* Assessment of Energy Metabolism in Health and Disease. *Columbus, OH: Ross Laboratories, 1980.)*

resting energy expenditure are seen in the well-nourished, heavily muscled young adult male. The lowest increases are seen in the female, the elderly, and the poorly nourished patient.

It is important to remember that the patient who has become depleted from simple starvation demonstrates a decrease in resting energy expenditure that, on a percentage basis, is greater than his decrease in body weight. The patient with weight loss during a long and complicated convalescence may show a "relative hypermetabolism" rather than the absolute increase in energy expenditure shown by the nondepleted patient. For example, the patient with major infection together with weight loss may have an oxygen consumption that is normal, or only slightly elevated, for the patient's normal weight. However, this represents significant hypermetabolism for the extent of tissue depletion that has occurred.

It is of interest that the resting energy expenditure (REE) and the nitrogen excretion on a given intake tend to increase in roughly parallel fashion with disease and injury, just as they both tend to decrease below normal in the presence of starvation. This parallel change led Cairnie and others [27] to suggest that the increased heat production of the rat after long-bone fracture could be accounted for by the increase in protein oxidation. They also noted that the expected increase in heat production and nitrogen excretion did not occur in rats fed a diet adequate in calories but containing no protein. Calculations in human cases of sepsis and burns suggest that increased protein oxidation is not sufficient to account for the

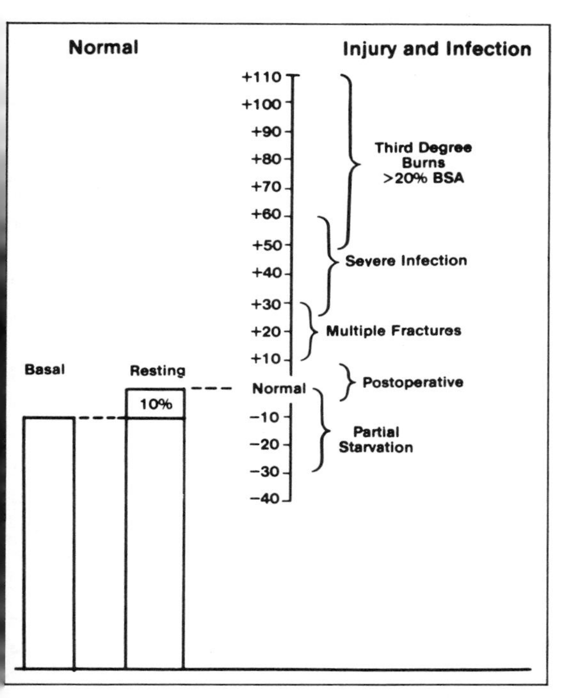

Figure 4-5. *The increases in resting energy expenditure that have been shown to occur during the acute catabolic phase of injury or infection, when compared with the decreases which develop during partial starvation. (J. M. Kinney, The Application of Indirect Calorimetry to Clinical Studies. In J. M. Kinney (Ed.),* Assessment of Energy Metabolism in Health and Disease. *Columbus, OH: Ross Laboratories, 1980.)*

measured increases in energy expenditure. An important aspect of surgical investigation over the coming years will be to define the level of resting hypermetabolism that is conducive to survival and recovery. This portion of hypermetabolism should be supported by adequate ventilation, circulation, and nutrition, but other hypermetabolism may be undesirable and justify the use of pharmacologic or physical means of abolishing this segment of the increased metabolism.

The measured increases in resting energy expenditure associated with major injury and infection are not well understood. The explanations may be related to alterations in intermediary metabolism and the oxidation of foodstuffs, the supply and demand for ATP, or problems related to thermal regulation and the underlying balance of the production and loss of heat.

Certain hormones, particularly the catecholamines and the thyroid hormones, cause an increase in resting energy expenditure. It is not clear whether this is the result of the influence of these hormones on pathways of intermediary metabolism or on the effectiveness of coupling between oxidation and the production of ATP in the mitochondria.

Major injury and sepsis may cause an increase in demands for ATP to support an increase in tissue and organ work (i.e., an increase in the work of breathing, the work of the left ventricle, or biochemical work in the liver). Various workers have suggested that the largest demand for cellular ATP utilization is to support protein synthesis and maintain the sodium-potassium pump across the cell membrane. Energy demands for each of these processes may be increased by injury or infection for reasons that are not clear at present. Also, there may be a reduction in the amount of ATP being produced for a given amount of substrate oxidation and heat production. In this loss of coupling efficiency, a given need for ATP would have to be met by a greater overall resting energy metabolism. An additional possibility has to do with various cyclic chemical reactions, in which one product is transformed to another product along pathway A and the second product can be converted back to the original product along pathway B [70]. The activity of these "futile cycles" requires energy, and there is some evidence that the hypermetabolic state associated with injury and illness may have an increased utilization of ATP to support these cycles without the production of corresponding work.

There may be an increase in the neuroendocrine stimulus for heat production, perhaps from alterations in the behavior of centers involved in thermoregulation, which are located in the brain stem. Maintaining the ambient temperature at higher than normal levels with the open treatment of the badly burned patient can reduce both the resting energy expenditure and the nitrogen loss of the patient. However, an unexplained difference exists between investigators regarding the role of surface heat loss in the hypermetabolism of the burn patient. Wilmore and associates [126] found that an increased surface heat loss was not the dominant factor in the hypermetabolism of the burn injury, whereas Arturson [2] and Caldwell and coworkers [28] have each presented studies supporting the primary role of surface heat loss in producing the hypermetabolic state of the burn patient.

Cuthbertson and coworkers [122] have reported that caring for patients with long-bone fractures at elevated ambient temperatures can reduce the daily urinary nitrogen excretion, although data are not available as to whether the resting energy expenditure can be decreased in such patients. It seems obvious that the major burn suffers from obligatory loss of both heat and water through the area of a third degree burn. Therefore, there must be a corresponding increase in heat production to maintain the body heat content (body temperature) within an acceptable limit. Why the patient with a major burn begins to run a low-grade fever by the second week after injury, when there is no evidence of infection, remains to be explained.

ENERGY EXPENDITURE WITH TOTAL PARENTERAL NUTRITION

The specific dynamic action of oral foodstuffs (SDA) appears to be seen with either bolus injection or constant infusion of intravenous diets. Giving amino acids by vein increases the energy expenditure at rest by approximately 10 percent over 24 hours in normal subjects and postoperative patients. The intravenous administration of glucose, or lipid, in amounts up to energy expenditure have little effect. Indeed, small amounts of glucose (approximately 100 gm per day) appear to decrease energy expenditure under certain circumstances, an effect that may be mediated by insulin [47]. When carbohydrate is given in excess of the energy expenditure, whether orally [35] or intravenously [48], it increases the energy expenditure. In the intravenous studies, 20 percent of the excess carbohydrate was used to increase energy expenditure, whereas 80 percent was converted to fat, suggesting that the increase in resting energy expenditure is related to lipogenesis. Thus, if an excess of 1,000 kcal is given, it will increase energy expenditure by 200 kcal, or roughly 10 to 20 percent of the BMR. A case was recently observed in which a carbohydrate intake of twice the resting energy expenditure, given to an infected hypermetabolic patient, resulted in a nonprotein RQ which remained below 1.0. This unexpected finding indicated a continued utilization of endogenous fat for energy, even though the high-carbohydrate intake would have been expected to abolish all net fat oxidation. The excess carbohydrate intake appeared to be associated with an increased oxygen consumption, an increased excretion of urinary norepinephrine, and, apparently, an increased glycogen deposition. The importance of such a response to intravenous carbohydrate led to a prospective clinical study of the response to parenteral nutrition, given as hypertonic glucose and amino acids, in depleted patients compared to those who were acutely injured or infected [5]. Eighteen depleted patients with a weight loss averaging 21 percent and a resting energy expenditure of minus 21 percent of predicted normal values were compared with a group of 14 acutely injured or septic patients, whose resting energy expenditure averaged 14 percent above predicted normal values, despite mild-to-moderate weight loss in certain patients. Resting energy expenditure was measured daily along with nitrogen balance. Beginning on the second day, total parenteral nutrition was started by central vein, and both groups were given an amount of TPN that varied from 1.35 to 2.25 times the daily energy expenditure at rest. The response of the acutely septic and injured patients to the high-glucose intake seemed to differ from the response of the nutritionally depleted patients (Figure 4-6). The depleted patients showed the expected response to a high-glucose intake by synthesizing fat from the excess carbohydrate, as

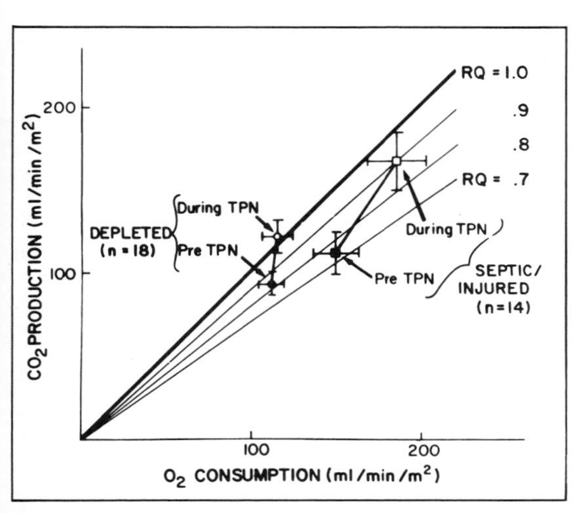

Figure 4-6. *Alterations in resting energy expenditure as indicated by values for gas exchange and respiratory quotient before and after a week of receiving high carbohydrate total parenteral nutrition. Note that the depleted patients did not increase their O_2 consumption while the acutely septic or injured patients had a thermogenic response. (J. Askanazi et al., Influence of total parenteral nutrition on fuel utilization in injury and sepsis.* Ann. Surg. *191:40, 1980.)*

indicated by a respiratory quotient that rose above 1.0 because of an increased CO_2 output, while the resting energy expenditure, as represented by O_2 consumption, was essentially unchanged. In contrast, when the acutely ill patients were given this same relative amount of hypertonic glucose and amino acids, there was not only a large increase in CO_2 production but a significant rise in O_2 consumption, with the RQ remaining below 1.0. These acutely ill patients responded to large infusions of glucose with a minimal reduction in net lipolysis [30], an increase in norepinephrine excretion and resting energy expenditure, and continuing fat oxidation [5].

In the acutely ill patients who were given total parenteral nutrition with fat partially replacing the glucose, there was essentially no increase of O_2 consumption. CO_2 production was increased, but not nearly to the extent seen in patients receiving glucose alone. The relationship of minute ventilation seems to bear a relatively constant relationship to the level of CO_2 production in the different clinical conditions in which total parenteral nutrition was used [6]. This suggests that the hyperventilation reported with TPN is largely related to the increased CO_2 production, more than to an increase in dead-space ventilation. An increased tidal volume accounts for most of the increase in minute ventilation. This increased tidal volume is secondary to an increased respiratory flow rate while the inspiratory time remains constant.

In both nutritionally depleted patients and acutely ill patients, the use of fat emulsions to provide part of the nonprotein calories results in a significant reduction in CO_2 production and, hence, in ventilatory requirements [7]. Additionally, in the acutely ill patients, the increased O_2 consumption or calorigenic response caused by high-carbohydrate intakes can be significantly minimized by the use of fat emulsions. Clinically, the increase in CO_2 production caused by the administration of a large carbohydrate load could be a critical factor in the patient with marginal pulmonary reserve. Likewise, parenteral nutrition with high-carbohydrate loads should be avoided at times of weaning a patient from mechanical ventilation. At this time, the patient's limited capacity for CO_2 excretion may easily be overwhelmed by an increase of 50 to 100 percent in the amount of CO_2 to be excreted as the result of giving a high-carbohydrate load as part of parenteral nutrition.

REFERENCES

1. Anand, B. K., and Brobeck, J. R. Hypothalamic control of food intake in rats and cats. *Yale J. Biol. Med.* 24:123, 1951.
2. Arturson, M. G. S. Metabolic changes following thermal injury. *World J. Surg.* 2:203, 1978.
3. Artz, C. P., and Reiss, E. *The Treatment of Burns.* Philadelphia: Saunders, 1957.
4. Ashworth, A. Metabolic rates during recovery from protein-calorie malnutrition: The need for a new concept of specific dynamic action. *Nature* 223:407, 1969.
5. Askanazi, J., Carpentier, Y. A., Elwyn, D. H., Nordenstrom, J., Jeevanandam, M., Rosen-

baum, S. H., Gump, F. E., and Kinney, J. M. Influence of total parenteral nutrition on fuel utilization in injury and sepsis. *Ann. Surg.* 191:40, 1980.
6. Askanazi, J., Rosenbaum, S. H., Hyman, A. I., Silverberg, P. A., Milic-Emili, J., and Kinney, J. M. Respiratory changes induced by the large glucose loads of total parenteral nutrition. *J.A.M.A.* 243:1444, 1980.
7. Askanazi, J., Nordenström, J., Rosenbaum, S. H., Elwyn, D. H., Hyman, A. I., Carpentier, Y. A., and Kinney, J. M. Nutrition for the patient with respiratory failure: Glucose vs. fat. *Anesthesiology* 54:373, 1981.
8. Atwater, W. O., and Rosa, E. B. Quoted in G. Lusk. *The Elements of the Science of Nutrition.* Philadelphia: Saunders, 1931. P. 61.
9. Atwater, W. O., and Benedict, F. G. Quoted in G. Lusk. *The Elements of the Science of Nutrition.* Philadelphia: Saunders, 1931. P. 61.
10. Ball, E. G. Some energy relationships in adipose tissue. *Ann. N.Y. Acad. Sci.* 131:225, 1965.
11. Behnke, A. R., Osserman, E. F., and Welham, W. C. Lean body mass: Its clinical significance and estimation from excess fat and total body water determinations. *Arch. Intern. Med.* 91:585, 1953.
12. Benedict, F. G. A study of prolonged fasting. *Carnegie Inst. Washington Publ.* No. 203, 1915.
13. Benedict, F. G., Miles, W. R., Roth, P., and Smith, H. M. Human vitality and efficiency under prolonged restricted diet. *Carnegie Inst. Washington Publ.* No. 280, 1919.
14. Benzinger, T. H., and Kitzinger, C. Gradient Layer Calorimetry-Human Calorimetry. In C. M. Herzfeld and J. D. Hardy (Eds.), *Temperature: Its Measurement and Control in Science and Industry.* New York: Rheinhold, 1963. Vol. 3, p. 87.
15. Bergström, J., and Hultman, E. A study of glycogen metabolism during exercise in man. *Scand. J. Clin. Lab. Invest.* 19:218, 1967.
16. Bergström, J., and Hultman, E. Nutrition for maximal sports performance. *J.A.M.A.* 221:999, 1972.
17. Black, J. Lectures on the Elements of Chemistry. In T. H. Benzinger (Ed.), *Temperature, Part I. Arts and Concepts.* Stroudsburg, PA: Dowden, Hutchinson, and Ross, 1977. P. 116.
18. Blackburn, G. L., Flatt, J. P., Clowes, G. H. A., and O'Donnell, T. E. Peripheral intravenous feeding with isotonic amino acid solutions. *Am. J. Surg.* 125:447, 1973.
19. Boothby, W. M., and Sandiford, I. Summary of the basal metabolism data on 8,614 subjects with especial reference to the normal standards for the estimation of the basal metabolic rate. *J. Biol. Chem.* 54:783, 1922.
20. Bray, G. A., and Gallagher, T. F. Manifestations of hypothalamic obesity in man: A comprehensive investigation of eight patients and a review of the literature. *Medicine* 54:301, 1975.
21. Brobeck, J. R. Food and Temperature. In G. Pincus (Ed.), *Recent Progress in Hormone Research.* New York: Academic, 1960. P. 439.
22. Brody, S. Basal Metabolism and Body Weight. In S. Brody, *Bioenergetics and Growth.* New York: Rheinhold, 1945. P. 368.
23. Buskirk, E. R., Iampietro, P. F., and Welch, C. E. Variations in resting metabolism with changes in food, exercise and climate. *Metabolism* 6:144, 1957.
24. Buskirk, E. R., Thompson, R. H., and Whedon, G. D. Metabolic response to cold air in men and women in relation to total body fat content. *J. Appl. Physiol.* 18:603, 1963.
25. Buskirk, E. R., Hodgson, J., and Blair, D. Assessment of Daily Energy Balance: Some Observations on the Methodology for Indirect Determinations of Energy Intake and Expenditure. In J. M. Kinney (Ed.), *Assessment of Energy Metabolism in Health and Disease.* Columbus, OH: Ross Laboratories, 1980. P. 113.
26. Cahill, G. F., Jr., and Aoki, T. T. Partial and Total Starvation. In J. M. Kinney (Ed.), *Assessment of Energy Metabolism in Health and Disease.* Columbus, OH: Ross Laboratories, 1980. P. 129.
27. Cairnie, A. B., Campbell, R. M., Pullar, J. D., and Cuthbertson, D. P. The heat production consequent on injury. *Br. J. Exp. Pathol.* 38:504, 1957.
28. Caldwell, F. T., Bowser, B. H., and Crabtree, J. H. The effect of occlusive dressings on the energy metabolism of severely burned children. *Ann. Surg.* 193:579, 1981.
29. Calloway, D. H., and Spector, H. Nitrogen balance of men with marginal intakes of protein and energy. *J. Nutr.* 105:914, 1975.
30. Carpentier, Y. A., Askanazi, J., Elwyn, D. H., Jeevanandam, M., Gump, F. E., Hyman, A. I., Burr, R., and Kinney, J. M. Effect of hypercaloric glucose infusion on lipid metabolism in injury and sepsis. *J. Trauma* 19:649, 1979.
31. Celesia, G. G., Archer, C. R., and Chung, H. D. Hyperphagia and obesity: Relationship to medial hypothalamic lesions. *J.A.M.A.* 246:151, 1981.
32. Christensen, E. H., and Hansen, O. Arbeitsfahigkeit und Ernahrung. *Scand. Arch. Physiol.* 81:160, 1939.

33. Cohn, C., and Joseph, D. Influence of body weight and body fat on appetite of "normal" lean and obese rats. *Yale J. Biol. Med.* 34:598, 1962.
34. Damask, M. C., Weissman, C., Hyman, A. I., Askanazi, J., Rosenbaum, S. H., and Kinney, J. M. A systematic approach to validation of gas exchange measurements during mechanical ventilation (abstract). *Crit. Care Med.* 9:270, 1981.
35. Danforth, E., Horton, E. S., O'Connell, M., Sims, E. A. H., Burger, A. G., Ingbar, S. H., Braverman, L., and Vagenakis, A. G. Dietary-induced alterations in thyroid hormone metabolism during overnutrition. *J. Clin. Invest.* 64: 1336, 1979.
36. Danforth, E. Nutritionally Induced Alterations in Metabolism. In J. M. Kinney (Ed.), *Assessment of Energy Metabolism in Health and Disease.* Columbus, OH: Ross Laboratories, 1980. P. 139.
37. DuBois, E. F. *Basal Metabolism in Health and Disease.* Philadelphia: Lea & Febiger, 1924.
38. DuBois, E. F. *Basal Metabolism in Health and Disease.* Philadelphia: Lea & Febiger, 1924. P. 108.
39. DuBois, E. F. *Basal Metabolism in Health and Disease.* Philadelphia: Lea & Febiger, 1924. P. 148.
40. DuBois, E. F. *Basal Metabolism in Health and Disease.* Philadelphia: Lea & Febiger, 1924. P. 237.
41. DuBois, E. F. *Basal Metabolism in Health and Disease.* Philadelphia: Lea & Febiger, 1924. P. 311.
42. Durnin, J. V. G. A. The use of surface area and of body weight as standards of reference in studies on human energy expenditure. *Br. J. Nutr.* 13:68, 1959.
43. Durnin, J. V. G. A., and Passmore, R. *Energy Work and Leisure.* London: Heinemann, 1967. P. 165.
44. Durnin, J. V. G. A., Edholm, O. G., Miller, D. S., and Waterlow, J. C. How much food does man require? *Nature* 242:418, 1973.
45. Edholm, O. G., Fletcher, J. G., Widdowson, E. M., and McCance, R. A. The energy expenditure and food intake of individual men. *Br. J. Nutr.* 9:286, 1955.
46. Edmundson, W. Individual variations in basal metabolic rate of mechanical work efficiency in East Java. *Ecol. Food Nutr.* 8:189, 1979.
47. Elwyn, D. H., Gump, F. E., Iles, M., Long, C. L., and Kinney, J. M. Protein and energy sparing of glucose added in hypocaloric amounts to peripheral infusions of amino acids. *Metabolism* 27:325, 1978.
48. Elwyn, D. H., Gump, F. E., Munro, H. N., Iles, M., and Kinney, J. M. Changes in nitrogen balance of depleted patients with increasing infusions of glucose. *Am. J. Clin. Nutr.* 32:1597, 1979.
49. Elwyn, D. H., Kinney, J. M., Jeevanandam, M., Gump, F. E., and Broell, J. R. Influence of carbohydrate intake on glucose kinetics in injured patients. *Ann. Surg.* 190:117, 1979.
50. Elwyn, D. H., and Kinney, J. M. A Unique Approach to Measuring Total Energy Expenditure by Indirect Calorimetry. In J. M. Kinney (Ed.), *Assessment of Energy Metabolism in Health and Disease.* Columbus, OH: Ross Laboratories, 1980. P. 54.
51. Farrar, K. R. *Dr. Joseph Priestley.* Birmingham, Eng.: North Western Museum of Science and Industry, 1976.
52. Felig, P. Starvation. In L. J. DeGroot (Ed.), *Endocrinology.* New York: Grune & Stratton, 1979. Vol. 3, p. 1927.
53. Garrow, J. W., and Hawes, S. F. The role of amino acid oxidation in causing "specific dynamic action" in man. *Br. J. Nutr.* 27:211, 1972.
54. Garrow, J. S. Problems in Measuring Human Energy Balance. In J. M. Kinney (Ed.), *Assessment of Energy Metabolism in Health and Disease.* Columbus, OH: Ross Laboratories, 1980. P. 2.
55. Garrow, J. S. *Energy Balance and Obesity in Man.* Amsterdam: Elsevier/North Holland, 1978.
56. Glick, Z., Teague, R. J., and Bray, G. A. Brown adipose tissue: Thermic response increased by a single low protein, high carbohydrate meal. *Science* 213:1125, 1981.
57. Grande, F., and Keys, A. Body Weight, Body Composition and Caloric Status. In R. S. Goodhart and M. E. Shils (Eds.), *Modern Nutrition in Health and Disease* (6th ed.). Philadelphia: Lea & Febiger, 1980. P. 3.
58. Grande, F. Energy Expenditure of Organs and Tissues. In J. M. Kinney (Ed.), *Assessment of Energy Metabolism in Health and Disease.* Columbus, OH: Ross Laboratories, 1980. P. 88.
59. Hegsted, D. M. Energy needs and energy utilization. *Nutr. Rev.* 32:33, 1974.
60. Hetherington, A. W., and Ranson, S. W. Hypothalamic lesions and adiposity in the rat. *Anat. Rec.* 78:149, 1940.
61. Himms-Hagen, J. Cellular thermogenesis. *Annu. Rev. Physiol.* 38:315, 1976.
62. Hirsch, J., and Han, P. W. Cellularity of rat adipose tissue: Effect of growth, starvation and obesity. *J. Lipid Res.* 10:77, 1969.

63. Hoebel, B. G., and Teitelbaum, P. Weight regulation in normal and hypothalamic hyperphagic rats. *J. Comp. Physiol. Psychol.* 16:189, 1966.
64. Howard, L. Dobbs, A., and Chodos, R. A comparison of administering protein alone and protein plus glucose on nitrogen balance. *Clin. Res.* 24:501A, 1976.
65. Hultman, E., Sjoholm, H., Sahlin, K., and Edstrom, L. Glycolytic and Oxidative Energy Metabolism and Contraction Characteristics of Intact Human Muscle. In R. Porter and J. Whelan (Eds.), *Human Muscle Fatigue: Physiological Mechanisms.* London: Pitman Medical, 1981. P. 19.
66. Janowitz, H. D., and Hollander, F. The time factor in the adjustment of food intake to varied caloric requirements in the dog: A study of the precision of appetite regulation. *Ann. N. Y. Acad. Sci.* 63:56, 1955.
67. Jeejeebhoy, K. M., Anderson, G. H., Nakhooda, A. F., Greenberg, G. R., Sanderson, I., and Marliss, E. B. Metabolic studies in total parenteral nutrition with lipid in man: Comparison with glucose. *J. Clin. Invest.* 57:25, 1976.
68. Jequier, E. Studies with Direct Calorimetry in Humans: Thermal Body Insulation and Thermoregulatory Responses During Exercise. In J. M. Kinney (Ed.), *Assessment of Energy Metabolism in Health and Disease.* Columbus, OH: Ross Laboratories, 1980. P. 15.
69. Johnson, R. E. Techniques for Measuring Gas Exchange. In J. M. Kinney (Ed.), *Assessment of Energy Metabolism in Health and Disease.* Columbus, OH: Ross Laboratories, 1980. P. 32.
70. Katz, J. Energy Balance and Futile Cycling. In J. M. Kinney (Ed.), *Assessment of Energy Metabolism in Health and Disease.* Columbus, OH: Ross Laboratories, 1980. P. 63.
71. Kennedy, G. C. The role of depot fat in the hypothalamic control of food intake in the rat. *Proc. R. Soc. Lond. Ser. B.* 140:578, 1953.
72. Keys, A., Brožek, J., Henschel, A., Mickelsen, O., and Taylor, H. L. *The Biology of Human Starvation.* Minneapolis: University of Minnesota Press, 1950. P. 303.
73. Keys, A., Brožek, J., Henschel, A., Mickelsen, O., and Taylor, H. L. *The Biology of Human Starvation.* Minneapolis: University of Minnesota Press, 1950. P. 1385.
74. Kinney, J. M., and Roe, C. F. Caloric equivalent of fever: I. Patterns of postoperative response. *Ann. Surg.* 156:610, 1962.
75. Kinney, J. M., Morgan, A. P., Domingues, F. J., and Gildner, K. J. A method for continuous measurement of gas exchange and expired radioactivity in acutely ill patients. *Metabolism* 12: 205, 1964.
76. Kinney, J. M., Long, C. L., Gump, F. E., and Duke, J. H. Tissue composition of weight loss in surgical patients: I. Elective operation. *Ann. Surg.* 168:459, 1968.
77. Kinney, J. M., Duke, J. H., Long, C. L., and Gump, F. E. Tissue fuel and weight loss after injury. *J. Clin. Pathol.* (Suppl. 4), (Royal College of Pathology). 23:65, 1970.
78. Kinney, J. M., Long, C. L., and Duke, J. H. Carbohydrate and Metabolism After Injury. In R. Porter and J. Knight (Eds.), *Energy Metabolism in Trauma.* London: Churchill, 1970. P. 103.
79. Kinney, J. M. The Application of Indirect Calorimetry to Clinical Studies. In J. M. Kinney (Ed.), *Assessment of Energy Metabolism in Health and Disease.* Columbus, OH: Ross Laboratories, 1980. P. 42.
80. Kleiber, M. Body size and metabolism. *Hilgardia* 6:315, 1932.
81. Kleiber, M. *The Fire of Life: An Introduction to Animal Energetics.* Huntington, NY: Krieger, 1975.
82. Krebs, H. A. The Metabolic Fate of Amino Acids. In H. N. Munro and J. B. Allison (Eds.), *Mammalian Protein Metabolism.* New York: Academic, 1964. Vol. 1, p. 125.
83. Lavoisier, A. L. *Elements of Chemistry in a New Systematic Order* (2nd ed., translated from the French by Robert Kerr). Edinburgh: Creech, 1793.
84. Lavoisier, A. L., and De LaPlace, P. S. Memoire sur la Chaleur, (translated excerpts). In T. H. Benzinger (Ed.), *Temperature, Part I. Arts and Concepts.* Stroudsburg, PA: Dowden, Hutchinson & Ross, 1977. P. 145.
85. Leslie, R. D. G., Isaacs, A. J., Gomez, J., Raggett, P. R., and Bayliss, R. Hypothalamo-pituitary-thyroid function in anorexia nervosa: Influence of weight gain. *Br. Med. J.* 2:526, 1978.
86. Liebig, J. Die organische Chemie in ihrer Anwendung auf Physiologie und Pathologie. *Braunschweig,* 1842.
87. Long, C. L., Kopp, K., and Kinney, J. M. Energy demands during ambulation in surgical convalescence. *Surg. Forum* 20:93, 1969.
88. Long, J. M., Wilmore, D. W., Mason, A. D., and Pruitt, B. A., Jr. Effect of carbohydrate and fat intake on nitrogen excretion during total intravenous feeding. *Ann. Surg.* 185:417, 1977.
89. Lusk, G. *The Elements of the Science of Nutrition* (4th ed.). Philadelphia: Saunders, 1928.
90. Mayer, J., and Bates, M. W. Blood glucose and food intake in normal and hypophysectomized,

alloxan-treated rats. *Am. J. Physiol.* 168:812, 1952.
91. Miller, D. S., and Mumford, P. Gluttony: I. An experimental study of overeating low- or high-protein diets. *Am. J. Clin. Nutr.* 20:1212, 1967.
92. Moore, F. D. Endocrine changes after anesthesia, surgery and unanesthetized trauma in man. *Recent Prog. Horm. Res.* 13:511, 1957.
93. Moore, F. D., et al. *The Body Cell Mass and Its Supporting Environment.* Philadelphia: Saunders, 1963.
94. Munro, H. N. Carbohydrate and fat as factors in protein utilization and metabolism. *Physiol. Rev.* 31:449, 1951.
95. Munro, H. N., Black, J. G., and Thomson, W. S. T. The mode of action of dietary carbohydrate on protein metabolism. *Br. J. Nutr.* 13:475, 1959.
96. Munro, H. N. General Aspects of the Regulation of Protein Metabolism by Diet and Hormones. In H. N. Munro and J. B. Allison (Eds.), *Mammalian Protein Metabolism.* New York: Academic, 1964. Vol. 1, p. 381.
97. Munro, H. N. Energy Intake and Nitrogen Metabolism. In J. M. Kinney (Ed.), *Assessment of Energy Metabolism in Health and Disease.* Columbus, OH: Ross Laboratories, 1980. P. 105.
98. Newsholme, E. A. The Glucose/Fatty Acid Cycle and Physical Exhaustion. In R. Porter and J. Whelan (Eds.), *Physiological Mechanisms.* Proceedings from a Ciba Foundation Symposium. London: Pitman Medical, 1981. P. 89.
99. Noltenius, F., and Hartmann, H. Das Verhalten der Korperfunktionen im Hungerzustande. *Dtsch. Med. Wochenschr.* 62:644, 1936.
100. Norton, A. C. Portable Equipment for Gas Exchange. In J. M. Kinney (Ed.), *Assessment of Energy Metabolism in Health and Disease.* Columbus, OH: Ross Laboratories, 1980. P. 36.
101. Owen, O. E., Morgan, A. P., Kemp, H. G., et al. Brain metabolism during fasting. *J. Clin. Invest.* 46:1589, 1967.
102. Pace, H., and Rathbun, E. N. Studies on body composition: III. The body water and chemically combined nitrogen content in relation to fat content. *J. Biochem.* 158:685, 1945.
103. Passmore, R., and Durnin, J. V. G. A. Human energy expenditure. *Physiol. Rev.* 35:801, 1955.
104. Peters, J. P., and Van Slyke, D. D. *Quantitative Clinical Chemistry: Interpretations* (2nd ed.). Baltimore: Williams & Wilkins, 1946. Vol. 1, p. 3.
105. Pettenkofer, M., and Voit, C. Quoted in G. Lusk, *The Elements of the Science of Nutrition.* Philadelphia: Saunders, 1931. P. 17.
106. Ramsay, W. *Joseph Black, M.D.: A Discourse.* Glasgow: MacLehose, 1904.
107. Rochelle, R. H., and Horvath, S. M. Metabolic responses to food and acute cold stress. *J. Appl. Physiol.* 27:710, 1969.
108. Roe, C. F., and Kinney, J. M. The caloric equivalent of fever: II. Influence of major trauma. *Ann. Surg.* 161:140, 1965.
109. Romsos, D. R. Efficiency of energy retention in genetically obese animals and in dietary-induced thermogenesis. *Fed. Proc.* 40:2524, 1981.
110. Rothwell, N. J., and Stock, M. J. A paradox in the control of energy intake in the rat. *Nature* 273:146, 1978.
111. Rothwell, N. J., and Stock, M. J. Regulation of energy balance. *Annu. Rev. Nutr.* 1:235, 1981.
112. Rubner, M. Quoted in M. Kleiber, *The Fire of Life: An Introduction to Animal Energetics.* Philadelphia: Wiley, 1961. P. 267.
113. Russek, M. Current Hypotheses in the Control of Feeding Behavior. In G. J. Mogenson and F. R. Calaresu (Eds.), *Neural Integration of Physiological Mechanisms and Behavior.* Toronto: University of Toronto Press, 1975. P. 128.
114. Seguin, A., and Lavoisier, A. L. Premier Memoire sur la Respiration des Animaux (an English summary). In T. H. Benzinger (Ed.), *Temperature, Part I. Arts and Concepts.* Stroudsburg, PA: Dowden, Hutchinson & Ross, 1977. P. 206.
115. Serog, P., Apfelbaum, M., Autissier, D., Brigant, L., and Baigts, F. Plasma Thyroid Hormones and Oxygen Consumption in 14 Healthy Volunteers on Low-Calorie and Weight-Maintaining Diets. A Preliminary Study. In L. E. Mount (Ed.), *Energy Metabolism.* London: Butterworth, 1980. P. 273.
116. Shaffer, P. A., and Coleman, W. Protein metabolism in typhoid fever. *Arch. Intern. Med.* 4:538, 1909.
117. Shapiro, B. In M. Apfelbaum (Ed.), *Energy Balance in Man.* Paris: Masson, 1973.
118. Sims, E. A. H., Goldman, R. F., Gluck, C. M., Horton, E. S., Kelleher, P. C., and Rowe, D. W. Experimental obesity in man. *Trans. Assoc. Am. Physicians* 81:153, 1968.
119. Sims, E. A. H., Danforth, E., Horton, E. S., Bray, G. A., Glennon, J. A., and Salans, L. B. Endocrine and metabolic effects of experimental obesity in man. *Rec. Prog. Horm. Res.* 29:457, 1973.
120. Stirling, J. L., and Stock, M. J. In M. Apfelbaum (Ed.), *Energy Balance in Man.* Paris: Masson, 1973.
121. Stolwijk, J. A. J. Partitional Calorimetry. In J. M. Kinney (Ed.), *Assessment of Energy Me-*

tabolism in Health and Disease. Columbus, OH: Ross Laboratories, 1980. P. 21.

122. Tilstone, W. J., and Cuthbertson, D. P. The Protein Component of the Disturbances of Energy Metabolism in Trauma. In R. Porter and J. Knight (Eds.), *Energy Metabolism in Trauma.* London: Churchill, 1970. P. 43.
123. Trenkle, A. Endocrine regulation of energy metabolism in ruminants. *Fed. Proc.* 40:2536, 1981.
124. Wassner, S. J., Orloff, S., and Holliday, M. A. Use of 3-methylhistidine to show cyclic variation of, and effects of starvation on, muscle protein catabolic rats. *Fed. Proc.* 35:497, 1976.
125. Webb, P. Energy Balance over a 45-Hour Period with a Suit Calorimeter. In J. M. Kinney (Ed.), *Assessment of Energy Metabolism in Health and Disease.* Columbus, OH: Ross Laboratories, 1980. P. 24.
126. Wilmore, D. W., Mason, A. D., Jr., Johnson, D. W., and Pruitt, B. A., Jr. Effect of ambient temperature on heat production and heat loss in burn patients. *J. Appl. Physiol.* 38:593, 1975.
127. Winslow, C.-E. A., Herrington, L. P., and Gagge, A. P. A new method of partitional calorimetry. *Am. J. Physiol.* 116:641, 1936.
128. Wolfe, B. M., Culebras, J. M., Tweedle, D., and Moore, D. F. Effect of glucose on the nitrogen-sparing effect of amino acids given intravenously. *Surg. Forum* 26:39, 1976.
129. York, D. A., Morgan, J. B., and Taylor, T. G. The relationship of dietary induced thermogenesis to metabolic efficiency in man. *Proc. Nutr. Soc.* 39:57A, 1980.

Intermediary Metabolism

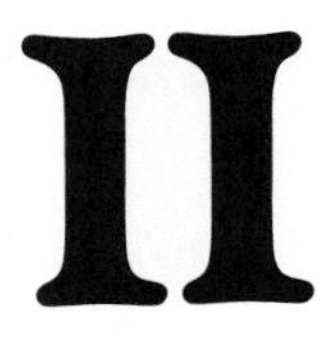

5

Protein and Amino Acid Metabolism

Katrin Valgeirsdóttir
Hamish N. Munro

The protein of the diet is normally the original source of the 20 amino acids used by the body for synthesizing tissue proteins. In order to make these amino acids accessible to the body, the dietary protein is hydrolyzed in the alimentary tract and absorbed into the circulation almost entirely as free amino acids. Once in the body, the free amino acids are used for the process of protein synthesis and for making many other nitrogenous tissue components such as creatine, purine, and pyrimidine bases. Protein and amino acid metabolism describes the history of dietary protein in the body, and the requirement for dietary protein can be related to the need of the body for individual amino acids.

AMINO ACID STRUCTURE AND CLASSIFICATION

The amino acids are so named from the presence of carboxyl and amino groups on the first (α) carbon atom of the amino acid skeleton, thus

$$R-CH\begin{cases} NH_2 \\ COOH \end{cases}$$

In the case of glycine, R is a hydrogen atom, but in the case of all other amino acids R consists of one or more carbon atoms. Consequently, there are four different groups attached to the α carbon atom of all amino acids except glycine, and these amino acids can accordingly exist as optically active isomers that rotate the plane of polarized light to the left (levorotatory) or to the right (dextrorotatory). Only one of each amino acid isomer pair is found in dietary and in body proteins. Since the amino and carboxyl groups of such naturally occurring amino acids occupy the same relative spatial relationship to one another, they are designated as the L-series, while those not usually found in proteins are the D-series, regardless of how they rotate the plane of polarized light. Many metabolic reactions, including protein synthesis and transport across cell walls, distinguish L- from D-forms. Some D-forms can be transformed by transamination into the L-form and thus made available to the body. Only certain D-amino acids, however, can become available to the body. In man, these are D-methionine and D-phenylalanine. Even so, recent studies [90] with intravenous infusion of D-methionine indicate that it is utilized less efficiently than the L-form. Hence, for practical purposes, synthetic mixtures of amino acids for oral or parenteral use should consist only of L-amino acids.

The chemical differences between amino acids are features of the carbon side-chain, R. Twelve are neutral amino acids, namely, glycine; alanine; the hydroxy-amino acids serine and threonine; the branched chain amino acids valine, leucine, and isoleucine; the sulfur-containing amino acids methionine and cysteine; and the aromatic amino acids phenylalanine, tyrosine, and tryptophan. Three amino acids are dibasic (arginine, lysine, histidine) and two diacidic (aspartic acid, glutamic acid). These features are important in determining the characteristics of amino acid transport across membranes.

The 20 common amino acids of dietary proteins are classified for nutritional purposes into *essential* and *nonessential.* An amino acid is an essential dietary constituent if its skeleton is not synthesized in the body. The other amino acids are nonessential if they can be made within the body from carbon and nitrogen precursors. All animal species from single-celled organisms through to mammals and man need the same 8 to 10 preformed amino acids (essential amino acids). The essential amino acids needed by man are histidine, isoleucine, leucine, lysine, methionine, phenylalanine, threonine, tryptophan, and valine; in addition, cysteine and tyrosine are synthesized in the body from the essential amino acids methionine and phenylalanine, respectively. The remaining nine amino acids used for protein synthesis (alanine, arginine, aspartic acid, asparagine, glutamic acid, glutamine, glycine, proline, and serine) are *not essential* in the diet, since the body is able to synthesize them from simple precursors.

In order to provide an account of protein metabolism appropriate for surgical nutrition, the subject will be presented in three sequential stages. First, an account of relevant aspects of amino acid metabolism will be given. Then, protein and amino acid metabolism in different organs and tissues of the body will be described and integrated, especially to illustrate how an influx of amino acids is dealt with. Finally, the needs of the body for dietary protein and amino acids will be assessed in the light of these mechanisms. Some further information on clinically relevant aspects of amino acid metabolism can be found in the proceedings of a recent symposium [35].

AMINO ACID METABOLISM

Protein present in the diet is enzymically hydrolyzed in the alimentary tract and is presented to the body as free amino acids passing into the portal vein for uptake by the tissues. In the tissues, the free amino acids undergo numerous metabolic reactions summarized in Figure 5-1. These reactions can be classified into three groups: (1) protein synthesis, which is accompanied by protein breakdown so that the amino acids are eventually returned to the free amino acid pool, (2) catabolic reactions leading to production of CO_2 and energy, or storage of the carbon as carbohydrate and fat, while the nitrogen is eliminated as urea, and (3) utilization of the nitrogen to synthesize nonessential amino acids and other nitrogenous small molecules such as purine and pyrimidine nucleotides and creatine. Presented in this section is a description of the free amino acid pools of the tissues, followed by discussion of the metabolic reactions in which they participate.

Free Amino Acid Pools

Free amino acid concentrations in the tissues average 0.01 M, which is only about 0.5 percent of the concentration of protein-bound amino acids in the body, namely, 2 M. Consequently, a small change in the amount of body protein will involve a much larger disturbance in free amino acid flux. In the body of the rat (Table 5-1), the concentrations of individual free amino acids do not reflect the average composition of the tissue proteins or of the dietary protein. In the tissues, the concentrations of free *essential* amino acids

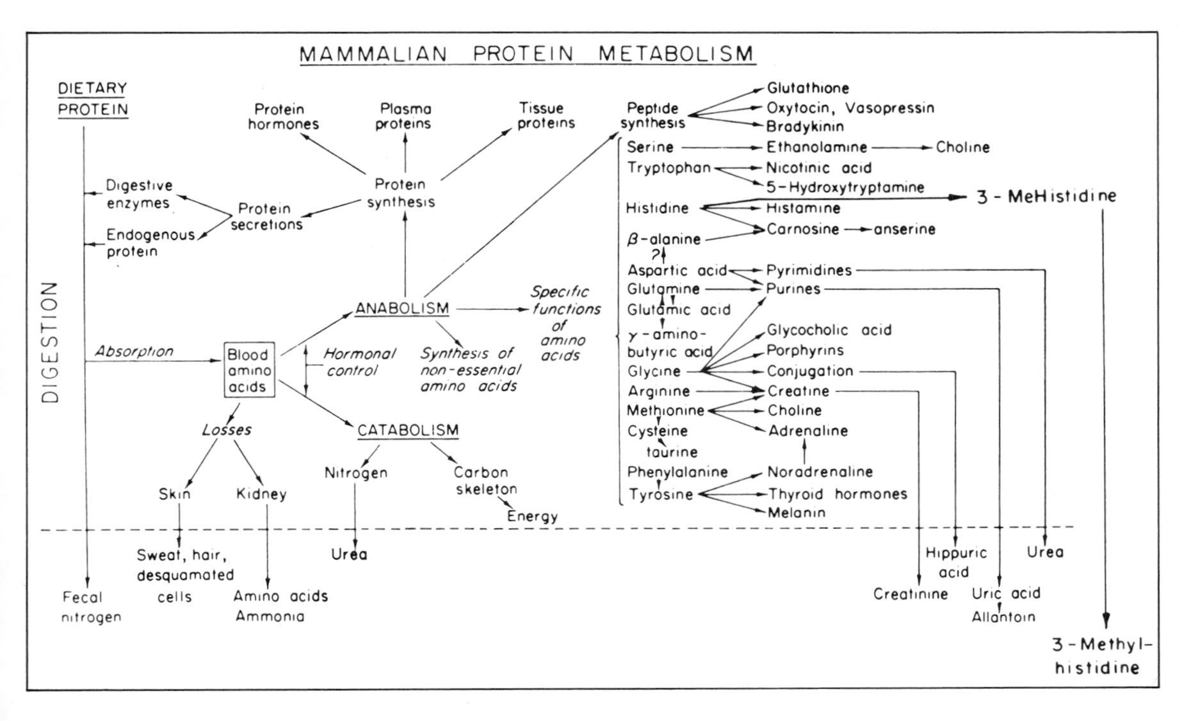

Figure 5-1. *Major pathways of mammalian protein metabolism. (Adapted from H. N. Munro, Biochemical Aspects of Protein Metabolism. In H. N. Munro and J. B. Allison (Eds.),* Mammalian Protein Metabolism. *New York: Academic, 1964. Vol. 1, p. 31.)*

are lower than those of the free *nonessential* amino acids, notably alanine, glutamic acid, glutamine, and glycine. The high tissue levels of these four amino acids are undoubtedly related to their participation in many metabolic reactions, so that they are readily and extensively synthesized. Table 5-1 shows that this large difference in concentration does not extend to the plasma, so that the tissue-to-plasma ratio is much greater for most nonessential amino acids than for essential amino acids.

Transport of free amino acids across cell membranes has been studied in detail, particularly in the case of intestinal mucosa, kidney tubules, and blood-brain barrier. Transport of individual amino acids into all these tissues can be assigned to one or more of several overlapping categories based on Christensen's [8] classification (Figure 5-2). Each category is presumably dependent on a carrier protein present in the cell membrane, but not yet purified from mammalian cells. Christensen's different systems listed below show competition between amino acids in each category, and less or no competition between amino acids belonging to different transport categories:

1. The A-system of Christensen has a high affinity for alanine and several other neutral amino acids including the synthetic model amino acid α-aminoisobutyric acid (AIB), which is not metabolized or incorporated into proteins and thus provides an uncomplicated measure of transport. The A-system is energy-dependent, that is, it is abolished by respiratory inhibitors.

2. The L-system of Christensen transports neutral branched-chain amino acids, such as leucine and aromatic amino acids. This system does not depend directly on energy, but is operated by

Table 5-1. *Concentration in the Body of the Fasting Rat of Protein-Bound Amino Acids and Free Amino Acids per 100 gm Body Weight, and of Free Plasma Amino Acids per 100 ml Plasma*

	Total Body Content (μmoles/100 gm)		Plasma Content (μmoles/100 ml)
Amino Acid	Protein-bound	Free	Free
Essential			
Arginine	8400	7	16
Histidine	3600	24	11
Isoleucine	8400	10	8
Leucine	16500	14	16
Lysine	8900	15	41
Methionine	4050	6	9
Phenylalanine	5800	9	9
Threonine	7550	20	24
Tryptophan	980	2	
Tyrosine	3550	8	9
Valine	9400	12	18
Nonessential			
Alanine	13500	100	32
Aspartic acid	11300	19	1
Glutamic acid	17700	132	15
Glutamine		223	55
Glycine	24700	323	45
Serine	12400	20	23

Source: Adapted from J. D. Herbert, R. A. Coulson, and T. Hernandez, Free amino acid in the caiman and rat. *Comp. Biochem. Physiol.* 17:583, 1966.

exchanging with intracellular amino acids, such as methionine, which is concentrated by the A-system.

3. Two distinguishable transport systems for basic amino acids, one of which is exclusive for this category of amino acids.

4. A system for transport of dicarboxylic (acidic) amino acids.

It has been proposed by Meister [58] that glutathione plays a major role in the mechanism of transport of amino acids across the cell membrane (Figure 5-2). He suggests that amino acids entering the cell, presumably through one of the aforementioned transport systems, are acted on by the cell membrane enzyme γ-glutamyltranspeptidase, which transfers the γ-glutamyl group of glutathione to the amino acid. This compound passes into a cell and is cleaved by γ-glutamylcyclotransferase to release the amino acid and glutamic acid cyclized in the form of 5-oxoproline. The latter is then returned by a series of reactions back to glutathione to complete the cycle. A small number of patients have been observed who lack the enzyme 5-oxo-prolinase and cannot complete the cycle; consequently, they excrete large amounts of 5-oxoproline in the urine.

Protein Synthesis and Degradation

The amount of protein in a cell is regulated by changes in the rates of either synthesis or break-

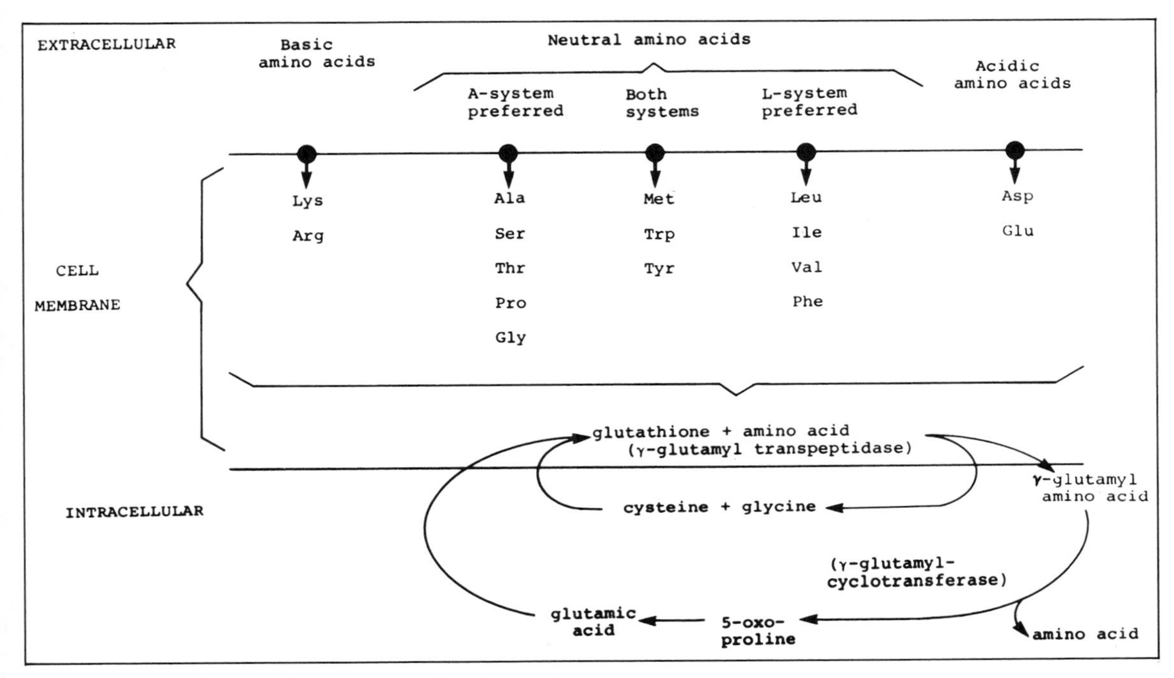

Figure 5-2. *Mechanisms for transport of amino acids into cells, based on the concepts of Christensen [8] for transport classes and of Meister [58] for the role of γ-glutamyl transpeptidation.*

down of the protein or by both. The term *turnover* refers to the combination of synthesis and breakdown, which in the steady state are equal in magnitude. Figure 5-3 shows that protein synthesis consists of two phases: *transcription,* in which messenger RNA (mRNA) is made on the DNA template, and *translation* of the mRNA in the cytoplasm with formation of the protein, often followed by *posttranslational modification* of the protein.

Transcription

In order to make the information in the chromosomes available, specific portions of chromosomal DNA are transcribed into mRNA, the structural RNA of the ribosomes (rRNA), and the transport RNA (tRNA), which recognizes individual amino acids for insertion into the growing peptide chain. Each of these RNA species is transcribed from the DNA as a precursor form. The rRNA is first made as a single long strand, which breaks into the two shorter strands (18S and 28S) found in the two ribosomal subunits. The messenger RNAs are first assembled as larger heterogeneous nuclear RNAs (HnRNAs), which are split within the nucleus to yield the mRNAs. These mRNAs then undergo addition of polyadenylic acid (poly-A) through the action of the nuclear enzyme poly-A polymerase and finally become associated with proteins for transport into the cytoplasm as messenger ribonucleoprotein particles (mRNP). Formation of these RNA species using the DNA template involves three RNA polymerases: polymerase I in the nucleolus transcribing rRNA, polymerase II in the nuclear sap for mRNA, and polymerase III to make tRNA and the small 5S RNA found as an additional component of the larger ribosomal subunit. Inhibitors of RNA synthesis can be used to explore these processes. Low doses of actinomycin D inhibit rRNA synthesis, whereas larger

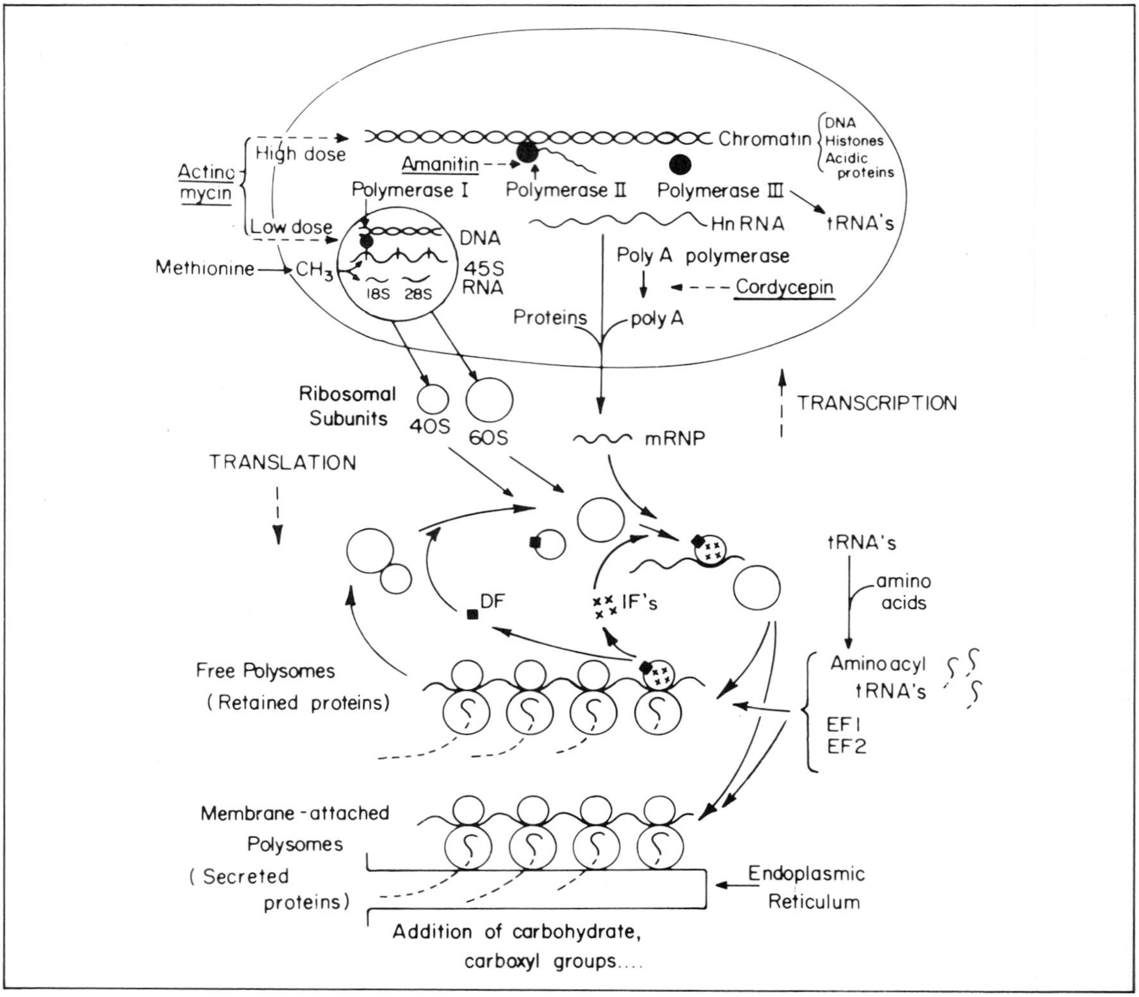

Figure 5-3. *Mechanism of protein synthesis in mammalian cells. (From T. S. Nowak and H. N. Munro. In R. J. Wurtman and J. J. Wurtman (Eds.),* Nutrition and the Brain, *Vol. 2. New York: Raven Press, 1977.)*

concentrations are needed to inhibit mRNA formation. Synthesis of mRNA can also be inhibited by the mushroom toxin, amanitine, which binds to polymerase II. Poly-A polymerase is sensitive to cordycepin. Accordingly, these various inhibitors can be used to determine whther changes in protein synthesis in the cytoplasm depend on a change in RNA synthesis in the nucleus.

The response of RNA synthesis to hormones and other factors is an important means of regulating protein synthesis. For example, rat liver RNA content increases after administration of large doses of corticosteroids [33]. Not only is this due to synthesis of more rRNA through activation of polymerase I [45], but the mRNAs for certain enzymes, such as tyrosine aminotransferase and tryptophan oxygenase [49], are transcribed in larger amounts, and in consequence more of these enzymes are made in the cytoplasm, an induction process that can be demonstrated by preventing transcription of mRNA with actinomycin D. The mechanism for such a hormonal effect has been elucidated by showing that steroid hormones bind to protein receptors in the cytoplasm of the target cell [2]. The receptor with steroid then enters the nucleus and attaches to the chromatin and alters the availability of template DNA, presumably by changing the configuration of the histones of acidic proteins of the chromosomes, and more mRNA is made.

TRANSLATION

Translation occurs in the cytoplasm in three stages: initiation, elongation, and termination. Initiation involves free ribosomal subunits, mRNA, methionyl initiator tRNA, GTP, and several protein initiator factors. Initiation is followed by elongation of the growing peptide chain by addition of amino acids, which are brought to the ribosome carrying the peptide chain by a series of 60 tRNA species, each of which recognizes the correct codon on the message for insertion of an amino acid. The processes of insertion of the amino acid and movement of the growing peptide chain are catalyzed by elongation factors 1 and 2, respectively, and GTP. After termination of the peptide chain, the ribosome separates from the mRNA and then dissociates into subunits by a mechanism requiring a dissociation factor (DF) (Figure 5-3).

Initiation by many ribosomes on the same mRNA strand results in a polyribosome. Figure 5-4 illustrates how the polyribosomes attached to membranes for protein secretion and those free in the cell sap, which synthesize retained proteins, can be separated according to size by rupturing the cell and then centrifuging the polyribosomes through a gradient of sucrose. The larger proteins are made by larger mRNAs, so that more ribosomes can be simultaneously translating the message. Thus polyribosome size is an indication of the size of the protein being synthesized. Balance between initiation and elongation determines the ratio of ribosomes in the form of polysomes to runoff ribosomes and subunits. If initiation is reduced, the ribosomes continue to pass along the mRNA strand and accumulate as runoff ribosomes. Polysomes diminish and runoff monosomes and subunits increase. For example, Figure 5-4 shows that fasting reduces the polyribosome population of the liver while increasing the number of inactive monoribosomes and subunits. Availability of tRNAs charged with the respective amino acids may be the factor underlying changes in liver polyribosome profiles in fasted and fed animals. If tRNA charged with a specific amino acid is not available in sufficient amounts, chain elongation is retarded at the points of insertion of this amino acid into the growing peptide chain [68].

POST-TRANSLATIONAL EVENTS

After the peptide chain has been synthesized and released from the ribosome, it often undergoes modifications to yield its biologically active form [71]. Thus, intrachain disulfide bond formation is a step in the folding process of many proteins. Phosphorylation of the polypeptide chain occurs as a means of activation of some enzymes, as in the case of interconversion between glycogen phosphorylase *a* and phosphorylase *b,* an enzyme in the pathway of glycogen breakdown. Many secreted proteins are modified by addition of sugars [71]. Such proteins are made on membrane-bound ribosomes, where the membrane is part of the endoplasmic reticulum. The endoplasmic reticulum in turn acts as a channel for secretion of these proteins, as well as the site for addition of sugars.

Some of these post-translational modifications aid in following the fate of the protein. In actin and myosin, some of the histidine components are methylated to form 3-methylhistidine. During intracellular turnover of these proteins, the 3-methylhistidine released is excreted quantitatively in the urine [73]. This can serve as a measure of muscle protein catabolism.

Degradative Pathways for Individual Amino Acids

Amino acids are important for general cell metabolism, because they serve not only as building blocks for protein synthesis but also as a source of

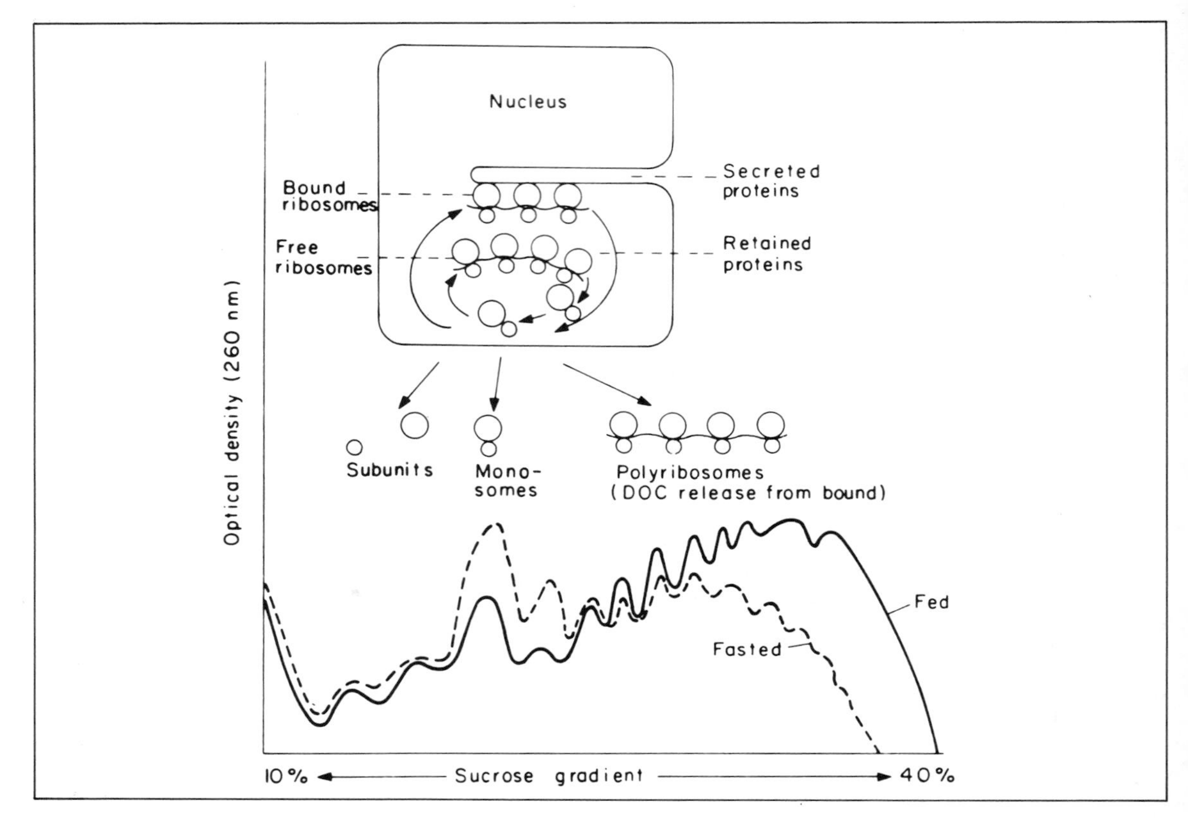

Figure 5-4. *Separation of polyribosomes, monoribosomes, and ribosome subunits on a sucrose gradient; comparison of relative amounts recovered from the livers of fed and fasted rats. (From H. N. Munro, C. Hubert, and B. S. Baliga, Regulation of Protein Synthesis in Relation to Amino Acid Supply: A Review. In M. A. Rothschild, M. Oratz, and S. S. Schreiber (Eds.),* Alcohol and Abnormal Protein Biosynthesis. *New York: Pergamon, 1975.)*

energy. The amount of amino acids used for energy production fluctuates, depending on availability of other fuels, need for amino acids in protein synthesis, and level of protein intake, in addition to other factors. The major degradative pathways [48] are outlined in Figure 5-5. Seven of the 10 essential amino acids are degraded in the liver, whereas the other three (the branched-chain amino acids, leucine, isoleucine, and valine) are mostly catabolized in muscle as well as in kidney and brain [59].

The first step in amino acid catabolism for at least 12 of the 20 amino acids is removal of the α-amino group by transamination to give a keto-acid. The remaining carbon skeleton is utilized in two major fashions: (1) conversion into glucose by gluconeogenesis or, (2) oxidation to CO_2 via the tricarboxylic acid cycle. A large part of the amino groups removed by transamination of the branched-chain amino acids in muscle is transferred to pyruvate and glutamate to produce alanine and glutamine, respectively. They are transported by way of the bloodstream to the liver (alanine) and the gut (glutamine). In the gut wall alanine and glutamic acid are formed, and the alanine passes through the portal system to the liver. This facilitates the transport of amino-N to the liver for urea formation, and the carbon of

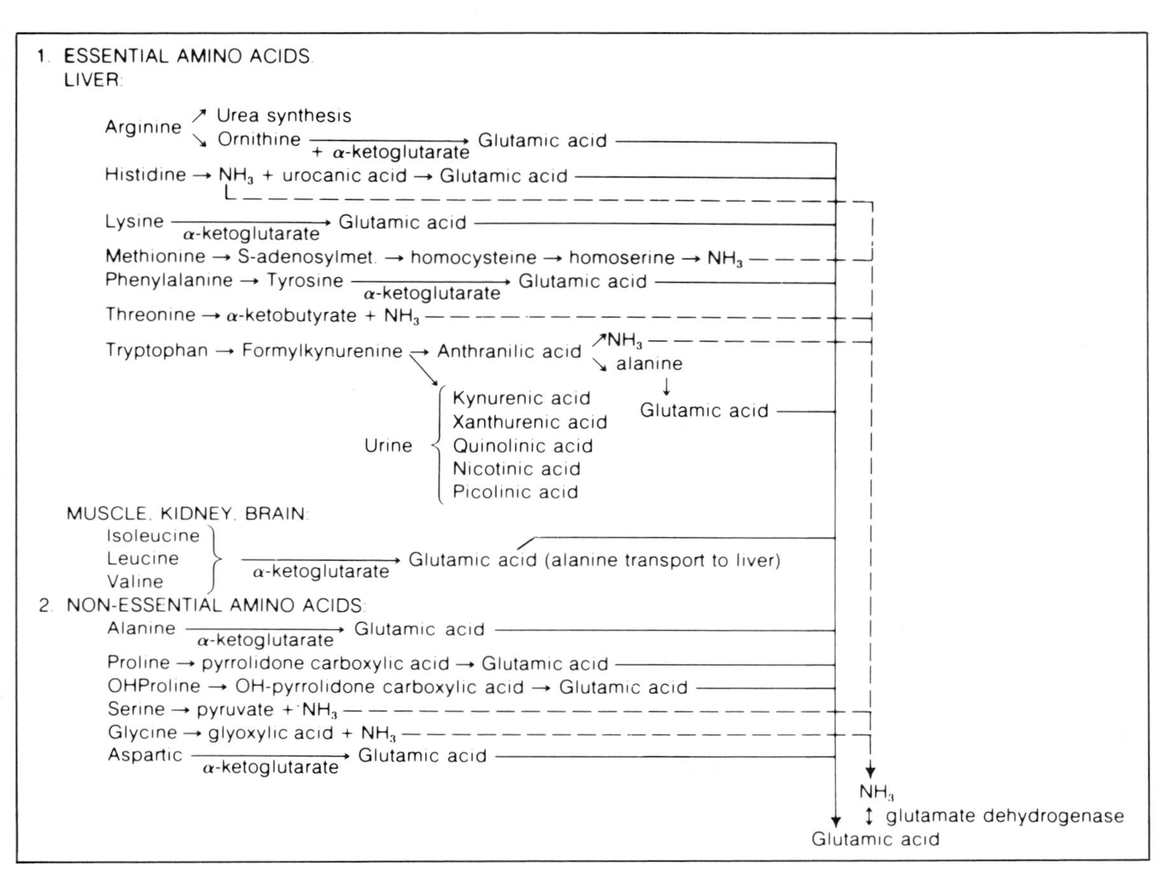

Figure 5-5. *Catabolic pathways for essential and non-essential amino acids. (From H. N. Munro and M. C. Crim, The Proteins and Amino Acids. In R. S. Goodhart and M. E. Shils (Eds.),* Modern Nutrition in Health and Disease *(6th ed.). Philadelphia: Lea & Febiger, 1980.)*

alanine becomes available for gluconeogenesis. The enzymes catalyzing the transaminations are called aminotransferases or transaminases. All of these enzymes have the same prosthetic group, pyridoxal phosphate, and their mechanism of reaction is the same [10].

A second type of deamination is oxidative deamination. This category is of secondary importance to general amino acid degradation. One of the most important reactions of this class is the conversion of glutamate to α-ketoglutarate and ammonia, which is catalyzed by glutamate dehydrogenase. Since this reaction is reversible, it represents the major pathway for taking up ammonia for amino acid synthesis (Figure 5-6). Oxidative deaminations occur in brain with the metabolism of catecholamine and serotonin [4].

As mentioned previously and illustrated in Figure 5-5, the carbon skeletons of the amino acids, after deamination, undergo a set of enzymatic reactions, ultimately to enter the tricarboxylic acid cycle, whereas the nitrogen is made available for urea synthesis through ammonia and glutamic acid.

Urea Synthesis

Ammonia formed in the body from the degradation of amino acids (see Figure 5-5) and from some other nitrogenous compounds is mostly transformed in the liver to urea for excretion in the urine. This centralization of urea formation implies that the extensive degradation of amino acids in other parts of the body requires transport of the resulting nitrogen to the liver. The release of alanine and glutamine from muscle and their metabolism by the gut and liver (see Figure 5-12) provide an important example of this transport process.

Figure 5-6 shows the urea cycle and the way in which it acquires nitrogen from amino acid degradation through ammonia and glutamic acid. The cycle begins with the reaction of the δ-amino group of ornithine with carbamyl phosphate, the latter formed from ammonia, CO_2, and ATP. This reaction produces citrulline. The second nitrogen for urea comes from the other major end product of amino acid degradation, glutamic acid, which transfers its amino group to aspartic acid. The latter condenses with citrulline to form argininosuccinate, which is resolved into arginine and fumarate by the enzyme argininosuccinase. Finally, the arginine so released is hydrolyzed by arginase to urea and ornithine, the latter becoming available to undergo another round of the urea cycle. The enzymes of the urea cycle are induced to increase by an increased amino acid load and to decrease by feeding a protein-deficient diet. The arginase activity can be increased by adding arginine to the low-protein diet [76].

Figure 5-6 also illustrates that some urea passes into the lumen of the lower intestine, where the urease of the gut bacteria releases ammonia. The latter passes back to the liver to form urea again. In cases of severe liver damage, failure to trap the ammonia is a cause of elevated peripheral blood ammonia levels. The magnitude of bacterial degradation of urea in the gut has been evaluated by Walser and Bodenlos [95], who administered ^{15}N- and ^{14}C-labeled urea parenterally to human subjects and recovered all the ^{15}N, but only 75 percent of the ^{14}C. Oral administration of neomycin raised urinary output of injected ^{14}C-urea to nearly 100 percent, confirming that gut bacteria were responsible for the hydrolysis of the administered ^{14}C-labeled urea.

Synthesis of Nonessential Amino Acids

When animals were fed ^{14}C-sucrose, none of the label was incorporated into the essential amino acids, whereas all the nonessential amino acids except tyrosine were extensively labeled [88]. The pathways of biosynthesis of the nonessential amino acids are shown in Figure 5-7. It is readily seen that all except tyrosine contain carbon atoms derived from glucose, thus accounting for the labeling pattern observed on feeding ^{14}C-labeled sugar.

Synthesis of Purine and Pyrimidine Nucleotides

The major pathways responsible for synthesis of purine and pyrimidine nucleotides are shown in outline in Figure 5-8. These pathways result in the formation of the nucleotides of adenine, guanine, uracil, and cytosine, leading to high-energy phosphate compounds (di- and triphosphates) in the cell, and to the formation of RNA and DNA.

Formation of purine nucleotides occurs by two routes: *de novo* and *salvage* pathways [16]. In de novo synthesis (Figure 5-8), glycine and phosphoribosylpyrophosphate (PRPP) initially react to form a series of intermediate compounds leading to the nucleotide inosine monophosphate (IMP) which contains the base hypoxanthine. Adenylic acid (AMP) and guanylic acid (GMP) are synthesized from this nucleotide by altering substituents on certain carbon atoms of the purine ring (see Figure 5-8). These mononucleotides can then be phosphorylated to make the high-energy compounds ADP, ATP, GDP, and GTP. The mononucleotides also can undergo degradation to adenosine and adenine or guanosine and guanine. The free bases adenine and guanine then are deaminated to hypoxanthine and xanthine, respectively, and finally, the hypoxanthine forms xanthine, which then is made

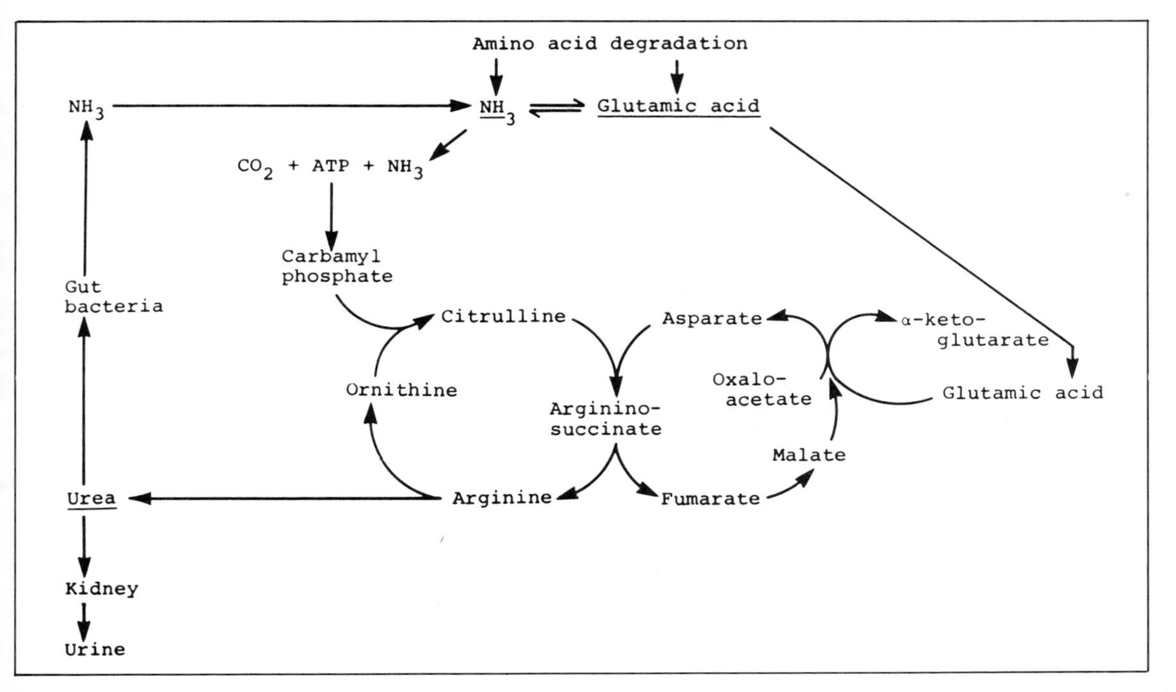

Figure 5-6. *Urea synthesis, showing also degradation of urea by gut bacteria and recycling of the ammonia to urea.*

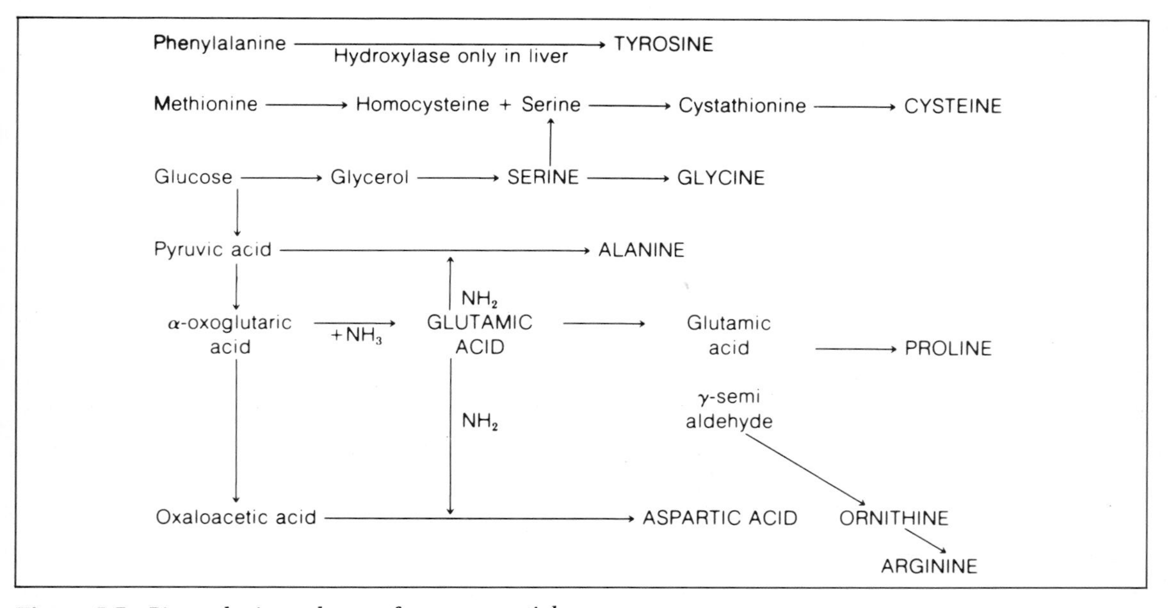

Figure 5-7. *Biosynthetic pathways for nonessential amino acids. (From H. N. Munro, The Evolution of Protein Metabolism in Mammals. In H. N. Munro (Ed.),* Mammalian Protein Metabolism, *Vol. 3. New York: Academic, 1969.)*

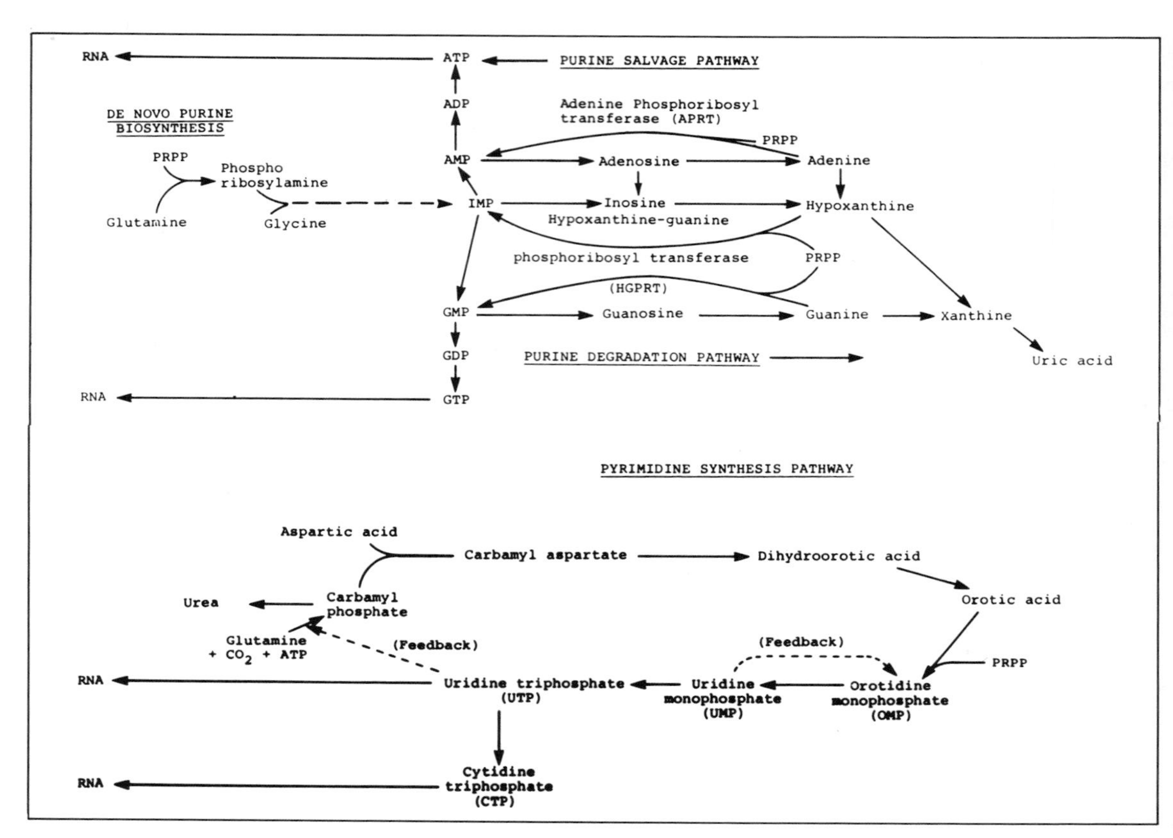

Figure 5-8. *Pathways of purine and pyrimidine nucleotide synthesis.*

into uric acid: both of the last two reactions are catalyzed by xanthine oxidase.

Purine nucleotides can also be made by salvage pathways, in which the free purine bases formed as already described react with PRPP to form the mononucleotides by a reaction involving a PRPP molecule (Figure 5-8). The salvage pathways are catalyzed by two enzymes, adenine-phosphoribosyl-transferase (APRT) and hypoxanthine-guanine phosphoribosyl-transferase (HGPRT), the latter enzyme being defective in the Lesch-Nyhan syndrome [84]. This defect leads to loss of salvage, and there is a consequent increased activity in the de novo pathway to compensate. This excessive synthesis of guanine results in formation of uric acid in large amounts and is thus a cause of gout.

Synthesis of the pyrimidine bases (Figure 5-8) also requires amino acids, the initial reaction in the pathway involving aspartic acid, which reacts with carbamyl phosphate, also a substrate for urea synthesis (see Figure 5-6). It has recently been shown [93] that lack of adequate amounts of dietary arginine to prime the urea synthesis cycle can result in diversion of carbamyl phosphate to the pyrimidine biosynthetic pathway. The pyrimidine pathway is subject to feedback regulation by the end product UTP and also to feedback regulation of the conversion of orotidine monophosphate to uridine monophosphate. Consequently, overproduction in this pathway is regulated by excretion of orotic acid and crotidine in the urine. Thus, one cause of high urinary output of orotic acid is arginine deficiency.

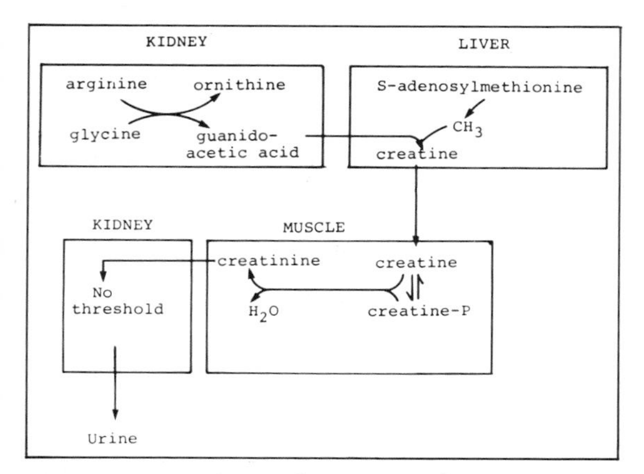

Figure 5-9. *Synthesis of creatine and creatinine.*

Creatine and Creatinine

Creatine is present in skeletal muscle both as creatine and as creatine phosphate. At rest, muscle creatine is present in the high-energy phosphate form, but after strenuous exercise the concentration of creatine phosphate can become very low, owing to conversion of creatine phosphate to creatine coupled with the synthesis of ATP. This allows muscle to generate additional ATP under anaerobic conditions.

Several organs participate in creatine synthesis (Figure 5-9). The first step occurs in the kidney and involves transamidination between the amino acids arginine and glycine, resulting in formation of glycocyamine (guanidoacetic acid) and ornithine. The guanidoacetic acid is methylated in the liver by S-adenosyl-methionine to form creatine. The creatine is then transported to muscle for active uptake. The first step in the pathway, synthesis of guanidoacetic acid in the kidney, is regulated by feedback control from the level of creatine. In muscle, both creatine phosphate and creatine undergo a nonenzymatic irreversible dehydration to creatinine, the reaction rate being faster for creatine phosphate. Unlike creatine, creatinine is not retained by muscle, but is distributed in body water and is removed by the kidney as a nonthreshold substance. The daily rate of creatinine formation from its creatine precursors averages 1.7 percent of the total creatine pool per day. Consequently, the amount of creatinine excreted daily reflects the size of the creatine pool. Studies by Crim et al. [11, 12] show that the body creatine pool can be increased by dietary creatine. This occurs by an increase in creatine content of muscle. Urinary creatinine has been used clinically as a measure of lean body mass or muscle mass. For group studies, this is fully justified. However, since the body pool of creatine for an individual depends on both dietary intake and synthesis, this use of urinary creatinine to assess muscle mass of individuals can be subject to appreciable error.

INTEGRATED PROTEIN METABOLISM

In the preceding section, the individual pathways of amino acid metabolism have been dealt with. Proteins are an integral part of the life processes, and therefore regulation of protein metabolism in an integrated fashion is necessary to maintain bodily functions. In this section we will discuss overall protein metabolism.

Digestion and Absorption

The initial step in protein digestion is breakdown by pepsin secreted in the gastric juice. This step is followed by attack of proteolytic enzymes originating in the pancreas and in the mucosa of the small intestine [32]. These enzymes are synthesized in a precursor form. When the pancreatic proenzymes meet the intestinal juice, an enterokinase activates trypsinogen by cleaving away a small peptide, and active trypsin is formed. This is followed by a cascade of activations of the other pancreatic proenzymes through proteolysis by trypsin of one specific peptide bond.

Dietary protein content in the gut seems to control secretion of proteolytic enzymes by the pancreas. It has been shown that, in the case of trypsin (Figure 5-10), the enzyme binds to protein in the gut lumen until an excess is present. The free enzyme then causes a feedback inhibition of trypsinogen synthesis in the pancreatic acinar

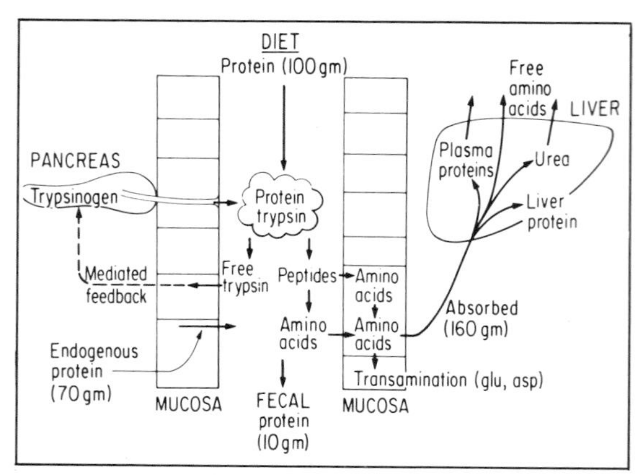

Figure 5-10. *Diagram illustrating the fate of dietary protein, the secretion of endogenous protein, and the transport of amino acids to the liver. (From M. C. Crim, and H. N. Munro, Protein and Amino Acid Requirements and Metabolism in Relation to Defined Formula Diets. In M. E. Shils (Ed.),* Defined Formula Diets for Medical Purposes. *Chicago: AMA, 1977. P. 5.)*

cells [34]. Some plants contain inhibitors of proteolytic enzymes, the best-known being the trypsin inhibitor present in soybeans. Feeding of unheated soybean to rats causes hypertrophy of the pancreas [83], presumably due to binding of trypsin by the inhibitor, which shuts off the feedback system and causes overproduction of enzymes.

The details of protein digestion can be found elsewhere [32]. The different proteolytic enzymes attack peptide bonds, the specificity being based on the amino acids on either side of the bond. Pepsin preferentially hydrolyses bonds adjacent to leucine and aromatic amino acids, whereas enzymes made in the pancreas have greater specificity for other bonds: trypsin for those adjacent to lysine and arginine, chymotrypsin for bonds adjacent to aromatic amino acids, and elastase for those next to neutral aliphatic amino acids. Finally, the free carboxy- and amino-ends of the peptide chains are attacked by carboxypeptidases secreted by the pancreas and aminopeptidases released from the intestinal mucosa, respectively. The dietary protein thus becomes resolved into free amino acids and small peptides.

It used to be thought that the end products of protein digestion absorbed into the mucosal cells of the small intestine were exclusively free amino acids. During the past decade, it has become evident that a considerable proportion enters the mucosal cells as small peptides, which are hydrolyzed to free amino acids by enzymes at the brush border and within the mucosal cell cytoplasm [50]. This process appears to result in complete resolution of the peptides, so that normally only free amino acids pass into the portal blood (Figure 5-10). Studies with various di- and tripeptides show that only a few, such as glycylglycine and peptides containing hydroxyproline, resist hydrolysis and enter the bloodstream, thus accounting for the excretion of hydroxyproline peptides in the urine after a meal containing gelatin [82].

The mucosal brush border transports both free amino acids and small peptides into the mucosal cells of the villi. Free amino acid uptake is mediated by mechanisms described earlier, in which amino acids fall into several transport classes (see Figure 5-2) within which they compete for uptake. Uptake of small peptides occurs by a separate series of transport mechanisms for which free amino acids are not competitors [50]. This is especially demonstrated by patients with genetic defects in uptake of free neutral amino acids (Hartnup disease) or basic amino acids (cystinuria). Such patients can nevertheless absorb adequate amounts of these amino acids when they are given in the form of dipeptides [55]. Since these patients grow normally despite almost complete inhibition of absorption of some free essential amino acids, we must conclude that peptide absorption by the mucosa is a major mechanism for providing the body with amino acids.

The mucosa metabolizes some of the amino acids entering from the gut. As shown in Figure 5-10, glutamic acid and aspartic acid undergo metabolic changes that are extensive enough to limit the amount passing into the portal circulation. Windmueller and Spaeth [97] have demonstrated that very little glutamic acid passes as such into the portal blood following absorption of moderate amounts from the gut. Instead, it undergoes transamination to alanine, with a smaller release into the portal blood of ornithine, citrulline, and proline. The pathways involved in synthesis of these nonessential amino acids have been described (see Figure 5-7). When the same investigators infused glutamine into the intestinal lumen, the same products appeared in the portal blood along with ammonia. Glutamine released from peripheral tissues such as muscle (see Figure 5-12) is removed from the mesenteric blood supply as it passes through the intestinal wall. This glutamine of peripheral origin also undergoes transamination with release of alanine. Whether arising from glutamic acid and glutamine absorbed from the gut, or from peripheral glutamine, the alanine formed in the mucosa is removed from the portal blood as it passes through the liver and is transaminated to release the amino-nitrogen to glutamic acid for transfer to urea. The carbon chain becomes pyruvate and thus enters the pool of intermediates available for oxidation in the tricarboxylic acid cycle, for fat synthesis, or, most importantly, for gluconeogenesis (see Figure 5-12).

Finally, the gastrointestinal tract also participates in protein metabolism by secreting protein into the gut [21]. This takes the form of enzymes and other proteins secreted in the digestive juices (about 17 gm protein daily in man) and a large number of epithelial cells shed from the intestinal villi, which have been rather insecurely estimated to account for 50 gm of protein daily [21]. Since the average American diet provides about 100 gm protein daily, the total protein entering the gut each day can be as large as 170 gm. Fecal output accounts for only 10 gm of this intake, so that daily absorption is about 160 gm (Figure 5-10). The efficiency of absorption probably benefits by the presence of bacteria in the lower part of the intestinal tract. Some studies on germ-free rats [53] show that more nitrogen is excreted in the feces by such animals than by animals with bacteria in the gut. In addition, gut bacteria metabolize nitrogenous small molecules, such as urea, which is hydrolyzed to ammonia (see Figure 5-6), and free amino acids, which are decarboxylated with formation of amines (see Figure 5-16). In both cases, these products of bacterial action are normally detoxified in the liver.

Role of the Liver

The portal vein is the route by which absorbed amino acids reach the liver. After a meal of protein, the amounts of amino acids in the portal vein increase to varying extents, whereas a lesser increase in amino acid levels occurs in the peripheral blood. The liver is the main or exclusive site of catabolism for seven of the essential amino acids; the remaining three (the branched-chain amino acids) are catabolized mainly in muscle and kidney [19]. Catabolism in the liver is adjusted to the needs of the body. Elwyn [19] fed dogs large amounts of meat, and showed that much of the incoming amino acids are degraded to urea as they pass into the liver, small proportions being used to make plasma proteins, whereas only about a quarter of the absorbed amino acids pass into the general circulation as such (Figure 5-11).

Elwyn's study [19] provides a balance sheet of glutamic acid, glutamine, and alanine exchange across the gut and liver (Table 5-2). The fed dogs transferred more of the intake of total glutamic acid (glutamate plus glutamine in meat protein) into the portal vein as glutamine than as glutamic acid; some of the missing glutamic acid could be accounted for by a considerable output of alanine from the gut, much greater than that in the meal. In contrast, the liver removed glutamic acid, glutamine, and alanine from the portal blood, so that the net result of passage of blood through the entire splanchnic area was a small reduction in the amount of the three amino acids entering the general circulation.

Similar studies have been made on sheep and man (Table 5-2). In fed sheep [3] it has been shown by cannulation of the appropriate vessels that glutamine and a small amount of glutamate are removed from the plasma as it perfuses the

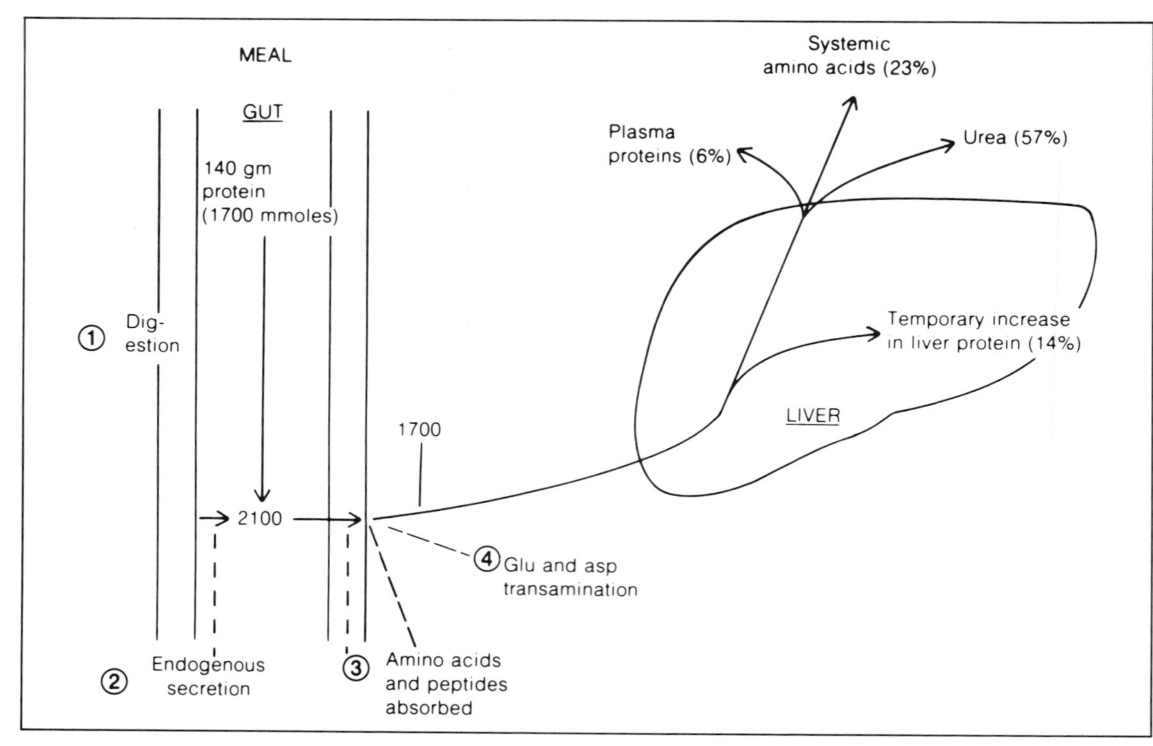

Figure 5-11. *Absorption and metabolism of amino acids after a meal of meat eaten by a dog, based on data of Elwyn [19]. (From H. N. Munro, and M. C. Crim, The Proteins and Amino Acids. In R. S. Goodhart, and M. E. Shils (Eds.),* Modern Nutrition in Health and Disease *(6th ed.). Philadelphia: Lea & Febiger, 1980.)*

Table 5-2. *Exchanges of Glutamic Acid, Glutamine, and Alanine Across the Viscera and Limb Muscles*

Species	Total Exchange During Period		
	Glutamic Acid	Glutamine	Alanine
Fed dog (mmoles/12 hr)			
Absorbed from gut lumen	160 (Glutamic Acid + Glutamine combined)		100
Gut output	+10	+50	+230
Liver output	−15	−70	−260
Total splanchnic output	−5	−20	−30
Fed sheep (mmoles/hr)			
Portal viscera output	−0.2	−1.5	+2.3
Liver output	+1.1	−2.1	−3.2
Total splanchnic output	+0.9	+3.6	−0.9
Hindquarters output	−11	+13	+14
Fasted human (μmoles/min)			
Total splanchnic output	+48	−59	−60
Leg output	−24	+50	+26

+ = output by organ; − = uptake by organ.

Source: H. N. Munro, Factors in the Regulation of Glutamate Metabolism. In L. J. Filer et al. (Eds.), *Glutamic Acid: Advances in Biochemistry and Physiology*. New York: Raven Press, 1979. P. 55.

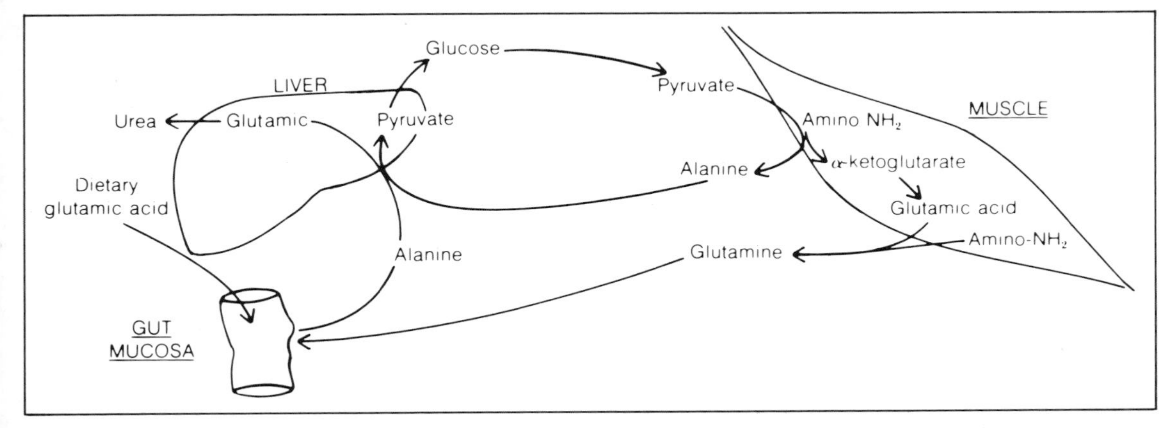

Figure 5-12. *Interchange of glutamic acid, glutamine, alanine, and glucose between muscle and viscera. (From H. N. Munro, Factors in the Regulation of Glutamic Metabolism. In L. J. Filer, et al. (Eds.),* Glutamic Acid: Advances in Biochemistry and Physiology. *New York: Raven Press, 1979. P. 55.)*

portal viscera; the liver removes further glutamine, but adds some glutamate to the plasma. On the other hand, the portal viscera put out alanine, while the liver takes it up. The general picture of the exchange across the splanchnic area, showing uptake of glutamine and alanine, with a smaller output of glutamic acid, is confirmed by studies on human subjects (Table 5-2).

These exchanges of amino acids across the viscera are related to complementary changes in the peripheral tissues, notably muscle (Figure 5-12). In the fasting human, muscle releases large amounts of alanine and glutamine, which are removed by the viscera. This balance between organs is seen in fasting human subjects (Table 5-2), who demonstrate net uptake of glutamic acid and release of glutamine and alanine as blood passes through the limb muscles, and a similar picture is seen for sheep (Table 5-2). In both cases, the output of glutamine and alanine by muscle is greater in the fasting state, thus providing carbon for gluconeogenesis.

The liver monitors the intake of amino acids and thus regulates the levels of individual essential amino acids available to the body. Progressive increase of dietary intake of an essential amino acid ultimately leads to induction of liver enzyme activity, at the point where intake exceeds requirement. This induction (e.g., threonine dehydratase in Figure 5-13) often shows a sudden increase at levels of intake beyond the needs of the body. This indicates that the liver accurately monitors intake in relation to the needs of the body and destroys only essential amino acids extensively above that critical level in the diet. In the case of nonessential amino acids, the levels of enzymes responsible for their metabolism do not show this inflection, but increase progressively with rising intake [37].

Conservation of essential amino acids is confirmed by studies in which varying quantities of lysine were fed to young growing rats [5]. Intake of 100 mg of lysine produces a maximal gain in body weight. At intakes beyond 100 mg daily, ^{14}C-carbon dioxide production from injected ^{14}C-lysine showed a rapid increase. This indicates that intake beyond a level producing maximal growth results in breakdown of excess lysine. The plasma level of lysine in the rat shows a similar response to lysine intake. Levels rise sharply when intakes of lysine exceed an amount sufficient for maximal growth [79]. This suggests that a rise in peripheral blood levels of essential amino acids signals enzyme induction in the liver.

Thus we find that degradative enzymes such as tyrosine aminotransferase and tryptophan pyr-

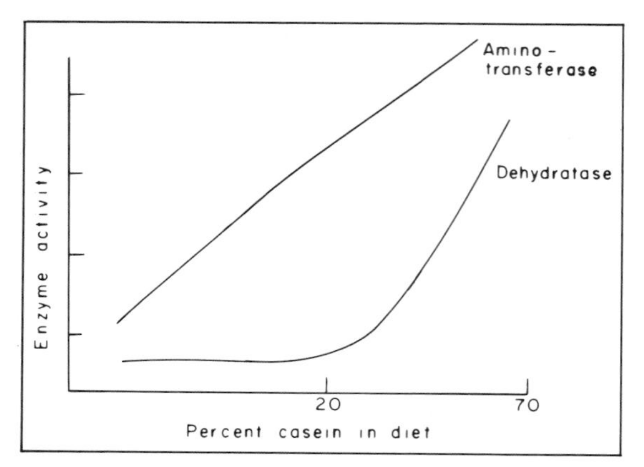

Figure 5-13. *Activities in rat liver of glutamate-oxaloacetate aminotransferase and threonine-serine dehydratase at different levels of protein intake. (Drawn from data of A. E. Harper, Diet and plasma amino acids.* Am. J. Clin. Nutr. *21:358, 1968.)*

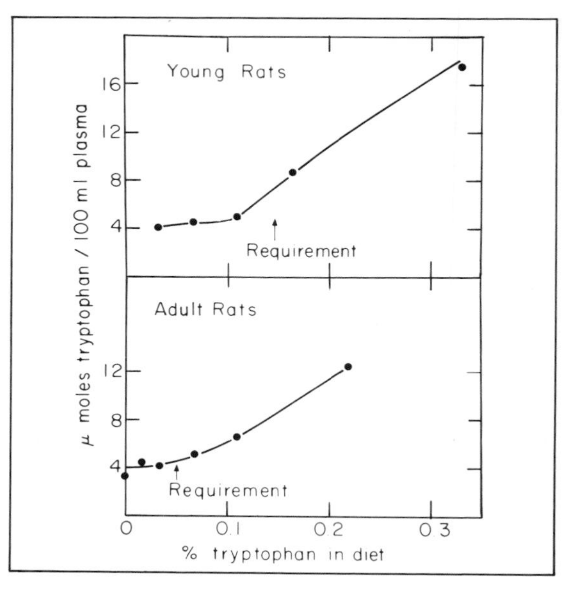

Figure 5-14. *Plasma tryptophan levels of young and mature rats fed amino acid diets containing various levels of tryptophan. The arrows indicate the requirement of tryptophan for maximal growth* (A) *and for weight maintenance* (B). *(Adapted from V. R. Young and H. N. Munro, Plasma and tissue tryptophan levels in relation to tryptophan requirements in weaning and adult rats.* J. Nutr. *103:1736, 1973.)*

rolase show diurnal variations related to meal consumption [99]. Furthermore, other metabolic events in the liver cell are subject to diurnal variations due to protein intake from the diet. Synthesis of RNA accelerates while RNA breakdown decreases. The latter leads to diminished purine nucleotide pools and, consequently, a stimulation of de novo purine biosynthesis (see Figure 5-8) after meals containing protein [9]. Some secreted proteins, such as albumin [68], do not appear to undergo diurnal rhythms in synthesis in normal animals, but synthesis does increase when protein is fed to protein-depleted animals, as is the case for most proteins. It has been suggested [68] that synthesis of albumin by the normal animal is regulated in relation to the plasma level and that response to protein intake in the depleted animal is due to the serum albumin level falling below this critical control level and then becoming regulated in relation to amino acid supply. Some secreted proteins, such as the $\alpha_{2\mu}$-globulin made by the liver of the mature male rat and excreted in the urine, show diurnal responses to protein intake even in well-nourished animals [18].

During the absorptive period, synthesis by the liver of degradative enzymes and other proteins is reflected by increased aggregation of polyribosomes (see Figure 5-4). Not only is there an elevation of synthesis due to absorption, but also a stabilization of the degradative enzymes by their respective substrates [63].

Regulation of Amino Acid Levels in the Blood

Although the liver monitors the passage of amino acids into the general circulation, this is insufficient to suppress some rise in blood amino acid levels after a meal. Plasma levels of many essential amino acids increase when dietary supply exceeds the requirements of the tissues. In some cases, the level of an essential amino acid in the peripheral blood rises quite abruptly when requirement is exceeded. For example, the response of plasma tryptophan concentration to different

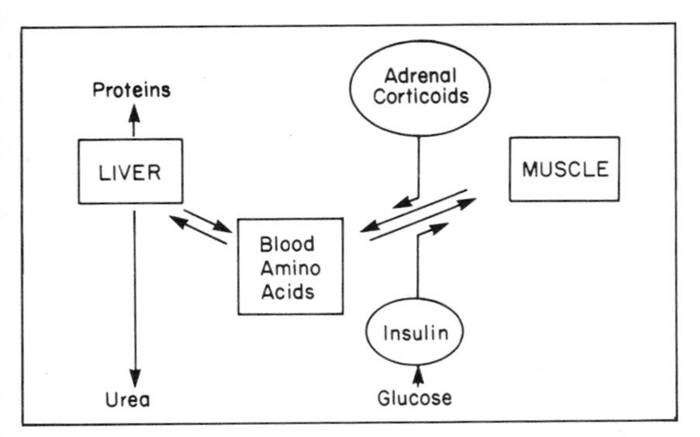

Figure 5-15. *Action of dietary carbohydrate on plasma amino acids, which, through the action of insulin, are preferentially deposited in muscle, with consequent reduction in amino acid availability for other tissues including urea formation by the liver. The opposite distribution occurs following adrenocortical steroid hormone administration. (From H. N. Munro, General Aspects of the Regulation of Protein Metabolism by Diet and by Hormones. In H. N. Munro and J. B. Allison (Eds.),* Mammalian Protein Metabolism, *Vol. 1. New York: Academic, 1964. P. 381.)*

levels of dietary tryptophan was examined in young rats and in mature rats (Figure 5-14). As the amount of tryptophan in the diet was increased from less than adequate to more than sufficient, the plasma tryptophan content rose sharply beyond the point of requirement at both ages. For rapidly growing rats, inflection occurred at 0.1 percent tryptophan in the diet, above which growth was not stimulated and plasma tryptophan started to rise. For the mature rats, 0.03 percent dietary tryptophan was sufficient to maintain weight, and above this intake, plasma tryptophan concentration rose. The response is thus sensitive to age-related changes in requirements. This method has been applied to human subjects, and in the case of tryptophan, the point of inflection agrees with the amount required for nitrogen balance of young adults [105]. In the case of other essential amino acids, such as lysine, less clear-cut points of inflection have been obtained.

The plasma levels of amino acids are also responsive to dietary carbohydrate through a mechanism involving insulin [61]. After a meal of carbohydrate, most plasma amino acids decrease in concentration because of deposition in muscle through the action of insulin-mediated transport (Figure 5-15). The greatest reduction is in branched-chain amino acids, whereas some other amino acids such as tryptophan are little affected [72].

Protein Metabolism in the Brain

These alterations in plasma free amino acid patterns due to the amounts of protein and carbohydrate in a meal affect the availability of amino acids to some peripheral tissues. The free tryptophan content of the brain of the rat can be elevated by feeding tryptophan, and this raises the serotonin content of the brain [25]. Tryptophan uptake by the brain is also determined by the plasma levels of competing neutral amino acids, especially the branched-chain amino acids (see Figure 5-2). The extensive reduction in plasma levels of branched-chain amino acids after a meal of carbohydrate thus promotes greater passage of tryptophan into the brain, and more serotonin is synthesized in consequence [25].

This mechanism is also important for brain function under pathologic conditions. In particular, hepatic cirrhosis results in a series of metabolic alterations relating to protein metabolism (Figure 5-16). Amines and ammonia generated by gut bacteria are no longer removed by the liver, but pass via the systemic blood to the brain. For example, phenethylamine produced from phenylalanine by bacterial action is probably transformed to octopamine and acts as a false neurotransmitter competing with catecholamines [17]. Amino acids normally regulated in the liver, notably tryptophan and phenylalanine, are no longer controlled and so their plasma levels rise. Finally, a large part of the insulin secreted by the pancreas is normally inactivated by the liver, but this no longer occurs in cirrhosis, so that postprandial insulin levels in the peripheral blood are very high [26]. This increases transport of branched-chain amino acids into muscle, ex-

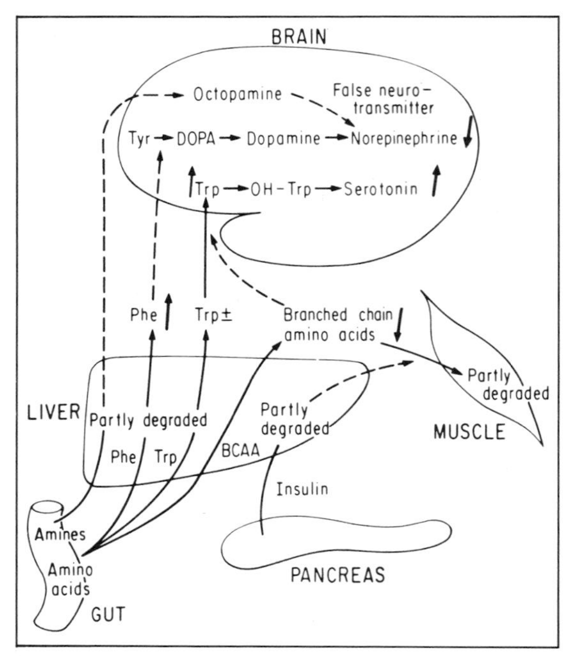

Figure 5-16. *Role of the branched chain amino acids in hepatic coma. Owing to unrestricted passage of insulin into the general circulation, branched chain amino acids are removed excessively by muscle. In consequence of this lowering of plasma branched chain amino acids, there is less competition with tryptophan for entry into the brain and thus more serotonin is made. (From M. C. Crim and H. N. Munro, Protein and Amino Acid Requirements and Metabolism in Relation to Defined Formula Diets. In M. E. Shils (Ed.),* Defined Formula Diets for Medical Purposes. *Chicago: A.M.A., 1977, P. 5.)*

plaining the depressed levels of amino acids in the blood of cirrhotics. The reduction in plasma levels of the branched-chain amino acids permits a larger proportion of the already elevated tryptophan content of the plasma to pass into the brain. In consequence, excessive serotonin is generated and contributes to hepatic coma [70]. This model of the role of excess serotonin formation in hepatic coma due to chronic liver damage receives some support from reversal of the comatose state following administration of branched-chain amino acids to patients with hepatic coma [27].

Role of Skeletal Muscle in Protein Metabolism

Skeletal muscle is the largest tissue in the body [62]. Thus, metabolism of amino acids in this tissue is of considerable significance for general protein metabolism [100]. Muscle is, in addition, the main site of catabolism of the branched-chain amino acids (leucine, isoleucine, and valine). Muscle is a major target for the action of insulin, which promotes entry of amino acids (especially the branched-chain amino acids). Insulin also induces synthesis of muscle protein and reduces muscle protein breakdown. Corticosteroids have the opposite effects (see Figure 5-15).

The effects of hormones and of nutrient intake on muscle protein metabolism have been examined by a variety of techniques, both in vivo and in vitro. In the human, two main methods have been employed: (1) measurement of the differences in amino acid levels of blood entering and leaving muscle (arteriovenous differences), and (2) measurement of the output of 3-methylhistidine, a urinary compound excreted in proportion to the rate of myofibrillar protein breakdown. The measurement of amino acid exchange with muscle (Table 5-2) shows that fasting human subjects release large amounts of alanine and glutamine into the blood (see Figure 5-12), equivalent to a loss of 75 gm of protein daily from the muscles of a 70 kg fasting man [81]. Pyruvate derived from glucose is transaminated, producing alanine, the amino groups coming from amino acids present in muscle. Consequently, alanine becomes a nitrogen carrier from muscle to liver, where its carbon skeleton is used in the gluconeogenic pathway and its amino group is converted into urea. Another carrier of nitrogen from muscle is glutamine, formed from glutamic acid (see Figure 5-12). This glutamine passes to the intestine where its amino group is transaminated to alanine, which now goes to the liver. These reactions comprise the mechanism by which transport of nitrogen and carbon from muscle to liver is facilitated. Some of the carbon is returned to muscle in the form of glucose, following gluconeogenesis in the liver, finalizing the *glucose-alanine cycle* between liver and muscle. Measurements of the arteriovenous differences across the forearm have shown that, if insulin or carbohydrate is administered, the release of alanine is reduced and, after a mixed meal, is completely reversed so that muscle actually gains protein [94]. This mechanism implies that, from the body mass of muscle (45 percent of body weight on the average), a considerable amount of carbon can be called upon for metabolism during fasting or other emergencies.

Recycling of amino acids within muscle cells obscures the interpretation of arteriovenous differences. Reduction in this difference after insulin administration could be due to either a decrease in protein breakdown or an increase in protein synthesis. In order to monitor release of amino acids from muscle protein breakdown without reutilization, we have used 3-methylhistidine output in urine [73]. Actin and myosin undergo methylation of histidine only after these proteins have been synthesized. When the protein in the myofibril is broken down, unlike other amino acids, 3-methylhistidine is not recycled, but is excreted in the urine, thus providing an index of myofibrillar protein breakdown (Figure 5-17). Several lines of evidence support this use of 3-methylhistidine. First, tRNA prepared from rat muscle is not charged with 3-methylhistidine [101], and therefore it is not recycled for muscle protein synthesis. Second, analysis of various tissues of the rat for 3-methylhistidine content shows that skeletal muscle is the major reservoir of this compound in the body [39]. Soon after administering $^{14}CH_3$-labeled 3-methylhistidine to rats [101] and to human subjects [54], essentially all of it was recovered in the urine over a short period.

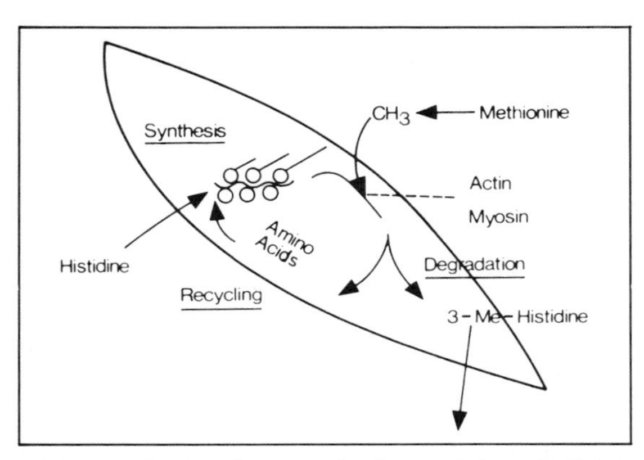

Figure 5-17. *Synthesis and release of 3-methylhistidine in muscle. (From H. N. Munro, In* Aromatic Amino Acids in the Brain. *Ciba Foundation Symposium 22, New York: Elsevier, 1974. P. 5.)*

The output of 3-methylhistidine has been used by us and by others to study dietary and hormonal effects on muscle protein breakdown. Changes in methylhistidine excretion have been demonstrated [38] in young rats receiving diets deficient in either protein alone or protein and calories. Protein deficiency caused a rapid reduction in output of 3-methylhistidine. In the case of protein-calorie deficiency, however, there was an initial rise followed by a fall in output. Thus muscle responds to protein depletion by shutting off breakdown. However, with semistarvation, breakdown at first increases and then diminishes. Malnourished children in India [75] and Guatemala [104] showed a similar low output of methylhistidine for weight, which rose during repletion. Similarly, grossly obese subjects treated by fasting over weeks showed a progressive reduction in 3-methylhistidine output [102].

Finally, 3-methylhistidine output is affected by age and by hormonal status. Table 5-3 shows that output per kilogram body weight is higher in neonates than in the mature adult and that it declines further in old age [73]. In the case of elderly adults, this is due to reduced muscle mass, which is consistent with a parallel reduction in their creatinine output. Unpublished data of Munro and Young show that output is increased by thyroxine secretion within the normal range of thyroid activity. On the other hand, adrenocortical steroids only affect output of 3-methylhistidine when the plasma level is excessive. Thus, we [91] observed that adrenalectomy of young rats did not result in a change in output of 3-methylhistidine, while administration of corticosterone to such animals in increasing doses did not affect

Table 5-3. *Urinary N^{τ}-Methylhistidine Excretion in Subjects at Various Ages and Consuming Flesh-Free Diets**

Group	No. of Subjects	N^{π}-Methylhistidine Excretion (μmoles) per: 24 hr	Body Wt (kg)	Creatinine (gm)
Neonate	10	8 ± 5	4.2 ± 1.3	253 ± 78
Young adults				
Men	4	245 ± 47	3.2 ± 0.6	126 ± 32
Women	2	112	2.1	92
Elderly				
Men	7	160 ± 47	2.2 ± 0.7	136 ± 25
Women	5	70 ± 17	2.2 ± 0.2	96 ± 18

*Based on unpublished data for neonates and on Uauy et al. [92] for adults.

Source: H. N. Munro and V. R. Young. Urinary excretion of N^{τ}-methylhistidine (3-methylhistidine): A tool to study metabolic responses in relation to nutrient and hormonal status in health and disease of man. *Am. J. Clin. Nutr.* 31:1608, 1978.

output until more than 1 mg/100 gm body weight was given daily. At levels of 5 and 10 mg daily, growth ceased, the gastrocnemius muscle lost weight, and there was an increased output of 3-methylhistidine in the urine. At such dose levels, plasma corticosterone concentrations were well above the normal range, being similar to those observed in severe trauma, such as burning with sepsis. We conclude that muscle protein breakdown rate is increased only by levels of blood corticosteroids equivalent to those found in stress. This conclusion has a bearing on the metabolic responses observed in various catabolic states associated with sepsis and injury.

Role of Kidney in Protein Metabolism

The major nitrogenous components of urine are urea, uric acid, creatinine, ammonia, and some amino acids including 3-methylhistidine. These represent end products of protein metabolism (see Figure 5-1), whose selective elimination from the body involves mechanisms of glomerular filtration followed by tubular reabsorption of some products and, in some cases, tubular secretion. In addition, the kidney performs two important functions in protein metabolism: ammoniagenesis and synthesis of arginine.

Ammonia is formed adaptively in the kidney in response to urinary acidification, as in starvation acidosis or in the ketoacidosis of diabetes. Thus, after starvation of human subjects for several weeks, more than 40 percent of the nitrogen output can be in the form of ammonia [78]. The secretion of ammonia allows the body to neutralize the acid without having to use fixed base (e.g., K^+) to perform the same function. The formation of ammonia is now known to be linked to another adaptive function of the kidney, gluconeogenesis.

The origin of the nitrogen for ammonia production is plasma glutamine, which is added to the blood by tissues such as muscle (see Figure 5-12). As shown in Figure 5-18, the amide-N is released as NH_3 by glutaminase, a second product of reaction being glutamic acid. A further molecule of ammonia is formed through the action of glutamic dehydrogenase on the glutamic acid. The other product of this reaction, α-ketoglutarate, enters the tricarboxylic acid cycle to become oxaloacetate. Through the action of the inducible enzyme phosphoenolpyruvate carboxykinase (PEPCK), the oxaloacetate forms phosphoenolpyruvate, an intermediate in the synthesis of glucose (gluconeogenesis). Studies on rats made acidotic show that,

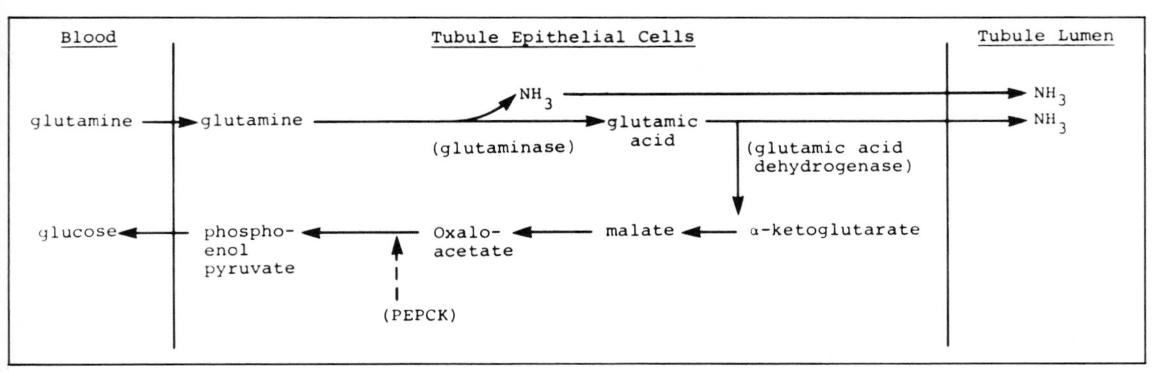

Figure 5-18. *Mechanism of ammonia formation by the proximal convoluted tubule of the kidney. PEPCK = phosphoenolpyruvate carboxykinase.*

in conjunction with the increased ammonia output, kidney glutaminase increases in activity [15] and there is also induction of the gluconeogenic enzyme PEPCK [36]. Thus, during starvation, the kidney becomes a source of blood glucose, as has been verified directly by arteriovenous differences across the kidneys of human subjects undergoing prolonged fasting [78]. These adaptive changes have been examined in different portions of the renal tubule. It has been shown with dissected rat kidney tubules that acidosis results in induction of glutaminase [15] and PEPCK [36] only in the proximal convoluted tubules, which are thus identified as the site of ammonia production.

The kidney also synthesizes arginine from the citrulline present in the plasma (see Figure 5-6 for pathway). Bergman and coauthors [3] measured the arteriovenous difference in blood levels of citrulline and arginine across the kidneys of sheep. They found a disappearance from the arterial blood passing through the kidney of 1.41 mmoles citrulline per hour and an addition to the blood of 1.46 mmoles of arginine in the same period. In order to evaluate the importance of this source of arginine to other organs, Featherstone et al. [22] injected rats with ^{14}C-ureido-citrulline and isolated labeled arginine from various tissues. When the blood supply to the kidneys was ligated, arginine labeling in muscle and brain was greatly reduced, indicating that the kidney is a significant source of arginine for these organs. On the other hand, ligation of the liver did not reduce the amount of labeled arginine found in muscle, brain, or kidney after labeled citrulline had been given, showing that little of the arginine made by the urea cycle in the liver becomes available to other organs.

Plasma Protein Metabolism

Plasma proteins provide a readily accessible component of protein metabolism in the human. Numerous studies have been made on pool sizes, intravascular and extravascular distribution, and turnover rates for individual proteins in the plasma, some of which are listed in Table 5-4. Together with other plasma proteins, they account for about 20 gm protein synthesized per day. Measurement [56] of turnover rate as well as pool size can be obtained by injecting the plasma protein labeled with ^{131}I or ^{125}I and measuring the rate of loss of label from the plasma. Alternatively, synthesis can be measured in the human by injection of $^{14}CO_2$, which labels arginine [47] in the guanido group. The labeling of free arginine in the liver can be monitored by measuring ^{14}C-labeling of urea formed from the same guanido group and excreted in the urine. We have adapted this procedure for continuous labeling with the heavy isotope ^{15}N, fed every 3 hours over a 60-hour period as ^{15}N-glycine [31]. The rates of

Table 5-4. *Turnover of Plasma Proteins*

Plasma Protein	Plasma Concentration (gm/100 ml)	Intravascular Pool (% total)	Fractional Catabolic Rate (% total mass/day)	Synthetic Mass (gm/day)
Albumin	4.2	45	4	11
Transferrin	0.2	49	8	1.1
IgC	1.1	58	4	2.1
IgM	0.1	74	8	0.3
Fibrinogen	0.4	84	21	2.2
Thyroxin-binding pre-albumin[a]	0.03	30	27	0.01
Retinol-binding protein[b]	0.006		120	

[a]From Socolow et al. [87].
[b]From Peterson [80].
Source: Adapted from S. Jarnum. In E. Vinnars (Ed.), *Metabolic Response to Trauma. Acta Anaesthesiol. Scand.*, [Suppl.] 55:87, 1974.

synthesis of albumin obtained by this procedure are similar to those provided by the other methods.

Plasma protein turnover responds to dietary and hormonal factors. Feeding rats on a diet low in protein has been found [51] to reduce albumin concentration in the plasma due entirely to a reduction in the rate of albumin synthesis. Restoration of protein to the diet rapidly stimulated synthesis which was followed by a more gradual restoration of plasma albumin concentration to normal. In clinical practice, reduction in plasma albumin concentration is too insensitive to be an indicator of subclinical protein depletion and repletion. Shetty [85] has suggested that plasma proteins with a more rapid rate of turnover, such as thyroxin-binding pre-albumin and retinol-binding protein (Table 5-4), should be more sensitive to dietary conditions, and he has shown this to be true for obese subjects on restricted caloric and protein intake.

Integrated Whole Body Protein Metabolism

The preceding analysis of the principles regulating amino acid metabolism in different organs and tissues of the body allows us to begin to assemble an overall picture of protein metabolism as a whole, and to analyze its responses to various factors.

Figure 5-19 assembles some data regarding whole body protein synthesis in a 70-kg young adult man and identifies some of the components of this. The total protein content of his body is taken at 10 kg, and his average daily turnover of this protein is 250 gm (2.5 percent). More than half of his daily turnover can be accounted for by secreted gut protein (70 gm), muscle turnover (50 gm), plasma proteins turnover (20 gm), white cell turnover (20 gm), and hemoglobin renewal (8 gm), all of which were measured by independent procedures. The extensive nature of this renewal of tissue proteins implies that the free amino acid pool of about 70 gm is in a dynamic state, in which the large-scale recycling of endogenous amino acids (250 gm daily) compares with the smaller dietary intake (100 gm), part of which will not ever reach the systemic circulation because of the intervention of the liver.

Age progressively diminishes turnover rate of body protein [74]. Protein synthesis per kilogram body weight per day diminishes from 25 gm in the neonate, through 7 gm in the infant of one year, to 3.2 gm in the adult male and 2.6 gm in the adult female. Table 5-5 provides data on turnover

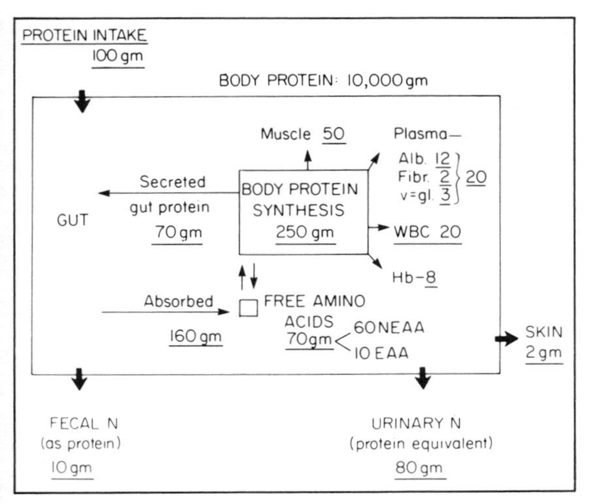

Figure 5-19. *Diagram to show the daily flux of amino acids on the body of a 70-kg man. (From H. N. Munro, Parenteral Nutrition: Metabolic Consequences of Bypassing the Gut and Liver. In* Clinical Nutrition Update: Amino Acids. *Chicago: A.M.A., 1977. P. 141.)*

of whole body protein compared with turnover of plasma albumin and of muscle protein for young and elderly adults. Both males and females show a small reduction with age in whole body protein turnover per kilogram body weight, but this becomes a small increase when turnover is computed per kilogram body cell mass. This increase occurs because of the reduced proportion of lean body mass with increasing age [30]. In contrast, muscle protein turnover, measured by 3-methylhistidine excretion, diminishes even when calculated per kilogram body cell mass, especially in females. However, 3-methylhistidine output is constant for young and old males or females when calculated per gram urinary creatinine. Creatinine output reflects the creatine pool in muscle. This demonstrates that the considerable reduction in 3-methylhistidine with advancing age is due to the extensive shrinkage of skeletal muscle mass with aging [52], which is much more severe than for other active tissues. This picture contrasts with the effects of aging on albumin metabolism. Table 5-5 shows that, although albumin synthesis per kilogram body weight declines slightly in both sexes, calculation per kilogram body cell mass causes this effect of aging on turnover to disappear. Thus, proteins of visceral origin, represented by albumin, continue to provide the same proportion of total turnover for the elderly as for the young, whereas the contribution of muscle to the total protein metabolism of the body diminishes as age advances.

This balance between muscle and viscera appears to be altered by a variety of factors. It is well known that insulin, secreted in response to an influx of dietary carbohydrate, diverts amino acids into muscle and stimulates muscle protein synthesis (see Figure 5-15). In a recent comparison of albumin synthesis rate postoperatively in patients receiving glucose or amino acids or glucose and amino acids parenterally, we [86] found that the inclusion of glucose in the infusion depressed synthesis, presumably by diverting available free amino acids into muscle.

A selective increase in muscle protein degradation rate is demonstrated by comparison of different types of trauma. Table 5-6 compares output of 3-methylhistidine and nitrogen balance in normal adults, in those undergoing an extensive planned operation (hip replacement), and in cases of accidental injury without ketosis. The planned operation caused only a slight negative nitrogen balance and a correspondingly small increment in 3-methylhistidine output above that of a normal adult, whereas the accidental injury produced a large loss of nitrogen and an increase in 3-methylhistidine output equivalent to loss of a similar amount of muscle protein. This suggests that increased muscle protein catabolism could account for the negative nitrogen balance associated with the injury, a conclusion that differs from that of the authors [96], who chose an incorrect value for the 3-methylhistidine content of muscle.

NUTRITIONAL NEEDS FOR PROTEIN AND AMINO ACIDS

The requirement of man for dietary protein has been recognized for more than a hundred years. During the current century, the need for certain

Table 5-5. *Comparison of Whole Body Protein Breakdown with Estimates of Muscle Protein Breakdown and Albumin Synthesis in Young and Old Adult Human Subjects*

		Whole Body Protein Breakdown[a] (gm/day)			Muscle Protein Breakdown[b] (gm/day)			Albumin Synthesis[c] (gm/day)		
Group	Mean Age (Yr)	Per kg Body Wt	Per kg BCM	Per gm Creatinine	Per kg Body Wt	Per kg BCM	Per gm Creatinine	Per kg Body Wt	Per kg BCM	Per gm Creatinine
Males										
Young	22	2.94	6.7	115	0.76	1.74	30	0.19	0.39	7.0
Old	70	2.64	7.5	163	0.53	1.50	32	0.15	0.40	8.4
Females										
Young	20	2.35	6.1	103	0.64	1.69	28			
Old	76	1.94	6.6	166	0.31	1.05	26			

[a] Measured by administration of ^{15}N-glycine [92].
[b] Measured as 3-methylhistidine output in urine and computed as muscle protein [92].
[c] Measured by administration of ^{15}N-glycine [31].

Table 5-6. *Excess Muscle Protein Breakdown Compared with Nitrogen Balance Following Planned Operations and Accidental Injuries*

Subjects	3-Methylhistidine Output: Total Output (μmoles/day)	3-Methylhistidine Output: Excess Over Controls	Equivalent Nitrogen Loss from Muscle Protein[a] (gm/day)	Observed Nitrogen Balance Change (gm/day)
Healthy adult controls[b]	220			
Orthopedic operation[c]	310	90	−3.5	−2.6
Fracture	650	430	−16.5	−12.4

[a]Based on 26 μmoles 3-methylhistidine per gm muscle protein nitrogen [104].
[b]From data given in Table 5-3, calculated for a 70-kg young male.
[c]From D. H. Williamson et al. [96] for hip replacement cases and for fractures without ketosis.

preformed amino acids (essential amino acids) was gradually established. A major advance was the demonstration in 1946, by Block and Mitchell, that various biologic measures of the quality of dietary proteins could be related to their content of essential amino acids expressed as a "chemical score," i.e., the concentration of the essential amino acid in least abundance relative to requirements. The emphasis on essential amino acids was further underlined in the 1950s by quantitative estimates of human requirements for individual amino acids. The protein and amino acid requirements of man have been reassessed periodically in publications of expert committees of the World Health Organization and of the Food and Agricultural Organization and also in *Recommended Dietary Allowances* for the United States, of which the Ninth Edition [29] has just appeared.

Protein Requirements

The amount of protein required in the diet to meet the needs of man can be estimated in two ways. One is to determine all losses of nitrogenous compounds from the body when the diet is free of protein and then to calculate how much high-quality dietary protein would be needed to replace these obligatory nitrogen losses, the so-called factorial method. The second method of estimating protein requirements is to determine directly the minimum amount of protein needed in the diet to keep the subject in nitrogen equilibrium. For infants and children, optimal growth and not nitrogen equilibrium is the criterion of adequacy.

The factorial method of measuring dietary protein needs requires measurement of all sources of nitrogen loss by a subject on a protein-free diet. When a protein-free diet is fed to an adult human subject, there is a rapid decrease in *urinary* nitrogen output for a few days, followed by a plateau [28]. Based on two sets of studies, this minimum output has been estimated to be 37 mg nitrogen per kilogram body weight. Even on a diet deficient in protein, there continues to be a loss of nitrogen in the *feces,* representing enzymes and desquamated intestinal cells that have not been fully reabsorbed, which averages about 12 mg nitrogen per kilogram body weight. Organic nitrogen is also lost from the skin as desquamated cells, hair, and sweat. This cutaneous nitrogen loss by adults on a normal protein intake is about 5 mg per kilogram body weight [7]. There are also minor routes of nitrogen excretion, such as ammonia in the breath, nasal secretions, menstrual flow in the female, and seminal fluid in the male. These minor routes approximate daily 2 mg nitrogen per kilogram body weight for men and 3 mg nitrogen per kilogram for women. Under pathologic conditions, each of these routes of nitrogen output can alter. In addition, the investigator should not forget that a change in the body urea pool of men (normally about 5 gm nitrogen) can affect nitrogen balance determinations.

The factorial approach predicts that protein requirements are the amounts needed in the diet to replace these nitrogen losses when the diet lacks protein. The sum of urinary, fecal, cutaneous and minor routes of nitrogen loss for the healthy adult on a protein-free diet is 54 mg nitrogen per kilogram body weight [28]. Expressed as body protein, these obligatory nitrogen losses represent a net daily loss of 0.34 gm body protein per kilogram body weight, which has to be replaced from the diet. By this method the daily protein requirement of the average adult would be 0.34 gm per kilogram of a dietary protein that is fully utilized. However, individuals show a coefficient of variation of 15 percent, so that the estimate of needs must be increased by 30 percent. In addition, adding increasing amounts of high-quality protein, such as whole egg protein, to the protein-free diet does not produce a linear response. As intake is increased, the efficiency of utilization falls off so that the amount needed to achieve nitrogen equilibrium is much greater than predicted (Figure 5-20). This loss of efficiency adds a further 30 percent to the amount of protein needed for nitrogen equilibrium, thus increasing the requirement for dietary protein to 0.59 gm protein per kilogram body weight. If the quality (amino acid pattern) of the dietary protein is less than that of egg protein, the amount needed to replace body protein will be correspondingly increased. Since the average protein of the Western diet has only 75 percent of the quality of egg protein, the requirement should be increased to 0.8 gm per kilogram body weight, or 56 gm protein daily for a 70-kg man [28].

It should be remembered that most men consume about twice this level of protein. In addition, the estimated need (0.8 gm/kg body weight)

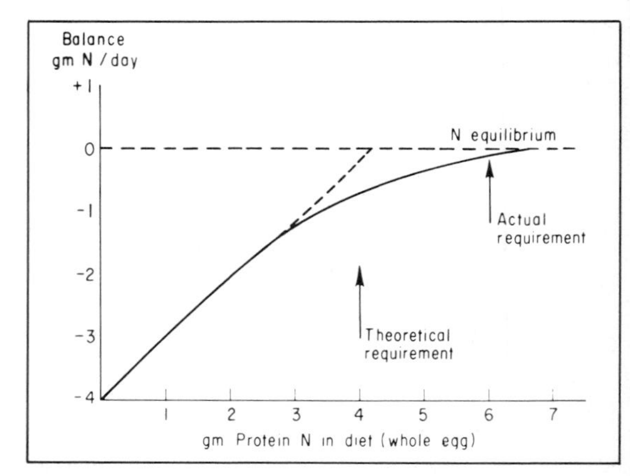

Figure 5-20. *Diagram to demonstrate how endogenous nitrogen (N) output on a protein-free diet would respond to stepwise addition of egg protein if utilization is 100% up to the point of requirements* (dotted line) *or if it becomes less well utilized as requirements are approached* (solid line).

has been determined for young adults, and it is possible that older adults, especially with their higher frequency of chronic illness, may have higher needs, as discussed elsewhere [74]. Finally, the patient under surgical treatment usually has needs that differ from normal, and the foregoing comments can only be regarded as a basis from which to begin.

Amino Acid Needs

For the adult human, the essential amino acids are isoleucine, leucine, lysine, methionine, phenylalanine, threonine, tryptophan, and valine. Histidine is needed by infants and probably in small amounts by adults. Amino acid needs of adults are primarily based on nitrogen balance determinations, and unfortunately, published estimates show a wide range of estimated needs even within a single study. Even so, a survey [44] of this evidence provides a striking picture (Figure 5-21). If the requirements taken selectively from the literature are compared with the needs for total protein, requirements for the essential amino acids add up to about 40 percent of the

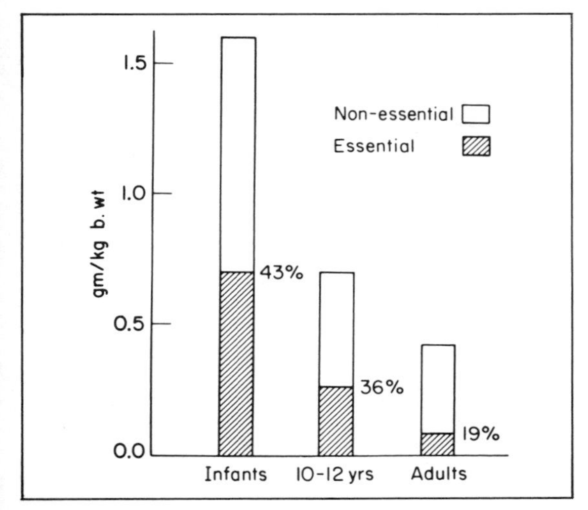

Figure 5-21. *Average requirements for total protein and essential amino acids by human subjects at various ages. (From H. N. Munro, In A. W. Wilkinson (Ed.),* Parenteral Nutrition. *London: Churchill Livingstone, 1972. P. 34.)*

total protein needs of the healthy infant, but they account for only 19 percent of the protein needs of the healthy adult. However, the adult depleted by disease or injury probably differs from a healthy person and, in order to repair tissue, may be considered to have amino acid needs that resemble those of the growing subject. This is supported by studies in which adult rats were depleted of protein and then repleted [89]. Repletion after depletion raised the requirement for each of the essential amino acids about threefold. This supports the conclusion that the demands of repletion are likely to be similar to those of growth in childhood.

These observations led to the conclusion that the most suitable amino acid pattern for administration orally or parenterally to patients is one approximating to that for infants, which will thus reflect the greater needs of depleted patients. Indeed, a mixture of synthetic amino acids resembling the foregoing (Table 5-7) has been administered parenterally by Anderson et al. [1] to adults depleted by gastrointestinal diseases. With this mixture, they obtained nitrogen retentions comparable to those observed when animal protein was given orally in comparable amounts. A casein hydrolysate was much less effective than the synthetic mixture. Further exploration of optimal mixtures for parenteral administration should include a wide range of indicators of repletion. Such formulations can be modified for use with cases of hepatic and renal failure.

Influence of Energy on Protein Needs and Utilization

In addition to quantity and quality of dietary protein, use of amino acids is influenced by the adequacy of energy intake. When energy intake is less than adequate, nitrogen balance becomes negative; whereas when extra energy is added above needs, nitrogen balance becomes positive [61]. The magnitude of the effect is about 2 to 3 gm nitrogen per 1,000 kcal change in energy intake. Consequently, it is not surprising that, on a diet adequate in protein, nitrogen balance can fluctuate around equilibrium dependent on energy intake [6]. Accordingly, nitrogen balance can only be defined in relation to energy intake as well as protein intake. This has been illustrated by Inoue [43], who showed that the requirement for protein could be altered significantly by changing the energy intake of a group of men. At an energy intake just sufficient for maintenance (45 cal/kg), the average requirement of egg protein for nitrogen equilibrium was 0.65 gm per kilogram body weight, whereas at a higher energy intake (57 cal/kg), protein requirement for nitrogen equilibrium fell to 0.46 gm per kilogram. Similarly, the requirement for rice protein changed from 0.87 gm per kilogram at the lower energy intake to 0.58 gm per kilogram at the higher level of energy.

The interaction of energy and protein intake is well illustrated in a study by us [33] on rats that received one of three levels of protein intake along with either a low or high intake of energy (Figure 5-22A). Nitrogen balance improved as protein intake or energy intake was raised. In the same study, animals on these six diets were also

Table 5-7. *Suggested Amino Acid Formula for Parenteral Intravenous Administration*

Amino Acid	Body Wt (mg/kg)	% to Mixture
Essential		
Histidine	60	2.4
Isoleucine	135	5.4
Leucine	200	8.0
Lysine	160	6.4
Methionine	55	2.2
Phenylalanine	110	4.4
Threonine	125	5.0
Tryptophan	35	1.4
Valine	155	6.2
		41.4
Nonessential		
Cystine	70	2.8
Tyrosine	100	4.0
Alanine	360	14.4
Arginine	200	8.0
Glycine	390	15.6
Proline	170	6.8
Serine	175	7.0
		58.6

Note: Glutamic acid, aspartic acid, glutamine, asparagine absent

Source: Adapted from Winters and Hasselmeyer by M. C. Crim and H. N. Munro, Protein and Amino Acid Requirements and Metabolism in Relation to Defined Formula Diets. In M. E. Shils (Ed.), *Defined Formula Diets for Medical Purposes.* Chicago: A.M.A., 1977. P. 50.

injected with large doses of cortisone (Figure 5-22B). At each level of protein and energy intake, the corticosteroid caused a loss of nitrogen from the body. Nevertheless, the addition of protein and/or energy to the diet still improved nitrogen balance. This demonstrates that, even under conditions of gross adrenocortical oversecretion in severe trauma, the administration of adequate amounts of protein and energy is still important. We [20] have illustrated the effect of parenteral energy intake on the nitrogen balance of trauma cases. Figure 5-23 shows that nitrogen retention became progressively more positive as increasing amounts of carbohydrate were added to the infusate.

Protein Depletion and Repletion

A major weakness in assessing the protein or amino acid needs of a patient is the availability of adequate tests of protein depletion and repletion. In chronic severe malnutrition in disadvantaged children in developing countries, a number of criteria have been used. In such cases, protein deficiency reduces plasma-essential amino acid levels, especially the branched-chain amino acids, with little or no effect on nonessential amino acid concentrations, so that the ratio of essential to nonessential amino acids is decreased [41]. However, this index is too easily altered by recent intake of protein to be a reliable

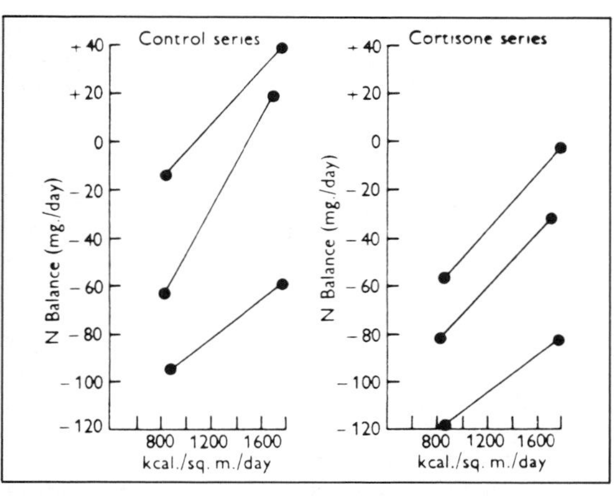

Figure 5-22. *Effect of cortisone administration over a four-day period on the nitrogen balance of rats receiving diets varying in protein and in energy content. Graphs* A *and* B *show the influence of energy intake on nitrogen balance at an adequate level of dietary protein* (upper line), *at a low level of dietary protein* (middle line), *and on a protein-free diet* (lower line). *Nitrogen balance was affected significantly ($P < 0.01$) by protein intake, by energy intake, and by cortisone administration. However, the action of cortisone on nitrogen balance was not significantly altered by diet. (From G. A. J. Goodlad, and H. N. Munro, Diet and the action of cortisone on protein metabolism.* Biochem. J. *73:343, 1959.)*

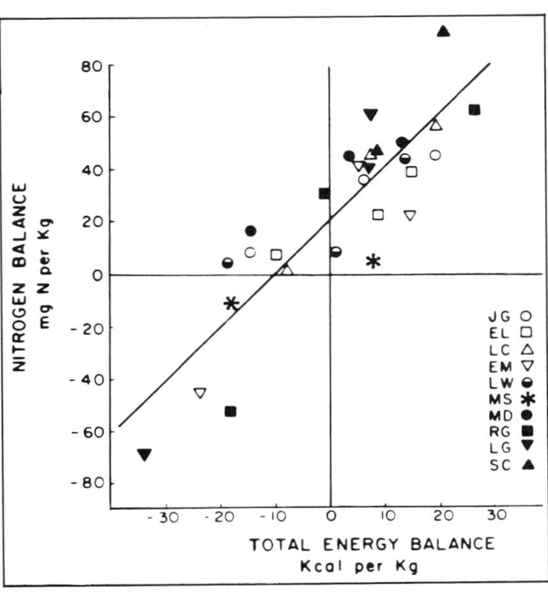

Figure 5-23. *Nitrogen balance as a function of total energy balance for 10 depleted patients on constant nitrogen (N) and variable glucose intake. The regression line had a slope of 1.7 mg nitrogen per kilocalorie and an intercept of 19.8 mg nitrogen per kilogram body weight. (From D. H. Elwyn, et al., Changes in nitrogen balance of depleted patients with increasing infusions of glucose.* Amer. J. Clin. Nutr. *32:1597, 1979.)*

indication of tissue depletion. In severely malnourished children, some plasma hormone levels undergo striking changes [14]. Thus, increments in growth hormone have been noted in kwashiorkor, but not in marasmus. A reduction in somatomedin level has been noted in kwashiorkor and might be a useful index of changes in liver function in response to diet. Cortisol is elevated in the marasmic patient, but not usually in the kwashiorkor case, whereas thyroid-stimulating hormone is a sensitive index of calorie deficiency. These alterations are obtained under extreme conditions of dietary deficiency, but suggest that endocrine changes deserve more attention in less severe malnutrition.

For hospital patients in more developed countries, anthropometric indices have been used, supplemented with measurements of plasma protein concentrations and loss of cellular response to cutaneous antigens. Although plasma albumin level is commonly used, the turnover rate of this protein (see Table 5-4) is too long to make it responsive to short-term changes in protein and energy intake [85]. Plasma transferrin levels are more severely reduced in severe malnutrition [42], but Shetty et al. [85] state it is insufficient for detecting subclinical malnutrition. In a study of obese subjects receiving calorie-poor reducing diets containing amounts of protein varying from 20 to 80 gm daily, they found that thyroxine-binding pre-albumin and retinol-binding protein were more sensitive indices of inadequate protein and energy intake, and attribute this to the more rapid turnover rate of these proteins (see Table 5-4). Finally, the effects of protein and energy insufficiency on 3-methylhistidine output of malnourished rats [38] and children [75] suggest that it may prove useful in following the course of depletion and repletion.

REFERENCES

1. Anderson, G. H., Patel, G. N., and Jeejeebhoy, H. N. Design and evaluation by nitrogen balance and blood aminograms of an amino acid mixture for total parenteral nutrition of adults with gastrointestinal disease. *J. Clin. Invest.* 53:904, 1974.
2. Baxter, J. D., and Funder, J. W. Hormone receptors. *N. Engl. J. Med.* 301:1149, 1979.
3. Bergman, E. N., and Heitmann, R. N. Metabolism of amino acids by the gut, liver, kidneys, and peripheral tissues. *Fed. Proc.* 37:1228, 1978.
4. Blaschko, H. Amine oxidase and amine metabolism. *Pharmacol. Rev.* 4:415, 1952.
5. Brookes, I. M., Owens, F. N., and Garrigus, V. S. Influence of amino acid level in diet upon amino acid oxidation by the rat. *J. Nutr.* 102:27, 1972.
6. Calloway, D. H. Nitrogen balance of men with marginal intakes of protein and energy. *J. Nutr.* 105:914, 1975.
7. Calloway, D. H., Odell, A. C. F., and Margen, S. Sweat and miscellaneous nitrogen losses in human balance studies. *J. Nutr.* 101:775, 1971.
8. Christensen, H. N. On the development of amino acid transport systems. *Fed. Proc.* 32:19, 1973.
9. Clifford, A. J., Riumallo, J. A., Baliga, B. S., Munro, H. N., and Brown, P. R. Liver nucleotide metabolism in relation to amino acid supply. *Biochim. Biophys. Acta* 277:443, 1972.
10. Committee on Dietary Allowances. *Human Vitamin B6 Requirements.* Washington, DC: National Academy of Sciences, National Research Council, 1978.
11. Crim, M. C., Calloway, D. H., and Margen, S. Creatine metabolism in men: Urinary creatine and creatinine excretions with creatine feeding. *J. Nutr.* 105:428, 1978.
12. Crim, M. C., Calloway, D. H., and Margen, S. Creatine metabolism in men: Creatine pool size and turnover in relation to creatine intake. *J. Nutr.* 106:371, 1976.
13. Crim, M. C., and Munro, H. N. Protein and Amino Acid Requirements and Metabolism in Relation to Defined Formula Diets. In M. E. Shils (Ed.), *Defined Formula Diets for Medical Purposes.* Chicago: AMA, 1977. P. 5.
14. Crim, M. C., and Munro, H. N. Protein-Energy Malnutrition and Endocrine Function. In L. J. DeGroot et al. (Eds.), *Endocrinology.* New York: Grune & Stratton, 1979. Vol. 3, p. 1987.
15. Curtoys, N. P., and Lowry, O. H. The distribution of glutaminase isoenzymes in the various structures of the nephron in normal, acidotic, and alkalotic rat kidney. *J. Biol. Chem.* 248:162, 1973.
16. Davidson, J. N. *The Biochemistry of the Nucleic Acids* (7th ed.). New York: Academic, 1972.
17. Dodsworth, J. M., James, J. H., Cummings, M. C., and Fischer, J. E. Depletion of brain norepinephrine in acute hepatic coma. *Surgery* 75:811, 1974.
18. Driscoll, H. K., Crim, M. C., Zahringer, J., and Munro, H. N. Hepatic synthesis and urinary excretion of $\alpha_2\mu$-globulin by male rats: Diurnal rhythm and response to fasting and refeeding. *J. Nutr.* 108:1691, 1978.
19. Elwyn, D. H. The Role of the Liver in Regulation of Amino Acid and Protein Metabolism. In H. N. Munro (Ed.), *Mammalian Protein Metabolism.* New York: Academic, 1970. Vol. IV, p. 523.
20. Elwyn, D. H., Gump, F. E., Munro, H. N., Iles, M., and Kinney, J. M. Changes in nitrogen balance of depleted patients with increasing infusions of glucose. *Am. J. Clin. Nutr.* 32:1597, 1979.
21. Fauconneau, G., and Michel, M. C. The Role of the Gastrointestinal Tract in the Regulation of Protein Metabolism. In H. N. Munro (Ed.), *Mammalian Protein Metabolism.* New York: Academic, 1970. Vol. IV, p. 481.
22. Featherstone, W. R., Rogers, Q. R., and Freedland, R. A. Relative importance of kidney and liver in synthesis of arginine by the rat. *Am. J. Physiol.* 224:127, 1973.
23. Felig, P., and Wahren, J. Amino acid metabolism in exercising man. *J. Clin. Invest.* 50:2703, 1971.
24. Felig, P. Wahren, J., Karl, I., Cerasi, E., Lufts, R., and Kipnis, D. M. Glutamine and glutamate metabolism in normal and diabetic subjects. *Diabetes* 22:573, 1973.
25. Fernstrom, J. D., and Wurtman, R. J. Brain serotonin content: Physiological regulation by plasma neutral amino acids. *Science* 178:414, 1972.
26. Fernstrom, J. D., Wurtman, R. J., Hammarström-Wiklund, B., Rand, W. M., Munro, H. N., and Davidson, C. S. Diurnal variations in plasma neutral amino acid concentrations among patients with cirrhosis: Effects of dietary protein. *Am. J. Clin. Nutr.* 32:1923, 1979.
27. Fischer, J. E., Rosen, H. M., Ebeid, A. M., James, J. K., Keane, J. M., and Soeters, P. B. The effects of normalization of plasma amino

acids on hepatic encephalopathy in man. *Surgery* 80:77, 1976.
28. Food and Agricultural Organization, World Health Organization Expert Committee Report. *Energy and Protein Requirements.* Geneva: Technical Report Series No. 522, WHO, 1973.
29. Food and Nutrition Board. *Recommended Dietary Allowances,* (9th ed.). Washington, DC: National Academy of Sciences—National Research Center, 1980.
30. Forbes, G. B., and Reina, J. C. Adult lean body mass declines with age: Some longitudinal observations. *Metabolism* 19:653, 1970.
31. Gersovitz, M., Young, V. R., Burke, J., and Munro, H. N. Albumin synthesis in young and elderly subjects using a new stable isotope methodology: Response to level of protein intake. *Metabolism* 29:1075, 1980.
32. Gitler, C. Protein Digestion and Absorption in Nonruminants. In H. N. Munro and J. B. Allison (Eds.), *Mammalian Protein Metabolism.* New York: Academic, 1964. Vol. I.
33. Goodlad, G. A. J., and Munro, H. N. Diet and the action of cortisone on protein metabolism. *Biochem. J.* 73:343, 1959.
34. Green, G. M., Olds, B. A., Matthews, B. A., and Lyman, R. L. Protein as a regulator of pancreatic enzyme secretions in the rat. *Proc. Soc. Exp. Biol. Med.* 142:1162, 1973.
35. Greene, H. L., Holliday, M. A., and Munro, H. N. (Eds.) *Clinical Nutrition Update: Amino Acids.* Chicago: AMA, 1977.
36. Guder, W. G., and Schmidt, U. The localization of gluconeogenesis in rat nephron. Determination of phosphoenolpyruvate carboxykinase in micro dissected tubules. *Z. Physiol. Chem.* 355: 273, 1974.
37. Harper, A. E. Diet and plasma amino acids. *Am. J. Clin. Nutr.* 21:358, 1968.
38. Haverberg, L. N., Deckelbaum, L., Bilmazes, C., Munro, H. N., and Young, V. R. Myofibrillar protein turnover and urinary N^{τ}-methylhistidine output: response to dietary supply of protein and energy. *Biochem. J.* 152:503, 1975.
39. Haverberg, L. N., Omstedt, P. T., Munro, H. N., and Young, V. R. N^{τ}-methylhistidine content of mixed proteins in various rat tissues. *Biochim. Biophys. Acta* 405:67, 1975.
40. Herbert, J. D., Coulson, R. A., and Hernandez, T. Free amino acid in the caiman and rat. *Comp. Biochem. Physiol.* 17:583, 1966.
41. Holt, L. E., and Snyderman, S. E. Anomalies of Amino Acid Metabolism. In H. N. Munro and J. B. Allison (Eds.), *Mammalian Protein Metabolism.* New York: Academic, 1964. Vol. 2, p. 321.
42. Ingenbleek, Y., VandenShrieck, H. G., De Nayer, P., and DeVisscher, M. Albumin, transferrin and the thyroxine-binding prealbumin/retinol-binding protein (TBPA-RBP) complex in assessment of malnutrition. *Clin. Chim. Acta* 63:61, 1975.
43. Inoue, G., Fugita, Y., and Niiyama, Y. Studies on protein requirements of young men fed egg protein and rice protein with excess and maintenance energy intakes. *J. Nutr.* 103:1673, 1973.
44. Irwin, M. I., and Hegsted, D. M. A conspectus of research on amino acid requirements of man. *J. Nutr.* 101:539, 1971.
45. Jacob, S. T., Sajdel, E. M., and Munro, H. N. Regulation of nucleolar RNA metabolism by hydrocortisone. *Europ. J. Biochem.* 7:449, 1969.
46. Jarnum, S. Plasma Protein Metabolism. In E. Vinnars (Ed.), *Metabolic Response to Trauma. Acta Anesth. Scand.,* Suppl. 55:87, 1974.
47. Jones, E. A., Carson, E., and Rosenoer, V. M. In M. A. Rothschild and T. Waldmann (Eds.), *Plasma Protein Metabolism.* New York: Academic, 1970. P. 11.
48. Kaplan, J. H., and Pitot, H. C. The Regulation of Intermediary Amino Acid Metabolism in Animal Tissues. In H. N. Munro (Ed.), *Mammalian Protein Metabolism.* New York: Academic, 1970. Vol. 4, p. 388.
49. Kenney, F. T. Hormonal Regulation of Synthesis of Liver Enzymes. In H. N. Munro (Ed.), *Mammalian Protein Metabolism.* New York: Academic, 1970. Vol. 4, p. 131.
50. Kim, Y. S., and Freeman, H. J. Digestion and Absorption of Protein. In H. L. Green, M. A. Holliday, and H. N. Munro (Eds.), *Clinical Nutrition Update: Amino Acids.* Chicago: AMA, 1977. P. 135.
51. Kirsch, R., Frith, L., Black, E., and Hoffenberg, R. Regulation of albumin synthesis and catabolism by alteration of dietary protein. *Nature* 217: 579, 1968.
52. Korenchevsky, V. In G. H. Bourne (Ed.), *Physiological and Pathological Aging.* New York: Hafner, 1961.
53. Levenson, S. M., and Tennant, B. Contributions of intestinal microflora to the nutrition of the host animal. *Fed. Proc.* 22:109, 1963.
54. Long, C. L., Haverberg, L. N., Kinney, J. M., Young, V. R., Munro, H. N., and Geiger, J. N. Metabolism of 3-methylhistidine in man. *Metabolism* 24:929, 1975.
55. Matthews, D. M., and Adibi, S. A. Peptide absorption. *Gastroenterology* 71:151, 1976.
56. McFarlane, A. S. In M. A. Rothschild and T.

Waldmann (Eds.), *Plasma Protein Metabolism.* New York: Academic, 1970. P. 51.

57. McGilvery, R. W. *Biochemistry—A Functional Approach.* Philadelphia: Saunders, 1970.
58. Meister, A., On the enzymology of amino acid transport. *Science* 180:33, 1973.
59. Miller, L. L. The Role of the Liver and the Nonhepatic Tissues in the Regulation of Free Amino Acid Levels in the Blood. In J. T. Holden (Ed.), *Amino Acid Pools.* Amsterdam: Elsevier, 1962. P. 708.
60. Munro, H. N. Biochemical Aspects of Protein Metabolism. In H. N. Munro and J. B. Allison (Eds.), *Mammalian Protein Metabolism.* New York: Academic, 1964. Vol. 1, p. 318.
61. Munro, H. N. General Aspects of the Regulation of Protein Metabolism by Diet and by Hormones. In H. N. Munro and J. B. Allison (Eds.), *Mammalian Protein Metabolism.* New York: Academic, 1964. Vol. 1, p. 381.
62. Munro, H. N. The Evolution of Protein Metabolism in Mammals. In H. N. Munro (Ed.), *Mammalian Protein Metabolism.* New York: Academic, 1969. Vol. 3.
63. Munro, H. N. Regulation Mechanisms in Protein Metabolism. In H. N. Munro (Ed.), *Mammalian Protein Metabolism.* New York: Academic, 1970. Vol. 4, p. 3.
64. Munro, H. N. In *Aromatic Amino Acids in the Brain.* Ciba Foundation Symposium 22, New York: Elsevier, 1974. P. 5.
65. Munro, H. N. Amino Acid Requirements and Metabolism and Their Bearing on Human Nutrition. In A. W. Wilkinson (Ed.), *Parenteral Nutrition.* London: Churchill Livingstone, 1972. P. 34.
66. Munro, H. N. Parenteral Nutrition: Metabolic Consequences of Bypassing the Gut and Liver. In *Clinical Nutrition Update: Amino Acids.* Chicago: AMA, 1977. P. 141.
67. Munro, H. N. Factors in the Regulation of Glutamate Metabolism. In L. J. Filer et al. (Eds.), *Glutamic Acid: Advances in Biochemistry and Physiology.* New York: Raven Press, 1979. P. 55.
68. Munro, H. N., Hubert, C., and Baliga, B. S. Regulation of Protein Synthesis in Relation to Amino Acid Supply: A Review. In M. A. Rothschild, M. Oratz, and S. S. Schreiber (Eds.), *Alcohol and Abnormal Protein Biosynthesis.* New York: Pergamon, 1975. P. 33.
69. Munro, H. N., and Crim, M. C. The Proteins and Amino Acids. In R. S. Goodhart and M. E. Shils (Eds.), *Modern Nutrition in Health and Disease.* Philadelphia: Lea & Febiger, 1980.
70. Munro, H. N., Fernstrom, J. D., and Wurtman, R. J. Insulin, plasma amino acid imbalance and hepatic coma. *Lancet* 1:722, 1975.
71. Munro, H. N., and Steinert, P. M. The Intracellular Organization of Protein Synthesis. In H. R. V. Arnstein (Ed.), *International Review of Science, Biochemistry Series.* Oxford: Med. Tech. Pub. Co., 1975. Vol. 7, chapter 9.
72. Munro, H. N., and Thomson, W. S. T. Influence of glucose on amino acid metabolism. *Metabolism* 2:354, 1953.
73. Munro, H. N., and Young, V. R. Urinary excretion of N^{τ}-methylhistidine (3-methylhistidine): A tool to study metabolic responses in relation to nutrient and hormonal status in health and disease of man. *Am. J. Clin. Nutr.* 31:1608, 1978.
74. Munro, H. N., and Young, V. R. Protein metabolism in the elderly: Observations relating to dietary needs. *Postgrad. Med.* 63:143, 1978.
75. Narasinga Rao, B. S., and Nagabhushan, V. S. Urinary excretion of 3-methylhistidine in children suffering from protein calorie malnutrition. *Life Sci.* 12:205, 1973.
76. Nettleton, J. A., and Hegsted, D. M. Reutilization of guanido labeled orginine in rat liver protein and the influence of diet. *J. Nutr.* 104:916, 1974.
77. Nowak, T. S., and Munro, H. N. Effects of Protein-Calorie Malnutrition on Biochemical Aspects of Brain Development. In R. J. Wurtman and J. J. Wurtman (Eds.), *Nutrition and the Brain,* Vol. 2. New York: Raven Press, 1977.
78. Owen, O. E. Morgan, A. P., Kemp, H. G., Sullivan, J. M. Herrera, M. G., and Cahill, G. F. Brain metabolism during fasting. *J. Clin. Invest.* 46:1589, 1967.
79. Pawlak, N., and Pion, R. *Ann. Biol. Anim. Biochem. Biophys.* 8:517, 1968.
80. Peterson, P. A. Demonstration in serum of two physiological forms of the human retinol binding protein. *Europ. J. Clin. Invest.* I:437, 1971.
81. Posevsky, T., Felig, P., Tobin, J., Soeldner, J., and Cahill, G. F. Amino acid balance across tissues of the forearm in postabsorptive man. Effects of insulin at two dose levels. *J. Clin. Invest.* 48:2273, 1969.
82. Prockop, D. J., and Sjoerdsma, A. Significance of urinary hydroxyproline in man. *J. Clin. Invest.* 40:843, 1961.
83. Rackis, J. J. Physiological properties of soybean trypsin inhibitors and their relationship to pancreatic hypertrophy and growth inhibition of rats. *Fed. Proc.* 24:1488, 1965.

84. Seegmiller, J. E. Biochemical and genetic studies of an x-linked neurological disease. *Harvey Lect. Series* 65:175, 1971.
85. Shetty, P. S., Jung, R. T., Watrasiewicz, K. E., and James, W. P. T. Rapid-turnover transport proteins: An index of subclinical protein-energy malnutrition. *Lancet* 2:230, 1979.
86. Skillman, J. J., Rosenoer, V. M., Pallotta, J. A., Young, J. B., Young, V. R., Long, R. C., Wilentz, K., and Munro, H. N. Albumin synthesis and nitrogen balance in postoperative patients. *Surgery* 87:305, 1980.
87. Socolow, E. L., Woeber, K. A., Purdy, R. H., Holloway, N. T., and Inghar, S. H. Preparation of I^{131}-labeled human serum prealbumin and its metabolism in normal and sick patients. *J. Clin. Invest.* 44:1600, 1965.
88. Steele, R. Formation of amino acids from carbohydrate carbon in mouse. *J. Biol. Chem.* 198:237, 1952.
89. Steffee, C. H., Wissler, R. W., Humphreys, E. M., Benditt, E. P., Woolridge, R. W., and Cannon, P. R. Studies in amino acid utilization: Determination of minimum daily essential amino acid requirements in protein-depleted adult male albino rats. *J. Nutr.* 40:483, 1950.
90. Stegink, L. D. D-Amino Acids. In *Clinical Nutrition Update—Amino Acids.* Chicago: AMA, 1977. P. 198.
91. Tomas, F. M., Munro, H. N., and Young, V. R. Effect of glucocorticoid administration on the rate of muscle protein breakdown in vivo in rats, as measured by urinary excretion of N tau-methylhistidine. *Biochem. J.* 178:139, 1979.
92. Uauy, R., Winterer, J. C., Bilmazes, C., Haverberg, L. N., Scrimshaw, N. S., Munro, H. N., and Young, V. R. The changing pattern of whole body protein metabolism in aging humans. *J. Gerontol.* 33:663, 1978.
93. Visek, N. J. Ammonia metabolism, urea cycle capacity and their biochemical assessment. *Nutr. Reviews* 37:273, 1979.
94. Wahren, J., Felig, P., and Hagenfeldt, L. Effect of protein ingestion on splanchnic and leg metabolism in normal man and in patients with diabetes mellitus. *J. Clin. Invest.* 57:987, 1976.
95. Walser, M., and Bodenlos, L. J. Urea metabolism in man. *J. Clin. Invest.* 38:1617, 1959.
96. Williamson, D. H., Farrell, R., Kerr, A., and Smith, R. Muscle-protein catabolism after injury in man as measured by urinary excretion of 3-methylhistidine. *Clin. Sci. Mol. Med.* 52:527, 1977.
97. Windmueller, H. G., and Spaeth, A. E. Intestinal metabolism of glutamine and glutamate from the lumen as compared to glutamine from blood. *Arch. Biochem. Biophys.* 171:662, 1975.
98. Winters, R. W., and Hasselmayer, E. G. (Eds.), *Intravenous Nutrition in the High Risk Infant.* New York: Wiley, 1975.
99. Wurtman, R. J. Diurnal Rhythms in Mammalian Protein Metabolism. In H. N. Munro (Ed.), *Mammalian Protein Metabolism.* New York: Academic, 1970. Vol. 4, p. 445.
100. Young, V. R. The Role of Skeletal and Cardiac Muscle in the Regulation of Protein Metabolism. In H. N. Munro (Ed.), *Mammalian Protein Metabolism.* New York: Academic, 1970. Vol. 4, p. 585.
101. Young, V. R., Alexis, S. D., Baliga, B. S., Munro, H. N., and Muecke, W. Metabolism of administered 3-methylhistidine. Lack of muscle transfer ribonucleic acid charging and quantitative excretion as 3-methylhistidine and its N-acetyl derivative. *J. Biol. Chem.* 247:3592, 1972.
102. Young, V. R. Haverberg, L. N., Bilmazes, C., and Munro, H. N. The potential use of 3-methylhistidine excretion as an index of progressive reduction in muscle protein catabolism during starvation. *Metabolism* 22:1429, 1973.
103. Young, V. R., and Munro, H. N. Plasma and tissue tryptophan levels in relation to tryptophan requirements in weaning and adult rats. *J. Nutr.* 103:1756, 1973.
104. Young, V. R., and Munro, H. N. N^{τ}-methylhistidine (3-methylhistidine) and muscle protein turnover: An overview. *Fed. Proc.* 37:2291, 1978.
105. Young, V. R., Tontisirin, R. K., Ozalp, I., Lakshmanan, and Scrimshaw, N. S. Plasma amino acid response curve and amino acid requirements in young men: Valine and lysine. *J. Nutr.* 102:1159, 1972.

Carbohydrates

John W. Vester
Harry Rudney

6

The study of the metabolism of carbohydrate by living cells began in earnest at the turn of this century and has played a central role in the evolution of biochemistry into a major science. Many of the key, fundamental discoveries were made by chemists who were trying to understand the mechanism of alcoholic fermentation in yeast. The most significant "break-through" observation was made by Buchner in 1897, who showed for the first time that sugars could be "fermented" by a cell-free extract. Progress was rapid from that point because studies were no longer restricted to intact cells. Soon the analogies between alcoholic fermentation and other fermentations, e.g., lactic acid, were discovered, and the essential role of phosphate was elucidated. A study of the chemical principles by which enzymes exerted their catalytic action originated from these observations. Space does not allow a full development of the exciting history of the role that the study of carbohydrate metabolism played in biochemistry, but some of the great names that stand out are Pasteur, Buchner, Harden, Embden, Meyerhof, Warburg, Neuberg, the Coris, and Krebs.

Carbohydrates account for a significant portion of the daily dietary intake in most human diets. The carbohydrate ingested takes many forms, most of which are broken down by digestion to the three major sugars: glucose, fructose, and galactose. Pentose sugars are also ingested, and their metabolism will be discussed in connection with the hexose monophosphate shunt pathway. The process of metabolism of six carbon sugars (hexoses) is referred to as glycolysis, and we will begin our discussion with the major sugar utilized by cells, i.e., glucose.

The word *metabolism* implies a state of change or flux. In the context of the major foodstuff that we will be considering in this chapter, metabolism consists of two major processes, catabolism and anabolism. With respect to carbohydrate, the first process is represented by equation 1:

$$\text{Glucose} + 6\ O_2 \rightarrow 6\ CO_2 + 6\ H_2O + \text{energy} \qquad (1)$$

The second process, anabolism, is represented by equation 2:

$$\text{Cellular energy} + \text{specific metabolic noncarbohydrate sources} \rightarrow \text{glucose} \qquad (2)$$

Let us examine further the nature of the energy released in equation 1 and the nature of the energy used in equation 2.

Living cells are chemical engines of a high degree of orderliness. They create and maintain their intricate orderliness in an environment that is relatively disordered and becoming more so with time. According to the laws of thermodynamics, order in an open system (negative entropy) can be maintained at the expense of creating disorder in the environment (i.e., positive entropy). The cell is in a highly ordered state and maintains itself in this way by taking in highly ordered material similar in composition to itself, i.e., foodstuffs, and breaks them down, i.e., creates disorder. The energy that went into making these foodstuffs is released by the cells in small increments, and the useful form of this energy, which can be used for cellular work, is conserved. This latter form of the energy generated by the cell, which is used for work, is called free energy.

The relationships between changes of free energy and entropy and the total energy of a system are given by the famous equation first elaborated by Gibbs:

$$\Delta G = \Delta E - T\Delta S \quad (3)$$

where ΔG = change in free energy
ΔE = change in total energy of the system, which closely approximates the total heat content of the system
ΔS = change in entropy
T = absolute temperature

The quantity $T\Delta S$ is the mathematical expression that describes the change in orderliness. In the example shown in Equation 1, the CO_2 and water produced contain less energy than the glucose and oxygen did. The energy released by the transformation of glucose to CO_2 and water consists simply of the difference between the amount of energy contained in the glucose and oxygen before the reaction and the amount of energy contained in the CO_2 and water after the reaction is completed. Not all the energy released in such a transformation is available for use by the cell or, indeed, by any engine. Some of the difference in energy content between products and reactants is accounted for by the difference in orderliness of the products as compared to the reactants. Six moles of CO_2 and water are more disordered than the mole of glucose and six moles of oxygen. The products, then, have more entropy than the reactants. The energy involved in increasing entropy cannot be used but all the other energy released by the change in heat content in converting reactants to products can be used and this is called free energy.

As stated above, the conversion of one mole of glucose to six moles of CO_2 and water will produce 686,000 calories. In biologic chemistry, use is made of the kilocalorie, i.e., 1,000 calories, so that the amount of free energy available from a mole of glucose is 686 kilocalories, and the kilocalorie is often abbreviated and symbolized by the word *Calorie* (with the C capitalized). Since the molecular weight of glucose is 180, simple calculation reveals that one gram of glucose will yield 3.81 Calories. In clinical parlance, this is rounded off to the well-known figure of 4 Calories per gram of carbohydrate.

ROLE OF ADENOSINE TRIPHOSPHATE

Now we may ask in what form the free energy produced in the breakdown of glucose is conserved and utilized. The substance adenosine triphosphate plays a universal role in all forms of life in acting as the medium for the collection, transfer and utilization of free energy in the cell. The structure of this molecule, abbreviated as ATP, is shown in Figure 6-1. Energy yielded from the degradation of fuel molecules (foodstuffs) is conserved by the phosphorylation of adenosine diphosphate (ADP) to form ATP according to equation 4.

$$ADP + H_3PO_4 + \text{energy} \rightarrow ATP \quad (4)$$

Energy is given off in exergonic reactions, and this energy is conserved in the ATP and can be transferred by donation of the terminal phos-

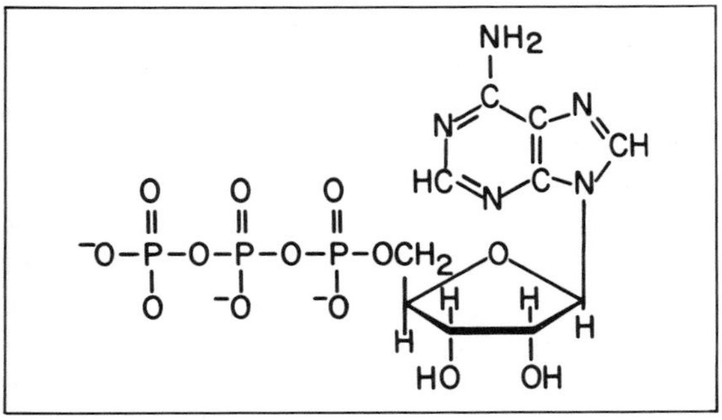

Figure 6-1. *The structure of adenosine triphosphate (ATP).*

phate of this molecule, popularly described as the high-energy phosphate group, to energy-requiring processes in the cell. Such energy-requiring processes are termed *endergonic reactions*.

When the terminal phosphates are referred to as high-energy bonds, what is really meant is that the energy does not reside in the bond between phosphorous and oxygen, but that there is a difference in the energy content of the reactants and the products, i.e., the ATP generally has a higher energy content than a product of the reaction of ATP with cellular constituents.

Other compounds in the cell also have high-energy phosphate with a standard free energy more negative than that of ATP, which is −7.3 Calories/mole, and some of these are produced in carbohydrate metabolism. Table 6-1 shows the standard free energies of some of these compounds.

A reaction with a high negative value for free energy has a greater tendency to react than one with a lower negative value. ATP occupies an intermediate position in this free energy scale of phosphate compounds, and this partly explains its central role. It can act as a linking system between compounds above it in high energy content (high-phosphate group transfer potential) and those below it (low-phosphate group transfer potential). Thus, the compounds above ATP can react with ADP to form ATP and nonphosphorylated derivatives. Nonphosphorylated derivatives of compounds below ATP in the table can

Table 6-1. *Standard Free Energy of Hydrolysis of Phosphate Compounds*

Phosphate Compounds	$\Delta G°$ (calories/mole)
Phosphoenolpyruvate	−14.8
1,3-Diphosphoglycerate	−11.8
Phosphocreatine	−10.3
Acetyl phosphate	−10.1
ATP	−7.3
Glucose-1-phosphate	−5.0
Fructose-6-phosphate	−3.8
Glucose-6-phosphate	−3.3
3-Phosphoglycerate	−2.4
Glycerol-3-phosphate	−2.2

react with ATP to form ADP plus the phosphorylated compound. It would not be possible, for example, for phosphoenolpyruvate ($\Delta G° = -14.8$ Calories) to react directly with glucose and the enzyme systems involved to form glucose-6-phosphate ($\Delta G° = -3.3$ Calories) without the intermediate intervention of ATP via the mechanism of coupled reactions. Thus, phosphoenolpyruvate will react with ADP to form ATP, and the ATP will react with glucose to form glucose-6-phosphate. Separate enzymes catalyze each of these reactions, as shown in equations 5 and 6.

$$\text{PEP} + \text{ADP} \rightarrow \text{ATP} + \text{pyruvate} \qquad (5)$$

$$\text{ATP} + \text{glucose} \rightarrow \text{glucose-6-phosphate} + \text{ADP} \qquad (6)$$

Net equation:

$$\text{PEP} + \text{glucose} \rightarrow \text{pyruvate} + \text{glucose-6-phosphate}$$

The foregoing illustrates one of the most basic principles of biochemistry, which is that of coupling two reactions by means of a common intermediate, e.g.,

$$A + B \rightarrow C + D \qquad (7)$$

$$C + E \rightarrow F + B \qquad (8)$$

The net reaction is

$$A + E \rightarrow F + D \quad (9)$$

The only way in which these reactions could have been linked is via the common intermediates B and C. Extending the analogy to equations 5 and 6, ATP then serves as a carrier of energy between high-energy donors and low-energy receptors. This may finally be summed up in general terms by the equations:

$$X \sim P + ADP \rightarrow X + ATP \quad (10)$$

$$ATP + Y \rightarrow ADP + YP \quad (11)$$

and the sum then represents $X \sim P + Y$ gives $X + YP$. The depiction of a high-energy phosphate bond has been symbolized by use of the symbol $\sim P$.

Since 686 Calories of free energy can be generated by the oxidation of 1 molecule of glucose to 6 molecules of CO_2 and 6 molecules of H_2O, we can begin to develop some efficiency calculations. In the complete oxidation of 1 molecule of glucose, as alluded to above, 38 molecules of adenosine triphosphate (ATP) can be produced. Since we know that each mole of ATP can yield 7.3 Calories, simple multiplication yields the information that 277.4 Calories of ATP-contained free energy are realized from the conversion of every mole of glucose to CO_2 and water. When we divide 686 Calories of free energy that can be shown to be released in a bomb calorimeter into 277.4 stored in the cell as ATP, we demonstrate that the cell oxidizes glucose to CO_2 and water at a thermodynamic efficiency of 40.4 percent. No man-made machine that depends on the burning of fuel even approaches this high degree of thermodynamic efficiency.

OXIDATIVE PHOSPHORYLATION

As already mentioned, it is the trick of harnessing coupled reactions that makes possible the orderly production of energy in the living cell and the equally orderly use of this energy to drive the myriad reactions that, in total, are the life process. As foodstuffs are oxidized, some of the energy that is yielded when the reduced form of a fuel is converted to the oxidized form is stored in the high-energy bond of the terminal phosphate of adenosine triphosphate. (We say *some* of the energy is stored because even in the superbly efficient living cell, some of the energy is lost as heat.) Under the conditions that exist in the intact living cell, about 12 Calories are necessary for the formation of one mole of ATP from one mole of ADP and one mole of inorganic phosphate. (Inorganic phosphate is hereinafter abbreviated as Pi.) Oxidative phosphorylation is the process whereby the cell traps the energy yielded in oxidation of foodstuffs as ATP.

The mitochondrion is the intracellular organelle in which oxidative phosphorylation takes place. These organelles are present in all cells that depend on oxygen for the oxidative derivation of chemical energy. There are about one thousand of them in a liver cell, and they make up 20 percent of the total cytoplasmic volume. In heart muscle cells, over 50 percent of the volume is occupied by mitochondria. The most extensively studied mitochondrion is that in the liver cell, and it is roughly football-shaped, about two microns long and one micron wide, with two membranes (Figure 6-2). The outer membrane is smooth and somewhat elastic, and the inner membrane has extensive inward folding called cristae.

The inner membrane is separated by 50 to 100 Å from the outer membrane. The outer membrane is about half lipid and half protein, whereas the inner membrane is denser and is about three-quarters protein and one-quarter lipid. Inside the inner compartment is the matrix. This is a gel-like phase and it contains about 50 percent protein. Some of this protein is organized into a reticular network that is apparently attached to the inner surface of the inner membrane. The matrix characteristically contains most of the tricarboxylic acid cycle enzymes, which will be described later. The interior surfaces of the cristae facing the matrix are studded with small protrud-

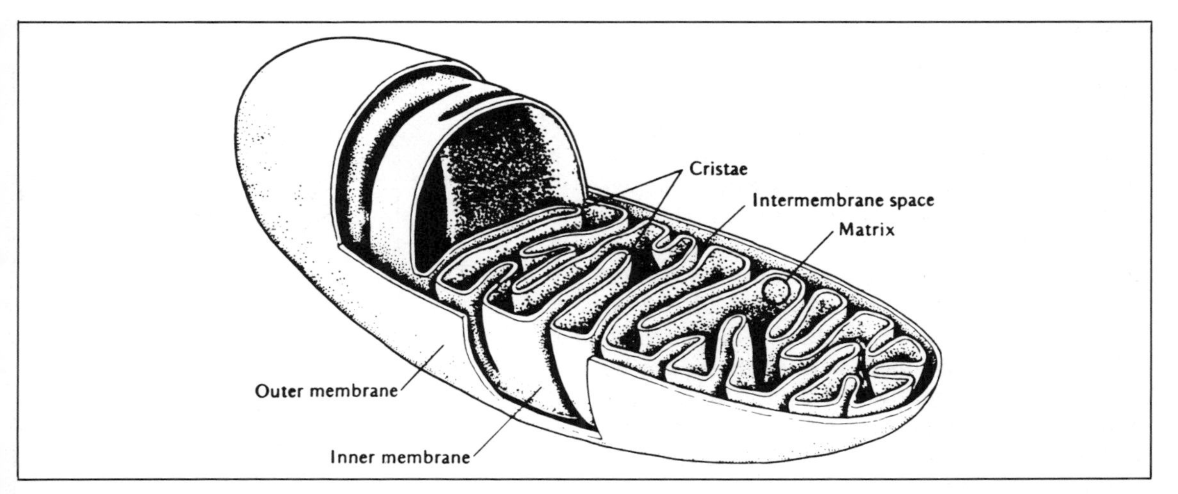

Figure 6-2. *Somewhat diagrammatic representation of a mitochondrion. The inner wall of the inner membrane faces the matrix contents and is studded with protrusions, largely the ATP synthetase. In the matrix are dissolved the dehydrogenases of the citric acid cycle. Suspended in the matrix are ribosomes and the mitochondrial DNA, inter alia. (From S. L. Wolfe,* The Biology of the Cell. *Belmont, CA: Wadsworth Publishing, 1972. Reprinted by permission, © 1972.)*

ing structures called elementary bodies or inner membrane particles. They consist of small spheres connected to the membrane through narrow stalks. The respiratory assembly, which is outlined later in this chapter and in which electron transport takes place, is an integral part of the inner mitochondrial membrane. The structure and function of the mitochondrion make it possible for the cell to extract the energy derived from food cell oxidation in an orderly fashion. If a metabolite (MH_2) were to react directly with oxygen, the reaction would be:

$$MH_2 + \frac{1}{2} O_2 \rightarrow M + H_2O \quad (12)$$

Such a reaction does not permit conservation of energy for synthesis of ATP. Instead, a class of enzymes defined as dehydrogenases catalyze electron transfer from substrate to acceptor molecules. When a reduced metabolite is oxidized in the living cell, it loses hydrogen and two electrons. The reaction that really occurs is as follows:

$$MH_2 + \text{acceptor} \rightarrow M + \text{acceptor } H_2 \quad (13)$$

In this reaction, two hydrogens and two electrons have been transferred to the acceptor. It is true that although this reaction is catalyzed by an enzyme, the function of the enzyme is to accelerate the reaction. It does not change its direction. What determines the direction of a biologic oxidation reaction of this general type is the difference in tendency to give off electrons and/or hydrogen between the substance that is oxidized, i.e., the donor, and the substance that oxidizes it, i.e., the acceptor. In the foregoing circumstance, the donor has a greater tendency than the acceptor to give off electrons and hydrogen.

This tendency to give up electrons can be looked upon as electron pressure. A substance that has a high electron pressure (a strong tendency to give up electrons) will give them up to a substance that has a lower electron pressure. If we were to catalyze electron transfer reactions between a series of acceptors arranged in decreasing order of electron pressure, we would transport the electrons from the substance that has the greatest tendency to give them off to the substance that has the least tendency to give them off. This flow of electrons is truly analogous to the flow of electric current in a wire. It is a transport of energy. Much as energy can be tapped from a wire carrying a current to operate devices such as lamps and motors, energy can be tapped from a chain of electron acceptor-donor compounds. One of the characteristics of the flow of electrons is voltage. When electrons flow from a substance with a greater tendency to give them off, to others with lesser tendencies to give them off, the voltage of this flow of electrons can be measured. In oxidative phosphorylation, the transfer of electrons from metabolite to electron acceptors is just the first step. The electrons are transferred through a sequence of electron acceptors or alternately referred to as electron carriers, arranged in decreasing order of electron pressure, finally reaching molecular oxygen. In the electron transport chain, this energy is tapped off at three discrete sites and used for the manufacture of ATP from ADP and Pi.

$FADH_2$ in flavoproteins ↓

NADH → NADH dehydrogenase → CoQ → Cyt *b* → Cyt c_1 → Cyt *c* → Cyt $(a + a_3)$ → O_2

ADP → ATP (Site 1) ADP → ATP (Site 2) ADP → ATP (Site 3)

The above is a schematic representation of the pathway of electron flow through the respiratory assembly. The three sites of generation of ATP are indicated. The molecule that is most frequently employed as acceptor of electrons from metabolites in biologic systems is nicotinamide adenine dinucleotide (NAD^+) (Figure 6-3).

On the dehydrogenase protein, a hydride ion is transferred from the substrate to the nicotinamide moiety and a proton is liberated into the medium (equation 14).

$$MH_2 + NAD^+ \rightarrow M + NADH + H^+ + 2e \qquad (14)$$

The electron chain in the mitochondrion, in most instances, begins with the $NAD^+/NADH + H^+$ oxidation-reduction pair.

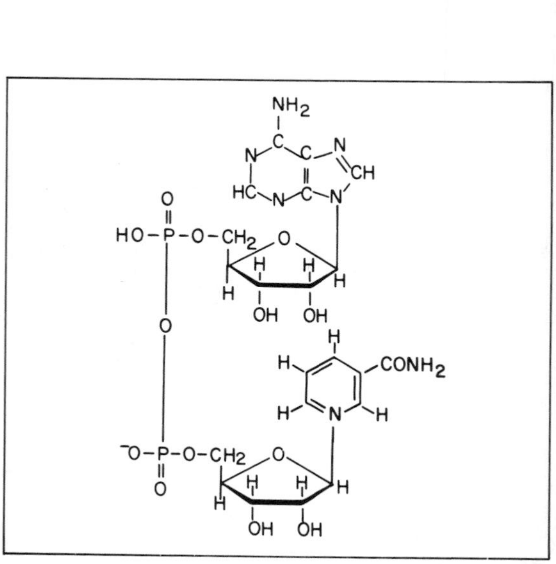

Figure 6-3. *The structure of nicotinamide adenine dinucleotide (NAD^+).*

There is a way to measure the electron donating tendency or electron pressure of such an oxidation-reduction pair. In a specially designed cell, such a pair can be compared with another oxidation-reduction pair that is used as a standard of reference. The formula for this reference pair oxidation-reduction reaction is as follows:

$$\tfrac{1}{2}H_2 \rightleftharpoons H^+ + e \qquad (15)$$

This reference electrode is the standard hydrogen electrode, and its potential is taken as zero for a solution containing hydrogen ions at unit activity in equilibrium with hydrogen gas at one atmosphere pressure. When we compare the $NAD^+/NADH + H^+$ pair with the standard hydrogen electrode, we will find that the $NAD^+/NADH + H^+$ is negative to the hydrogen electrode by 320 millivolts or that it has an electrode potential of -0.32 volt. Remember that the final oxidation-reduction reaction of the electron transport chain is as follows:

$$\tfrac{1}{2}O_2 + 2H^+ + 2e \rightarrow H_2O \qquad (16)$$

The electrode potential for the reduction of oxygen to water, still compared to the standard

(17) $MH_2 + NAD^+ \rightleftharpoons M + NADH + H^+ + 2e$

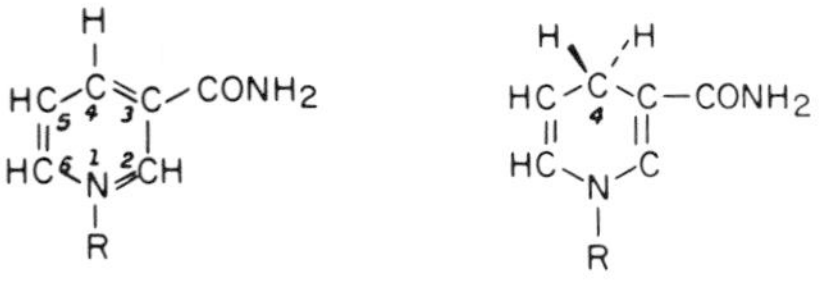

(18) $2e + NADH + H^+ + FMN \longrightarrow FMNH_2 + NAD^+$

Figure 6-4. *The stereospecific reduction of the pyridine ring of NAD⁺. R represents the remaining structure.*

hydrogen electrode, is +0.82 V. Simple algebraic calculation indicates then that the voltage difference between the $NAD^+/NADH$ and ½ O_2/H_2O pairs is 1.14 V.

By a rather complex calculation, it can be shown that the transfer of electrons from one mole of $NADH + H^+$ to one mole of ½ O_2, traversing a voltage drop of 1.14 V, will yield about 52.7 Calories. In a biologic system it takes about 12 Calories to make one mole of ATP from a mole of ADP and Pi. This can be calculated to require a voltage drop of only 0.25 V. It is immediately obvious that it is quite possible to make three moles of ATP by tapping off energy across the voltage drop of 1.14 V. Before we leave this subject, it should be pointed out that another term for the "electrode potentials," about which we have been speaking, is oxidation-reduction potential. Often this term is shortened to "redox potential." The designation for redox potential under standard conditions is E'_o.

ELECTRON TRANSPORT CHAIN

In mitochondrial oxidative phosphorylation, the first step is intramitochondrial dehydrogenation of the substrate (equation 17).

$$MH_2 + NAD^+ \rightleftharpoons M + NADH + H^+ + 2e \quad (17)$$

Mitochondrial NAD is largely restricted to the matrix fluid. The gel contains the dehydrogenases, and the NAD is the coenzyme that links the substrates that are to be oxidized with the electron transport chain. It is the pyridine ring of the NAD that is reduced enzymatically by a dehydrogenase. The structural consequences are shown in Figure 6-4.

NADH is then re-oxidized to NAD by an NADH dehydrogenase. This enzyme is a flavoprotein that contains tightly bound flavin mononucleotide (FMN) as its prosthetic group. Two electrons are transferred from NADH to FMN to give the reduced form, $FMNH_2$ (equation 18 and Figure 6-5).

$$2e + NADH + H^+ + FMN \rightarrow FMNH_2 + NAD^+ \quad (18)$$

This NADH dehydrogenase also contains iron, and the iron, more than likely, plays a role in electron transfer. It is to be borne in mind that this iron is not part of a heme group. Thus, NADH dehydrogenase is a flavoprotein, but it is also a nonheme iron protein. The oxidation reduction potential difference between NADH and FMN is quite large. The E'_o for the NAD/NADH pair is −0.320 V and the E'_o of the $FMN/FMNH_2$ pair is −0.03 V. Thus, the $FMN/FMNH_2$ pair is positive to the NAD/NADH pair by 0.29 V. This is quite enough of a potential drop to generate an ATP, and indeed the first ATP of oxidative phosphorylation is generated at this step. The reaction that is coupled to the dehydrogenation of NADH is the phosphorylation reaction:

$$ADP + Pi \rightleftharpoons ATP \quad (19)$$

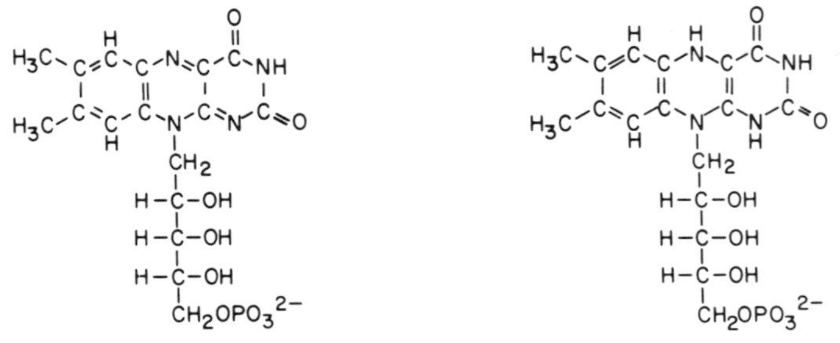

$$ADP + Pi \rightleftharpoons ATP$$

$$FMNH_2 \rightarrow FMN + 2H^+ + 2e$$
$$CoQ + 2H^+ + 2e \rightarrow CoQH_2$$

$$(14)\ SUM: FMNH_2 + CoQ \rightarrow CoQH_2 + FMN$$

Figure 6-5. *The structure of oxidized and reduced flavin mononucleotide.*

The proposed mechanisms whereby this coupling takes place will be discussed briefly in the next section.

The next moiety in the chain is known as coenzyme Q (CoQ). It is a quinone derivative with a long isoprenoid tail (Figure 6-6). It is also known as ubiquinone because it is so ubiquitous in biologic systems. It is reduced by $FMNH_2$ via the following series of reactions (equation 20).

$$\begin{array}{l} FMNH_2 \rightarrow FMN + 2H^+ + 2e \\ CoQ + 2H^+ + 2e \rightarrow CoQH_2 \\ \hline SUM: FMNH_2 + CoQ \rightarrow CoQH_2 + FMN \end{array} \quad (20)$$

The nonheme iron in the NADH dehydrogenase complex is associated with a sulfur molecule and is one of several such centers known as iron-sulfur proteins. The precise mechanism of the function of these iron-sulfur proteins has not been defined, but it clearly must be related to electron transport. The iron atoms seem to function in the electron transport system by reversible oxidation and reduction between the Fe^{2+} and Fe^{3+} states.

The electron carriers between ubiquinone and O_2 are cytochromes. There is probably also one iron-sulfur protein involved in this part of the chain as well. The cytochromes are electron-transporting proteins that contain a heme prosthetic group. The iron atom in cytochromes alternates between a reduced and oxidized state Fe^{2+}/Fe^{3+}. Another special aspect of this latter part of the chain is that each cytochrome molecule now only transfers one electron. From NAD through CoQ, the coenzymes carry two electrons per molecule. Since this is no longer the case and two electrons are released in the re-oxidation of reduced ubiquinone, the high-potential electrons must be transferred to two molecules of cytochrome b, the next member of the electron transport chain. There are five cytochromes between ubiquinone and oxygen in the electron transport chain.

$$CoQ \rightarrow Cyt\ b \rightarrow Cyt\ c_1 \rightarrow Cyt\ c \rightarrow Cyt\ (a + a_3) \rightarrow O_2$$

These cytochromes have distinctive structures and properties, the details of which are beyond the purview of this discussion.

The oxidation-reduction potential of cytochrome b is +0.07 V. The next cytochrome on the chain is cytochrome c_1, which has an E'_0 of +0.215 V. This voltage drop is about 0.15 V and is the site of the generation of the next molecule of ATP from one molecule each of ADP and Pi.

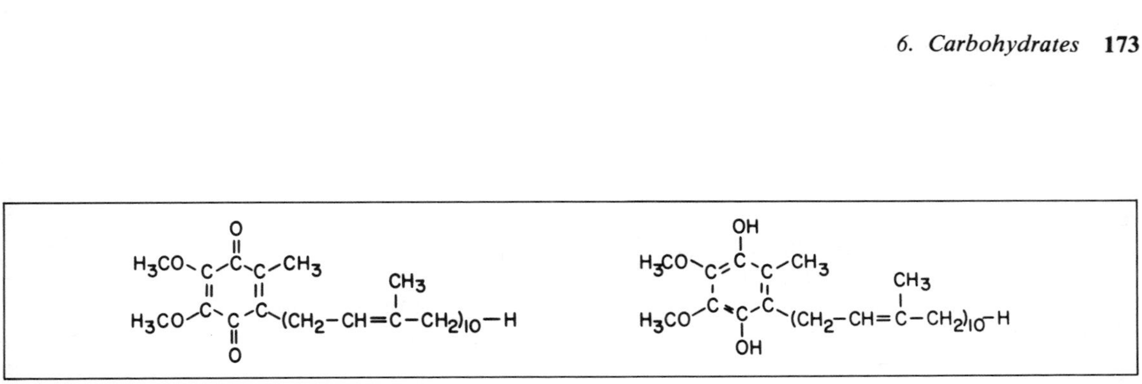

Figure 6-6. *The structure of coenzyme Q_{10} (ubiquinone$_{10}$).*

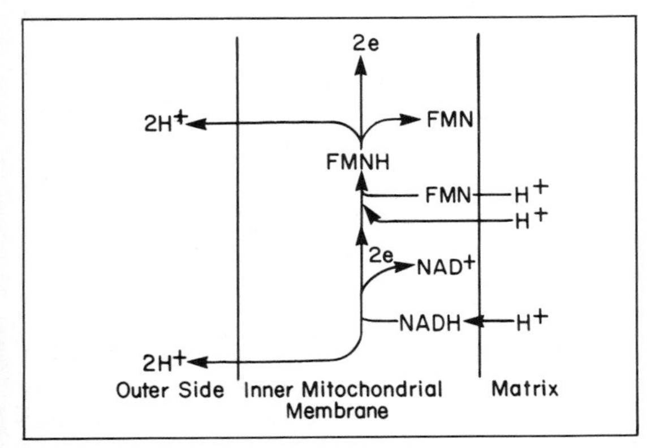

Figure 6-7. *The chemiosmotic mechanism, proposed by Mitchell, for coupling oxidation and phosphorylation.*

Cytochromes a and a_3 are the final members of the respiratory chain. They exist as a complex that is sometimes called cytochrome oxidase. Electrons are transferred to the cytochrome a part of the complex, and then to cytochrome a_3, which contains copper. This copper atom also alternates between a reduced and an oxidized form Cu^{+1}/Cu^{+2}. Dissolved oxygen, in the form of O_2 accepts four electrons and reacts with four protons to form two molecules of water (equation 21).

$$O_2 + 4\ H^+ + 4e^- \rightarrow 2\ H_2O \qquad (21)$$

There are some unique aspects to the foregoing mechanisms of electron transport. There is a vectorial factor resulting from the location of these carriers in the inner membrane, which allows for a separation of the protons from the electrons, resulting in protons being discharged to the space between the inner and outer membrane. Thus, in the preceding example of oxidation of $NADH_2$, the electrons are passed from one carrier of the membrane to the next, whereas the protons from the matrix side, which are used for the reduction reaction, are essentially expelled externally to the inner membrane. The net result is a large concentration gradient of protons from the intermembrane space to the matrix (Figure 6-7). This concentration gradient is an essential part of the chemiosomotic mechanism proposed by Mitchell to explain oxidative phosphorylation.

COUPLED PHOSPHORYLATION

The precise details of the mechanism whereby the energy derived from the transport of electrons is transferred in such a fashion as to make possible the generation of ATP from ADP and Pi have not been definitively elucidated. There are, currently, three hypotheses.

The chemical-coupling hypothesis postulates the formation of a covalent high-energy intermediate that serves as a precursor of ATP. Let us suppose, for a moment, that we designate one of the three sites in the electron transport chain where phosphorylation is known to occur as the reaction between A_r and B_o. The intermediate that has been reduced is designated A_r, and the intermediate with which it will react is designated B_o. The reaction will then be:

$$A_r + B_o \rightarrow A_o + B_r \qquad (22)$$

In the chemical coupling hypothesis there is a postulated high-energy compound formed designated as $A \sim C$. The theory is that this $A \sim C$ is formed when the reduced form of A transfers its electrons to the oxidized form of B. Then, the high-energy bond in $A \sim C$ is split as ADP is phosphorylated to ATP, according to the following series of reactions (equation 23).

$$\begin{array}{l} A_r + B_o + C \rightarrow A_o \sim C + B_r \\ A_o \sim C + ADP + Pi \rightarrow A_o + C + ATP \\ \hline \text{SUM: } A_r + B_o + ADP + Pi \rightarrow A_o + B_r + ATP \end{array} \quad (23)$$

Despite the best efforts of a number of investigators, it has not been possible to demonstrate the existence of C or $A \sim C$.

The conformational hypothesis is simply a variant of the above. Here, the idea is that A_o is coupled to a protein in the carrier whose conformation is so altered as to be activated and thereby contain the energy released. This combination of A_o with a conformationally activated state of an electron carrier is designated by A_o^*. These reactions would then be summarized as follows (equation 24):

$$\begin{array}{l} A_r + B_o \rightarrow A_o^* + B_r \\ A_o^* + ADP + Pi \rightarrow A_o + B_r + ATP \\ \hline \text{SUM: } A_r + B_o + ADP + Pi \rightarrow A_o + B_r + ATP \end{array} \quad (24)$$

The theory now currently in vogue is the chemiosmotic hypothesis. Peter Mitchell was awarded the Nobel Prize for his contribution to the development of this hypothesis, even though the hypothesis has not been finally and completely proved to be the correct mechanism. Nonetheless, it appears to account most satisfactorily for most of the observed phenomena. The essentials of this concept, as described in the preceding section, are that protons are pumped out of the inner mitochondrial membrane and accumulate on the outer face of the membrane during electron transport. The resulting proton concentration gradient and membrane potential drive the synthesis of ATP via a mechanism whereby the return of protons to the matrix drives the reaction:

$$ADP + Pi \rightarrow ATP + H_2O \quad (25)$$

This process is under active investigation at present and involves a complex array of many factors whose relationships to each other are gradually becoming known. For further discussions of these three theories, the reader is referred to Lehninger [14a].

In the normal mitochondria of most tissues, phosphorylation is tightly coupled to electron transport and substrate oxidation. As long as electrons can be transported down the electron transport chain to their final recipient, O_2, ATP continues to be generated and substrate continues to be oxidized. This occurs only if there is adequate ADP and Pi to accept the energy released at the three phosphorylation sites. If anything interferes with the supply of ADP or Pi or both, phosphorylation stops because of lack of acceptors for the oxidatively-derived energy. When this stops, electron transport stops. When electron transport stops, oxidation of substrate stops and oxygen uptake stops.

This close interdependence is what we mean when we say that oxidative phosphorylation is tightly coupled. For every pair of electrons that has been transported down the chain, one-half of a molecule of O_2 is reduced. As a consequence of this transport of two electrons, three molecules of ATP are generated. Thus, for every ½ O_2 taken up and converted to water, three ATPs are generated. It is this ratio that is expressed as follows:

$$P:O = 3 \quad (26)$$

Early in the research into mitochondrial oxidative phosphorylation, it was discovered that 2,4-dinitrophenol (DNP) and some other acidic aromatic compounds could uncouple oxidative phosphorylation. In the presence of these compounds, electron transport proceeds normally from $NADH + H^+$ to O_2, but ATP is not formed by the respiratory assembly. The consequence of this is that electron transport now proceeds at an increased rate, oxygen consumption is increased, and NADH is oxidized at an increased rate. ATP is not formed because electron transport is now no longer coupled to phosphorylation. The energy derived from electron transport is now lost as heat since it cannot be stored by the formation of ATP. Whether or not uncoupling of oxidative phosphorylation ever plays a role in clinical disease states has not been proved. The data supporting any such hypothesis are scant.

This concludes our overview of basic thermodynamic concepts that are important in any discussion of carbohydrate metabolism. For those who wish to explore these matters in more detail, there are several summaries and reviews that should prove useful [14a, 23, 24].

GLYCOLYSIS

In this part of the chapter we will review the pathway from glucose to pyruvate. The overall pattern of this transformation involves several steps. First of all, the glucose must enter the cell from the extracellular fluid. Once inside it must be phosphorylated. Once phosphorylated, it undergoes a rearrangement to a fructose phosphate derivative and then is once again phosphorylated to a fructose diphosphate derivative. This hexose diphosphate is then split into two triose phosphates. Both halves of this molecule, in the final analysis, traverse the same pathway, ultimately becoming pyruvic acid. For each pyruvate formed there is a net gain of one molecule of ATP, or two ATPs generated for each molecule of glucose that is converted to two molecules of pyruvate. In addition, for each molecule of pyruvate formed, there is one conversion of NAD^+ to $NADH + H^+$. We will, of course, direct our attention to the fate of this reduced coenzyme and the reducing equivalents it carries.

CELL MEMBRANE CONCEPTS

In the series of sequential reactions in processes whereby glucose is converted in the cell to CO_2 and H_2O, a number of rate-limiting steps serve as control points. The first of these is the cell membrane barrier itself. In the matter of glucose entry through cell membranes to reach the interior of the cell, tissues in the body vary in their permeability to glucose and their response to insulin. In cardiac and skeletal muscle, for example, there is a membrane blockade to the entry of glucose that allows for comparably slow passive diffusion. The concentration of glucose in the extracellular fluid is many times higher than it is in the intracellular space. In fact, the rate of entry of glucose into the cell, through the cell membrane, is so much slower than the mechanisms for converting glucose to its metabolic products that the concentration of free glucose inside these cells is extremely low, close to zero. The rate of conversion of glucose to its metabolic products is so much faster than the rate of entry of glucose into the cell through the cell membrane that little free glucose can ever be found inside the cell. In cardiac and skeletal muscle, the entry of glucose into the cell through the cell membrane is facilitated by the presence of insulin, i.e., at a faster rate than would be the case if simple passive diffusion due to a concentration gradient is present. Even though the entry of glucose into cardiac and skeletal muscle cells is markedly accelerated by the presence of insulin, the rate in the insulin-facilitated state is still so slow, when compared to metabolic turnover rates, that no free glucose can be found inside the cell. Thus, the term for the entry of glucose into muscle cells is facilitated transport, inasmuch as insulin facilitates the passive diffusion of glucose into these cells.

Adipose tissue is similar to muscle in this respect. The rate of glucose entry into fat cells is so much slower than the rate of its turnover that little free glucose can be found in this tissue, much the same as in muscle. Also, entry of glucose into adipose tissue cells is facilitated by the presence of insulin, and the process of facilitated transport pertains here, as well.

The liver is quite another matter. It has been conclusively demonstrated that the concentration of free glucose inside the liver cell is the same as in the extracellular fluid. Accordingly, membrane transport is not a rate-limiting step in the metabolism of glucose in the liver.

The role of the cell membrane in controlling the rate of glucose entry into brain cells is still debated. Numerous investigators have studied the matter, and their results are not in agreement.

It does appear that the brain cell membrane does, indeed, present some blockade to the entry of glucose. No investigator has reported that free glucose inside brain cells is equal to that in the circulating blood, as obtained in the liver. On the other hand, the question now centers around how much of a blockade the cell membrane presents. Some observers have reported data indicating that the concentration of free glucose inside the brain cell is very low, resembling the situation that obtains in muscle and adipose tissue. Other, more recent, studies suggest that this is not the case. The concentration of free glucose inside the cell is, as already stated, not equal to that in the circulating blood, but appears to be considerably higher than in muscle and fat. The best synthesis of observations made to date indicates that free glucose concentrations inside the brain cell are somewhat less than half that in the circulating blood, within the normal ranges of physiologic variations.

The matter of the effect of insulin on glucose entry into brain cells is likewise still one of controversy. Both human and animal data do indicate that insulin, under appropriately set conditions, can increase the extraction of glucose by the brain, i.e., increase the entry of glucose into brain cells. Since no change of oxygen uptake occurs as a consequence of this increased glucose extraction by the brain, it is postulated that facilitated entry of glucose into the brain as a consequence of insulin action probably is directed into pathways other than oxygen-dependent oxidizing systems, such as glycogen synthesis. The best recent summary of these matters can be found in the treatise by Seisjo [20].

In summary, then, the role of the cell membrane as a control point governing the rate of glucose metabolism in cells varies from organ to organ. In adipose tissue, skeletal muscle, and cardiac muscle, the cell membrane is a primary rate-limiting step, and the concentration of free glucose in the cell is extremely low. In liver, the concentration of free glucose inside the cell is equal to that in the circulating blood. The situation in the brain probably is somewhere between that of liver and the other tissues. In all likelihood, membrane transport of glucose would be a significant rate-limiting step in the brain only in the circumstance of extremely low blood glucose levels, i.e., below 40 mg/dl.

METABOLISM OF GLUCOSE

Under ideal conditions, the resting cell, adequately supplied with oxygen and glucose, will convert that substance completely to carbon dioxide and water as in equation 1.

This process forms the central core of our understanding of fuel metabolism in the living cell. Its intricacies have been the bane of students of medicine for as long as it has been taught. In actual fact, however, it is easily understood if viewed in its totality.

In the set of circumstances alluded to at the beginning of this section, the process has three major divisions. The first involves the conversion of the 6-carbon hexose, glucose, into phosphorylated derivatives; the second involves splitting of the phosphorylated 6-carbon chain into two molecules of glyceraldehyde phosphate; and the third is the conversion of the latter to pyruvic acid accompanied by the conservation of energy. This sequence is known as glycolysis. The set of reactions that make up the glycolytic sequence occurs in the cytosol. The remainder of the reactions, the other division of the overall process, occurs in the mitochondrion, and it is here that the two molecules of pyruvic acid enter into reactions with a net yield of 6 molecules of carbon dioxide and water.

GLYCOLYTIC REACTIONS

In this process the 6-carbon glucose molecule is rearranged in such a fashion that it can be cleaved to produce, eventually, 2 identical molecules of pyruvic acid. In the first step, the glucose is phosphorylated. All the reactions in the glycolytic scheme involve phosphorylated derivatives of 6-carbon and 3-carbon compounds. We call on ATP as our source of phosphate, and we rely on

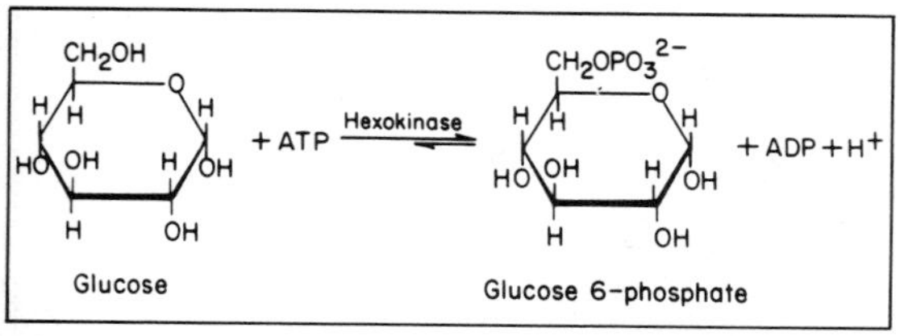

Figure 6-8. *The reaction catalyzed by hexokinase.*

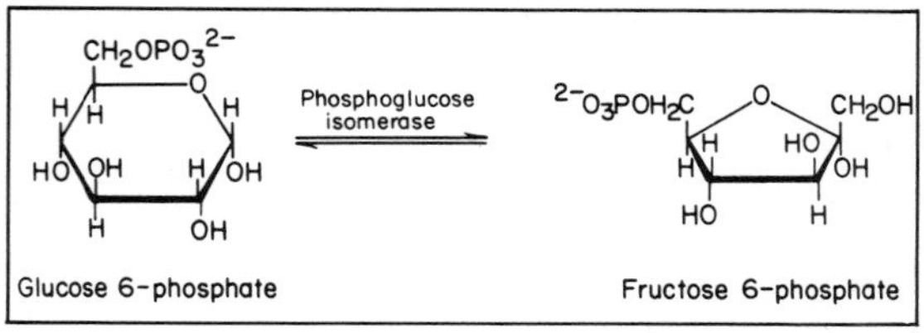

Figure 6-9. *The isomerization of glucose-6-phosphate.*

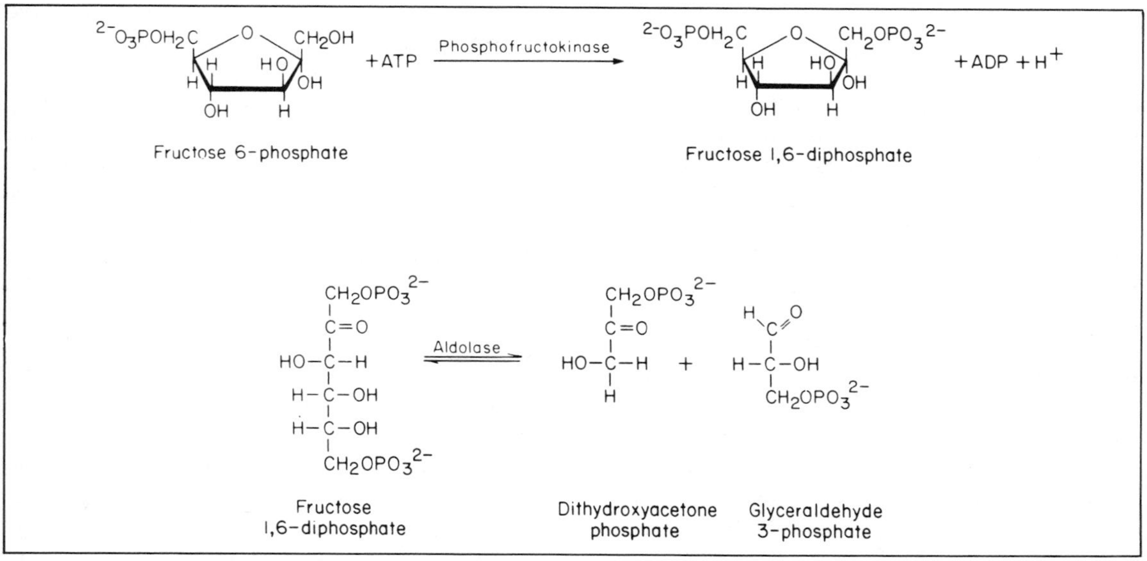

Figure 6-10. *The formation of fructose 1,6-diphosphate and its cleavage and isomerization to glyceraldehyde-3-phosphate.*

the high-energy content of the terminal phosphate bond of ATP to provide the energy that drives the reaction of phosphorylation. This reaction is catalyzed by the enzyme hexokinase and adds the phosphate moiety to the sixth carbon of glucose to form a phosphate ester (Figure 6-8).

With the glucose molecule phosphorylated at the 6 carbon, a line of cleavage that would make for a symmetrical split of the molecule is not readily apparent. In order to get ready for this split, we simply isomerize the glucose-6-phosphate to fructose-6-phosphate (Figure 6-9). The further reactions in glycolysis necessitate that the derivatives be phosphorylated. This requirement is met by adding another phosphate on the first position of the fructose-6-phosphate. This reaction is catalyzed by a key enzyme of the pathway, phosphofructokinase, thus completing the first stage (Figure 6-10).

Both the hexokinase step and the phosphofructokinase step are worthy of further comment at this point. First, it is to be emphasized that, because of energy considerations, both reactions are irreversible. When we consider the matter of gluconeogenesis, later in this chapter, we will have to provide a different type of reaction to get around this irreversibility. Furthermore, both reactions are important control points in governing the rate of flow of carbon through the glycolytic scheme. Phosphofructokinase appears to be

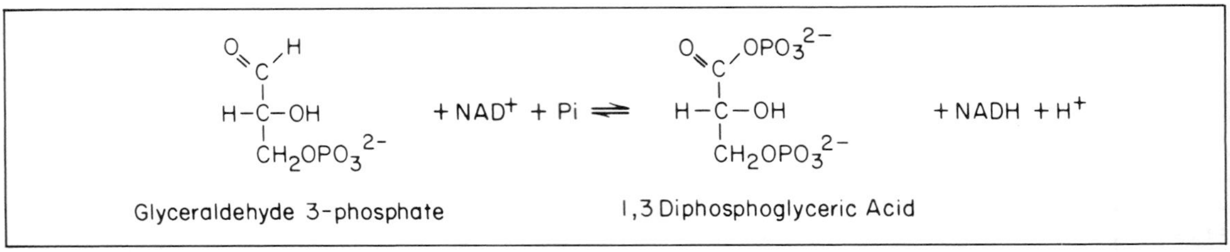

$$\underset{\text{Glyceraldehyde 3-phosphate}}{\begin{array}{c} O\!=\!C\!-\!H \\ | \\ H\!-\!C\!-\!OH \\ | \\ CH_2OPO_3^{2-} \end{array}} + NAD^+ + Pi \rightleftharpoons \underset{\text{1,3 Diphosphoglyceric Acid}}{\begin{array}{c} O\!=\!C\!-\!OPO_3^{2-} \\ | \\ H\!-\!C\!-\!OH \\ | \\ CH_2OPO_3^{2-} \end{array}} + NADH + H^+$$

Figure 6-11. *The generation of 1,3-diphosphoglycerate.*

pivotal in this regard. It has been shown to be inhibited by increasing concentrations of ATP and activated by increasing concentrations of ADP, AMP, and Pi, especially AMP. In a cell that has a high ambient level of ATP, phosphofructokinase will be inhibited, and that reaction will slow down. As a consequence, fructose-6-phosphate will accumulate. The reaction that converts glucose-6-phosphate to fructose-6-phosphate is easily reversible, so that glucose-6-phosphate will accumulate as well. As an indirect consequence of the initial inhibition of phosphofructokinase by ATP, elevated levels of glucose-6-phosphate in the cytosol will result. The elevated levels of glucose-6-phosphate inhibit the hexokinase, further damping the flow of carbon through the glycolytic scheme. This concept is important in reviewing the effect of adequacy of oxygen supply on the rate of glycolysis.

Now that we have formed fructose-1,6-diphosphate, a line of cleavage is readily apparent and the second stage can begin. It is an easy matter to split this molecule, at the point indicated, to produce two triose phosphates (Figure 6-10).

It is to be emphasized that glyceraldehyde 3-phosphate is on the main stream of glycolysis, whereas dihydroxyacetone phosphate is not. A look at the structures will show that isomerization is an easy matter and that is indeed what happens. The dihydroxyacetone phosphate is isomerized to glyceraldehyde 3-phosphate, and we now have two molecules of glyceraldehyde 3-phosphate resulting from our split of the doubly phosphorylated hexose.

Let us stop to reflect for a moment. We have described glycolysis as part of the fuel metabolism of the cell. Implied in such a concept is the hope that a net yield of usable chemical energy will result from any such series of transformations. At this point, we are far from that eventuality. In fact, we are in debt. We have used two molecules of ATP to perform the necessary phosphorylations. So far, then, instead of producing a net energy yield, we have produced a net deficit of two ATPs.

In the third stage we now begin to return toward a redress of this deficit and to generate a surplus. Glyceraldehyde 3-phosphate is oxidized to 1,3-diphosphoglyceric acid (Figure 6-11). The phosphate that we have added at the first position to make 1,3-diphosphoglycerate is a high-energy phosphate. We can, therefore, react this substance with ADP to produce 3-phosphoglycerate and a molecule of ATP (Figure 6-12). Since this has happened to both of the two halves of the original glucose, we have now produced two ATPs to balance out the initial investment of two ATPs in the earlier two phosphorylation steps. Any further yield of ATP will be on the plus side.

Next, we move the phosphate from the third position to the second position and remove the elements of water (Figure 6-13). The product of this set of reactions is phosphoenolpyruvate, and the phosphate on the second position is also a high-energy phosphate (Figure 6-14). We now react phosphoenolpyruvate with ADP to produce pyruvate and a net yield of one molecule of ATP. Since this ATP yield will happen with both of the two fragments, we have a net yield of two ATPs in the process of converting one molecule of glucose to two molecules of pyruvic acid.

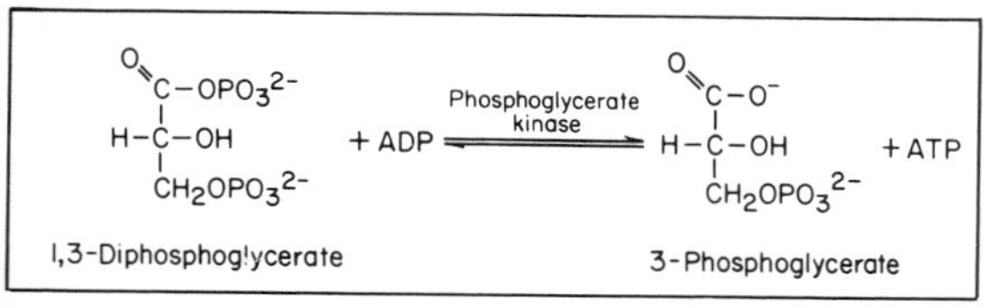

1,3-Diphosphoglycerate + ADP ⇌ (Phosphoglycerate kinase) 3-Phosphoglycerate + ATP

Figure 6-12. *The formation of ATP from 1,3-diphosphoglycerate.*

3-Phosphoglycerate ⇌ (Phosphoglyceromutase) 2-Phosphoglycerate

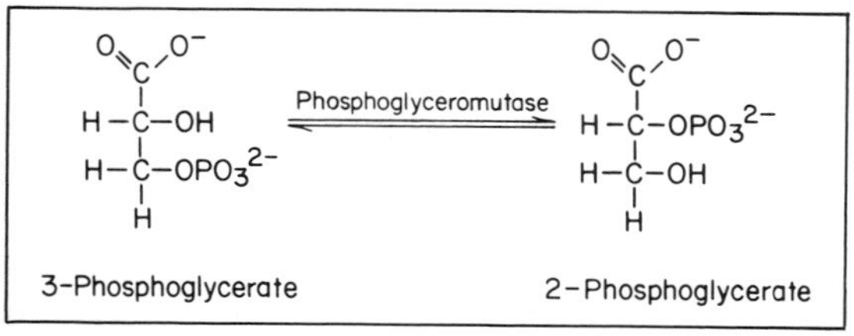

Figure 6-13. *The action of phosphoglyceromutase.*

2-Phosphoglycerate ⇌ (Enolase, H_2O) Phosphoenolpyruvate + ADP → (Pyruvate kinase) Pyruvate + ATP

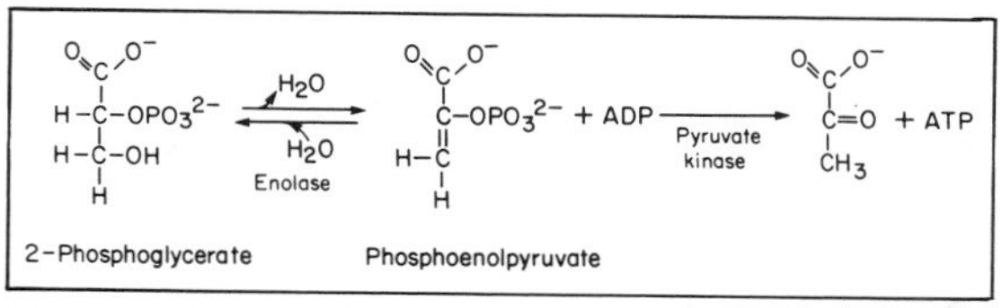

Figure 6-14. *The formation of pyruvate and ATP.*

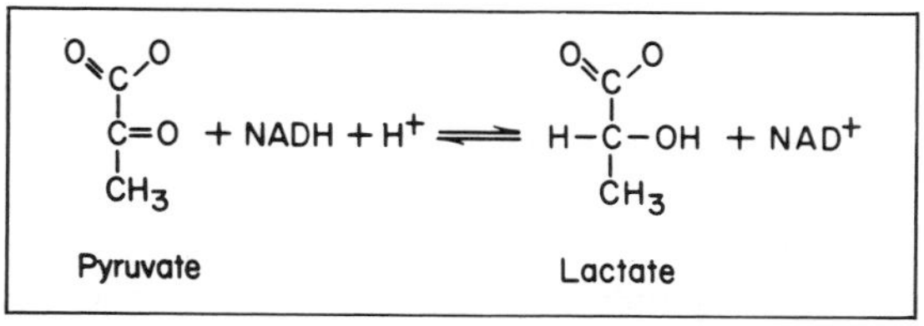

Pyruvate + NADH + H^+ ⇌ Lactate + NAD^+

Figure 6-15. *The reduction of pyruvate to lactate.*

The reader will remember the reaction whereby we oxidized glyceraldehyde 3-phosphate, adding a phosphate, to produce 1,3-diphosphoglycerate. A necessary substrate for that reaction was NAD (nicotinamide adenine dinucleotide), and it was reduced to NADH + H^+. The total amount of NAD^+ + NADH in the cytosol does not vary widely, and if it is all converted to NADH, then glycolysis will stop. If the flow of glucose to pyruvic acid is to continue, we must find a means of regenerating the NAD. When we consider the mitochondrion and the final steps in the conversion of pyruvic acid to CO_2 and water, it will become apparent how this is done in the intact cell. However, some cells do not have mitochondria (the red blood cell), and other cells are sometimes subjected to varying degrees of relative or absolute hypoxia, rendering these mitochondrial mechanisms diminished or absent. What then? In this circumstance, the pyruvate is converted to lactate by the enzyme lactate dehydrogenase. This conversion requires NADH and produces NAD^+ (Figure 6-15).

Lactate is essentially an end product. It can only re-enter a metabolic sequence by being reconverted to pyruvate. In states of excessive production of pyruvate, the conversion to lactate is favored, and this end product of glycolysis leaves the cell as such. When it leaves the cell in this fashion, it leaves it as lactic acid. Accumulation of lactic acid inside the cell can rapidly lead to intracellular acidosis, which impairs function and, ultimately, structure. On the other hand, when it leaves the cell, it places a burden on the acid-base buffering mechanism of the blood that must be dealt with. Rapid accumulation of lactic acid in the bloodstream is the principal reason for the extreme degrees of metabolic acidosis seen in hypoxic states.

This method of disposition of pyruvic acid with its accompanying regeneration of NAD allows glycolysis to proceed when there is no mode of aerobic disposition of pyruvate or regeneration of NAD. Since it can proceed in the absence of oxygen, it is termed anaerobic glycolysis. It must be borne in mind that the energy yield of glycolysis alone is very small when compared to the total possible energy yield, to which we alluded early in this chapter, available from the aerobic cellular conversion of one molecule of glucose to CO_2 and water. In anaerobic glycolysis, the production of two molecules of lactic acid from each molecule of glucose results in a net production of two molecules of ATP or 7.3 Calories. This is far from the potential realization of 270 Calories, of which an intact, fully oxygenated cell is capable. Thus, anaerobic glycolysis makes it possible for the cell to supply a small amount of net energy from glucose oxidation, but it is an inefficient process.

CITRIC ACID CYCLE

In the intact cell, the remainder of the steps necessary for the conversion of pyruvic acid to carbon dioxide and water, and the generation of the maximum possible amount of ATP occur in the mitochondrion. Pyruvic acid enters the mitochondria and is decarboxylated and combined with coenzyme A to produce acetyl CoA. It is the acetyl CoA that enters the citric acid cycle, the discussion of which will form the bulk of this section.

Pyruvic acid is converted to acetyl CoA in a reaction catalyzed by the pyruvate dehydrogenase complex. This large, multi-enzyme complex is a highly integrated array of three kinds of enzymes. The reaction catalyzed by this complex (equation 27) involves thiamine pyrophosphate, lipoamide, and FAD, which serve as catalytic cofactors in addition to CoA and NAD^+, the stoichiometric cofactors.

$$\text{Pyruvate} + \text{CoA} + \text{NAD}^+ \rightarrow \text{acetyl CoA} + \text{CO}_2 + \text{NADH} \qquad (27)$$

A detailed description of this complex series of reactions is beyond the scope of this presentation. Interested readers are referred to the elegant description of this process to be found in Stryer [23].

In terms of conversion of pyruvic acid to CO_2 and water, we are now one-third of the way down the road. The terminal carboxyl group of pyruvic acid has been released as carbon dioxide. Furthermore, we have produced an $NADH + H^+$. This enters into the electron transport chain of oxidative phosphorylation and yields three molecules of ATP.

The citric acid cycle is regarded by most observers as complex, but the basic principle is indeed simple. However, an overview of the process will illustrate (Figure 6-16): A 2-carbon molecule combines with a 4-carbon molecule to form a 6. Two carbons from the 6 are sequentially removed to regenerate a 4-carbon fragment, available to begin the cycle all over again. This now simple concept of a catalytic cycle reaction to achieve the oxidation of acetic acid was the great achievement of H. A. Krebs, and this cycle is often called the Krebs cycle. The 2 carbons of acetyl CoA react with the 4-carbon compound, oxaloacetate, to form citrate. The steps that make up the citric acid cycle result in the loss of first one, and then another, carbon as carbon dioxide and the regeneration of a molecule of oxaloacetate capable of combining with another acetyl CoA to begin the cycle again. Three molecules of NADH are produced from NAD^+ in the process, and each molecule of NADH can give rise to three ATPs by the oxidative-phosphorylation electron-transport chain. One molecule of another high-energy phosphate, guanosine triphosphate, is also generated. In addition, one molecule of the reduced form of flavin adenine dinucleotide is also produced, and this compound enters into the electron transport chain in such a fashion as to give rise to 2 molecules of ATP. Thus, in one turn of the cycle, we have generated 12 ATPs and 2 CO_2s.

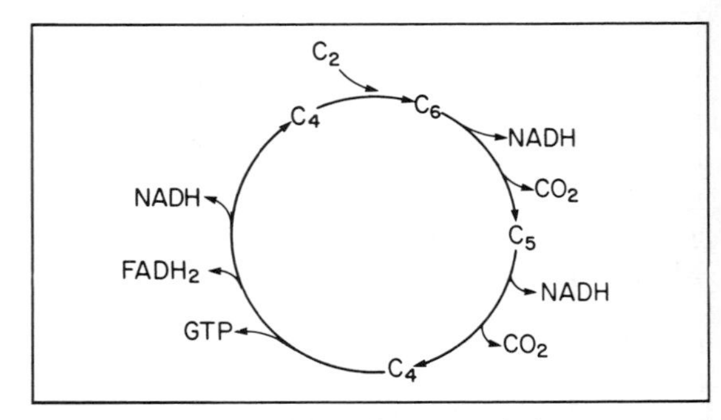

Figure 6-16. *Overall mechanism of the citric acid cycle.*

The first reaction is the one catalyzed by citrate synthetase. It will be noted that citryl CoA is an intermediate in this reaction (Figure 6-17). The hydrolysis of this intermediate coenzyme A ester is highly exergonic and makes the formation of

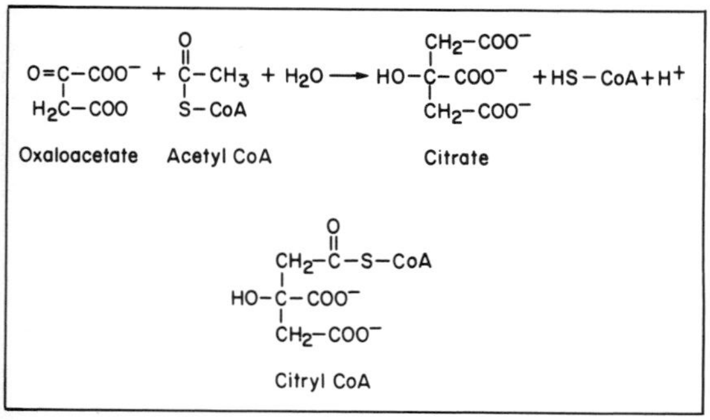

$$O{=}C(COO^-){-}H_2C{-}COO \;+\; O{=}C(CH_3){-}S{-}CoA \;+\; H_2O \longrightarrow HO{-}C(COO^-)(CH_2{-}COO^-)(CH_2{-}COO^-) \;+\; HS{-}CoA + H^+$$

Oxaloacetate　Acetyl CoA　Citrate

$$CH_2{-}C(=O){-}S{-}CoA$$
$$HO{-}C{-}COO^-$$
$$CH_2{-}COO^-$$

Citryl CoA

Figure 6-17. *The condensation of oxaloacetate and acetyl CoA to form citrate.*

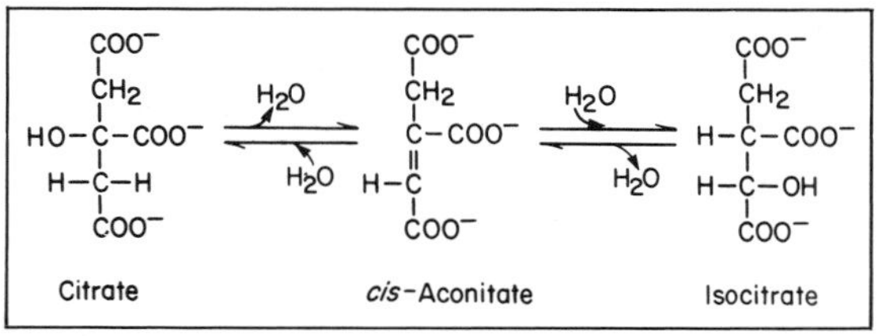

$$COO^-{-}CH_2{-}C(OH)(COO^-){-}CH_2{-}COO^- \underset{H_2O}{\overset{H_2O}{\rightleftharpoons}} COO^-{-}CH_2{-}C(COO^-){=}CH{-}COO^- \underset{H_2O}{\overset{H_2O}{\rightleftharpoons}} COO^-{-}CH_2{-}CH(COO^-){-}CH(OH){-}COO^-$$

Citrate　*cis*-Aconitate　Isocitrate

Figure 6-18. *The isomerization of citrate to isocitrate.*

citrate an almost irreversible reaction. It is true, though, that oxaloacetate and acetate, by themselves, will combine to form citrate. For this to happen, however, relatively high concentrations of the starting materials will be needed, at levels beyond those ordinarily seen in the mitochondria. With the involvement of the coenzyme A ester, the reaction proceeds readily even when the intramitochondrial concentration of oxaloacetate falls to four micromolar or lower. We have now produced our initial six carbon compound, citrate. For oxidation to proceed, we must rearrange the citrate molecule a bit. The alcohol in citrate is a tertiary alcohol and cannot be oxidized without breaking a carbon bond. The alcohol group is moved to the next carbon atom where it is now a secondary alcohol that can be oxidized. This is a two-step sequence catalyzed by the enzyme aconitase. The elements of water are removed from citrate to form cis-aconitate and then put back to form isocitrate (Figure 6-18).

The next set of reactions are catalyzed by the enzyme isocitrate dehydrogenase. It should be noted that, in the cell, isocitrate dehydrogenase occurs in two forms. The one that is important in this instance, in the mitochondrion, is dependent upon NAD^+ as a substrate. There is another one that is dependent on NADP, which functions in another context. Isocitrate is first oxidized to the presumed intermediate, oxalosuccinate. Next a CO_2 is lost to produce α ketoglutarate (Figure 6-19). This step is β-decarboxylation and requires Mn^{++} or Mg^{++}. We have now lost one of the carbon atoms from the original molecule of oxaloacetate that entered the beginning of the citric acid cycle, and we have produced three molecules of ATP by virtue of the interaction of the NADH with the electron transport chain. This reaction catalyzed by isocitrate dehydrogenase is an oxidative decarboxylation.

The next step is the oxidation of α-ketoglutarate (Figure 6-20). This reaction is catalyzed by α-ketoglutaric dehydrogenase and is extremely complex. It is similar to the reaction sequence in the conversion of pyruvate to acetyl CoA. It uses the same cofactors, and the α-ketoglutaric dehydrogenase complex has structural features in common with the pyruvate dehydrogenase complex. We have now lost the second carbon atom that we were to lose from the original oxaloacetate molecule and have generated three more ATP by virtue of the interaction of NADH with the electron transport chain.

The thioester bond of succinyl coenzyme A is energy-rich and is used to generate another molecule of high-energy phosphate. Here, the substrate is not ADP, as in the electron transport chain, but guanosine diphosphate (GDP) (equation 28).

$$\text{Succinyl CoA} + \text{Pi} + \text{GDP} \rightleftharpoons \text{succinate} + \text{GTP} + \text{CoA} \qquad (28)$$

The phosphoryl group in guanosine triphosphate (GTP) is readily transferred to ADP to form ATP in a reaction catalyzed by nucleoside diphosphokinase.

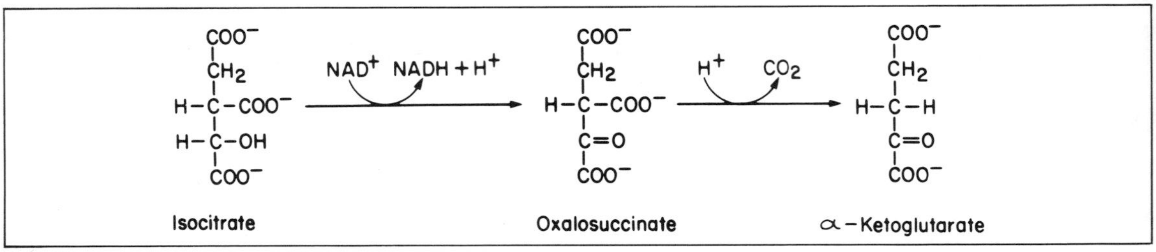

Isocitrate ($NAD^+ \rightarrow NADH + H^+$) → Oxalosuccinate ($H^+ \rightarrow CO_2$) → α-Ketoglutarate

Figure 6-19. *The conversion of isocitrate to* α-ketoglutarate.

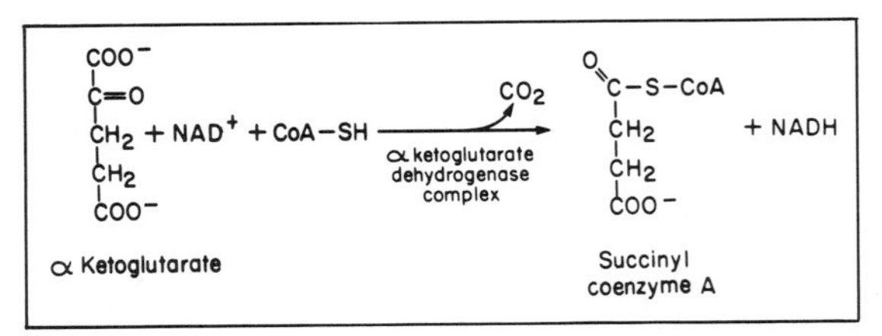

Figure 6-20. *The oxidative decarboxylation of* α-ketoglutarate.

This generation of a high-energy phosphate bond from succinyl CoA is a substrate-level phosphorylation and is the only one of its kind in the citric acid cycle. All the rest of the high-energy phosphate bonds are generated from the transfer of reducing equivalents through the electron transport chain.

Succinate, the product of this reaction, is a 4-carbon molecule, but the cycle is not complete yet. The next steps involve conversion of succinate to oxaloacetate in three steps (Figure 6-21).

Succinate, as shown in Figure 6-21, is oxidized to fumarate by the enzyme succinate dehydrogenase. Here the hydrogen acceptor is flavin adenine dinucleotide (FAD). Succinate dehydrogenase is directly linked to the electron transport chain. The reoxidization of the $FADH_2$ does not yield three molecules of ATP, but only two.

Next, a molecule of water is introduced in a reaction catalyzed by the enzyme fumarase to produce malate. This reaction is NAD^+-dependent and, as such, generates three more molecules of high-energy phosphate. The product of the reaction is oxaloacetate, which is now available to begin the cycle once again. Interestingly enough, this circumstance avoids the accumulation of oxaloacetate, which is a powerful inhibitor of succinate dehydrogenase, but it also limits the possible rate of citrate synthesis. Because the concentration of oxaloacetate is kept low by this circumstance, we are even more dependent on the direction given to the citrate synthetase reaction by the free energy of hydrolysis of the thioester.

We have now completed one turn of the cycle and generated 12 molecules of ATP and produced 2 molecules of CO_2. Oxaloacetate is regenerated to begin the cycle once again.

REGULATION OF GLUCOSE OXIDATION

The glycolytic and citric acid cycle processes are absolutely central to the life of an organism. It is not only necessary, then, that the process be continuous, but that the processes also be capable of change in rate to meet demands. The requirement for energy of a muscle, as it passes from rest to maximum exertion, increases by several hundred-fold. How is this requisite regulation, so that energy supply meets demand, accomplished? Several of the more important sites and mechanisms of rate control are worthy of note. First, it is safe to say that ATP as the coin of exchange for energy supply occupies a prominent position in regulation of cellular activities. As cellular activity increases, ATP supplies decrease. As ATP is used, ADP and Pi are produced. When ATP supplies are exhausted and large amounts of ADP are present, myokinase (adenylate kinase)

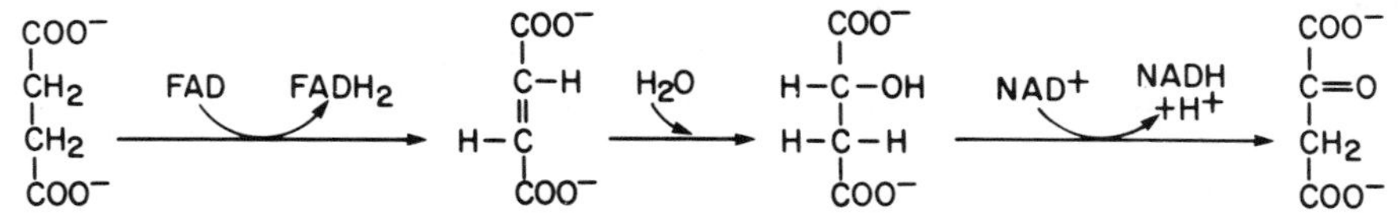

$$\begin{array}{c} COO^- \\ | \\ CH_2 \\ | \\ CH_2 \\ | \\ COO^- \end{array} \xrightarrow{FAD \; \to \; FADH_2} \begin{array}{c} COO^- \\ | \\ C{-}H \\ \| \\ H{-}C \\ | \\ COO^- \end{array} \xrightarrow{H_2O} \begin{array}{c} COO^- \\ | \\ H{-}C{-}OH \\ | \\ H{-}C{-}H \\ | \\ COO^- \end{array} \xrightarrow{NAD^+ \; \to \; NADH + H^+} \begin{array}{c} COO^- \\ | \\ C{=}O \\ | \\ CH_2 \\ | \\ COO^- \end{array}$$

Figure 6-21. *The conversion of succinate to oxaloacetate.*

catalyzes the reaction that generates ATP and produces adenosine monophosphate (AMP).

$$2\ ADP \rightleftharpoons ATP + AMP \qquad (29)$$

As ATP is used to provide energy when demand increases, there will be a drop in the level of ATP and a rise in the levels of ADP, AMP, and Pi. Changes in the concentration ratios of these substances regulate the rate of combustion of glucose to meet changes in demands for energy. As muscle activity increases, ATP is used up and the store of high-energy phosphate in the cell declines. Coincident with the drop in the ATP concentration are increases in the concentrations of ADP, AMP, and Pi. We can examine the control points and the modes whereby those controls are effected by retracing our steps along the path from glucose to CO_2 and water.

Hexokinase in all cells is inhibited by increasing concentrations of the product of its reaction, glucose-6-phosphate (in the liver, a specific hexokinase, known as glucokinase, is not inhibited by glucose-6-phosphate). If glucose-6-phosphate accumulates and is not removed in the formation of fructose-6-phosphate and fructose-1,6-diphosphate, hexokinase will be inhibited and the entry of glucose into the metabolic scheme will diminish. On the other hand, if glucose-6-phosphate is removed by an increase in the rate of formation of fructose-6-phosphate and fructose-1,6-diphosphate, its level will drop and the activity of hexokinase will increase because of removal of inhibition. The level of glucose-6-phosphate in cells is markedly affected by the activity of phosphofructokinase, the enzyme that catalyzes the formation of fructose-1,6-diphosphate from fructose-6-phosphate.

The activity of phosphofructokinase is directly affected by changes in concentrations of ATP, ADP, and AMP. This enzyme is a critical control point. The potential for high rates of activity when fuel demand is high is a consequence of rapid energy expenditure. If the activity of this enzyme remained high at rest, however, it would continue to use ATP and hexose phosphates until one or the other was exhausted. Accordingly, it is kept in an inhibited state until demands for its product develop. ATP occupies a key role in this mechanism. ATP is, of course, a substrate for the enzyme and absolutely necessary for the formation of fructose-1,6-diphosphate from fructose-1-phosphate. Phosphofructokinase is, however, almost totally inhibited by physiologic concentrations of ATP. This inhibition is accomplished by the combination of ATP with allosteric sites on the enzyme that render it inactive. This results in low activities of phosphofructokinase when muscles are at rest and ATP concentrations are high, and ADP and AMP concentrations are low. In activity, ATP concentration drops and levels of ADP and AMP rise. The allosteric binding of ATP to the inhibitory site on the enzyme is blocked by ADP and AMP, especially the latter. As a consequence, increasing muscle activity causes a blockade of the ATP inhibitory site on the enzyme by AMP and ADP, so phosphofructokinase activity increases. This increases the supply of fructose-1,6-diphosphate and decreases the level of glucose-6-phosphate in the cell. Therefore, the decrease in the ATP level, with the concomitant rise in the levels of ADP and AMP, results in acceleration of the action of phosphofructokinase and hexokinase, thus increasing the rate of combustion of glucose.

There are further effects of these ratio changes on the glycolytic sequence beyond hexokinase and phosphofructokinase. The conversion of 1,3-diphosphoglycerate to 3-phosphoglycerate is ADP-dependent, and the rate of this reaction will accelerate as ADP concentrations rise. Similarly, the conversion of phosphoenol-pyruvate to pyruvate is ADP-dependent and accelerated by rising ADP concentrations. The foregoing are the major control points that make possible the regulation of combustion of glucose so that energy supply meets demand. Any situation that drops the ATP concentration in the cell will result in a corresponding increase in levels of ADP and AMP. The rate of combustion of glucose is thereby accelerated to meet the demand for greater supplies of ATP.

It is quite clear, then, how increased muscular activity increases the rate of glucose combustion. It should be similarly apparent that decrease in the oxygen supply will have similar effects. Since by far the greatest percentage of the ATP made in the cell is manufactured in the mitochondrion by oxidative phosphorylation, any impairment of the latter process will produce a marked drop in the ATP supply. Decreased availability of oxygen will decrease the rate of flow along the entire respiratory chain with a consequent decrease in ATP production. One of the immediate results will be increased rate of glucose combustion and increased rate of formation of pyruvate from glucose. This is the Pasteur effect. If pyruvate accumulates at a rate greater than can be disposed of by mitochondrial oxidative phosphorylation, a large portion of it will be converted to lactate by the enzyme lactic dehydrogenase, and lactate production will increase. This explains the increased glucose utilization and increased production of lactate in states of oxygen deprivation. There are more sites at which effects of changes in concentrations of ATP, ADP, and AMP affect combustion rate. These can be seen in the citric acid cycle and in the respiratory chain as well as in glycolysis.

Quantitatively, the citric acid cycle generates the major portion of the formation of reducing equivalents that are involved in the formation, via oxidative phosphorylation, of ATP from ADP and Pi in the cell. We must be able to slow this cycle when demand is low and to accelerate it at an appropriate rate when demand increases. It is the concentration of ADP that is usually limiting in animal tissues. Electrons will not be transferred along the respiratory chain unless the ATP that is formed by this electron flow can be used, ensuring continued production of ADP. When ATP concentrations are high and ADP levels correspondingly low, oxygen consumption diminishes in resting cells, and the electron carriers accumulate in their reduced form. Thus, NADH accumulates and the level of NAD drops. Those citric acid cycle reactions that depend on NAD as a substrate will slow as a consequence of any decrease in the level of NAD. Accordingly, the oxidations of isocitrate, α-ketoglutarate, and malate will diminish in rate. This accumulation of reduced barriers also effects FAD and $FADH_2$ accumulations, so that succinate oxidation is similarly decreased in rate. It is worth remembering, however, that inorganic phosphate is also necessary for the formation of ATP. Nutritional disease states accompanied by a decrease in the supply of inorganic phosphorous may well be characterized by muscular weakness or impaired cardiac performance, as a consequence.

CITRATE

The product of the citrate synthase reaction is a competitive inhibitor of the binding of oxaloacetate, one of the substrates of the enzyme; hence, the rate of the citrate synthase reaction is critically dependent on oxaloacetate concentration. If the citric acid cycle is slowed as a consequence of accumulation of ATP, citrate inhibits the binding of oxaloacetate and, furthermore, traps oxaloacetate as citrate. If the ADP level rises and the entire cycle accelerates, citrate levels drop and oxaloacetate levels rise, accelerating the citrate synthase reaction.

Isocitrate dehydrogenase is another control point. ADP is a specific activator of this enzyme and increases its affinity for its substrate, isocitrate. Hence, increased energy utilization resulting in a rise in ADP concentration will specifically increase the rate of isocitrate dehydrogenase function by its activator role. This enzyme, isocitrate dehydrogenase, is also inhibited by one of the products of its reaction, NADH, that binds at an allosteric site. If ADP concentrations are low and NADH correspondingly accumulates, isocitrate dehydrogenase is inhibited and the rate of the reaction slows.

One final control point worthy of consideration is α-ketoglutarate dehydrogenase. If this reaction were not controlled, coenzyme A could be trapped as succinyl coenzyme A. The latter compound does tend to accumulate at rest because the supply of GDP and Pi is low. This situation is prevented from going to extremes by the fact that α-ketoglutaric dehydrogenase is inhibited by succinyl coenzyme A, which is a competitive inhibitor of the binding of coenzyme A, itself. When activity increases and GDP and Pi accumulate, α-ketoglutaric dehydrogenase is removed from the inhibition by succinyl coenzyme A because the latter is converted to succinate.

GLUCONEOGENESIS

Rapidly contracting muscles produce lactate and a lesser amount of pyruvate that diffuse into the circulating blood. These incompletely oxidized residues of glucose are used by other tissues, and these mechanisms improve the overall efficiency of fuel metabolism.

One way of disposing of lactate is to convert it to pyruvate by the action of lactate dehydrogenase. It must be remembered that lactate itself is a metabolic dead end. In order for anything further to happen to it, it must be converted to pyruvate. Tissues with a high oxidative capacity, such as red muscle fibers and heart, do convert lactate extracted from the circulating blood to pyruvate, which is then further oxidized in mitochondria in the usual way.

Only part of the lactate in the circulating blood can be burned in this fashion. The remainder is reconverted to glucose, and this is accomplished primarily by two organs, the liver and the kidney. The total amount of glucose formed from lactate in the kidney is only about one-tenth the amount formed in the liver because of the much smaller mass of the kidneys. The process of converting circulating lactate and pyruvate to free glucose is known as gluconeogenesis. Thus, there is a cycle in which glucose is converted to lactate in skeletal muscles by glycolysis and the lactate is converted back to glucose in the liver and kidneys by the gluconeogenic pathway. This cycle is known as the Cori cycle, named for the Nobel laureates Carl F. and Gerty T. Cori, who first described it.

Glycolysis, as we have previously described it, is an irreversible process. The reason glycolysis is irreversible is that there are three reaction sequences that are essentially irreversible because of thermodynamic considerations. These irreversible reactions are those catalyzed by hexokinase, phosphofructokinase, and pyruvate kinase. In order to convert pyruvate, the oxidation product of lactate, to glucose, there are distinctive reactions of gluconeogenesis that make possible the flow from pyruvate to glucose.

The pathway around pyruvic kinase involves several steps. The first step is the pyruvate carboxylase reaction which, itself, has two stages. First, CO_2 from bicarbonate is bound to a complex of the enzyme and biotin, in an activated form. ATP supplies the energy for this activation. Next, the activated carboxyl group is transferred from carboxy-biotin to pyruvate to form oxaloacetate (Figure 6-22). This pyruvate carboxylase reaction is also a key control point. The enzyme is totally inactive unless acetyl CoA is bound to it. It must be emphasized that acetyl CoA is not a reactant in this process, but it is necessary that it be bound to the enzyme for the enzyme to be activated. Here is how this allosteric activation of pyruvate carboxylase by acetyl CoA works: When there is a high level of acetyl CoA in the mitochondrion, it is a signal of the need for more oxaloacetate. The activation of pyruvate carboxylase makes possible the formation of more oxaloacetate from pyruvate. If there is a surplus of ATP, the oxaloacetate will be di-

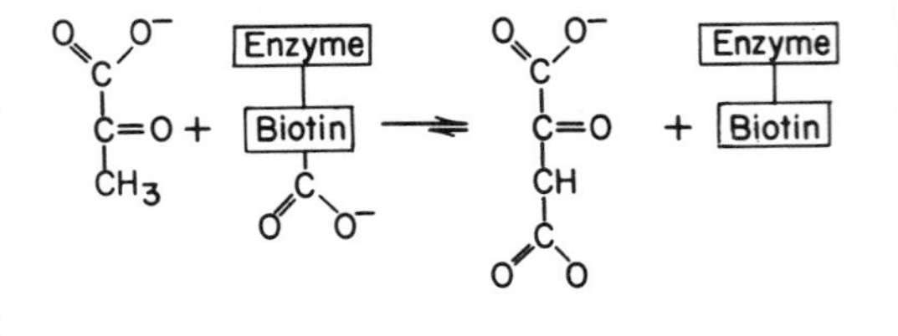

Pyruvate Oxaloacetate

Figure 6-22. *The role of biotin in the carboxylation of pyruvate.*

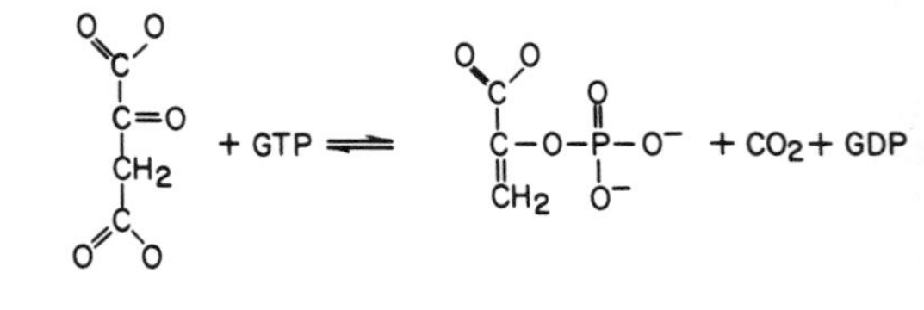

Oxaloacetate Phosphoenolpyruvate

Figure 6-23. *The conversion of oxaloacetate to phosphoenolpyruvate.*

verted to gluconeogenesis. If, on the other hand, there is a deficiency of ATP, the oxaloacetate will enter the citric acid cycle upon condensing with some of the abundant acetyl CoA that turned on the pyruvate carboxylase reaction. It is worth reminding those who are interested in nutrition that biotin is an essential nutrient and must be supplied in the diet. Mammals are not capable of synthesizing this vitamin.

Now we face another barrier. Oxaloacetate is formed in the mitochondrion and cannot diffuse out of it. All the remaining enzymes of gluconeogenesis are in the cytosol. Accordingly, oxaloacetate is converted to malate, which can diffuse across the mitochondrial membrane. Oxaloacetate is reduced to malate inside the mitochondrion by the NADH-linked malate dehydrogenase. The malate diffuses into the cytosol and is reoxidized to oxaloacetate by an NAD^+-linked malate dehydrogenase in the cytoplasm.

The next reaction accomplishes two processes at the same time. Oxaloacetate is simultaneously decarboxylated and phosphorylated by the enzyme phosphoenol-pyruvic-carboxykinase. Here the necessary energy is supplied by GTP, not ATP (Figure 6-23).

The product is phosphoenol-pyruvate which then can traverse up the glycolytic cycle to the next irreversible step. The CO_2 that was added to pyruvate by pyruvate carboxylase comes off in this step. This decarboxylation, in fact, makes the reaction energetically feasible.

The next irreversible step on the pathway from pyruvate to glucose is encountered at phosphofructokinase. Here we rely on a phosphatase to produce fructose-6-phosphate from fructose 1,6-diphosphate. The enzyme fructose-1,6-diphosphatase catalyes the exergonic hydrolysis of the phosphate ester at C-1, producing fructose-6-phosphate.

The final irreversible step, at hexokinase, is circumvented by a microsomal enzyme, glucose-6-phosphatase. This enzyme hydrolyzes off the phosphate at carbon six to produce free glucose. It is to be borne in mind that only liver and kidney possess this last enzyme. Accordingly, only liver and kidney are capable of producing free glucose from lactate and pyruvate.

It is worthy of note here that amino acids are also capable of serving as substrates for gluconeogenesis. Quantitatively, alanine and glutamine are most important in this regard. Both of these amino acids must have their amino groups removed by transamination before entering into the gluconeogenic process. Alanine becomes pyruvate and follows the pathway just discussed. Glutamate becomes α-ketoglutarate and enters the Krebs cycle. We will look at the importance of amino acids as gluconeogenic substrates and their role in total body economy in more detail later on in this chapter.

GLYCOLYSIS AND GLUCONEOGENESIS: ENERGY CONSIDERATIONS

If simple reversal of glycolysis were possible, it would be energetically highly unfavorable, requiring an input of 20 Calories per mole of glucose formed. Gluconeogenesis, as it actually occurs, requires the input of six high-energy phosphate bonds to synthesize one molecule of glucose from two of pyruvate. With this input of six high-energy phosphates, gluconeogenesis is now energetically favored and is exergonic.

This extremely useful mechanism is still not without its cost, however. The reader will remember that the production of two molecules of pyruvate from one molecule of glucose results in the net generation of two molecules of ATP. Gluconeogenesis requires the input of six molecules of ATP. Therefore, it is obvious that it costs four more ATPs to make a molecule of glucose from two of pyruvate than one can derive by the conversion of one molecule of glucose to two of pyruvate. This price is worth paying, however. It is a necessary reaction to deal with the lactate produced when muscles contract rapidly. Although the yield of ATP from glycolysis in muscle is very much lower than the yield from complete oxidation of glucose to CO_2 and water, glycolysis is capable of proceeding some 25 times faster than the full oxidation scheme. Therefore, muscles can make twice as much ATP per second by converting glycogen to lactate as they can by oxidizing it completely. The extra energy cost of reconverting the lactate to glucose is worth it when one reflects that this scheme makes possible the very rapid supplies of energy needed for quick and forceful muscle action.

It must also be remembered that gluconeogenesis makes possible the continuing supply of the glucose so necessary for the brain during times of fasting and starvation. In these circumstances, mobilization of body fat provides fuel in the form of acetyl CoA to generate ATP. This ATP is used as the energy input for the manufacture of glucose from lactate and amino acids in the kidney and in the liver.

HEXOSE MONOPHOSPHATE SHUNT

Prior to this time, we have concerned ourselves with the formation of glucose-6-phosphate as the first committed step in glycolysis or as the immediate substrate for the glucose-6-phosphatase reaction, whereby free glucose is produced in liver and kidney. In glycolysis, NAD^+ was the cofactor and acceptor of reducing equivalents, and the coin of exchange of chemical energy was ATP. In the hexose monophosphate shunt, we see that $NADP^+$ is the acceptor of reducing equivalents and ATP is not involved. Cells have developed another mechanism whereby glucose-6-phosphate is metabolized according to equation 30.

$$\text{Glucose-6-PO}_4 + 7\ H_2O + 12\ NADP^+ \rightarrow 6\ CO_2 + H3PO_4 + 12\ NADPH + 12\ H^+ \quad (30)$$

There are two major functions of this pathway. One is to provide a source of reducing equivalents for biosynthetic purposes and the other, which will become apparent as the pathway is described, is to provide a source of five carbon sugars (pentoses) required for nucleic acid metabolism. We will be able to understand this pathway better if we realize that in order to bring about the complete conversion of glucose-6-phosphate to CO_2, we require six molecules of glucose-6-phosphate. In the first two steps, the reducing equivalents are generated and the 6-carbon chain is decarboxylated, so that six molecules of pentose-phosphate are obtained. The six molecules of pentose-phosphate are rearranged and reassembled so that we generate five moles of glucose-6-phosphate. When all of these reactions are summed, we end up with the reaction shown.

In mammalian striated muscle, there appears to be no hexose monophosphate shunt. In liver, however, in the neighborhood of 30 percent or more of the CO_2 arising from glucose is generated in this shunt. Mammary gland, testis, adipose tissue, leukocytes, and adrenal cortex catabolize an even larger proportion of glucose by this mechanism. Red cells also have an active shunt mechanism, and disorders or deficiencies of hexose monophosphate shunt enzymes are associated with clinical hemolytic anemias. Liver, mammary gland, testis, adrenal cortex, and adipose tissue are active sites of fatty acid and/or steroid synthesis requiring large amounts

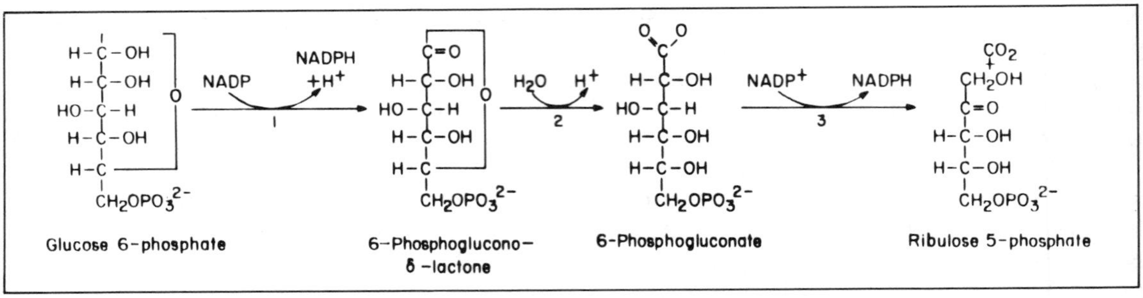

Figure 6-24. *The oxidative portion of the hexose monophosphate shunt pathway.*

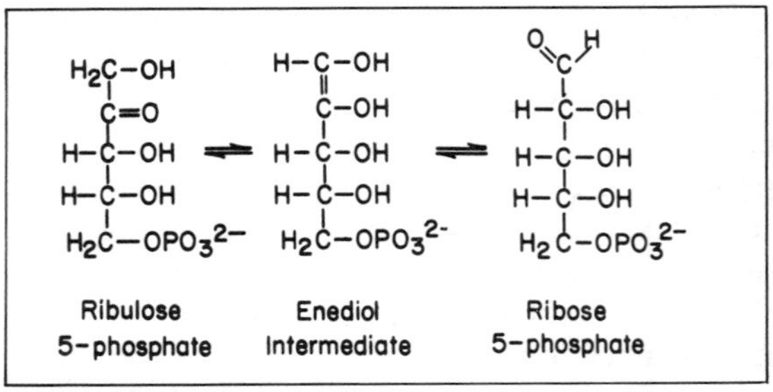

of reducing power as NADPH. This pathway starts with glucose-6-phosphate and therefore requires no further input of ATP. The first series of reactions (Figure 6-24) generates two NADPH and a CO_2, as 6-phosphogluconate is decarboxylated to ribulose 5-phosphate.

The pentose phosphate pathway starts with the dehydrogenation of glucose-6-phosphate at C-1. This reaction involves $NADP^+$ as a cofactor and is catalyzed by the enzyme glucose-6-phosphate dehydrogenase. The product of this reaction, a lactone derivative of 6-phosphogluconate, is hydrolyzed to 6-phosphogluconate. This latter 6-carbon sugar is oxidatively decarboxylated by 6-phosphogluconate dehydrogenase, yielding ribulose 5-phosphate, NADPH, and CO_2.

Ribulose 5-phosphate is then isomerized to ribose 5-phosphate by the formation of an enediol intermediate (Figure 6-25).

So far we have produced NADPH and one ribose 5-phosphate for each glucose-6-phosphate oxidized. Many cells require much more NADPH than ribose 5-phosphate for nucleotide and nucleic acid synthesis. Under these conditions, ribose 5-phosphate is converted into glyceraldehyde 3-phosphate and fructose-6-phosphate, allowing re-entry of the pentose phosphate product of the initial reactions into the mainstream of glycolysis. First, some of the ribulose 5-phosphate is epimerized to form xylulose 5-phosphate (Figure 6-26).

Then a molecule of xylulose 5-phosphate reacts with a ribose 5-phosphate, in a reaction catalyzed by transketolase, to form glyceraldehyde 3-phosphate and sedoheptulose 7-phosphate (Figure 6-27). Transaldolase then catalyzes the reaction between sedoheptulose 7-phosphate and glyceraldehyde 3-phosphate to form erythrose 4-phosphate and fructose-6-phosphate (Figure 6-28). Next, transketolase is again employed to catalyze the reaction between xylulose 5-phosphate and erythrose 4-phosphate, yielding glyceraldehyde 3-phosphate and fructose-6-phosphate (Figure 6-29). The net result is that we have provided a pathway where three ribose 5-

Figure 6-25. *Isomerization steps among pentose phosphates.*

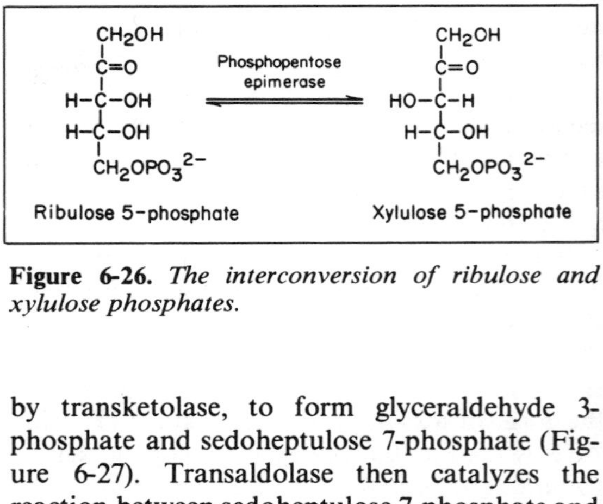

Figure 6-26. *The interconversion of ribulose and xylulose phosphates.*

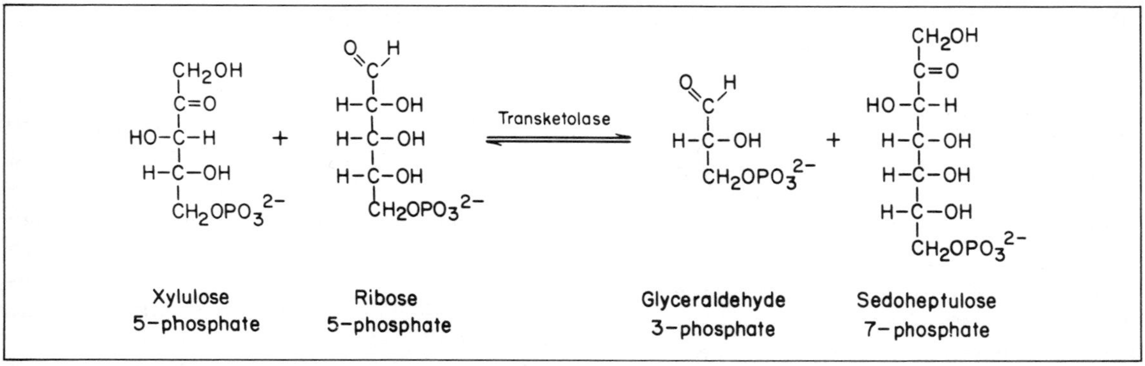

Xylulose 5-phosphate + Ribose 5-phosphate $\xrightleftharpoons{\text{Transketolase}}$ Glyceraldehyde 3-phosphate + Sedoheptulose 7-phosphate

Figure 6-27. *The formation of sedoheptulose phosphate catalyzed by transketolase.*

Sedoheptulose 7-phosphate + Glyceraldehyde 3-phosphate $\xrightleftharpoons{\text{Transketolase}}$ Erythrose 4-phosphate + Fructose 6-phosphate

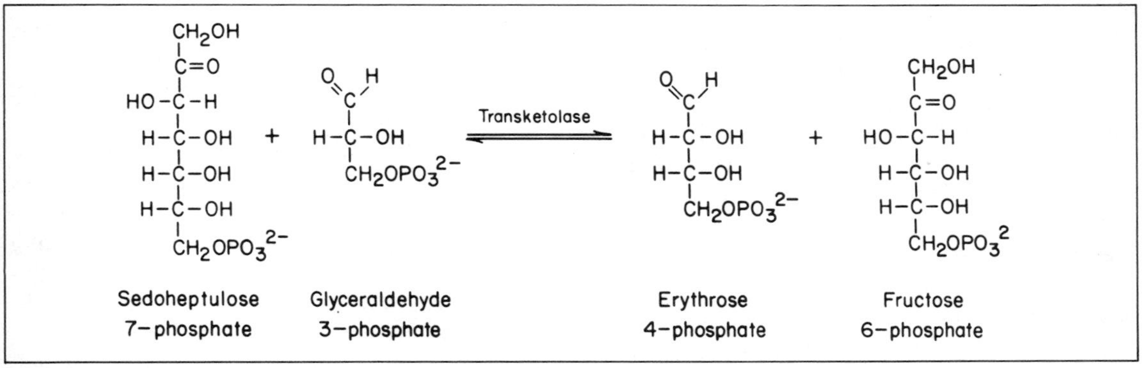

Figure 6-28. *The formation of fructose-6-phosphate via transaldolase.*

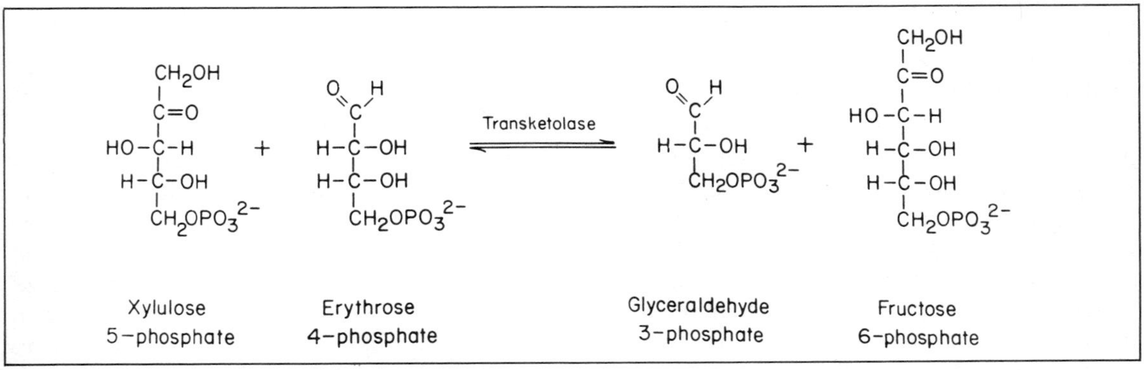

Xylulose 5-phosphate + Erythrose 4-phosphate $\xrightleftharpoons{\text{Transketolase}}$ Glyceraldehyde 3-phosphate + Fructose 6-phosphate

Figure 6-29. *The formation of fructose-6-phosphate catalyzed by transketolase.*

phosphate moieties can produce two fructose-6-phosphates and one glyceraldehyde 3-phosphate moiety. Accordingly, excess ribose 5-phosphate can be quantitatively converted to glycolytic intermediates, either for glycolysis or reconversion to glucose-6-phosphate to begin the cycle again. Depending on the requirements of the cells for NADPH and ribose 5-phosphate, different relative amounts of these two substances can be produced. We have already shown the possibility of reconversion of fructose-6-phosphate to glucose 6-phosphate and the conversion of glyceraldehyde 3-phosphate to fructose diphosphate. Thus, if instead of three moles of ribose 5-phosphate we have six, then we can readily reconvert them to five moles of glucose-6-phosphate.

Transketolase is an enzyme of special importance to those interested in nutrition. The reason for this is that it contains a tightly bound thiamine pyrophosphate as its prosthetic group. Its activity, therefore, depends on the amount of thiamine available to the organism in its diet. It is the only thiamine-dependent enzyme that is present in cytosol, rather than in mitochondria, and can therefore be measured in red cells, which have no mitochondria.

Assessment of thiamine nutritional status in the laboratory is now accomplished by measuring the degree of thiamine pyrophosphate saturation of transketolase. In brief, a hemolysate of washed red cells is incubated with and without added thiamine pyrophosphate. Then ribulose 5-phosphate is added to both incubation media. The step from phosphogluconate to ribulose 5-phosphate is irreversible, and so any ribulose 5-phosphate that becomes glucose-6-phosphate has to do so by traversing transketolase, not once, but twice. After a standardized period of time, the amount of glucose-6-phosphate formed from the added ribulose 5-phosphate is measured in the two incubation vessels. If the vessel to which thiamine pyrophosphate was added shows 15 percent or greater augmentation of glucose-6-phosphate formation from ribulose 5-phosphate, clinically significant thiamine undernutrition is present.

REGULATION OF THE HEXOSE MONOPHOSPHATE SHUNT

Often, the mechanism of regulation of a metabolic pathway can be readily recognized by examination of the products of that pathway and invoking the concept of negative feedback inhibition, i.e., the products of a sequence of reactions will generally interact in some manner with the first committed step of the pathway to regulate its activity. Applying these criteria to the HMP shunt, we find that, as one would expect, the ratio of NADPH to $NADP^+$ controls the activity of the first enzyme in the pathway, i.e., the glucose-6-phosphate dehydrogenase. When the ratio of NADPH/NADP exceeds ten, then various degrees of inhibition occur. The inhibition can be reversed by oxidized glutathione. This relationship has important implications in red cell metabolism of which there is an excellent account in Stanbury et al. [22].

The HMP shunt, especially glucose-6-phosphate dehydrogenase, is responsive to changes in carbohydrate intake. For example, as carbohydrate intake increases and more of it is being converted to fat, we find large increases in glucose-6-phosphate dehydrogenase activity. In view of its function in supplying reducing equivalents for synthetic purposes, the HMP shunt will be most active in those tissues where a high level of biosynthetic activity is required, i.e., adipose tissue, liver, and lactating mammary gland.

GLYCOGEN

Synthesis

Reflect for a moment on the extraordinary flexibility of the fuel economy of the human. He can meet his energy requirements by the usual three meals a day, by frequent small snacks, or by no food intake at all, and often for long periods of time. Much as he can adapt to wide ranges in food intake, he is capable of meeting wide ranges of demand for energy. He is capable of going rapidly from complete rest to maximal physical exertion, and fuel supply is seldom limiting.

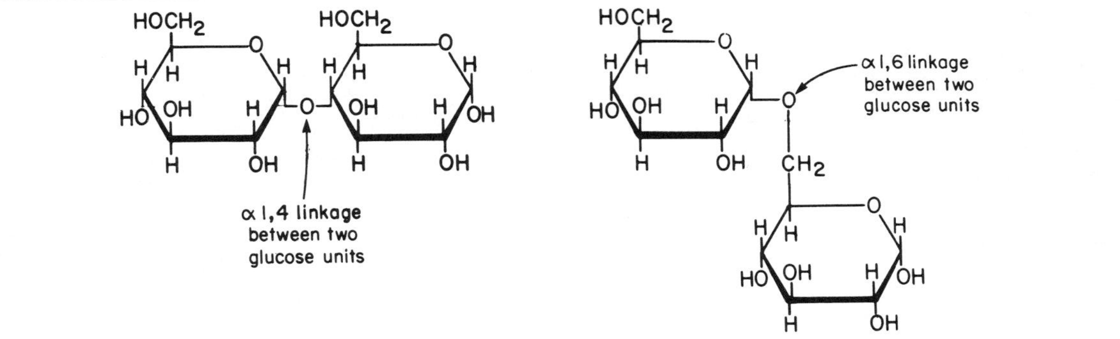

Figure 6-30. *The types of glycosidic bonds in glycogen.*

Glycogen is the fuel depot that is first called upon when fuel demands of any sort arise.

Glycogen is the storage form of glucose and it can be readily mobilized. It is a high-molecular-weight polymer arranged in linear arrays, connected to each other to form a branching system of glucose residues. These glucose residues in the chains are linked by α-1,4-glycosidic bonds. The branches are created by α-1,6-glycosidic bonds and they occur, on the average, about once in 10 residues (Figure 6-30).

Glycogen can be considered as a storage polysaccharide and is deposited in the cytosol of cells as granules with a diameter ranging from 100 to 400 Å. The granules contain not only the glycogen, but the enzymes that carry out its synthesis and degradation and some of the enzymes that regulate these processes. Because of the storage function, glycogen in the liver plays a key role in the regulation of blood glucose level in periods of brief fast. Glycogen in muscle is a readily available fuel form that makes it possible for the muscles to increase abruptly their rate of activity by 100- or even 1,000-fold.

We have previously alluded to the facts that glucose-6-phosphate can be degraded by glycolysis, can enter into the hexose monophosphate shunt, or can be converted to free glucose in liver and kidney by the action of glucose-6-phosphatase. Entry into glycogen synthesis is yet another possible fate for glucose-6-phosphate. When glycogen stores are low and glucose is available, glucose-6-phosphate is diverted into restoration of glycogen stores. The first step is a conversion of glucose-6-phosphate to glucose-1-phosphate through the action of phosphoglucomutase. This reaction takes place through an intermediate, glucose-1,6-diphosphate. A continuing supply of glucose-1,6-diphosphate is assured by the action of the enzyme phosphoglucokinase, which catalyzes the reaction whereby glucose-1-phosphate reacts with ATP to yield glucose-1,6-diphosphate and ADP. Glucose-1-phosphate then reacts with uridine triphosphate to form an activated form of glucose, UDP-glucose (Figure 6-31).

This reaction is readily reversible, but is pushed in the direction of the formation of UDP-glucose by the action of an inorganic pyrophosphatase that rapidly hydrolyzes the pyrophosphate formed, preventing reversal of the foregoing reaction. This reaction introduces us to a key mechanism for activation of many different sugars in the cell, i.e., by conversion to a UDP derivative according to the following general reaction:

$$\text{Sugar} - PO_4 + \text{UTP} \rightleftharpoons \text{UDP sugar} + \text{pyrophosphate} \qquad (31)$$

Next, the activated glucosyl unit of UDP-glucose is transferred to the hydroxyl group at a C-4 terminus of glycogen to form an α-1,4-glycosidic linkage (Figure 6-32).

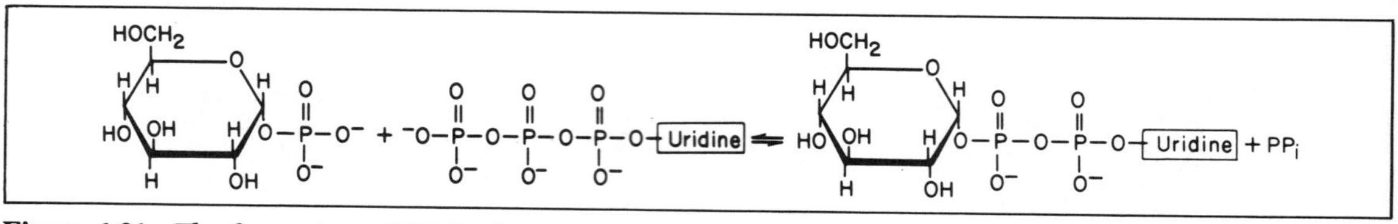

Figure 6-31. *The formation of UDP-glucose.*

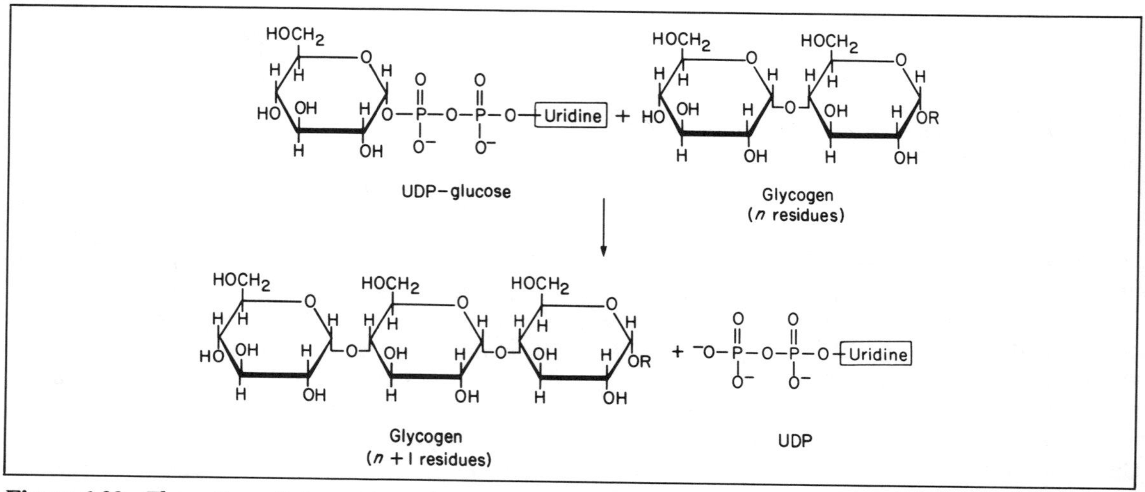

Figure 6-32. *The action of glycogen synthetase.*

The UDP that is formed can be reconverted to UTP by reacting with ATP in a reaction catalyzed by nucleoside diphosphokinase. The addition of a glucosyl residue to an amylose chain is catalyzed by the enzyme glycogen synthetase, and this addition can only occur if the polysaccharide chain already contains at least four residues.

After a number of glucosyl residues are joined in α-1,4 linkage by glycogen synthetase, a branch is created by the breaking of an α-1,4 link and the formation of an α-1,6 link. This branching enzyme, glycosyl-4:6-transferase, catalyzes the transfer of a segment of amylose chain onto the C-6 hydroxyl of a neighboring chain. The enzyme moves a block of seven 1,4-residues from a chain at least 11 residues in length and transfers it onto another segment of amylose chain at a point at least four residues removed from the nearest branch (Figure 6-33).

Branching is important because it increases the solubility of glycogen and creates a large number of nonreducing terminal residues from which glucosyl moieties can be mobilized, one at a time. The more branches, the larger the number of nonreducing terminal residues, which are the sites of addition of glucosyl moieties. Thus, branching increases the potential rate of both glycogen synthesis and glycogen degradation.

Several points about glycogen in the body need to be made here. First, there is an energy cost for laying down glycogen. Because of the need for UTP to activate glucose as UDP-glucose, there is an expenditure of one high-energy phosphate for every glucosyl moiety converted to glycogen. Thus, glycogen is formed in times of plentiful supply of exogenous fuel in the form of food. In the well-fed state, the concentration of glycogen in the liver is higher than in the muscle.

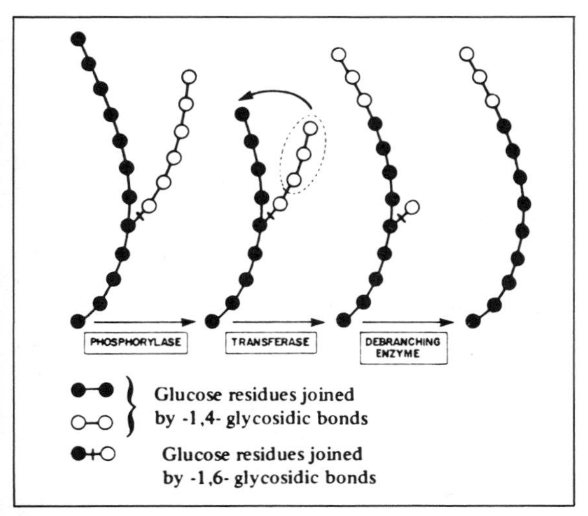

Figure 6-33. *Steps in glycogenolysis. (From D. W. Martin, Jr., P. A. Mayes, and V. W. Rodwell,* Harper's Review of Biochemistry *(18th ed.). Los Altos, CA: Lange Medical Publications, 1981. P. 172.)*

The maximum concentration of glycogen in the liver is in the neighborhood of 400 millimoles of glucosyl residues (65 gm dry weight) per kilogram. Considering that the liver of the 70-kg man weighs about 1.6 kg, the total liver store of glycogen is 0.6 moles of glucosyl residues. Glycogen concentration in muscle ranges widely. Usually, it is in the neighborhood of 85 millimoles per kilogram of muscle tissue. After an hour or two of heavy work, the muscle content of glycogen can fall to as low as one millimole per kilogram. After muscle has been depleted in this fashion, several subsequent days of high-carbohydrate diet can raise the level to as high as 300 millimoles of glucosyl residues per kilogram of muscle. Long-distance runners appear to have discovered this fact independently, and part of the routine preparation for a marathon race is several days of high-carbohydrate feeding immediately preceding the contest. In the ordinary state of things, however, the 70-kg man with 28 kg of skeletal muscle will have 2.4 moles of glucosyl residues as glycogen in muscle.

The preceding statements underline the fact that glycogen synthesis and, as we shall see later, glycogen breakdown, are controlled processes. The major site of regulation of rate of synthesis is the reaction catalyzed by glycogen synthetase.

Degradation

In the breakdown of glycogen, the main reaction is a simple phosphorolysis of the 1,4-glucosidic bonds, by inorganic phosphate, to form glucose-1-phosphate. This primary reaction which, by the way, is the main site of control of glycogen breakdown, cleaves the terminal 1,4-glucosidic bond at the nonreducing end of a glycogen chain to produce one molecule of glucose-1-phosphate and shorten the chain by one residue. In vitro, this reaction is freely reversible and at equilibrium the ratio of Pi to glucose-1-phosphate is about 3.5. In vivo, the concentration of Pi is some 30-fold greater than the concentration of glucose-1-phosphate, and so the reaction always proceeds in the direction of glucose-1-phosphate. Although the Coris were able to demonstrate synthesis of glycogen by simple reversibility of the phosphorylase reaction in vitro, such a synthetic pathway does not take place in the intact body. Two other bits of information emphasize the fact that the phosphorylase reaction, in vivo, must proceed in the direction of glycogen degradation. Hormones, to be discussed later, that lead to an increase in phosphorylase activity always elicit glycogen breakdown, not synthesis. Finally, patients with McArdle's disease, who lack muscle phosphorylase entirely, are able to synthesize muscle glycogen.

Glucose residues can be successively removed by phosphorolysis in the manner just described. This proceeds until the reaction approaches a branch point in the glycogen residue. Phosphorylase will only attack 1,4-bonds that are at least four residues removed from a 1,6-branch. If there is no debranching activity, glycogen will be completely sheared by phosphorylase to four residue stubs, and the product is called limit dextrin.

For further degradation to continue, a second enzyme, amylo-1,6-glucosidase, catalyzes two successive reactions. First, it acts as a glucosyl transferase reminiscent of the branching enzyme that functions during glycogen synthesis. This enzyme transfers three glucosyl residues from a branch onto a chain terminus so as to lengthen it. When this enzyme acts on limit dextrin, for example, it will remove three residues of the four-residue stub and add it to another four-residue stub. The second stub is now seven residues long and can be attacked again by phosphorylase. The single residue remaining on the C-6 at the branch is now hydrolyzed to yield free glucose, not glucose-1-phosphate. This action, then, has removed the single-branched residue to expose another straight chain of 1,4-linked residues down to the next branch, so that phosphorylase can continue to act once again. The sequence of glycogen degradation by the action of glycogen phosphorylase and amylo-1,6-glucosidase acting in concert produces a continuous stripping of glucosyl residues. Those released by phosphorylase are in the form of glucose-1-phosphate and those released by the glucosidase are as free glucose. The degree of branching is such that 11 to 14 molecules of glucose-1-phosphate are formed for each molecule of free glucose released.

The glucose-1-phosphate is converted to glucose-6-phosphate by the action of phosphoglucomutase, at no energy cost. The other 10 percent or so of glucosyl moieties that are cleaved at branch points to produce free glucose must be phosphorylated and will cost a molecule of ATP for each free glucose converted to glucose-6-phosphate.

In any event, the glucose-6-phosphate produced by glycogen degradation is now available to the cellular engine. In muscle, this is used to provide a quick burst of energy via glycolysis for sudden activity before sufficient oxygen is available for the aerobic generation of ATP. In liver and kidney, the enzyme glucose-6-phosphatase can produce free glucose to bolster the blood glucose level in times of fasting.

Regulation of Glycogen Metabolism

The processes of synthesis and degradation of glycogen must be tightly and smoothly regulated to meet the demands of body economy. Glycogen must be laid down when glucose supply is plentiful, as during absorption from a meal. When a cell has laid down the maximum amount of glycogen appropriate to its structure and function, the process must be shut off. Furthermore, both muscle and liver must be able to respond to demands for quick energy or free glucose supply for regulation of blood glucose levels. A stimulus that initiates glycogen synthesis must be able to shut off glycogen degradation, or a futile cycle wastefully expending ATP would be set in motion. The main control points, as already defined, are glycogen synthetase and phosphorylase. The changes in activity of these two enzymes result from their existence in both active and inactive conformations. Although these conformations may be made to change by direct interaction of the enzymes with some metabolites, the principal cause of a shift in conformation and, hence, activity is a phosphorylation of the respective enzymes. Basically, phosphorylation activates glycogen phosphorylase and increases glycogen degradation. At the same time, phosphorylation of glycogen synthetase decreases its activity and diminishes the rate of glycogen synthesis. Let us first direct our attention to muscle phosphorylase and its response to epinephrine. As we all know, confrontation of a stressful situation causes a surge of epinephrine in the bloodstream that rapidly mobilizes large amounts of muscle glycogen. Epinephrine activates muscle phosphorylase by means of a reaction cascade that involves cyclic AMP and provides a high degree of amplification of the epinephrine signal (Figure 6-34).

When epinephrine binds to the plasma membrane of a muscle cell, it activates the enzyme adenyl cyclase (Figure 6-34). This enzyme catalyzes an intramolecular rearrangement of ATP to produce cyclic AMP and pyrophosphate. Cyclic AMP is the widely known second messenger discovered and defined by Earl Sutherland, for which he received the Nobel Prize. The action of adenyl cyclase causes an increase in the intracellular level of cyclic AMP. This substance then binds with a cyclic AMP protein kinase, in a fashion that is rather complex, but deserves some

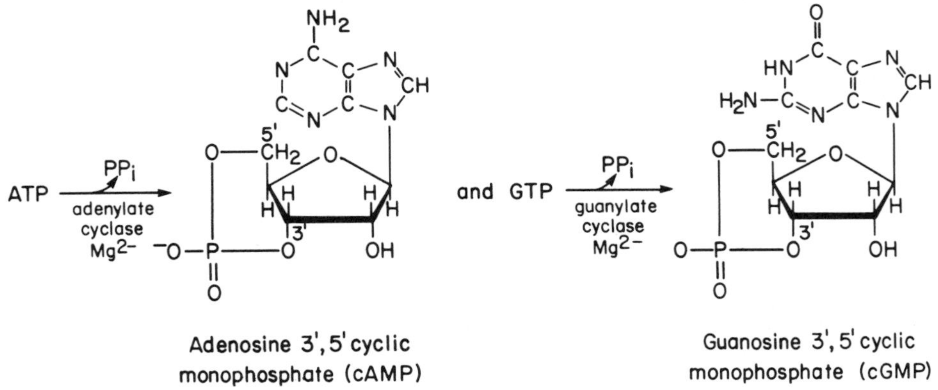

$$ATP \xrightarrow[\text{adenylate cyclase, } Mg^{2-}]{PP_i} \text{Adenosine 3',5' cyclic monophosphate (cAMP)} \quad \text{and} \quad GTP \xrightarrow[\text{guanylate cyclase, } Mg^{2-}]{PP_i} \text{Guanosine 3',5' cyclic monophosphate (cGMP)}$$

Figure 6-34. *The action of adenyl and guanyl cyclases.*

description here because it is undoubtedly prototypical. Protein kinase consists of two pairs of polypeptide chains, a C-peptide and an R-peptide. The C-peptide is a catalytic one and the R-peptide is a regulator peptide. When the two are bonded together, the C-peptide is inactive. When cyclic AMP concentration rises, it binds allosterically with the R-peptide and releases active, free, C-peptide (equation 32). When the cyclic AMP concentration falls the R-peptide is now able to bind with the C-peptide and inactivate it.

$$R_2C_2(\text{Mg-ATP})_2 \underset{+2\text{Mg-ATP}}{\overset{-2\text{Mg-ATP}}{\rightleftharpoons}} R_2C_2 \underset{\text{protein kinase}}{\overset{+2\text{cAMP}}{\rightleftharpoons}} R_2(\text{cAMP})_2 + 2C \qquad (32)$$

The active, free, C-polypeptide catalyzes the phosphorylation of the enzyme, glycogen phosphorylase kinase, in an ATP-dependent reaction (Figure 6-35). The phosphorylated glycogen phosphorylase kinase, is much more active than the nonphosphorylated free enzyme. Active glycogen phosphorylase kinase (phosphorylated) now is capable of catalyzing the phosphorylation of glycogen phosphorylase itself, again in an ATP-dependent reaction. Thus, the relatively inactive glycogen phosphorylase is converted to the fully active, phosphorylated, glycogen phosphorylase that now catalyzes the degradation of glycogen by acting at the 1,4-bonds of glycogen, as described. The active muscle phosphorylase is called phosphorylase *a,* and the usually inactive form is called phosphorylase *b*. Phosphorylase *b* is a dimer, and the activated phosphorylase *a* (phosphorylated) is a tetramer.

Once this cascade is turned on by epinephrine, how is it turned off when the epinephrine stimulus disappears? When the epinephrine stimulus is removed, adenyl cyclase is no longer activated, and its formation shuts down. The cyclic AMP already formed is hydrolyzed by cyclic AMP phosphodiesterase to produce ordinary 5′-AMP. As the intracellular concentration of cyclic AMP falls, the R-peptide of protein kinase is now released and able to bind the C-peptide, inactivating it. The activated, phosphorylated, phosphorylase kinase is now dephosphorylated by the action of phosphorylase kinase phosphatase, and rendered less active. The active, phosphorylated tetramer, phosphorylase *a,* is converted to the nonphosphorylated, relatively inactive, phosphorylase *b* by the action of phosphorylase phosphatase. Thus, the epinephrine-stimulated cascade is shut off as soon as the epinephrine stimulus disappears.

When the epinephrine stimulus turned on phosphorylase, how did it simultaneously turn off glycogen synthetase? Quite simply, the very same series of events phosphorylated glycogen

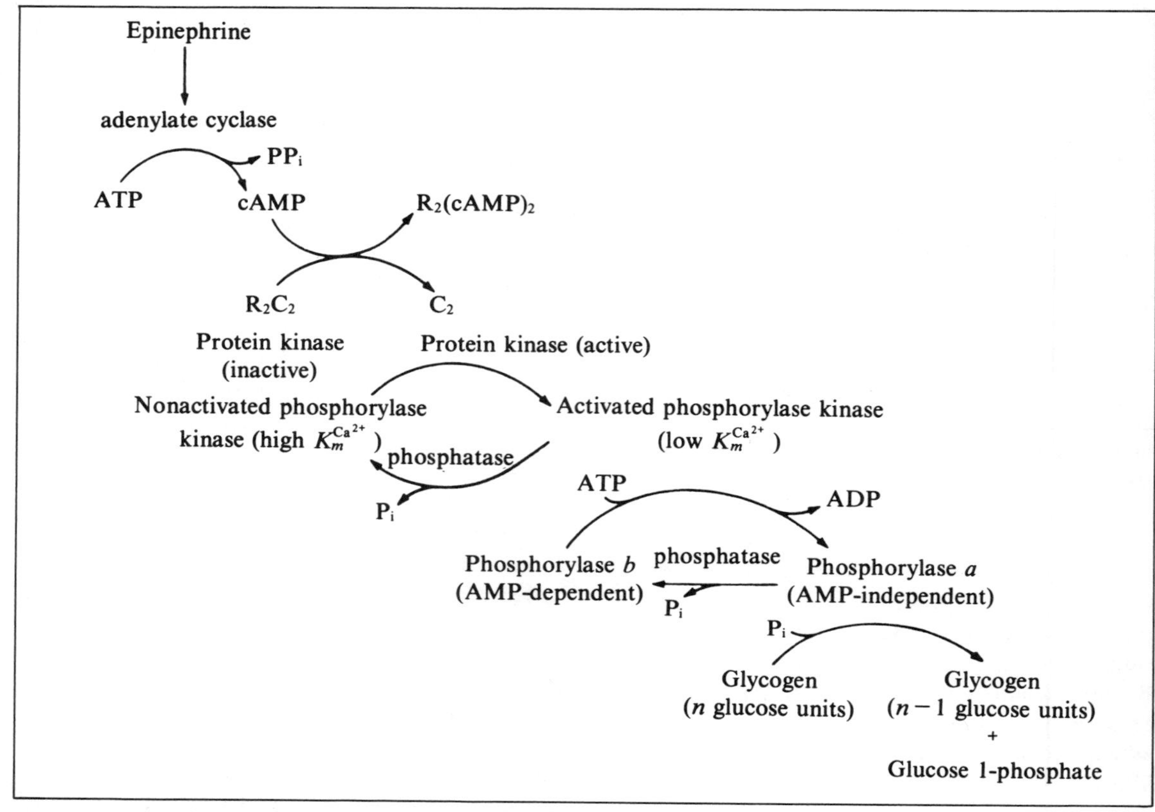

Figure 6-35. *Schematic representation of the cascade of the activation and deactivation of glycogen phosphorylase in skeletal muscle. At each lower level of the activating cascades, the number of molecules involved increases by at least one order of magnitude. (From A. White, P. Handler, E. L. Smith, et al.* Principles of Biochemistry *(6th ed.). New York: McGraw-Hill, 1978.)*

synthetase at the same time that it phosphorylated phosphorylase (Figure 6-36). Nonphosphorylated glycogen synthetase is active and is independent of glucose-6-phosphate levels. Hence, the active form of glycogen synthetase is called the independent form (I-form). When the epinephrine-stimulated cascade activates protein kinase so that the I-form of glycogen synthetase is phosphorylated, the product is the D-form. This form is less active and requires high levels of glucose-6-phosphate for activity. Therefore, the epinephrine stimulus turned off glycogen synthetase activity at the same time that it turned on phosphorylase activity. When the epinephrine stimulus disappears, a glycogen synthetase phosphatase dephosphorylates the relatively inactive D-form, converting it to the active I-form, which can now promote glycogen synthesis (Figure 6-37).

Each step in the foregoing cascade amplifies the effect of epinephrine. Thus, a minute amount of epinephrine has a large effect. It has been estimated that a rise in the concentration of cyclic AMP to one micromole per kilogram of muscle causes the formation of 25,000 times as much glucose-1-phosphate per minute.

It is to be borne in mind that phosphorylase kinase can be partially activated in a fashion independent of the cyclic AMP system. When

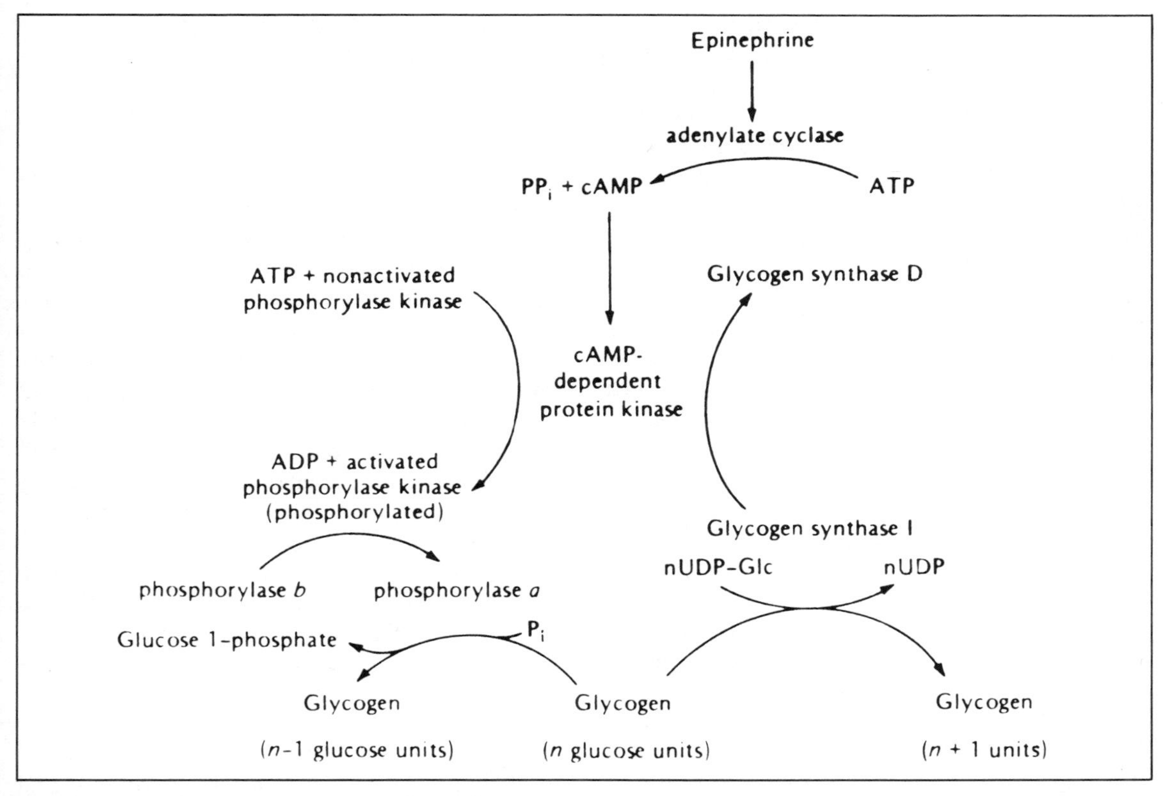

Figure 6-36. *The schematic series of coupled reactions in skeletal muscle, showing reciprocal control of glycogenolysis and glycogen synthesis, mediated by stimulation of adenylate cyclase by epinephrine. (From A. White, P. Handler, E. L. Smith, et al.* Principles of Biochemistry *(6th ed.). New York: McGraw-Hill, 1978.)*

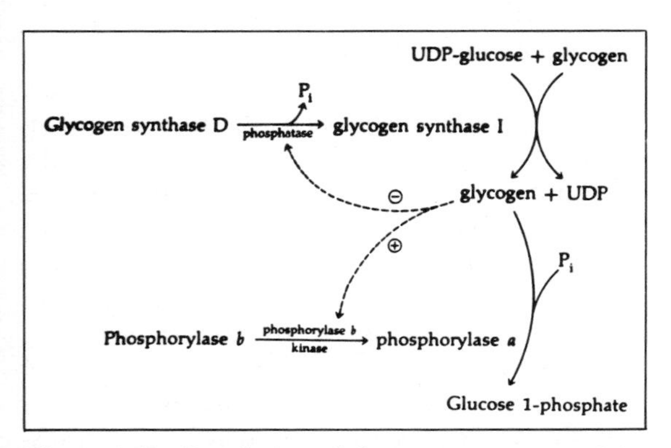

Figure 6-37. *Regulation of the interconversion of the I and D forms of glycogen synthase.*

muscle contraction is triggered by the release of calcium ions, these same calcium ions are capable of partial activation of phosphorylase kinase without phosphorylating it. Thus, glycogen breakdown and muscle contraction are linked by a transient increase in the level of calcium ions in the cytoplasm. In this instance, calcium ions have partially activated phosphorylase kinase, increasing the rate of phosphorylation of phosphorylase itself and, hence, the phosphorylase activity.

One of the consequences of the use of fuel in muscle contraction is a rise in the concentration of ordinary 5′ AMP. The relatively inactive nonphosphorylated form of glycogen phosphorylase can form a complex with AMP that is more active than the nonphosphorylated form that is not bound with AMP. Accordingly, a rise in AMP levels has stimulated the mobilization of fuel by increasing the activity of phosphorylase.

Now, how is glycogen synthesis shut down when appropriate amounts of glycogen have been synthesized in the resting state? Remember that glycogen synthetase can occur in the active, nonphosphorylated form and in the relatively inactive, phosphorylated form. Glycogen synthetase phosphatase dephosphorylates glycogen synthetase, converting the relatively inactive form to the active form. This phosphatase is inhibited by rising concentrations of glycogen. Therefore, as glycogen accumulates in the muscle, it inhibits the protein phosphatase, and more and more of the glycogen synthetase is present as the relatively inactive phosphorylated form. Hence, the accumulation of glycogen in muscle shuts off its own production.

We have discussed the action of epinephrine on glycogen mobilization in muscle. In larger concentrations, epinephrine is also capable of stimulating the mobilization of glycogen from liver, apparently by a different, as yet undefined, mechanism. First, epinephrine does not bind to β-receptors in the liver. Accordingly, the once feared possibility of hypoglycemia as a consequence of the administration of β-blockers, such as propranolol, does not occur. Second, the mechanism of epinephrine activation of phosphorylase in liver does not involve the cyclic AMP cascade. Administration of epinephrine does not produce measurable changes in intracellular levels of cyclic AMP in liver. Glucagon, which has no effect on muscle, has a marked effect on phosphorylase activity in liver. It does so by activating exactly the same cascade as was described for epinephrine in muscle.

At the conclusion of this section reviewing glycogen metabolism and its controls, it must be mentioned that there are a number of human disease states associated with inherited lack of one or more of the enzymes of glycogen metabolism. Discussion of these disease states is beyond the scope of this treatise, and the reader is referred to Stanbury et al. [22].

DISACCHARIDE METABOLISM AND HEXOSE INTERCONVERSION

More than half the carbohydrate in the human diet is ingested in the form of plant starch. There are two forms of starch, amylose and amylopectin. Amylose is the unbranched type of starch, and it consists of glucose residues in α-1,4 linkage. Amylopectin is more branched in that it has an α-1,6 linkage per 30 or so α-1,4 linkages. α-Amylase is the digestive enzyme that breaks these starches down to maltose and isomaltose. Maltose is two glucose residues in α-1,4 linkage. In isomaltose, the linkage is α-1,6. The breakdown of dietary starch to maltose and isomaltose occurs in the lumen of the intestine. Salivary α-amylase probably is of little importance, but pancreatic amylase is essential.

The intestinal mucosal cells are presented with two other common disaccharides, in addition to maltose and isomaltose. These latter are sucrose, a disaccharide of glucose and fructose, and lactose, a disaccharide of glucose and galactose.

All these disaccharides are broken into monosaccharides in the brush border of the mucosal epithelium of the small intestine. Maltase and isomaltase are specific for maltose and isomaltose. There is also a specific sucrase for sucrose. Lactose is hydrolyzed to glucose and galactose by several enzymes, the principal of which is a true lactase. Lactase deficiency is a well-defined clinical condition and patients afflicted with this disorder develop gastrointestinal disturbances following ingestion of milk. Galactose and glucose are absorbed most rapidly by active transport mechanisms. They can be concentrated against a 10-fold gradient, and the transport system requires that sodium ions be present in the lumen and be moving across the brush border in the same direction. Since the sodium ion concentration in the cytosol of the mucosal epithelium is low, the sodium is moving with a gradient and thereby providing the energy to drive the sugar against a gradient. Fructose appears to be absorbed by a facilitated transport, but cannot be concentrated against a gradient. The efficiency of fructose absorption,

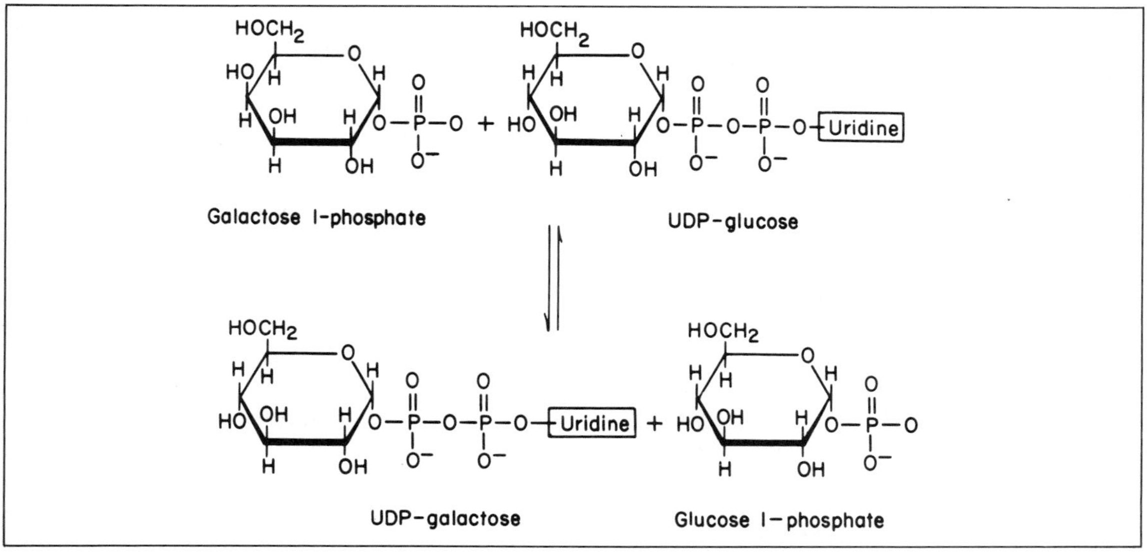

Figure 6-38. *The action of galactose 1-phosphate uridyl transferase.*

therefore, depends on its rate of removal by outward diffusion from the serosal site of the cell into the circulation.

Fructose comprises a significant portion of the carbohydrate in the human diet. Typically, the daily intake approaches 100 gm, both as the free sugar and as part of sucrose. It is worthwhile examining the mechanism whereby fructose enters into glycolysis. Most of this operation is accomplished in the liver. First, fructose is phosphorylated to fructose-1-phosphate by a specific enzyme, fructokinase. This fructokinase, unlike glucokinase, is not dependent on insulin for its induction. As a consequence, patients with diabetes mellitus can metabolize fructose as well as nondiabetics. Obviously, the same is not true for glucose. Fructose 1-phosphate is then split into glyceraldehyde and dihydroxyacetonephosphate by fructose 1-phosphate aldolase. Glyceraldehyde is then phosphorylated to glyceraldehyde 3-phosphate by a triose kinase and ATP, so that it, too, can enter glycolysis.

The liver also possesses hexokinase, which is not specific for glucose, in addition to glucokinase, which is. Hexokinase has an affinity for glucose 20 times as high as it does for fructose. In the liver, because glucose freely diffuses across the liver cell membrane, the glucose level is quite high at all times and there is little phosphorylation of fructose by hexokinase to fructose-6-phosphate.

The situation in adipose tissue is somewhat different. Fructose can enter adipose tissue cells in such a fashion that the level of fructose inside adipose tissue cells is higher than that of glucose. As a consequence, fructose-6-phosphate can be formed by hexokinase activity in adipose tissue. Most of the fructose in adipose tissue, then, is metabolized by way of fructose-6-phosphate.

Galactose is metabolized differently from fructose. As expected, the first reaction is a phosphorylation on the number one carbon. Galactokinase and ATP produce galactose 1-phosphate. Next, galactose 1-phosphate reacts with UDP-glucose, catalyzed by galactose 1-phosphate uridyl transferase. The products of this reaction are UDP-galactose and glucose-1-phosphate (Figure 6-38). The glucose-1-phosphate enters glycolysis by way of the phosphoglucomutase catalyzed conversion to glucose-6-phosphate.

An epimerization of UDP-galactose at the four position converts it to UDP-glucose. This UDP-glucose–UDP-galactose interconversion is important. First of all, when it goes in the direction we just described, it regenerates UDP-glucose to react with another molecule of galactose-1-phosphate. In the other direction, this epimerization converts UDP-glucose to UDP-galactose, which is essential for the synthesis of galactosyl residues in complex polysaccharides and glycoproteins if the amount of galactose in the diet is inadequate to meet these needs.

All are familiar with the disease galactosemia, which is due to the inherited deficiency of galactose-1-phosphate uridyl transferase. This disease is treated, of course, by the exclusion of galactose from the diet. Because the epimerase is present, patients with galactosemia can meet their requirements for galactosyl residues from UDP-glucose.

METABOLIC INTERRELATIONS

No discussion of carbohydrate metabolism would be complete without consideration of body fuel metabolism in general. Protein and fat metabolism have been looked at separately and extensively elsewhere in this volume, but this section is devoted to a review of the interrelationships that exist among all three types of fuel. Because of the precisely regulated interplay among these processes, the human body is capable of departing from its usual three meals a day to brief fasts and even to prolonged starvation, with surprisingly little impairment of ability to perform work without loss of structural integrity.

In 1970, George Cahill published an influential article [5] and we will here look at the subject of metabolic interrelations following his general format as it is a most useful one. Table 6-2 is taken from that article of Cahill's and summarizes the fuel composition of a normal 70-kg man.

We have already discussed glycogen as a carbohydrate storage form. Considering that the normal caloric requirement of a middle-aged, sedentary, 70-kg man is around 2,000 to 2,200 calories, the 900 calories as glycogen is really quite a small storage depot. Even though glycogen is a macromolecule, it requires water for its storage to maintain isotonicity, about one or two grams of water for every gram of carbohydrate stored as glycogen. Therefore, glycogen is a relatively inefficient storage depot on a weight basis.

Protein is a much larger storage depot, but use of protein for fuel ultimately compromises function. The reason for this is that each protein molecule is present in the body for a function other than fuel, be it enzyme, contraction, structure, or others. Protein is not accumulated as a storage depot. When the body has all the protein that it needs for function, extra protein ingested is metabolized. Consideration of protein as a fuel must contend with the fact that it also involves a weight factor. Body protein is generally an aqueous solution, and a gram of normal, wet-weight body protein contains only one-quarter to one-fifth protein by dry weight.

Fat, on the other hand, is stored in a nonaqueous environment and therefore does not involve the extra aqueous addition to weight that is characteristic of protein and glycogen. Ninety percent of depot fat is actually lipid, so that one gram of adipose tissue yields very close to the theoretical 9.4 calories per gram of pure triglyceride.

On a caloric basis, it would seem a simple matter to tolerate the assault of brief fasting and even prolonged starvation. If there are 141,000 calories available, stored as fat, in the 70-kg man, and we assume a basal caloric requirement of 1,800 calories per day, reliance on fat should make it possible to tolerate 78 days without food. It is not as simple as that, however. A large part of the human body can indeed use fatty acids or the partial oxidation products of fatty acids, the ketone bodies, directly as fuel. The heart, kidney, adrenal cortex, and skeletal muscle are examples of such organs. On the other hand, there are other organs that require glucose. For instance, in a 24-hour fasted man, nervous tissue (mainly brain) would use 144 grams of glucose. There are other glycolytic tissues such as erythrocytes,

Table 6-2. *Fuel Composition of Normal Man*

Fuel	Weight (kg)	Calories
Tissues		
Fat (adipose triglyceride)	15	141,000
Protein (mainly muscle)	6	24,000
Glycogen (muscle)	0.150	600
Glycogen (liver)	0.075	300
Total		165,900
Circulating fuels		
Glucose (extracellular fluid)	0.020	80
Free fatty acids (plasma)	0.0003	3
Triglycerides (plasma)	0.003	30
Total		113

Source: From G. F. Cahill, Starvation in man. *N. Engl. J. Med.* 282: 668, 1970. Reprinted by permission.

leukocytes, bone marrow, adrenal medulla, and others that specifically need glucose as well, requiring 36 gm of glucose per day. When we remember that there is no net synthesis of glucose from fat, we begin to outline the problem of starvation metabolism. The only storage reserve of carbohydrate that can be converted to blood glucose is liver glycogen; there is very little of this and it is used only sparingly. Thus, the only mechanism that can be used to supply glucose in times of starvation is gluconeogenesis from protein. As protein is used to supply essential glucose, function will be impaired, as all protein is present in the body primarily to serve a nonfuel function. Now the problem of dealing with starvation becomes more clearly defined. The body must decrease, to the absolute minimum, its need for glucose, thereby sparing protein breakdown to the greatest degree possible. How the body accomplishes this can best be understood by comparing fuel metabolism in brief fasting and after prolonged starvation.

Figure 6-39 summarizes the pattern of fuel supply in use after a brief fast. In a 24-hour fast, a normal man with basal caloric use of 1,800 calories will derive one-sixth of his calories by burning about 75 gm of protein. The remainder of the caloric need is made up by 160 gm of triglyceride from adipose tissue. A look at the right side of Figure 6-39 will show where the fuel goes, and in what form. The glycolytic tissues require a total of 180 gm of glucose. This is supplied for them by the liver and is derived from liver glycogen, augmented by gluconeogenesis. The requirement of 144 gm for the brain and other nervous tissue is a complete drain. Glucose metabolized by these tissues is oxidized all the way to carbon dioxide and water, and this accounts for 144 gm of the total 180. The other glycolytic tissues, such as erythrocytes and white blood cells, require about 36 gm of glucose during this 24-hour period, but they metabolize it to lactate and pyruvate, which return to the liver to be reconstituted into glucose. This is the Cori cycle discussed earlier in this chapter. As mentioned, another substrate for the manufacture of glucose by the liver is amino acid released by protein degradation. Converting amino acids, lactate, and pyruvate to glucose in the liver is an energy-requiring process, and the liver derives the energy necessary for that process by burning some of the fat released from the adipose tissue. Fatty acids are oxidized in two stages. The long chains are broken down, by an oxidative process, into two carbon fragments, acetyl CoA, and this process produces about a third of the total energy stored

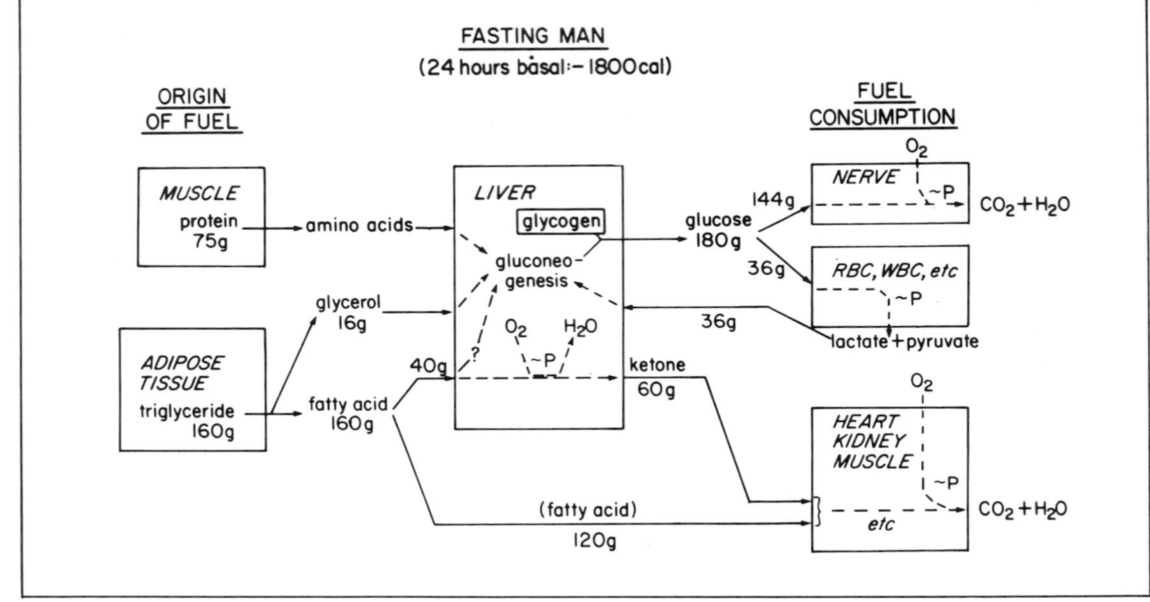

Figure 6-39. *General scheme of fuel metabolism in a normal fasted man, showing the two primary sources, muscle and adipose tissue, and the three types of fuel consumers, nerve, pure glycolyzers (such as the red cells [RBC] and white cells [WBC]) and the remainder of the body (composed of heart, kidney, and skeletal muscle) that use fatty acids and ketones. (From G. F. Cahill, Starvation in man.* N. Engl. J. Med. *282:668, 1970. Reprinted by permission.)*

in fat. The second stage of fatty acid oxidation is the terminal combustion of acetyl CoA to CO_2 and water in the tricarboxylic acid cycle. The acetyl CoA produced from fat in times of fasting exceeds the amount that can enter the tricarboxylic acid cycle. The excess acetyl CoA is condensed into ketone bodies, acetoacetate, and β-hydroxybutyrate, which are then released into the circulation. Thus, of the 160 gm of fat released from the adipose tissue depot, 40 gm are used in the liver to provide energy and to generate 60 gm of ketone bodies. These ketone bodies can be used as energy by such organs as heart, kidney, and muscle. One-hundred and twenty grams of fatty acid are used directly by the same tissues.

Let us now summarize the processes whereby the human body has adapted to a 24-hour fast and is using its fuel reserves. Remember, we have certain demands that must be met. First, we must mobilize 1,800 calories for the 24-hour period. Second, we must be able to provide 180 gm of glucose.

Five-sixths of the caloric requirement is met by adipose tissue lipolysis. One hundred and sixty grams of triglyceride are split by lipase activity to yield 160 gm of fatty acid and 16 gm of glycerol. The glycerol helps the liver in its job of making the 180 gm of glucose because it can be converted to glucose. Seventy-five grams of muscle protein are mobilized to aid in the manufacture of glucose by the liver by supplementing the glucose that can be derived from glycogenolysis and gluconeogenesis from glycerol, lactate, and pyruvate. What are the signals that the body uses to ensure that this supply of fuel and glucose precursors is smooth and uninterrupted?

In the fasting state, probably the first signal that reserves must be mobilized is the drop in blood glucose consequent upon termination of food intake. As blood glucose levels drop, release of insulin by the pancreatic β cells also drops.

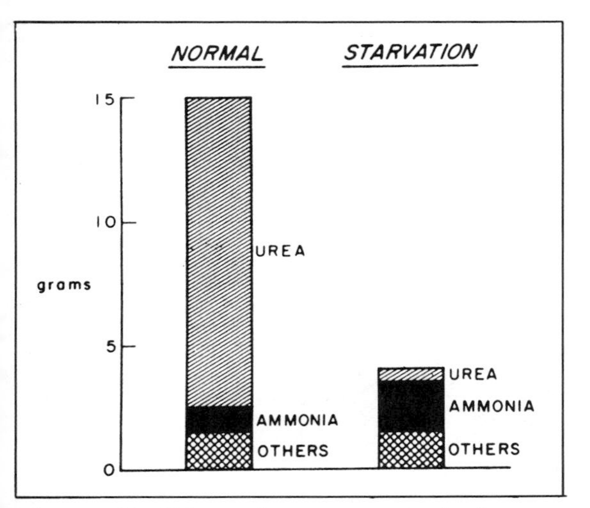

Figure 6-40. *Urinary nitrogen excretion in the postabsorptive state after a standard diet of 90 to 100 gm of protein after five to six weeks of starvation, showing the marked reduction in total nitrogen, the relative increase in ammonia, and the relatively unchanged excretion of the sum of uric acid, creatinine, and so forth. (From G. F. Cahill, Starvation in man.* N. Engl. J. Med. *282:668, 1970. Reprinted by permission.)*

Furthermore, low insulin levels, coupled with low glucose levels, trigger the release of glucagon. It appears most likely that it is the low levels of insulin and the rising levels of glucagon that are the primary messengers that facilitate mobilization of fuel depots.

First, what are the results of decreasing insulin levels? Glucose uptake by muscle, heart, and adipose tissue will decrease as blood insulin levels continue to drop. The effect of that hormone in lowering cyclic AMP levels in adipose tissue is abated. As the cyclic AMP-lowering effect of insulin in adipose tissue diminishes, the hormone-sensitive lipolytic enzyme in adipose tissue becomes more active. As a consequence of the increased activity of the hormone-sensitive lipase in adipose tissue, breakdown of triglycerides into fatty acids and glycerol increases. Since insulin also suppresses gluconeogenesis in the liver, decreasing levels of this hormone in the plasma allow for increasing rates of gluconeogenesis in the liver. In summary, decreasing insulin levels cause a diminution of glucose uptake by heart, skeletal muscle, and adipose tissue, an increase in release of fatty acid and glycerol from adipose tissue, and an increase in gluconeogenesis by the liver. Insulin has been shown to promote uptake of amino acids by skeletal muscle and incorporation of amino acids into protein. Furthermore, insulin infusions have been shown to decrease rate of amino acid release by perfused limbs. As insulin levels decrease, then, the stimulus to protein synthesis is diminished and protein breakdown continues, unbalanced by protein synthesis. The net result is a marked increase in release of amino acids for use by the liver in the manufacture of glucose.

What of the effects of the elevation in glucagon levels? First of all, glucagon causes a marked augmentation in glycogenolysis by the liver. Furthermore, there are data that suggest that glucagon may inhibit protein synthesis and increase protein degradation in muscle. Glucagon has been shown to stimulate hepatic gluconeogenesis, especially from alanine.

The fuel fluxes seen in Figure 6-39 illustrate the well-controlled processes whereby the body adapts to brief fasting. It is obvious that some of the 180 gm of glucose needed must come from liver glycogen, in all likelihood. The gluconeogenic precursors are not capable of making up the total amount of glucose required. Examination of the rate of protein depletion, however, indicates that this type of overall process cannot be tolerated for very long. If it were, about one-third of the total body protein would be depleted in three weeks, and man cannot survive this degree of protein loss. Figure 6-40 indicates that this amount of nitrogen wasting does not occur in prolonged starvation. It can be seen that urea loss has shrunk to a small fraction of that seen in the normal postabsorptive state. Ammonia excretion has increased, and the other nitrogenous substances in the urine have remained constant.

Figure 6-41 shows the fuel fluxes seen in a man adapted to starvation, after about five to six weeks. First, total caloric demand has dropped to 1,500 calories, probably related to diminished activity. Triglyceride mobilization remains essen-

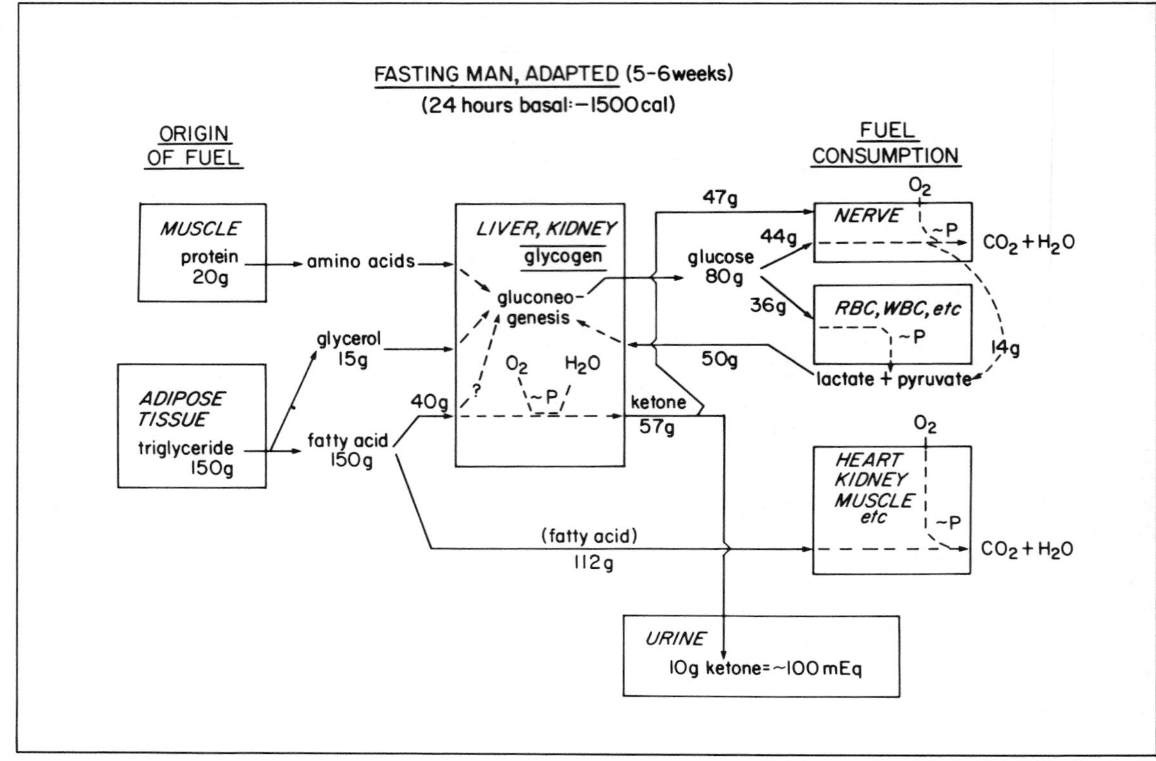

Figure 6-41. *General scheme of fuel metabolism after five or six weeks of starvation, showing the diminished rate of mobilization of muscle protein. (From G. F. Cahill, Starvation in man.* N. Engl. J. Med. *282:668, 1970. Reprinted by permission.)*

tially the same, but protein breakdown has dropped to 20 gm per day, a marked decrease. The obligatory glucose requirement by the glycolytic tissues that produce lactate and pyruvate remains the same. The amount of glucose used by brain and nerve, all of which is lost as CO_2 and water, has dropped from 144 gm to 47 gm. The fuel deficit that this drop in glucose consumption engenders is now made up by ketone bodies. Owen [17] has shown that β-hydroxybutyrate and acetoacetate displace glucose oxidation in prolonged fasting and enable sparing of body protein. As much as one-third to over one-half of the caloric requirements of brain and nerve can be made up by ketone body oxidation. Liver gluconeogenesis has decreased, and more than three-fourths of the glucose made by the liver is from lactate, pyruvate, and glycerol. The kidney has now adapted to this prolonged fast by increasing its gluconeogenesis to about 40 gm of glucose per day. The relationship between increased gluconeogenesis and ammoniagenesis is suggested by the increased ammonia excretion seen in Figure 6-40. In the ketotic fasting state, the kidney is excreting about 10 gm of ketone bodies per day. The amino acids that come to the kidney are deaminated and deamidated to produce the ammonia necessary to neutralize the acid ketone bodies being excreted in such large amounts. The carbon residues, after removal of the nitrogen for ammonia formation, are incorporated into glucose resulting in the increased renal gluconeogenesis.

In the concerted effort to conserve protein, two major changes have taken place. Since a large

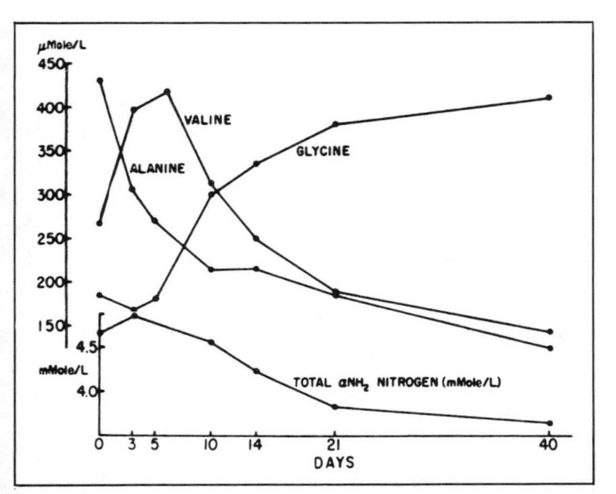

Figure 6-42. *Levels of total alpha-amino nitrogen and three representative amino acids in man during prolonged starvation. The marked fall in alanine concentration is of major importance since this appears to be the principal substrate used for hepatic gluconeogenesis. (From G. F. Cahill, Starvation in man.* N. Engl. J. Med. *282:668, 1970. Reprinted by permission.)*

amount of the brain and nerve fuel requirement is made up by ketone bodies, the liver can decrease its manufacture of glucose from amino acids, and muscle can decrease the rate at which it releases amino acids into the circulation. These changes are absolutely essential to make possible prolonged starvation without rapidly fatal depletion of protein reserves. How are they accomplished?

Let us first direct our attention to the liver. What is the signal that results in a decrease in gluconeogenesis from protein by this organ? Gluconeogenesis is limited by limitation of the substrate for the manufacture of glucose. More specifically, it is limitation of amino acid substrate that decreases the rate of formation of glucose by the liver. A comparison of Figure 6-39 and Figure 6-41 indicates that the lactate-pyruvate supply does not decrease in prolonged starvation. In fact, the amount of lactate and pyruvate returned to the liver for gluconeogenesis is slightly augmented by an increased production of these substances by brain and nerve. It is the amino acid supply that diminishes. Furthermore, it is specifically diminution in release of alanine that limits hepatic gluconeogenesis by substrate limitation. A look at Figure 6-42 reveals that alanine levels in the bloodstream behave uniquely, falling off sharply early in a fast and decreasing to less than a third of the postabsorptive level. Felig and his colleagues studied amino acid levels in the plasma in prolonged starvation [11] and demonstrated that although total plasma α amino nitrogen levels fell only 12 percent, alanine levels decreased by 70 percent. Furthermore, alanine in both the postabsorptive and prolonged-fast states is the principal amino acid extracted by the liver for gluconeogenesis. There is even more convincing evidence for the role of alanine in the regulation of gluconeogenesis. Felig and his colleagues [10] showed that the infusion of small amounts of alanine to a fasting patient resulted in a rapid rise in plasma glucose concentration, confirming that the rate-limiting step to gluconeogenesis in fasting man is the concentration of alanine coming to the liver.

Now these observations allow us to formulate the concept of a glucose-alanine cycle. Glucose taken up by muscle from the bloodstream serves directly, or indirectly via glycogen, as a glycolytic source of pyruvate for alanine synthesis. Alanine is released into the circulation, taken up by the liver, and converted by gluconeogenesis into glucose, which is then returned to the bloodstream. This scheme involves a constant recycling of glucose carbon between muscle and liver and complements the carbon recycling via lactate and pyruvate of the Cori cycle. Much has been written about this cycle and the reader is referred to an excellent recent review [21]. There are some complexities in this cycle and its regulation that require further examination. The striking feature of amino acid release from muscle is that more than 50 percent of the total amino acid released by skeletal muscle is as alanine and glutamine. This percentage is considerably more than their relative abundance in muscle proteins but not as free amino acids. The implication of these findings is that alanine and glutamine release involves not only muscle proteolysis, but also the synthesis de novo of these amino acids within the muscle. Early in the course of these investigations, it was postulated that the alanine, released from muscle in amounts greater than its presence in muscle, arose from transamination of pyruvate formed from glucose taken up from the muscle. It was hinted that decreasing insulin supplies, as a fast progressed, decreased the uptake of glucose by muscle, thus limiting the production of pyruvate and, hence, the production of alanine. The increasing reliance of muscle, in the starved state, on fatty acid as its major fuel source provided a further limitation of pyruvate synthesis. As increasing amounts of fatty acids are oxidized, increasing amounts of citrate are formed and citrate inhibits phosphofructokinase allosterically. Therefore, a further damper of pyruvate production is seen in advancing starvation, with dependence upon fatty acid oxidation for muscle fuel. Further observations, however, summarized by Snell [21], cast serious doubt on the concept that the rate of glycolysis is rate-limiting for alanine formation. Stimulation of glucose uptake and glycolysis by the addition of insulin to muscle incubations or to hind limb perfusions have been shown to have a negligible or slightly inhibitory effect on alanine release despite a stimulation of lactate and pyruvate release. Furthermore, the addition of dibutyryl cyclic AMP to muscle homogenate, or β-adrenergic agonists to intact muscle preparations (which would increase pyruvate formation by stimulating glycogenolysis) actually decreased alanine release while increasing lactate and pyruvate release.

Now, what do we know about the pathways and controls of amino acid release from muscle? We stated above that alanine and glutamine together account for more than 50 percent of the total amino acids released by skeletal muscle. Alanine is the prime substrate for hepatic gluconeogenesis. In contrast, glutamine is not removed from the circulation by the liver, but by the small intestine and the kidney. The mucosal epithelial cells of the small intestine apparently utilize glutamine as a major source of respiratory fuel. In addition, glutamine contributes both carbon and nitrogen for alanine formation and release by the intestine, so that glutamine is indirectly involved in gluconeogenesis insofar as it serves as a precursor of circulating alanine. Extraction of glutamine by the kidney is elevated in starvation and under acidotic conditions, in which the amino acid nitrogen is removed to produce ammonia for the neutralization of acid urine. The carbon of glutamine may be oxidized by the kidney or used for the synthesis of glucose. Renal gluconeogenesis becomes of increasing significance as starvation continues.

Now, how does muscle produce so much more alanine and glutamine, in proportion to other amino acids released, than it can be shown to contain on a percentage composition basis? Currently, it appears that these two amino acids are synthesized from other amino acids within the muscle.

Alanine is formed in the muscle by transamination of pyruvate. The other reactant is glutamate and the enzyme that catalyzes the reaction is alanine aminotransferase. The products of this reaction are alanine and α-ketoglutarate. Glutamate can be reconstituted by transamination of α-ketoglutarate by other amino acids. The formation of glutamate is essential, since it is only glutamate that can transaminate pyruvate to make alanine. Glutamate is also essential for the production of glutamine. It is postulated that the glutamine, which is the other amino acid released in large amounts by muscle, is synthesized from glutamate and NH_3 by way of the glutamine synthetase reaction. This is an endergonic reaction and requires an ATP so that glutamate + NH_3 + ATP will yield glutamine + ADP + Pi. Now, where does the glutamate come from? It is possible that some of it comes from other amino acids, e.g., proline, arginine, histidine, although the capacity of the pathways for converting these amino acids to glutamate may be very small in muscle. The reader is referred to another excellent review of the subject by Eric Newsholme [15]. Newsholme postulates that it is more likely that glutamate is produced by transamination of α-ketoglutarate and the latter is obtained from the citric acid cycle. It is known that muscle can oxidize a number of amino acids, including leucine, valine, isoleucine, and aspartate. When these amino acids give up their nitrogen via transamination, the resultant ketoacid gives rise to intermediates of the citric acid cycle such as succinate and α-ketoglutarate. Eventually, these intermediates produce malate and oxaloacetate. It appears likely, then, that the continuing supply of glutamate is by transamination of α-ketoglutarate. The further metabolism of the carbon skeletons of the donor amino acids gives rise to a continuing supply of α-ketoglutarate. The problem remaining is that of identifying the source of NH_3 in muscle for the glutamine synthetase reaction. At present, this is unknown. There is yet another contribution of the other amino acids to the synthesis of alanine. Valine, isoleucine, aspartate, and glutamate are all theoretically able to supply pyruvate carbon for alanine synthesis by contributing net carbon to the citric acid cycle. Four-carbon fragments in the citric acid cycle can produce pyruvate via oxaloacetate and phosphoenol-pyruvate, catalyzed by phosphoenol-pyruvate carboxykinase. Support for this concept is provided by the finding that incubation of hemidiaphragms with glutamate or isoleucine, in the absence of glucose, increased alanine output and increased the intracellular concentration of pyruvate.

Thus, other amino acids contribute to the large formation of alanine and glutamine by providing both the nitrogen and, to some degree, the carbon skeletons. The branched-chain amino acids appear to play a special role, and muscle is believed to be the major body site of branched-chain amino acid metabolism, while most other amino acids are predominantly metabolized by the liver. In contrast to glutamine and alanine, the release of branched-chain amino acids by muscle is less than would be expected from their relative frequency in muscle protein, and it can be calculated that their intracellular metabolism is sufficient to account for the observed rate of alanine synthesis. Intracellular protein breakdown is probably the major source of the branched-chain amino acids. In vitro, the branched-chain amino acids are among the most effective precursors for alanine formation. Protein feeding results in a continuous output of alanine and glutamine by leg muscles, and it is likely that this is due, in a large part, to metabolism of the branched-chain amino acids taken up by the muscle. Dietary supplementation of rats with branched-chain amino acids results in increased alanine output by muscle in vitro. Starvation, which results in increased alanine release by muscle, is also accompanied by increased branched-chain amino acid metabolism.

The branched-chain amino acids have another effect besides acting as precursors for alanine synthesis. They have been shown, and especially so in the case of leucine, to stimulate protein synthesis and to independently inhibit protein degradation in the muscle. At present, though, the mechanisms of these effects on protein turnover are not known. The potential importance of this observation is highlighted by the work of Rannels et al. [18], who showed that the addition of branched-chain amino acids to the perfused rat heart increases the rate of protein synthesis. Buse and Reid [3] showed that leucine, but not valine or isoleucine, increases the incorporation of amino acids into protein in the isolated rat diaphragm preparation.

That concept, that branched-chain amino acids can decrease the rate of protein degradation and increase the rate of protein synthesis, takes us one step closer to unraveling the mystery of the mechanism of decreasing alanine production in prolonged starvation as a mechanism of muscle protein conservation.

Blackburn [2] et al. first showed that infusions of amino acids into patients recovering from surgery caused an elevation in the level of ketone bodies in the blood while reducing nitrogen loss. Next, Sherwin [19] showed that infusion of ketone bodies into human subjects resulted in a specific decline in plasma alanine comparable to that observed in starvation, accompanied by a decrease in urinary nitrogen excretion in starved subjects. Furthermore, the addition of ketone bodies to incubated rat diaphragm in vitro resulted in decreased protein breakdown and a decrease in alanine release. The final key to the puzzle may well be found in the work of Buse and her collaborators [4]. They found that ketone bodies inhibit branched-chain amino acid oxidation in muscle tissue in vitro. Inhibition of branched-chain amino acids by ketone bodies could produce an accumulation of branched-chain amino acids in the muscle, leading to inhibition of protein degradation and/or the stimulation of protein synthesis. This would diminish the flow of amino acid precursors for alanine formation. If branched-chain amino acid metabolism is inhibited in this fashion by ketone bodies, it could also decrease alanine formation by blocking the flow of carbon skeletons to pyruvate.

It now appears that the answer to our second question is at hand. The elevated levels of ketone bodies in the blood, as occur in prolonged starvation, in addition to serving as fuel for brain and nerve to conserve glucose, exercise a regulatory function. They inhibit the oxidation of branched-chain amino acids and the result is a decreased rate of release of alanine. As alanine release decreases, the prime substrate for gluconeogenesis from protein by the liver also decreases, and the rate of gluconeogenesis falls to the low level seen in Figure 6-41. The human body, then, is able to tolerate prolonged fasts because of this marvelously efficient mechanism for preserving body protein.

We must not overlook the fact that insulin, in the normal person, plays a role in restricting gluconeogenesis. The amount of insulin circulating in a state of prolonged starvation is small, but it appears to be essential. Felig, in a recent review [9], calls attention to the fact that gluconeogenesis in diabetes is increased, even though alanine levels are low. It appears that the insulin-deficient liver increases its fractional extraction two- to threefold to support increased gluconeogenesis in the face of low blood alanine levels.

A brief recapitulation is in order. In a brief fast, man mobilizes fuel from muscle and adipose tissue. Fatty acid oxidation provides the bulk of the calories needed. Some of the fatty acids are oxidized directly by many tissues of the body, and some are partially oxidized in the liver to ketone bodies. Fatty acid oxidation by the liver provides the energy source necessary to drive the formation of glucose from glycerol, lactate, pyruvate, and amino acids. The large amount of glucose required by brain and nerve is supplied by a combination of glycogenolysis in the liver and gluconeogenesis derived from alanine released by muscle protein degradation.

As the fast becomes prolonged, adaptive mechanisms that decrease potentially lethal rapid muscle wasting come into play. The absolute requirement of brain and nerve for glucose is diminished by deriving a large percentage of the calories for those tissues from ketone bodies. Fatty acid oxidation continues to supply the caloric needs of the body. Muscle protein degradation is diminished as the need for glucose by brain and nerve decreases. It appears that the ketone bodies not only meet a large portion of the caloric requirement of brain and nerve, but they also decrease the oxidation of branched-chain amino acids by muscle. The consequence of diminished degradation of branched-chain amino acids by muscle is a stimulation of protein synthesis or, at least, a decrease in the rate of protein degradation, leading to a drop in alanine release.

It is certain that hormonal signals contribute to this regulatory process. Decreased insulin levels allow continued mobilization of fatty acids from triglycerides and continue ketogenesis. Low insulin levels cause the gluconeogenic pathways to be wide open, but the gluconeogenesis is damped by diminished availability of alanine. One indicator of the importance of insulin levels comes from the old observation that administration of small amounts of glucose to the fasting person decreases the excretion of nitrogen in the urine of a fasting man. The infusion of 100 to 150 gm of glucose per day spares about 50 gm of protein. In all likelihood, this is due to stimulation of insulin release by the glucose and the meeting of the brain's need for glucose. Insulin spares nitrogen by inhibiting muscle proteolysis and inhibiting hepatic gluconeogenesis.

Glucagon undoubtedly plays a role, as well. Fasting produces elevations in glucagon levels and glucagon stimulates both glycogenolysis and gluconeogenesis. The details and significance of the insulin-glucagon interrelationship in the control of substrate flux in fasting and starvation have yet to be fully delineated.

SEPSIS AND TRAUMA

In the modern era, Cuthbertson pioneered in the studies of the impact of trauma and sepsis on human substrate metabolism. His long series of publications on the subject are summarized in a recent symposium [7]. He and many other workers who followed pointed out that extensive trauma is characterized by increased nitrogen excretion, which is believed to reflect mainly the breakdown of muscle protein. The quantity of muscle breakdown and nitrogen excretion is in excess of what could be explained merely on the basis of inactivity and starvation, though both may play a partial role. In general, it can be stated that extensive trauma and, to an even greater degree, sepsis somehow override the adaptive mechanisms that decrease potentially lethal, rapid muscle wasting in prolonged fast.

A landmark study of the problem was performed during the Korean War and published by Captain John Howard of the United States Army Medical Corps [14]. He described the appearance of a diabetic glucose tolerance curve and increased insulin resistance as a consequence of serious injury. One part of this study suggested that the resistance to insulin persisted longer in the face of severe infection.

A surgical metabolic balance study published in 1970 [8] confirmed the widely held impression that any form of severe injury (including sepsis, trauma, and burns) impairs the mechanisms by which protein breakdown and nitrogen excretion are reduced. Clowes and his colleagues published the results of their studies of the effect of sepsis on energy metabolism in 1974 [6]. In this study, they introduced a new determinant in evaluating patients assaulted by sepsis. They showed that there is a difference in the pattern of energy production in septic patients, depending on whether cardiac output is elevated or depressed. Septic patients and septic experimental animals with a high cardiac output are characterized by having high blood insulin levels (3 times normal). In these subjects, blood sugar is found to be normal or high and lipolysis is suppressed. Experimental measurements of limb substrate utilization showed that oxygen and glucose uptake were the same as in fasting normals, whereas net fat utilization is almost zero. There is, of course, negative nitrogen balance in these subjects. Part of this state of affairs is relatively easy to understand. Since adipose tissue is known to be much more sensitive to insulin than muscle, elevated insulin levels would indeed suppress lipolysis and, therefore, release of nonesterified fatty acids. Such a subject, if fasting, would therefore have very little in the way of fatty acid substrate to offer to muscle as a fuel, and therefore fatty acid substrate utilization by muscle could be expected to be zero, as it indeed was. Since there was a tendency for blood glucose levels to be normal or on the high side, and a similar tendency for insulin levels to be elevated, any peripheral resistance to insulin action could be overcome by the combination of easy availability of glucose and high insulin levels so that glucose utilization could be expected to be normal as it, indeed, also was. In those septic subjects and septic experimental animals with low cardiac output, the blood insulin level was found to be low or lower than in starvation. The authors postulated intense catecholamine activity in at least partial explanation for this phenomenon. In this circumstance, peripheral oxygen uptake is unaltered and net fat utilization is normal. Without elevated levels of insulin to counteract lipolysis and the presence of increased catecholamine activity, as postulated, lipolysis would certainly not be suppressed, and fatty acid substrate would be available for muscle for utilization, as the data indicated. Peripheral glucose uptake was found to be normal in these subjects, and there was again a severe negative nitrogen balance.

A paper published in 1976 by essentially the same observers [16] presented data derived from the study of 16 seriously ill septic patients. Once again, cardiac output was a determinant. Those septic patients with high cardiac output had arterial free fatty acid levels markedly below those seen in fasting normals. It is not surprising that the low arterial free fatty acid level resulted in a markedly diminished peripheral utilization of free fatty acid substrate. Furthermore, nitrogen balance was markedly negative. The patients with low cardiac output did not show elevated insulin levels. Their plasma free fatty acid levels were somewhat lower than those seen in fasting normals but, in this study, there was no demonstrable net peripheral utilization of free fatty acids as fuel. Once again, there was a markedly negative nitrogen balance. It is of great interest that there was little in the way of ketone body production in either the high-flow or the low-flow septic patient. Both groups of patients had levels of alanine production markedly higher than that seen in fasting normals, lending further substance to the concept of increased proteolysis.

Reflecting upon the fact that the data cited in the previous section of the review suggest that ketone body production plays an important role in suppressing proteolysis in prolonged fast, a possible mechanism explaining the rapid wastage of muscle nitrogen reserves in sepsis begins to emerge. On the other hand, the explanation for these potentially explanatory low arterial ketone body levels does not appear to be forthcoming. In a high-flow state, with high insulin levels, one would expect diminished lipolysis and therefore diminished substrate availability for hepatic ketone body production. In the low-flow state, low insulin levels, coupled with a postulated high catecholamine level, could be expected to lead to elevated levels of free fatty acids. They are not elevated, however, and indeed are lower than the levels seen in fasted normals. One would expect, then, in a low-flow state, high free fatty acids and high ketone body production. In actual fact, ketone body levels were observed to be low and free fatty acid levels were seen to be also low in both high-flow and low-flow states.

In summary, then, the high insulin levels of the high-flow septic patient suppressed free fatty acid release, and ketone body production is depressed because of low substrate availability. In the absence of ketone bodies, the usual conservation of muscle protein that is seen in prolonged fasting does not occur. The low-flow patient, on the other hand, has low insulin levels, but still has relatively low free fatty acid levels and very low ketone body levels. The reason for the low ketone body levels in the low-flow septic patient remains unexplained. What *is* understandable, however, is that the low ketone body level in both groups of patients results in continued high wastage of muscle protein.

In 1978, attention was directed to specific amino acid patterns in both muscle and plasma as a consequence of inactivity, starvation, and injury [1]. Total hip replacement patients were studied preoperatively and four days postoperatively, during which four days they had received 90 gm of glucose/day as sole nutrient. Normal control patients were studied and then placed on four days of bed rest. One group received a regular diet and one group received only 90 gm of glucose/day. The total hip replacement patients showed increases in muscle levels of branched-chain amino acids, aromatic amino acids (phenylalanine and tyrosine), and methionine. Plasma levels of essential amino acids tended to increase. It was the author's analysis that this pattern differed from starvation and from inactivity to a significant degree.*

It must be noted, at this point, that the matter of peripheral insulin resistance in sepsis and/or trauma is not without some debate. Wichterman and his colleagues [25] published a study of the effects of sepsis on glucose metabolism in rats. They could demonstrate no peripheral insulin resistance and postulated that there might be impairment of hepatic response to insulin as a consequence of sepsis.

Fischer and his colleagues have published two studies of plasma glucose, hormone, amino acid, and amino acid metabolic byproduct levels in septic patients [12, 13]. In the first of these papers, insulin levels were found to be elevated in septic

**Editor's Note:* The hypothesis put forth by the authors, places, in my opinion, too high a priority on data that other workers have not confirmed. In addition, the mechanism proposed, does not, in my opinion, explain the observations.

patients as were the insulin/glucagon ratios. Total plasma amino acid level was elevated, owing mainly to high levels of the aromatic amino acids (phenylalanine and tyrosine) and the sulfur-containing amino acids taurine, cystine, and methionine. Alanine, aspartic acid, glutamic acid, and proline were also elevated to a lesser degree. The branched-chain amino acids (valine, leucine, and isoleucine) were within normal limits. The patients who did not survive sepsis had higher levels of aromatic-sulfur containing amino acids than those who did. Further, the patients who survived sepsis had higher levels of alanine and branched-chain amino acids. In five of the patients in the first study, septic encephalopathy occurred and was treated with a parenteral nutrition solution consisting of 23 percent dextrose and an amino acid formulation enriched with branched-chain amino acids to the level of 35 percent. In these five patients, normalization of the plasma amino acid pattern and reversal of the encephalopathy was observed.

The second study demonstrated increased levels of the same amino acids shown to occur in increased amounts in the plasma in the first study. Furthermore, high levels of aromatic and sulfur-containing amino acids helped to identify those patients who did not survive sepsis, and high levels of branched-chain amino acids were associated with survival of sepsis. The authors also concluded that statistical analysis of amino acid patterns in septic patients could distinguish between patients with and without hepatic encephalopathy, with a high level of predictability.

The study of metabolic derangement resulting from trauma and sepsis is proceeding rapidly at present. It appears that these states are characterized by insulin resistance and impaired ability to oxidize glucose. In contradistinction to the fasting normal, there is a decreased lipolysis and diminished use of endogenous free fatty acids as a source of fuel. There is markedly increased proteolysis and negative nitrogen balance. Branched-chain amino acids appear to be used to meet muscle fuel requirements. Alanine production, as a source of hepatic glucose, appears to be unimpaired. Serious derangements in plasma amino acid patterns are present that appear to be useful in identifying clinical characteristics and eventual outcome. It may well be that the striking diminution of ketone body production in septic and traumatized patients is a major factor in the etiology of the resultant dangerous proteolysis.

REFERENCES

1. Askanazi, J., et al. Muscle and plasma amino acids after injury. *Ann. Surg.* 188:797, 1978.
2. Blackburn, G. L., et al. Protein sparing therapy during periods of starvation with sepsis in trauma. *Ann. Surg.* 125:588, 1973.
3. Buse, M. G., and Reid, S. S. Leucine. A possible regulator of protein turnover in muscle. *J. Clin. Invest.* 56:1250, 1975.
4. Buse, M. G., et al. The oxidation of branched chain amino acids by isolated heart and diaphragms of the rat. *J. Biol. Chem.* 247:8085, 1972.
5. Cahill, G. F. Starvation in man. *N. Engl. J. Med.* 282:668, 1970.
6. Clowes, G. H. A., et al. Energy metabolism in sepsis: Treatment based on different patterns in shock and high output stage. *Ann. Surg.* 179:684, 1974.
7. Cuthbertson, D. P. Post-traumatic metabolism: A multidisciplinary challenge. *Surg. Clin. North Am.* 58:1045, 1928.
8. Duke, J. H., et al. Contribution of protein to calorie expenditure following injury. *Surgery* 68: 168, 1970.
9. Felig, P. Amino acid metabolism in man. *Annu. Rev. Biochem.* 44:933, 1975.
10. Felig, P., Marliss, E., Owen, O. E., and Cahill, G. F., Jr. Role of substrate in the regulation of hepatic gluconeogenesis. *Adv. Enzyme Regul.* 7:41, 1969.
11. Felig, P., Owen, O. E., Wahren, J., and Cahill, G. F. Amino acid metabolism during prolonged starvation. *J. Clin. Invest.* 48:584, 1969.
12. Freund, H., Ryan, J. A., and Fischer, J. E. Amino acid derangements in patients with sepsis: Treatment with branched chain amino acid rich infusions. *Ann. Surg.* 188:423, 1978.
13. Freund, H., et al. Plasma amino acids as predictors of the severity and outcome of sepsis. *Ann. Surg.* 190:571, 1979.
14. Howard, J. M. Studies of the absorption and metabolism of glucose following injury. *Ann. Surg.* 141:321, 1955.

14a. Lehninger, A. L. *Biochemistry* (2nd ed.). New York: Worth, 1975.

15. Newsholme, E. A. Carbohydrate metabolism in vivo: Regulation of the blood glucose level. *J. Clin. Endocrinol. Metab.* 5:543, 1976.
16. O'Donnell, T. F., et al. Proteolysis associated with a deficit of peripheral energy fuel substrates in septic man. *Surgery* 80:192, 1976.
17. Owen, O. E., et al. Brain metabolism during fasting. *J. Clin. Invest.* 46:1589, 1967.
18. Rannels, E. D., Hyalmarson, A. C., and Morgan, H. E. Effects of non-carbohydrate substrates on protein synthesis in muscle. *Am. J. Physiol.* 226: 528, 1974.
19. Sherwin, R. S., Handler, R. G., and Felig, P. Effect of ketone infusions on amino acid and nitrogen metabolism in man. *J. Clin. Invest.* 55: 1382, 1975.
20. Siesjo, B. K. *Brain Energy Metabolism.* New York: Wiley, 1978.
21. Snell, K. Muscle alanine synthesis and hepatic gluconeogenesis. *Biochem. Soc. Trans.* 8:205, 1980.
22. Stanbury, J. B., Wyngaarden, J. B., and Fredrickson, D. S. *The Metabolic Basis of Inherited Disease.* 5th Ed. New York: McGraw-Hill, 1982.
23. Stryer, L. *Biochemistry.* 2nd Ed. San Francisco: Freeman, 1981.
24. White, A., et al. *Principles of Biochemistry* (6th ed.). New York: McGraw-Hill, 1978.
25. Wichterman, K. A., Chaudry, I. H., and Baue, A. E. Studies of peripheral glucose uptake during sepsis. *Arch. Surg.* 114:740, 1979.

7

Lipid and Lipoprotein Metabolism

Jane L. H. C. Third
W. Fraser Bremner

Lipids are ubiquitous constituents of body tissues and fluids with two major functions to perform. First, they are a major source of energy for the body and, as triglycerides (or, more properly triacylglycerols), function as the major energy source for many tissues. Triacylglycerol is the storage form of energy in preference to carbohydrate or protein. Its caloric value of 9.0 kcal/gm is more than twice that of the other two potential energy sources, and it requires less water as a storage form, so that it has advantages both in terms of energy per unit stored and in terms of space required for storage. The second important function of lipids is as major structural components of every cell and tissue in the body. For example, 44 percent of the red cell membrane is lipid, compared with 48 percent protein and only 8 percent carbohydrate [16]. Both surface area and shape of the red cell depend on the cholesterol content of the membrane and upon the membrane cholesterol:phospholipid molar ratio. Normally this ratio ranges from 0.83 to 0.95 [8]. Membrane cholesterol is in dynamic equilibrium with the cholesterol in the surrounding plasma, and if the plasma concentration is abnormal, red cell cholesterol and membrane function are consequently distorted. Such a consequence may arise in the course of cholestatic jaundice [9].

Although most cells have the capacity to synthesize and degrade lipids, the arrangement of tissues into organs has necessitated a specific transport system for lipids in the form of the lipoproteins. These components are particularly important because of their intrinsic function as a transport system, because they are subject to many metabolic defects [14, 44], and particularly because they play an important role in the development of atherosclerotic heart disease [5].

FATTY ACID OXIDATION

The degradation of fatty acids requires initial enzyme-mediated oxidation with ATP before degradation can occur (Figure 7-1) [15]. The enzyme thiokinase (acyl CoA synthetase) catalyzes production of acyl CoA by expenditure of the high-energy bonds in ATP.

$$\text{Fatty acid} + \text{CoASH} \xrightarrow[\text{synthetase}]{\text{ATP} \searrow \text{ acyl CoA } \nearrow \text{AMP}} \text{fatty acyl CoA} + \text{PPi}$$

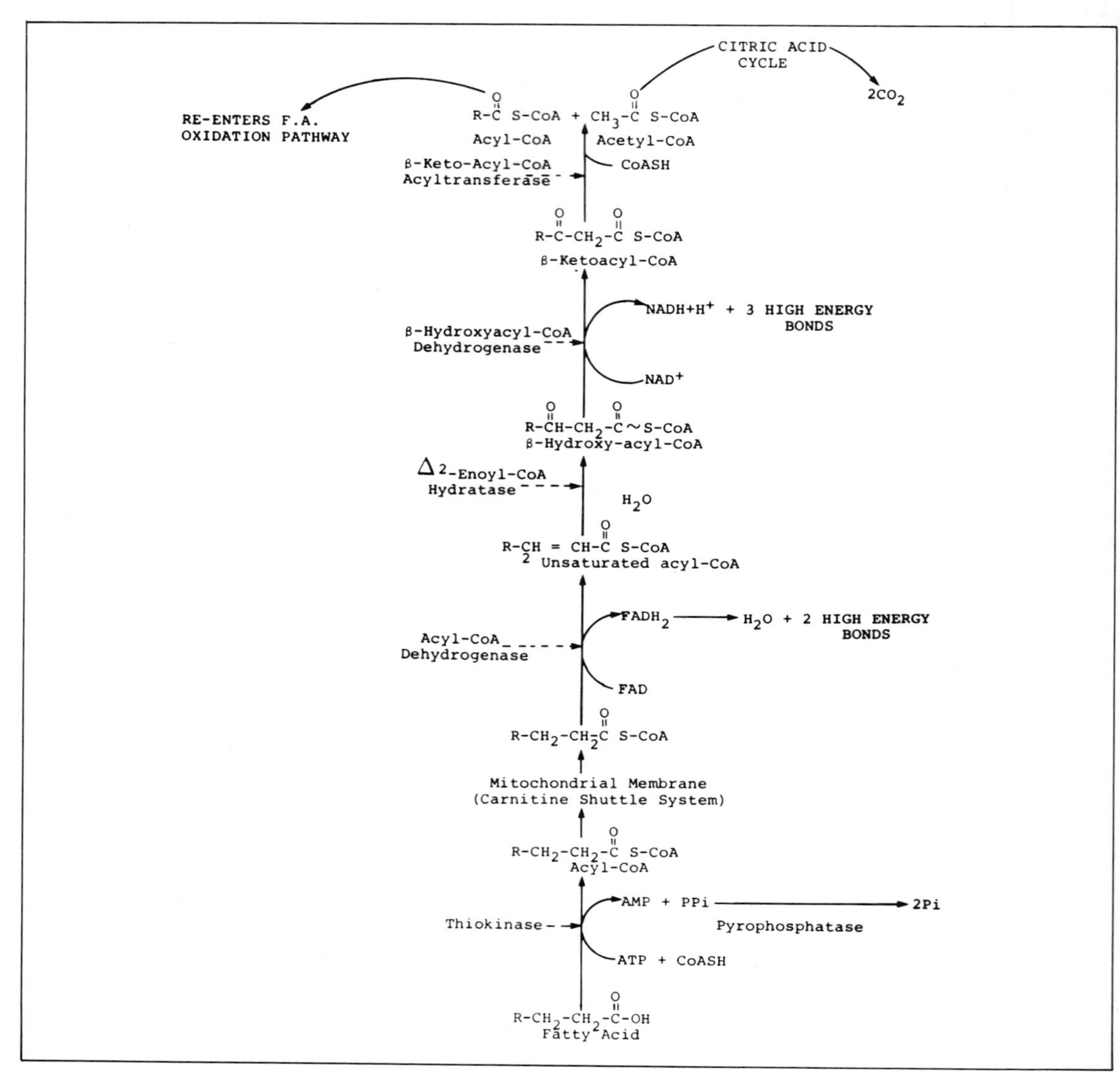

Figure 7-1. *Fatty acid oxidation. Note: ~ denotes a "high energy" bond, and FAD = flavoprotein.*

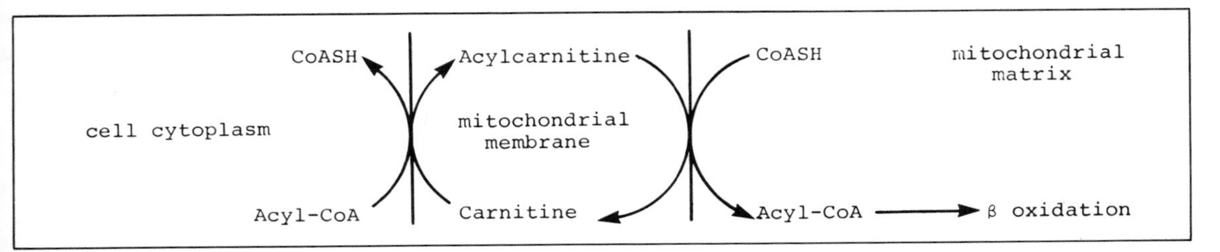

Figure 7-2. *The carnitine shuttle.*

$$PPi + H_2O \xrightarrow[\text{pyrophosphatase}]{\text{inorganic}} 2Pi$$

Coenzyme A is an essential cofactor in fatty acid oxidation. This reaction is driven to the right by pyrophosphatase, which breaks down pyrophosphate so that the net energy utilization is two high-energy bonds for activation of one fatty acid molecule. Thiokinases are intra- and extra-mitochondrial and are specific for fatty acids of different chain lengths.

Shorter-chain fatty acids can be activated inside the mitochondria, but longer-chain fatty acids undergo activation in the microsomes and on the outer mitochondrial membrane. Since subsequent degradation proceeds inside the mitochondria, a means of transferring activated fatty acids to the inner surface of the membrane is required, and this is accomplished by the carrier compound carnitine [β-OH-γ-trimethylammonium butyrate, $(CH_3)\ N^+\text{-}CH_2\text{-}CH\ (OH)\text{-}CH_2\text{-}COOH$] [31]. This compound is found in most tissues, particularly in muscle, where energy utilization is obviously of major significance. The enzyme carnitine palmitylacyltransferase forms acylcarnitine with release of coenzyme A, and the acylcarnitine can then penetrate the mitochondria. The carnitine appears to act as a shuttle mechanism residing in the inner mitochondrial membrane, as in Figure 7-2. In addition, there is another enzyme, carnitine-acetylacyltransferase, which appears to function in the transfer of short-chain acylgroups between coenzyme A and carnitine. Congenital defects in carnitine production result in a cardiomyopathy that may be fatal. Prolonged dialysis can induce carnitine deficiency and this may play a role in cardiomyopathy in uremic subjects on dialysis. Addition of carnitine to the dialysate lowers serum triglyceride levels.

Subsequent degradation of fatty acids is by way of the β-oxidation pathway, as originally described by Knoop. Figure 7-1 outlines this degradative pathway. In brief, an enzyme complex termed fatty acid oxidase, which resides in the mitochondrial matrix, catalyzes a sequence of chemical reactions. Once the acyl CoA moiety has reached the inner region of the mitochondrion by way of the carnitine shuttle system, two hydrogen atoms are removed from the α and β carbons under the action of acyl CoA dehydrogenase to produce an αβ-unsaturated acyl CoA. This dehydrogenase utilizes a flavin group as cofactor. Next, the double bond is saturated by the addition of the constituents of water to form β-hydroxy acyl CoA; the reaction is catalyzed by Δ^2-enoyl-CoA-hydratase. This is followed by further dehydrogenation of the B-carbon to form the corresponding B-keto-acyl CoA compound, this time using nicotinamide adenine dinucleotide (NAD) as coenzyme. In the final reaction the β-keto-acyl CoA acyl transferase utilizes another molecule of coenzyme A to produce acetyl CoA and an acyl CoA derivative, which has two carbon atoms less than the original acyl CoA molecule entering this reaction sequence. Thus, the pathway results in the breakdown of fatty acids in 2-carbon steps. For even-numbered fatty acids, the end-result is the production of C_2 units as acetyl coenzyme A, which can then be oxidized, and water by way of the citric acid cycle, which is also found within the mitochondria. For odd-numbered fatty acids, the end-result is loss of

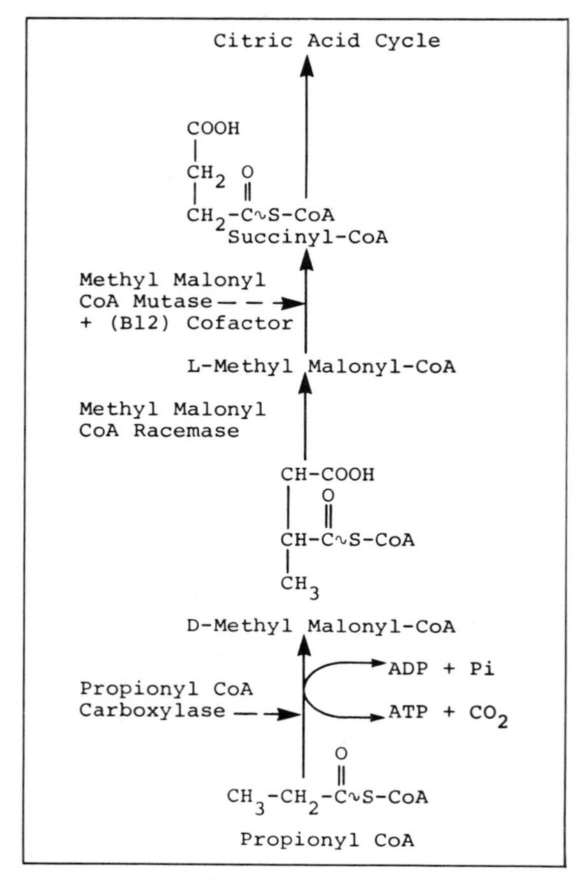

Figure 7-3. *Metabolism of propionyl residues.*

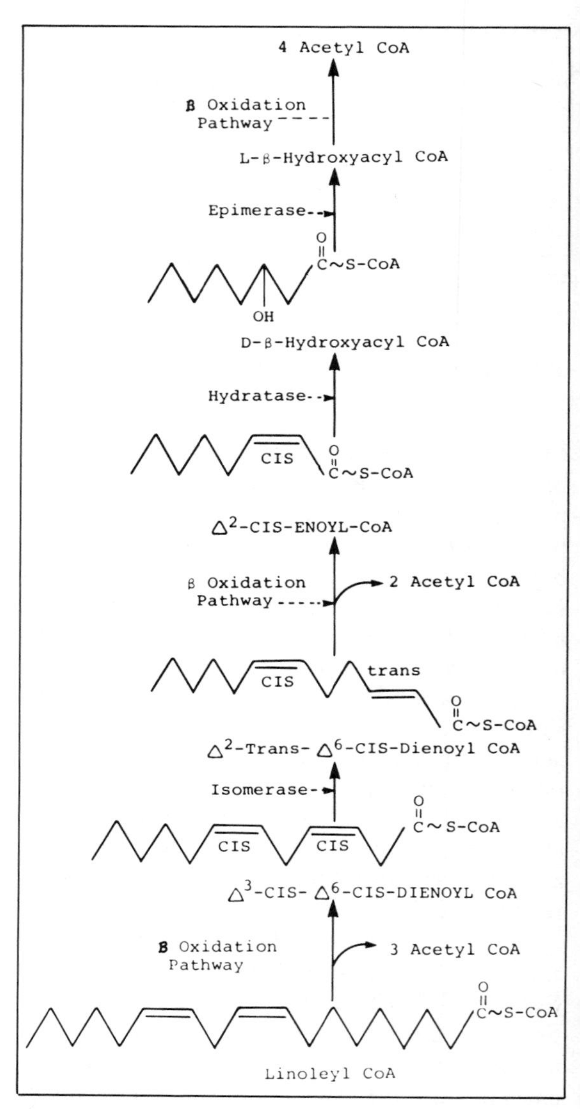

Figure 7-4. *Oxidation of unsaturated fatty acids.*

sequential 2-carbon moieties and their eventual oxidation by way of the citric acid pathway, with an additional 3-carbon propionyl CoA residue remaining. Propionyl CoA carboxylase, a biotin-dependent enzyme, then catalyzes carboxylation of propionyl CoA at the expense of a high-energy bond from ATP to form methylmalonyl CoA which, after racemization to the l form by a B_{12}-dependent isomerase, is converted to succinyl CoA, an intermediate of the citric acid cycle (Figure 7-3). Propionic acid can also be utilized by adipose tissue and by the mammary gland, where the synthesis of odd-chain fatty acids into longer odd-chain fatty acids is a significant route. Although the β-oxidative pathway is by far the most important degradative pathway utilizing fatty acids, there are two other minor pathways that utilize α- and ω-oxidation. Alpha-oxidation occurs principally in the brain and involves the carboxyl end of the molecule. It does not occur by way of coenzyme A intermediates and does not generate high-energy phosphate bonds. Hydroxylase enzymes in microsomes can perform ω-oxidation by conversion of the methyl group to a CH_2OH group, which can then be oxidized to a carboxyl group to yield a dicarboxylic acid. This minor pathway is of clinical significance in Refsum's disease, in which subjects lack the enzyme that performs α-oxidation on the methyl group of phytanic acid and consequently this compound, which is produced from phytol, a plant sterol, accumulates and produces central nervous system dysfunction.

The β-oxidation pathway will also sequentially degrade unsaturated fatty acids until the stage of a Δ^3- or Δ^2-cis-acyl CoA compound is produced. The Δ^3 compounds undergo isomerization with subsequent hydration to β-hydroxy acyl CoA, whereas the Δ^2 compound is first hydrated and then undergoes epimerization again to form β-hydroxy acyl CoA, which compound is one of the intermediates in β-oxidation (Figure 7-4).

ENERGY BALANCE OF FATTY ACID METABOLISM

If we consider the utilization of palmitic acid as an energy source, it can be seen from Figure 7-1 that electrons can flow from NAD and FAD in the reduced state down the respiratory chain to produce five high-energy phosphate bonds for each of the seven acetyl CoA molecules initially produced by β-oxidation of palmitate. Each acetyl coenzyme A molecule formed will produce 12 high-energy bonds from oxidation in the citric acid cycle. In total this will produce $7 \times 5 + 8 \times 12$ high-energy bonds with the initial two being required for the activation of the fatty acid to acyl CoA. The net gain will be 129 high-energy bonds per molecule. If one accepts a value of 7.6 kcal per bond, this will produce 9,804 kcal per molecule. This represents an efficiency of energy utilization of approximately 40 percent, since oxidation of palmitic acid in a bomb calorimeter yields 24,000 kcal/mol.

BIOSYNTHESIS OF FATTY ACIDS

Although reversal of the β-oxidation sequence is feasible, it appears to be little used, functioning in the main only to elongate fatty acid chains. This evolutionary development of separate systems for biosynthesis and degradation, one in the cytoplasm and the other in the mitochondrion, facilitates efficient hormonal and substrate regulation. The biosynthetic route appears to involve a specific extramitochondrial system complex found in many tissues including liver, kidney, brain, lung, mammary gland, and adipose tissue. This multi-complex has been separated into subunits in lower forms of life, particularly plants and bacteria, but in mammalian systems the complex loses activity if it is split up [17]. It appears to function as a dimeric complex of several enzymes, which utilizes sulfhydryl groups in common. Separation of separate enzyme functions renders the whole complex inactive.

The initial reaction utilizes bicarbonate to carboxylate acetyl coenzyme A to malonyl coenzyme A, using a high energy bond from ATP and the vitamin biotin as essential cofactors. The enzyme complex requires that the malonyl CoA then reacts with a central sulfhydryl group while further acetyl CoA reacts with a peripheral sulfhydryl group. Subsequently these components are condensed together by the acetyl group attacking the methylene group of the malonyl residue, with liberation of carbon dioxide and production of acetoacetyl enzyme, the acetoacetyl component being attached to the central sulfhydryl group. The reaction is driven to completion by the decarboxylation. The acetoacetyl group subsequently undergoes reduction, dehydration, and further reduction to form the saturated acyl enzyme. The saturated acetoacetyl group transfers to the peripheral sulfhydryl group, a further malonyl residue is taken up by the central sulfhydryl group, and the process is repeated to produce a saturated acyl radical of appropriate length. The saturated fatty acid most commonly produced is palmitic, which is liberated from the enzyme complex by hydrolysis and is then usually esterified into acylglycerols. The net equation for synthesis of palmitate from acetyl CoA and malonyl CoA is:

$$\text{Acetyl CoA} + 7\ \text{malonyl CoA} \xrightarrow[14\ \text{NADPH} + H^+ \ \rightarrow\ 14\ \text{NADP}^+]{} \text{palmitate} + 7\ CO_2 + 8\ \text{CoASH} + 6\ H_2O$$

Mammalian liver and mammary gland may also utilize butyryl coenzyme A as primer molecule. Two reduction steps utilize NADPH, and this comes largely from the hexose monophosphate shunt pathway. It follows that tissues active in lipogenesis, such as liver, adipose tissue, and lactating mammary gland, will also have active hexose monophosphate shunt pathways. But since both metabolic pathways occur outside the mitochondria, there are no membrane barriers to hinder transfer of NADPH from one pathway to another. Thus malic enzyme, which converts malate to pyruvate, can function as a source of NADPH.

A major source of acetyl coenzyme A, the basic unit for fatty acid synthesis, is from carbohydrate by way of oxidation of pyruvate inside the mitochondria. Acetyl coenzyme A, however, does not diffuse easily out of mitochondria to reach fatty acid synthetase in the cell cytoplasm. The route that is believed to function is as follows: Pyruvate carboxylase oxidatively decarboxylates pyruvate to acetyl coenzyme A, which then condenses with oxaloacetate to form citrate within the mitochondria. The citrate then translocates into the extramitochondrial compartment, where the enzyme ATP-citrate lyase (citrate cleavage enzyme) splits the citrate into acetyl CoA and oxaloacetate. The acetyl CoA can then be converted to malonyl CoA and eventually to palmitate. Oxaloacetate forms malate by way of malate dehydrogenase (NADH-dependent) with subsequent production of NADPH by malic enzyme, which produces pyruvate and NADPH. NADPH then becomes available for lipogenesis. In other words, this pathway functions as a means of transferring reducing equivalents from extramitochondrial NADH to NADP. Malate may also be transported into the mitochondrion to form oxaloacetate. An alternative pathway is for decarboxylation of oxaloacetate to phosphoenol-pyruvate, but this pathway is insignificant in mammalian lipogenesis.

Chain elongation utilizes the C_{10}-C_{16} series as primer molecules and possibly some unsaturated fatty acids. This pathway is found in the microsomal system and uses malonyl CoA as acetyl donor and NADPH as the source of reducing equivalents. This system virtually stops with starvation. This pathway becomes important when specific demands have to be met. For example, elongation of stearoyl coenzyme A in the brain rises dramatically during myelination to produce C_{22} and C_{24} fatty acid constituents of sphingolipids. An elongation pathway also functions in mitochondria. General reference texts are available [2, 48].

ESSENTIAL FATTY ACIDS

The human organism has a massive capacity to produce several unsaturated fatty acids, such as palmitoleic or oleic acid. It cannot, however, produce three fatty acids—linoleic, linolenic, and arachidonic—and these are therefore known as essential fatty acids, since they must, of necessity, be supplied by the diet. However, the body can add acetate groups to dietary linoleic acid to form arachidonic acid. The importance of linolenic acid as an essential dietary component is uncertain: it will maintain growth in rats, but does not cure skin lesions due to deficiency of linoleic or arachidonic acids. Linoleic acid, therefore, can be regarded as *the* essential fatty acid. Experimental studies of deficiency of these particular fatty acids in animals demonstrate, as signs of deficiency, reduced growth, dermatitis, decreased reproductive capacity, and abnormalities of lipid transport. The skin is particularly susceptible to infection. Since only a small proportion of the total caloric intake has to be of essential fatty acids (1 to 2 percent), the dietary complement of these particular compounds is usually excessive, and deficiency is rare except in unusual circumstances. However, lack of essential fatty acids in subjects being maintained long-term by parenteral hyperalimentation has produced deficiency syndromes. Also, some infants receiving formula diets low in these fats developed skin problems that required essential fatty acids for cure. Monounsaturated fatty acids are produced by an enzymatic system, found in liver microsomes, that catalyzes the conversion of

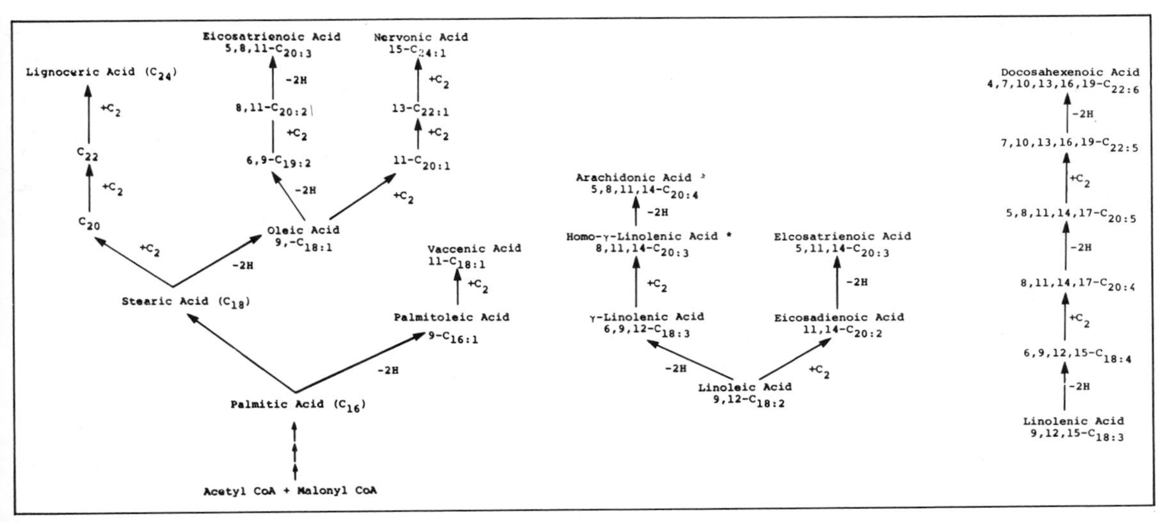

Figure 7-5. *Origins of polyenoic fatty acids in humans. * = source of prostaglandins.*

compounds such as stearoyl coenzyme A to oleyl coenzyme A using oxygen and NADPH or NADH for the reaction. The enzyme is a monooxygenase and utilizes cytochrome B5. Polyunsaturated fatty acids are produced by a combination of chain elongation and desaturation, but animals cannot produce the ω6 and ω3 series. Arachidonic acid, one of the ω6 series can, however, be produced from linoleic acid, another of the ω6 series, by a pathway utilizing dehydrogenation of the coenzyme A ester to α-linolenate, with the addition of a 2-carbon unit as malonyl CoA in the microsomal system, with chain elongation to eicosatrienoate and subsequent dehydrogenation to arachidonic acid. The capacity to produce polyunsaturated fatty acids is reduced by starvation and by insulin deficiency.

Figure 7-5 outlines the four series of polyunsaturated fatty acids in humans. Two necessarily come from dietary intake; the other two can be synthesized from oleic and palmitoleic acids. Linoleic acid is found in high concentration in edible vegetable oil such as corn, peanut, sunflower, soybean, and cottonseed, but not in olive or coconut oils. Arachidonic acid occurs in animal fats, but only in small amounts. Fatty acids are particularly common in phospholipids, mainly in the 2-position, and are essential components of the structural lipids of cell membranes, particularly mitochondrial membranes. They occur in high concentration in the reproductive organs. It should be noted that the essential fatty acids are *cis* in configuration. In consequence, transpolyunsaturated fatty acids lack essential fatty acid equivalence. These trans fatty acids are produced in margarine and may accumulate in tissues to form approximately 15 percent of fatty acid concentrations. They are metabolized as saturated fatty acids.

SPECIFIC FATTY ACID GROUPS

Acylglycerols

Triacylglycerols are the major constituents of adipose tissue, which is found distributed throughout the body and particularly in the subcutaneous tissue. Triacylglycerols are stored in the cytoplasm of adipose cells as fat droplets. They function as the body's major source of energy, as well as thermal and mechanical insulation for the body core.

The triacylglycerol stores of adipose tissues are constantly in flux as a result of a continuous process of lipolysis and re-esterification. These processes utilize two separate pathways, which facilitate control over the flux of the components of triacylglycerol. Acylglycerols undergo lipolysis (hydrolysis) to fatty acids and glycerol, with subsequent release of free fatty acids into the plasma, where they circulate combined with serum albumin to the tissues that have the capacity to utilize these compounds. Such tissues include liver, heart, kidney, muscle, lung, testis, and adipose tissue. The brain can also oxidize long-chain fatty acids, but cannot extract them from the blood. Catabolism of glycerol is dependent on tissues possessing the necessary activating enzyme glycerokinase. This enzyme is found in liver, kidney, intestine, and lactating mammary gland, as well as in brown adipose tissue. Metabolism of liver and muscle is particularly dependent on the level of plasma-free fatty acids, and this in turn is regulated by the mechanisms controlling release of these compounds from adipose tissue.

Synthesis of acylglycerols utilizes ATP for activation of both glycerol and fatty acids. The enzyme glycerokinase in liver, kidney, intestinal mucosa, and lactating mammary gland phosphorylates glycerol to glyceryl 3-phosphate. In tissues where the enzyme level is low, such as muscle or adipose tissue, glycerol 3-phosphate is produced from an intermediate of the Embden-Meyerhof glycolytic pathway, dihydroxyacetone phosphate, by an NADH-dependent reduction catalyzed by glycerol 3-phosphate dehydrogenase.

Fatty acids are activated to acyl CoA derivatives by thiokinase utilizing ATP and coenzyme A. Two molecules of acyl CoA (usually saturated and unsaturated C_{16} and C_{18} acids) combine with glycerol 3-phosphate to form 2-diacylglycerol phosphate (phosphatidate). This is a two-stage process with lysophosphatidate being formed first, the step being catalyzed by glycerol 3-phosphate acyl transferase and by the 1-acylglycerol 3-phosphate acyl transferase. Phosphatidate is converted to 1,2-diacylglycerol and undergoes further esterification with another molecule of acyl CoA to form a triacylglycerol.

Phospholipids [4] are produced from phosphatidate or from 1,2-diacylglycerol. Thus, in the production of phosphatidylinositol, CTP reacts with phosphatidate to form a cytidinediphosphate diacylglycerol. This compound then reacts with inositol under the influence of the enzyme CDP diacylglycerol inositol transferase to form a phosphatidyl inositol. For the biosynthesis of phosphatidyl choline and phosphatidyl ethanolamine (lecithins and cephalins), choline and ethanolamine are first activated by a two-step process involving first a reaction with ATP to produce the corresponding monophosphate, then a further reaction with CTP to produce CDP choline or CDP ethanolamine. These compounds can then react with 1,2-diacylglycerol to produce transfer of phosphorylated base to the diacylglycerol producing phosphatidyl choline or phosphatidyl ethanolamine.

Glycerol Ether Phospholipids and Plasmalogens

Dihydroxyacetone phosphate combines with acyl coenzyme A to form 1-acyl-dihydroxyacetone phosphate. This compound then exchanges the acyl group for a long-chain alcohol to form a 1-alkyldihydroxyacetone phosphate, which contains an ether link. In the presence of NADPH this is converted to 1-alkylglycerol 3-phosphate. Further acylation in the 2-position produces a 1-alkyl-2-acylglycerol 3-phosphate, which is then hydrolyzed to give the free glycerol derivative. Plasmalogens are formed by desaturation of the analogous glycerol-ether lipid. These compounds are the major structural phospholipid components of mitochondria.

The ester bond in position 2 of glycerophospholipids is hydrolyzed by phospholipase A_2 to produce a lysophospholipid, which may then be attacked by lysophospholipase (phospholipase B) with removal of the remaining 1-acyl group to produce glyceryl phosphoryl base, which may then go on to further hydrolysis with liberation of glycerol 3-phosphate plus base. Phospholipase A_1 attacks the ester bond in position 1 of phos-

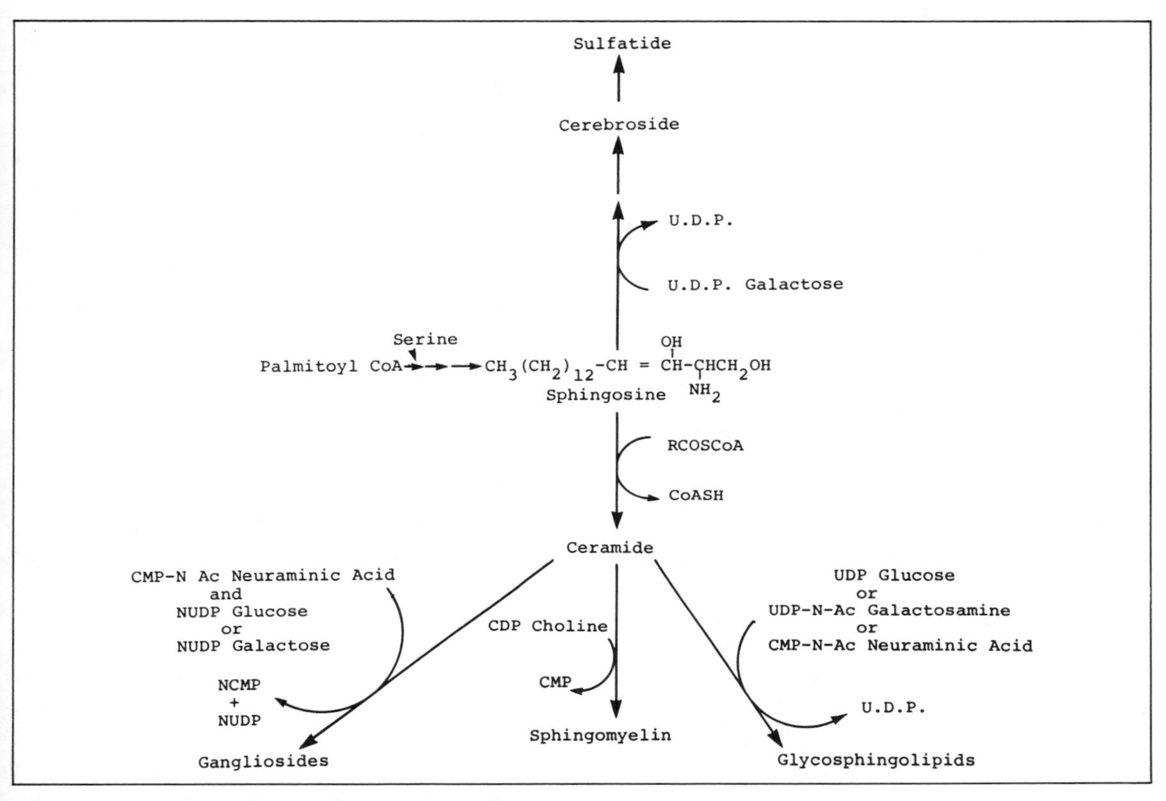

Figure 7-6. *Outline of biosynthetic routes to formation of complex lipids.*

pholipids. Phospholipase C splits the ester bond in position 3, with liberation of 1,2-diacylglycerol and a phosphoryl base. Lysolecithin is also formed by lecithin cholesterol acyltransferase (LCAT), an enzyme occurring in plasma and liver, which will transfer the fatty acid residue from the 2-position of lecithin to cholesterol to produce cholesterol ester. LCAT is responsible for the production of most of the cholesterol ester in plasma lipoproteins and exerts a protective role, since free unesterified cholesterol is toxic to tissue.

SPHINGOLIPIDS [45]

Sphingomyelins are complex phospholipids composed of a fatty acid, phosphoric acid, choline, and the amino alcohol sphingol (sphingosine). Synthesis is initiated with activation by pyridoxyl phosphate, resulting in the combination of serine with palmityl coenzyme A to produce 3-ketodihydrosphingosine, with a concomitant decarboxylation. Two reductive steps subsequently produce sphingosine. Sphingosine then reacts with CDP choline to produce sphingosine phosphoryl choline, which is then acylated at the amino group by a long-chain fatty acid acyl coenzyme A derivative to produce sphingomyelin. Sphingomyelin can also be synthesized from sphingosine by way of the production of a ceramide (an N-acyl sphingosine derivative), which can then react with CDP choline to produce CMP and sphingomyelin. Sphingomyelin is a major component of nerve myelin. Figure 7-6 outlines the major biosynthetic routes to formation of complex lipids.

CEREBROSIDES, SULFATIDES, AND GANGLIOSIDES

Cerebrosides are glycolipids composed of sphingosine, fatty acid, and galactose. These compounds characteristically contain C_{24} fatty acids such as lignoceric, cerebronic, and nervonic acids. Lignoceric acid is synthesized from acetate; cerebronic acid, the 2-hydroxy derivative of lignoceric acid, is formed from lignoceric acid. Nervonic acid, a monounsaturated acid, is produced by stepwise elongation of oleic acid. The galactose moiety is derived from glucose utilizing an epimerase enzyme, which requires uridine-diphosphate-glucose as substrate. The reaction occurs in the brain, liver, and mammary gland. Cerebrosides form a significant component of the myelin sheaths of nerves.

Sulfatides are derived from cerebrosides, using active sulfate (3^1-phosphoadenosine-5^1-phosphosulfate). Gangliosides are produced from ceramide by a stepwise addition of activated sugars, such as UDP galactose or UDP glucose and N-acetyl neuraminic acid. Glycosphingolipids function as constituents of cell membranes and are particularly involved in immunologic reactions that form the basis for current systems of classifying the various blood groups.

Degradation of complex sphingolipids utilizes specific enzymes, and several enzyme deficiencies and their clinical consequences have been described as specific syndromes [47]. For example, in Tay-Sachs disease there is a deficiency of hexoseaminidase A, with the resultant accumulation of ganglioside GM_2. This results in mental retardation, blindness, and muscular weakness. The enzyme deficiency can be detected in heterozygotes by a serum enzyme assay. The abnormality can also be detected in cultured skin fibroblasts, and amniocentesis can now assist in prenatal diagnosis of this abnormality. Many of these sphingolipidoses have been delineated.

TISSUE SPECIALIZATION IN LIPID METABOLISM AND INTER-ORGAN CONTROL

Most lipid is derived from the diet, mainly as triglyceride, and, initially, this is transferred mostly in the form of large particles called chylomicrons, to the liver, which then processes these compounds and dispatches them to peripheral tissues. In the periphery, the main storage site is adipose tissue, and there are regulatory means for controlling the uptake and release of triglyceride components and the transfer of these components back to the liver or other tissues such as muscle. Obviously, with this sort of functional specialization, a fairly complex control system is required, and there are many regulatory mechanisms that respond to dietary intake and to organ requirements.

DIGESTION OF FATS

Dietary lipid is a major component of the American diet, supplying one-third to one-half of the caloric value. Most dietary lipid is taken in as triacylglycerol, and in the gut a significant proportion is hydrolyzed by lipases to fatty acids and glycerol [39]. This hydrolysis is rarely complete, so that the end-result is a mixture of mono- and diacylglycerols as well as free glycerol and fatty acids. There is a lipase in the stomach, but its optimum pH is around neutrality, so its significance in regard to lipid digestion is uncertain. It may play a more significant role in the infant, who has a much higher gastric pH and in whom the lipid of milk is highly emulsified, thus offering a particularly large surface area to a water-soluble enzyme such as gastric lipase. The major site of lipid digestion occurs in the small intestine, where ingested food meets bile and the pancreatic secretions. Lipids are insoluble in water, and the process of emulsification occurs in the gut. This breaks down the lipid into multiple small droplets, thus exposing the maximum surface area to the lipid/water interface, which is the only point at which aqueous enzymes can attack lipid [35]. Bile and pancreatic juice, being alkaline, produce a largely neutral environment in the duodenum, thus permitting the bile acids, taurocholic and glycoholic acids, which are amphiphiles, to emulsify the lipid content of food. Emulsification is also facilitated by protein and by mechanical mixing produced by peristalsis. Bile salts are not, in fact, essential for digestion, since diversion of bile in the experimental animal results in the appearance of largely hydrolyzed lipid residues in the feces. However, subjects with biliary obstruction cannot tolerate large lipid loads, and this would suggest that bile is a significant mechanism in the digestion of lipids [46]. Some monoacylglycerols produced from partial hydrolysis of fats act as detergents and augment the role of the bile salts. Entry of gastric chyme into the duodenum results in hormonally-mediated stimulation of pancreatic juice and release of lipase into the intestinal lumen. Lipase is activated in the lumen and proceeds to hydrolyze triglycerides, although the hydrolysis is incomplete, yielding a mixture of free glycerol, fatty acids, and 1,2-diacyl- and 2-monoacylglycerols. Calcium accelerates lipolysis, as it forms insoluble soaps with liberated fatty acids and so moves the equilibrium toward hydrolysis. In addition, pancreatic juice contains esterases, which will not function in the absence of bile salts. They catalyze the hydrolysis of short-chain fatty acid esters, such as tributyrin and cholesterol esters. Phospholipase A_2 is secreted by the pancreas in an inactive form and is then activated by trypsin in the gut to phospholipase A_2, which will function only in the presence of bile salts and calcium to produce lysophosphatidylcholine from phosphatidylcholine. The enzyme is also found in the intestinal mucosa. Lysophosphatidylcholine is an effective detergent and accelerates emulsification of dietary lipid.

In general, about 40 percent of dietary triacylglycerols are hydrolyzed to glycerol and fatty acids. Three to 10 percent are absorbed as triacylglycerol, and the remainder are partially hydrolyzed mainly to the monoacylglycerols.

Short-chain fatty acids (less than 10 carbon atoms in length) are absorbed in a nonesterified form and transferred by the portal route directly to the liver. This route is particularly relevant to the absorption of milk, which is the major dietary constituent for infants.

Long-chain fatty acids (more than 14 carbon atoms in length) enter chyle as regenerated triacylglycerols in the form of large particles, about one micrometer in diameter, termed *chylomicrons*. These particles are extremely rich in lipid, with a small amount of carrier protein. Chylomicrons travel to the thoracic duct and enter the circulation through the jugular and subclavian veins, mainly on the left side. Bile plays a major role in efficient absorption of lipids and in the absorption of such lipid-soluble substances as vitamins A, D, and K. In extrahepatic biliary obstruction, loss of bile results in deficiency of these components, which is frequently of clinical significance. The bile acids return to the liver from the portal blood, and are reprocessed back into bile and form an enterohepatic circulation.

In addition, the intestinal mucosa itself is rich in enzymes capable of converting free fatty acids and mono- and diacylglycerols to triacylglycerols. Of the dietary sterols, only cholesterol is absorbed in any significant quantity. Disruption of the supply of bile or pancreatic juice or defects in intestinal mucosa give rise to lipid excess in the stools or steatorrhea.

Lipids are virtually insoluble, so a carrier system is essential for their transfer to various organs. The transfer system is composed of specific lipoproteins, which are synthesized in the intestinal mucosa and the liver. Table 7-1 gives an outline of the various lipoproteins and their constituents [11, 27, 38, 42].

Following a meal, normal human plasma contains about 500 mg of total lipid per 100 ml, of which 125 mg will be triacylglycerol and 220 mg will be cholesterol, with two-thirds of the cholesterol being esterified and one-third being the free sterol. Phosphoglycerides form about 160 mg/100 ml, with a higher concentration of phosphatidylcholine than phosphatidylethanolamine. Free (i.e., unesterified) fatty acids are found complexed to albumin and occur only in low concentrations. Lipoproteins can be fractionated by ultracentrifugation into various families, and this also divides them into classes of different functions. The fractions of lowest density are richest in triacylglycerols and poorest in protein.

The structure of lipoproteins, in general, is a central core of hydrophobic lipids, triacylglyc-

Table 7-1. *Major Plasma Lipoproteins: Characteristics and Constituents*

Lipoprotein Class	Diameter (Å)	Density (gm/ml)	Electrophoretic Mobility	Composition (%) Chol.	Trig.	Phospholipid	Protein
Chylomicrons	750–4000	0.93	α_2	5	90	3	2
VLDL	300–800	0.95–1.006	pre-β	12	60	18	10
LDL	220	1.019–1.063	β	50	10	15	25
HDL	75–100	1.063–1.085	α	20	5	25	50

VLDL = very low density lipoprotein; LDL = low density lipoprotein; HDL = high density lipoprotein.

erols, and cholesterol esters, with outer regions, in direct contact with plasma, containing the hydrophilic lipids such as phosphatidyl choline. The protein components are arranged so that the hydrophobic portions of the chain are in the interior, while the hydrophilic parts lie predominantly on the outside of the particles; thus the plasma proteins play a major role in the stabilization and transport of the water-insoluble lipids. Dietary triacylglycerols are transported in the form of chylomicrons mainly to the liver and adipose tissue, but also to the heart, lung, and other organs. The enzyme lipoprotein lipase is situated in the capillary beds perfusing these organs, and it hydrolyzes triacylglycerols, producing fatty acids and glycerol, which are absorbed by adjacent cells. Thereafter, fatty acids and glycerol may be directly metabolized or resynthesized to triacylglycerols for storage. Only the brain does not utilize fatty acids for oxidation. Lipoprotein lipase is sensitive to regulation by hormones and by protein cofactors that circulate on the various lipoproteins. Thus, apo C_{II} activates the enzyme from adipose tissue. Phosphatidylcholine also activates the enzyme. Serum albumin is essential as a receptor for liberated fatty acids if the enzyme is to function. Plasma-free fatty acids are present in a concentration of 8 to 30 mg/100 ml and exhibit a rapid metabolic turnover rate. Absence of lipoprotein lipase is responsible for the condition of familial hyperchylomicronemia (type I hyperlipoproteinemia) [34], in which there is a major reduction in the rapidity of clearance of chylomicrons, and levels of plasma triacylglycerols usually reach over 2 gm/100 ml, with the production of gross lipemia. The condition predisposes to acute pancreatitis, but probably not to atherosclerosis because these particles are so large that they cannot easily penetrate the arterial wall.

The amount of triacylglycerol stored in depot sites is dependent on dietary intake. There is some capacity for regulation of fatty acid deposition through control of the appetite by hunger and satiety centers in the brain, but in the face of a prolonged exposure to excess caloric intake, this mechanism is in general somewhat inadequate, and obesity is the most common nutritional disorder in Western countries. Conversely, in cases of severe starvation, it is possible for depot fat to disappear virtually completely, leaving the subject with less than his lean body mass and no reserves.

LIPID AND CARBOHYDRATE INTERRELATIONSHIPS

Carbohydrate is a prime carbon source for fatty acid synthesis. If the body is presented with a caloric excess of fatty acids, these will be deposited in tissue primarily as triacylglycerols. There will also be production of more complex lipids, but these are minor pathways in comparison to the huge amounts of triacylglycerol that can be deposited in adipose tissue and in other sites. Conversion of glucose to glycogen is controlled at the level of entry to the cell by insulin, but the capacity to store glycogen is a limited one.

Acetyl CoA carboxylase in liver and adipose tissue consists of inactive subunits, which are activated by citrate and isocitrate to a multi-unit filamentous form [2]. Citrate and isocitrate, which are metabolites of carbohydrate metabolism, thus regulate lipogenesis by activating acetyl CoA carboxylase, a biotin cofactor-requiring enzyme that is the rate-limiting step in fatty acid biosynthesis. Malonyl CoA serves only as an intermediary in fatty acid biosynthesis. Formation of carboxybiotin inactivates the carboxylase, unless citrate or isocitrate is present. These effectors act allosterically to modify V_{max}. Citrate passes freely through the mitochondrial membrane when present in excess to activate acetyl CoA carboxylase in the cytoplasm. The enzyme is depressed by fasting or high-fat diets, and is increased by a high-carbohydrate fat-free diet, which is therefore a lipogenic one.

Isocitrate dehydrogenase regulation facilitates a balance between carbohydrate and fatty acid metabolism, since it is allosterically regulated by ATP and AMP. High ATP levels inhibit the dehydrogenase, and citrate accumulates and passes out of the mitochondria, stimulating fatty acid biosynthesis at the carboxylase level as well as providing citrate for degradation in the cytoplasm, by citrate lyase, to acetyl CoA for lipogenesis. Conversely, when AMP accumulates in the mitochondria, isocitrate dehydrogenase is activated by the positive allosteric effector AMP, and citric acid cycle activity is augmented with consequent decline in citrate efflux into the cytoplasm. Since the cellular capacity for glycogen storage is limited, it is economical for citrate and isocitrate, as they accumulate, to move out of the mitochondria and activate fatty acid biosynthesis. Thus, insulin enhancement of cellular carbohydrate uptake and storage eventually leads to fatty acid biosynthesis and more efficient energy storage. Conversely, glucagon preserves cyclic AMP levels, thus leading to hepatic release of free fatty acids and loss of acetyl CoA for citrate synthesis, so that the resultant fall of cytoplasmic citrate shuts off fatty acid synthesis.

The triacylglycerols stored in adipose tissue can be mobilized, distributed, and oxidized sufficiently to support about 50 percent of the oxidative metabolism of the body. This occurs under such circumstances as starvation, cold exposure, exercise, reproduction, and growth. The stimulus in these situations is largely hormonal [18, 49].

The hormones that mobilize lipids from adipose tissue include epinephrine and norepinephrine, adrenal steroids, glucagon, and the hormones from the hypophysis—vasopressin, thyrotropin, adrenocorticotropin, luteotropin, somatotropin, and the β- and α-lipotropins. In stress situations, serotonin is released and also induces adipose tissue release of fatty acid. The general effect of these hormones and serotonin is to stimulate lipolysis. Lipid-mobilizing hormones activate hormone-sensitive lipoprotein lipase and increase glucose utilization, through stimulation of esterification by increased production of free fatty acids. For optimal lipid-mobilizing effect, most of the lipolytic process requires the presence of thyroid hormone and glucocorticoids. These particular hormones alone are not potent augmentors of lipolysis, but they do act in a permissive capacity with regard to other lipid-mobilizing endocrine agents. Hormones that promote lipolysis do so by stimulation of adenylate cyclase, which converts ATP to cyclic AMP. Cyclic AMP in turn activates a protein kinase, which converts inactive hormone-sensitive triacylglycerol lipase into the active lipase. Lipolysis is controlled largely by the amount of cyclic AMP present in a particular tissue. The degradation of cyclic AMP to 5′AMP is controlled by the enzyme cyclic 3′, 5′-nucleotide phosphodiesterase. This particular enzyme is inhibited by methyl xanthines, such as caffeine and theophylline, and drinking coffee results in markedly prolonged elevation of plasma-free fatty acids in humans.

Insulin has a potent antilipolytic effect and antagonizes the effect of the lipolytic hormones. Lipolysis is particularly sensitive to changes in the concentration of insulin, much more so than glucose utilization and esterification. Just how thyroid hormones facilitate lipolysis is unclear, but thyroid hormones do appear to augment the level of cyclic AMP and may inhibit phosphodiesterase activity. Growth hormone requires the presence of glucocorticoids to promote lipolysis, and it does so by inducing new formation of the enzymes involved in the formation of cyclic AMP.

The sympathetic nervous system, by way of norepinephrine liberation in adipose tissue, plays a central role in mobilization of free fatty acids. Denervation of adipose tissue or chemical blockade reduces or abolishes the increased lipolysis induced by many of the aforementioned factors.

Human adipose tissue is responsive to the catecholamines, but less responsive to most of the lipolytic hormones.

FREE FATTY ACIDS

Free fatty acids circulate combined with serum albumin in concentrations between 0.1 and 2.0 microequivalents per milliliter of plasma. They comprise the long-chain fatty acids found in adipose tissue, that is, palmitic, stearic, oleic, palmitoleic, linoleic, and other polyunsaturated acids, as well as smaller quantities of other long-chain fatty acids. (The binding of free fatty acids to albumin has been discussed in detail by Spector [43].) Plasma levels are lowest in the fully fed condition. In uncontrolled diabetes mellitus, levels may rise to 2 microequivalents per milliliter. The levels vary with meals, falling just after a meal and rising again prior to the next meal. Removal of free fatty acids from the blood is fast. Estimates indicate that free fatty acids supply one-quarter to one-half of the energy requirements in the fasting subject. A fatty acid binding protein has been described in the cytoplasm of the cells of most tissues, and presumably its role is to function as the intracellular equivalent of extracellular albumin.

METABOLISM OF LIPOPROTEINS
(Figure 7-7) [11, 42]

Chylomicron formation fluctuates with the amount of triacylglycerol absorbed from the diet. Chylomicrons are synthesized by the intestinal cells and then released into the spaces between the cells, eventually making their way into the lymphatic system that drains the intestine. From there they traverse the lymphatic system to the thoracic duct and enter the circulation on the venous side. Production of chylomicrons and their release into the bloodstream is somewhat similar to the production of very low-density lipoprotein (VLDL) by hepatic parenchymal cells. These somewhat smaller units are secreted by the hepatic parenchymal cells into the space of Disse and then into the hepatic sinusoids. Both chylomicrons and VLDL require apoprotein synthesis, and in abetalipoproteinemia, there is a lack of chylomicrons and VLDL. Lipid droplets accumulate in the intestine and liver, and red cell membranes show a particular abnormality, in addition to the neurofunctional disorder which characterizes this condition.

Chylomicrons are rapidly cleared from the bloodstream with a half-time of about one hour. Liver does not metabolize chylomicrons or native VLDL to any great extent, but it does receive a large proportion of their lipid moiety through recycling from the extrahepatic tissues. These lipoproteins undergo degradation of the triacylglycerol moiety by lipoprotein lipase, also known as clearing factor lipase, in the walls of blood capillaries. The enzyme requires phospholipids and the apoprotein CII as cofactors for optimal activity [21]. Both chylomicrons and VLDL carry substrate and cofactor to the enzyme, and hydrolysis occurs while the lipoproteins are attached to the enzyme on the endothelial lining. The activity of lipoprotein lipase is regulated by the balance between CII (activator) and CIII (and CI) (inhibitor). With increasing triglyceride concentration, this balance moves progressively toward enhanced transfer of CII to chylomicrons and VLDL. Triacylglycerols undergo progressive hydrolysis through the diacylglycerol stage to a monoacylglycerol, which is finally hydrolyzed by a discrete monoacylglycerol hydrolase. Some of the released free fatty acids enter the circulation, but most are transported into the tissues. Lipoprotein lipase can remove about 90 percent of the triacylglycerol of chylomicrons, and apoprotein CII components return to high-density lipoprotein (HDL). The end-result of this sequential process of degradation is to produce a lipopro-

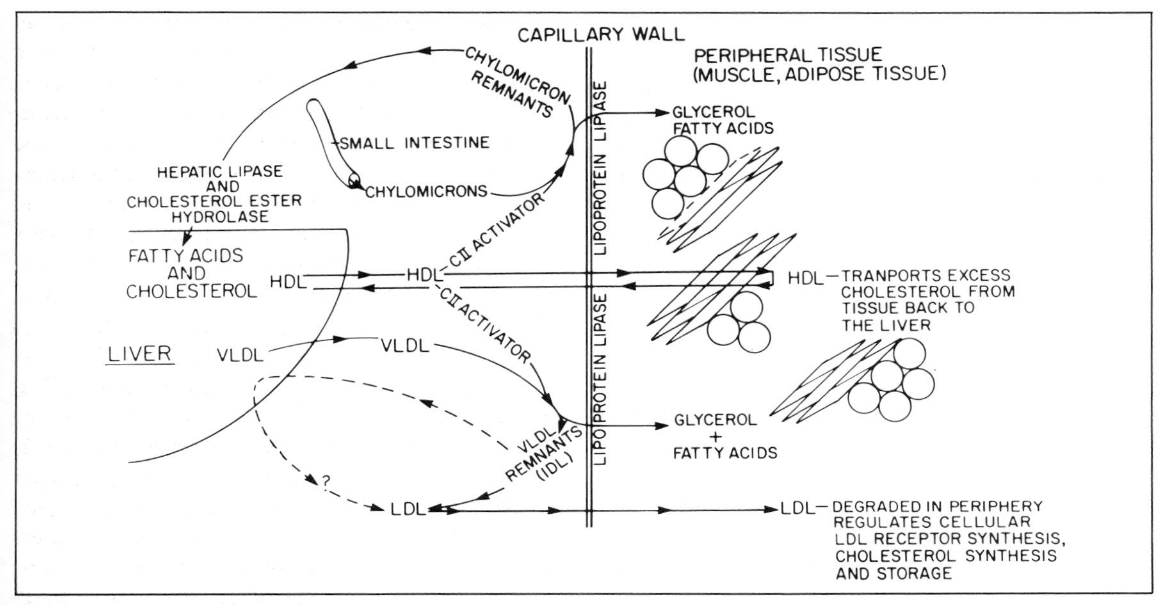

Figure 7-7. *Lipoprotein interrelationships.*

tein remnant that is about half the diameter of the parent chylomicron, but carries much more in the way of cholesterol and cholesterol esters proportionately through the loss of triacylglycerol. These remnants are then taken up by the liver, which hydrolyzes the cholesterol esters and the remains of the triacylglycerol acids. The fatty acids are incorporated mainly into phospholipids, which are then released from the liver as a phospholipid lipoprotein, the subsequent degradation of which is not clearly delineated. The degradation of VLDL eventually produces a smaller lipoprotein, low-density lipoprotein (LDL), which may be regarded as an end-stage in lipoprotein metabolism. The half-time of disappearance from the circulation of apoprotein B in LDL is about 2½ days. Classic work by Goldstein and Brown [14] has delineated the presence of specific receptor sites for apoliprotein B on human fibroblasts, lymphocytes, and arterial smooth muscle cells. Most of the work has been performed using in vitro tissue culture techniques.

The implication of this large body of work is as follows: LDL is taken up by peripheral cells and the protein moiety is degraded to amino acids in lysosomes. However, the cholesterol is released, and it has three effects inside the cell. First, it suppresses the activity of hydroxymethylglutaryl CoA reductase, so that cell production of cholesterol is cut off. This is obviously economical, since the cell is receiving its cholesterol (for membrane maintenance and the like) from the liver as a component of LDL. Second, when sufficient cholesterol has accumulated through the LDL pathway to meet the cell requirement for membrane synthesis, the excess cholesterol is re-esterified and stored in the cell as cholesterol ester. This re-esterification process is catalyzed by the microsomal enzyme acyl CoA cholesterol acyltransferase, the activity of which is stimulated by the cholesterol derived from LDL. This reaction appears to be important because free cholesterol is toxic to tissue and so rapid esterification of cholesterol is important. A third effect of the delivery of cholesterol to the cell by the LDL pathway is that the cholesterol exerts a feedback effect on the synthesis of LDL receptor sites, that is, as the cellular cholesterol content rises, the number of sites is reduced, again protecting the cell from excessive uptake of cholesterol. Much of the evidence that supports the foregoing has come from studies of cells from subjects who are homozygous and heterozygous for abnormalities of the LDL receptor site. These subjects, if homozygotes, have no receptors, and if heterozygous, have only one-half the normal complement of receptors, with the result that LDL accumulates in plasma. The LDL percolates into the walls of arteries, where the cholesterol component is deposited, exciting the proliferation of cells in the vicinity, particularly smooth muscle cells. These cells produce collagen and other components, and the net result is a fibrous response to the presence of cholesterol, which eventually produces severe atherosclerosis. Homozygotes are notorious for developing severe problems with coronary atherosclerosis before the age of twenty, and heterozygotes run into the same problems in the fourth and fifth decades [41]. The other broader implication of this work by Goldstein and Brown [14] is that the plasma levels of LDL found in Western man are unphysiologically high. A further implication of this suggestion is that the Western diet is unhealthy in that it induces unduly high levels of LDL, with a consequent increased propensity to atherosclerosis because of infiltration of LDL into arterial walls [25].

High-density lipoprotein (HDL) is synthesized by both liver and intestine, and HDL is the cofactor for the enzyme lecithin cholesterol acyl transferase (LCAT). Newly formed or rascent HDL is discoid in shape, and it is thought that LCAT converts surface phospholipid and free cholesterol into cholesterol esters and lysolecithin. The nonpolar cholesterol esters penetrate into the hydrophobic interior of the HDL discoid bilayer, whereas lysolecithin is transferred to plasma albumin. The reaction eventually generates a nonpolar core that pushes the bilayer apart to produce a spherical HDL protein covered by a surface film of polar lipids and apoproteins. The LCAT system is considered to be primarily concerned with removal of excess unesterified cholesterol from lipoproteins. In LCAT deficiency [44] a large particle accumulates that is rich in unesterified cholesterol. HDL apoproteins appear to undergo final degradation in the liver and possibly to some extent in the intestine. The role of HDL has recently been extended, with the suggestion that HDL functions primarily as a means of collecting excess cholesterol from peripheral tissues and transporting it back to the liver. Thus, LDL would appear to function as a cholesterol delivery mechanism and HDL as a protective return pathway for removal of cholesterol back to the liver. There is extensive epidemiologic evidence [5] implicating high levels of circulating LDL as being atherogenic, whereas high levels of HDL are anti-atherogenic, possibly as a result of the scavenging mechanism that is proposed as a role of HDL. In the inherited condition of Tangier disease [44], HDL is absent in its normal functional form. Huge amounts of cholesterol esters accumulate in the reticuloendothelial system. The tonsils are grossly swollen, and peripheral neuropathy develops. The cholesterol ester deposition appears to be due to phagocytosis of abnormal lipoprotein particles. LDL is abnormally rich in triglycerides, and hypertriglyceridemia also ensues because the VLDL particles are deficient in C-apoproteins.

KETONE BODIES

When there is a high rate of fatty acid oxidation, the liver produces a large amount of acetoacetate and β-hydroxy butyrate, which enters the blood by simple diffusion. Peripheral tissue can convert acetoacetic acid to its CoA derivative because these tissues possess a specific thiophorase unlike liver. The enzyme thiophorase transfers a CoA residue to acetoacetate from succinyl CoA. Thiolases can convert acetoacetyl CoA to two molecules of acetyl CoA. Acetoacetate spontaneously (and enzymatically) decarboxylates to acetone, and these three substances are known as the ketone bodies (Figure 7-8). Normally the total concentration of ketone bodies of the blood of well-fed mammals does not exceed 1 mg/dl measured as acetone equivalents. In the human less than 1 mg is lost in the urine in 24 hours. Abnormally high quantities of ketone bodies in

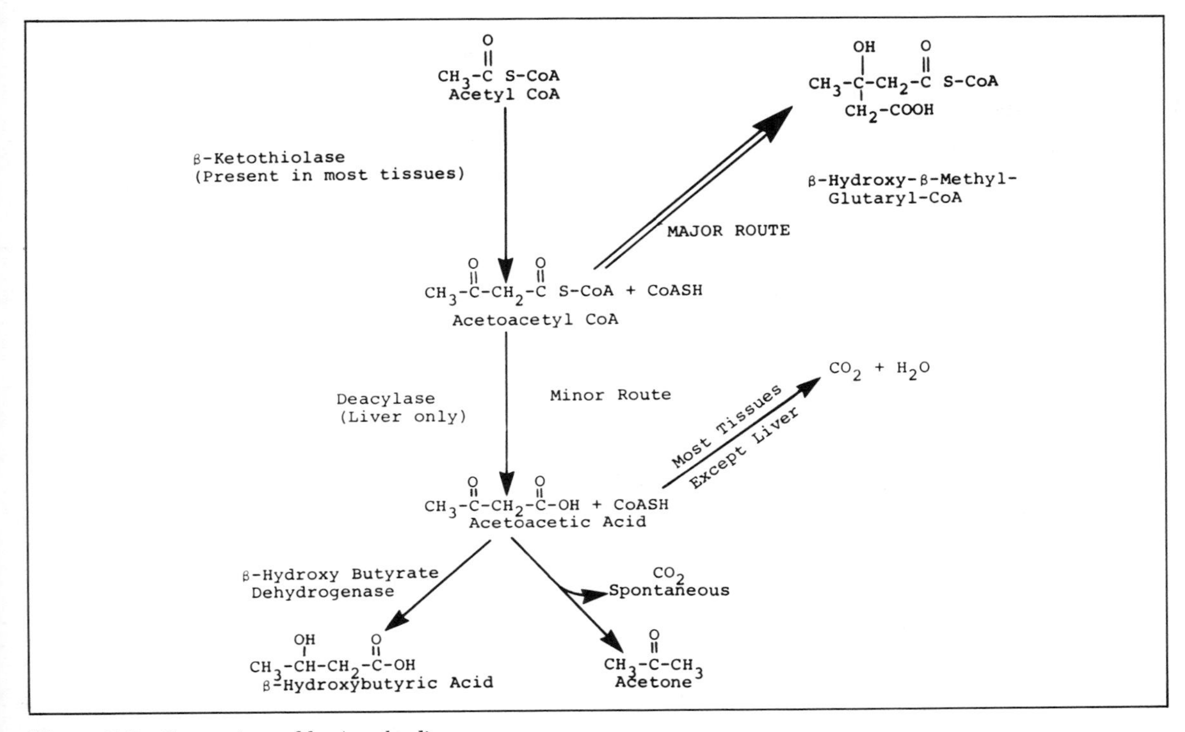

Figure 7-8. *Formation of ketone bodies.*

blood or urine constitute ketonemia or ketonuria, and the overall condition is called ketosis. Acetoacetic and β-hydroxybutyric acids are strong acids, and they need to be buffered if produced in excess. Continued production of these compounds in excess depletes the body's alkaline reserve, causing a frequent terminal acidosis in uncontrolled diabetes mellitus. The urinary excretion of ketone bodies may reach as high as 500 mg/24 hr, whereas the blood concentration can reach 90 mg/100 ml. Excretion of the salts of acetoacetic and β-hydroxybutyric acid leads to loss of large quantities of fluid in the urine. Fluid loss may be exacerbated by vomiting and result in severe dehydration and acidosis.

ETHANOL AND LIPID METABOLISM

Consumed in moderate amounts, ethanol merely adds additional calories to the diet by virtue of its metabolism to acetate, conversion to acetyl CoA, and further metabolism down the usual pathways for this substance (Figure 7-9). In high doses, ethanol acts as a metabolic poison and produces particular derangements of lipid metabolism [25]. Alcohol is water-soluble and is rapidly absorbed from the stomach and intestines. Alcohol, once absorbed, reaches and affects all organs. Thus, it produces inflammation of the stomach, intestines, and pancreas, with upsets in digestion. It affects all of the central nervous system, usually in combination with nutritional deficiencies resulting from the low consumption of protein and vitamins. The classic syndrome of alcoholism is the Wernicke-Korsakoff syndrome of polyneuropathy, which is largely due to associated dietary thiamine deficiency. Alcohol excess in general is associated with various nutritional deficiencies because generally the individual consuming a consistently large amount of alcohol has a low protein and vitamin intake. Alcohol is largely metabolized in the liver by ethanol dehydrogenase, which converts ethanol

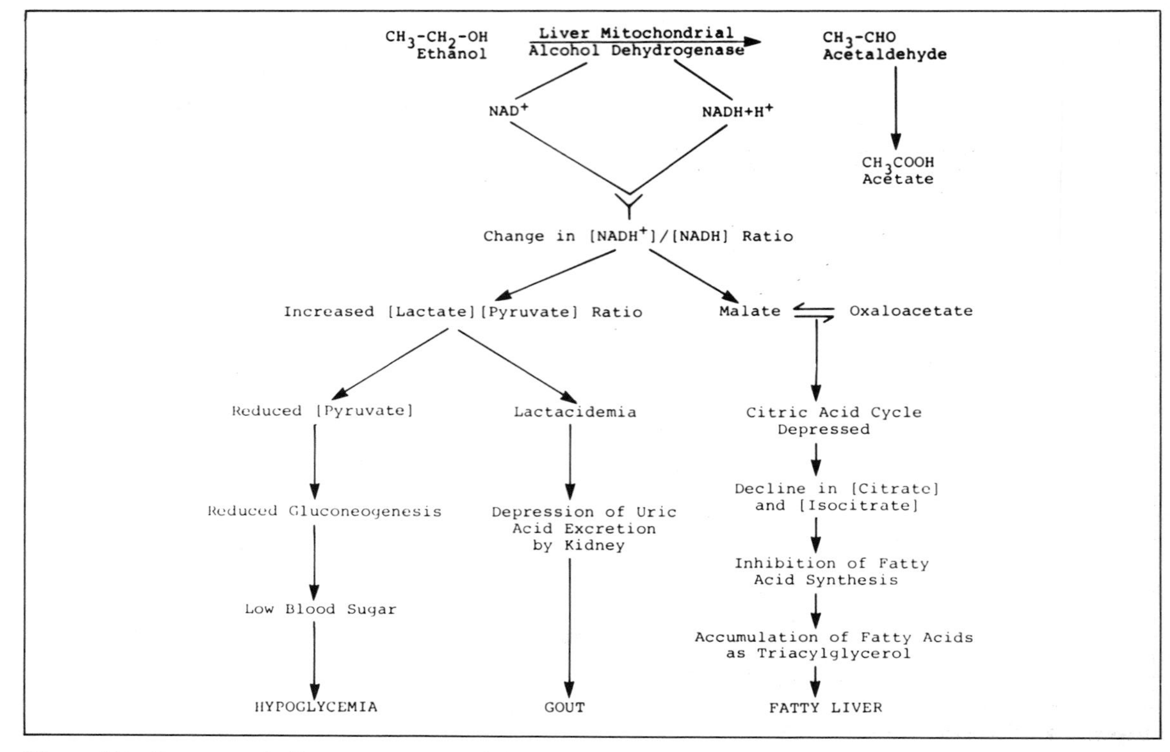

Figure 7-9. *Some metabolic consequences of chronic ethanol ingestion.*

to acetaldehyde (Figure 7-9). Acetaldehyde is subsequently oxidized to acetate by at least three different enzymes. The acetyl CoA that is produced by these enzymes is then utilized in the usual way. The production of both NADH and acetyl CoA, with consequent formation of ATP, spares fatty acids, which in turn accumulate and together with the high levels of NADH stimulate the conversion of pyruvate to lactate. A mild lactic acidosis results, along with a lowered blood sugar concentration, since gluconeogenesis from pyruvate is suppressed. As the availability of glucose is reduced, ketone bodies may be produced in excess and mimic the ketosis of diabetics.

In chronic alcoholics, lipid mobilization is excessive, and eventually a fatty liver develops. The actual mechanism of production is not clear, but several factors appear to be interrelated: (1) There is sparing action of ethanol oxidation on the utilization of liver triacylglycerols; (2) there is excessive mobilization of triacylglycerols from adipose tissue to liver, due in part to ethanol triggering release of lipid-mobilizing hormones; and (3) there is an inadequate synthesis of sufficient lipoproteins to transport triacylglycerols because of disruption of amino acid availability. In a significant proportion of alcoholics with fatty liver, the damage proceeds to a fibrotic reaction, with eventual cirrhosis and major disturbance of hepatic function. In moderate amounts, however, ethanol may be of value as a source of calories in parenteral nutrition. While the caloric value of ethanol is high, 7 calories/gm, the association of ethanol with pancreatitis in patients receiving parenteral nutrition has led most units to discontinue the use of ethanol in parenteral nutrition solutions.

STEROL METABOLISM AND REGULATION

Cholesterol is the most abundant sterol of animal tissues. It is a common constituent of the diet since it is present in all animal and some plant tissues. Cholesterol may undergo some bacterial degradation in the intestine to compounds such as cholestanol and coprostanol, but these are poorly absorbed from the gut. The major part of the cholesterol that is absorbed appears in lymphatic chylomicra as cholesterol esters. Cholesterol may also be synthesized endogenously, and nearly all tissues possess the enzymes for this cholesterol production. The work by Goldstein and Brown [14], however, suggests that in many tissues cholesterol production is minimal or absent, and most of the cholesterol required for tissue needs is supplied by the liver.

All the carbon atoms of endogenously produced cholesterol derive from acetyl CoA. The enzymes of the biosynthetic pathway of cholesterol reside in the microsomes of the cytoplasm. The initial step involves head-to-tail condensation of two molecules of acetyl CoA, a reaction catalyzed by acetyl CoA acetyl transferase, a mitochondrial enzyme. Further condensation of the acetoacetyl CoA with another molecule of acetyl CoA is achieved by the enzyme β-hydroxy β-methyl-glutaryl CoA synthase. Next, this compound is converted to mevalonic acid by a sulfhydryl-containing NADPH-dependent enzyme 3-hydroxy 3-methyl-glutaryl CoA reductase. This reaction is the rate-controlling step in the biosynthetic pathway of cholesterol. Sterol biosynthesis then proceeds by condensation of six 5-carbon units, each of which derives from mevalonic acid. Figure 7-10 outlines the reaction mechanisms. Production of cholesterol is by way of squalene and lanosterol. About 80 percent of the cholesterol formed by the liver is converted to various bile acids. The major components are cholic and chenodeoxycholic acids. The cholesterol nucleus is hydroxylated and the side-chain degradation is completed. The bile acids are then conjugated to glycine or taurine by way of the coenzyme derivatives of the bile acids to produce the bile salts. The bile salts are excreted in concentrations of 0.5 to 1.5 percent in the bile and participate in an enterohepatic circulation that minimizes loss of bile acids in the stools.

Cholesterol is the source of steroid hormones formed in the gonads and adrenal cortex. Some cholesterol is also dehydrogenated to 7-dehydrocholesterol by the intestinal mucosa and skin. The 7-dehydrocholesterol stored in the skin can be converted by the action of sunlight to vitamin D. Endogenous and exogenous cholesterol are interrelated. Both fasting and cholesterol feeding markedly reduce the activity of HMG CoA reductase in the liver. There is a definite feedback mechanism controlling endogenous cholesterol synthesis, since both synthesis and the activity of this particular enzyme are inhibited by cholesterol. An increase in dietary carbohydrate or triacylglycerol will stimulate cholesterol synthesis from acetyl CoA. There is also some suggestion of a further feedback mechanism whereby dietary cholesterol exerts some regulatory effect at the cyclization step of squalene to lanosterol. There is evidence that the blood cholesterol level is increased by dietary intake of more saturated fatty acids. The mechanism for this increase is not known, but it is suggested that it is an important element in the production of atherosclerosis. It is also suggested that impurities (oxidation products) of dietary cholesterol are particularly atherogenic [23].

THE PROSTAGLANDINS

The prostaglandins are ubiquitous C_{20} carboxylic acids containing a cyclopentane ring [32, 37]. The prostaglandins have multiple actions, but appear to be the primary regulatory compounds involved in the control of local metabolic processes. There are two main series of prostaglandins, the E and F series, each having three members. The series differ from each other in that the E series has a keto oxygen at C_9 and a hydroxyl group at C_{11}, whereas the F series has a hydroxyl group in both positions in the cyclopentane ring. The series are further described

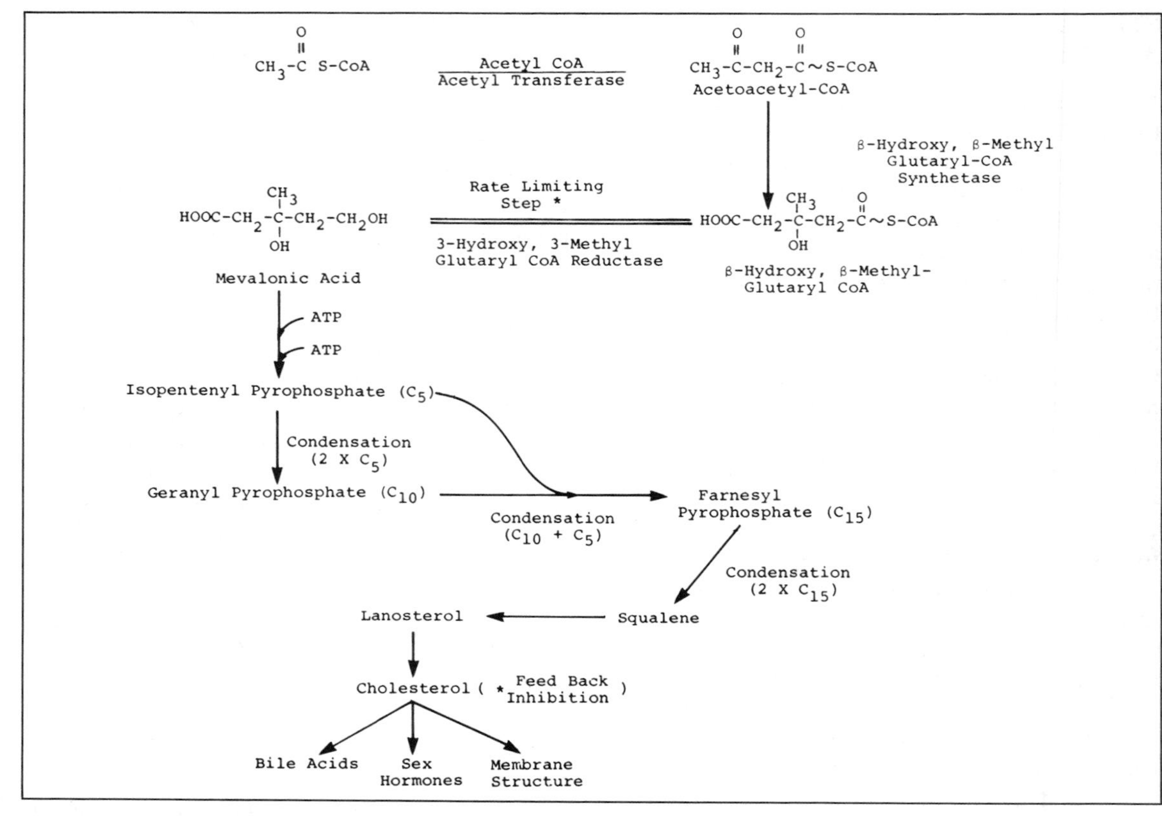

Figure 7-10. *Cholesterol biosynthesis.*

by subscript numerals 1, 2, and 3 which denote the number of double bonds in the R_1 and R_2 side chains. Prostaglandins with one, two, or three double bonds in the side chains in the E and F series are synthesized from the unsaturated fatty acids eicosa-8,11,14-trienoic, eicosa-5,8,11, 14-tetraenoic, and eicosa-5,8,11,14,17-pentaenoic acids, respectively. Primary prostaglandins contain two fewer double bonds than the fatty acids from which they are synthesized so that the precursor of PGE_1 and $PGF_{2\alpha,\alpha}$ is eicosatrienoic acid, of PGE_2 and PGF_2 is arachidonic acid and of PGE_3 and $PGF_{3\alpha}$ is eicosapentaenoic acid. The C_{20}, tri, tetra, and pentaenoic fatty acids that are the precursors of the prostaglandins come largely from intracellular phosphoglycerides, from which they are released by the action of phospholipase C_2. This step probably regulates prostaglandin biosynthesis by controlling the quantity of substrate available to prostaglandin synthase, which is a membrane-bound multienzyme complex in the microsomes. A sequence of reactions is initiated by fatty acid cyclooxygenase, eventually resulting in the production of various prostaglandins. The final products of the prostaglandin biosynthetic pathway differ in various organs. In most of the organs the prostaglandin endoperoxides are converted into PGEs and PGFs. In addition, only platelets, spleen, and lung form thromboxanes from PGG_2 and PGH_2. The intimal lining of blood vessels, in addition, forms PGI_2. The biosynthetic prostaglandin pathway is regulated at several steps. The initial oxidation proceeds only for a short time, and the extent of the reaction is limited by the quantity of enzyme. The cyclo-oxygenase undergoes a self-catalyzed destruction, and this type of

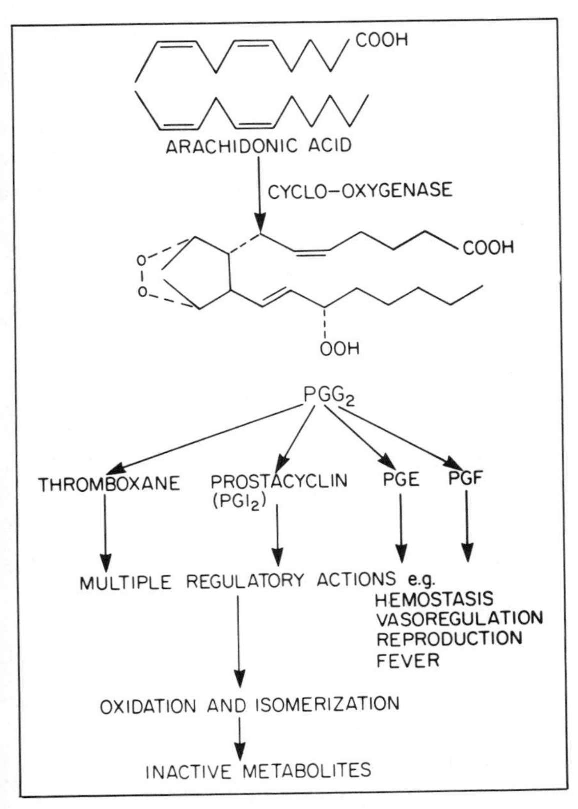

Figure 7-11. *Outline of prostaglandin metabolic routes.*

control permits a finite response that is self-limiting and not dependent on the diffusion of an end product to a regulatory site. In other words, de novo protein synthesis exerts a major regulatory effect upon the prostaglandin pathway. Since this depends on the production of messenger RNA, hormonally mediated control may be introduced at this point. In addition, cyclo-oxygenase exists in inactive forms that can be activated by such compounds as catecholamines. There are well-known interactions between the enzyme and certain drugs, such as aspirin, which inhibit prostaglandin biosynthesis and appear to exert their anti-inflammatory effects by this method [26].

The half-life of the primary prostaglandins is extremely short, frequently less than one minute, and metabolism exerts a major regulatory control upon tissue concentrations. Metabolism is largely the result of 15-hydroxy-prostaglandin dehydrogenase and Δ-13-reductase. Figure 7-11 outlines the biosynthetic and degradative pathways for the prostaglandins. The variety and multiplicity of the effects of prostaglandins deserves emphasis. For example, prostaglandins of the E series inhibit lipolysis by adipose tissue in vitro; low doses of PGE in human subjects tend to stimulate lipolysis, possibly by an indirect stimulation of catecholamine release, which is also reflected in hyperglycemia. The prostaglandins have major actions upon platelet aggregation, and there appears to be a balance between thromboxane, which is produced by platelets in response to such stimuli as catecholamines and predisposes to aggregation, and prostacyclin, which is produced by endothelial tissue lining arterial walls and inhibits platelet aggregation. A genetic effect that leads to absence of prostacyclin and thromboxane has been described. In this "balanced deficiency" situation, there appear to be no major consequences [29]. Prostaglandins have been shown to be vasodilators, and there is some evidence that they may play a significant role in control of coronary artery blood flow. Prostaglandins enhance ion flux across epithelial membranes, and it has been suggested that they are important local regulators in regard to renal function and urine production. Prostaglandins have been shown to exert important effects on the gut and will produce diarrhea partly by an effect on intestinal motility, which is enhanced, and partly by augmentation of water production. It is well known that they have major effects on the reproductive system, and prostaglandin derivatives are extensively studied and used clinically in the termination of pregnancy. In addition, they have important effects on inflammation, smooth muscle constriction, the immune system, and many other biologic processes.

LIPIDS, MEMBRANE STRUCTURE, AND FUNCTION

The original unit structure proposed for cell membranes by Davson and Danielli has, by and large, stood the test of time [10]. Basically, it envisaged cell membranes as being composed of a lipid bilayer, with the polar component of the lipids pointing to the exterior and interior of the cells, and the hydrophobic tail elements forming the central part of the lipid bilayer. This structure was incorporated into the fluid mosaic model proposed by Singer and Nicolson in 1972 [40]. In this model phospholipids are arranged in a lipid bilayer to form a sheet two molecules thick and 45 Å wide. Cholesterol is intercalated between molecules, and the phospholipid bilayer forms a liquid crystalline matrix as the basis of the cell membrane. Even more recently, Rothman and Lenard have described a degree of asymmetry in the bilayer membrane, with phosphatidyl choline and sphingomyelin being concentrated primarily in the outer leaflet, and phosphatidyl ethanolamine and phosphatidyl serine in the cytoplasmic component of the lipid bilayer [36].

The phospholipids are in a dynamic state in the intact membrane with significant lateral movement being permitted to these components, but little or no movement between the inner and outer monolayers. Transfer through or within membranes depends to a great extent on the fluidity of the membrane. This relates to the degree of resistance a particle encounters if it enters the interior of the lipid bilayer. Fatty acids with short chains are more fluid than longer-chain fatty acids. The greater the degree of unsaturation of a fatty acid, the greater the fluidity of the bilayer at a lower temperature. To maintain normal fluidity of a membrane, a certain cholesterol/phospholipid ratio is required. This ratio may be disturbed in various diseases, such as obstructive jaundice or other forms of liver disease. The erythrocytes from subjects with significant hepatocellular damage have increased membrane cholesterol levels. This produces distortion of the red cell structure, appearing as spur cells. In abetalipoproteinemia, the total phospholipid content of the red cell membrane is decreased owing to lack of lecithin, and so the cholesterol/phospholipid ratio is increased. There is also an increase in membrane sphingomyelin. The net effect of these abnormalities is to produce cells with spiky projections on the surface, termed *acanthocytes.* Evidence suggests that the convex portion of the red cell membrane is richer in cholesterol than the concave portion, implying that cholesterol molecules serve to wedge the membrane into its classic biconcave shape. In hereditary elliptocytosis, cholesterol appears to be condensed at the convex tips of these abnormal erythrocytes [1].

Plasma-free fatty acids, unesterified cholesterol (contained in serum lipoproteins), and phospholipids can exchange with their respective membrane counterparts. Exchange studies indicate that about 30 percent of membrane sphingomyelin and 60 percent of membrane phosphatidyl choline can exchange rapidly with their plasma equivalents. In addition to lipid components, cell membranes contain significant protein elements, which function in part as a matrix that helps to anchor the lipids and so reduce their lateral mobility and in part as discrete components of the membrane performing specific functions, such as enzymatic systems, among which is the Na-K-ATPase pump. Lipids are probably essential in the organizational structure of these components and play a significant role as a component of the various channels involved in transfer of materials from the exterior to the interior of the cells.

LIPID: ENTERAL AND PARENTERAL

Dietary Fat

For some time, the disadvantages of taking fat in the diet have taken precedence over the advantages because of the relationships between dietary fat, increased caloric intake, and obesity, and because of the epidemiologic and experimental animal studies that relate excessive dietary cholesterol intake, or more correctly, cholesterol precursor intake, to acceleration of atherosclerosis [22, 24, 33]. In general, the last decade or so has seen a trend away from foodstuffs rich in cholesterol precursors [24]. However, these arguments have little relevance to the use of fat in the maintenance of patients, whether they be used orally or parenterally, since atherosclerosis is a chronic disease requiring years to become manifest.

In the preparation of food, fat acts primarily as a means of enhancing flavor. Thus, butter or margarine can be added to cooked vegetables, cream is commonly served with desserts, and oils are widely used as dressing for salad. Fats are, of course, frequently used to fry food because this is a particular method of producing an attractive flavor and appearance. Here, there has been a trend away from saturated fat to polyunsaturated fat.

Most edible fat and oils consist largely of triglycerides with a very small fraction of other fats, such as mono- and diglycerides, fatty acids, or phospholipids. In general, it is rare to find completely saturated dietary fat in large amounts. Exceptions to this are beef fat and lard. Chicken fat is less saturated than beef fat, though this will depend, in part, upon the food with which the chickens are fed. Oils, unlike fats, are liquid at room temperature, and they contain more unsaturated fatty acids. In general, the most common saturated fatty acids are stearic, palmitic, and myristic. Oleic acid is the most common unsaturated fatty acid. The principal sources of linoleic acids are vegetable oils. Lard contains a small amount of arachidonic acid.

Most naturally occurring fatty acids are in the *cis* form, with a molecule folded back on itself at the double bond. The *trans* form is, however, produced by hydrogenation of fat or oil. This technique is used to render the fat or oil firmer and more palatable. Margarine is particularly rich in *trans* unsaturated fatty acids compared to butter. These *trans* fatty acids cannot substitute for essential fatty acids in the diet, as they are not metabolized in the same fashion as *cis* fatty acids. The number of double-bond fatty acids in a compound is expressed as the iodine number. The higher the iodine number, the greater the degree of unsaturation. For example, corn oil has a range of 115 to 124, whereas lard has a range of 50 to 65. Methods of animal husbandry may alter quite significantly the fat content of the meat from animals. Thus, the fatty acid content of cow's milk may be altered by controlling the animals' feed.

Human and cow's milk contain about the same amount of fat, but human milk contains more linoleic acid, whereas cow's milk is richer in low-molecular-weight fatty acids. An extensive evaluation of the relative proportions of saturated and unsaturated fats, as well as essential fatty acids, in various foodstuffs may be found in *Fat in Food and Diet,* USDA Agricultural Information Bulletin No. 361 [12].

In addition to changes in the type of fat produced by commercial processing, there are other materials sometimes added to prevent rancidity. It is common to add antioxidants to potato chips, peanut butter, and other fatty food mixtures. Lecithin may also be added because it is an effective emulsifier and improves the palatability.

It is interesting to note that the dietary intake in the United States has changed over the last 70 years. The USDA [12] has produced estimates of nutrient intakes from the turn of the century until today. Figures would indicate that per capita fat consumption per day has increased from 125 gm in the period 1909–1913 to around 159 gm by 1977. In the 1909–1913 period, 83 percent of total fat came from animal sources and only 17 percent from plant sources. By 1977, 33 percent of the total available fat came from meat, fish and poultry while 14 percent came from dairy products, excluding butter. Four percent was produced from eggs, while 39 percent came from fats and oils, including butter. The remainder came from other foods.

Because of the strong emphasis on the relationship between cholesterol and cholesterol precursors in the diet and premature coronary atherosclerosis, dietary alterations have been recommended and supported by a large body of opinion. At present, it is recommended that the typical American diet be reduced in content of cholesterol, total fat, saturated fatty acids, and calories, and the polyunsaturated fatty acid component be increased [33]. The optimal ratio of polyunsaturated to saturated fats is considered to be around one. This has led to emphasis on eating margarine instead of butter, the use of oils for cooking, an increased intake of poultry and fish with less fatty meat, the use of low fat milks and less intake of eggs and total calories. It has recently been demonstrated that cardiovascular mortality has dropped by some 20 percent over the last decade or so. The reason for this decrease is not clear, but it does appear to be a true decline. This decline is unique to a few countries including the United States and Australia. A recent conference convened to assess the implications of this decline, related it to changes in dietary habits of Americans, treatment of hypertension, and possibly to an increasing tendency to more physical activity [19].

Parenteral Administration of Lipids

Parenteral administration of lipids may be necessary on two counts: (1) as a source of essential fatty acids, that is, of fatty acids that the body is unable to synthesize for itself, and (2) as a source of caloric energy. At least one, and possibly two, polyunsaturated fatty acids are essential for proper health maintenance, adequate growth, and cell membrane integrity in the human. The fatty acids involved are linoleic, linolenic, and arachidonic acid. Arachidonic acid is the major essential fatty acid for the human, but since human tissue can convert linoleic to arachidonic acid, linoleic and linolenic can be supplied as the only essential fatty acids necessary in the diet. If dietary supplementation lacks an adequate supply of these polyunsaturated fatty acids, there will be a decrease in linoleic and arachidonic acid and an increase in oleic and eicosatrienoic acids in the plasma. Arachidonic acid has four double bonds and eicosatrienoic has three double bonds. They are classed as tetra- and trienoic compounds, respectively. One test for detecting, at a biochemical level, essential fatty acid deficiency, is the measurement of the ratio of plasma triene to plasma tetraene. The ratio is normally 0.1:0.3 and in severe deficiency can rise as high as 5:0. The clinical consequences of essential fatty acid deficiency were described initially in rats fed a fat-free diet [6]. The animals developed scaly skin, loss of hair, and skin sores. A similar syndrome has been described in human infants, in whom the prominent feature is usually eczematous dermatitis. The syndrome was also reported in subjects who received prolonged parenteral nutrition and in addition who were observed to suffer from poor wound healing. Other reported consequences in experimental animals included decreased fertility, altered cell membrane function, and decreased prostaglandin production. Prostaglandin deficiency due to essential fatty acid deficiency has not been reported in humans to date.* Precise data for assessing the daily requirements of essential fatty acids in man is scanty. Collins et al. considered that a minimum of 7.5 gm of linoleic acid per day was required to correct essential fatty acid deficiency in one particular adult patient [7]. In another study, Jeejeebhoy et al. concluded that the amount of linoleic acid required to prevent essential fatty acid deficiency in a patient who had undergone total small bowel resection was approximately 25 gm per day [20]. A more recent study has suggested that lower requirements may be more accurate. A study by Press et al. involved three adults with essential fatty acid deficiency [30]. They were given 120 mg of linoleic acid by topical application in the form of 230 mg of sunflower oil each day, and this treatment reversed the essential fatty acid deficiency. This implies that the daily requirement for linoleic acid in the adult may be as low as 2 to 3 mg/kg/day. In younger subjects, the generally recommended amount for linoleic acid is 4 percent of the caloric intake. The USDA suggests that 1 to 2 percent of daily caloric intake should be in the form of saturated fat. While the exact human requirements are unknown, it is a relatively simple matter to administer the necessary daily requirements to meet either of the foregoing suggested levels in the human, using parenteral preparations of lipid. One unit of Intralipid or

**Editor's Note:* Prostaglandin deficiency in fat-free total parenteral nutrition has been reported [12a]. Normal plasma concentrations of prostaglandins were obtained when fat was given.

liposyn 10 percent will supply these requirements. Intralipid is composed of 100 gm of soybean oil, while liposyn consists of safflower oil together with 12 gm of egg yolk phospholipids (75 to 80 percent fatty acids), 25 gm of glycerol, and the emulsion suspended in distilled water.

The optimal amount of fat that should be administered to meet caloric requirements in relation to carbohydrate administration is unclear. Fat administration, however, offers significant advantages in the management of the patient dependent on parenteral nutrition. In particular, a high concentration of calories can be given in a relatively small volume of solute, and the calories can be delivered in isosomotic form, thereby greatly reducing problems of thrombophlebitis and sometimes obviating the necessity for placement of central venous catheters. However, lipid emulsions such as Intralipid are irritant to subcutaneous tissues and produce soap deposition if they extravasate. The general tendency of animal and human studies has been to suggest that a certain amount of calories should be given in the form of fat. The evidence for this conclusion rests in part on animal studies showing enhanced growth and weight gain on diets that contain fat, compared to isocaloric diets low or lacking in fat.* In general, few studies have recommended that more than 50 percent of the total daily energy requirements be provided by fat emulsions. Given in high dosage, fat emulsions carry a risk of certain complications, in particular they may induce significant lipemia, particularly in premature infants, in whom the necessary lipolytic mechanisms may be unable to deal with a concentrated load of substrate.

In a one-week-old infant, approximately 50 percent of the total caloric intake is obtained as fat from human milk. On this basis, many young infants, particularly premature infants, have been treated with fairly high doses of Intralipid or its equivalent, by both the intragastric and the parenteral routes, and significant weight gain and salvage of at-risk subjects has been reported.* When fat emulsions are given by the parenteral route, they are broken down and degraded by lipoprotein lipase and fed down the metabolic pathway that normally deals with chylomicrons. Care should be taken not to overload the system, and it is a relatively simple matter to observe plasma samples for the presence of lipemia or to measure the plasma total triglyceride in the laboratory. The rate of clearance of emulsion lipid is probably slowed in preterm infants and appears to be accelerated by fasting. In general, it appears advisable to keep the plasma triglyceride levels below 250 mg/100 ml. A further conclusion from this general guideline is that subjects with abnormalities of lipid and lipoprotein metabolism may be at particular risk from the complications of parenteral lipid administration. Thus a subject with type I hyperlipoproteinemia who lacks lipoprotein lipase and routinely has hyperchylomicronemia will rapidly develop severe hyperlipidemia following parenteral administration of lipid, and this hyperlipidemia will persist for hours. The particular problem with high circulating levels of lipid particles is the precipitation of acute abdominal pain or frank acute pancreatitis. Other abnormalities attributed to the use of this material include abnormalities of lung perfusion, subnormal lipase levels, and derangement of the clotting system. Subjects with type V hyperlipoproteinemia who have defective clearance rates of triglyceride are probably similarly at risk, and subjects with type IV hyperlipoproteinemia may also be at risk, though this is less certain.

Following infusion of Intralipid, the removal of infused triglyceride follows an exponential curve. If very high doses are given (e.g., >500 mg/kg), removal is delayed significantly. Administration of Intralipid intravenously has been used in a test devised by Boberg to measure lipo-

**Editor's Note:* Some recent animal studies suggest that between 15 and 50% of calories as intravenous fat may enhance hepatic protein synthesis [6a]. Similar studies utilizing oral intake have also been published [28a].

**Editor's Note:* Infants may be capable of utilizing such high amounts of fat because infants consist largely of viscera, which utilize fat as a caloric source.

protein lipase activity [3]. The enzyme is activated by an intravenous dose of heparin, which releases the enzyme into the circulation as well as activating it; a fixed amount of Intralipid per kg is given; and the clearance rate is measured as the clearance of turbidity due to the induced particulate lipemia. Some studies suggest that heparin should be given to enhance the uptake of administered lipid, but heparin increases plasma free-fatty acid levels and, if given in large doses, may lead to bleeding problems. In general, heparin administration is not usually necessary, and if it is considered to be required, a relatively small amount is needed.

There is only scanty evidence [13] that long-term administration results in serious accumulation of lipid material in the body, and the few studies available show no evidence of long-term complications such as carcinoma. Some complications that were reported in the earlier days of the use of lipid emulsions, such as the so-called overloading syndrome, or deposition of fat pigment in hepatic Kupffer cells, appear to be specific for particular emulsions and are not encountered in current usage [28]. Lipid emulsions have been used in subjects with diabetes mellitus, various hepatic diseases, and blood coagulation defects. There is little evidence of significant toxic effects in these situations, but careful monitoring of serum parameters, particularly by hepatic function tests, is strongly advisable.

Care should be taken to store solutions such as Intralipid correctly. Maintenance of strict asepsis is essential, and prolonged contact with infusion sets should be avoided to prevent leaching of plasticizers by the fat solution.

REFERENCES

1. Ballas, S. K., and Krasnow, S. H. Structure of erythrocyte membrane and its transport functions. *Ann. Clin. Lab. Sci.* 10:209, 1980.
2. Bloch, K., and Vance, D. Control mechanisms in the synthesis of saturated fatty acids. *Annu. Rev. Biochem.* 46:263, 1977.
3. Boberg, J., and Hallberg, D. The intravenous fat tolerance test. *Scand. J. Clin. Lab. Invest.* 24:47, 1969.
4. van den Bosch, H. Phosphoglyceride metabolism. *Annu. Rev. Biochem.* 43:243, 1974.
5. Bremner, W. F., and Third, J. L. H. C. The hyperlipoproteinemias and atherosclerosis. Current understanding of their interrelationships (Monograph). New York: Eden Press/Churchill Livingstone, 1979.
6. Burr, G. O., and Burr, M. M. New deficiency disease produced by rigid exclusion of fat from the diet. *J. Biol. Chem.* 82:345, 1929.

6a. Buzby, G. P., Mullen, J. L., Stein, T. P., et al. Optimal TPN caloric substrate for correction of protein malnutrition. *Surg. Forum* 30:64, 1979.

7. Collins, F. D., et al. Plasma lipids in human linoleic deficiency. *Nutr. Metab.* 13:150, 1971.
8. Cooper, R. A. Lipids of human red cell membrane. Natural composition and variability in disease. *Semin. Hematol.* 7:920, 1970.
9. Cooper, R. A. Abnormalities of cell membrane fluidity in the pathogenesis of disease. *N. Engl. J. Med.* 297:371, 1977.
10. Davson, H., and Danielli, J. F. *The Permeability of Natural Membranes.* Cambridge: Cambridge University Press, 1952.
11. Eisenberg, S., and Levy, R. I. Lipoprotein metabolism. *Adv. Lipid Res.* 12:1, 1975.
12. Food and Nutrition Board, Committee on Dietary Allowances, Committee on Interpretation of Recommended Dietary Allowances. *Recommended Dietary Allowances.* NAS-NRC: Washington, DC, 1974.

12a. Freund, H., Floman, N., Schwartz, B., and Fischer, J. E. Essential fatty acid deficiency in total parenteral nutrition. *Ann. Surg.* 190:139, 1979.

13. Freund, U., et al. Iatrogenic lipidosis following prolonged intravenous hyperalimentation. *Am. J. Clin. Nutr.* 28:1156, 1975.
14. Goldstein, J. L., and Brown, M. S. The low-density lipoprotein pathway and its relation to atherosclerosis. *Annu. Rev. Biochem.* 46:897, 1977.
15. Greville, G. D., and Tubbs, P. K. The Catabolism of Long Chain Fatty Acids in Mammalian Tissues. In P. N. Campbell and G. D. Greville (Eds.), *Essays in Biochemistry.* New York: Academic, 1968. Vol. 4.
16. Guidotti, G. The composition of biological membranes. *Arch. Intern. Med.* 129:194, 1972.
17. Guy, P., Law, S., and Hardie, G. Mammalian fatty acid synthetase. *FEBS Lett.* 96:33, 1978.
18. Harper, H. A., Rodwell, V. W., and Mayes, P. A. *Review of Physiological Chemistry.* Los Altos, CA: Lange, 1979.
19. Havlik, R. J., and Feinleib, M. *Proceedings of the conference on the decline in coronary heart*

disease mortality. NIH Publication No. 79-1010. Bethesda, MD, 1979.
20. Jeejeebhoy, K. N., et al. Total parenteral nutrition at home for 23 months without complication and with good rehabilitation. A study of technical and metabolic features. *Gastroenterology* 65:811, 1973.
21. Kashyap, M. L., et al. The role of high density lipoprotein apolipoprotein C_{II} in triglyceride metabolism. *Lipids* 13:933, 1978.
22. Keys, A. Coronary heart disease—the global picture. *Atherosclerosis* 22:149, 1975.
23. *Lancet* Editorial. 1:964, 1980.
24. Levy, R. I., et al. *Nutrition, Lipids and Coronary Heart Disease. A Global View*. New York: Raven Press, 1979.
25. Lieber, C. S., et al. Differences in hepatic and metabolic changes after acute and chronic alcohol consumption. *Fed. Proc.* 34:2060, 1975.
26. Masotti, G., et al. Differential inhibition of prostacyelin production and platelet aggregation by aspirin. *Lancet* 2:1213, 1979.
27. Morrisett, J. D., Jackson, R. L., and Gotto, A. M., Jr. Lipoproteins: Structure and function. *Annu. Rev. Biochem.* 44:183, 1975.
28. Mueller, J. F., and Viteri, F. E. Clinical studies in patients receiving long-term infusions of fat emulsions. *J. Okla. State Med. Assoc.* 53:367, 1960.
28a. Munro, H. N., Naismith, D. J., and Wikramanayake, T. W. Influence of energy intake on ribonucleic acid metabolism. *J. Biochem.* 54: 198, 1953.
29. Pareti, F. I., Mannucci, P. M., and D'Angelo, A. Congenital deficiency of thromboxane and prostacyclin. *Lancet* 1:898, 1980.
30. Press, M., Hartop, P. J., and Protley, C. Correction of essential fatty acid deficiency in man by the cutaneous administration of sunflower-seed oil. *Lancet* 1:597, 1974.
31. Ramsay, R. F. The role of carnitine, the carnitine acyltransferases and the carnitine exchange system. *Biochem. Soc. Trans.* 6:72, 1978.
32. Ramwell, P. W. *The Prostaglandins*. New York: Plenum, 1973-1979.
33. Rifkind, B. M., Goor, R. S., and Levy, R. I. Current status of the role of dietary treatment in the prevention of and management of coronary heart disease. *Med. Clin. North Am.* 63: 911, 1979.
34. Rifkind, B. M., and Levy, R. I. *Hyperlipidemia: Diagnosis and Therapy*. New York: Grune & Stratton, 1977.
35. Rommel, K., and Bohmer, R. *Lipid Absorption: Biochemical and Clinical Aspects*. Baltimore: University Park Press, 1976.
36. Rothman, J. E., and Lenard, J. Membrane asymmetry. *Science* 195:743, 1979.
37. Samuelsson, E., et al. Prostaglandins. *Annu. Rev. Biochem.* 47:997, 1978.
38. Scanu, A. M., and Wisdom, C. Serum lipoproteins: Structure and function. *Annu. Rev. Biochem.* 41:703, 1972.
39. Senior, J. R. Intestinal absorption of fats. *J. Lipid Res.* 5:495, 1964.
40. Singer, S. J., and Nicholson, G. L. The fluid mosaic model of the structure of cell membranes. *Science* 175:720, 1972.
41. Slack, J. Risks of ischaemic heart disease in familial hyperlipoproteinaemic states. *Lancet* 2:1380, 1969.
42. Smith, L. C., Pownall, H. J., and Gotto, A. M., Jr., The plasma lipoproteins: Structure and metabolism. *Annu. Rev. Biochem.* 47:751, 1978.
43. Spector, A. A. Fatty acid binding to plasma albumin. *J. Lipid Res.* 16:165, 1975.
44. Stanbury, J. B., Wyngaarden, J. B., and Frederickson, D. S. *The Metabolic Basis of Inherited Disease* (4th ed.). New York: McGraw-Hill, 1978.
45. Sweeney, C. C. *Chemistry and Metabolism of Sphingolipids*. Amsterdam: North Holland, 1970.
46. Taylor, W. *The Hepatobiliary System*. New York: Plenum, 1972.
47. Volk, B., and Schneck, L. *Sphingolipids, Sphingolipidoses and Allied Disorders*. New York: Plenum, 1972.
48. Volpe, J. J., and Vagelos, P. R. Mechanisms and regulation of biosynthesis of saturated fatty acids. *Physiol. Rev.* 56:339, 1976.
49. White, A., et al. *Principles of Biochemistry* (6th ed.). New York: McGraw-Hill, 1978.

8

Vitamins*

Bengt Jeppsson
Zvi Gimmon

A vitamin may be broadly defined as a substance that is essential in minute amounts for the maintenance of normal metabolic functions, but cannot be synthesized by the body and therefore must be furnished from an exogenous source. The importance of vitamins for maintenance of metabolic functions in response to stress, trauma, or sepsis; or in the presence of certain degrees of protein-calorie malnutrition; or in different degrees of hepatic and renal failure cannot be overemphasized.

The routine use of vitamins in parenteral nutrition formulas is well established, although needs are less well known. The dosage frequency and routes of administration are different for the water-soluble and fat-soluble vitamins. Requirements for vitamins change with different underlying conditions, which may result in increased requirements for vitamins as well as decreased tolerance.

In the following discussion, the different aspects of the use of vitamins in nutritional support and parenteral nutrition will be reviewed.

WATER-SOLUBLE VITAMINS

B-Complex

THIAMINE (VITAMIN B_1)

Recognition of vitamin B_1 activity dates back to 1890, when the Dutch physician Eijkman observed that chickens fed a diet consisting mainly of polished rice developed polyneuritic symptoms similar to those common to beriberi patients. Subsequent studies showed that these symptoms could be relieved by adding rice polishings to the diet. Some time later, Funk isolated from rice polishings and yeast a crystalline substance that was effective in the prevention and cure of experimental beriberi. The compound was believed to be an amine and was essential to life. Therefore, Funk called the substance vitamine. In 1926, vitamin B_1 was isolated in crystalline form by Jansen and Donath, and in 1926 Williams determined its structure [46].

**Editor's Note:* Although knowledge of vitamins has increased in the past decades, our knowledge of altered metabolism and requirements remains marginal at best. In this chapter, the authors have developed a rationale for needs during nutritional repletion and TPN. These are admittedly imprecise, but the reader should be able to derive enough information to draw independent conclusions.

Chemistry. Thiamine is a complex organic molecule containing a pyrimidine and a thiazole nucleus. The pyrimidine structure is common in nature, but the thiazole nucleus is unique and appears, so far as is known, only in thiamine. Thiamine carries out its function in the body in the form of the coenzyme thiamine pyrophosphate [46].

Source. Thiamine is found in yeast, rice husk, and wheat germ (which contain more than 1 mg/100 gm), but many fruits and vegetables also contain thiamine. Small amounts of vitamin B_1 are also found in meats, but liver and kidney are particularly rich in thiamine. Freezing does not affect the vitamin, but prolonged cooking destroys a large portion of food's vitamin content [46, 116].

Diet is not the only source of vitamin B_1. Some normal intestinal saprophytes (e.g., *Bacillus bifidus*) synthesize large amounts of the vitamin, which may be reabsorbed by the intestines. The availability of this source, however, has been questioned [46].

Function. The primary function of thiamine is to act as a cofactor for three enzymes involved in carbohydrate metabolism (pyruvate dehydrogenase, α-ketoglutarate dehydrogenase, and transketolase). Possibly the most important function of thiamine pyrophosphate (TPP) is in oxidative decarboxylation of α-keto acids, pyruvate, and α-ketoglutarate, as well as in the utilization of pentose in the hexose monophosphate shunt. In animal cells the coenzyme thus plays a critical role in the attainment of energy. In thiamine deficiency the oxidation of α-keto acids is impaired, with increased plasma concentration of pyruvic acid one of the diagnostic signs of the deficiency state. An additional important TPP requiring enzyme in plants and animals is transketolase. The measurement of transketolase activity in erythrocytes is also used as a diagnostic test for thiamine deficiency.

Thiamine pyrophosphate is also used in protein metabolism, e.g., during decarboxylation of ketoacid analogues of branched-chain amino acids [46, 74]. Besides the function as a coenzyme, several studies support a specific role of thiamine in neurophysiology. It has been demonstrated that TPP is involved in the metabolism and function of excitable membranes, although the precise mechanism of action is not known [6].

Thiamine also has a role in the conversion of the amino acid tryptophan to nicotinic acid and nicotinamide [3].

Absorption, Metabolic Fate, Excretion. Absorption of thiamine occurs in the duodenum and small intestine by two mechanisms. At high concentration thiamine is absorbed by passive diffusion, whereas at low or physiologic concentrations it is absorbed by an active process [91]. Alcohol often depresses thiamine absorption, and this may be related to a folic acid deficiency as well [54].

The maximum daily absorption of thiamine is 8 to 15 mg. Absorption following intramuscular administration is rapid and complete. Serum levels of thiamine range from 25 to 72 ng/ml in normal individuals. The best assay for determining metabolically active thiamine in man is a microbiologic assay method utilizing *Ochromonas danica* [5]. As with most of the water-soluble vitamins, the body is unable to store thiamine in any great quantity. The adult human body contains about 30 mg of thiamine. Approximately 1 mg of thiamine per day is completely degraded by the tissues, and this amount is roughly the minimal daily requirement. Thiamine is excreted in the urine. The administration of diuretics may cause excessive loss of the vitamin in the urine [42].

Deficiency. A thiamine deficiency in animals and humans is called *beriberi.* There is impairment of nervous, cardiovascular, and gastrointestinal systems. In the Western world the disease is rarely seen except in alcoholics, food faddism, and sometimes in the malabsorption syndromes. Clinically, beriberi presents a spectrum of manifestations. Their presence seems, in part, to be determined by the chronicity of the deficiency, its severity, and stress factors. Thus, individuals subsisting on a thiamine intake of 0.2 to 0.3 mg/1000 kcal, which is slightly less than the thiamine requirement, may gradually become depleted and develop peripheral neuropathy. Paresthesia, hyperesthesia, anesthesia, formication, and weakness are experienced. The muscles are often tender and may atrophy. Fatigue, decreased attention span, and impaired capacity to work are striking. This type of beriberi is called dry beriberi.

If the patient has been subsisting on less than 0.2 mg of thiamine per 1000 kcal, the deficiency is more severe, and he will develop wet beriberi. In addition to neurologic manifestations, cardiovascular signs appear. Dependent edema may be seen. The heart is often enlarged and the patient complains of palpitation and precordial pain. Digestive disturbances with anorexia and constipation commonly occur. Fulminant cardiac failure may be precipitated by physiologic stress in the aforementioned types of patients [3, 42, 45]. The most acute type of thiamine deficiency, Wernicke's encephalopathy, occurs primarily in alcoholics, but has recently also been described in several cases of severe malnutrition or in patients with total parenteral nutrition (TPN) with inadequate vitamin B_1 administration [8, 45, 63, 73, 75]. Manifestations range from mild confusion to coma.

A third type of beriberi is infantile beriberi, which is rarely seen in the Western world. The clinical onset may appear as acute cardiac failure in a previously healthy-appearing child. In other babies, the signs may be primarily neurologic, with aphonia or features suggestive of meningitis [74].

Toxicity. True toxicity of thiamine has not been described in the human. Intravenous doses of 500 mg have been well tolerated by thiamine-deficient individuals [74]. In rare instances, however, 100 mg or less thiamine has caused nearly fatal anaphylactic-type reaction. The nature of this toxicity or so-called thiamine shock is not understood [51].

Human Requirements. Thiamine requirement is a function of metabolic rate. The minimal requirement in humans approximates 0.33 mg/1000 kcal. However, to provide a margin of safety the National Research Council recommends a daily allowance of 0.5 mg/1000 kcal [38] (Table 8-1). The recommended daily intakes of thiamine for infants and children are: 0 to 6 mo, 0.3 mg; 6 mo to 1 yr, 0.5 mg; 1 to 3 yr, 0.7 mg; 4 to 6 yr, 0.9 mg; 7 to 10 yr, 1.2 mg; boys 11 to 14 yr, 1.4 mg; and girls 11 to 14 yr, 1.2 mg (Table 8-1).

There is an increased demand for thiamine in conditions with hypermetabolism, e.g., febrile conditions, hyperthyroidism, and trauma [42].

Determinations of thiamine levels in patients with chronic renal failure have shown normal values [62]. Little is known about thiamine turnover in these patients, but the recommended daily allowance of thiamine for normal subjects is probably adequate.

Requirements During TPN. Since thiamine is necessary for decarboxylation of α-keto acids, its requirement is directly proportional to the percentage of carbohydrate in the diet. Fat and protein have a thiamine-sparing effect. Since TPN in this country often is based on carbohydrate as the main caloric source, increased requirements for thiamine may be seen during TPN [42, 45]. A carbohydrate load can precipitate Wernicke's encephalopathy in the thiamine-deficient individual because of the prompt consumption of the remaining vitamin as a cofactor in the carbohydrate metabolism [8, 63, 73, 75]. In three studies in patients undergoing TPN, thiamine status was evaluated by determining the erythrocyte transketolase activity [9, 61, 107a]. In one study [61], a daily administration of 5 mg thiamine to patients on TPN was found sufficient. In another study [9], 50 mg thiamine was given daily to critically ill surgical patients. This dose raised the erythrocyte transketolase

Table 8-1. *Water-Soluble Vitamin Requirements during TPN*

	RDA[a]			Recommended Daily Doses during TPN[b]			Suggested Composition for Intravenous Multivitamin Preparation for Daily Maintenance of Adequate Vitamin Status[c]	
Vitamin	Infants	Children 1–10	Adults	Infants	Children 1–10	Adults	Infancy to 10 Years	Adults
Thiamine B_1 (mg)	0.3–0.5	0.7–1.2	1.0–1.5	1.2–10	1.2–10	1.2–50	1.2	3.0
Niacin (mg)	5–8	9–16	12–20	8–20	8–20	10–150	17.0	40.0
Riboflavin B_2 (mg)	0.4–0.6	0.8–1.2	1.1–1.8	0.6	2.0	1.8–10	1.4	3.6
Pantothenic acid B_3 (mg)				3–6	3–6	5–25	5.0	15.0
Biotin (μg)				0–20	0–20	0–200	20.0	60.0
Pyridoxine B_6 (mg)	0.3–0.4	0.6–1.2	1.6–2.0	0.4–3.0	0.4–3.0	2.0–15.0	1.0	4.0
Folic acid (μg)	50	100–300	400	100–140	100–140	200–5000	140.0	400.0
Vitamin B_{12} (μg)	0.3	1.0–2.0	3.0	0.7–2.0	0.7–2.0	2–50	1.0	5.0
Ascorbic acid (mg) vitamin C	35	40	45	35–100	35–100	30–700	80.0	100.0

[a]From Food and Nutrition Board [38].
[b]From Bradley et al. [9], Broviac and Scribner [12], Dudrick et al. [29], Gruppo and Fraham [47], Jeejeebhoy et al. [57], Kishi et al. [61], Lorch and Lay [70], Lowry et al. [71], Nichoalds, Meng, and Caldwell [77], Shils [99], and Stromberg et al. [107a].
[c]From American Medical Association [2], and Nutritional Advisory Group on Total Parenteral Nutrition [78].
Source: RDA on vitamins from *Recommended Daily Allowances,* 8th ed., Publication No. 2216, National Academy of Sciences, 1974; and Table on recommended doses of vitamins during TPN from Nutritional Advisory Group: Vitamin preparations for parenteral use, Appendix A in symposium of Total Parenteral Nutrition. Chicago: AMA, 1972. Pp. 457–464.

activity, indicating its adequacy for these patients. There were no signs of toxicity. In the third study [107A], 2 of 39 patients requiring TPN for postsurgical complications became deficient 7 and 17 days after the start of TPN. The daily dose of vitamin B_1 in this study was 1.2 mg.

The Nutrition Advisory Group of the American Medical Association, Department of Food and Nutrition [2, 78], recommends a daily intake of 3.0 mg thiamine for adults and 1.2 mg from infancy to 11 years (Table 8-1).

Several centers recommend daily doses of 10 to 50 mg vitamin B_1 for patients undergoing TPN [12, 29, 47, 57, 77, 99] and 1.2 to 10 mg in children [70] (Table 8-1). Our current practice is to administer 15 mg thiamine daily. Patients with acute renal failure receiving TPN with essential amino acids receive 50 mg thiamine daily [1]. In the presence of significant liver disease, we administer 50 mg thiamine daily. In this group we also supplement folate and vitamin B_{12} immediately in the course of TPN, since the combination of deficiencies is common [40, 74]. In cases of deficiency, 50 to 100 mg thiamine should be administered daily intramuscularly or intravenously. This dose usually results in reversal of neurologic symptoms within hours. This initial treatment should then be followed by the regular daily dose [42, 46].

Preparations and Incompatibility. Thiamine hydrochloride is a part of all multivitamin preparations (see Table 8-2). It is compatible in amino acid and dextrose solutions with electrolytes [95].

Niacin (Nicotinic Acid, Nicotinamide)

Pellagra was recognized as early as 1735 by Don Gaspar Casal, physician to King Philip V of Spain. Although largely unknown in the United States until the twentieth century, as many as 170,000 cases of pellagra were reported annually from 1910 to 1935 in the southeastern part of the United States. Pellagra was established as a deficiency disease by Joseph Goldberger, who also recognized its similarity to canine black tongue, and it was thought to result from an inadequate intake of vitamin B_2. This observation made possible the identification of nicotinic acid as the responsible factor by Elvehjem, Woolley, and their associates in 1937 [3, 46]. Nicotinic acid and nicotinamide are biologically equivalent as vitamins, and both are referred to as niacin, which is the official designation for this vitamin [46]. Niacin is unique as a vitamin in that it can be synthesized by the liver. Its precursor is the essential amino acid tryptophan.

Chemistry. Niacin is β-pyridine carboxylic acid. This is easily converted to the physiologically active nicotinic acid amide (nicotinamide) [46].

Source. Niacin is widely distributed in plants and in animal foods, but in most cases in small amounts. Meat products, particularly liver, are the richest dietary sources. Milk and eggs are almost devoid of niacin; their pellagra-preventive action is probably related to their tryptophan content. Milling procedures used in production of white flour remove most of the niacin, which is replaced by the addition of synthetic nicotinic acid. The human body has the ability to convert tryptophan to niacin. It is believed that about 60 mg dietary tryptophan is equivalent to 1 mg niacin. Diets in the United States often contain 600 mg or more tryptophan, and this provides a substantial contribution to the niacin pool [3].

Function. Niacin carries out its function in the body by being converted either into niacin adenine dinucleotide (NAD) or niacin adenine dinucleotide phosphate (NADP). These participate in oxidation-reduction reactions in cooperation with a large number of dehydrogenases, and thus serve as part of intracellular respiratory mechanism of all cells. They are involved in glycolysis, aerobic oxidation, fatty acid oxidation, and glucuronide, pyrimidine, amino acid, and steroid biosynthesis. Therefore, it is not surprising that niacin deficiency leads to a complex pathologic picture [46, 74, 116]. In addition to these reactions, pharmacologic doses of nicotinic acid (but

Table 8-2. *Some Multivitamin Preparations for Parenteral Use*

Vitamin	MVI-12 USV Laboratories (Vial 1; 5 ml)	MVI-12 USV Laboratories (Vial 2; 5 ml)	MVI USV Laboratories (10 ml; 5 ml conc)	Berroca-C Roche (2 ml)	Bejectal Abbott (10 ml)	Bejectal-C Abbott (10 ml)	Bejex Abbott (5 ml)	Betalin Complex Lilly (1 ml)	Betalin Complex/Fortified C Lilly (1 ml)	Folbesyn Lederle (2 ml)	Solu B with C Upjohn (2 ml)
Vitamin A (IU)	3,300		10,000								
Vitamin D (IU)	200		1,000								
Vitamin E (IU)	10		5								
Vitamin C (mg)	100		500	100		1,000	500		75.0	300	500
Thiamine (B_1) (mg)	3.0		50	10	100	200	10	5	12.5	10	10
Riboflavin (B_2) (mg)	3.6		10	10	20	30	10	2	3.0	10	10
Niacin (mg)	40.0		100	80	750	750	250	75	50	75	250
Pyridoxine (B_6) (mg)	4.0		15	20	50	50	5	5	5	15	5
Pantothenic acid (mg)	15.0		25	20	50	50	50	2.5	2.5	10	50
Biotin (mcg)		60		0.2							
Vitamin B_{12} (mcg)		5				20	25	2.5		15	
Folic acid (mcg)		400								1,000	

not the amide) have two other actions for which the mechanism has not been clearly defined: peripheral vasodilation and a tendency toward reduction of serum cholesterol levels.

Absorption, Metabolic Fate, Excretion. Niacin is readily absorbed from all portions of the intestinal tract and from parenteral sites of administration. The vitamin is distributed in all tissues. Normal serum levels of niacin range from 3.5 to 7.0 μg/ml. Deficiency levels are below 2.8 [5]. Several microbial assay methods for niacin are used, employing *Lactobacillus plantarum* and *Tetrahymena thermophila.*

When therapeutic doses of niacin are administered, only small amounts of the unchanged vitamin appear in the urine. When extremely high doses of the vitamin are given, the unchanged vitamin represents the major urinary component. Excretion of niacin takes place after hepatic conversion of NAD to N′-methyl niacinamide (N′-ME) and N′-methyl-3-pyridone-5-carboxylamide (2-pyridone). Measurement of excretion in urine of these two metabolites is also used in assessment of niacin nutriture [74].

Deficiency. Lack of niacin in the diet may lead to pellagra. Early, mild niacin deficiency may have as its only manifestation redness of the tongue with a slight atrophy or hypertrophy of the papillae.

Pellagra is characterized by signs and symptoms involving skin, gastrointestinal tract, and central nervous system.

The skin lesions consist of erythematous cutaneous eruptions resembling sunburn. Blebs and blisters may develop. The dermatitis is symmetrical and is most often found on the face and neck, back of the hand, and forearm. The chief symptoms referable to the digestive tract are stomatitis, enteritis, and diarrhea. The tongue becomes very red and swollen and may ulcerate. Diarrhea is recurrent. Stools are watery and may occasionally be bloody.

The psychic manifestations are variable. Early findings are anxiety, irritability, and depression. In more advanced deficiency, confusion, disorientation, delusions, and hallucinations may appear. As the disease progresses, delirium ensues, and the patient may die in coma.

A syndrome of acute encephalopathy with clouding of consciousness and motor abnormalities has been described that appears to be due to acute severe niacin deficiency. It has been observed in malnourished subjects following intravenous administration of glucose without concomitant administration of niacin [42].

Diet-induced pellagra is now seen in the United States largely in chronic alcoholics, food faddists, and patients with malabsorption. It is also occasionally seen in patients with neoplasms or prolonged febrile illness [74].

Alterations in the metabolic pathways of niacin and tryptophan may produce secondary pellagra. In functional carcinoid syndrome, some patients develop pellagra presumably because of the deviation of significant amounts of ingested tryptophan into serotonin production [42]. Pellagra is also seen in patients receiving isoniazid, which is thought to interfere with the conversion of tryptophan to niacin [45].

Toxicity. Niacin is essentially nontoxic. Toxic effects of nicotinic acid when used in large doses (3 to 10 gm/day) for hyperlipemia induce flushing, dryness of the skin, dizziness and nausea. Common gastrointestinal complaints are diarrhea, abdominal pain, and aggravation of symptoms of peptic ulcer [74]. The most common serious toxicities are abnormal liver function and jaundice, which are reversible at discontinuation of the drug [110, 120].

Human Requirements. Since the dietary requirement can be satisfied not only by niacin, but also by tryptophan, the requirement is influenced by the quantity and the quality of dietary protein. The minimal requirement of niacin (including that formed from tryptophan) to prevent pellagra averages 4.4 mg/1000 kcal [46]. As noted, an average of 60 mg tryptophan is converted to 1 mg niacin, but this equivalence varies from individual to individual, e.g., the conversion is reduced in diabetics and increased in pregnant women and those taking oral contraceptives [116]. It should be noted that a simple approximation of the tryptophan content of a protein can be made by assuming that one percent of the protein is tryptophan.

There are few data on the niacin requirements of children from infancy through adolescence.

The RDA is 6.6 mg/1000 kcal or not less than 12 mg at caloric intakes of less than 2000 kcal [38] (see Table 8-1). Corresponding doses for infants are 5 to 8 mg and for children 9 to 16 mg [70].

Requirements During TPN. There is little information available on increased requirements for niacin in different diseases or during TPN. The Nutrition Advisory Group on Total Parenteral Nutrition [2, 78] recommends 17 mg niacin from infancy to 11 years and 40 mg for adults (see Table 8-1).

Most centers recommend daily doses of 20 to 150 mg of niacin to patients undergoing TPN [51, 57, 61, 77, 99] (see Table 8-1). No instances of pellagra have been reported using these doses during long-term parenteral nutrition. Acute niacin deficiency has been seen in malnourished patients following intravenous administration of glucose, as noted.

We use 100 mg niacin daily in patients on standard TPN. The same doses are used for patients in acute renal failure and liver failure [1, 40].

In acute pellagra, it is customary to give 300 to 500 mg niacin per day. Niacin should be administered orally if possible, since that is the most efficient route. In the treatment of mild deficiency, administration of 50 mg niacin three times daily should be sufficient [42].

Preparations and Interaction. All multivitamin preparations contain niacin in amounts well above the RDA and the recommendations by the AMA [2, 38, 78] (Table 8-2). There are no reports of incompatibilities of niacin in TPN solutions [95].

RIBOFLAVIN (VITAMIN B_2)

In 1879, Blythe, an English chemist, extracted a yellow pigment from milk. Its physiologic significance was not appreciated at that time. At a later date similarly pigmented compounds were isolated from a variety of sources and designated as flavins. It was soon demonstrated that these various flavins were identical in chemical composition. In the meantime, water-soluble vitamin B had been separated into a heat-labile antiberiberi factor and a heat-stable growth-promoting factor. The two factors were called vitamins B_1 and B_2. The heat-stable fraction did not have the antipellagra properties ascribed to vitamin B_2, e.g., curing black tongue in dogs, and it was clear, therefore, that this factor was just another of several factors present in the heat-stable fraction of the B-complex. In 1935, riboflavin was synthesized by two independent groups, Kuhn and his colleagues in Heidelberg and Karrers' group in Basel [3, 46, 116].

Chemistry. The riboflavin molecule consists of an isoalloxazine nucleus with a ribityl side-chain attached to the middle ring (6,7-dimethyl-9-(dl'-ribityl)isoalloxazine). It is water-soluble, especially in acid solutions, and heat stable, but is easily decomposed by light [3, 116].

Source. Riboflavin is widely distributed in plant and animal tissue. The best food sources include milk, eggs, liver, kidney, heart, and green leafy vegetables. Fortunately, the relative heat stability of riboflavin in the absence of light favors its preservation in ordinary cooking procedures [3].

Function. Riboflavin carries out its functions in the body in the form of one or the other of two coenzymes, riboflavin-5'-phosphate (called mononucleotide, FMN) and flavin adenine dinucleotide (FAD). The riboflavin coenzymes are essential parts of a number of oxidative enzyme systems involved in electron transport. These include the amino acid oxidases, xanthine oxidase, the succinic dehydrogenase complex, glutathione reductase, and many others. It is axiomatic that cellular growth cannot evolve in the absence of riboflavin [3, 116].

Absorption, Metabolic Fate, Excretion. Riboflavin is readily absorbed from the upper gastrointestinal tract, but the rate of this process is reduced in patients with hepatitis or hepatic cirrhosis and in those receiving probenecid. The vitamin is also readily absorbed following parenteral administration [46]. Circulating riboflavin values range from 100 to 500 ng/ml in normal individuals. Values below 80 ng/ml are seen in deficiency states [5].

Several chemical assays of riboflavin are used, relying on the fluorescence of riboflavin; paper and column chromatography [5] are also used.

The vitamin is distributed in all tissues, but little is stored. The liver and kidney usually contain more than other tissues. Excretion of riboflavin is by the urine, although some is eliminated in bile and recirculated via enterohepatic circulation. Urinary excretion is quantitatively variable and is affected by nutritional intake and disease. In conditions such as acute starvation or trauma, urinary excretion is increased, but the increased excretion is temporary because of depletion of riboflavin stores [74]. Riboflavin is always present in the feces and probably represents vitamin synthesized by intestinal microorganisms. There is no evidence that this riboflavin can be absorbed [46]. During intravenous administration there is an increased loss from urinary excretion as compared to oral administration of the vitamin. The same holds true for vitamin B_6 (pyridoxine) [45].

Deficiency. Riboflavin deficiency is characterized by cheilosis, angular stomatitis, seborrheic dermatitis, and glossitis. Ocular symptoms have also been described. Cheilosis begins with redness and denudation of the lips along the line of closure. Fissures may develop. The seborrheic dermatitis has a red, scaly, greasy appearance and often involves the areas around the nose, mouth, ears, and eyes. The glossitis is indistinguishable from that seen with deficiency of niacin, folic acid, or vitamin B_{12}. Riboflavin deficiency may also lead to anemia, which is normochromic and normocytic; this is associated with diminished reticulocytosis [46].

The problem in the clinical recognition of riboflavin deficiency is that most of the symptoms may be seen with deficiencies of other vitamins as well. Recognition of riboflavin deficiency is also difficult because it rarely occurs as an isolated finding.

Riboflavin deficiency is relatively common in all parts of the world, and occurs primarily as the result of an inadequate dietary intake. It is frequently observed in association with pellagra.

Deficiency is more frequent during periods of physiologic stress, such as rapid growth in childhood, or during pregnancy and lactation. It may be the result of pathologic stress, including burns, surgical procedures, and other types of trauma. It occurs also in chronic debilitating illness and malignancy [42].

Toxicity. Toxicity to riboflavin has not been demonstrated in man or animals. Equivalent doses of 20 gm/day for a man have been administered to animals without any apparent toxic effects [74].

Human Requirements. The requirement for riboflavin is fairly closely related to energy expenditure, but is also markedly affected by alterations in nitrogen balance. The requirement for riboflavin is increased during periods of stress, such as trauma, burns, or debilitating illnesses and malignancies, as already mentioned. Patients with second- and third-degree burns excrete twice the normal intake of riboflavin [116]. It is assumed that the increased excretion results from decreased utilization and that the massive nitrogen loss that occurs in extensive burns is responsible for the decreased vitamin consumption.

The minimal requirement for riboflavin to prevent clinical signs of deficiency appears to be about 0.3 mg/1000 kcal [46]. To provide a margin of safety, the Food and Nutrition Board of the National Research Council recommends a somewhat higher riboflavin allowance, which is calculated on the basis of metabolic body size [38]. The RDAs are 0.4 to 0.6 mg for infants, 0.8 to 1.2 mg for children, and 1.1 to 1.8 mg for adults (see Table 8-1).

Elevated plasma levels of riboflavin have been reported in patients undergoing hemodialysis. There is considerable loss during dialysis, suggesting that the recommended daily allowance for riboflavin is adequate [62]. Treatment of riboflavin deficiency consists of daily administration of 1 to 3 mg of the vitamin to infants and children and 10 to 20 mg to adults [74].

Requirements During TPN. The Nutrition Advisory Group on TPN of the American Medical Association (AMA) suggests a daily maintenance dose of 1.4 mg from infancy to 11 years and 3.6 mg for adults [2, 78]. Bradley and coworkers administered 10 mg riboflavin daily to 26 critically ill surgical patients on TPN. This dose maintained the distribution of red cell riboflavin [9]. In the study by Stromberg et al. [107a] a daily dose of 1.8 mg was found sufficient in patients with postsurgical complications undergoing TPN.

Several centers administer daily doses of riboflavin to patients on TPN varying from 3 to 10 mg [29, 47, 57, 61, 77] (see Table 8-1). The recommendations for pediatric use range from 0.6 to 2.0 mg daily [70].

Our current practice is to administer 10 mg riboflavin daily to patients on standard TPN, as well as to patients in acute renal or hepatic failure [1, 40].

Preparations and Incompatibility. Riboflavin is contained in all multivitamin preparations (Table 8-2). Direct light, particularly sunlight, may induce rapid deterioration of the dissolved vitamin.

There is no known incompatibility with TPN solutions [95].

Pantothenic Acid (Vitamin B_3)

Pantothenic acid was identified in 1933 by Williams and associates as a growth factor for yeast. The role of pantothenic acid in animal nutrition was first defined in chicks.

Pantothenic acid is of such widespread distribution in foods that an occurrence of a deficiency of the vitamin is exceedingly rare [46].

Chemistry. Pantothenic acid consists of α,γ-dihydroxy-β,β'-dimethyl butyric acid and β-alanine joined by an amide linkage. The vitamin is stable in neutral solution, but is readily destroyed by heat at either alkaline or acid pH [46]. Pantothenic acid is converted in the body via pantetheine to coenzyme A.

Source. Pantothenic acid is widely distributed in food, especially in foods from animal sources. It is probably synthesized by intestinal bacteria. In most cooking and baking procedures there is little loss of the vitamin, but temperature above the boiling point may cause considerable loss [3].

Function. Pantothenic acid is an integral part of coenzyme A, a critical molecule for acetylation reactions. Coenzyme A is involved in the intermediary metabolism of carbohydrates, fat, and protein, leading to energy release, synthesis of fatty acids and sterols, gluconeogenesis, and many other essential reactions. Because of its role in energy metabolism, it can be considered to be vital to all energy-requiring processes within the cell [74, 116].

Absorption, Metabolic Fate, Excretion. Pantothenic acid is readily absorbed from the gastrointestinal tract. It is distributed in all tissues. Normal serum values range from 200 to 800 ng/ml with values below 160 deficient [5]. Pantothenic acid is measured by microbiologic procedures or chemical methods, including gas chromatography. The vitamin is apparently not destroyed in the body, since the intake and the excretion of the vitamin are approximately equal. The major route of excretion is the urine [46].

Deficiency. In the human, pantothenic acid deficiency has been produced in volunteers by the use of a purified diet and a specific antagonist [3]. Evidence of a dietary deficiency has not been clinically recognized in the human, and the administration of a metabolic antagonist appears to be necessary to produce clinical symptoms. Symptoms developed during the second to third week and consisted of headache, fatigue, impaired motor coordination, paresthesia, muscle cramps, and intermittent vomiting and diarrhea. There was also a loss of antibody formation [3, 74]. All symptoms were cured by the administration of the vitamin.

Deficiency of pantothenic acid is found in generalized malnutrition, but it is often difficult to distinguish specific features occasioned by each factor. Low serum and urine levels of pantothenic acid have also been observed in poorly nourished alcoholics [74].

Toxicity. Toxic reactions to pantothenic acid have not been found in man, but when administered in mice at doses of 5 to 7.5 gm/kg body weight, it kills 50 percent of the animals [116].

Human Requirements. There is insufficient evidence on which to base recommended allowance for pantothenic acid. The Food and Nutrition Board has not established a recommended dietary allowance for pantothenic acid, but states that a daily intake of 5 to 10 mg is probably adequate for children and adults [38].

Requirements During TPN. There is little information available for the need of pantothenic acid in patients on TPN. The Nutrition Advisory Group of AMA recommends daily doses of 5 mg pantothenic acid to children and 15 mg to adults [2, 78]. Most centers give average daily doses of pantothenic acid varying from 5 to 25 mg to adults and 3 to 6 mg to children [47, 57, 61, 70, 71, 77, 99] (see Table 8-1). We administer 20 mg pantothenic acid daily in patients on TPN; the same dose is used in renal and hepatic failure [1, 40].

Preparations. Calcium pantothenate is available in all multivitamin preparations (Table 8-2).

BIOTIN

In 1916, Bateman observed that a high concentration of egg white in experimental diets was toxic. In 1927, Boas confirmed the fact that rats fed a diet containing raw egg white as the sole source of protein developed a syndrome characterized by neuromuscular disorders, severe dermatitis, and loss of hair. She also demonstrated that it could be prevented by cooking the protein or by the administration of yeast, liver, or other food. György also investigated the syndrome and was convinced that it was a vitamin deficiency. He called the protective substance vitamin H. In 1936, Kögl and Tönnis isolated an essential factor from egg yolk that was called biotin. This substance was later demonstrated to be identical to vitamin H. In 1942, du Vigneaud established the structural formula of biotin. In the meantime, the nature of the antagonist to biotin was studied. The compound is a glucoprotein and called avidin [3, 46].

Chemistry. Biotin is a complex, optically active organic acid. It is water-soluble, and labile to alkali and oxidation. Biotin is partly destroyed by cooking [3].

Source. Biotin is present in almost all foods; liver, kidney, milk, egg yolk, and yeast are the richest sources. Biotin is obtained not only from the diet, but also from synthesis by intestinal bacteria. The availability from this source in humans has been questioned, however [74].

Function. Biotin acts as a coenzyme in numerous carboxylation reactions in intermediary metabolism of carbohydrates, proteins, and fats. The identified biotin-requiring enzymes are: pyruvate carboxylase, β-methyl crotanyl CoA carboxylase, propionyl CoA carboxylase, geranolyl CoA, and acetyl CoA carboxylase. It has also been shown to participate in the activation of folate to its coenzyme forms [74].

Absorption, Metabolic Fate, Excretion. Biotin is rapidly absorbed from the gastrointestinal tract after ingestion and is excreted in the urine predominantly in the form of free biotin. Achlorhydria may be accompanied by decreased biotin absorption. It has been suggested that biotin levels below 10 mμg/100 ml of whole blood may be indicative of biotin deficiency [5, 74].

Deficiency. Biotin deficiency is seldom observed in humans mainly because of its wide distribution in almost all foods and its bacterial synthesis in the gut, although the contribution of the latter is still questionable. However, biotin deficiency has apparently been observed in patients without gut on long-term total parenteral nutrition.

Biotin deficiency has been observed in children under four years of age. It has been produced in adults by feeding raw egg-white diets. It causes a scaling seborrheic dermatitis affecting mainly the chest, neck, umbilicus, and groin. Other symptoms include muscle pain, paresthesia, anorexia, nausea, hypercholesterolemia, and electrocardiographic changes [3, 46, 74, 116].

Toxicity. Although no studies of biotin toxicity in human beings have been conducted, toxicity appears to be low.

Human Requirements. The human daily requirement for biotin is unknown. Diets providing a daily intake of 150 to 300 μg of biotin are considered adequate by the Food and Nutrition Board [38].

Requirements During TPN. Little is known about the need for biotin during TPN. The Nutrition Advisory Group on TPN of AMA recommends 20 μg from infancy to 11 years and 60 μg biotin for children above 11 years and adults [2, 78]. Several centers do not give biotin to patients undergoing TPN. Broviac and Scribner [12] administer 100 μg daily to patients on long-term TPN. Shils recommends a daily dose of 60 μg biotin [99]. Jeejeebhoy and coworkers did not administer biotin to patients on TPN and observed low blood levels of biotin [57]. In several patients with TPN without oral intake and antibiotic treatment, there is a risk for development of biotin deficiency, and the vitamin should be administered regularly in long-term TPN patients without significant gastrointestinal tract function [28]. We administer 200 μg biotin daily to all patients on TPN.

Preparations and Incompatibility. Several multivitamin preparations do not contain biotin (Table 8-2). Among the more commonly used preparations only Berocca C (Roche) and MVI-12 (USV Laboratories) contain biotin. No information is available about incompatibilities of biotin in TPN solutions [95].

PYRIDOXINE (VITAMIN B_6)

Vitamin B_6 was first identified as essential in the nutrition of the cat for preventing a dermatitis called acrodynia. Pyridoxine was isolated from liver and yeast in 1938 and synthesized in the same year. The vitamin was found essential also for man and many other species, including several microorganisms [3, 46].

Chemistry. Pyridoxine owes its name to its structural resemblance to the pyrimidine ring. Pyridoxine is biologically converted into two other compounds: (1) pyridoxal (an aldehyde) and (2) pyridoxamine (an amide). All three of these compounds are active biologically as the vitamin, and pyridoxine is often used as the collective term for all three. Pyridoxine is quite stable in acid solutions, but rapid destruction by light occurs in neutral and alkaline solutions.

Source. Pyridoxine is widespread in nature, but frequently occurs in very small amounts. Good sources of the vitamin are yeast, wheat and corn, egg yolk, liver, kidney, and muscle meats.

Food appears to be the only source of the vitamin, because most of the vitamin produced by the bacterial flora of the intestine is excreted in the feces [3, 116].

Function. Vitamin B_6 is rapidly converted by the liver into the metabolically active forms, pyridoxal phosphate (PLP) and pyridoxamine phosphate. These compounds are distributed throughout the tissues. The function of vitamin B_6, primarily as PLP, is to act as a coenzyme for a wide variety of metabolic transformations of amino acids, including decarboxylation, transamination, and racemization, as well as for enzymatic steps in the metabolism of tryptophan, sulfur-containing amino acids, and hydroxy amino acids. PLP is also required for the synthesis of δ-aminolevulinic acid, a precursor of heme. A large percentage of body vitamin B_6 is found in the phosphorylase, the enzyme that converts glycogen to glucose 1-phosphate. Pyridoxine also appears to be involved in the metabolism of the central nervous system [3, 46, 74, 116].

Absorption, Metabolic Fate, Excretion. Pyridoxine is absorbed in the upper part of the small intestine. Once absorbed, all three forms are converted to pyridoxal phosphate, the coenzyme form. Following absorption, the vitamin phosphate is distributed throughout the body tissues, and approximately half of it is found in skeletal muscle.

Plasma levels of PLP correlate with tissue content of the vitamin and represent a meaningful indicator of vitamin B_6 nutriture. Plasma levels range from 30 to 80 ng/ml [5].

Pyridoxine is excreted in the urine chiefly as 4-pyridoxic acid. Measurement of this metabolite by a fluorometric method has been useful in studies on vitamin B_6 nutrition [5].

During intravenous administration of the vitamin there is a greater waste by increased urinary excretion as compared with oral administration [46].

Deficiency. Primary vitamin B_6 deficiency in man is rare. It generally occurs with the following three conditions:

1. Severe dietary deprivation or malabsorption, as is seen in celiac sprue.
2. Underlying illness, such as chronic liver disease, alcoholism, or uremia.
3. Use of drugs that affect absorption or metabolism of vitamin B_6 (e.g., isonicotinic acid hydrazide [INH], hydralazine, and cycloserine) [46].

Pyridoxine deficiency causes central nervous system, skin, and erythropoietic symptoms and signs. Central nervous system symptoms include irritation, depression, and somnolence. Deficiency may lead to convulsive seizures, most often observed in infants. Some patients may develop peripheral neuritis, especially during treatment of tuberculosis. Skin symptoms consist of a seborrheic dermatitis, mainly involving the face. Glossitis, cheilosis, and angular stomatitis indistinguishable from the lesions of niacin and riboflavin deficiency sometimes occur. Several reports of pyridoxine-responsive anemia, classified as microcytic, hypochromic anemia have been published [42].

High intakes of protein appear to hasten the onset of pyridoxine deficiency because of the active role the vitamin plays in protein metabolism.

Toxicity. Toxicity has been described in patients receiving 300 mg/day. This dose far exceeds any recommended for treatment, however [116].

Human Requirements. The requirement for pyridoxine increases with the amount of protein in the diet. The average adult minimal requirement for pyridoxine is about 1.25 mg per day in individuals ingesting 100 gm of protein per day. To provide a reasonable margin of safety, an intake of 2.0 mg per day is recommended for adults by the Food and Nutrition Board [38].

There is little information available on additional vitamin B_6 requirement in certain disease states. The requirement is increased in patients with hyperthyroidism and in patients undergoing treatment with certain drugs (see above). During pregnancy the need for the vitamin increases to 4 to 10 mg/day [74].

Patients with chronic renal failure undergoing maintenance hemodialysis have been found to be vitamin B_6-deficient [62]. The minimum quantity of vitamin B_6 necessary to correct biochemical evidence of the deficiency is not known, but the requirement probably exceeds the recommended daily allowance for normal people.

Requirements During TPN. The requirement of pyridoxine in patients with TPN has not been well studied. The Nutrition Advisory Group on TPN of AMA recommends 1.0 mg for intravenous use in children under 11 years of age and 4.0 mg to children over 11 years and to adults [2, 78].

Kishi and collaborators compared daily administration of 3 mg and 102 mg pyridoxine in a study of patients with malignant disease of the gastrointestinal tract or with chronic diseases of the liver and small bowel who were receiving TPN. They found that 3 mg per day of pyridoxine was a sufficient and safe level as opposed to 102, which was too high [61]. Bradley and coworkers, in a study of critically ill surgical patients on TPN, administered 15 mg pyridoxine daily [9]. This dose raised values of red cell vitamin B_6 significantly during treatment. Jeejeebhoy gave 5.5 mg pyridoxine daily to patients on long-term TPN [57]. Plasma pyridoxine levels in this study were slightly reduced in 2 of 6 patients. In the study by Stromberg et al. [107a] a daily dose of 2 mg pyridoxine was found sufficient in patients with postsurgical complications on TPN. Other centers give daily doses of 3.0 to 15.0 mg to adults on TPN and 0.4 to 0.3 mg to infants and children [29, 47, 70, 77, 99]. We administer 20 mg daily of pyridoxine to patients on standard TPN. The same dose is used for patients in renal and hepatic failure [1, 40]. In the treatment of established deficiency, 10 to 150 mg/day of pyridoxine has been used [42].

Preparations and Incompatibility. Pyridoxine is contained in all multivitamin preparations (Table 8-2). There is no known incompatibility of pyridoxine in TPN solutions [95].

Folic Acid (Folacin)

The discovery of folacin (or folic acid) began with the studies of Dr. Wills in India in 1931, when she called attention to a megaloblastic anemia found in pregnant women. She could also produce the anemia in monkeys by feeding them a diet similar to that eaten by her patients—primarily polished rice. In 1941, Mitchell and coworkers in the United States obtained a factor from spinach that was a growth factor for *Lactobacillus casei.* They called the material folic acid because it came from foliage plants such as spinach. Folic acid was found to be effective in curing the dietary anemia of monkeys. In 1945, Spies found folic acid effective in the treatment of the megalocytic anemias of pregnancy and also of tropical sprue [3, 116].

Chemistry. Folic acid (pteroylglutamic acid) consists of a pteridine moiety linked by a methylene bridge to a para-aminobenzoic acid, which is joined by a peptide linkage to glutamic acid. Folic acid is sparingly soluble in water and stable in acid solutions. When heated in neutral or alkaline solution it is rapidly destroyed.

Source. Good sources of folic acid are green leafy vegetables, liver, kidney, lima beans, asparagus, whole grain cereals, nuts, legumes, and yeast. Folate is highly susceptible to oxidative destruction; 50 to 95 percent of the folate content of foods may be destroyed by protracted cooking or other processing [3].

Function. Folate coenzymes are concerned with mammalian metabolic systems involving transfer of a 1-carbon unit. In this role it receives 1-carbon radicals from such amino acids as serine, glycine, histidine, and tryptophan and transfers them at two steps in purine synthesis.

In pyrimide synthesis it is essential in the insertion of the methyl group in deoxyuridylic acid to form thymidylic acid, the characteristic nucleotide of DNA. Failure in this synthetic step is responsible for the megaloblastosis seen in folate deficiency and in vitamin B_{12} deficiency.

Folic acid is needed for thymidylate synthesis as 5.10-methylenetetra-hydrofolate. This molecule is made from tetrahydrofolate via methyl-tetrahydrofolate, the principal form of folate in the human liver. The distinction between a folic acid deficiency and vitamin B_{12} deficiency appears to lie in the fact that when vitamin B_{12} is deficient, most of the folate is trapped in the methyl-tetrahydrofolate, which cannot then be used in the subsequent necessary reactions for the formation of thymidylate for DNA synthesis [3, 116].

Absorption, Metabolic Fate, Excretion. Food folate is absorbed primarily from the proximal third of the small intestine, although it is capable of being absorbed from the entire length of the small bowel. Folate in food is present primarily in polyglutamate form. The small intestine has a conjugase in the intestinal epithelium, which hydrolyzes the polyglutamate forms to free folic acid. This is then absorbed, and during absorption it is believed that folic acid is reduced and methylated to methyl-tetrahydrofolic acid [3]. This is the principal form of folate present in serum.

Normal human serum contains 7 to 16 ng of folic acid activity per ml of serum [5]. The most reliable methods for detecting these tiny quantities are microbiologic or radioisotopic. Folic acid can also be measured in erythrocytes, where normal levels are 160 to 650 ng/ml [42]. Indirect methods for determining folate status have been used. One depends on estimating the formiminoglutamic acid (FIGLU) arising from histidine catabolism. FIGLU is normally converted into glutamic acid by donating its formimino groups to tetrahydrofolate. In severe folate deficiency no acceptor tetrahydrofolate is available; hence, large amounts of FIGLU are excreted. The test is, however, nonspecific for folate deficiency [5]. Normal total-body folate stores are in the range of 5 to 10 mg, of which approximately half is in the liver.

Folate is excreted in urine and bile in metabolically active and inactive forms. There is an enterohepatic circulation of about 100 μg folate daily. Alcohol seems to interfere with this cycle [3, 116].

Deficiency. Folic acid deficiency is probably the most common hypovitaminosis of man. In the United States it has been estimated that 45 percent of adult patients who are indigent or in the low income group are deficient in folic acid [45]. Deficiency is often found during pregnancy because of substantially increased folate requirements. Folic acid deficiency often occurs in chronic alcoholism. This is probably caused not only by poor dietary intake, but also by decreased hepatic affinity and stores, and increased requirements for folic acid in chronic alcoholism.

Anorexia in a number of chronic diseases may result in deficiency. Folic acid deficiency may also be associated with certain disorders of the gastrointestinal tract, including chronic inflammatory diseases, diverticulosis, Whipple's disease, stricture, and anastomoses following extensive small bowel resections, and in sprue and gluten-induced enteropathy. Deficiency may be encountered following the administration of drugs, particularly anticonvulsant drugs, antimalarials, oral contraceptives, and folic acid antagonists in the treatment of malignant disease [42].

Folic acid deficiency is characterized not only by macrocytic anemia, megaloblastosis of the bone marrow, but also thrombocytopenia and leukopenia. Besides these most common findings, diarrhea, glossitis, and weight loss frequently occur.

In healthy humans, megaloblastic anemia develops after five months of administration of a folic acid-deficient diet, suggesting that it takes that long to deplete the body of its folic acid reserves or sources [45]. Recently several reports have described early appearance of folic acid deficiency with pancytopenia in certain disease states or during TPN. TPN with amino acid-sorbitol-ethanol (ASE) solutions in patients with gastrointestinal tract diseases caused a reduction of serum folate levels within 48 hours [118]. This was followed by pancytopenia in some patients after one week. In a control group receiving same TPN with folate supplements (0.5 mg folic acid daily), folate levels remained normal. The ethanol may be the major factor in causing the fall in serum folate concentration, but it has not been proved to be the sole cause, and other regimens for parenteral nutrition may contribute to a similar syndrome.

Ibbotson et al. report the onset of folic acid deficiency with megaloblastosis in two patients 8 and 17 days after start of TPN without folic acid [55]. Both patients had severe infections and were being dialyzed. Infection affects folate metabolism (see below) and folic acid is dialyzable, and both facts probably contributed to the rapid deficiency. Shah and coworkers found folic acid deficiency in two alcoholic patients supported with hyperalimentation therapy after 10 and 14 days [96]. Steinberg found folic acid deficiency in two patients on TPN without folic acid after 16 and 66 days [108]. In both instances, there was sepsis and hepatic failure. Recently, acute onset of folate deficiency was described in four patients with ruptured abdominal aortic aneurysm under intensive care [6a]. All patients had postoperative infections and developed acute renal failure.

Greene reports two patients who developed folic acid deficiency 7 and 27 days after the onset of intravenous nutrition without folic acid [44]. In both patients jaundice was a striking feature, and the jaundice was more severe than is usual for uncomplicated megaloblastic anemia. The jaundice disappeared rapidly after the start of folate supplementation. All the reported patients have as common features not only TPN therapy, but also a high incidence of sepsis, extensive surgical trauma, chronic inflammatory bowel disease, liver failure, renal failure, and chronic alcoholism.

Toxicity. No toxic reactions to folic acid have been seen when doses up to 15 mg have been taken daily for one month. There have been a few reports of hypersensitivity to folic acid, especially when given intravenously [80].

Human Requirements. The exact human requirements for folic acid are unknown, but it is estimated that 100 to 300 μg of folic acid is required daily in adults and 50 μg in infants.

The Nutrition Board's RDA for total folate is 400 μg for adults and children over 11 years of age, and it ranges from 50 μg for infants to 300 μg for children 7 to 11 years (see Table 8-1) [38].

Certain patient groups have increased requirement for folic acid or are particularly likely to develop early and severe deficiency of folic acid. These include:

1. Patients who may have malabsorption of folic acid, such as patients with inflammatory bowel disease.
2. Patients with increased folate requirements by the tissues as in malignant diseases, burns, surgical trauma, pregnancy, and sepsis.
3. Patients with decreased hepatic stores or decreased ability to convert dietary folic acid.
4. Patients with chronic alcoholism.
5. Patients undergoing hemodialysis.

Dialysis depresses folic acid levels and folic acid is dialyzable. Supplements of approximately 1 mg/day of folic acid are probably sufficient for patients undergoing hemodialysis [62].

Requirements During TPN. The Nutrition Advisory Group on TPN of AMA recommends the intravenous administration of 140 μg folacin to children under 11 years and 400 μg to adults [2, 78] (see Table 8-1).

Several studies have been undertaken to determine the efficacy of folic acid administration in patients with TPN. In his study, Bradley administered 15 mg folic acid as an intramuscular preparation on the first day of intravenous nutrition and thereafter once weekly [9]. This regimen maintained red cell folate and serum folate within normal limits. Nichoalds and associates gave 300 and 600 μg folate respectively in two TPN programs [77]. The daily dose of 300 μg was found insufficient to maintain serum folate levels. When the dose was doubled, serum folate was normalized. Lowry et al. studied vitamin levels of 40 patients undergoing TPN [71]. A majority of the patients had malignant diseases. One miligram of folate was administered daily, and this dose was found adequate to maintain or improve serum folate levels. Stromberg, finally, administered 200 mg daily to patients with postoperative complications on TPN and found this dose adequate for maintenance, but inadequate for correction of a deficiency state [107a]. Other groups administer 0.4 to 5.0 mg daily to adults and 100 to 140 μg to children during TPN [12, 29, 47, 57, 70, 99] (see Table 8-1).

Since deficiency may appear early, especially in the aforementioned patients at risk, it is recommended that administration of folic acid should start early in the course of TPN, particularly in patients with chronic alcoholism. The indiscriminate use of folic acid can interfere with the clinical diagnosis of vitamin B_{12} deficiency, however, and may be harmful. It is therefore advisable to measure vitamin B_{12} levels when giving folic acid or to routinely administer both to patients at risk.

Our group administers 5 mg folic acid weekly to patients receiving standard TPN, starting after one week. To high-risk patients, and especially patients with renal and hepatic failure, 1 mg folic acid is given daily, starting at once. We always give folate as a separate injection, not admixed with the TPN solution because of the inactivation of folate in glucose amino acid solutions [1, 40].

Preparations and Incompatibility. Few multivitamin preparations contain folic acid (Table 8-2). Folbesyn (Lederle) has 1,000 μg folic acid and MVI-12 (USV Laboratories) contains 400 μg.

The information on the incompatibility of folic acid in TPN solutions is scarce. Although folic acid is easily soluble in TPN solutions and causes no physical changes of the solution [95], the retrieval of folic acid added to TPN solutions has not been well studied, and most centers recommend giving folic acid either orally or intramuscularly and not adding it to TPN solutions because of possible oxidation.

VITAMIN B_{12} (COBALAMIN, CYANOCOBALAMIN)

Thomas Addison, a physician working in Guy's Hospital, London, discovered an anemia in 1849 that occurred mostly in elderly patients and led to death in two to five years. So inevitable was death that the disease became known as pernicious anemia. Later, in 1926, Minot and Murphy in Boston found that a remission in pernicious anemia occurred when patients were fed large amounts of whole liver.

At about the same time, W. B. Castle observed that pernicious anemia patients had an abnormal gastric secretion. He demonstrated that normal human gastric juice contains an intrinsic factor that combines with an extrinsic factor found in animal protein to result in absorption of the antipernicious anemia principle. When vitamin B_{12} was isolated in 1948 almost simultaneously in the United States and England, Berk and his associates showed that this vitamin has both extrinsic factor and antipernicious anemia principle [3, 116].

Chemistry. The two major portions of vitamin B_{12} are corrin nucleus (a planar group) and a nucleotide lying in a plane nearly at right angles to the corrin nucleus and linked to it by D-1-

amino-2-propanol. The nucleotide (5,6-dimethylbenzimidazole) is attached to ribose by an alpha-glycoside linkage. A second bond between the two major parts of the molecule is the coordinate linkage of the cobalt atom to one of the nitrogen atoms of the nucleotide. In cyanocobalamin the anionic group in coordinate linkage with the cobalt is cyanide.

Coenzyme B_{12} and methylcobalamin are the two vitamin B_{12} coenzymes known to be active in man, and constitute the dominant form of B_{12} in mammalian tissues. Both are unstable in light and undergo photolysis with formation of aquacobalamin, or cyanocobalamin.

Cyanocobalamin is a semisynthetic name for vitamin B_{12}. However, the term is also found in the literature as a generic term for all the cobalamins active in man [116].

Source. Vitamin B_{12} can be found only in food of animal origin. Microorganisms in the human gastrointestinal tract can synthesize the vitamin, but the site of synthesis in the colon does not permit absorption [3].

Function. Vitamin B_{12} is essential to the proper functioning of all mammalian cells.

DNA SYNTHESIS. Both vitamin B_{12} and folic acid (see above) are required for synthesis of thymidylate, and therefore of DNA. A vitamin B_{12}-containing enzyme removes a methyl group from methyl folate and delivers it to homocysteine, thereby converting homocysteine to methionine and regenerating tetrahydrofolic acid (THFA), from which the 5,10-methylene THFA involved in thymidylate synthesis is made. Since methyl folate is the dominant form of folate in human serum and liver, and since methyl folate may only return to the body's folate pool via a vitamin B_{12}-dependent step, when a patient suffers from vitamin B_{12} deficiency, much of this folate is trapped as methyl folate and thus is metabolically useless. The hematologic damage results from lack of adequate 5,10-methylene THFA, which delivers its methyl group to deoxyuridylate to convert that substance to thymidylate, and thus makes DNA during the S-phase [116].

FAT AND CARBOHYDRATE METABOLISM. Coenzyme B_{12} is required for the hydrogen transfer and isomerization whereby methylmalonate is converted to succinate, and thus B_{12} is involved in both fat and carbohydrate metabolism [3]. One possible explanation for the neurologic damage of patients with vitamin B_{12} deficiency is inability to make the lipid portion of the lipoprotein myelin sheath (related to inadequate interconversion of methylmalonate to succinate) [3].

PROTEIN AND FAT METABOLISM. Vitamin B_{12} is involved in protein synthesis through its role in the synthesis of the amino acid methionine. Since methionine is involved in making available more of the lipotropic substances choline and betaine, this is another point where cobalamin may play a role in lipid metabolism.

VITAMIN B_{12} AS A REDUCING AGENT. Vitamin B_{12} appears to be involved in the maintenance of sulfhydryl (SH) groups in the reduced form necessary for the functioning of many SH-activated enzyme systems. A deficiency of the vitamin is characterized by a decrease in reduced glutathione of erythrocytes and liver [3].

Absorption, Metabolic Fate, Excretion. There are two separate and distinct mechanisms for the absorption of vitamin B_{12}. The physiologic mechanism, the derangement of which accounts for much human vitamin B_{12} deficiency, is capable of handling 1.5 to 3.0 μg of free vitamin B_{12} at any one time. Vitamin B_{12} requires a heat-labile glycoprotein-intrinsic factor for intestinal absorption. This substance is secreted from the parietal cells of the stomach during the normal secretion of gastric juice. The intrinsic factor is believed to help attach the vitamin to a receptor in the intestinal mucosa of the lower ileum. In the intestinal cell membrane, vitamin B_{12} is released from the intrinsic factor and absorbed into the blood.

The pharmacologic mechanism of vitamin B_{12} absorption appears to be diffusion. It accounts for the absorption along the entire length of the small intestine of approximately one percent of any quantity of free vitamin B_{12} in the small bowel.

Vitamin B_{12} in human serum is bound to three different vitamin B_{12}-binding proteins, transcobalamin I, II, and III.

Normal human serum levels of vitamin B_{12}, as measured by radioassay, range from 200 to 900 pg per ml; values below 80 pg represent B_{12} deficiency [5].

Vitamin B_{12} is stored in the body in amounts ranging from 1 mg to 10 mg, with the liver containing 50 to 90 percent of the total stored vitamin. There is normally an enterohepatic circulation of vitamin B_{12}, which may account for approximately 0.6 to 6 μg of the vitamin being excreted in the bile and reabsorbed in the ileum [74]. This almost total conservation of vitamin B_{12} explains why it takes a long time to develop deficiency of the vitamin.

Deficiency. Dietary deficiency of vitamin B_{12} is rare, occurring almost exclusively in vegetarians. Pernicious anemia is the most important condition resulting from vitamin B_{12} deficiency. In this disease, deficiency is caused by failure of absorption of vitamin B_{12} from the intestinal tract due to lack of intrinsic factor in the gastric juice. It is common following gastrectomy and after resections of lower ileum, as well as in a number of malabsorption syndromes.

Acquired vitamin B_{12} deficiency may also follow the chronic ingestion of alcohol or may result from folic acid deficiency because folate is required for absorption of B_{12}. A deficiency may also follow the administration of neomycin, para-aminosalicylic acid, or colchicine. The most important manifestations of vitamin B_{12} deficiency are macrocytic anemia, megaloblastosis of the bone marrow, glossitis, and neurologic abnormalities. The mean corpuscular volume is greater than normal, and nucleated red cells may be seen in the peripheral blood smear. The white cells and platelets are usually reduced in number.

The earliest neurologic complaints are paresthesias involving the hands and feet. Progress of the deficiency leads to loss of vibratory and position sense, muscle weakness, and loss of deep tendon reflexes. Mental changes such as irritability, memory disturbances, and depression may occur. Anorexia, nausea, vomiting, and diarrhea are common [42, 116].

Toxicity. Vitamin B_{12} has no known toxicity.

Human Requirements. The human needs very small amounts of vitamin B_{12}. The Food and Nutrition Board has set the RDA for vitamin B_{12} at 3 μg per day for adolescents and normal adults, assuming that at least 50 percent of quantities up to 3 μg of food vitamin B_{12} is absorbed [38] (see Table 8-1). The requirement is increased if the body metabolic rate is raised, as in fever or hyperthyroidism [3]. Patients undergoing maintenance hemodialysis usually show no significant changes in serum B_{12} concentrations [62].

In the treatment of deficiencies with macrocytic anemia or neurologic abnormalities, vitamin B_{12} is given in amounts of 50 to 100 μg three times daily until findings have returned to normal [42].

Requirements During TPN. Little information is available about the requirements of vitamin B_{12} during TPN. The AMA Nutrition Advisory Group recommends 1.0 μg vitamin B_{12} for infants and children under 11 years and 5.0 μg for adults as maintenance doses for intravenous use [2, 78] (see Table 8-1).

Lowry and co-authors gave 5 μg of vitamin B_{12} daily to patients receiving TPN [71]. This dose maintained serum B_{12} levels within normal range and raised serum B_{12} in 3 of 30 patients. Nichoalds et al. used 15 μg of vitamin B_{12} daily in a similar study and found that this dose maintained serum vitamin levels adequately [77]. Patients receiving long-term TPN were given 12.5 μg vitamin B_{12} daily by Jeejeebhoy [57], and he could not detect any abnormalities of vitamin B_{12} levels. Stromberg gave 2 μg daily and found this dose adequate in patients studied [107a]. Several other centers administer 15 to 50 μg

vitamin B_{12} per day or 1,000 μg per week to adults on TPN and 50 μg daily to children [12, 29, 47, 61, 70, 99] (see Table 8-1). Our group administers vitamin B_{12} in a dose of 1,000 μg intramuscularly once weekly to patients receiving TPN.

Preparations and Incompatibility. Most multivitamin preparations do not contain vitamin B_{12} (see Table 8-2). There are some indications that vitamin B_{12} is incompatible with mixture in most TPN solutions, although it has not been fully investigated [95]. Most centers recommend that the vitamin be given as an intramuscular injection weekly.

Non-B-Complex

L-Ascorbic Acid (Vitamin C)

Scurvy has plagued seamen and explorers since antiquity. It was responsible for some of the ghost ships that wandered on the sea with their dead crew. The use of oranges was proposed as a cure for scurvy as early as 1593. In 1795, Lind, a Scottish physician, revived the use of lime as a preventive of scurvy and introduced an admirality rule prescribing the use of orange and lemon juice in the Royal Navy. From then on, scurvy disappeared from the Royal Navy. Funk suspected that scurvy resulted from a vitamin deficiency. In the early 1930s, Szent-Györgyi crystallized hexuronic acid from an adrenal preparation, and several years later the compound was shown to be identical to the vitamin contained in the fruits [13, 116].

Chemistry. L-ascorbic acid is a simple 6-carbon organic compound ($C_6H_8O_6$) closely related to glucose. It is an ene-diol lactone of an acid whose chemical configuration is analogous to L-glucose. The D-form of ascorbic acid has very little antiscorbutic activity. Ascorbic acid is stable to acid, but easily destroyed by oxidation, alkali, and heat. In aqueous solution and in the presence of copper it is readily destroyed. This is of interest in connection with cooking utensils [3, 116].

Source. Fruits, especially citrus fruits, and tomatoes are rich sources of vitamin C.

Function. It was initially assumed that the metabolic role of ascorbic acid relates to its reversible oxidation and reduction. No biologic oxidation system has yet been described in which ascorbic acid serves as a specific coenzyme. Nevertheless, ascorbic acid is essential to a variety of biologic oxidation processes [3].

One of the most prominent aspects of ascorbic acid is its role in collagen synthesis. It plays a key role in the hydroxylation of proline and lysine, necessary for normal collagen synthesis.

Ascorbic acid is also essential for normal protein and amino acid metabolism. Deficiency results in lowering of plasma albumin and disturbance of tyrosine metabolism [13]. In vitamin C-deficient individuals, there is also an alteration of various amino acid concentrations in muscle (e.g., an increase of glutamic acid, leucine, valine, and methionine, and a decrease of glutamine and aspartic acid) and in blood (e.g., a decrease of most amino acids, with a small rise of phenylalanine, leucine, and histidine). There is no definite explanation for these changes [116]. Ascorbic acid is also involved in carbohydrate metabolism, as evidenced by the fact that scorbutic animals exhibit hyperglycemia, reduced glucose tolerance, and low hepatic glycogen content, and they are resistant to insulin. There are increased levels of pyruvic and lactic acid levels in blood [13].

Ascorbic acid occurs in high concentration in both the cortex and the medulla of the adrenals. It has been proposed that vitamin C is concerned with the synthesis of adrenocorticosteroids, but there is no direct evidence to support this. The ascorbic acid content of the glands rapidly disappears following stress [3].

Absorption, Metabolic Fate, Excretion. Ascorbic acid is readily absorbed from the upper part of the intestinal tract. Under special circumstances, as in diarrhea, absorption may be limited [13].

There are several chemical methods for determining ascorbic acid values. The methods of choice for determination of ascorbic acid status involve plasma or serum ascorbic acid concentration and white blood cell-blood platelet ascorbate concentration, which is more closely related to tissue stores. Normal serum values in adults range from 0.4 to 1.5 mg/100 ml, and values below 0.2 mg/100 ml indicate deficiency [5].

The body pool of vitamin C of healthy adults averages 1500 mg, and the rate of metabolism of ascorbic acid is about 3 percent per day of the existing body pool.

The human kidney handles ascorbic acid in much the same way as it handles glucose. There is renal threshold for vitamin C, and the vitamin is excreted by the kidneys in large amounts only when the plasma concentration exceeds this threshold, which is approximately 1.4 mg/100 ml [13].

Deficiency. Ascorbic acid deficiency-scurvy occurs in infants in many parts of the world, but is far less frequent than in former years. Scurvy is also seen in adults, particularly in persons living alone on very restricted diets. It may be found in chronic alcoholism and in diarrheal diseases. Early symptoms in infants include poor appetite, increased irritability, and minimal growth failure. Then, tenderness of the legs and pseudoparalysis, usually involving the lower extremities, appears. Bleeding into the skin or gums is a fairly frequent manifestation. In adults, nonspecific findings appear first: weakness, lassitude, irritability, and vague aching pain in the joints and muscles. Weight loss may occur. In more advanced deficiency, the tendency to hemorrhage becomes marked. Anemia is common, secondary to blood loss. Wound healing is impaired since ascorbic acid is necessary for the formation of collagen.

A decrease of plasma ascorbic acid occurs following trauma or surgical procedures, apparently due to a shift of ascorbic acid from serum to the site of the wound [3, 42, 116].

An abrupt decrease in dietary ascorbic acid from a regular intake of 2 to 3 gm/day to doses equivalent to the recommended dietary allowance may precipitate ascorbic acid deficiency.

Toxicity. Although serious toxicity from the administration of vitamin C is uncommon, untoward effects have been reported.

Acidification of the urine by ascorbic acid may cause precipitation of cystine or oxalate stones in the urinary tract and will alter the excretion of certain other drugs administered concurrently [13].

Human Requirements. The human requirement for vitamin C has been studied extensively, but there is disagreement on optimal intake. The recommended dietary allowances by the Food and Nutrition Board range from 45 to 80 mg in adults and 35 to 40 mg in children (see Table 8-1) [38].

Under certain circumstances, the rate of destruction and, consequently, the requirements for Vitamin C are significantly increased:

1. Patients suffering from certain infectious diseases have increased requirements. An individual with tuberculosis may need 100 percent more vitamin C than does a normal subject [13].
2. Patients with thyrotoxicosis [74].
3. Patients with neoplastic diseases. It has been argued that as ascorbic acid is necessary for collagen synthesis, it might be required in increased amounts for the protective encapsulation of tumors [17]. It has been shown that cancer patients in general have low plasma ascorbic acid levels. There are some indications of a beneficial effect of increased survival in cancer patients by increasing intake of ascorbic acid [16]. Contradictory findings have been reported from animal studies [18], and the issue is still surrounded by controversy.
4. Patients with trauma, extensive burns, or surgical stress. Vitamin C requirements may increase as much as a hundredfold with major burns and extensive trauma, and normal body

stores can be exhausted often as early as 24 to 48 hours after injury [13].

5. Patients with chronic pressure sores. Paraplegic patients with chronic ulcers had lower leukocyte ascorbic acid concentrations than controls. When this was corrected by vitamin C supplementation, the ulcers healed [14].

6. Patients in renal failure undergoing hemodialysis. Vitamin C is extracted continuously throughout dialysis [62, 111]. Supplements of 100 mg per day of ascorbic acid are probably sufficient for patients undergoing hemodialysis.

Requirements During TPN. The Nutrition Advisory Group of AMA recommends 80 mg of ascorbic acid daily for infants and children under 11 years and 100 mg for adults [2, 78] (see Table 8-1).

The requirement for vitamin C in surgical patients undergoing TPN has been studied by some investigators. Nichoalds and coworkers administered 465 mg vitamin C to patients on TPN, and this dose raised serum levels slowly over the five weeks of the study [77]. A lowering of the dose to 210 mg daily maintained normal serum levels of the vitamin. In another study by Lowry and associates, approximately 700 mg ascorbic acid was administered daily to patients on TPN [71]. This massive dose did not yield elevated serum levels, probably because the renal threshold for ascorbic acid was exceeded. Bradley and coworkers gave 500 mg vitamin C to the 26 critically ill surgical patients in their study [9]. Most patients had normal white blood cell vitamin C before the study, and this was elevated during the time of the study.

Several other groups administer vitamin C in daily doses of 170 to 700 mg to adults and 35 to 100 mg to children on TPN [29, 47, 57, 70, 99] (Table 8-1). Most centers administer higher doses than recommended, and this probably reflects an estimation of increased need for vitamin C in many disease states.

Our group administers 500 mg ascorbic acid daily to patients on regular TPN. Patients in acute renal failure treated with essential amino acids are given 1.5 gm ascorbic acid daily to compensate for increased need in this condition [1, 62].

Preparations and Interactions. Most multivitamin preparations contain ascorbic acid (Table 8-2). There is no known incompatibility of ascorbic acid in TPN solutions [95]. It is important to remember that the excretion of ascorbate in the urine of patients receiving vitamin C may cause analytic errors of readings for glycosuria by a reduction of colorimetric agents or the activation of glucose oxidase.

FAT-SOLUBLE VITAMINS

VITAMIN A

The symptomatology of vitamin A deficiency, namely nightblindness, xerophthalmia, and keratomalacia, has been known for some time in different parts of the world, mainly in undernourished populations [72, 116]. In 1913, two groups independently reported retardation of growth in rats fed an artificial diet based on lard, which could be corrected by addition of egg yolk, cod liver oil, or butter. In 1919, Steenbock discovered the empiric formula of xerophitol and pointed to the relation between degree of yellow pigmentation of plants and their vitamin A activity content.

Chemistry. The structure of vitamin A was elucidated first by Karrer in 1931. Vitamin A exists in a variety of forms. It consists of a benzoyl ring, with one double bond, three methyl groups, and a long 9-carbon aliphatic chain, which is unsaturated and has four double bonds. The sidechain, theoretically, may exist as 32 different geometric isomers and ends in an alcoholic group. The primary alcohol, retinol (vitamin A_1), may be oxidized to the aldehyde, retinal, or the related acid, retinoic acid. Vitamin A_2 is found in freshwater fish and has an additional double bond in the benzoyl ring, 3 dehydroretinol (retinol$_2$). Of all the isomers, the greatest biologic activity is exhibited by the all-trans retinol and its aldehyde.

Vitamin A does not exist in bacteria and plants. They provide provitamin A, carotene. The β-carotene is the most active carotenoid. Its structure is like two retinol molecules attached through a double bond.

Source. Carotenes are abundant in carrots, tomatoes, maize, peas, and other yellow-pigmented vegetables. Vitamin A is found in cod liver oil, and in dairy products, mainly butter, and egg yolk [72].

Function. Vitamin A has several important functions: It participates as a constituent of the visual pigment in the visual cycle, it is an important factor in conserving integrity of epithelial membranes, and it stabilizes lysosomal membranes.

VITAMIN A AND THE VISUAL CYCLE. Human photoreceptor cells contain light-sensitive pigments. These are arranged in protein-lipid discs, one molecule per disc, with each rod and cone containing approximately 700 discs. Each of the light-absorbing proteins (opsins) is tightly bound to 11-*cis*-retinal. The retinal is bound, most probably, by a Schiff base-like linkage to the e-NH_2 group of lysine of opsin. Rhodopsin is the photopigment of the 120 million rods, and it has its maximum absorption at about 507 nm wavelength, which is suitable for dim light. The 6 million cones contain three different photopigments at about 440 nm (blue-sensitive), 535 nm (green-sensitive), and 570 nm (red-sensitive) wavelengths, respectively [34, 76, 116].

When the visual pigment absorbs light, the bound 11-*cis*-retinal undergoes isomerization to all-trans retinal and dissociation from the bleached photopigment yielding free opsin and the all-*trans*-retinal. The change in the shape of rhodopsin releases Ca^{2+}, which is sequestered within the disc and closes the Na^+ channels in the membrane, thus hyperpolarizing the membrane and triggering graded nervous potentials. Since 11-*cis*-retinal is in a higher energy state than all-*trans* retinal, its recovery for further light perception needs energy. The resynthesis of 11-*cis*-retinal is carried out in the photoreceptor cells, by light, or in the darkness in the retinal pigment epithelium, by a chain of enzymatic reactions involving $NAD/NADH + H^+$ as coenzyme for retinal reductase, which is identical to alcohol dehydrogenase [76, 116].

Dark adaptation is the process of increase in sensitivity of the eye to detection of light during darkness (scotopic vision). The sensitivity increases in two exponential steps following exposure to bright light: The first step reaches plateau after 5 to 9 minutes and is attributed to regeneration of the pigment in the cones; the second step reaches plateau after 30 to 45 minutes and is attributed to regeneration of the photopigment in the rods. Vitamin A deficiency can be detected clinically by deranged dark adaptation and by electroretinogram (ERG) changes with dampening of ERG tracing.

VITAMIN A ACTION ON EPITHELIAL MEMBRANES. The action of vitamin A on mammalian epithelial membranes is more difficult to elucidate than its role in the visual cycle. From morphologic data considering effects of deficiency and excess of vitamin A, it was concluded that it enhances mucous secretion and inhibits keratinization of epithelial membranes. Further intensive work elucidated vitamin A as an important cofactor in glycosyl transfer reactions in glycoprotein synthesis in the epidermis, cornea, respiratory tract epithelium, intestinal tract epithelium, and liver [26, 60].

An alternative proposed mechanism for the action of vitamin A is by influencing DNA transcription, similar to the action of steroid hormones: Binding to specific receptors present in the cytosol, the ligand-protein couple translocates into the nucleus, changes the expression of the genome, which changes nuclear RNA synthesis, and results in changed epithelial differentiation. This assumption is supported by finding of specific uptake of the retinol-RBP-prealbumin complex by plasma membrane, and by finding of an intracellular retinol binding protein and an intracellular retinoic acid binding protein [21].

The finding that retinoic acid may be an active form of retinol in maintaining growth and in its antikeratinizing action, but not in the visual cycle and not in the reproductive system, is exciting [21, 26]. Since conversion of retinol to retinoic acid is performed in the proximal tubule of the kidney, an analogy to vitamin D conversion to its active form, 1.25 $(OH)_2D_3$, exists [26, 114].

The presence of the cellular retinol and retinoic acid-binding protein in fetal tissue and in malignant tissue [21] implies the association of vitamin A with development of cancer, squamocarcinoma in particular. Since vitamin A protects against squamous metaplasia and controls differentiation of epithelial cells, intensive investigations of the prophylactic capacity of vitamin A and its analogues, the retinoids, for developing epithelial cancer have been carried out [32, 106].

Absorption, Metabolic Fate, Excretion. The diet contains vitamin A esters, which are hydrolyzed in the lumen of the intestine or in the brush border. Retinol is re-esterified before absorption in the lymph and then into the venous system; it is then transported to the tissues in the esterified form. The absorption of vitamin A and carotene is dependent on the presence of bile and lipase. Carotenes are split to vitamin A in the intestine. Such tissues as lung, kidney, and liver split the carotene if it is administered intravenously. The breakdown of carotene to vitamin A is not by splitting the molecule into two equal halves, but by splitting one half of the molecule in different sites and oxidizing the other half to vitamin A. Carotene is much less effective than vitamin A. Although 50 to 70 percent of carotene is absorbed in the intestine, only 30 percent can be recovered in the liver as vitamin A. The remainder results in different fatty chains and sterol rings [116].

Vitamin A is stored in the liver with average content 149 ± 132 mg/gm liver. Other organs such as adrenal, adipose tissue, testis, kidney, and heart contain about 1 to 1.5 mg/gm tissue [94]. Vitamin A is stored, mainly in the Kupfer cells, as a palmitate ester and is bound to protein [116]. The maximal storage capacity of the liver is 300 mg/gm, which can supply the body's needs for a year [30].

Vitamin A is mobilized from the hepatic stores as an unesterified retinol, bound to the specific carrier-retinol binding protein (RBP). The protein has a molecular weight of 21,000 daltons and has a single binding site for one molecule of retinol. RBP circulates normally bound in a protein complex with prealbumin (MW 55,000 daltons), which is identical with the thyroxine-binding prealbumin [10, 103, 104, 114]. The interaction between these two proteins is specific, and the affinity is high.

RBP is synthesized by the liver. Its synthesis is very much dependent upon the nutritional status of the patient, and is very much impaired in protein-calorie malnutrition [66, 88, 104] and in patients with chronic liver disease [93, 103]. Its synthesis requires zinc [10, 105], which seems to be important for vitamin A mobilization. The RBP is present as free form in small amounts in the normal plasma and is in equilibrium with the prealbumin RBP complex. Plasma concentration of free RBP is about 5 μg/ml and the concentration of the bound RBP is 45 μg/ml.

The biologic half-life of the free RBP is very short (about 4 hours), and the bound RBP, 11 hours. Its synthetic rate is about 190 mg/day/m^2 [103]. The corresponding figure for albumin, which is the predominant plasma protein, on a molar basis, is only tenfold higher [114]. The prealbumin synthetic rate is about 300 mg/d/m^2, 40 percent lower than that of RBP calculated on a molar basis.

Being a low-molecular-weight protein, the RBP passes easily through the glomerular barrier, and is subsequently reabsorbed and catabolized by the cells of the proximal tubuli. About one-third of the plasma vitamin A is deposited in the proximal tubuli of the kidneys, where it is oxidized to retinoic acid [114].

Plasma vitamin A level is constant over a wide range of storage in the liver. Plasma vitamin A levels reflect the total body vitamin A status only in severe depletion or huge toxic doses [66, 89, 104]. Vitamin A levels in plasma drop only after hepatic reserves fall below 6 to 10 μg/gm tissue [66].

Since the indicator of low vitamin A levels below 20 mg/100 ml has not proved to be a reliable indicator of vitamin A deficiency, and since it is dependent on RBP levels, which are reduced at protein-calorie malnutrition and stress condition [88], loading with a single dose of vitamin A and its effect on blood vitamin A was used as an indicator for deficiency [66, 107]. Relative dose response (RDR) of 50 percent or above indicated that vitamin A storage in the liver was below 8 to 10 μg/gm.

The excretion of vitamin A is in a conjugated form to β-glucoronide after being oxidized to retinoic acid [72, 122]. It is excreted mainly in the bile, but part of vitamin A can be recovered from the urine.

Deficiency. Vitamin A deficiency is still prevalent in many parts of the world and is secondary, as an isolated nutritional deficiency disease, only to protein-calorie malnutrition. The problem is of particular concern in tropical and subtropical regions and in developing countries [72, 94]. Even in the United States and Western Europe, where animal fats constitute a significant portion of the diet, a marginal supply of vitamin A, iron, and calcium in the diet, mainly in black and Mexican-American children, was found by the ten-state Nutrition Survey of the United States [71, 94].

Vitamin A deficiency may be detected subclinically by measuring vitamin A levels in the blood, though these values are influenced both by stores of vitamin A in the liver, by disease states affecting RBP levels, and by drugs. Values below 20 mg/100 ml are considered as indicating hypovitaminosis A.

Vitamin A stores may be estimated by studying liver samples obtained by biopsy or at autopsy [89, 94]. Depending on the geographic area of the United States, 11.8 to 35 percent of the livers analyzed were low or deficient in vitamin A [94].

The clinical symptomatology of vitamin A deficiency is multisystemic:

1. Night blindness (nyctalopia) [76, 116].
2. Xerophthalmia due to scaling, keratinization, desiccation, and ulceration of the conjunctivae and cornea, and scaling and occlusion of the lacrimal ducts, which prevents normal flow of tears. These may lead to keratomalacia and blindness [116].
3. Transformation of the epithelium to a keratinizing epithelium, which may predispose to bronchitis and impairment of pulmonary function [72].
4. The intestinal mucosa show a reduction in goblet cells, but no keratinization. The low levels of vitamin A found in premature neonates implicated the association of necrotizing enterocolitis with hypovitaminosis A [10]. The same association was drawn to higher incidence of stress ulcerations in post-traumatic and burned patients [19, 86].
5. The keratinization of urinary cellular debris serving as a nidus for stone formation and urinary tract infection [72, 116].
6. The skin shows typical inflammatory follicular-conical keratotic lesions, with hyperkeratosis of hair follicles, obstruction of sebum glands by horny plugging, perivascular dermal inflammatory reaction [116, 119], and sweat gland keratinization [72].
7. Changes in smell and taste senses and hearing loss are associated with keratinization of the naso- and oropharynx epithelium [52, 105].
8. Anemia is associated with vitamin A deficiency. Its mechanism has not yet been completely elaborated, although some data implicate shortened life span of erythrocytes due to defective cellular membrane [52].

In animals other lesions occur: bone growth retardation, central nervous system lesions, hydrocephalus, impaired spermatogenesis with testicular atrophy, congenital teratogenic anomalies such as cleft lip, cleft palate, accessory ears, and increase in intrauterine death rate [116].

Some of the symptoms of vitamin A deficiency are present in any of the conditions which may produce vitamin A deficiency, such as cirrhosis of the liver, cystic fibrosis of the pancreas, sprue [72], malabsorption following small bowel bypass for obesity [119], and premature birth [10]. A fall in plasma levels of vitamin A is associated with acute catabolic state, as is seen in burned and post-traumatic stressed patients [19], but may in turn be due to low RBP rather than to absolute depletion of vitamin A [71, 99].

An investigation conducted by the Medical Research Council of Great Britain, commonly referred to as the Sheffield study, demonstrated a fall in plasma values of vitamin A in volunteers who consumed a vitamin A-deficient diet. The subjects manifested impaired dark adaptation, dryness of skin, and hearing impairment prior to detection of decreased plasma values [94].

In another study, vitamin A in plasma fell during the first 184 days of vitamin A depletion, from 57 to 78 mg/100 ml to 20 to 32 mg/100 ml [94], but clinical symptomatology of deficiency may precede the fall in plasma vitamin A levels. Follicular hyperkeratomas and dark adaptation impairment occurred when plasma vitamin A levels were about 30 mg/100 ml. Abnormal ERG was obtained only when plasma level fell below 11 mg/100 ml. During repletion with vitamin A and β-carotene, clinical improvement occurred prior to the return of plasma vitamin A levels to normal. In order to restore plasma vitamin A to normal, 2 to 4 times the dose is required; 1200 μg daily as compared with the 300 to 600 μg daily maintenance [94].

Toxicity. Excessive continuous intake of vitamin A produces distinct toxic manifestations: anorexia, nausea, vomiting, headache, pseudotumor cerebri, muscle and bone pain, muscle fasciculation, pruritus, peripheral paresthesia, desquamative dermatitis, alopecia, dry skin, and hepatotoxicity [30, 35, 101, 104]. It may develop in patients who consume high doses of vitamin A, 25,000 IU or more daily, for several months.

Patients in chronic renal failure are vulnerable to hypervitaminosis A [43, 101, 103, 114, 122]. These patients have elevated plasma vitamin A and carotenoid levels of 5.9 ± 0.9 IU/ml (normal 1.5 ± 0.04) and 3.9 ± 1.0 IU/ml (normal 1.9 ± 0.1) respectively; these are little affected by hemodialysis [43]. Two cases have been reported with increased concentration of vitamin A in the liver, 600 μg/gm liver, which is five times the normal [122]. Hypervitaminosis A may contribute to vulnerability to fractures in patients with renal osteodystrophy, owing to the effect of vitamin A on the bone matrix [101, 122] and on the parathyroid glands. Vahlquist et al. [114] found a longer half-life of free RBP (60 hrs—10 to 15 times the normal) and higher plasma free RBP levels in patients with renal failure. Smith et al. [103] showed the same increase in free RBP with higher ratios of RBP to vitamin A and RBP to prealbumin in plasma.

The loss of renal parenchyma may impair oxidation of retinol to retinoic acid by the proximal tubule cells [101, 114, 122] and may decrease vitamin A excretion as retinoyl glucoronide via the bile. Patients in chronic renal failure consume excesses of vitamin A together with the recommended higher intake of vitamin D.

Smith et al. [104] emphasize the importance of several measurements: the higher percentage of retinyl esters as of total vitamin A in plasma, the higher retinol:RBP ratio, and the higher total vitamin A:RBP ratio. Association of total vitamin A level in the plasma of 100 to 300 μg/100 ml (normal 50 μg/100 ml) with normal RBP and prealbumin values and increase in the ratio of total vitamin A:RBP imply that the excess vitamin A is in the form of retinyl esters. The esters are not bound to RBP, but to plasma lipoproteins, which are less protective against toxicity. The binding of retinol to RBP seems to be protective in nature, since the toxic effects of vitamin A elaborated by causing lysosomal membrane instability are more easily produced by non-RBP-bound vitamin A.

Although the liver is the main storage organ for vitamin A, its function is impaired by hypervitaminosis A. Hepatocellular damage with portal fibrosis is apparent on histologic examination [30, 35]. Specific features are hypertrophied fat-storing cell of Ito, with lipofuscin and lipid droplet accumulation and hypertrophy of smooth endoplasmic reticulum [35]. Studies in rats demonstrated increased gluconeogenic enzyme activity, decrease in glycolytic enzyme activity, and enhancement of glycogen deposition.

The symptoms of hypervitaminosis A subside within a few weeks after cessation of vitamin A intake [101, 104]. The high levels of retinyl esters clear within months [104]. Since mobilization of the hepatic stores of vitamin A lasts years, the possibility of continuous hepatic damage exists.

Unitage and Bioassay. Bioassay depends on the ability of vitamin A to support growth of vitamin A-depleted rats. The USP reference standard refers to the purified all-trans vitamin A acetate in vegetable oil. Each gram contains 100,000 units. One USP unit has the specific biologic activity of 0.3 μg retinol, 0.34 μg retinyl acetate, or 0.6 μg of β-carotene. New nomenclature refers to retinol equivalent, which represents one μg of retinol (3.3 USP units) or 6 μg of β-carotene (10 USP units) [72].

Human Requirements. The recommended daily allowances for normal adult male and female are 1,000 and 800 retinol equivalents (5,000 and 4,000 IU), respectively. It is assumed that half of dietary vitamin A is derived from β-carotene [72]. The conclusions from the British Medical Council study were that 390 mg retinol daily represents the minimal protective dose of vitamin A, but 750 mg of retinol was accepted as daily vitamin A requirements for the adult human. Subsequently the aforementioned 1,000 retinol equivalents daily was adopted by the Food and Nutrition Board [38].

In vitamin A-depleted patients, supplementation with retinol is much more effective than β-carotene in alleviating symptoms and restoring vitamin A levels in plasma to normal [94]. To prevent dark adaptation impairment, 150 to 300 μg of retinol are required (300 to 600 mg of β-carotene). Prevention of skin lesions requires 600 mg/day retinol. Restoration of plasma levels to above 30 mg/dl requires 1,200 mg retinol (2,400 mg β-carotene) daily [94].

The requirement of infants is 420 retinol equivalents (RE) (as vitamin A in milk) during the first 6 months, 400 RE up to 3 years of age, 500 RE up to 6 years of age, and 700 RE up to 10 years of age, assuming that one quarter of intake is a β-carotene. Pregnant women require 1,000 mg and lactating women 1,200 mg vitamin A [38, 70]. Premature neonates require a relatively higher dose of vitamin A because their stores are minimal [10, 49].

Patients with liver disease have marginal levels of vitamin A [93, 103]. Their plasma vitamin A levels are markedly decreased. Hepatic content of vitamin A is depressed, and their ability to synthesize RBP and prealbumin is impaired.

Requirements During TPN. Patients who require TPN are marginal as far as their vitamin A status is concerned (Table 8-3). They may have low levels of vitamin A and RBP [71, 88, 99].

Lowry et al. [71] indicate the prevalence of hypovitaminosis A in the malnourished American population and their need for high doses of administered vitamin A, 1,300 to 2,900 IU daily. Some of the malnourished patients may require up to 4,500 IU daily to reverse subnormal levels. They claimed that when vitamin A is administered intravenously, toxicity is a rarity.

Low carotene levels (37 ± 6 mg/100 ml) were found during TPN, but they were unrelated to plasma vitamin A levels. They may just reflect low enteral intake [71]. Nichoalds et al. [77], administering 3,300 IU vitamin A daily, found lower than normal (40 mg/100 ml) plasma levels of vitamin A. Jeejeebhoy et al. administered 2,500 IU daily (5,000 IU every other day) and found vitamin A values within normal limits [57]. The same dose was used by Stromberg et al. [107a] and was found adequate in their study of patients with postoperative complications. Our

Table 8-3. *Fat-Soluble Vitamin Requirements During TPN*

	RDA [38]						Recommended Daily Doses During TPN [2, 77]			Suggested Composition for Intravenous Multivitamin Preparation for Daily Maintenance of Adequate Vitamin Status [2, 78]	
Vitamin	Infants		Children 1–10		Adults		Infants	Children 1–10	Adults	Infancy to 10 Years	Adults
Vitamin A RE/IU	0–6 mo	420 RE 400 IU	1–3 yr	400 RE 2,000 IU	Males	1,000 RE 5,000 IU*	2,000 [70]	2,300	3,300 IU [2, 77]	2,300	3,300
	6–12 mo	400 RE 2,000 IU	4–6 yr 7–10 yr	500 RE 700 RE 3,300 IU	Females	800 RE 4,000 IU*					
Vitamin D IU		400		400		400	200 [70]	400	200	400	200
Vitamin E IU	0–6 mo 6–12 mo	4 5	1–3 yr 4–6 yr 7–10 yr	7 9 10	Males Females	15 12	1 [70]	7	10 [2] 1.65–2.1 [77] 525 [57]	7.0	10.0
Vitamin K	0.5–5 μg/day [2]		1 mg/day–1 mg/week [2]		0.03–1.5 μg/kg/day [70]		10–20 μg/kg up to 0.2 mg/day [2]	0.2 mg/day [2] 0.2 mg–1.5 mg/week	2–4 mg/week [2]		

*Assumes 50 percent intake as carotene, which is less readily available than vitamin A.

Source: RDA on vitamins from *Recommended Daily Allowances* (8th ed.), Publication No. 2216, National Academy of Sciences, 1974; and Table on recommended daily doses of vitamins during TPN from Nutrition Advisory Group: Vitamin preparations for parenteral use, Appendix A in symposium of Total Parenteral Nutrition, Chicago: American Medical Association, 1972. Pp. 457–464.

current practice is to administer a 5,000 to 20,000 IU vitamin A total per week, or 700 to 3,000 IU/day.

The Nutrition Advisory Group of the AMA Department of Food and Nutrition [2, 78] recommended 3,300 IU vitamin A for adults and children above the age of 11 years. For children under 11 years, 2,300 IU are recommended. This dose may be too high if administered intravenously, but further data are required.

Preparations and Incompatibility. The commonly used preparation during TPN is MVI (USV Laboratories), which contains 10,000 IU/vial.

No chemical incompatibilities with TPN solution have been demonstrated [95]. Hartline et al. [49] pointed to a decrease in delivery of vitamin A administered to the patient by the TPN solution, owing to absorption by the chamber and tubing of about two-thirds of the vitamin A in solution. Vitamin A is photosensitive, but protection of the TPN solution by aluminum foil did not change the percentage absorbed [49].

VITAMIN D

Vitamin D was recognized as a vitamin in 1920 by Mellanby and Huldschinsky, who demonstrated the antirachitic action of both cod liver oil and exposure to sunlight [109]. Vitamin D, a common ingredient of the Western diet, is found in dairy products, meat, and any of the lipid components of food. The detailed elucidation of the metabolism of the vitamin, its conversion into a hormone, and its mechanism of action have only recently become available by means of sophisticated radiochemical techniques.

Chemistry. Vitamin D is a sterol that must be metabolically activated before functioning at the target organ. It is derived either from the diet or by the action of solar ultraviolet irradiation on 7-dehydrocholesterol. This photometabolic step involves cleavage of the carbon bond between C-9 and C-10 of the sterol B ring. The resulting product is vitamin D_3 (cholecalciferol) [50]. Vitamin D_2 (ergocalciferol) is found in yeast and fungi. It differs from vitamin D_3 by a double bond at the side-chain between C-22 and C-23. In man there are no practical differences between the two [84, 109].

Vitamin D, from either source, is hydroxylized at C-25 site by liver microsomal fraction of all species studied, by a vitamin D_3-25-hydroxylase enzyme (25-OH-ase) to form 25-(OH)-D_3. This compound has two to five times more effective antirachitic action than the parent vitamin D [24, 25, 50].

The crucial hydroxylation in vitamin D_3 activation is performed exclusively in the renal mitochondria. The compound enzymatic system 25-(OH)-D_3-1-α hydroxylase is made up of flavoprotein, renal ferredoxin, cytochrome P 450, molecular oxygen, and NADPH. It introduces a hydroxyl group in 1 position to form the active form of 1,25-dihydroxy vitamin D_3. This compound is 1,000 to 5,000 times more active than vitamin D in the mobilization of calcium from cultures of embryonic bone, and three to five times more active and faster in promoting calcium absorption from the intestine [24, 25, 50, 84]. The active form of vitamin D, 1,25-$(OH)_2$-D_3, functions in a classic endocrine fashion. It is produced in the kidney and is physiologically active in the intestine and bone, and its level is modulated according to the calcium and phosphorus needs of the organism.

The control of the production of 1,25-$(OH)_2$-D_3 in the kidney seems to be very stringent at the 1-alpha hydroxylase step [39], whereas the preceding step of 25-hydroxylation in the liver is not tightly controlled. 1-alpha hydroxylation of 25-(OH)-D_3 is regulated by an interplay of factors: low phosphorus and low calcium, which act through the parathyroid glands with parathyroid hormone (PTH) acting as mediator. Other hormones—such as calcitonin, prolactin, estrogen, cortisol, and growth hormone—are postulated modulators [24, 25, 50].

Function. Vitamin D_1, through its active hormone 1,25-$(OH)_2$-D_3, is involved in calcium metabolism affecting its intestinal absorption, its mobilization from bone, and its reabsorption in the renal tubuli.

In the intestine, vitamin D enhances absorption of both calcium and phosphorus. This is done at the brush border as an active process requiring energy utilizing a specific carrier. Its mode of action is by conformational specific ligation of the tri-hydroxy sterol to an intestinal cytoplasmic receptor, migration to the nucleus, biosynthesis of a new mRNA, which induces synthesis of new functional proteins, such as Ca-binding protein, which enhances calcium and phosphate translocation [50].

Vitamin D mobilizes calcium and phosphate from previously formed bone by increasing osteocytic osteolysis [87]. This seems to somewhat contradict the expected action of vitamin D, which is to enhance bone mineralization. Actually, vitamin D, through its different metabolites, enhances the bidirectional transfer of calcium from bone to plasma and calcification of newly formed hydroxyapatite [24, 50, 87, 109]. This action is not exerted by simply increasing the mineral ion product in the plasma and the extracellular fluid, but by an orderly well-controlled mineralization by the osteoid osteocytes at the mineralization front [87]. In addition, vitamin D has a presumptive modulating effect in the parathyroid glands, since specific macromolecular receptors for 1,25-$(OH)_2$-D_3 have been found in these glands [24, 50].

Vitamin D functions in concert with PTH on bone, but in the kidney it enhances phosphate absorption, in contrast to PTH, which enhances phosphaturia [87]. Vitamin D affects only one percent of the total filtered calcium load in the tubuli, 99 percent of which is reabsorbed independent of the action of vitamin D [24, 25, 50, 109].

Absorption, Metabolic Fate, Excretion. Vitamin D is absorbed adequately from the small bowel. It appears first in the lymph and primarily in the chylomicron fraction [109]. Hepatobiliary dysfunction, as well as abnormalities of the gastrointestinal tract, may interfere with proper absorption of vitamin D.

Absorbed vitamin D circulates in the blood in association with a specific alpha-globulin which acts as a vitamin D-binding protein. The 25 (OH) D_3, which is the hepatic hydroxylation product, circulates bound to the same carrier as the parent vitamin, but has higher affinity. It can be measured in blood [100] (normal 29.5 ± 9.9 ng/ml), and its half-life is estimated to be 19 to 20 days [50, 100], or shorter (5 to 6 days) in acute renal failure [81].

Vitamin D is stored in the adipose tissue in its unaltered form and is released slowly, according to the needs for 25-hydroxylation in the liver. The vitamin D stores are estimated to be sufficient for four months [92].

The main excretory route is the bile. It is not quite clear in which form vitamin D is excreted, but it does participate in an enterohepatic circulation [24, 50, 100, 109]. Less than 4 percent is excreted in the urine.

Deficiency. The clinical symptomatology of rickets due to vitamin D deficiency in childhood is well known [50, 100, 109], and includes skeletal malformations caused by bowing of the rachitic bones with specific radiologic and biochemical histopathologic features. In adults, vitamin D deficiency results in osteomalacia, with decrease in bone density, and abnormal bone formation, with excessive amounts of uncalcified matrix [50, 109, 115].

Toxicity. Excessive acute or chronic intake of vitamin D may result in hypervitaminosis D, vitamin D intoxication. In England, following World War II, food supplementation was used in excess of the requirements, and infantile hypercalcemia occurred [109]. The occurrence of intoxication indicates that storage is limited, and the conversion to 1,25-$(OH)_2$-D_3 is not under absolute control [50]. It is conceivable that intoxication is due to increased 25-(OH)-D_3 levels.

Clinical symptomatology consists of weakness, fatigue, lassitude, headache, nausea, vomiting, and diarrhea. Renal impairment is manifested by polyuria, polydipsia, and decreased ability to concentrate the urine. In patients with chronic renal failure, further deterioration of renal function follows hypervitaminosis D [20]. Nephrolithiasis and nephrocalcinosis occur, as well as metastatic soft tissue calcification, with generalized osteoporosis due to enhanced mobilization of calcium from the bones [50, 109].

Unitage. The USP unit is equivalent to the specific biologic activity of 0.025 μg of vitamin D_3, i.e., 1 mg equals 40,000 units [109].

Human Requirements. Human requirements differ depending on age, pregnancy, and lactation. The recommended dietary allowance by the Food and Nutrition Board, National Academy of Sciences is 400 IU daily [38] for all ages. The American Academy of Pediatrics (AAP) suggested an allowance of 55 IU/kg (range 44 to 66 IU) for infants, or 40 IU/100 kcal for infants under the age of one year [2, 78].

In certain conditions the requirements are changed. Since premature babies have negligible stores of vitamin D, and since their ability for 25-hydroxylation in the liver begins only at 36 to 38 weeks of gestation and is probably suboptimal, they require more vitamin D. The few reported cases of rickets in premature babies [48, 65] indicate the lack of complete knowledge of the requirements for premature babies.

Patients with intestinal malabsorption or jejunoileal bypass [100] have reduced absorption of vitamin D and manifest lower blood levels (12 $\mu g/L$) of 25-(OH)-D_3 (normal 33 ± 11.5 $\mu g/L$) [100].

Patients with chronic liver disease show impairment in vitamin D metabolism, manifested clinically as hepatic osteodystrophy [33, 67, 68]. The decreased bile salt excretion and the use of drugs, such as cholestyramine, impair absorption and change the enterohepatic circulation of vitamin D. In patients with hepatic failure, a low blood level of 25-(OH)-D_3 implies defective 25-hydroxylation. To overcome these defects, increased doses of vitamin D_3 or its more potent analogues are utilized.

Patients in renal failure develop renal osteodystrophy, both because of reduced 1-α hydroxylation and because of target organ resistance to vitamin D [22, 37, 39]. Patients in acute renal failure have normal blood values of 25-OH-D_3 during the first week (10.5 $\mu g/L$) but after two weeks of oliguria levels decrease to a mean 5.8 $\mu g/L$ with an apparent shortened half-life to 5.6 days [81]. The reduced plasma level of 25-(OH)-D_3 may be due to hypercatabolism of 25-(OH)-D_3 binding protein, as well as increased tissue uptake. The requirements of patients in chronic renal failure for vitamin D can be met either by mega-doses of vitamin D (100,000 to 300,000 IU/day) or by the use of potent analogues: 1 to 2 μg/day of 1,25-$(OH)_2$-D_3 (40 to 80 IU) or 0.1 mg/day of 25-(OH)-D_3 (4,000 IU) [22], or 1 μg/day of 1-α hydroxy cholecalciferol [20, 112] combined with calcium. The treatment with vitamin D analogues, though proved to be beneficial in normalizing blood calcium, was found to decrease further creatinine clearance in those patients. This finding, together with recent evidence of the effect of calcium and phosphorus product on decreased renal function in chronic renal disease, suggests caution in the use of vitamin D in renal failure. *

Requirements During TPN. The requirements for vitamin D during TPN (Table 8-3) are not well established, although different schedules and guidelines are used. Our own practice is to administer vitamin D intravenously to all our patients in doses of 1,000 to 2,000 IU/week. Utilizing this schedule, we have encountered neither vitamin D deficiency nor toxicity. Since most of our patients receive total parenteral nutrition for only two to four weeks, the stores of vitamin D are generally sufficient.

**Editor's Note:* An increasing body of evidence suggests that Vitamin D, or its analogues, may contribute to the deterioration of renal function in patients with renal failure.

In patients with liver failure receiving hepatic failure formulation (F080), we have not increased the dosage [40], but these depleted patients with impaired liver function may ultimately be shown to require higher doses of vitamin D [67, 68].

Patients in acute renal failure and who are supported by our renal failure formulation [1] receive vitamin D daily (as 2.5 ml MVI, 500 IU of vitamin D per bottle). This may change if vitamin D is clearly shown to be deleterious.

Lowry et al. [71] and Nichoalds et al. [77] point out that blood vitamin D levels do not reflect tissue levels. The levels of vitamin D in serum in patients on TPN were found at the lower margin of normal 17.8 ± 1.9 μg/L 25-(OH)-D_3 (normal 26.8 ± 4.2 μg/L). The efficacy of assimilation and storage of parenterally administered vitamin D remains uncertain [71]. Their schedule includes administration of fat-soluble vitamins once a week (1,000 IU/week), which is below the daily recommended allowance. Nichoalds et al. [77] suggested higher doses of 330 to 420 IU daily.

Few cases of rickets occurring in premature infants on TPN had been reported [48, 65]. Lorch and Lay [70] recommended a dose of 200 IU vitamin D daily as MVI and did not report any complication.

Jeejeebhoy et al. [57] studied the nutritional requirements of patients on total parenteral nutrition at home. Their patients' daily input of vitamin D was 250 IU. The serum values were 34.4 ± 1.9 ng/ml 25-(OH)-D_3 (normal 28 to 42 ng/ml). In a recent report, Shike et al. [98] drew attention to a metabolic bone disease occurring in patients on long-term parenteral nutrition (7 to 89 months). The disease is characterized by hypercalciuria, intermittent hypercalcemia, reduced skeletal calcium, reduced circulating parathormone, normal levels of 25-OH-vitamin D (9.1 to 23.9 μg/L), and a bone biopsy compatible with osteomalacia. These findings improved within one or two months after withdrawal of vitamin D from the solution. The explanation of this TPN-associated metabolic bone disease is not clear yet, but again clearly calls for caution in using this vitamin.

Preparation and Interaction. The most common preparation used is the multivitamin infusion product (MVI) of USV Laboratories. This preparation is water-soluble. It has no overt incompatibility with TPN formula [95]. Its composition follows the guidelines of the Nutrition Advisory Group on Total Parenteral Nutrition of the Department of Foods and Nutrition, American Medical Association [2, 78].

Vitamin E

Vitamin E was first described by Evans and Bishop in 1922 [116]. It is not a single compound, but is composed of seven naturally occurring tocopherols. The alpha tocopherol (2,5,7,8 tetramethyl-2-(4′8′12 trimethyl-decyl)-6-chromanol) comprises about 90 percent of the tocopherols in animal tissues and displays the greatest biologic activity. The isomers differ in number and position of methyl groups. Optical isomers affect activity, the D-forms being more active than L-forms [23, 116]. All isomers of tocopherol have identical side chain.

Vitamin E is widely distributed among plants and animals. It is derived from vegetable oil, margarine, bean, and seeds. The normal Western diet contains 4 to 9 mg alpha tocopherol (6 to 13.5 IU). Vitamin E intake is low in poor countries, where diet contains less than 5 mg (7.5 IU) of alpha tocopherol equivalent. In spite of the low intake, deficiency of vitamin E is not seen, but this is due in part to the lack of a recognizable syndrome of clinical deficiency.

Function. The exact role of vitamin E is still unknown despite attribution of antioxidation properties to it [7, 23, 116]. However, the antioxidant properties and biologic activities are inversely related among the different isomers of tocopherols.

The primary action of vitamin E is considered to be prevention of in vivo peroxidation of lipids, and it would seem as if an increased intake of polyunsaturated fatty acids raises the requirements for tocopherols [7, 53]. Vitamin E suppresses lipid oxidation and formation of ceroid and lipofuscin. Other systems, glutathione reductase and *p*-phenylenediamine peroxidase, share control of free-radical formation with vitamin E. Vitamin E is a cofactor in maintaining the integrity of the erythrocyte membrane, mainly in the newborn and in hemolytic disorders like thalassemia. The effects of peroxidation, which inhibit specific enzymes and alter the permeability properties of structural membranes, were seen in vitamin E-deficient animals [7]. Several enzymes, such as muscle creatine kinase and liver xanthine oxidase, double their activity and their turnover in vitamin E-deficient animals [7].

Vitamin E, like other fat-soluble vitamins, is absorbed through the small intestine to the lymph [7]. In the blood, it is associated up to 65 percent with the LDL fraction, 24 percent with HDL, and 8 percent with VLDL. Plasma levels are about 1.05 mg/100 ml (0.5 to 1.6 mg/100 ml) in adults, and 0.64 mg/100 ml (0.2 to 1.3 mg/100 ml) in infants. Circulating tocopherols are taken up rapidly by most tissues, the adipose tissue being the main site of storage [7]. Vitamin E is excreted in the bile and urine after conversion to a dimer or trimer in the form of conjugated hydroxyquinone or tocopheronic acid [116].

Deficiency. Vitamin E deficiency may occur in specific clinical conditions:

PREMATURE INFANTS. These infants have an average plasma tocopherol of 0.25 mg/100 ml [7]. They have reduced stores of vitamin E, since they are devoid of adipose tissue and have increased requirements for growth; they sustain intestinal immaturity and may show failure to absorb vitamin E enterally. Vitamin E deficiency was related to retrolental fibroplasia in premature infants and had been documented to be prevalent in the outer segment of the vertebrate eye [7, 59]. Hemolytic anemia presents another aspect of vitamin E deficiency in premature infants. The physiologic rapid transformation of erythrocyte population from fetal hemoglobin to adult hemoglobin is decreased by addition of vitamin E. A debate still exists as to whether the improvement in hematologic variables is completely the result of vitamin E administration.

MALABSORPTION STATES. Low levels of plasma tocopherol were found in different patients with steatorrhea, cystic fibrosis of pancreas, and other malabsorption disorders. Some of the neuromuscular symptoms associated with elevated creatine phosphokinase (CPK) and aldolase activities may be associated with vitamin E deficiency. These patients show shortened half-life time of labeled erythrocytes, but no clinical evidence for hemolysis [7, 23]. In some of these patients, accumulation of an acid-fast pigment, ceroid or lipofuscin, was found in the smooth muscle along the gastrointestinal tract. The contribution of these pigments to organic disease has not yet been determined.

Toxicity. The existence of hypervitaminosis E is still a matter of dispute. In studies using megavitamin E supplementation (100 to 800 IU/day for 3 years), no signs of toxicity could be detected [36]. When the serum level of vitamin E was doubled (from 0.65 mg/100 ml to 1.34 mg/100 ml), no changes in liver, renal, thyroid, muscular, erythrocyte, leukocyte, and coagulation function were noted. Prasad [83], in a similar study, found depression of bactericidal activity of the leukocyte. He attributed it to the increased stability of leukocyte membrane.

Briggs [11] summarized adverse effects of high doses of vitamin E in both laboratory animals and man. Rats fed high doses of vitamin E showed cholesterol and triglyceride accumulation in liver as well as intimal sclerosis of the aorta.

Fatigue, weakness, striking creatinuria, and raised serum creatine kinase were reported in man as side effects of overdosage.

Unitage and Dosage. An IU is equivalent to the activity of 1 mg of the racemate d-1 α tocopheryl acetate. The 3-α tocopherol has activity of 1.49 IU/mg [22].

Human Requirements. The human requirements of vitamin E vary according to age, sex, and unsaturated fatty acid dietary intake.

The RDAs are 15 IU for adults, 5 IU for infants, and 7, 9, 10, and 12 IU for children aged 3, 6, 10, and 14 years, respectively [38]. Horwitt [53] elaborated a formula to calculate requirements of tocopherol equivalent according to the amount of polyunsaturated fatty acids (PUFA) in the diet: d-α tocopherol in mg/day = 0.25 (percent PUFA + gm PUFA) + 4. The minimal requirement is 10 IU/day, the range being up to 30 IU/day.

Witting and Lee [121] reevaluated the recommendation for 0.6 mg alpha tocopherol/gm dietary PUFA. They suggested that the requirement of vitamin E be related to the PUFA composition of adipose tissue rather than to dietary fat. They recommended 0.6 IU per gram of linoleate in 100 gm adipose tissue.

Requirements During TPN. The data for vitamin E requirements during TPN (Table 8-3) are few. Their evaluation is difficult, since plasma vitamin E values do not represent the amount stored.

The Nutrition Advisory Group of AMA suggested the administration of 7 IU daily to children under 11 years of age and 10 IU to adults and children above 11 years of age [2].

Nichoalds et al. [77] found low plasma values of vitamin E, 0.2 to 0.4 mg/100 ml (normal 1.0 ± 0.5 mg/100 ml), in patients on TPN, despite a daily vitamin E intake of 1.65 or 2.1 IU/day.

Shils [99] recommended 10 IU/week obtained as 2 ampules MVI/week. Lorch et al. [70] used 1 ml MVI (1 IU/day) in neonates who required TPN and did not detect any deficiency. Johnson et al. [58], administering 0.5 mg tocopherol daily in TPN schedule based on fibrin hydrolysate, found low plasma tocopherol values and increased hemolysis, which responded well to additional daily supplementation of 100 IU vitamin E orally.

The increasing incorporation of fat emulsions, rich with PUFA, in both pediatric TPN and adult TPN increases the requirements for vitamin E.

Jeejeebhoy et al. [57] measured vitamin E levels in patients on home TPN who were getting 52.5 IU vitamin E daily (50 mg of which were in the Intralipid emulsion) and found low levels, 0.65 ± 0.07 mg/100 ml (normal 0.8 to 1.2 mg/100 ml). They suggested a further increase in vitamin E intake.

Most of our adult patients are receiving short-term TPN (two to four weeks), and our dose of 5 to 10 IU vitamin E per week seems to be sufficient. Our general use of three to seven bottles of 500 ml 10 percent fat emulsion weekly does not dictate an increased dose of vitamin E.

Preparation and Compatibility. The water-soluble MVI (USV Laboratories) is commonly used. It contains 5 IU vitamin E in an ampule as d-1 α tocopherol. It has no incompatibilities with TPN solutions [95] and is in accordance with the guidelines of the Nutrition Advisory Group of AMA Department of Foods and Nutrition [2].

Vitamin K

In 1929, H. Dam discovered an essential vitamin for normal biosynthesis of several factors required for blood coagulation [79, 117] and named it vitamin K for *Koagulation.* Its structure was subsequently elucidated; at least two distinct fat-soluble substances, vitamin K_1 and vitamin K_2, were isolated [23, 79]. Vitamin K_1, phylloquinone, was defined as 2-methyl-3-phytyl-1,4-naphthoquinone. It is found in certain plants and is the only naturally occurring vitamin K for clinical use. Vitamin K_2, menaquinone, was defined as 2-methyl-3-difarnesyl-1,4-naphthoquinone. The menaquinones are synthesized by intestinal bacterial flora, mainly in the colon [97]. Other substances have been synthesized and tested for their vitamin K activity.

Function. Vitamin K is required for the hepatic synthesis of four blood clotting factors: prothrombin, and Factors VII, IX, and X.

In 1974, gamma-carboxyglutamate was isolated from bovine prothrombin, and a significant clarification of the mode of action of vitamin K took place [56, 64, 79, 85, 90, 117]. Vitamin K functions in the post-ribosomal, post-translational carboxylation of several glutamic acid residues in the liver microsomal precursor proteins to form biologically active prothrombin and the other vitamin K-dependent plasma clotting Factors VII, IX, and X. The carboxylation requires reduced form of vitamin K, oxygen, and CO_2. Vitamin K is converted by the microsomal fraction of liver to 2,3 epoxide vitamin K. This epoxidation reaction is coupled to the carboxylation reaction [64] and is the presumptive site for the anticoagulant reaction [56, 79, 90].

The modification of the peptide chain by γ carboxylation of 10 out of 43 glutamate residues in prothrombin convert the prothrombin to a biologically active substance. This carboxylation allows Ca^{2+} binding by the biologically active K-dependent proteins and further binding to the phospholipid. The abnormal hypo or α-carboxylated prothrombins are not able to bind Ca^{2+}.

These PIVKA proteins (acronym for Protein Induced by Vitamin K Absence or Antagonism) can be determined quantitatively by immunologic assays in vitamin K-depleted rats or in anticoagulant-treated rats. They can be activated to thrombin by snake venoms, but are inactive in the normal coagulation process.

The four known vitamin K-dependent clotting factors are not the only ones dependent on γ carboxylation of glutamate for activation. A 10,000 to 12,000 dalton Ca^{2+} binding bone protein, osteocalcin, was found to be vitamin K-dependent for gamma carboxylation [79, 85].

Three plasma proteins (the exact role of which has not yet been clarified), C, S [79], and Z [85], share similar peptide chain sequence and the presence of γ-carboxylated glutamate as the known blood clotting factors.

Absorption, Metabolic Fate, Excretion. Man and other animals with similar clotting mechanism require an exogenous source of vitamin K. Vitamin K is absorbed, like other fat nutrients, in the proximal jejunum. Its absorption is highly dependent on the presence of bile salts and pancreatic lipase, and it efficiently absorbs 80 percent of the administered dose [23, 113]. The menaquinones are more lipophilic than phylloquinone, and the presence of bile salts for absorption is mandatory. Since bile salts are absorbed in the terminal ileum, it is difficult to conceive the mechanism by which menaquinones, produced by the bacterial flora in the colon, will be absorbed [97]. Udal demonstrated lack of vitamin K absorption when administered to the cecum of warfarin-treated patients [113]. The lymph is the major route of transport for the absorbed phylloquinone.

The clearance of vitamin K from the circulation is rapid (t½—20 minutes) [113], and the vitamin is probably taken up by the liver. The stores of vitamin K in liver and other tissues are small [2]. Phylloquinone is rapidly metabolized to more polar metabolites and is excreted in the urine and via the bile into the intestine [97].

Deficiency. Vitamin K deficiency may be purposely and iatrogenically induced by anticoagulant medications. Newborns have hypoprothrombinemia for a few days after birth—the time required to obtain an adequate dietary intake and to establish a normal intestinal bacterial flora [23, 31].

Vitamin K deficiency must be suspected in certain conditions: decreased food intake, cancer anorexia, prolonged postoperative course, concomitant antibiotic therapy, renal failure, decreased intestinal absorption as in biliary obstruction, malabsorption condition, or inadequate utilization as in hepatocellular liver disease [4, 31, 82].

Starvation alone will not induce vitamin K deficiency in normal volunteers, but if it is associated with three to four weeks of antibiotic therapy, clinical deficiency does occur [41].

Pineo [82] found 27 patients with vitamin K deficiency, 22 of whom were on antibiotic therapy. Traditionally, the vitamin K produced by intestinal bacteria was considered an important source, but evidently vitamin K produced in the colon is poorly absorbed there [113]. The exact mode of action of antibiotics in inducing vitamin K deficiency should be considered whether it is due to induction of malabsorption or to change of bowel flora [15, 31]. The reason for the high incidence of vitamin K deficiency with renal failure is not clear [4, 82]. It may be due to decreased activity of vitamin K-dependent clotting factors in renal disease rather than any change in vitamin K itself [4].

Toxicity. Phylloquinone and menaquinones are nontoxic to animals. Since the rate of metabolism and excretion is more rapid for vitamin K than for vitamins A and D, the danger of toxicity is less, though present. In patients with severe hepatic disease, the administration of large doses of vitamin K may depress hepatic function further. Vitamin K may induce hemolysis in G-6-PD deficiency patients. In premature infants, menadione causes hemolytic anemia, presumably because of its reaction with free sulfhydryl groups of proteins [2].

Administration of 10 mg vitamin K daily for three days to premature infants causes hyperbilirubinemia, whereas a higher single dose of 25 mg intravenously is not associated with increased bilirubin levels [2].

Human Requirements. The human requirements of vitamin K are extremely small. Frick and Riedler [41] found that starvation associated with antibiotic therapy for three to four weeks induced hypoprothrombinemia, which can be reversed by as little as 0.03 μg/kg/day of vitamin K (up to 1.5 μg/kg/day) [31]. In infants, 1.25 mg/day lowers elevated prothrombin time [2].

Requirements During TPN. Requirements during TPN (Table 8-3) depend on the associated disease of the patient, and hepatic function. Our usual schedule is 10 mg vitamin K in intramuscular injections once weekly. Broviac et al. [12] administer 10 mg of vitamin K weekly with the TPN solution. Jeejeebhoy et al. [42] and Shils [99] suggest 5 mg vitamin K once a week.

The Nutrition Advisory Group of AMA suggests that vitamin K not be included in the regular TPN formulation in order to allow flexibility for administration of anticoagulants. Their recommended dose is 2 to 4 mg once a week [2, 78].

Shils pointed out [2] the wide range of proposed dose in infancy. Normal prothrombin levels were maintained in infants by administering from 25 to 250 μg/kg/day for weeks. Older children maintained normal prothrombin levels without evidence of toxicity at dosages ranging from 1 mg/day to 1 mg/week. The Nutrition Advisory Group [2] suggested 0.02 mg of vitamin K_1/kg of body weight up to 0.2 mg/day or 0.2 to 1.5 mg weekly as safe and effective doses at infancy and childhood.

Preparations and Compatibility. Vitamin K is prepared as phytonadione, Aquamephyton, and is insoluble in water but occurs in emulsion, either in polysorbate (Konakion) or in polyethylated fatty acids derivative and dextrose. Aquamephyton may be used intravenously and intramuscularly.

Menadione, vitamin K_3, is insoluble in water, but its sodium bisulfite (Hykinone) derivative is highly soluble in water and can be administered parenterally [23].

Addition of phytonadione to parenteral nutrition solutions is not done routinely in most centers. There is physical compatibility of phytonadione in the solution, but the chemical stability is questionable, as is decomposition of phytonadione by cyanocobalamine [95]. Longe [69] claims that vitamin K is unstable on exposure to light, and as a result, the patient may receive an inactive ingredient if it is administered by slow intravenous drip. Jeejeebhoy et al. [57] and Broviac et al. [12], who administer vitamin K with the TPN solution once a week, do not report any incompatibility.

The Nutrition Advisory Group suggested incorporation of 0.2 mg/day of vitamin K as part of intravenous multivitamin preparation for TPN solutions for use in infants and children under the age of 11 years [2].

REFERENCES

1. Abel, R. M., et al. Improved survival from acute renal failure after treatment with intravenous essential L-amino acids and glucose. *N. Engl. J. Med.* 288:695, 1973.
2. American Medical Association, Department of Foods and Nutrition. Multivitamin preparations for parenteral use, a statement by the nutrition advisory group. *J.P.E.N.* 3:258, 1979.
3. Anderson, C. E. Vitamins. In H. A. Schneider, C. E. Anderson, and D. B. Coursin (Eds.), *Nutritional Support of Medical Practice.* Hagerstown, MD: Harper & Row, 1977. Pp. 24–56.
4. Ansell, J. E., Kumar, R., and Deykin, D. The spectrum of vitamin K deficiency. *J.A.M.A.* 238:40, 1977.
5. Baker, H., Frank, D., and Hutner, S. H. Vitamin Analyses in Medicine. In R. S. Goodhart and M. E. Shils (Eds.), *Modern Nutrition in Health and Disease* (6th ed.). Philadelphia: Lea & Febiger, 1980. Pp. 611–640.
6. Barchi, R. L. The Non-Metabolic Role of Thiamine in Excitable Membrane Function. In C. Guble, M. Fujiwara, and P. Dreyfuss (Eds.), *Thiamine.* New York: Wiley, 1976. Pp. 283–305.

6a. Beard, M. E. J., Hatipov, C. S., and Hamer, J. W. Acute onset of folate deficiency in patients under intensive care. *Crit. Care Med.* 8:500, 1980.

7. Bieri, J. G., and Farrell, P. M. Vitamin E. *Vitam. Horm.* 34:31, 1976.
8. Blennow, G. Wernicke encephalopathy following prolonged artificial nutrition. *Am. J. Dis. Child.* 129:1456, 1975.
9. Bradley, J. A., et al. Vitamins in intravenous feeding: A study of water-soluble vitamins and folate in critically ill patients receiving intravenous nutrition. *Br. J. Surg.* 65:492, 1978.
10. Brandt, R. B., et al. Serum vitamin A in premature and term neonates. *J. Pediatr.* 92:101, 1978.
11. Briggs, M. H. Vitamin E in clinical medicine. *Lancet* 1:220, 1974.
12. Broviac, J. W., and Scribner, B. H. Prolonged parenteral nutrition in the home. *Surg. Gynecol. Obstet.* 139:24, 1974.
13. Burns, J. J. Water-Soluble Vitamins. Ascorbic Acid (Vitamin C). In P. L. White, M. E. Nagy, and D. C. Fletcher (Eds.), *Total Parenteral Nutrition.* Acton, MA: Publishing Sciences Group, 1974. Pp. 1564–1569.
14. Burr, R. G., and Rajan, K. T. Leucocyte ascorbic acid and pressure sores in paraplegia. *Br. J. Nutr.* 28:275, 1972.
15. Calvin, B. T., and Lloyd, M. J. Severe coagulation defect due to dietary deficiency of vitamin K. *J. Clin. Pathol.* 30:1147, 1977.
16. Cameron, E., and Pauling, L. Supplemental ascorbate in the supportive treatment of cancer: Re-evaluation of prolongation of survival times in terminal human cancer. *Proc. Natl. Acad. Sci. USA* 75:4538, 1978.
17. Cameron, E., Pauling, L., and Leibovitz, B. Ascorbic acid and cancer: A review. *Cancer Res.* 39:663, 1979.
18. Cameron, I., Grubbs, B., and Rogers, W. High-dose methylprednisolone, vitamin A, and vitamin C in rats bearing the rapidly growing Morris 7777 hepatoma. *Cancer Treat. Rep.* 63:477, 1979.
19. Chernov, M. S., Hale, H. W., Jr., and Wood, M. Prevention of stress ulcers. *Am. J. Surg.* 122:674, 1971.
20. Christiansen, C., et al. Deterioration of renal function during treatment of chronic renal failure with 1,25-dihydroxycholecalciferol. *Lancet* 2:700, 1978.
21. Chytil, F., and Ong, D. E. Cellular vitamin A binding proteins. *Vitam. Horm.* 36:1, 1978.
22. Coburn, J. W., Hartenbower, D. L., and Brickman, A. S. Advances in vitamin D metabolism as they pertain to chronic renal disease. *Am. J. Clin. Nutr.* 29:1283, 1976.
23. Cohn, V. H. Fat-Soluble Vitamins: Vitamin K and Vitamin E. In L. S. Goodman and A. Gilman (Eds.), *The Pharmacological Basis of Therapeutics* (5th ed.). New York: Macmillan, 1975. Pp. 1591–1595.
24. DeLuca, H. F. Metabolism of vitamin D: Current status. *Am. J. Clin. Nutr.* 29:1258, 1976.
25. DeLuca, H. F. Vitamin D endocrinology. *Ann. Intern. Med.* 85:367, 1976.
26. DeLuca, L. M. The direct involvement of vitamin A in glycosyl transfer reactions of mammalian membranes. *Vitam. Horm.* 35:1, 1977.
27. Dileepan, K. N., Singh, V. N., and Ramachandran, C. K. Early effects of hypervitaminosis A on gluconeogenic activity and amino acid metabolizing enzymes of rat liver. *J. Nutr.* 107:1807, 1977.
28. Dudrick, S. J. Personal communication, 1980.
29. Dudrick, S. J., et al. Parenteral nutrition techniques in cancer patients. *Cancer Res.* 37: 2440, 1977.
30. Eaton, M. L. Chronic hypervitaminosis A. *Am. J. Hosp. Pharm.* 35:1099, 1976.

31. Editorial. Vitamin K deficiency in adults. *Nutr. Rev.* 26:165, 1968.
32. Editorial. Vitamin A and cancer prophylaxis. *Br. Med. J.* 2:2, 1976.
33. Editorial. Bone biopsy and vitamin D in primary biliary cirrhosis. *Lancet* 1:1138, 1978.
34. Faigenbaum, S. J., and Leopold, I. H. Opthalmology. In H. A. Schneider, C. E. Anderson, and D. B. Coursin (Eds.), *Nutritional Support of Medical Practice.* Hagerstown, MD: Harper & Row, 1977. Pp. 422–428.
35. Farrell, G. C., Bhathal, P. S., and Powell, L. W. Abnormal liver function in chronic hypervitaminosis A. *Dig. Dis. Sci.* 22:724, 1977.
36. Farrell, P. M., and Bieri, J. G. Megavitamin E supplementation in man. *Am. J. Clin. Nutr.* 28:1381, 1975.
37. Farrington, K., et al. Hepatic metabolism of vitamin D in chronic renal failure. *Lancet* 1: 321, 1979.
38. Food and Nutrition Board, National Research Council. *Recommended Daily Allowances* (8th ed.), publication #2216. Washington, DC: National Academy of Sciences, 1974.
39. Fraser, D. R., and Kodicek, E. Unique biosynthesis by kidney of a biologically active vitamin D metabolite. *Nature* 228:764, 1970.
40. Freund, H., et al. Infusion of branched-chain enriched amino acid solution in patients with hepatic encephalopathy. *Ann. Surg.* Submitted for publication, 1982.
41. Frick, P. G., Riedler, G., and Brögli, H. Dose response and minimal daily requirements of vitamin K in man. *J. Appl. Physiol.* 23:387, 1967.
42. Goldsmith, G. A. Curative Nutrition: Vitamins. In H. A. Schneider, C. E. Anderson, and D. B. Coursin (Eds.), *Nutritional Support of Medical Practice.* Hagerstown, MD: Harper & Row, 1977. Pp. 101–123.
43. Gotloib, L., Sklan, D., and Mines, M. Hemodialysis. Effect on plasma levels of vitamin A and carotenoid. *J.A.M.A.* 239:751, 1978.
44. Green, P. J. Folate deficiency and intravenous nutrition. *Lancet* 1:814, 1977. Letter.
45. Greene, H. L. Vitamins. In *Symposium of Total Parenteral Nutrition.* Chicago: AMA, 1972. Pp. 241–256.
46. Greengard, P. Water-Soluble Vitamins. The Vitamin B Complex. In P. L. White, M. E. Nagy, and D. C. Fletcher (Eds.), *Total Parenteral Nutrition.* Acton, MA: Publishing Sciences Group, 1974. Pp. 1549–1563.
47. Gruppo, R. A., and Fraham, G. G. Total parenteral alimentation solution. *Hopkins Med. J.* 127:352, 1970.
48. Gutcher, G. R., and Chesney, R. W. Iatrogenic rickets as a complication of a total parenteral nutrition program. *Clin. Pediatr.* 17:817, 1978.
49. Hartline, J. V., and Zachman, R. D. Vitamin A in total parenteral nutrition solution. *Pediatrics* 58:448, 1976.
50. Haussler, M. R., and McCain, T. A. Basic and clinical concepts related to vitamin D metabolism and action. *N. Engl. J. Med.* 297:974 (Part I), 1041 (Part II), 1977.
51. Herman, R. H., Stifel, F., and Greene, H. L. Vitamin-Deficient States and Other Related Diseases. In J. M. Dietschy (Ed.), *Disorders of the Gastrointestinal Tract, Disorders of the Liver, Nutritional Disorders.* New York: Grune & Stratton, 1976. Pp. 390–393.
52. Hodges, R. E., et al. Hematopoietic studies in vitamin A deficiency. *Am. J. Clin. Nutr.* 31:876, 1978.
53. Horwitt, M. K. Status of human requirements for vitamin E. *Am. J. Clin. Nutr.* 27:1182, 1974.
54. Howard, L., Wagner, C., and Shecker, S. Malabsorption of thiamine in folate-deficient rats. *J. Nutr.* 104:1024, 1977.
55. Ibbotson, R. M., Colvin, B. T., and Colvin, M. P. Folic acid deficiency during intensive therapy. *Br. Med. J.* 2:145, 1975.
56. Jackson, C. M., and Suttie, J. W. Recent developments in understanding the mechanism of vitamin K and vitamin K-antagonist drug action and the consequences of vitamin K action in blood coagulation. *Prog. Hematol.* 10:333, 1977.
57. Jeejeebhoy, K. N., et al. Total parenteral nutrition at home: Studies in patients surviving four months to five years. *Gastroenterology* 71:943, 1976.
58. Johnson, A. M., and Morriss, M. A. W. Can vitamin E deficiency occur in an infant receiving total parenteral nutrition? *Pediatrics* 59: 789, 1977.
59. Johnson, L., Schaffer, D., and Boggs, T. R. The premature infant, vitamin E deficiency and retrolental fibroplasia. *Am. J. Clin. Nutr.* 27:1158, 1974.
60. Kiorpes, T. C., Kim, Y. C. L., and Wolf, G. Stimulation of the synthesis of specific glycoproteins in corneal epithelium by vitamin A. *Exp. Eye Res.* 28:23, 1979.
61. Kishi, H., et al. Thiamine and pyridoxine requirements during intravenous hyperalimentation. *Am. J. Clin. Nutr.* 32:332, 1972.

62. Kopple, J. D., and Swendseid, M. E. Vitamin and nutrition in patients undergoing maintenance hemodialysis. *Kidney Int.* (Suppl) 7:79, 1975.
63. Kramer, J., and Goodwin, J. A. Wernicke's encephalopathy. Complications of intravenous hyperalimentation. *J.A.M.A.* 238:2176, 1977.
64. Larson, A. E., and Suttie, J. W. Vitamin K dependent carboxylase: Evidence for a hydroperoxide intermediate in the reaction. *Proc. Natl. Acad. Sci. USA* 75:5413, 1978.
65. Leape, L. L., and Valaes, T. Rickets in low birth weight infants receiving total parenteral nutrition. *J. Pediatr. Surg.* 11:665, 1976.
66. Loerch, J. D., Underwood, B. A., and Lewis, K. C. Response of plasma levels of vitamin A to a dose of vitamin A as an indicator of hepatic vitamin A reserves in rats. *J. Nutr.* 109:778, 1979.
67. Long, R. G., et al. Parenteral 1,25-dihydroxycholecalciferol in hepatic osteomalacia. *Br. Med. J.* 1:75, 1978.
68. Long, R. G., et al. Clinical, biochemical and histological studies of osteomalacia, osteoporosis, and parathyroid function in chronic liver disease. *Gut* 19:85, 1978.
69. Longe, R. L. Stability of phytonadione in hyperalimentation fluid. *Am. J. Hosp. Pharm.* 31:1039, 1974.
70. Lorch, V., and Lay, S. A. Parenteral alimentation in the neonate. *Pediatr. Clin. North Am.* 24:547, 1977.
71. Lowry, S. F., et al. Parenteral vitamin requirements during intravenous feeding. *Am. J. Clin. Nutr.* 31:2149, 1978.
72. Mandel, H. G. Fat-Soluble Vitamins—Vitamin A. In L. S. Goodman and A. Gilman (Eds.), *The Pharmacological Basis of Therapeutics* (5th ed.). New York: Macmillan, 1975. Pp. 1570–1578.
73. Meyers, C. C., Schocher, S. S., and McCormick, W. F. Wernicke's encephalopathy in infancy. Development during parenteral nutrition. *Acta Neuropathol. (Berl.)* 43:267, 1978.
74. Moran, J. R., and Greene, H. L. The B vitamins and vitamin C in human nutrition. *Am. J. Dis. Childh.* 133:192, 308, 1979.
75. Nadel, A. M., and Burger, P. C. Wernicke encephalopathy following prolonged intravenous therapy. *J.A.M.A.* 235:2403, 1976.
76. Newell, F. W. *Ophthalmology, Principles and Concepts* (4th ed.). St. Louis: Mosby, 1978. Pp. 80–112.
77. Nichoalds, G. E., Meng, H. C., and Caldwell, M. D. Vitamin requirements in patients receiving total parenteral nutrition. *Arch. Surg.* 112:1061, 1977.
78. Nutrition Advisory Group on Total Parenteral Nutrition. Vitamin Preparations for Parenteral Use, Appendix A. In *Symposium of Total Parenteral Nutrition.* Chicago: AMA, 1972. Pp. 457–464.
79. Olson, R. E., and Suttie, J. W. Vitamin K and 8-carboxylglutamate biosynthesis. *Vitam. Horm.* 35:59, 1977.
80. Perrillo, R. P., Tedesco, F. J., and Wise, L. The role of additives in allergic vasculitis during intravenous hyperalimentation. *Dig. Dis.* 20: 1191, 1975.
81. Pietrek, J., Kokot, F., and Kuska, J. Kinetics of serum 25-hydroxyvitamin D in patients with acute renal failure. *Am. J. Clin. Nutr.* 31: 1919, 1978.
82. Pineo, G. F., Fallus, A. S., and Hirsh, J. Unexpected vitamin K deficiency in hospitalized patients. *Can. Med. Assoc. J.* 109:880, 1973.
83. Prasad, J. S. Effect of vitamin E supplementation on leukocyte function. *Am. J. Clin. Nutr.* 33:606, 1980.
84. Procsal, A., Okamara, W. H., and Norman, A. W. Vitamin D, its metabolites and analogs, a review of the structural requirements for biological activity. *Am. J. Clin. Nutr.* 29:1271, 1976.
85. Prydz, H. Vitamin K dependent clotting factors. *Semin. Thromb. Hemostas.* 4:1, 1977.
86. Rai, K., and Courtemanche, A. D. Vitamin A assay in burned patients. *J. Trauma* 15:419, 1975.
87. Rasmussen, H., and Bordier, P. Vitamin D and bone. *Metab. Bone Dis. Rel. Res.* 1:7, 1978.
88. Reddy, V., Mohanram, M., and Raghranulu, N. Serum retinol binding protein and vitamin A levels in malnourished children. *Acta Pediatr. Scand.* 68:65, 1979.
89. Reitz, P., Wiss, O., and Weber, F. Metabolism of vitamin A and the deterioration of vitamin A status. *Vitam. Horm.* 32:237, 1974.
90. Ren, P., et al. Mechanism of action of anticoagulants: Correlation between the inhibition of prothrombin synthesis and the regenerating of vitamin K from vitamin K epoxide. *J. Pharmacol. Exp. Ther.* 201:541, 1977.
91. Rindi, G., and Ventura, U. Thiamine intestinal transport. *Physiol. Rev.* 52:817, 1972.
92. Rosentreich, S., Rich, C., and Volwiler, W. Deposition in and release of vitamin D_3 from

body fat: Evidence for a storage site in the rat. *J. Clin. Invest.* 50:679, 1971.
93. Russell, R. M., et al. Vitamin A reversal of abnormal dark adaptation in cirrhosis. Study of effects on the plasma retinol transport system. *Ann. Intern. Med.* 88:622, 1978.
94. Sauberlich, H. E., et al. Vitamin A metabolism and requirements in the human. Studies with the use of labeled retinol. *Vitam. Horm.* 32:251, 1974.
95. Schuetz, D. H., and King, J. C. Compatibility and stability of electrolytes, vitamins and antibiotics in combination with 8% amino acid solutions. *Am. J. Hosp. Pharm.* 35:33, 1978.
96. Shah, P. C., Zafar, M., and Patel, A. R. Folate deficiency during intravenous hyperalimentation. *J. Med.* 8:383, 1977.
97. Shearer, M. J., McBurney, A., and Barkham, P. Studies on the absorption and metabolism of phylloquinane (vitamin K_1) in man. *Vitam. Horm.* 32:513, 1974.
98. Shike, M., et al. Metabolic bone disease in patients receiving long-term total parenteral nutrition. *Ann. Intern. Med.* 92:343, 1980.
99. Shils, M. E. Parenteral Nutrition. In R. S. Goodhart and M. E. Shils (Eds.), *Modern Nutrition in Health and Disease* (6th ed.). Philadelphia: Lea & Febiger, 1980. Pp. 1125–1152.
100. Shoen, M. S., et al. Significance of serum level of 25-hydroxy-cholecalciferol in gastrointestinal disease. *Dig. Dis.* 23:137, 1978.
101. Shumens, E. Hypervitaminosis A in a patient with alopecia receiving renal dialysis. *Arch. Dermatol.* 115:882, 1979.
102. Singh, V. N., Singh, M., and Dileepan, K. N. Early effects of vitamin A toxicity on hepatic glycosis in rat. *J. Nutr.* 108:1959, 1978.
103. Smith, F. R., and Goodman, D. S. The effect of diseases of the liver, thyroid, and kidneys on the transport of vitamin A in human plasma. *J. Clin. Invest.* 50:2426, 1971.
104. Smith, F. R., and Goodman, D. S. Vitamin A transport in human vitamin A toxicity. *N. Engl. J. Med.* 294:805, 1976.
105. Smith, J. C., et al. Zinc: A trace element essential in vitamin A metabolism. *Science* 181:954, 1973.
106. Sporn, M. B. Retinoids and carcinogenesis. *Nutr. Rev.* 35:65, 197.
107. Srikantia, S. G., and Reddy, V. Effect of a single massive dose of vitamin A on serum and liver levels of the vitamin. *Am. J. Clin. Nutr.* 23:114, 1970.
107a. Stromberg, P., Shenkin, A., Campbell, R. A., Spooner, R. J., Davidson, J. F., and Sim, A. J. W. Vitamin status during total parenteral nutrition. *J.P.E.N.* 5:295, 1981.
108. Steinberg, D. Folic acid deficiency: Early onset of megaloblastosis. *J.A.M.A.* 222:490, 1972. Letter.
109. Straw, J. A. Fat-Soluble Vitamins: Vitamin D. In L. S. Goodman and A. Gilman (Eds.), *The Pharmacological Basis of Therapeutics* (5th ed.). New York: Macmillan, 1975. Pp. 1579–1590.
110. Sugarman, A. A., and Clark, C. G. Jaundice following the administration of niacin. *J.A.M.A.* 228:202, 1974.
111. Sullivan, J. F., and Eisenstein, H. B. Ascorbic acid depletion in patients undergoing chronic hemodialysis. *Am. J. Clin. Nutr.* 23:1339, 1970.
112. Tougaard, L., et al. Controlled trial of hydroxycholecalciferol in chronic renal failure. *Lancet* 1:1044, 1976.
113. Udal, J. A. Human sources and absorption of vitamin K in relation to anticoagulation stability. *J.A.M.A.* 194:127, 1965.
114. Vahlquist, A., Peterson, P. A., and Wibell, L. Metabolism of the vitamin A transporting complex: I. Turnover studies in normal persons and in patients with chronic renal failure. *Eur. J. Clin. Invest.* 3:352, 1973.
115. Van Lancker, J. L. Calcium and Phosphorous Metabolism: Rickets. In J. L. Van Lancker (Ed.), *Molecular and Cellular Mechanisms in Disease*. New York: Springer-Verlag, 1976. Pp. 341–345.
116. Van Lancker, J. L. Vitamin Deficiency. In J. L. Van Lancker (Ed.), *Molecular and Cellular Mechanisms in Disease.* New York: Springer-Verlag, 1976. Pp. 266–317.
117. Wallin, R., and Prydz, H. Studies on a subcellular system for vitamin K dependent carboxylation. *Thromb. Hemostas.* 41:529, 1979.
118. Wardrop, C. A., et al. Acute folate deficiency associated with intravenous nutrition with amino acid-sorbitol-ethanol: Prophylaxis with intravenous folic acid. *Br. J. Haematol.* 37: 521, 1977.
119. Wechsler, H. L. Vitamin A deficiency following small bowel bypass surgery for obesity. *Arch. Dermatol.* 115:73, 1979.
120. Winter, S. L., and Boyer, J. L. Hepatic toxicity from large doses of vitamin B_3 (nicotinamide). *N. Engl. J. Med.* 289:1180, 1973.
121. Witting, H. A., and Lee, L. Recommended dietary allowance for vitamin E: Relation to

dietary, erythrocyte and adipose tissue linoleate. *Am. J. Clin. Nutr.* 28:577, 1975.
122. Yatzidis, H., Digenis, P., and Koutsicos, D. Hypervitaminosis A accompanying advanced chronic renal failure. *Br. Med. J.* 2:352, 1975.

Trace Metals*

Ronald G. Kay
Grant S. Knight

9

ZINC

History

Although the importance of zinc for the normal growth and development of plants has been known for over 100 years [199], an understanding of its wider significance in nature is much more recent. In 1934, Todd, Elvehjem, and Hart [252] reported that the metal was an essential nutrient in the rat, thus establishing a role for zinc in mammalian biology, which was later confirmed in a wide variety of other animal species. Poor growth and development are standard features of deficiency, and they may be accompanied by severe dermatitis, alopecia, and diarrhea, particularly in swine [255], dogs [205], and calves [150].

In 1940, Keilin and Mann [123] established that zinc was an essential component of the enzyme carbonic anhydrase. In 1954, a second enzyme, bovine pancreatic carboxypeptidase A, was also found to contain zinc in an essential biologic role, and Vallee and Neurath [260] dramatically demonstrated that although zinc formed only one of 4,790 atoms in the molecule, it was vital to its ultimate function.

Since then progress has been rapid, and if related enzymes from different animal species are included, almost 100 zinc metalloenzymes have now been reported.

Biochemistry of Zinc

Zinc metalloenzymes are diverse, both in their catalytic function and in the role played by the metal atom [182]. The metal is located at the active site, and although it usually participates in the actual catalytic process, it may also have a regulatory role [208] or serve to stabilize structure [261].

Zinc is now known to be essential for the function and/or structure or regulation of several dehydrogenases, aldolases, peptidases, phosphatases, an isomerase, a transphosphorylase, and aspartate transcarbamylase [262], and there are, in fact, zinc metalloenzymes in each of the

**Editor's Note:* The trace metals represent an area of nutritional support about which comparatively little is known. This chapter represents our current state of knowledge in this area. Investigations currently underway will undoubtedly expand what we know about the trace metals reviewed and will add new trace metals.

six categories of enzymes designated by the International Union of Biochemistry [203].

Zinc enzymes are present throughout all phyla, in which they play a widely diverse role in carbohydrate, lipid, and protein metabolism and in nucleic acid synthesis or degradation. Zinc has been identified in both DNA [228] and RNA polymerase and thymidine kinase [125], enzymes that have a central role in nucleic acid metabolism [196]. Recent studies of *Euglena gracilis* [58], an alga that requires zinc for growth, confirm the important and sensitive role of zinc in growth and show that the metal is essential for each step in the growth cycle.

In addition to its varied enzymic role, it has also been suggested that zinc may influence nonenzymic free-radical reactions, protecting against iron-catalyzed free-radical damage [282]. Other trace elements, however, particularly copper and selenium, and the antioxidant vitamin E, appear to be more actively involved in this area.

The wide role of zinc in biology is due to its position in the periodic table of the elements. The zinc cation has a d10 electronic configuration, and it always exists in the 2+ oxidation state. This chemical stability is probably essential to its role in diverse biologic processes, such as hydrolysis, transfer and addition to double bonds, even oxidoreduction. In redox enzymes, however, such as alcohol dehydrogenase, it does not donate or accept electrons; instead it serves as a Lewis acid [204].

Metabolism of Zinc in Humans

The human body contains between 1 and 2 gm of zinc, and the adult human requirement has been estimated to be between 15 and 20 mg daily [289]. Higher levels are recommended during pregnancy and lactation, and for infants and children, to cover the requirements for physical growth.

Zinc is widespread in nature, and although it is abundant in many foodstuffs [259], the bioavailability of zinc in the diet has been poorly defined. There is increasing evidence, for example, that zinc in human milk has greater bioavailability than in cow's milk, possibly owing to a different zinc-binding ligand in human milk [53, 86]. The amount of zinc in the diet depends largely on the protein content. The bioavailability of zinc from animal products is greater than from plants; meat and fish provide the best sources [63], and the zinc content of vegetarian diets is said to be very low [12]. One recent analysis of a good-quality hospital diet revealed a zinc content between 7 and 16.3 mg a day [178], and it is possible that some communities, even affluent ones, do not achieve the recommended level of dietary intake. This view is supported by the Denver study, which reported unexpected evidence of symptomatic zinc deficiency with poor growth, anorexia, and impaired taste acuity (hypogeusia) in a number of otherwise normal children who had no recent or chronic illness [85]. In fact, suboptimal zinc nutrition has recently been calculated to pose a risk for substantial sections of the population of the United States, particularly those on low-income diets and those experiencing rapid growth [211].

Zinc Absorption

Studies in the rat suggest that the pancreas secretes a ligand that is similar to the low-molecular-weight zinc-binding ligand found in rat and human milk [103]. In the intestinal lumen, the pancreatic ligand complexes with zinc and transfers it to binding sites on the basolateral plasma membrane of the epithelial cell, from which it is removed by albumin or transferrin and transported to the liver. Intestinal metallothioneins probably regulate this process by sequestering excess zinc in the mucosal cells [202].

The percentage of zinc absorbed from the diet is variable and is influenced by such factors as the zinc status of the organism and the presence or absence of chelating agents, such as phytate, in the diet [169].

Distribution in the Body

In the human body the distribution of zinc is nonuniform, with high concentrations reported in the pancreas, the skin and its appendages, the prostate, the liver, and the choroid and retina [249].

Muscle is also rich in zinc [192]. In our laboratory the muscle zinc level in normal subjects is 227 ± 20.2 μg/gm, and if the large body muscle mass is taken into consideration, muscle contains a high percentage of the total body zinc [191]. Hair is a useful index of body zinc status, but only in states of chronic deficiency. The zinc content in normal hair is 193 ± 18 μg/gm.

Zinc in Plasma and Red Cells

In blood 80 percent of zinc is bound to erythrocytes, 16 percent is present in plasma, and 3 percent in leukocytes [172]. The normal plasma level, determined by AA spectrophotometry, is 12 to 20 μmoles/L, about 60 percent of which is loosely bound to albumin [134]. This is in equilibrium with a much smaller amount of zinc in the form of micromolecular complexes with amino acids, especially histidine and cysteine, and lesser amounts of threonine, glycine, and asparagine [67, 194]. Such zinc-amino acid complexes may, nevertheless, play an important role in biologic transport [194]. Thirty to forty percent of the plasma zinc is more firmly bound to $\alpha 2$ macroglobulin, although the high zinc content previously reported, 320 to 770 μg/ml [182], may be inaccurate, as a recent report accords to $\alpha 2$ macroglobulin a zinc content of only 150 to 180 μg/gm and a lessened biologic role [2].

The zinc content of the red cell, 10 to 14 μg/ml [144], is, like the white cell, six to eight times higher than plasma. Such zinc is stably bound, chiefly as a component of such enzymes as carbonic anhydrase and alkaline phosphatase, and shows little variation, even in severe deficiency when plasma levels may fall below 5 μmoles/L.

Plasma zinc is dynamic, and a circadian periodicity has been detected in normal man [93]. Much larger fluxes occur in states of stress, and in acute inflammatory states, for example, the plasma zinc level falls. This is due to internal shifts, which have been shown by studies with ^{65}Zn to be mainly into the liver [184]. These abrupt alterations of plasma zinc are believed to be mediated by a hormone-like substance termed leukocyte endogenous mediator (LEM), which is liberated from polymorphonuclear leukocytes under certain conditions, including some infections and bacterial, endotoxic, and tissue damage [114].

Zinc Excretion

On an oral intake the major route of zinc excretion is fecal. Part of this is comprised of unabsorbed zinc, but the remainder is due to secretion into the intestine, chiefly by way of the pancreatic juice [138]. The intestinal route of excretion remains important, even when zinc is given intravenously. Studies in man with ^{65}Zn show that intestinal secretion may be as high as 18 percent of the administered zinc tracer [236].

Under normal circumstances the urinary excretion of zinc is small and less than 10 μmoles per day. ^{65}Zn studies have shown that 2 to 8 percent of total serum zinc is ultrafiltrable [194], and this percentage is strikingly reduced if the serum is predialyzed, removing amino acids, particularly histidine, glutamine, threonine, cystine, and lysine, with which zinc, as a loosely bound zinc-amino acid complex, passes across the renal glomerulus. Most of the glomerular filtered zinc is reabsorbed [93], but the intrarenal mechanisms controlling the renal handling of zinc are unclear and differ markedly from other divalent cations [239].

In association with catabolic states, however, urinary excretion becomes much more significant. Total starvation doubles the daily urinary zinc loss [235], and a similar increase in urinary zinc excretion, which follows injury and surgical procedures, has been ascribed to loss of muscle tissue, as there is a good correlation between the urinary zinc/creatine ratio and the urinary excretion of nitrogen [60].

Disorders of Zinc Metabolism

Hypogonadal Dwarfism

Although disorders of growth and development were well recognized in a variety of animal species, in the human, because of the widespread presence of zinc in food and water supplies, zinc deficiency was thought impossible until 1961, when Prasad and his colleagues [193] linked zinc deficiency to a syndrome comprising anemia, hepatosplenomegaly, and hypogonadal dwarfism, initially in a group of Iranian boys and then in a number of young Egyptians from the Kharga Oasis in southwest Egypt [195]. Zinc deficiency in these subjects was believed to be related to the high dietary intake of phytate (inositol hexaphosphate) and the habit of clay eating, or geophagia [25], which tend to cause zinc malabsorption [165]. The high fiber content of the diets of these subjects may also be a contributory factor by interfering with zinc absorption [201].

Complete acceptance of an association between zinc and the syndrome described by Prasad has not been universal [30]. In a later study, a randomly selected group of subjects with normal growth and development from the Kharga Oasis were also found to have low plasma zinc levels comparable to the values found in the group with retarded maturation. In addition, vitamin A levels in the Egyptian group were nearly all normal whereas, at least in rats, zinc deficiency is associated with markedly diminished vitamin A levels [231].

Dark Adaptation

The enzymatic activity of retinol alcohol dehydrogenase is significantly reduced in the zinc-deficient rat [101]. This enzyme is essential for the oxidation of vitamin A alcohol (retinol) to the photochemically active vitamin A aldehyde (retinaldehyde), which must be supplied constantly to the rods for the formation of visual pigment (rhodopsin) and the prevention of night blindness [200].

In 1939, Patek and Haig [183] showed that some cirrhotic patients had night blindness that did not improve with vitamin A therapy. This has been confirmed [155] and extended in a study of six stable alcoholic cirrhotics with low serum zincs, in whom dark adaptation was improved by the addition of zinc [156]. Animal experiments using zinc-deficient swine, rats, and lambs have confirmed the interrelationship between zinc and vitamin A. These animals have in general exhibited low plasma vitamin A and retinol binding protein (RBP), adequate concentrations of liver vitamin A and depressed liver RBP. Zinc repletion restored plasma vitamin A levels to normal [230].

Zinc deficiency in cirrhotics is probably due to a combination of reduced intake and increased urinary excretion. The urinary loss is caused by a shift in binding of zinc from macromolecular ligands, particularly zinc bound to albumin, to micromolecular amino-acid bound zinc, especially histidine and cysteine, resulting in increased filtration of zinc at the renal glomerulus. This hypothesis is supported by the fact that increased urinary excretion of several amino acids, including histidine, has been observed in some patients with acute viral hepatitis and in others with cirrhosis [95, 273].

Prenatal and Neonatal Development

The teratogenic effect of zinc deficiency is now well documented in animal experiments [102]. Approximately 50 percent of embryos are resorbed in pregnant rats fed severely zinc-depleted diets, and 90 to 100 percent of the offspring are malformed at term [104]. Such malformations affect every organ system with about 40 percent affecting the central nervous system. A similar percentage showed lung abnormalities. These wide-ranging anomalies are probably not linked to individual enzyme deficiencies, but to impaired synthesis of nucleic acids.

The evidence for a relationship between maternal zinc deficiency and congenital abnormalities in humans is at present only circumstantial, but it is perhaps of significance that the highest rates of congenital malformations of the central nervous system are found in countries where zinc deficiency has been described in human beings. There is also increasing evidence that zinc deficiency may be more common than previously suspected, even in children from middle and upper income families [85]. A third piece of circumstantial support is the report of multiple congenital anomalies in each of 8 children born of alcoholic mothers [110], a group in whom a low serum zinc and hyperzincuria may occur even in the absence of cirrhosis [243].

Zinc deficiency in pregnancy may have additional deleterious effects. In 1968, Apgar [6] reported that female rats had a prolonged and difficult parturition and failed to gather and nurse their young if fed a low-zinc diet during gestation. It has also been suggested that a zinc-deficient pregnant rat may be unable to make normal hemodynamic adjustments, leading to hemoconcentration at a time when blood volume should be increasing [7]. The effects are similar to those obtained by administration of aspirin, and it is possible that the common feature of the two conditions may be reduced prostaglandin biosynthesis or effectiveness [168].

Taste and Smell

Abnormalities of taste and smell (hypogeusia and hyposmia) with, at times, perversion of these senses, have also been associated with zinc deficiency [92]. The effect of zinc on taste perception is mediated through a salivary zinc protein, gustin, and low salivary zinc levels were recorded in the group of patients reported by these authors [96].

Abnormalities of taste and smell have been described in a variety of clinical disorders. Not all of them may be due to trace element deficiency, but there is considerable evidence for a relationship to zinc in hepatitis, cirrhosis of the liver, and individuals treated with penicillamine which, acting as a chelating agent, increases zinc excretion [126].

Some of the Denver children reported by Hambidge in 1979 [85] also had loss of taste and smell, and assessment of taste acuity may be useful in the diagnosis of subtle zinc deficiency.

Wound Healing

Pories and his colleagues, in 1966 [190], were the first to suggest that zinc stimulated the healing process of human surgical wounds. This relationship is controversial [8], and many of the earlier studies were uncontrolled. In zinc-deficient animals, however, there is good experimental evidence supporting the value of zinc therapy in the enhancement of the healing process. In the rat, zinc-deficiency is associated with decreased tensile strength [198, 212] and decreased DNA, protein, and collagen synthesis in surgically wounded skin [240]. Recent controlled studies in patients with venous and ischemic leg ulcers demonstrated accelerated wound healing with supplemental zinc therapy in those patients with decreased serum zinc levels, but no effect if the serum concentration was normal [79, 80].

Zinc in Trauma

The urinary excretion of zinc rises quite sharply after trauma, and although in normal subjects the daily excretion of 7.5 ± 4.5 μmoles is not a major source of loss, two- to fourfold increases have been frequently reported in response to various forms of injury [40, 81, 97]. The extent and duration of such an increase seems to be related to the severity and nature of the injury [59], which is also associated with parallel increases in urinary potassium and creatine, indicative of the importance of muscle in the protein metabolic response to trauma. Isotope studies with ^{65}Zn have confirmed muscle as a major source of the post-traumatic urinary zinc loss, and urinary zinc excretion may be regarded as a useful index of the metabolic state [60].

Zinc in Total Parenteral Nutrition

Because patients supported by total parenteral nutrition (TPN) are also frequently seriously ill, they constitute a metabolic group in whom major

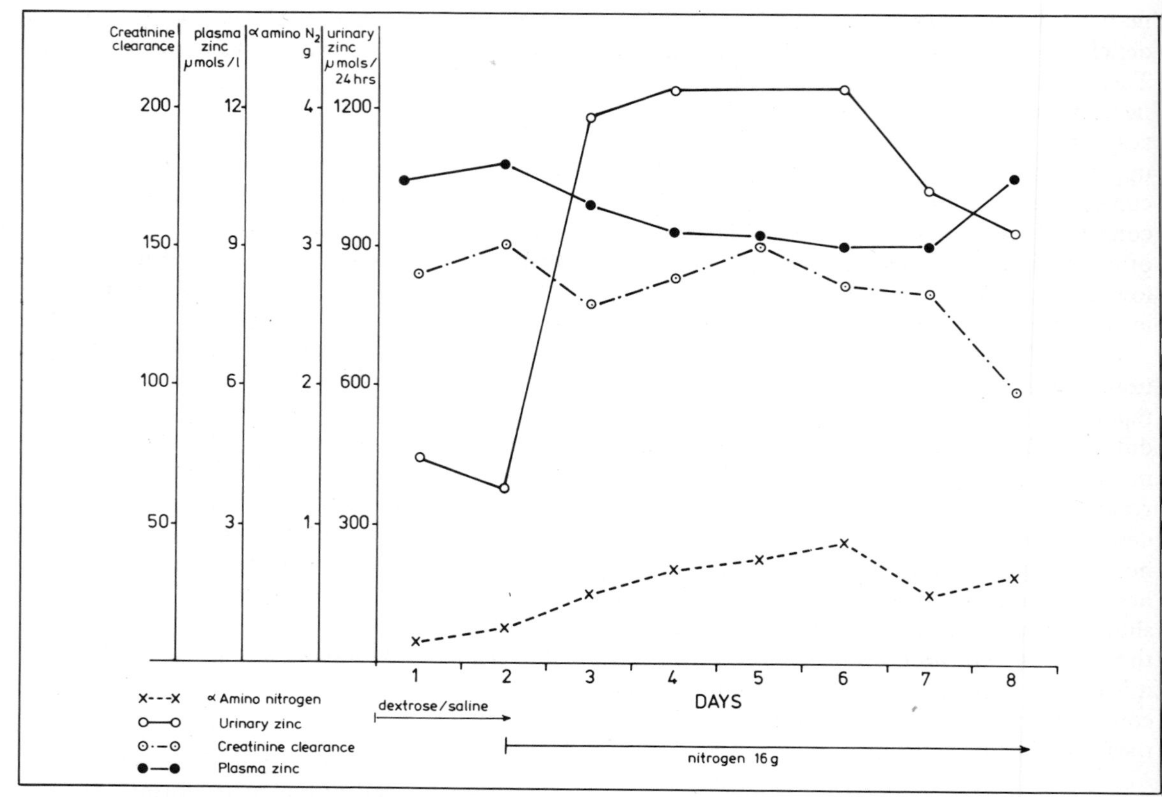

Figure 9-1. *Effect of amino acid loading on urinary zinc excretion.*

zinc losses might occur. In addition, apart from casein hydrolysate, which has a zinc content of 2.5 to 3.5 mg/L, the fibrin hydrolysate and crystalline amino acid preparations are low in zinc, ranging from 0.24 to 1.24 mg/L [14, 263], whereas the contribution from the various glucose and saline solutions is negligible. During TPN the need for zinc and other trace metals has certainly been recognized [62, 88, 107, 232, 285], but the recommendations for supplementation have generally been limited to the addition of only basal requirements. Although usually accepted as 20 µg/kg body weight for adults and 40 µg/kg body weight for infants, Wretlind, in 1975 [286], indicated that these might be insufficient for some patients.

In studies of more than 80 adult patients receiving TPN by standard techniques using the crystalline amino acid preparation Aminofusin and, as caloric sources, 25 percent and 50 percent dextrose and 10 percent and 20 percent Intralipid, daily urinary zinc losses between 60 and 120 µmole (4,000 to 8,000 µg) have been frequently observed. In some patients, urinary zinc has been much higher, peaking at 343 µmoles (22,400 µg/24 hours) in one patient (see Figure 9-9), and at close to 700 µmole in another, almost 100 times normal.

Although the infusion of amino acids promptly increases the urinary loss of zinc (Figure 9-1) [264], due to an increase in the amino acid-bound ultrafiltrable fraction [194], this is not the only explanation for the hyperzincuria frequently observed in the early severe catabolic phase. In our

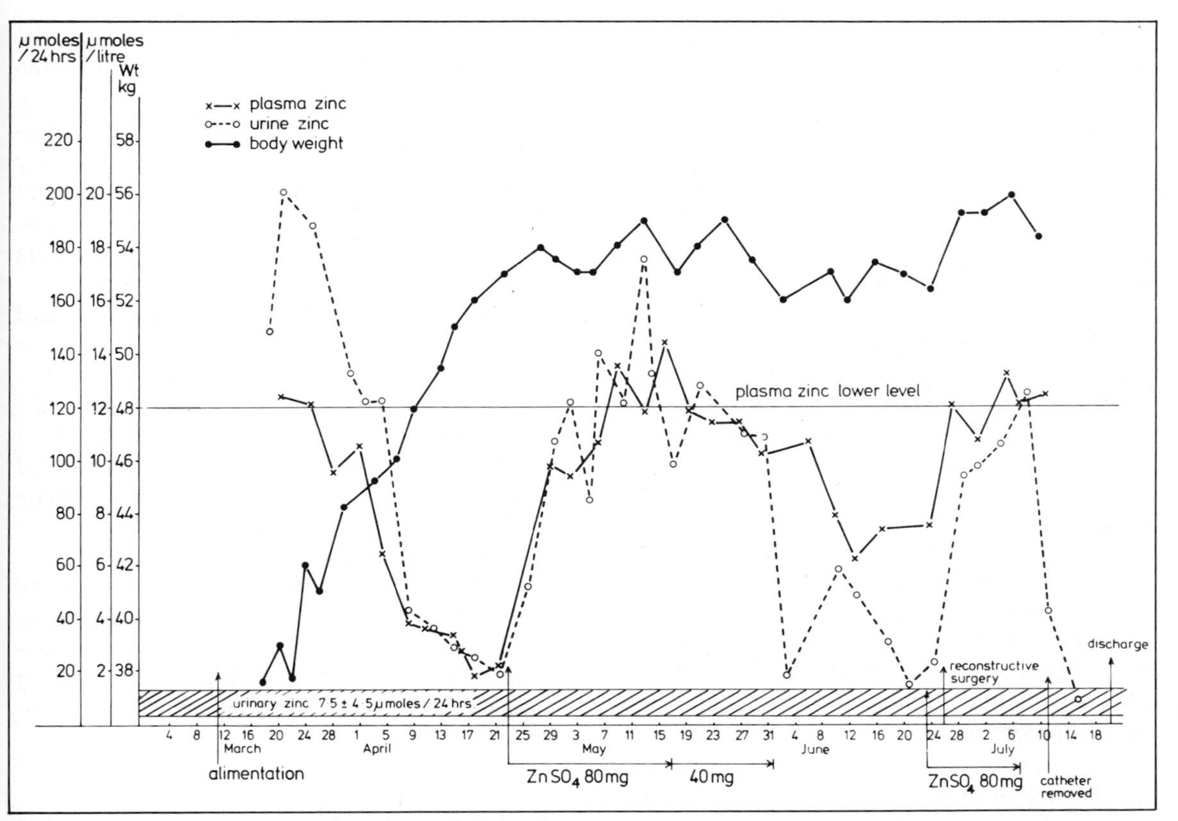

Figure 9-2. *Near normal urinary zinc excretion at peak amino acid loading (32 gm N/day) during sustained anabolism. The fall in plasma zinc during this phase is striking.*

studies, for example, the urinary excretion of alpha amino nitrogen has never exceeded 10 percent of the total amount infused, and urinary zinc excretion almost always returns to normal, or low levels, during sustained anabolism, despite the fact that this is also the phase of peak amino acid infusion (Figure 9-2).

Excessive urinary zinc losses may also occur during TPN owing to the complexing of zinc with sugar amine compounds [64]. This only occurs, however, if the protein hydrolysate or crystalline amino acid solutions are heat-sterilized with dextrose when the sugar-amino compounds, slowly formed by the Maillard reaction, act as chelating agents. The possibility of free amino acid binding as an explanation for the observed increase in urinary zinc was also considered, but no difference could be found in amino acid excretion between two groups of patients given protein solutions that were identical except that one of them contained sugar-amine compounds.

The fecal zinc in patients on TPN is generally insignificant, particularly during periods of total bowel rest when pancreatic secretion diminishes.

A number of measurements have also been made on small bowel fistulous fluid, but apart from one patient with severe pseudomembranous ileitis, even high output states have not been associated with a loss of zinc in excess of 15 µmole/L.

Plasma zinc constitutes less than 1 percent of the total body zinc content, and its value as an index of body zinc status has recently been questioned, particularly at moderate levels of depression [234]. Our experience during TPN, not only with patients in acute catabolism who may have massive zincuria, but also in those with long-term debilitating illnesses, in which zincuria is much less striking, supports this view. In both groups the plasma zinc, prior to nutritional support, is usually in the low normal, or modestly subnormal, range. Striking changes occur, however, as the catabolic phase is arrested and converted to anabolism. Plasma zinc falls at a rate inversely proportional to the improvement in nutrition, as reflected by weight gain and positive nitrogen balance (Figures 9-2, 9-3). This decline may be precipitous during rapid sustained anabolism, and it is not due to an assocaited hyperzincuria, since urinary zinc excretion during this phase is never prominent and may be close to normal. Our studies suggest that there is a tissue demand for zinc during anabolism, which leads to a rapid depletion of the available plasma zinc, unless there is concomitant exogenous supplementation.

In a recent group of patients, the zinc content of skeletal muscle has also been measured at various stages of the illness.

In one patient on long-term TPN (Figure 9-4), the urinary zinc losses were initially very high, reflecting the serious nature of the illness, hemorrhagic pancreatitis with infection, secondary hemorrhage, and a duodenal fistula. In this metabolic setting and despite a high calorie/nitrogen intake, catabolism, reflected by a persistently negative weight gain and nitrogen balance, was merely slowed but never reversed.

Despite this, plasma zinc was generally maintained in the normal range, probably because of continued leaching from the skeletal muscle mass, the major tissue reservoir, as skeletal muscle zinc declined steadily throughout the illness to well below the normal range.

Figure 9-5 illustrates the zinc metabolic data on a second patient who was referred for nutritional support with an upper small bowel fistula following repeated surgical procedures during which he had lost 15 kg in weight.

At the start of TPN, muscle zinc was at the lower limit of normal, but increased during the first three weeks of intravenous nutrition, despite the absence of exogenous zinc supplementation. This was a phase of slow but steady weight gain, and it is reasonable to conclude that the declining plasma values reflect transfer of zinc into muscle, and presumably other tissues, during this anabolic phase.

A brief catabolic period at the end of the third week was associated with a sharp fall in muscle zinc, which then stabilized as metabolism improved. Such stabilization appears to be at the expense of the plasma zinc, which declined to a low point of 3.2 μmole/L. The introduction of intravenous zinc therapy, 80 mg of zinc sulphate daily, quickly restored both plasma and muscle zinc values into the normal range.

The role of muscle as a zinc reservoir is well supported in this patient because the sharp fall in body weight, which occurred as TPN was discontinued, was associated with a parallel fall in muscle zinc, despite continued supplementation.

Acute Zinc Deficiency

Figure 9-6 shows the severe facial dermatitis that developed during the third week of TPN in a 23-year-old man with severe Crohn's colitis. By the fifth week of treatment, the facial rash was severe, and there was also involvement of the perineum and scrotum, the extensor aspects of the elbows, the back, and the fingers and toes (Figure 9-7). During the sixth week he showed obvious loss of scalp hair, which progressed to almost total alopecia (Figure 9-8).

Plasma zinc, measured at the end of the seventh week, was found to be very low at 1.8 μmole/L. Accordingly, treatment with oral zinc sulfate was begun and within one week, a marked improvement in the skin rash was clearly apparent. Restoration of hair loss proceeded more slowly, but was eventually complete.

A similar facial rash developed in a 58-year-old man during a period of TPN in July, 1974. The initial illness was severe, with a peak urinary

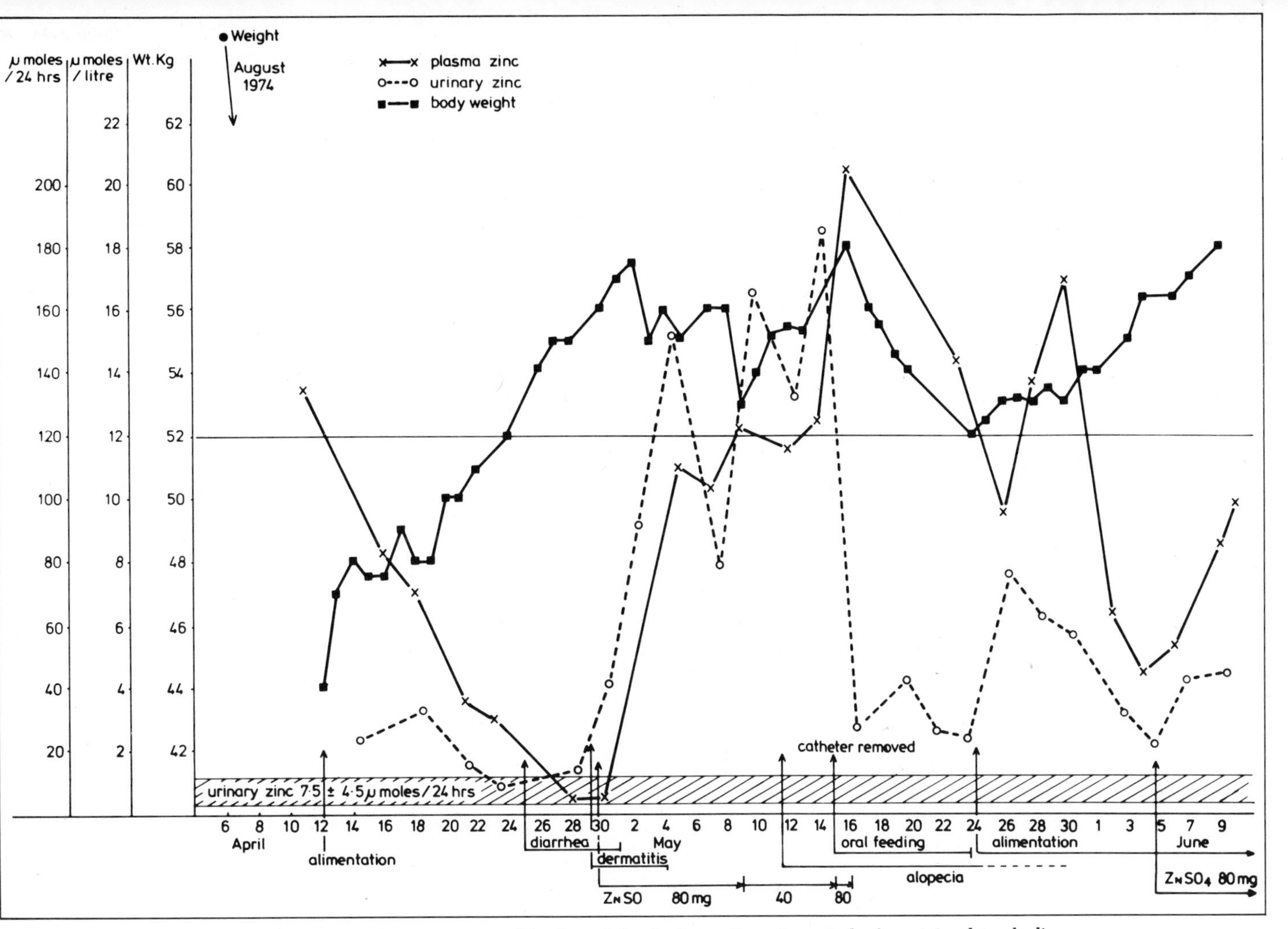

Figure 9-3. *Inverse relationship between plasma zinc and body weight during a 3-week period of sustained anabolism.*

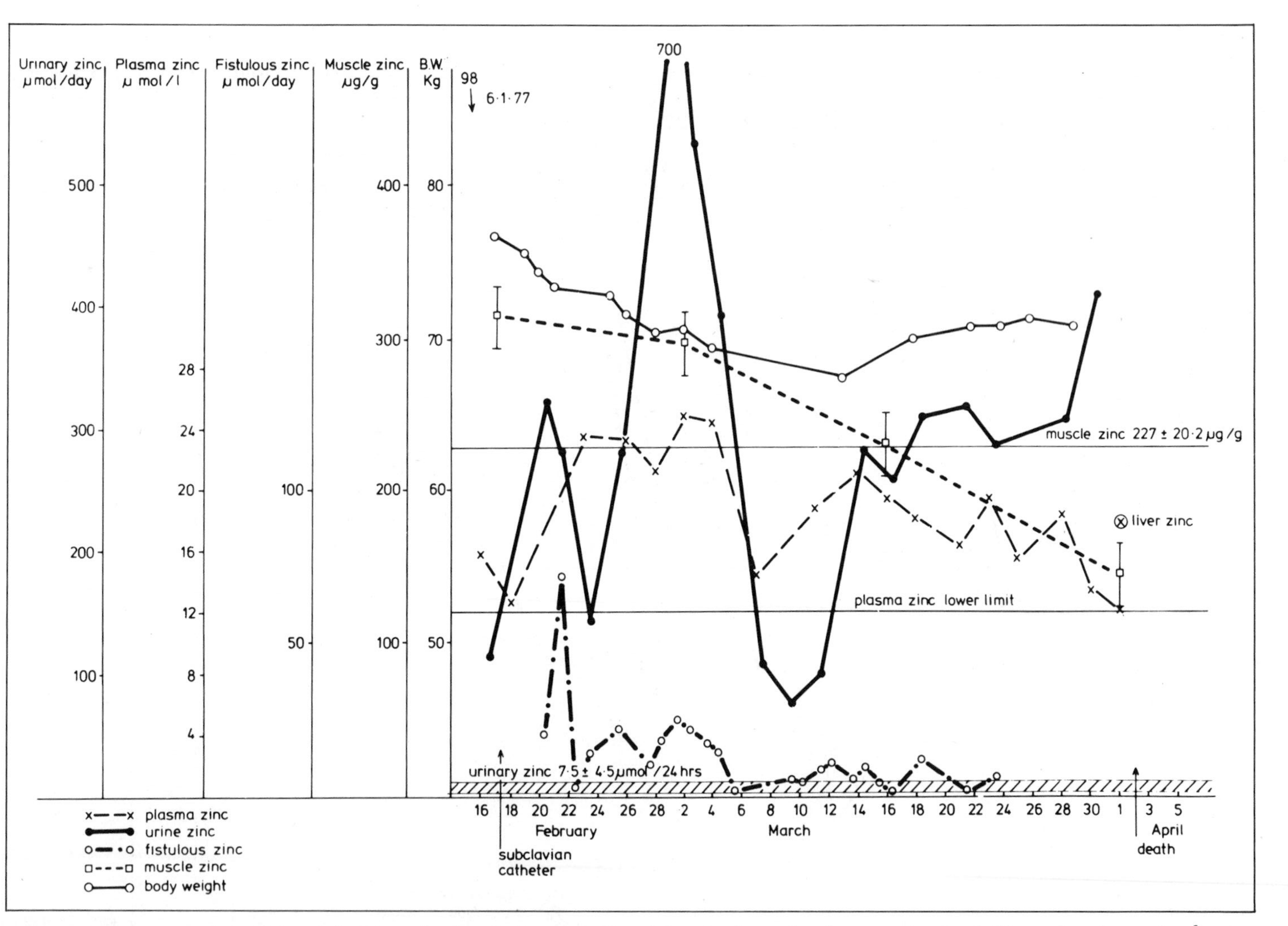

Figure 9-4. *During prolonged catabolism muscle zinc declines steadily, although plasma levels are maintained. The early urinary zinc losses are very high.*

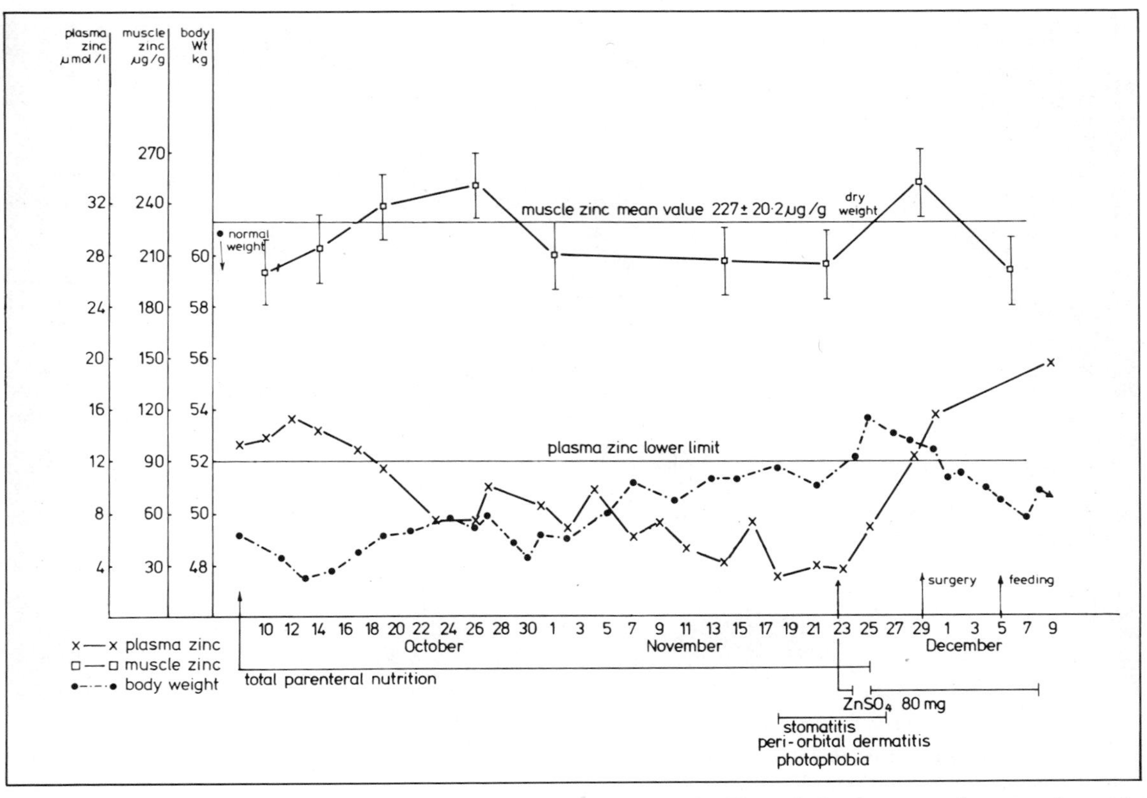

Figure 9-5. *Flux of zinc between plasma and muscle reflects the metabolic state.*

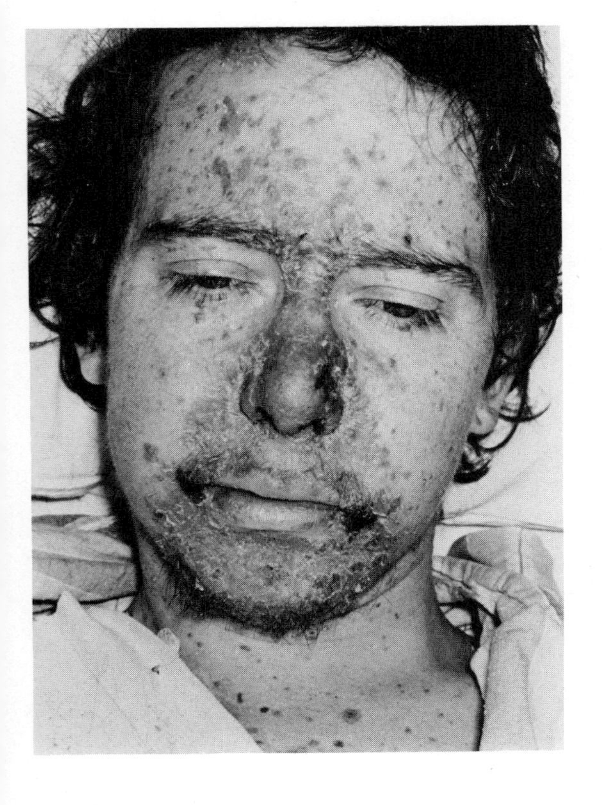

Figure 9-6. *Severe facial rash of acute zinc deficiency. (From R. G. Kay, A syndrome of acute zinc deficiency during total parenteral alimentation in man.* Ann. Surg. *183:331, 1976.)*

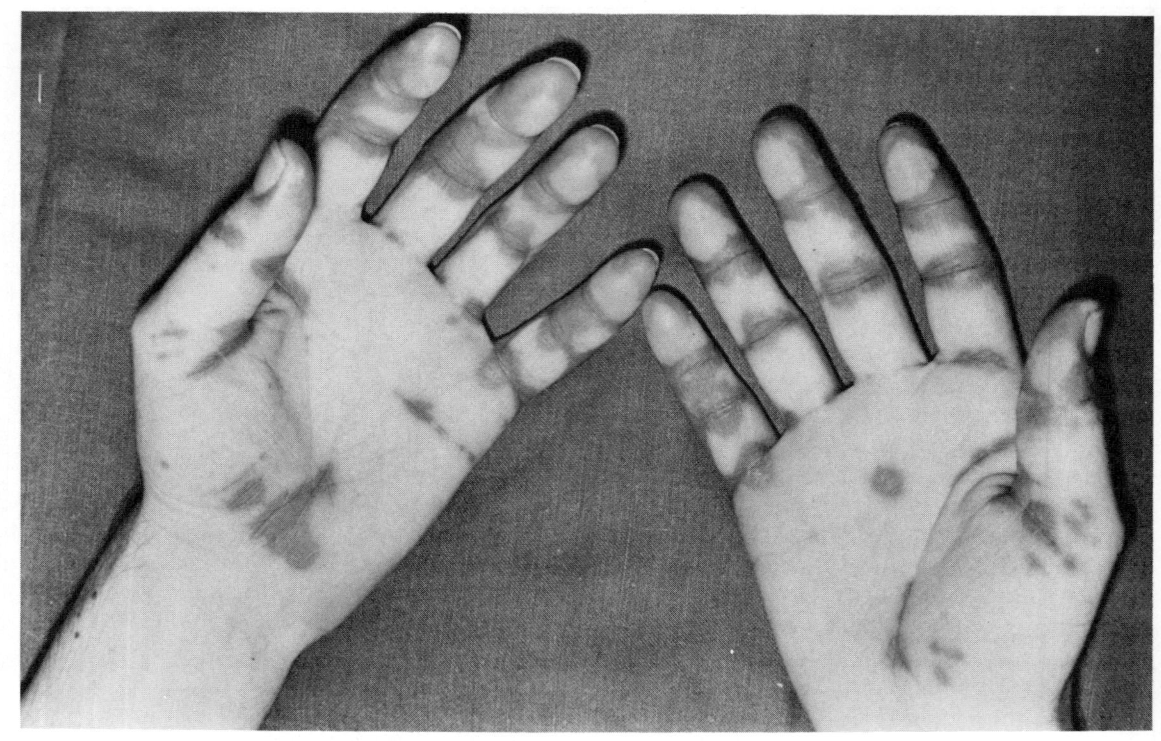

Figure 9-7. *Distribution of the skin lesions of acute zinc deficiency on the fingers. (From R. G. Kay, A syndrome of acute zinc deficiency during total parenteral alimentation in man.* Ann. Surg. *183:331, 1976.)*

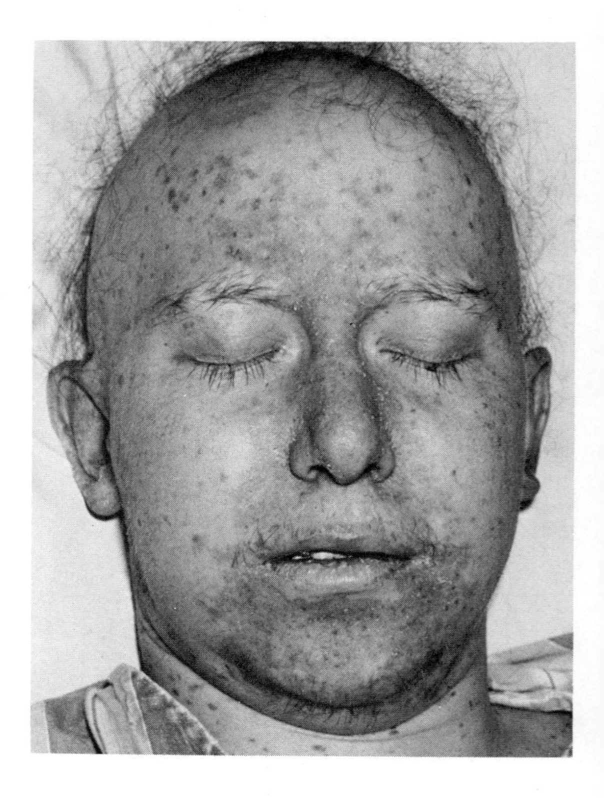

Figure 9-8. *Alopecia due to acute zinc deficiency. (From R. G. Kay, A syndrome of acute zinc deficiency during total parenteral alimentation in man.* Ann. Surg. *183:331, 1976.)*

zinc loss of 342 μmole/day, more than 50 times normal. Nevertheless plasma zinc levels were not significantly below normal during this phase, and a serious decline occurred only when a second course of nutritional support achieved a weight gain of 10 kg over three weeks (Figure 9-9). In parallel with this decline, he became confused and depressed and then, as the plasma concentration of zinc reached its lowest point, 1.2 μmole/L, he developed a severe moist eczematoid rash involving the scrotum, oral mucosa, and perioral skin (Figure 9-10).

The response to intravenous zinc therapy, 80 mg zinc sulfate daily, was striking. Improvement of the rash and mental state was apparent within two days, and within 10 days the facial and scrotal changes had cleared completely (Figure 9-11).

These two cases and others previously reported [118, 119, 171] confirm that zinc is an essential element in human metabolism. The decline in plasma zinc can be precipitous in a sustained anabolic phase and may be associated with the development of overt signs of acute zinc deficiency.

Diarrhea

Diarrhea, which may be severe, is the first manifestation of this syndrome, which may occur at plasma zinc levels not seriously depleted below normal—further evidence that plasma zinc is a poor index of the total body zinc status. The pathogenesis of the diarrhea is unclear, but the response to zinc therapy is usually rapid, with complete control in three to four days. Recognition and prompt treatment at this stage can prevent the onset of the more florid manifestations of acute deficiency.

Disturbance of Mood

Apathy, confusion, and mental depression are also early features, although their precise relationship to acute zinc deficiency is more difficult to define. Nevertheless, the marked improvement in mood that follows zinc therapy is impressive. Severe depression and suicidal tendencies were also reported by Henkin in 1971 [92] in some of his group of adult patients with viral hepatitis and zinc deficiency, and disturbance of mood is a feature of acrodermatitis enteropathica at all ages [158].

Zinc is present in abundance in the brain, particularly in the hippocampus, the cortex, the striatum, and the cerebellum [38, 49], and there is speculation that zinc is related to schizophrenia in that 30 percent of the schizophrenic population excrete a zinc and vitamin B_6 binding substance in the urine called kryptopyrole [186].

Skin Lesions

The most severe manifestations of acute zinc deficiency occur at plasma levels below 3 μmole/L. Inflammatory changes start in the oral mucosa and nasolabial folds (Figure 9-12), and are similar to those first described by Tucker and Salmon in 1955 in dietary-induced acute zinc deficiency in pigs and subsequently reported in a variety of other animal species. The skin lesions, which also resemble those seen in acrodermatitis enteropathica [246], progress rapidly, in the absence of treatment, to involve, in particular, the periorificial areas and the extremities.

Skin biopsies were taken from two patients in the acute phase. One showed hyperkeratosis with layers of keratin infiltrated by large numbers of neutrophils. Apart from acanthosis, the epidermis showed no other abnormality. In the second case the epidermis showed spongiosis and parakeratosis. No acantholysis was present. The dermis showed solar elastosis and a mild chronic inflammatory infiltrate. The appearances were those of a nonspecific subacute dermatitis.

Alopecia

Loss of hair is a well-recognized phenomenon in animal models of acute zinc deficiency [82, 179], and in the chick the degeneration of the feather follicles is due to hyperkeratosis [167]. Hair loss,

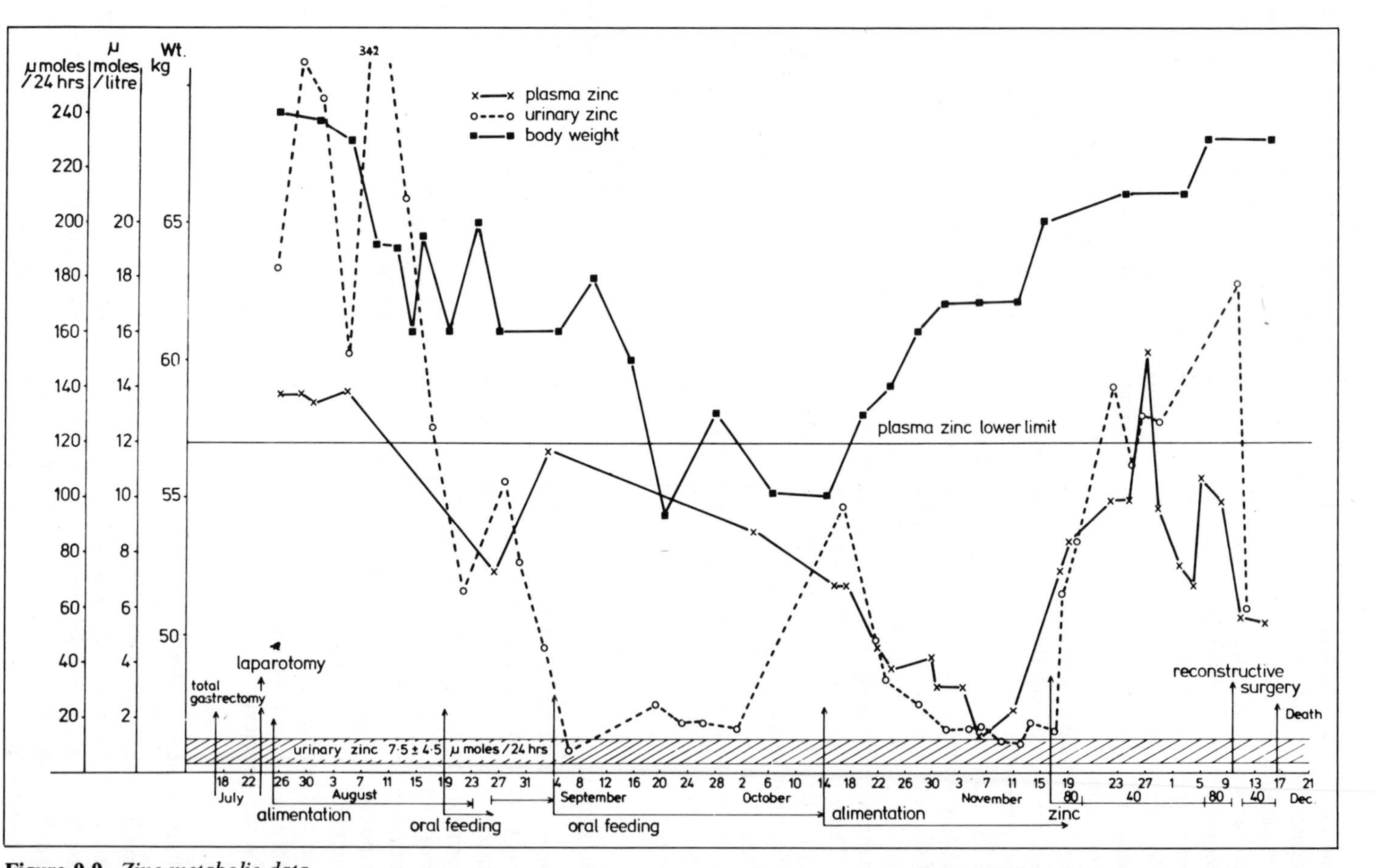

Figure 9-9. *Zinc metabolic data.*

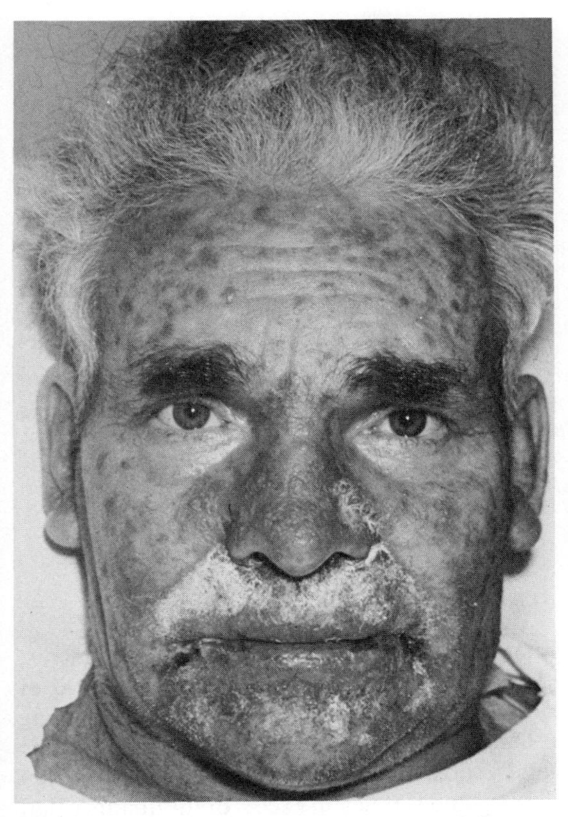

Figure 9-10. *The facial rash of acute zinc deficiency. (From R. G. Kay, A syndrome of acute zinc deficiency during total parenteral alimentation in man.* Ann. Surg. *183:331, 1976.)*

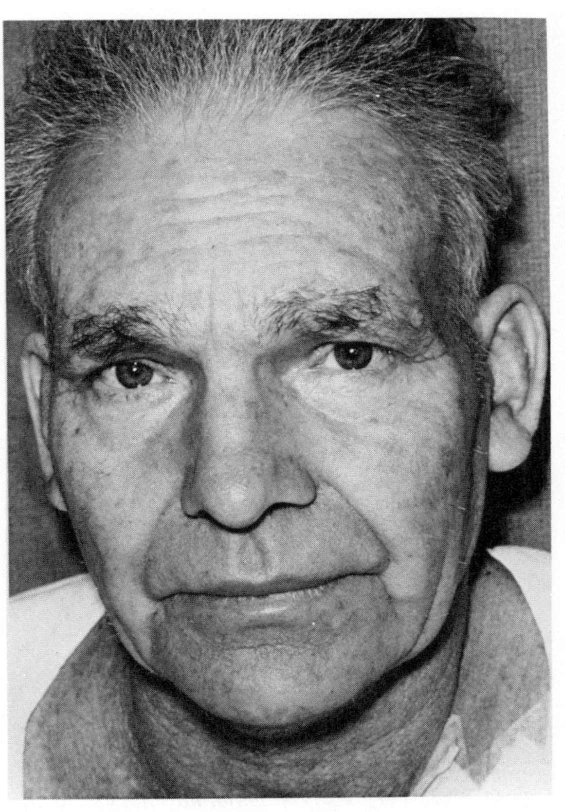

Figure 9-11. *Marked improvement after 10 days of intravenous zinc therapy. (From R. G. Kay, A syndrome of acute zinc deficiency during total parenteral alimentation in man.* Ann. Surg. *183:331, 1976.)*

which may be severe, has also occurred in association with acute zinc deficiency during TPN [119, 245, 256].

Alopecia in this group is slower to develop than the epidermal manifestations, but major hair loss may be expected unless the early skin changes are recognized and promptly treated. Zinc-associated alopecia appears to be completely reversible, although full regrowth of scalp hair may take some months.

Acute Growth Arrest

An association between chronic zinc deficiency and disturbances of growth is now well recognized in both animals and man. Growth arrest, however, also occurs in acute deficiency and is well illustrated by the Beau's lines (Figure 9-13), indicative of nail growth arrest, which developed at the height of illness in the young man with Crohn's colitis. Similar changes in the nails, in association with the classic skin changes, have also been reported by Weismann (1977) [274] in a patient with acrodermatitis enteropathica, in whom the serum zinc fell to a low point of 5.4 μmole/L.

Acrodermatitis Enteropathica

This autosomal recessive, inherited, potentially fatal disorder is characterized by severe chronic

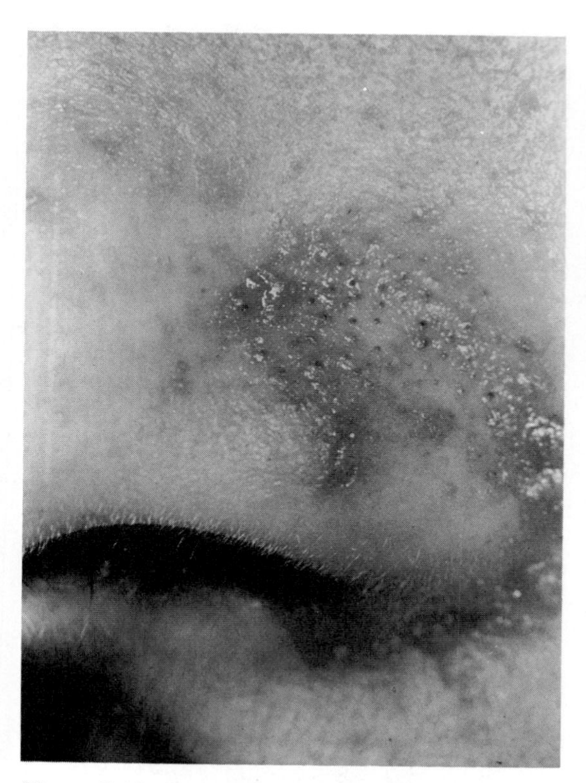

Figure 9-12. *Very early eczematoid changes in the nasolabial fold. (From R. G. Kay, A syndrome of acute zinc deficiency during total parenteral alimentation in man.* Ann. Surg. *183:331, 1976.)*

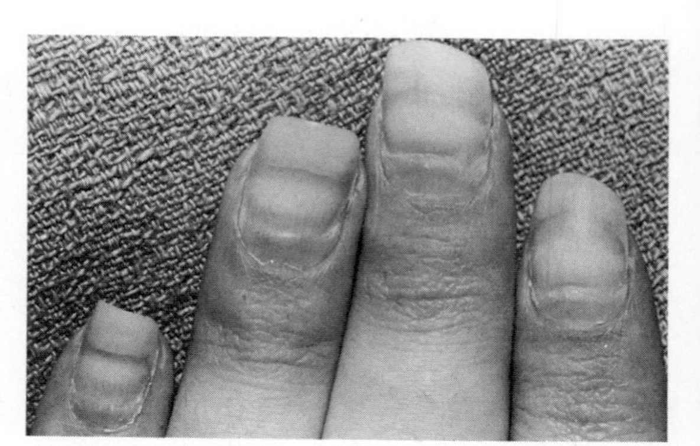

Figure 9-13. *Beau's lines. Nail growth arrest during the phase of acute zinc deficiency. (From R. G. Kay, A syndrome of acute zinc deficiency during total parenteral alimentation in man.* Ann. Surg. *183:331, 1976.)*

diarrhea, loss of weight, alopecia, and periorificial dermatitis, features that parallel those recognized as being associated with zinc deficiency in animals and are strikingly similar to those now reported as zinc-related in man during TPN.

The crucial role of zinc in this disorder was first recognized by Moynihan in 1974 [157], who successfully treated a series of infants with daily supplements of 35 mg zinc sulfate.

The underlying mechanism of zinc deficiency in these patients is probably malabsorption, which may be related to an abnormality of Paneth cells [137].

Zinc Toxicity

Zinc, in comparison with other trace elements, is relatively nontoxic. The usual oral dose of zinc sulfate, 220 mg three times daily, providing 150 mg of zinc a day, is empirically based on the similar dose of ferrous sulfate used in iron deficiency and is much in excess of the quantity that Halsted reported effective in the treatment of severe zinc deficiency. By contrast, the recommendations for intravenous supplementation during TPN have generally been very tentative and have failed to appreciate the potentially severe total body zinc deficit that may develop during a catabolic illness of any length or severity. In our experience a daily intravenous supplement of 40 mg of zinc sulfate is well tolerated on a long-term basis and 80-mg boluses have been safely and regularly administered for periods of two to three weeks, although caution is advisable if there is impairment of renal function, the main route of excretion in this group of patients.

Zinc poisoning has been described after oral administration, but the lethal dose is unknown, and the symptoms of ingestional poisoning are nonspecific: vomiting, diarrhea, fever, and muscle pain [188].

Acute intravenous zinc poisoning, however, has recently been reported in a 72-year-old woman on TPN who accidentally received 46 mmol (7.4 gm) of zinc sulfate over a 60-hour period. The toxic effects, which were ultimately fatal, were characterized by hypotension, pulmonary edema, diarrhea, cholestatic jaundice, and progressive oliguric renal failure. Cardiac arrhythmias, hyperamylasemia without evidence of acute pancreatitis, and acute anemia and thrombocytopenia were other features of an illness that casts zinc in the role of a diffuse cellular toxin that can produce multi-system failure [15].

COPPER

History

Although the presence of copper in almost all forms of living tissue was recognized early in the nineteenth century, a key physiologic role in vertebrate metabolism was not established until 1928, when copper was found to be essential, together with iron, for normal erythropoiesis [89]. In 1934 copper was found to be essential for the formation of heme A, a component of cytochrome oxidase [31], and in 1938 an important cuproprotein was isolated from bovine erythrocytes [143], although an actual function for this enzyme, superoxide dismutase, was not recognized until 1969 [140].

Body Distribution

The total body content of copper in the adult is little more than 100 mg [214]. The highest concentration is found in the liver, then the brain, the heart, and the kidneys [248]. The concentration in muscle is low, 5.4 μg/gm (SD 2.8), but the large muscle-bone mass contains approximately 50 percent of the total body copper, whereas only 10 percent is located in the liver. Eight percent is present in the brain, particularly in pigmented areas, where a concentration as high as 1,000 μmole/kg has been recorded in the locus ceruleus [52].

Absorption

The normal daily diet contains 2 to 5 mg of copper. The exact consumption varies according to the geographic area and varying soil content. This affects the copper content of grain and, consequently, diets fed to sheep and cattle. Shellfish, legumes, dried vegetables, and cocoa contain relatively large amounts of copper [17].

Copper is absorbed from the stomach and upper small intestine, and two mechanisms appear to be involved. One probably represents the absorption of copper complexes of amino acids, but the major mechanism involves the binding of copper to two protein fractions in the intestinal mucosa, superoxide dismutase and a protein rich in sulfhydryl groups similar to metallothionein [55]. The absorption of copper from the gut is adversely affected by the presence of molybdenum and sulfate radicals, although the mechanism of this antagonism is unclear. Other transition elements in the diet—such as cadmium, mercury, and silver—also interfere with copper absorption by competing for the binding sulfhydryl groups [17].

Copper in Blood

The normal plasma copper is 13 to 22 μmole/L, but in blood, copper is also found in the erythrocyte, mainly as the enzyme superoxide dismutase. The erythrocyte copper concentration of 15.4 μmole/L [17] tends to remain constant despite deficiencies of dietary intake or changes in the plasma level.

After absorption and transport from the intestinal cells into the blood plasma, copper is initially bound to albumin [9]. This is a labile fraction that rapidly disappears in parallel with the appearance of up to 90 percent of the absorbed copper in the liver [177].

Studies with ^{64}Cu show that after oral administration a secondary plasma peak occurs after 1 to 2 days. This is due to the incorporation of copper into ceruloplasmin, a protein, which is synthesized by the liver and which contains a major portion of the plasma copper in health.

A small part of the total blood copper is also complexed to amino acids, and this amino acid-bound fraction may be important in the entry of copper into cells.

Excretion

Radioactive copper studies show that of the 32 percent of orally ingested copper that is absorbed, more than 80 percent is excreted through the bile, about 15 percent is excreted back directly into the bowel, and about 1 to 5 percent, 0.6 to 1.2 μmole/day, is excreted into the urine [20, 24]. Up to 98 percent of the orally ingested copper is thus recovered in the stools, and only about 1 to 2 percent in the urine [20].

Copper excretion through the biliary tract is complex and not well understood, but much of it is probably derived from a subcellular lysosomal fraction. In bile, copper is mainly associated with macromolecules, although a limited amount is excreted as copper-amino acid complexes. Macromolecular copper is fairly inert and undergoes essentially no reabsorption; the enterohepatic circulation is minimal [24].

Copper Proteins

The functions of copper are related to the enzymatic action of specific complexes that are formed with a limited number of enzyme proteins. During these enzymatic reactions it is believed that copper undergoes a valency change between the Cu (I) and Cu (II) states.

Cytochrome Oxidase

This cuproprotein catalyzes the final and irreversible step in the mitochondria electron transport chain. It is therefore of key importance in energy production for protein biosynthesis and muscle work. There is, at present, no specific disease in man attributed to decreased activity, although lack of cytochrome oxidase in motor neurons is thought to be the basic biochemical deficit in neonatal ataxia, or sway back, which occurs in copper deficient lambs [257]. These animals show myelin aplasia, and in advanced copper deficiency, hepatic mitochondria become progressively enlarged and deformed [66].

Superoxide Dismutase

This enzyme contains both copper and zinc, and although it was the first cuproprotein isolated, in 1938, its function has only recently been identified [140]. Superoxide dismutase is located in the cell cytosol and appears to be an important protective catalyst. For example, it is now known that oxidation of some substrates by molecular oxygen gives rise to the superoxide anion (O_2^-), a free radical that is both highly reactive and toxic. Superoxide dismutase is believed to play a protective role in this type of reaction catalyzing the conversion of the superoxide anion radicals to peroxide and oxygen.

No disease in higher animals has so far been attributed to a lack of this copper protein, but it is known that anaerobic microorganisms contain no superoxide dismutase, whereas all the aerobes surveyed by Fridovich in 1972 [65] contained relatively high levels of the enzyme.

δ-Aminolevulinate-Dehydratase

δ-Aminolevulinate-dehydratase is an enzyme essential for the condensation of two molecules of δ-aminolevulinate into porphobilinogen, one of the important compounds required for heme formation. Copper is therefore necessary for the formation of hemoglobin.

Ceruloplasmin

This protein belongs to the family of dark blue copper proteins that show oxidase activity in the presence of oxygen. Ceruloplasmin is an α 2 globulin that is formed in the liver, but the mechanisms of control are not known. Elevated levels, however, are found in association with inflammatory states and diseases of the reticuloendothelial system, whereas subnormal values are characteristic of Wilson's disease. Ceruloplasmin has a biologic half-life of one week, but following release into the plasma, where it has a normal concentration of about 15 μM/L, it stably binds almost all the plasma copper, and the half-life then falls to 13 hours. It is not, however, the transport protein for the movement of copper from the gut to the liver, but it does provide transport for the delivery of copper to extrahepatic tissues. Ceruloplasmin is an oxidase that catalyzes the oxidation of aromatic and other amines, such as norepinephrine and epinephrine, but it also oxidizes ferrous ion into the ferric state, and this function has led to its designation by the alternate name of ferro-oxidase [175].

The precise role of ceruloplasmin in iron metabolism is still unclear. One suggested hypothesis is that ceruloplasmin catalyzes the oxidation of Fe^{2+} to Fe^{3+}, an essential step for the binding of iron to transferrin, the transport protein that supplies iron to the bone marrow cells. Copper-depleted animals, unable to sustain a ferrous to ferric conversion, fail to transfer iron efficiently from the mucosa and other storage sites, and abnormally large iron stores may accompany an iron-deficiency anemia [176].

In the human, however, the ferrous-oxidase activity of ceruloplasmin is less than in the pig, and there is some doubt about its role in the regulation of iron metabolism [229]. Patients with Wilson's disease, for example, have low plasma ceruloplasmin levels, but maintain a normal hemoglobin and plasma iron turnover [164]. This may be due to the fact that there are at least two other nonceruloplasmin peroxidases in plasma that may be responsible for alternate pathways of iron flow in this disease [131, 281], and there is evidence that one of these, ferro-oxidase II, contains copper [253].

Tyrosinase

Tyrosinase, a copper enzyme, is essential for pigmentation processes and, through two initial catalytic reactions, the synthesis of melanin [189]. A genetic absence of this enzyme leads to albinism, and a distinguishing feature of copper deficiency in animals with pigmented hair, wool, or feathers is achromotrichia, a failure of melanin formation.

Monoamine Oxidase

Monoamine oxidase enzymes are widely distributed and catalyze the oxidative deamination of a variety of monoamines by molecular oxygen, giving rise to an aldehyde and hydrogen peroxide. One particular one, lysyl oxidase, is essential for the structural integrity of both vascular and bone tissue through its role in the maturation of the connective tissue proteins, collagen and elastin [21].

Another important function of amine oxidase is the inactivation, by deamination, of the nerve transmitters epinephrine and norepinephrine.

Dopamine β-Hydroxylase

This enzyme has similarities to tyrosinase and is involved in the synthesis of biogenic amines such as norepinephrine and epinephrine. There are then three copper enzymes—tyrosinase, dopamine β-hydroxylase, and amine oxidase—that are involved in the synthesis, transformation, and inactivation of nerve cell transmitters. This probably accounts for the high concentration of copper in brain tissues.

Copper Deficiency in Animals

Not all the cuproenzymes so far identified have defined physiologic roles, but the following associations have been recognized in animals and, some at least, in man.

Disorders of Bone

Bone defects have been observed in a variety of domestic animals consuming copper-deficient diets [257]. The bone cortices are thin, trabeculae are deficient, and spontaneous fractures are frequent occurrences. Studies in the chick [210] show that these defects are due to impaired collagen cross-linking [163].

Cardiovascular Defects

Failure of collagen and elastin cross-linking also accounts for at least the majority of the defects that affect the cardiovascular system in copper-deficient animals. Sudden death due to heart failure, on a basis of myocardial atrophy and replacement fibrosis, has been recognized in cattle [257] and pigs [22].

Structural defects, due to deficiencies in collagen and elastin, also occur in major arteries. Pigs [227] and chicks [166] fed copper-deficient diets have been known to die suddenly from massive internal hemorrhage, which is commonly preceded by aneurysmal dissection.

These disorders of cross-linking of the connective tissue proteins are believed to be due to a deficiency of the amine oxidase cuproenzyme, lysyl oxidase.

Disorders of the Central Nervous System

Neonatal ataxia, a nervous disorder of neonatal lambs characterized by a lack of muscular coordination, is associated with both primary and molybdenum-induced copper deficiency [61]. Locomotor incoordination is associated with myelin aplasia, and cell necrosis and fiber degeneration in the brain stem and spinal cord [257]. Early severe cases also show neuronal damage and cerebral cavitation. Nervous disorders caused by dietary copper deficiency have also been observed in the offspring of several other domestic animals including goats, rats, and pigs [257], and in neonatal guinea pigs of copper-deficient dams, the cerebellum is severely damaged and there is lack of myelination throughout the brain [56].

The basic cause of these changes is believed to be low levels of the cuproenzyme cytochrome oxidase in motor neurons. The similarities between neonatal ataxia in lambs and Parkinson's disease in man also raises the possibility that copper deficiency affects the dopaminergic system in the caudate nucleus. Brain dopamine, norepinephrine, and serotonin levels are depressed in ataxic lambs, but although dopamine levels can be significantly increased by copper supplementation, the locomotor disorder remains unchanged [170].

Melanin Formation

The cuproenzyme tyrosinase catalyzes two reactions leading to the formation of melanin—hydroxylation of tyrosine to 3,4-dihydroxyphenylalanine (dopa) and the oxidation of dopa to the quinone [189]. Lack of tyrosinase is thought to account for the failure of melanin formation, achromotrichia, in animals with pigmented hair, wool, or feathers. Such depigmentation is frequently associated with lack of crimp and a steely texture due to failure of oxidation of sulfhydryl groups to disulfide bonds, which normally predominate in hair and wool. An enzyme that catalyzes this oxidation has not so far been described [257].

Iron Metabolism and Anemia

In all the experimental animal studies, copper deficiency leads to anemia, although the precise role of copper in hemopoiesis is still unclear. Ceruloplasmin is believed to catalyze the oxidation of ferrous iron to the ferric form, essential for the binding of iron to transferrin, and in the pig, copper deficiency is associated with impaired release of iron from the duodenal mucosa, the reticuloendothelial system, and the hepatic parenchymal cell. The result is a severe, hypochromic, microcytic anemia and a low serum iron, which responds rapidly to copper administration [132]. In the human, however, the ferrous-oxidase activity of ceruloplasmin is much less clearly established.

Copper may have other functions in hemopoiesis. It seems to be essential for the development of the reticulocyte [164], and in copper-depleted rats, the persistence of iron in the normoblasts of the bone marrow suggests that iron-limited erythropoiesis is not the basic limiting factor in the accompanying anemia, but that there is an additional defect involving the incorporation of iron into hemoglobin [69].

Copper Deficiency in Humans

Copper is so widely distributed that in humans consuming a normal varied diet with normal absorption, copper deficiency has long been regarded as unlikely. In a recent study of the nutritional status of adolescent girls, only 3 to 4 percent could be classified as being in a "marginal" nutritional status with regard to both zinc and copper, and the group was asymptomatic [72].

In 1964, however, hypocupremia was reported in malnourished Peruvian infants given milk-based, low-copper diets. If not present on admission, anemia soon developed in these children, who also showed both neutropenia and bone demineralization [70]. Oral copper quickly resolved these features, whereas iron alone was ineffective.

As the serum copper and ceruloplasmin fell in these children, the earliest manifestation of deficiency was a persistent neutropenia, although the neutrophil response to infection was unimpaired. Bone demineralization, and failure of erythropoiesis with anemia, were later features.

In 1962, Menkes and his colleagues [147] described an X-linked recessively inherited disease in which affected infants exhibited symptoms similar to those seen in copper-deficient animals. Serum copper, ceruloplasmin, and the copper content of the brain and liver were very low in these children, in whom copper deficiency was characterized by progressive cerebral degeneration, pili torti, depigmentation of hair, arterial changes, and death within three years. This disorder is probably due to a defect in the release of copper from the epithelium of the gut and/or the binding of copper to albumin [43, 44], and a recent report suggests a frequency of one in every 35,000 live births [42].

The underlying arterial abnormality in Menkes' syndrome, disruption and fragmentation of the internal elastic lamina [45], is similar to that found in the aorta of copper-deficient swine, and it is probably due to a deficiency of lysyl oxidase, essential for the integrity of both elastic tissue and collagen [21].

Lack of other copper proteins has been linked to the other features of the disease. Copper is needed for the disulfide bridging of wool keratin and presumably serves a similar function in human hair. Tyrosinase is required for pigmentation, and brain damage probably results from a combination of the vascular lesions, the low concentration of cytochrome oxidase, and impaired synthesis of the transmitter substances dopamine, norepinephrine, and epinephrine.

The long-term support of seriously ill patients by total parenteral nutrition (TPN), using solutions containing minimal amounts of copper, has defined a further group who may be at risk with respect to copper deficiency. Indeed this possibility has now been confirmed, and Karpel and Peden [116], in 1972, reported one case in an infant characterized by anemia, leukopenia, and neutropenia, together with scorbutic type bone lesions. Administration of copper rapidly corrected the hematologic abnormalities, but the bone defects were slower to respond, although they eventually returned to normal.

Copper-related bone changes consisting of osteoporosis, metaphyseal spur formation, and soft tissue calcification have subsequently been reported in two other infants on prolonged TPN. The bone lesions are similar to those seen in scurvy, in which abnormal collagen is due to deficient hydroxylation of peptidyl lysine and proline. In copper deficiency, however, they develop in the presence of normal ascorbic acid levels and are characterized by a decrease in the cross-links that normally form aldehyde groups along the peptide chain [91].

Anemia, leukopenia, and neutropenia, associated with hypocupremia, and similarly responsive to copper supplementation, have also been reported in a number of adults during TPN [50, 62, 180, 270, 288].

The anemia in these patients is probably due to a combined deficiency of ceruloplasmin and δ-aminolevulinate dehydratase, enzymes that affect both iron metabolism and heme formation. It may also be influenced by the effect of copper deficiency on the development of the reticulocyte.

The mechanism responsible for leukopenia and neutropenia is not known with certainty, but Zidar and his colleagues (1977) [288] found that the bone marrow in severe deficiency showed no evidence of granulocytic maturation beyond the myelocyte stage, and abnormal granulopoiesis could be demonstrated using the in vitro granulocyte colony assay.

In a personal series of more than 60 adult patients receiving TPN, plasma copper, urinary copper excretion, ceruloplasmin, and serum iron have been measured twice weekly. Urinary copper does increase during a catabolic phase, but the loss is not striking, seldom exceeding 20 μmole/day, and is usually closer to 4 to 5 μmole (normal 0.6 to 1.2). In addition, copper losses from external fistulas are unimpressive and have never exceeded 5 μmole/day, even in high-output states (Figure 9-14). Such data, together with the fact that the copper content of the solutions infused during TPN is generally below 1.5 μmole/day, support the view that declining plasma copper values during TPN reflect long-term inadequate intake, rather than renal or extrarenal losses.

The development of hypocupremia in this setting of prolonged negative copper balance is nevertheless unpredictable, probably because of the complex effects of inflammatory processes on this cation. Leukocyte endogenous mediator (LEM), released by polymorphonuclear leukocytes in response to certain infections, bacterial endotoxin, and tissue damage [18], will, for example, induce the hepatic synthesis of acute phase reactants, including ceruloplasmin, and plasma copper then rises in association with inverse effects on zinc and iron.

Hypocupremia has been seen in a small number of patients in this series, but it is always slow to develop and, unlike zinc, appears largely uninfluenced by the rate and duration of anabolism. Declining copper values are invariably associated with a parallel fall in ceruloplasmin, but both indices respond rapidly to intravenous copper supplementation given as either the sulfate or the chloride, 2 to 4 mg per day.

Figure 9-15 illustrates the neutropenia associated with severe copper deficiency and the rapid response to intravenous copper therapy. It also supports the concept that copper is essential for the proper utilization of iron because serum iron remained below normal during the period of copper depletion, despite regular iron dextran injections.

The inference from these studies is that some caution should probably be exercised in the administration of iron in patients who are potentially copper-depleted. Evidence of excessive iron in Kupffer cells, together with some iron in hepatocytes, in a number of liver biopsies, adds further support to the view that serum iron, in copper-depleted subjects, may be an inaccurate index of total body iron stores.

Ferritin, the major iron storage protein, has usually been regarded as an intracellular protein identifiable in histologic sections, together with its insoluble derivative hemosiderin, by the blue color seen after staining by the Prussian Blue reaction. The development of a sensitive immunoradiometric assay [1] has, however, revealed ferritin as a normal constituent of serum [106] with a normal range between 20 and 250 μg/L, the higher levels being found in men [34].

The relationship between serum iron, ferritin, and plasma copper has recently been studied in a small number of patients during medium- to long-term TPN. The results are inconsistent and frequently paradoxical (Figure 9-16), and ferritin cannot be regarded as a reliable guide to iron therapy in this group of patients, who are fre-

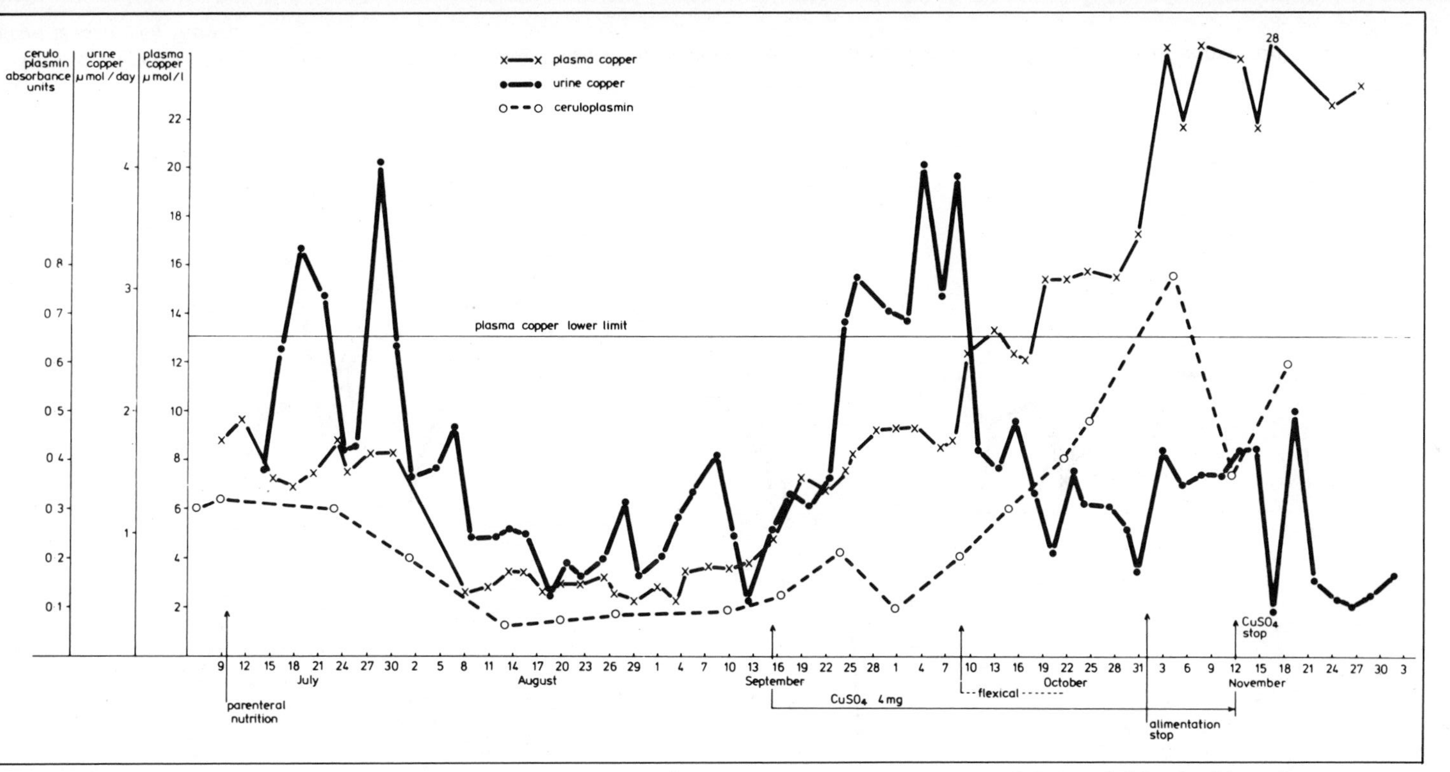

Figure 9-14. *Copper metabolic data. Urinary copper excretion is not impressive and has not exceeded 4µmole/day in this patient.*

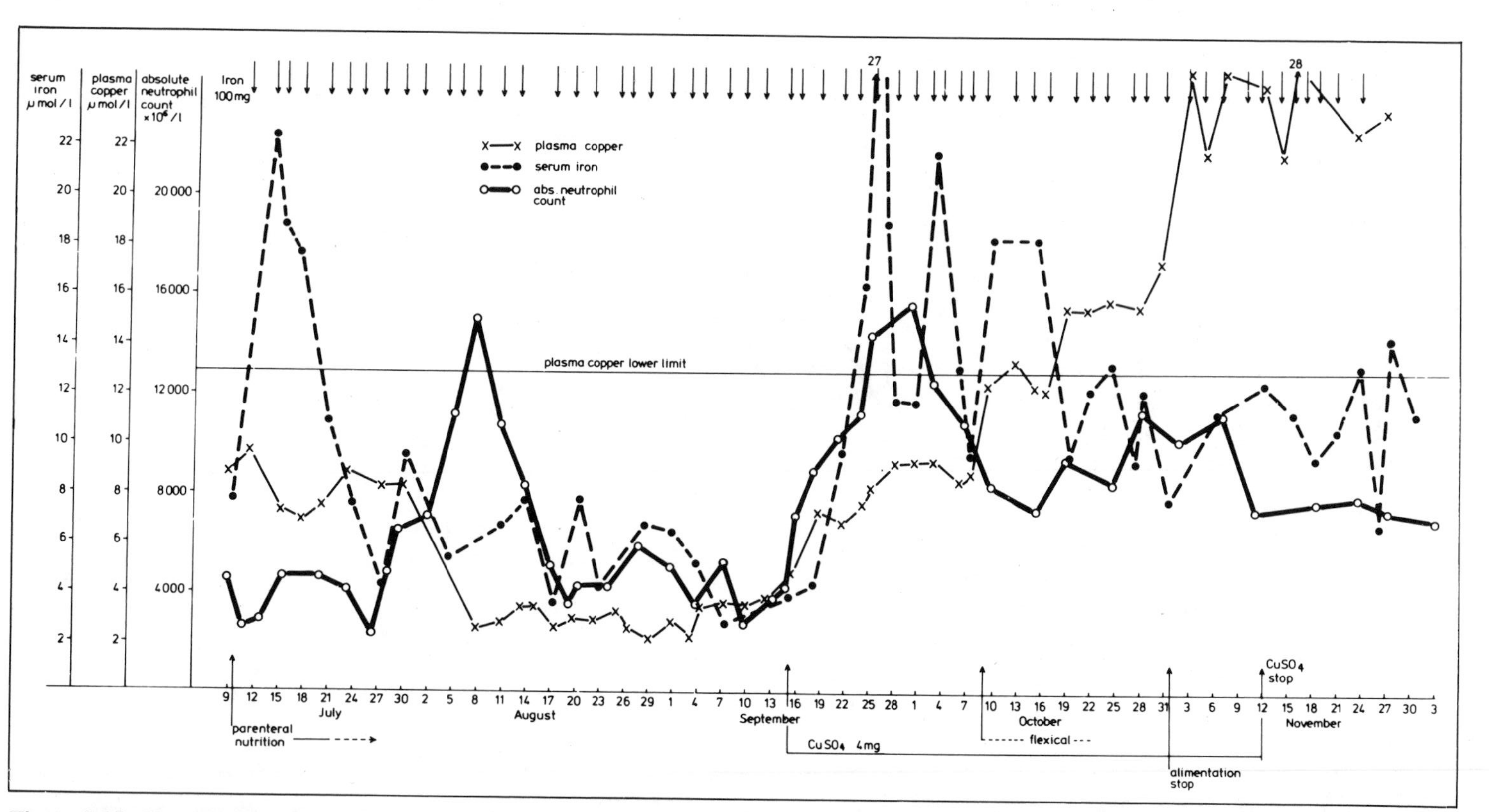

Figure 9-15. *Neutropenia of copper deficiency has responded well to intravenous copper supplementation. The influence of copper on iron metabolism is also well shown.*

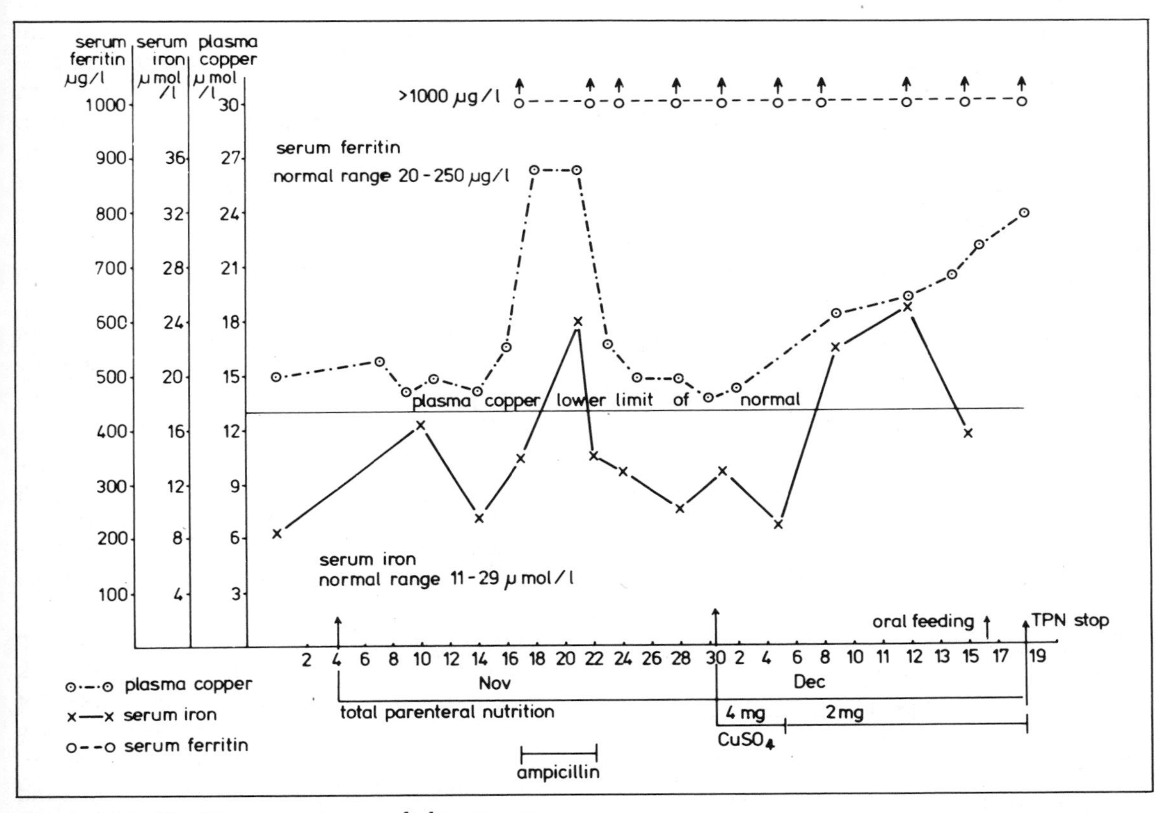

Figure 9-16. *Ferritin, serum iron, and plasma copper relationships. Ferritin is a poor guide to iron therapy in these patients.*

quently seriously ill with widespread metabolic derangements. High serum ferritin levels, inappropriate to the amount of storage iron, have also been found in acute and chronic liver disease [197], leukemia [284], and Hodgkin's disease [111]. In some cases this may be due to ferritin release from degenerating cells, but in other conditions high concentrations may be due to increased production of the protein, for all cells have the capacity to synthesize ferritin, and in mononuclear phagocytic cells that capacity is particularly marked [244].

Copper Toxicity

Copper toxicity is uncommon in humans, although in India the suicidal ingestion of copper sulfate is not infrequent [29]. Copper poisoning has also occurred in renal dialysis units and after consumption of liquids into which copper has leaked from containing vessels or plumbing. Symptoms such as nausea, vomiting, diarrhea, and intestinal colic will follow the ingestion of more than 15 mg of elemental copper; more severe cases may show intravascular hemolysis due to the inhibiting effect of copper on a number of enzyme systems such as glucose 6-phosphate dehydrogenase [57].

In humans, significant copper toxicity is also seen in individuals with Wilson's disease, a congenital disorder with a familial tendency that is believed to be due to a failure of normal copper excretion in the bile [241]. Serum copper and ceruloplasmin are low, but copper accumulates in the tissues, particularly the liver, kidney, and brain, causing progressive degeneration. Copper deposits in the cornea, Kayser-Fleischer rings, are diagnostically important as they are always present in those affected patients who show characteristic neurologic signs or symptoms [214], such as tremor and muscular rigidity, suggestive of a corpus striatum lesion of the Parkinsonian type.

Treatment with chelating agents such as penicillamine, which bind and excrete tissue copper via the urine, can reverse the early toxic manifestations of Wilson's disease, and Kayser-Fleischer rings become much less prominent and may disappear. Successfully treated patients may become asymptomatic and remain so indefinitely.

SELENIUM

History

Selenium, first isolated in 1817 by J. J. Berzelius [11], is widely distributed in the earth's crust with an abundance that approximates that of cadmium and antimony. The photoconductive properties of this element have been important in the development of the physics of semi-conductors, but in biology, interest in selenium was initially confined to its toxic effects on animals. These were first observed in 1842 [108], but not clarified in veterinary science until 1933, when two diseases of livestock known as "blind staggers" and "alkali disease," occurring in certain areas of the Great Plains of North America, were identified as manifestations of acute [10] and chronic [206] selenosis.

It is now known that the soils in these regions contain high levels of selenium, which is readily taken up by plants and consumed by grazing animals. Signs of chronic poisoning are poorly defined, but include growth depression, loss of hair, cracking of the hooves, impaired reproduction, anemia, and fatty liver degeneration.

In 1957, the classic paper of Schwarz and Foltz [223] focused attention on the physiologic role of selenium following work on dietary necrotic liver degeneration in the rat. This fatal deficiency disease is complex and can be produced by a variety of diets, all of which, however, are lacking in vitamin E, low in sulphur amino acids, and deficient in a third factor, Factor 3, an organic but still uncharacterized form of selenium, which, independently of the other two agents, prevents the disease.

In the late 1950s, veterinary scientists in both New Zealand [90] and the United States [160] linked selenium deficiency with a widespread naturally occurring form of muscular dystrophy in sheep and cattle known as white muscle disease. Subsequently, areas of selenium deficiency associated with impaired animal health were identified in many countries, but particularly in New Zealand [275] and Scandinavia [71].

Selenium deficiency disorders were later identified in various other animal species, but many of the diverse manifestations were also found to be responsive to vitamin E. The interrelationship is complex, but based on studies in the chick [247], it is now clear that vitamin E does not simply replace selenium as a nutrient. Dietary selenium is not effective against all vitamin E-related effects, such as fetal resorption in rats and encephalomalacia in chicks [233], and in the rat, selenium supplements produce independent growth effects [222]. Vitamin E, on the other hand, was more effective in preventing white muscle disease in recent experiments in sheep fed purified diets [277].

In 1954, selenium was found to be an essential biologic component of the bacterial enzyme formate dehydrogenase [187]. In animal biology, on the other hand, almost 20 years were to elapse before selenium was similarly recognized as the active component of the enzyme glutathione peroxidase [209], an active catalyst in peroxide metabolism.

Dietary Intake

A well-balanced American diet provides an average selenium intake of about 150 μg per day. By contrast, the daily intake in New Zealand is only 6 to 70 μg [74]. This significant difference reflects the striking influence of locality and variable topsoil content on the important dietary contributors, grains and cereal products. The contribution of most fruits, vegetables, and sugars to the selenium intake is small [154], but all seafood is rich in this element, and in North America fresh meat is also an excellent source.

Absorption and Excretion

Animal studies with ^{75}Se indicate that the duodenum is the main site of absorption of selenium [287], and absorption is better in monogastric animals than in ruminants.

Similar isotope studies in young New Zealand women show that the intestinal absorption of food selenium varies between 0.76 and 0.83 with a mean of 0.79 (ratio of dietary intake). In this same group, on a 14-day ad lib diet, with a mean selenium content of 24.2 μg/day, the mean urinary selenium was 13.1 μg/day, approximately half the oral intake, and the mean fecal loss 10.8 μg/day [242]. Whether a similar distribution holds for higher intakes of selenium is uncertain, but the available data suggest that urinary selenium is controlled, as in the rat, by the dietary intake.

Blood Levels

Whole blood levels of selenium show wide regional differences in parallel with the topsoil selenium content and dietary intake. In the United Kingdom, for example, the mean level is 0.32 μg/ml [13], in the United States it is 0.21 μg/ml [3] and in Sweden 0.12 μg/ml [16]. Whole blood levels in New Zealand residents are much lower, 0.068 μg/ml in the South Island [75] and 0.079 μg/ml in the Auckland area of the North Island, the variation being due to regional differences in the topsoil content and dietary intake [117]. The importance of these factors is well illustrated by the decline in whole blood selenium, observed in sequential samples taken over a 12-month period, from four adults who arrived in New Zealand from the United States [75].

Biochemistry

The enzyme glutathione peroxidase (GSH-Px) was first discovered in 1957 when Mills [151] reported that bovine erythrocytes contained, in addition to catalase, another enzyme that prevented oxidative denaturation of hemoglobin by hydrogen peroxide. Purification confirmed that the peroxidase and catalase activities of the red cell were independently served by two different enzymes [153].

In 1963, Cohen and Hockstein compared the activity of these two erythrocyte enzymes in the catalytic destruction of hydrogen peroxide and showed that GSH-Px played the predominant role [32].

The existence of GSH-Px in other organs—notably the liver, lung, and kidney [152]—suggested a wider role for this enzyme, and this was confirmed when GSH-Px was also shown to catalyze the reduction of hydroperoxides formed from fatty acids or other substances, as well as hydrogen peroxide [28, 136].

The discovery that selenium was an active constituent of glutathione peroxidase, made by Rotruck and his coworkers at the University of Wisconsin in 1972, constituted a major advance in the understanding of the biologic role of this element [210].

These workers showed that peroxide-induced hemolysis was greatly enhanced in red blood cells of selenium-deficient rats. Subsequent studies have shown that GSH-peroxidase is also an enzyme of great importance in the metabolism of the liver, kidney, and endothelial lining of vessels and the lens of the eye [224]. The liver is one of the richest sources, and GSH-Px constitutes about 0.25 percent of the soluble protein of normal human and rat liver [238]. This level falls substantially during the development of dietary induced liver necrosis, adding strong support to the relationship [224].

It is now apparent that GSH-Px has a broad role in protecting tissues from oxidative damage. It utilizes peroxides, normal products of intermediary metabolism, to reoxidize reduced glutathione, formed in large amounts during electron transfer reactions in mitochondria and microsomes.

Selenium—Vitamin E

The relationship between selenium and tocopherol is not fully understood, but it is clear that these two agents do not merely substitute for each other, but are essential for alternate pathways of intermediary metabolism [219].

A metabolic explanation for the interrelationship, recently proposed, suggests that selenium, as GSH peroxidase, guards against oxidative damage to the cell membrane by converting organic hydroperoxides to less damaging alcohols, whereas vitamin E, in a similar protective role, prevents the formation of lipid hydroperoxides [98]. It is also suggested that the sulfur-containing amino acids may interact with this metabolic system by serving as precursors of GSH, thus potentially sparing both vitamin E and selenium.

Peroxides are usually considered as harmful by-products of metabolism, and enzymes such as catalase and the cuproprotein, superoxide dismutase, probably function as detoxifying agents. Some cells, however, such as the erythrocyte, tolerate hydrogen peroxide well, and the seleno-enzyme GSH peroxidase actually uses peroxides as the immediate source of oxidative energy.

Peroxide derivatives with important metabolic functions are being increasingly recognized. Glutathione peroxidase appears to play an important role in the biosynthesis of prostaglandins. Prostaglandin G contains hydroperoxide groups at the 15 position, and reduced glutathione is essential for the conversion to prostaglandin E and F. These endoperoxide forms of prostaglandin are important physiologically, being potent inducers of platelet aggregation and stimulants of arterial and bronchial musculature [220].

Selenium Deficiency in Animals

Selenium responsive diseases occur in a wide variety of animal species, and the responsible dietary deficiency is usually linked to a low topsoil content. Topsoils in New Zealand, for example, have selenium concentrations between 0.1 and 4.0 $\mu g/gm$ and in many regions, including most of the arable land of the South Island, the soil selenium is less than 0.5 $\mu g/gm$ [275]. In such localities there is, in the absence of selenium dosing, a high incidence of selenium responsive disorders in farm livestock characterized by decreased fertility, increased perinatal mortality, and the type of muscular dystrophy called white muscle disease [5]. Muscle lesions occur in both skeletal muscle and the heart and consist of Zenker's necrosis, interstitial fibrosis, and foci of dystrophic calcification, particularly of the endocardium [218]. These changes are accompanied by elevated plasma levels of creatine phosphokinase (CPK), lactic dehydrogenase (LDH), and glutamic oxaloacetic transaminase (GOT). Creatine phosphokinase is the most specific of these enzymes [277], although the activity of fructose diphosphate aldolase may also be valuable in evaluating the severity of the disease [276].

Muscular dystrophy is usually the major feature of selenium deficiency in most species, but in chicks and other fowl an exudative diathesis is predominant [221], while selenium-deficient, but vitamin E-supplemented, rats grow slowly, lose their hair, develop cataracts, and have aspermatogenesis [237]. In mice, deficiency is also accompanied by severe kidney damage, together with pronounced degeneration and fibrosis of the exocrine pancreas [220], a feature of deficiency that is also prominent in the chick [73].

Ultrastructural alterations in both skeletal and cardiac muscle have been extensively studied by Van Vleet and his associates in a variety of animal species with nutritionally induced selenium-vitamin E deficiency [266–268]. In the skeletal muscle of the pig, myofibrillar alterations are a major early feature, and morphologic alterations in mitochondria, sarcoplasmic reticulum, and plasma membranes only become apparent in fibers with advanced myofibrillar lysis and disruption. In rabbits [265] and chicks [27], however, the earliest ultrastructural evidence of muscle damage is morphologic alteration in the mitochondria.

Selenium Deficiency in the Human

Selenium deficiency in the human has not yet been clearly established, although the pancreatic changes in chicks and mice are similar to those seen in children suffering from protein malnutrition (kwashiorkor). Decreased plasma and whole blood selenium levels have been reported in protein-calorie malnutrition, and although plasma proteins rapidly returned to normal after the institution of an adequate diet, the selenium response was much slower, taking many months to reach the normal range [19].

SELENIUM DURING TOTAL PARENTERAL NUTRITION (TPN)

Because of low topsoil content and dietary intake, whole blood levels of selenium in New Zealand residents are only one-third of those found in North America. For this reason, there must be concern about the potential for very severe deficiency, which may develop during TPN in New Zealand residents, because the solutions infused in that program have been found to contain less than 1 μg of selenium per day. This is much lower than the daily dietary intake in this country, 6 to 70 μg [74], which itself is low by international standards.

Figure 9-17 demonstrates the changes in red cell, whole blood, and plasma selenium in one such patient. All three indices decline steadily, but packed cell transfusion is followed by a sharp rise in red cell selenium concentration and delayed effects on the whole blood and plasma values. The lowest plasma selenium recorded, 23 ng/ml, is well below the normal range (64.09 ± 14.04) for an adult in this area.

Studies have now been carried out on more than 20 adult patients during TPN. All have shown a similar pattern of declining blood values, transiently influenced by red cell transfusion, and effectively reversed, in one recent patient, by the intravenous infusion of 50 μg of selenium on a daily basis. The average peak daily urinary excretion in this group, 16.04 μg/day, is only slightly above the normal mean of 12.2 μg, and urinary losses do not appear to be significantly altered by the metabolic state. In one severely catabolic patient, for example, the maximum excretion of selenium did not exceed three times normal, whereas the urinary excretion of zinc reached a peak of 700 μmole/day, 100 times the normal mean value.

Ileostomy and fistulous selenium have also been measured in a number of patients in this group. Such losses, however, have never been impressive (Figure 9-18), and it is evident that the declining blood levels during TPN reflect long-term inadequate intake rather than the sum of the measured renal and extrarenal losses.

The low levels of selenium that have been regularly observed in patients on TPN are of some concern. Plasma selenium in one patient fell to 8 ng/ml and levels below 20 ng/ml have not been infrequent. These are well below the normal range for New Zealand residents (64 ± 14 ng/ml) and they are strikingly deficient by American, and some European, standards. Nevertheless, overt evidence of deficiency has not been recognized. This may be due to the protective effect of vitamin E, regularly infused as a component of the multivitamin preparation, MV1, or contained in the soybean oil fraction of the intravenous fat preparation, Intralipid.

In two recent studies, however, ultrastructural examination of sequential skeletal muscle biopsy samples has shown basement and plasma membrane degeneration, extensive fat droplet formation, and some evidence of myofibrillar de-

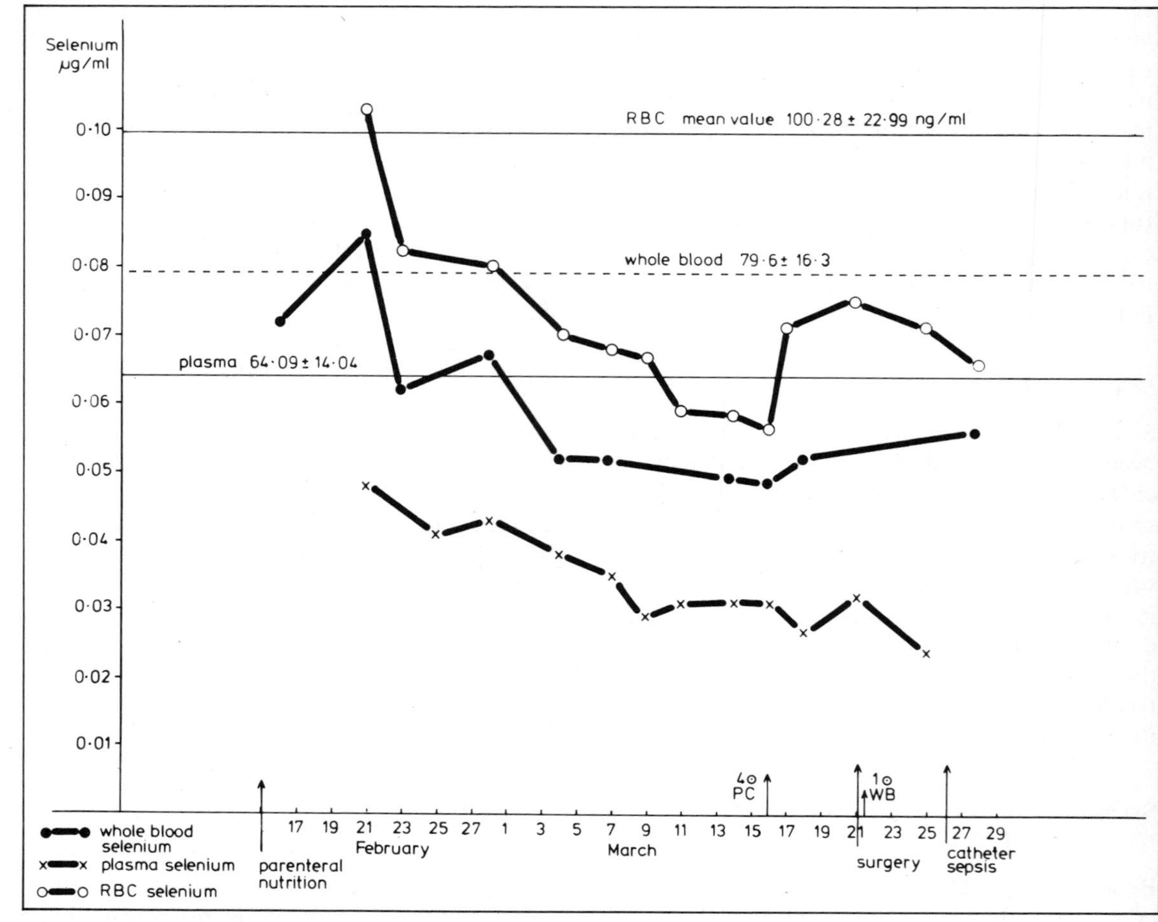

Figure 9-17. *Red cell, whole blood, and plasma selenium during total parenteral nutrition.*

generation with separation of fibrils and loss of density in Z-bands. These changes have some similarities to those described by Van Vleet in various animal species, and they support the increasing evidence for the importance of selenium and vitamin E in the human.

CHROMIUM

History

Chromium is a ubiquitous element found in all soils and waters in a concentration ranging from trace levels to 3,750 μg/gm for soils [207] and 0 to 1 μg/ml for most water [51]. The intake from drinking water is insignificant and in an inorganic form that is particularly poorly absorbed [148], so that the bulk of the intake is directly from plants or indirectly from animal products.

A major problem, still only partly solved, is the difficulty in accurate analysis of the minute levels of chromium present, and estimates have tended to follow the detection levels of methods and equipment. Plasma estimations of 20 to 50 ng/ml in 1969 [148] have been reduced to as low as 0.14 ng/ml by 1978 [122]. Currently the widely accepted analytic methods are flameless atomic absorption and neutron activation.

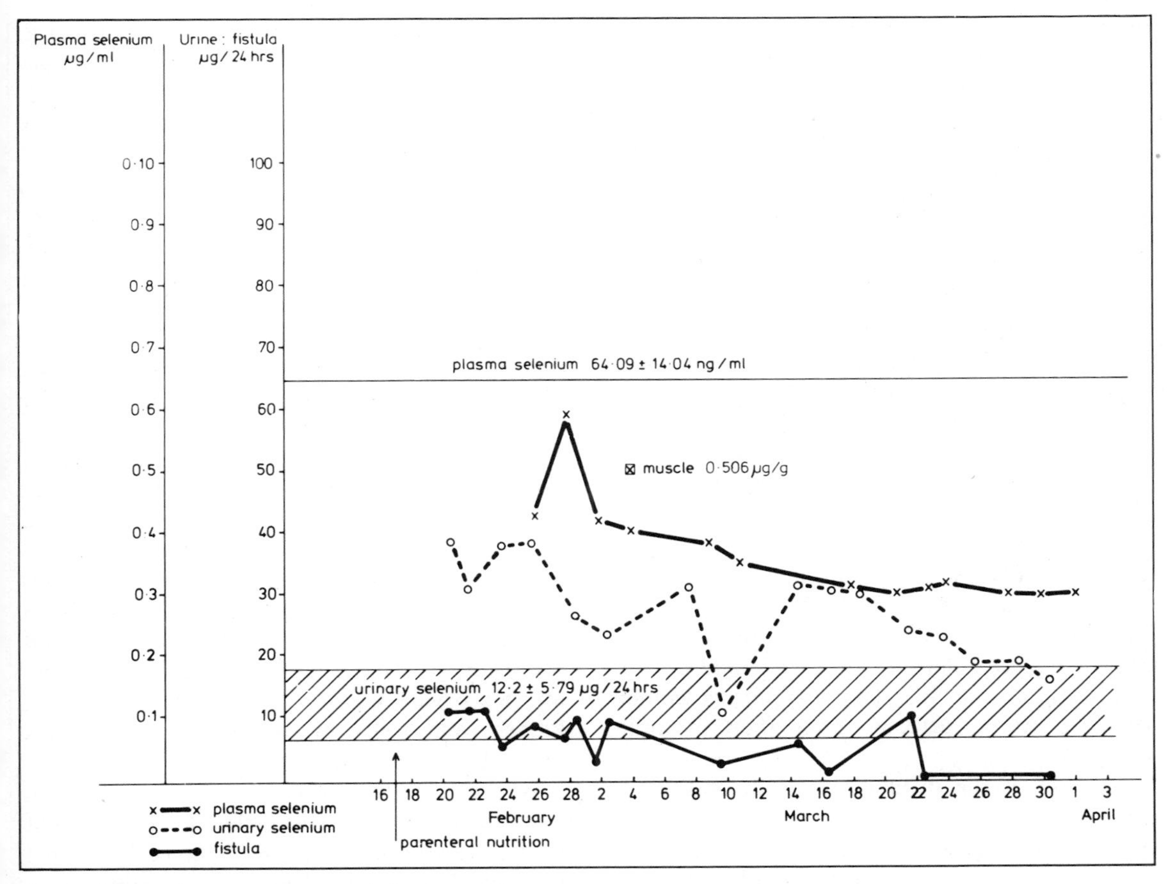

Figure 9-18. *Plasma, urinary, and fistulous selenium during total parenteral nutrition.*

Although it was originally considered unlikely, evidence for deficiency in humans and domestic animals has steadily accumulated [84] and has been widely linked to impaired glucose tolerance [148]. Such deficiency may be accentuated by refining of food, especially sugar and flour.

The biochemical function of chromium is not well known, and no firm biologic role other than in glucose tolerance factor, an organic Cr complex, has been found. No enzymes are specifically activated by chromium, but several show increased action in the presence of Cr^{++} (as well as numerous other metallic ions).

Normal Requirements

The average American diet has been found to contain from 50 to 80 µg of chromium per day, with a range of 5 to 115 µg [133]. This is regarded as low and is further depressed by large losses of Cr in food refining. Up to 90 percent of Cr is lost during sugar refining, so that pure sugar contains only 0.08 µg/gm, whereas the level in molasses is 1.2 µg/gm. Much of the Cr content is also lost in white flour production, and white bread may contain only 0.14 µg/gm [215, 216]. Even these levels have been challenged by Schroeder [215] as too high due to inadequate sample preparation and inaccurate analyses.

The predisposition to deficiency, caused by the low chromium content of processed foods, is further aggravated if there is a heavy consumption of carbohydrate, which increases the urinary chromium excretion [214].

Intakes in other countries show a wide global variation. In Italy the range is 64 to 120 μg/gm/day, Japan 130 to 140 μg [159], and India 7 to 172 μg [112]. In Nigeria less than 10 μg of Cr is obtained from one liter of the staple diet, maize pap.

More important than the absolute quantity of Cr absorbed daily is the form in which the Cr is bound. Biologically the most useful form is as glucose tolerance factor (GTF) [250]. Mertz has suggested an intake of 10 to 30 μg of GTF-chromium per day to meet man's daily requirements, but if the intake is mainly inorganic, at least 270 μg would be necessary [148].

In pregnancy only Cr bound in GTF may pass across the placenta. As a result of heavy fetal demand, it has been shown that breeding rats have low liver Cr levels and frequently show impaired glucose tolerance [48]. It has also been demonstrated that hair levels in parous women were up to 66 percent lower than in nulliparae [87].

Because of the diversity of form and availability of dietary Cr, no accurate minimum daily intake can be given. All the suggestions of deficiency have been based in fact on the apparent decline in body stores with age and the marked biochemical response of elderly subjects to oral supplement of Cr. These responses appear as improved glucose tolerance, especially in maturity-onset diabetics, and a lowering of plasma cholesterol [47] and triglycerides.

Transport and Distribution

Chromic acetate and citrate are rapidly absorbed from the gastrointestinal tract, and up to 64 and 92 percent, respectively, of the dose is excreted within 4 days [271]. However, excretion of chromic chloride or chromate, either colloidal- or protein-bound, is very much slower because of the strong uptake by the reticuloendothelial system, liver, spleen, and bone marrow. Because all chemical forms, with the exception of chromate, clear the blood rapidly, and because no positive equilibrium exists between tissue and blood, plasma levels are not a reliable indication of tissue stores [23].

Hexavalent Cr is rapidly absorbed into the erythrocyte but the trivalent form does not penetrate the cellular membrane. Instead, it is rapidly bound to proteins and may be readily recovered from plasma precipitate. Small amounts are bound to transferrin [99], the iron-binding protein, but these binding sites are easily saturated. The removal from blood to tissue depends on the chemical form of administration.

Very little injected chromium is taken up in skeletal muscle or brain tissue [24], and the bone marrow is by far the largest reservoir. In the marrow Cr is not intracellular but associated with a trichloroacetic acid-precipitatable fraction. Vittorio et al., in 1961 [272], found that tissue incorporation was maximal in young mice and decreased to almost half with aging. The most affected organs were the liver, stomach, thymus, kidney, and testes. They considered that this paralleled the human situation.

At the subcellular level, 49 percent of the total Cr is concentrated in the nucleus [26], 23 percent in the supernatant, and the balance is divided between the mitochondria and microsomes.

Excretion

Urinary excretion accounts for at least 80 percent of total losses, with the balance appearing in the feces. The site of excretion of Cr into the intestine is not known, and the importance of this route is not well understood. The portion of the Cr that is bound to small molecules, and is therefore in a dialyzable form, is filtered at the glomerulus, but up to 63 percent of such Cr is reabsorbed in the tubules [27].

The rate of removal of injected $^{51}Cr^{3+}$ follows the normal exponential curve [33], with the three main components in the rat having a half-life of 0.5, 5.9, and 83.4 days. These were found to hold true for both large and small doses of Cr. This may be interpreted as suggesting that the metabolism of Cr is not strongly controlled by the nutritional status. This contrasts with the uptake and retention of iron and manganese.

Glucose Tolerance Factor

Glucose tolerance factor (GTF) is a low-molecular-weight complex of Cr^{3+} liganded to nicotinic acid, glycine, glutamic acid, and cysteine [250]. In contrast to the poor absorption from the intestine of trivalent Cr (0.5 to 1 percent) [9] and tetravalent Cr (2.1 percent) [48], at least 10 percent of orally administered GTF is taken up [84]. GTF Cr is a far more potent form than inorganic Cr^{3+}, and glucose metabolism has been found to be greatly increased in insulin-dependent mammalian systems, particularly in adipose tissue. Tenfold increases in CO_2 output were recorded by Mertz in 1969, compared to 50 to 80 percent increases with Cr^{3+} administration [149].

The action of GTF is closely associated with insulin, and no systems have been found where supplementation with Cr^{3+} or GTF has any effect in the absence of insulin. The interaction of insulin and GTF is considered to be taking place at the cell membrane in insulin-sensitive tissues, where Cr enhances the initial reaction with insulin and its receptor, possibly forming a ternary complex. This effect has been described in the rat [149] and diabetic mouse [254]. After an oral glucose challenge there is a temporary increase in the plasma chromium. This effect does not appear in Cr deficiency and is not normally detectable in maturity-onset diabetics [68]. Such subjects only show a rise following dietary supplementation with Cr^{3+} or GTF. The influence of GTF uptake by the fetus is illustrated by the fact that there is a plasma Cr^{3+} response to oral glucose in those 58 percent of pregnant women who showed evidence of impaired glucose tolerance.

There is no relationship between the Cr content of a wide variety of foods and the GTF biologic activity, but if foods are extracted with 50 percent ethanol, the GTF fraction may be separated [250]. Foods showing little or no GTF activity include most fruits and vegetables and egg yolk. Those containing the highest concentrations of ethanol extractable GTF were brewer's yeast, black pepper, liver, beef, bread, and, on a dry weight basis, beer and mushrooms. Low levels were recorded from skim milk, haddock, flour, and chicken flesh [84]. In addition to absorbing GTF from food, the human body may manufacture a limited amount using inorganic Cr^{3+}. This is considered to be inadequate, and it has been suggested that GTF be regarded as a vitamin. This may be particularly true in adults showing diabetes mellitus when Cr^{3+} brings about a marked improvement in glucose tolerance. These subjects may have partially lost the ability to manufacture GTF and/or absorb adequate Cr^{3+}.

Synthetic preparation of GTF has not yet been entirely successful, but preparations of Cr^{3+}, combined with nicotinic acid, glycine, cysteine, or glutamic acid, have been found to show limited activity, and it is likely that the active portion of the molecule is the niacin-Cr^{3+}-niacin axis. A preparation of nicotinic acid, Cr^{3+}, and glutathione was found to bind strongly to porcine insulin and give good GTF activity [4].

Chromium Deficiency in Humans and Animals

In many countries, tissue levels of chromium have been shown to fall steadily throughout life. This is the only element that shows this trend. Repeated pregnancies produce a more rapid decline, as shown by hair concentrations. This suggests that a finite store is being depleted faster than absorption from food can replace it. Opposed to this is the possibility that the decline is a natural phenomenon, with the largest amount being required during the period of rapid growth. Studies on wild animals, however, do not support this [21], nor do the high Cr levels found in mature humans in Middle Eastern countries.

In the United States, the probable intestinal absorption of chromium, based on a urinary output of 5μg/L, is 7 to 8 μg/day. Unfortunately, there is little information about the proportion of naturally occurring Cr complexes that are absorbed, and so whether the estimated daily dietary intake of 52 μg is adequate cannot be decided. A study of children 0 to 10 years of age and of adults over 30 years of age in this dietary environment showed hepatic ash Cr levels of 17.2 μg/gm and 1 to 2 μg/gm, respectively [47].

Maturity-onset diabetics have been the subject of intense study and, in many cases, have shown dramatic improvement of plasma glucose levels after supplementation with inorganic Cr^{3+}. In four elderly patients, Doisey and his colleagues showed that doses as small as 50 μg of Cr^{3+} three times daily produced a significant fall in plasma glucose levels. A parallel test in young volunteers, however, showed negligible change [47].

In cases of protein-calorie malnutrition [76] and kwashiorkor [23] in children, a Cr^{3+} supplement of 250 μg/day in milk formula rapidly restored glucose tolerance tests to normal. In a similar group in Egypt, no benefit could be shown by supplement, since this is a region of high Cr dietary intake [23], the hospital diet having a mean Cr^{3+} level of 129 μg/day, and a range from 75 to 1057 μg [145].

Realization of the importance of chromium in glucose metabolism has stimulated attempts to supplement GTF using alcohol extracts of brewer's yeast. In such a test conducted on an elderly institutionalized group of 31 patients over 65 years of age, 45 percent had an abnormal glucose tolerance test (GTT). After 2 months of daily supplement, the GTT in 50 percent had returned to the normal range. The results were highly significant: $p = 0.001$.

GTF is only active in the presence of insulin, but supplementation with GTF promotes more efficient use of circulating insulin and reduces insulin output in response to sudden glucose loading. After glucose ingestion, the peak insulin response is lowest and most rapid in children, intermediate in adults, and very high and delayed in elderly patients [105]. The magnitude of the insulin peak may be correlated with tissue chromium levels [47], and it is possible that the body stores, as GTF, influence the degree of insulin response to glucose loading.

As well as reducing insulin requirements, supplementation with GTF also reduces fasting serum cholesterol and triglyceride levels [47]. Fasting cholesterol levels in young normal patients showed a mean decrease of 36 mg/100 ml after one month's supplementation of the diet with brewer's yeast. The content of GTF was not determined. Similarly, Schroeder, in 1968 [215], showed a 14 percent drop in serum cholesterol using oral Cr^{3+}. The effect is considerably greater if the fasting levels are 240 mg/100 ml or higher. The mechanism involved in these decreases is not known. It is possible that the nicotinic acid content of the brewer's yeast may be aiding the effect, but since the usual dose of nicotinic acid for reduction of elevated cholesterol levels is 1 to 2 gm three times daily, the 10 mg received daily from the yeast supplement is unlikely to be very effective. It is also possible that therapeutic doses of nicotinic acid derive their effect by conversion to GTF, if there are adequate chromium stores.

In insulin-requiring diabetics there is also a response to oral GTF. McKay [139], in 1952, reported a reduction in daily requirement of insulin of 20 to 45 units/day in diabetics whose daily requirement ranged from 60 to 130 units/day. Since most of these subjects have little endogenous insulin production, elimination of the requirement is not likely, but patients who require small amounts of insulin may recover entirely. The insulin requirement is usually reduced within 24 hours and may be associated with hypoglycemia. It then progressively decreases 1 to 2 units every 48 to 72 hours.

Chromium Deficiency in Total Parenteral Nutrition

Deficiency of chromium during total parenteral nutrition (TPN) would seem rather unlikely in the light of recent work by Seeling and his associates [226], who found relatively high Cr levels in a number of parenteral fluids, particularly plasma protein solution and human albumin. Using non-glucose carbohydrates, human albumin 20 percent, and Aminofusin L 600 S and L 600 X, these workers found that serum chromium rose rapidly in the first 7 days of TPN. The mean serum Cr concentration of 16 patients increased from a mean of 1 ng/ml to 11.3 ± 0.26 ng/ml. During the same period, urinary excretion rose from the normal level of 1.8 ± 1.1 μg/L to 37.7 ± 4.1 μg/L. Of the approximately 160 to 250 μg Cr supplied per day, 111 ± 2.0 μg were excreted, with large amounts being retained and stored.

In one case, however, reported by Jeejeebhoy and his colleagues [109], low levels of chromium in blood and hair developed after 3 years of home TPN in a 40-year-old woman who had undergone complete enterectomy for mesenteric thrombosis. This deficiency was associated with glucose intolerance, peripheral neuropathy, and inexplicable weight loss, all of which responded to chromium supplementation, 20 μg per day.

MANGANESE

History

Manganese, first isolated in 1774, is widely distributed in terrestrial and marine environments. It is found in trace amounts in most living systems, but particularly in animal cells. Within tissues, the highest levels of manganese have been found in liver, bone, and lactating mammary tissue. Its essentiality for growth and reproduction was first shown in rats and mice by Kemmerer et al. [124] and Orent and McCollum [174] in 1931. In 1936, a well-known skeletal abnormality in chickens, termed perosis, was also shown to be due to manganese deprivation [280].

Manganese deficiency has never been recognized in humans on normal diets, but has been induced accidentally under metabolic ward conditions, when a purified diet lacking manganese was supplied [46].

Experimentally induced manganese deficiency in domestic animals produces numerous physical and biochemical symptoms, such as poor growth, decreased testicular and ovarian function leading to sterility, accumulation of fat, hypocholesterolemia, and diabetes-like glucose tolerance curves.

Biochemical Function

The bulk of intracellular manganese is found associated with the mitochondria, the site of many enzymatic reactions. The metal may act as part of a metalloenzyme in which the Mn is an integral part of the molecule, or it may act as a dissociable cofactor. Here the metal ion is free to detach, but must be present for the activity of the enzyme. There are very few proven Mn metalloenzymes, but a large range of enzymes may be activated by Mn, as well as by other metallic ions such as Fe^{2+}, Co^{2+}, N_1^{2+}, and Mg^{2+}. Categories of enzymes that may be stimulated in this fashion include phosphatases, kinases, thioesterases, some peptidases and dehydrogenases, decarboxylases, glycotransferases, and adenyl cyclase [258]. In 1969, Leach and his coworkers [128] compared the effectiveness of Mn, Mg, Co, and Ni in the activation of the enzymes polysaccharide polymerase and galactose transferase in vitro. They found that cobalt was almost equally as effective as manganese with polysaccharide polymerase, but considerably more so with galactose transferase. However, when additional cobalt was provided for Mn-deficient animals, the symptoms caused by inactivation of these enzymes were not relieved. They concluded that the specificity of the metal cofactor effect varied in vivo. This highlights the problem of relating in vitro results to in vivo effects.

Further studies [129] showed that at least one group of enzymes, the glycosyl transferases, all of which require metal ions, performed at their optimum when Mn was utilized. These enzymes are important in the biosynthesis of polysaccharides and glycoproteins. They are found in abundance in the microsomal fraction of epiphyseal cartilage homogenate [128], and a deficiency is considered to account in part for the severe skeletal abnormalities and postural defects in experimental animals.

Manganese is also associated with the synthesis of RNA, DNA, and protein. Both the DNA and RNA polymerase systems have been shown to be affected by Mn [278], but only one of the two possible RNA polymerases has been shown to require Mn specifically [279]. The details of the in vivo role of Mn in protein synthesis is not understood. Manganous ions have been shown to stimulate the enzymatic coupling of monoiodotyrosine forming diiodotyrosine in vitro [17], but there is little evidence for the reaction occurring in vivo. However, rats given Mn have shown an increase in iodinated tyrosine in their tissues [113]. Kehoe [121] and his colleagues, in 1969, found that cortisol regulated the Mn-activated RNA polymerase activity within mice lymphocyte nuclei.

Manganese Metalloenzymes

Two Mn metalloenzymes have been identified. The first, pyruvate carboxylase, originally found in avian liver [224], is now considered to be present in all species. The second, superoxide dismutase, has been confirmed in avian liver and some bacteria.

Pyruvate carboxylase catalyzes the first step in carbohydrate synthesis from pyruvate, particularly in the liver and kidney, but also in the brain and adipose tissue. In animal cells the enzyme is large (MW 500,000), and contains biotin in four subunits. In some cases the enzyme may also contain magnesium as the activator, and this is a complicating factor when assessing the effect of manganese lack. Superoxide dismutase catalyzes the oxidation of the superoxide radical, formed by partial reduction of oxygen, to molecular oxygen and peroxide. The superoxide radicals are considered to arise by incomplete reduction of oxygen by flavin oxidase.

Other manganoproteins that have been found include transmanganin [35], a protein specially devoted to the transport of manganese in blood, although this has been disputed [16, 26]. Concanavalin A and manganin are both considered to be structural manganoproteins and have been isolated from the Jack bean and peanut, respectively.

Manganese and Brain Function

Manganese may affect the nervous system, and in particular the brain, with respect to deficiency [258] and excess [146]. A mutant gene affecting the coat color in mice, pallid, also produces a congenital ataxia identical to that seen in manganese-deficient mice. Supplementation of the mutant individuals during pregnancy produces normal offspring, but the mutant gene may again be expressed in the second generation in the absence of supplementation. Axatic pallid mice were found to have low manganese in their brains and a diminished production of cerebral dopamine and serotonin after the administration of the respective precursors [37].

Excess manganese, seen in workers exposed to manganese ores and fumes, produces a self-limiting psychiatric syndrome similar to schizophrenia and precedes a permanent neurologic phase, which closely resembles clinical Parkinson's disease. The condition is improved by levodopa medication, suggesting that dopamine is involved. Primates chronically poisoned with manganese develop similar permanent neurologic symptoms, and autopsy shows low striatal dopamine similar to that of Parkinsonian patients.

Experiments in which mice were fed supplements of ^{55}Mn showed that there was a rapid increase in brain manganese from the normal 1.85 ± 0.03 μg/gm to 5.86 ± 0.16 μg/gm. This was followed by a slow fall [37]. Concurrently, the level of brain dopamine rose from 0.47 ± 0.02 μg/gm to 0.80 ± 0.07 μg/gm. This corresponds to the situation in exposed human subjects in which the self-limiting psychiatric phase shows similarities to the mental effects in increased cerebral dopamine [146]. This temporary elevation is followed by a fall and the onset of a permanent neurologic disorder.

Normal Intake and Tissue Levels

A 70-kg adult human contains approximately 12 to 20 mg of Mn. The daily intake varies widely, but is generally considered to lie within 0.7 to 22 mg. The highest levels of manganese are found in plant products, particularly nuts, grains, and cereals. Lowest amounts occur in dairy products, meat, fish, poultry, and most seafoods. Manganese levels of full cream and skim milk from New Zealand were 2.1 μg/gm and 1.1 μg/gm, respectively, and for mixed vegetables, 8 μg/gm [141]. These correspond well to other estimations [257].

The recommended dietary intake for Mn is based on the minimum adequate intake given by the World Health Organization (1973) [283] and the National Research Council Food and Nutrition Board (1974) [162], of 2 mg/day and 2.5 mg/day, respectively. A New Zealand study of adults on a normal diet showed an intake of 2.7 mg/day [78], whereas the intake by babies during their first six months ranged from 2.5 to 75 μg/kg/day.

Metabolic balance studies of Mn suggest that about 20 μg of Mn per day would be retained under conditions of minimum intake and that this is adequate to prevent the deficiency in humans [17]. In food Mn is in the form of specific organic complexes, although these have not been clearly defined, and the changes that occur with cooking are unknown.

In early childhood, when the diet is mainly mother's milk, the low intake of about 7 μg/day produces a temporary negative Mn balance. After the first week, a progressively increasing intake raises the body stores, and from the age of two years a very constant level of Mn is maintained in the body [269].

Manganese Homeostatis

The level of Mn in the blood and tissue is closely regulated by excretion via the bile. Absorbed Mn, surplus to immediate requirement, rapidly appears in the bile and is excreted in the feces. Excretion also takes place in pancreatic secretion, but this is normally reabsorbed in the duodenum, jejunum, and ileum [17]. Very little Mn is lost through the urine. In subjects on normal diets, the fecal loss ranges from 0 to 8.3 mg/24 hr [26] and the urinary excretion from 0.2 to 1.4 μg/L [115].

Whereas in the gut there is an interaction between manganese and iron, once Mn is absorbed the pathway is particularly specific, and only manganese will accelerate the excretion of radiomanganese from the body [129]. The mechanism is considered to be capable of preventing deficiency under most conditions, except possibly where heavy demands are placed on reserves in rapid growth, pregnancy, or diabetes.

Observed values of manganese for plasma range from 0.38 to 1.04 ng/ml [269] and for whole blood from 8.6 to 16.5 ng/ml.

Manganese Deficiency in Animals and Humans

The most striking outward sign of manganese deficiency in animals shows as postural and skeletal defects, combined with a reduced growth rate. Sterility occurs at maturity, and the life span may be considerably shortened.

In poultry, perosis, or slipped tendon, appears because of failure of collagen and mucosaccharide formation. A similar failure accounts for the lack of otolith growth in the inner ears of rats, and subsequent ataxia.

Biochemically, a universal symptom of Mn deficiency is hypocholesterolemia [46]. It has been suggested that Mn is necessary in the formation of cholesterol at several stages [173]. This may also explain sterility, since lack of cholesterol and its precursors limits production of sex hormones and other steroids [46].

In humans, deficiency of Mn was found to cause reddening of normally black hair, mild evanescent dermatitis, slowed growth of hair and nails, occasional nausea, a decrease in serum phospholipids and triglycerides, and a moderate weight loss. Protein synthesis is not severely affected, since hemoglobin, red blood cells, and serum proteins are readily replaced [46].

Blood clotting time is increased due to lack of vitamin K activity. Of the four clotting proteins under the control of vitamin K, prothrombin, a glycoprotein, is depressed. Manganese may be necessary for the action of glycosyl transferases to complete terminal carbohydrate units converting preprothrombin to prothrombin.

REFERENCES

1. Addison, G. M., et al. An immuno-radiometric assay for ferritin in the serum of normal subjects and patients with iron deficiency and iron overload. *J. Clin. Pathol.* 25:326, 1972.
2. Adham, N. F., Song, M. K., and Rinderknecht, H. Binding of zinc to alpha-2-macroglobulin and its role in enzyme binding activity. *Biochim. Biophys. Acta* 495:212, 1977.
3. Allaway, W. H., et al. Selenium, molybdenum and vanadium in human blood. *Arch. Environ. Health* 16:342, 1968.
4. Anderson, R. A., and Brantner, J. H. Binding of chromium by porcine insulin. *Fed. Proc.* 36: 1123, 1977.
5. Andrews, E. D., Hartley, W. J., and Grant, A. B. Selenium responsive diseases of animals in New Zealand. *N.Z. Vet. J.* 16:3, 1968.
6. Apgar, J. Effect of zinc deficiency on parturition in the rat. *Am. J. Physiol.* 215:160, 1968.
7. Apgar, J. Effects of some nutritional deficiencies on parturition in rats. *J. Nutr.* 105:1553, 1975.
8. Barcia, P. J. Lack of acceleration of healing with zinc sulphate. *Ann. Surg.* 172:1048, 1970.
9. Bearn, A. G., and Kunkel, H. G. Localisation of Cu^{64} in serum fractions following oral administration: Alterations in Wilson's disease. *Proc. Soc. Exp. Biol. Med.* 85:44, 1954.
10. Beath, O. A., Eppson, H. F., and Gilbert, C. S. *Wyoming Agr. Exp. Sta. Bull.* No. 206, 1935.
11. Berzelius, J. J. *Ann. Chim. Phys.,* Paris, Serie 2, Tome 7:199, 1817.
12. Bodzy, P. W., Freeland, J. H., Eppright, M. A., and Tyree, A. Zinc status in the vegetarian. *Fed. Proc.* 36:1139, 1977.
13. Bowen, H. J. M., and Cawse, P. A. The determination of selenium in biological material by radioactivation. *Analyst* 88:721, 1963.
14. Bozian, R. D. Copper, zinc and manganese contents of four amino acid and protein hydrolysate preparations. *Am. J. Clin. Nutr.* 29:1131, 1976.
15. Brocks, A., Reid, H., and Glazer, G. Acute intravenous zinc poisoning. *Lancet* 1:1390, 1977.
16. Brune, D., Samsahe, K., and Wester, P. O. A comparison between the amounts of As, Au, Br, Cu, Fe, Mo, Se and Zn in normal and uraemic whole blood by means of nutron activation analysis. *Clin. Chim. Acta* 13:285, 1966.
17. Burch, R. E., Hahn, H. K., and Sullivan, J. F. Newer aspects of the roles of zinc, manganese and copper in human nutrition. *Clin. Chem.* 21: 501, 1975.
18. Burch, R. E., and Sullivan, J. F. Clinical and nutritional aspects of zinc deficiency and excess. *Med. Clin. North Am.* 60:675, 1976.
19. Burk, R. F., Peason, W. N., Wood, R. P., and Viteri, F. Blood-selenium levels *in vitro* red blood cell uptake of ^{75}Se in kwashiorkor. *Am. J. Clin. Nutr.* 20:723, 1967.
20. Bush, J. A., Mahoney, J. P., Markowitz, H., Gubler, C. J., Cartwright, G. E., and Wintrobe, M. M. Studies on copper metabolism: XVI. Radioactive copper studies in normal subject and in patients with hepatolenticular degeneration. *J. Clin. Invest.* 34:1766, 1955.
21. Carnes, W. H. Role of copper in connective tissue metabolism. *Fed. Proc.* 30:995, 1971.
22. Carnes, W. H., Cartwright, G. E., and Wintrobe, M. M. Copper and connective tissue metabolism. *Int. Rev. Connect. Tissue Res.* 4:197, 1969.
23. Carter, J. P., Kattab, A., Abd-el-Hadi, K., Davis, J. T., El Cholmy, A., and Patuwardhen, V. N. Chromium III in hypoglycemia and in impaired glucose utilisation in kwashiorkor. *Am. J. Clin. Nutr.* 21:195, 1968.
24. Cartwright, G. E., and Wintrobe, M. M. Copper metabolism in normal subjects. *Am. J. Clin. Nutr.* 14:224, 1964.
25. Cavdar, A. O., and Arcasoy, A. Haematologic and biochemical studies of Turkish children with pica. A presumptive explanation for the syndrome of geophagia, iron deficiency anaemia, hepatosplenomegaly and hypogonadism. *Clin. Pediatr.* 11:215, 1972.
26. Chapman, B. E., MacDermott, T. E., and O'Sullivan, W. J. Studies on manganese complexes of human serum albumin. *Bioinorg. Chem.* 3:27, 1973.
27. Cheville, N. F. The pathology of vitamin E deficiency in the chick. *Pathol. Vet.* 3:208, 1966.
28. Christopherson, B. O. Formation of monohydroxy-polyenic fatty acids from lipid peroxides by a glutathione peroxidase. *Biochim. Biophys. Acta* 164:35, 1968.
29. Chuttani, H. K., Gupta, P. S., Gulatti, S., and Gupta, D. N. Acute copper sulphate poisoning. *Am. J. Med.* 39:849, 1965.

30. Coble, Y. D., Schulert, A. R., and Farid, Z. Growth and sexual development of male subjects in an Egyptian oasis. *Am. J. Clin. Nutr.* 18:421, 1966.
31. Cohen, E., and Elvehjem, C. A. The relation of iron and copper to the cytochrome oxidase content of animal tissue. *J. Biol. Chem.* 107: 97, 1934.
32. Cohen, G., and Hochstein, P. Glutathione peroxidase: The primary agent for the elimination of hydrogen peroxide in erythrocytes. *Biochemistry* 2:1420, 1963.
33. Collins, R. J., Fromm, P. O., and Collings, W. D. Chromium excretion in the dog. *Am. J. Physiol.* 201:795, 1961.
34. Cook, J. D., Lipschitz, D. A., Miles, L. E., and Finch, C. A. Serum ferritin as a measure of iron stores in normal subjects. *Am. J. Clin. Nutr.* 27: 681, 1974.
35. Cotzias, G. C., and Bertinchamps, J. Transmangin, the specific manganese-carrying protein of human plasma. *J. Clin. Invest.* 39:979, 1960.
36. Cotzias, G. C., Millar, S. T., Papavasiliou, P. S., and Tang, L. C. Interactions between manganese and brain dopamine. *Med. Clin. North Am.* 60:429, 1976.
37. Cotzias, G. C., and Papavasiliou, P. S. State of binding of natural manganese in human cerebrospinal fluid, blood and plasma. *Nature* 195:823, 1962.
38. Crawford, I. L., and Connor, J. D. Zinc in maturing rat brain: Hippocampal concentration and localisation. *J. Neurochem.* 19:1451, 1972.
39. Cross, J. D., Leslie, A. C. D., and Smith, H. Copper levels in human tissue. *J. Forens. Sci. Soc.* 16:311, 1976.
40. Cuthbertson, D. P., Fell, G. S., Smith, C. M., and Tilstone, W. J. Metabolism after injury: I. Effects of severity, nutrition, and environmental temperature on protein, potassium, zinc and creatine. *Br. J. Surg.* 59:925, 1972.
41. Czerniejewski, C. P., Shank, C. W., Bechtel, W. G., and Bradley, W. B. The minerals of wheat, bread and flour. *Cereal Chem.* 41:65, 1964.
42. Danks, D. M., Campbell, P. E., Stevens, B. J., Mayne, V., and Cartwright, E. Menkes' kinky hair syndrome. An inherited defect in copper absorption with widespread effects. *Pediatrics* 50:188, 1972.
43. Danks, D. M., Campbell, P. E., Walker-Smith, J., Stevens, B. J., Gillespie, J. M., Blomfield, J., and Turner, B. Menkes' kinky hair syndrome. *Lancet* 1:1100, 1972.
44. Danks, D. M., Cartwright, E., Stevens, B. J., and Townley, R. R. W. Menkes' kinky hair disease: Further definition of the defect in copper transport. *Science* 179:1140, 1973.
45. Danks, D. M., Cartwright, E., and Stevens, B. J. Menkes' steely hair (kinky hair) disease. *Lancet* 1:891, 1973.
46. Doisy, E. A., Jr. Micronutrient Control on Biosynthesis of Clotting Proteins and Cholesterol. In D. D. Hemphill (Ed.), *Proceedings of the University of Missouri's 6th Annual Conference on Trace Substances in Environmental Health, 1973.* Columbia, MO: University of Missouri Press, 1973.
47. Doisy, R. J., Streeter, D. H. P., Frieberg, J. M., and Schneider, A. J. Chromium Metabolism in Man and Biochemical Effects. In A. S. Prasad (Ed.), *Trace Elements in Human Health and Disease.* New York: Academic, 1976.
48. Donaldson, R. M., and Barreras, R. F. Intestinal absorption of trace quantities of chromium. *J. Lab. Clin. Med.* 68:484, 1966.
49. Donaldson, J., Pierre, T. S., Minnich, J. L., and Barbeau, A. Determination of Na^+, K^+, $Mg2^+$, $Cu2^+$, $Zn2^+$ and $Mn2^+$ in rat brain regions. *Can. J. Biochem.* 51:87, 1973.
50. Dunlap, W. M., Hames, E. W., III, and Hume, D. M. Anaemia and neutropenia caused by copper deficiency. *Ann. Intern. Med.* 80:470, 1974.
51. Durum, W. H., and Hafty, J. Occurrence of minor elements in water. *Geochim. Cosmochim. Acta* 27:1, 1963.
52. Earl, C. J. In J. M. Walshe and J. N. Cumings (Eds.), *Wilson's Disease: Some Current Concepts.* Oxford: Blackwell, 1961. P. 18.
53. Eckhert, C. D., Sloan, M. V., Duncan, J. R., and Hurley, L. S. Zinc binding: Difference between human and bovine milk. *Science* 195:789, 1977.
54. Edwards, C., Olson, K. B., Heggen, G., and Glenn, J. Intracellular distribution of trace elements in liver tissue. *Proc. Soc. Exp. Biol. Med.* 197:94, 1961.
55. Evans, G. W. The biological regulation of copper homeostasis in the rat. *World Rev. Nutr. Diet.* 17:225, 1973.
56. Everson, G. J., Shrader, R. E., and Wang, T. Chemical and morphological changes in the brains of copper-deficient guinea-pigs. *J. Nutr.* 96:115, 1968.
57. Fairbanks, V. F. Copper sulphate induced haemolytic anaemia. *Arch. Intern. Med.* 120: 428, 1967.
58. Falchuk, K. H., Fawcett, D. W., and Vallee, B. L. Role of zinc in cell division of euglena gracilis. *J. Cell. Sci.* 17:57, 1975.

59. Fell, G. S., Cuthbertson, P. P. C., Queen, K., and Morrison, C. IVth Int. Cong. Nutr., Mexico, 1972. Abstract. P. 138.
60. Fell, G. S. Cuthbertson, D. P., Morrison, C., Fleck, A., Queen, K., Bessent, R. G., and Husain, S. L. Urinary zinc levels as an indication of muscle catabolism. *Lancet* 1:280, 1973.
61. Fisher, G. L. Function and homeostasis of copper and zinc in mammals. *Sci. Total Environ.* 4:373, 1975.
62. Fleming, C. R., Hodges, R. E., and Hurley, L. S. A prospective study of serum copper and zinc levels in patients receiving total parenteral nutrition. *Am. J. Clin. Nutr.* 29:70, 1976.
63. Freeland, J. H., and Cousins, R. J. Zinc content of selected foods. *J. Am. Diet. Ass.* 68:526, 1976.
64. Freeman, J. B., Stegink, L. D., Meyer, P. D., Fry, L. K., and Denbesten, L. Excessive urinary zinc losses during parenteral alimentation. *J. Surg. Res.* 18:463, 1975.
65. Fridovich, I. Superoxide radical and superoxide dismutase. *Accounts Chem. Res.* 5:321, 1972.
66. Gallagher, C. H., Reeve, V. E., and Wright, R. Copper deficiency in the rat. Effect on the ultrastructure of hepatocytes. *Aust. J. Exper. Biol. Med. Sci.* 51:181, 1973.
67. Giroux, E. L., and Henkin, R. I. Competition for zinc among serum albumin and amino acids. *Biochim. Biophys. Acta* 273:64, 1972.
68. Glinsman, W. H., Feldman, F. J., and Mertz, W. Plasma chromium after glucose administration. *Science* 152:1243, 1966.
69. Goodman, J. G., and Dallman, P. R. Role of copper in iron localisation in developing erythrocytes. *Blood* 34:747, 1969.
70. Graham, G. C., and Cordano, A. Copper depletion and deficiency in the malnourished infant. *Johns Hopkins Med. J.* 124:139, 1969.
71. Grant, C. A., and Thafvelin, B. *Nord. Veterin. Med.* 10:657, 1958.
72. Greger, J. L., Higgins, M. M., Abernathy, R. P., Kirksey, A., De Corso, M. B., and Baligar, P. Nutritional status of adolescent girls in regard to zinc, copper and iron. *Am. J. Clin. Nutr.* 31:269, 1978.
73. Gries, C. L., and Scott, M. L. Pathology of selenium deficiency in the chick. *J. Nutr.* 102: 1287, 1972.
74. Griffiths, N. M. Dietary intake and urinary excretion of selenium in some New Zealand women. *Proc. Univ. Otago Med. School* 51:8, 1973.
75. Griffiths, N. M., and Thomson, C. D. Selenium in whole blood of New Zealand residents. *N.Z. Med. J.* 80:199, 1974.
76. Gürson, C. T., and Saver, G. Effect of chromium or glucose utilisation in marasmic protein-calorie malnutrition. *Am. J. Clin. Nutr.* 24: 1313, 1971.
77. Gürson, C. T., and Saver, G. Effect of chromium supplementation on growth in marasmic protein calorie malnutrition. *Am. J. Clin. Nutr.* 26:988, 1973.
78. Guthrie, B. E., and Robinson, M. F. The nutritional status of New Zealanders with respect to manganese, copper, zinc and cadmium. *N.Z. Med. J.* 87:3, 1968.
79. Haeger, K., and Lanner, E. Oral zinc sulphate and ischaemic leg ulcers. *J. Vasc. Dis.* 3:77, 1974.
80. Hallbook, T., and Lanner, E. Serum zinc and healing of venous leg ulcers. *Lancet* 2:780, 1972.
81. & 82. Halsted, J. A., Smith, J. C., and Irwin, M. I. A conspectus of research on zinc requirements of man. *J. Nutr.* 104:347, 1974.
83. Hambidge, K. M. Chromium nutrition in man. *Am. J. Clin. Nutr.* 27:505, 1974.
84. Hambidge, K. M. Zinc and chromium in human nutrition. *J. Hum. Nutr.* 32:99, 1978.
85. Hambidge, K. M., Hambidge, C., Jacobs, M., and Baum, J. D. Low levels of zinc in hair, anorexia, poor growth and hypogeusia in children. *Pediatr. Res.* 6:868, 1972.
86. Hambidge, K. M., Nelder, K. H., Walravens, P. A., Weston, W. L., Silverman, A., Sabol, J. L., and Brown, R. M. Zinc and Acrodermatitis Enteropathica. In K. M. Hambidge and B. L. Nichols (Eds.), *Zinc and Copper in Clinical Medicine*. New York: Spectrum, 1977.
87. Hambidge, K. M., and Rodgerson, D. P. A comparison of the hair chromium levels of nulliparous and parous women. *Am. J. Obstet. Gynecol.* 103:320, 1969.
88. Harkins, D. A., Riella, M. C., Scribner, B. H., and Babb, A. L. Whole blood trace element concentrations during total parenteral nutrition. *Surgery* 79:674, 1976.
89. Hart, E. B., Steenbock, H., Waddell, J., and Elvehjem, C. A. Iron in Nutrition: VII. Copper as a supplement to iron for haemoglobin building in the rat. *J. Biol. Chem.* 77:797, 1928.
90. Hartley, W. J., and Grant, A. B. A review of selenium responsive diseases of New Zealand livestock. *Fed. Proc.* 20:679, 1961.
91. Heller, R. M., Kirchner, S. G., O'Neill, J. A., Hough, A. J., Howard, L., Kramer, S. S., and Green, H. L. Skeletal changes of copper deficiency in infants receiving prolonged total parenteral nutrition. *J. Pediatr.* 92:947, 1978.
92. Henkin, R. I., Schechter, P. J., Hoye, R., and Mattern, C. F. T. Ideopathic hypogeusia, with

dysgeusia, hyposmia and dysosmia. A new syndrome. *J.A.M.A.* 217:434, 1971.
93. Henkin, R. I. Metal-albumin-amino acid interactions: Chemical and physiological interrelationships. *Adv. Exp. Med. Biol.* 48:299, 1974.
94. Henkin, R. I. Newer Aspects of Copper and Zinc Metabolism. In W. Mertz and W. E. Cornatzer (Eds.), *New Trace Elements in Nutrition.* New York: Dekker, 1972. P. 255.
95. Henkin, R. I., and Smith, F. R. Zinc and copper metabolism in acute viral hepatitis. *Am. J. Med. Sci.* 264:401, 1972.
96. Henkin, R. I., Lippoldt, R. E., Bilstad, J., et al. Zinc protein isolated from human parotid saliva. *Proc. Nat. Acad. Sci. USA* 72:488, 1975.
97. Henzel, J. H., De Weese, M. S., and Lichti, E. L. Zinc concentrations within healing wounds. *Arch. Surg. (Chic.)* 100:349, 1970.
98. Hoekstra, W. G. Biochemical function of selenium and its relation to vitamin E. *Fed. Proc.* 34:2083, 1975.
99. Hopkins, L. L., Jr., and Price, M. G. Effectiveness of chromium III in improving the impaired glucose tolerance of middle-aged Americans. *Proc. 2nd West. Hemisphere Nutr. Congr.,* 1968. Abstract. Vol. 2, p. 40.
100. Hopkins, L. L., Jr., and Schwarz, K. Chromium (III) binding to serum proteins, specifically siderophilin. *Biochim. Biophys. Acta* 90:484, 1964.
101. Huber, A. M., and Gershoff, S. N. Effects of zinc deficiency on the oxidation of retinol and ethanol in rats. *J. Nutr.* 105:1486, 1975.
102. Hurley, L. S. Zinc deficiency in prenatal and neonatal development. *Prog. Clin. Biol. Res.* 14:47, 1977.
103. Hurley, L. S., Duncan, J. R., Sloan, M. V., and Eckhert, C. D. Development of zinc binding ligands during the post-natal period. *Fed. Proc.* 36:1138, 1977.
104. Hurley, L. S., Gowan, J., and Swinerton, H. Teratogenic effects of short-term and transitory zinc deficiency in rats. *Teratology* 4:199, 1971.
105. Jackson, R. L., Guthrie, R. A., and Murthy, D. Y. N. Oral glucose tolerance tests and their reliability. *Metabol. Clin. Exp.* 22:237, 1973.
106. Jacobs, A., Miller, F. M., Worwood, M., Beamish, M. R., and Wardrop, C. A. Ferritin in the serum of normal subjects and patients with iron deficiency and iron overload. *Br. Med. J.* 4:206, 1972.
107. James, B. E., and MacMahon, R. A. Trace elements in intravenous fluid. *Med. J. Aust.* 2: 1161, 1970.
108. Japha, A. Dissertation Halle, 1842. Quoted by A. L. Moxon and M. Rhian. *Physiol. Rev.* 23: 305, 1943.
109. Jeejeebhoy, K. N., Chu, R. C., Marliss, E. B., Greenberg, G. R., and Bruce-Robertson, A. Chromium deficiency, glucose intolerance, and neuropathy reversed by chromium supplementation, in a patient receiving long-term total parenteral nutrition. *Am. J. Clin. Nutr.* 30:531, 1977.
110. Jones, K. L., Smith, D. W., Ulleland, C. N., and Streissguth, A. P. Pattern of malformation in offspring of chronic alcoholic mothers. *Lancet* 1:1267, 1973.
111. Jones, P. A. E., Miller, F. M., Worwood, M., and Jacobs, A. Ferritinaemia in leukaemia and Hodgkin's disease. *Br. J. Cancer* 27:212, 1973.
112. Joseph, K. T., Panday, V. K., Raut, S. J., and Soman, S. D. Per capita daily intake of trace elements from vegetables, fruits and drinking water in India. *At. Absorption Newsletter* 7:25, 1968.
113. Kaellis, E. Effect of manganous ions on thyroidal iodine metabolism in the rat. *Proc. Soc. Exp. Biol. Med.* 135:216, 1970.
114. Kampschmidt, R. F., Upchurch, H. F., Eddington, C. L., and Pulliam, L. A. Multiple biological activities of a partially purified leucocyte endogenous mediator. *Am. J. Physiol.* 224: 530, 1973.
115. Kanabrocki, E. C., Case, L. F., and Fields, T. Manganese and copper levels in human urine. *J. Nucl. Med.* 6:780, 1965.
116. Karpel, J. T., and Peden, V. H. Copper deficiency in long-term parenteral nutrition. *J. Pediatr.* 30:32, 1972.
117. Kay, R. G., and Knight, G. S. Blood selenium values in an adult Auckland population group. *N.Z. Med. J.* 90:11, 1979.
118. Kay, R. G., and Tasman-Jones, C. Acute zinc deficiency in man during intravenous alimentation. *Aust. N.Z. J. Surg.* 45:325, 1975.
119. Kay, R. G., Tasman-Jones, C., Pybus, J., Whiting, R., and Black, H. A syndrome of acute zinc deficiency during total parenteral alimentation in man. *Ann. Surg.* 183:331, 1976.
120. Kayne, F. J., Komar, G., Laboda, H., and Vanderlinde, R. E. Atomic absorption spectrophotometry of chromium in serum and urine with a modified Perkin Elmer 603 atomic absorption spectrophotometer. *Clin. Chem.* 24: 2151, 1978.
121. Kehoe, J. M., Lust, G., and Beisel, W. R. Lymphoid tissue-corticosteroid interaction: An early effect on both Mg^{+2} and Mn^{+2} activated RNA polymerase activities. *Biochim. Biophys. Acta* 174:761, 1969.

122. Kehoe, R. A., Cholak, J., and Storey, R. V. Spectrochemical study of normal ranges of concentrations of certain trace metals in biological materials. *J. Nutr.* 19:579, 1940.
123. Keilin, D., and Mann, T. Carbonic anhydrase. Purification and nature of the enzyme. *Biochem J.* 34:1163, 1940.
124. Kemmerer, A. R., Elvehjem, C. A., and Hart, E. B. Studies on the relation of manganese to the nutrition of the mouse. *J. Biol. Chem.* 92:623, 1931.
125. Kirchgessner, M., Roth, H. P., and Weigand, E. Biochemical changes in zinc deficiency. In A. S. Prasad (Ed.), *Trace Elements in Human Health and Disease.* New York: Academic, 1976. Vol. 1, p. 189.
126. Klingsberg, W. G., Prasad, A. S., and Oberleas, D. Zinc Deficiency Following Penicillamine Therapy. In A. S. Prasad (Ed.), *Trace Elements in Human Health and Disease.* New York: Academic, 1976. P. 51.
127. Kraintz, L., and Talmage, R. V. Distribution of radio-activity following the i.v. administration of trivalent chromium[51] in the rat and rabbit. *Proc. Soc. Exp. Biol. Med.* 81:490, 1952.
128. Leach, R. M., Jr., Muester, A. M., and Wien, E. M. Studies on the role of manganese in bone formation: II. Effect upon chondroitin sulphate synthesis in chick epiphyseal cartilage. *Arch. Biochem. Biophys.* 133:22, 1969.
129. Leach, R. M., Jr. Metabolism and Function of Manganese. In A. S. Prasad (Ed.), *Trace Elements in Human Health and Disease.* New York: Academic, 1976. P. 235.
130. Leach, R. M., Jr. Role of manganese in mucopolysaccharide metabolism. *Fed. Proc. Am. Soc. Exp. Biol.* 30:991, 1971.
131. Lee, G. R., Nacht, S., Christensen, D., Hansen, S. P., and Cartwright, G. E. The contribution of citrate to the ferroxidase activity of serum. *Proc. Soc. Exp. Biol. Med.* 131:918, 1969.
132. Lee, G. R., Nacht, S., Lukens, J. N., and Cartwright, G. E. Iron metabolism in copper-deficient swine. *J. Clin. Invest.* 47:2058, 1968.
133. Levine, R. A., Streeten, D. H. P., and Doisy, R. J. Effects of oral chromium supplementation on the glucose tolerance of elderly human subjects. *Metabol. Clin. Exp.* 17:114, 1968.
134. Li, T. K., and Vallee, B. L. The Biochemical and Nutritional Role of Trace Elements. In R. S. Goodhart and M. E. Shils (Eds.), *Modern Nutrition in Health and Disease.* Philadelphia: Lea & Febiger, 1973. P. 372.
135. Lin, V. J. K., Nordstrom, J., Kohrs, M. B., Corah, E., and Dewdy, R. Effect of high-chromium yeast-extract supplementation on serum lipid, serum insulin, and glucose tolerance in older women. *Fed. Proc.* 36:1123, 1977.
136. Little, C., and O'Brien, P. J. An intracellular GSH-peroxidase with a lipid peroxidase substrate. *Biochem. Biophys. Res. Commun.* 31: 145, 1968.
137. Lombeck, I., Bassewitz, D. B., von Becker, K., Tinschamann, P., and Kastner, H. Ultrastructural findings in acrodermatitis enteropathica. *Pediatr. Res.* 8:82, 1974.
138. McCance, R. A., and Widdowson, E. M. The absorption and excretion of zinc. *Biochem. J.* 36:692, 1942.
139. McCay, C. M. Chemical Aspects of Ageing and the Effect of Diet on Ageing. In A. J. Lansing (Ed.), *Cowdry's Problems of Ageing* (3rd ed.). Baltimore: Williams & Wilkins, 1952. Chap. 6.
140. McCord, J. M., and Fridovich, I. Superoxide dismutase. An enzymic function for erythrocuprein (haemocuprein). *J. Biol. Chem.* 244: 6049, 1969.
141. McLeod, B. A., and Robinson, M. F. Dietary intake of manganese by New Zealand infants during the first six months of life. *Br. J. Nutr.* 27:229, 1972.
142. Mahoney, J. P., Sargent, J. P., Greland, M., and Small, W. Studies on manganese: I. Determination in serum by atomic absorption spectrophotometry. *Clin. Chem.* 15:313, 1969.
143. Mann, T., and Keilin, D. Haemocuprein and hepatocuprein, copper protein compounds of blood and liver in mammals. *Proc. Roy. Soc. Ser. B.* 126:303, 1938.
144. Mansouri, K., Halsted, J., and Gombos, E. A. Zinc, copper, magnesium and calcium in dialysed and non-dialysed uremic patients. *Arch. Intern. Med.* 125:88, 1970.
145. Maxia, V., Meloni, S., Rollier, M. A., Brandone, A., Patwarden, V. N., Waslien, C. I., and Said-El-Shami. Selenium and Chromium Assay in Egyptian Foods and Blood of Egyptian Children by Activation Analysis. In *Nuclear Activation Techniques in the Life sciences.* IAEA-SM 157/ 67, p. 527. Vienna: IAEA, 1972.
146. Mena, I., Marin, O., and Fuenzalida, S. Chronic manganese poisoning. Clinical picture and manganese turnover. *Neurology* 17:128, 1967.
147. Menkes, J. H., Alter, M., Steigleder, G. K., Weakley, D. R., and Sung, J. H. A sex-linked recessive disorder with retardation of growth, peculiar hair and focal cerebral and cerebellar degeneration. *Pediatrics* 29:764, 1962.
148. Mertz, W. Chromium occurrence and function in biological systems. *Physiol. Rev.* 49:163, 1969.

149. Mertz, W., Roginski, E. E., and Reba, R. C. Biological activity and fate of intravenous chromium: III. In the rat. *Am. J. Physiol.* 209: 489, 1965.
150. Miller, J. K., and Miller, W. J. Experimental zinc deficiency and recovery of calves. *J. Nutr.* 76:467, 1962.
151. Mills, G. C. Haemoglobin catabolism: I. Glutathione peroxidase, an erythrocyte enzyme which protects haemoglobin from oxidative breakdown. *J. Biol. Chem.* 229:189, 1957.
152. Mills, G. C. Glutathione peroxidase and the destruction of hydrogen peroxide in animal tissues. *Arch. Biochem.* 86:1, 1960.
153. Mills, G. C. The purification and properties of glutathione peroxidase of erythrocytes. *J. Biol. Chem.* 234:502, 1959.
154. Morris, V. C., and Levander, O. A. Selenium content of foods. *J. Nutr.* 100:1383, 1970.
155. Morrison, S. A., Russell, R. M., Carney, E. A., and Oaks, E. V. Failure of cirrhotics with hypovitaminosis A to achieve normal dark adaptation performance on vitamin A replacement. *Gastroenterology* 71:922, 1976.
156. Morrison, S. A., Russell, R. M., Carney, E. A., and Oaks, E. V. Zinc deficiency: A cause of abnormal dark adaptation in cirrhotics. *Am. J. Clin. Nutr.* 31:276, 1978.
157. Moynahan, E. J. Acrodermatitis enteropathica: A lethal inherited human zinc deficiency disorder. *Lancet* 2:399, 1974.
158. Moynahan, E. J. Zinc deficiency and disturbance of mood and visual behaviour. *Lancet* 1:91, 1976.
159. Murakami, Y., Suzuki, Y., Yamagata, T., and Yamagata, N. Cr and Mn in Japanese diet. *J. Radiat. Res.* (Tokyo) 6, 1965.
160. Muth, O. H., Oldfield, J. E., Remmert, L. F., and Schubert, J. R. Effects of selenium and vitamin E on white muscle disease. *Science* 128: 1090, 1958.
161. Nandekar, A. K. N., Nurse, C. E., and Friedberg, F. Mn^{2+} binding by plasma proteins. *Int. J. Pept. Protein Res.* 5:279, 1973.
162. National Research Council, Food and Nutrition Board. *Recommended Dietary Allowances* (8th ed.). Washington, DC: National Academy of Sciences, 1974.
163. O'Dell, B. L. Biochemistry and Physiology of Copper in Vertebrates. In A. S. Prasad and D. Oberleas (Eds.), *Trace Elements in Human Health and Disease. Vol. I. Zinc and Copper.* New York: Academic, 1976.
164. O'Dell, B. L. Biochemistry of copper. *Med. Clin. North Am.* 60:687, 1976.
165. O'Dell, B. L. Dietary factors that affect biological availability of trace elements. *Ann. N.Y. Acad. Sci.* 199:70, 1972.
166. O'Dell, B. L., Hardwick, B. C., Reynolds, G., and Savage, J. E. Connective tissue defect resulting from copper deficiency. *Proc. Soc. Exp. Biol. Med.* 108:402, 1961.
167. O'Dell, B. L., Newberne, P. M., and Savage, J. E. Significance of dietary zinc for the growing chicken. *J. Nutr.* 65:503, 1958.
168. O'Dell, B. L., Reynolds, G., and Reeves, P. G. Analogous effects of zinc deficiency and aspirin toxicity in the pregnant rat. *J. Nutr.* 107:1222, 1977.
169. O'Dell, B. L., and Savage, J. E. Effect of phytic acid on zinc availability. *Proc. Soc. Exp. Biol. Med.* 103:304, 1960.
170. O'Dell, B. L., Smith, R. M., and King, R. A. Effect of copper status on brain neurotransmitter metabolism in the lamb. *J. Neurochem.* 26:451, 1976.
171. Okada, A., Takagi, Y., Itakura, T., Satani, M., Manabe, H., Iida, Y., Tanigaki, T., Inasaki, M., and Kasahara, N. Skin lesions during intravenous hyperalimentation: Zinc deficiency. *Surgery* 80:629, 1976.
172. Olehy, D. A., Schmitt, R. A., and Bethard, W. F. Neutron activation analysis of magnesium, calcium, strontium, barium, manganese, cobalt, copper, zinc, sodium and potassium in human erythrocytes and plasma. *J. Nucl. Med.* 7:917, 1966.
173. Olsen, J. A. The biosynthesis of cholesterol. *Rev. Physiol. Biochem. Exptl. Pharmacol.* 56: 173, 1965.
174. Orent, E. R., and McCollum, E. V. Effects of deprivation of manganese in the rat. *J. Biol. Chem.* 92:651, 1931.
175. Osaki, S., Johnson, D. A., and Frieden, E. The possible significance of the ferrous oxidase activity of ceruloplasmin in normal human serum. *J. Biol. Chem.* 241:2746, 1966.
176. Osaki, S., Johnson, D. A., and Frieden, E. The mobilization of iron from the perfused mammalian liver by a serum copper enzyme, ferroxidase I. *J. Biol. Chem.* 246:3018, 1971.
177. Osborn, S. B., Roberts, C. N., and Walshe, J. M. Uptake of radiocopper by the liver. A study of patients with Wilson's disease and various control groups. *Clin. Sci.* 24:13, 1963.
178. Osis, D., Kramer, L., Wiatrowski, E., and Spencer, H. Dietary zinc intake of man. *Am. J. Clin. Nutr.* 25:582, 1972.
179. Ott, E. A., Smith, W. H., Stob, M., and Beeson,

W. M. Zinc deficiency syndrome in the young lamb. *J. Nutr.* 82:41, 1964.
180. Palmisano, D. J. Nutrient deficiencies after intensive parenteral alimentation. *N. Engl. J. Med.* 291:799, 1974.
181. Parisi, A. F., and Vallee, B. L. Isolation of a zinc $\alpha 2$ macroglobulin from human serum. *Biochemistry* 9:2421, 1970.
182. Parisi, A. F., and Vallee, B. L. Zinc metalloenzymes: Characteristics and significance in biology and medicine. *Am. J. Nutr.* 22:1222, 1969.
183. Patek, A. J., and Haig, C. The occurrence of abnormal dark adaptation and its relation to vitamin A metabolism in patients with cirrhosis of the liver. *J. Clin. Invest.* 18:609, 1939.
184. Pekarek, R. S., and Beisel, W. R. Redistribution and sequestering of essential trace elements during acute infection. *Nutr. Proc. Int. Congr. IX,* 1972. P. 183.
185. Pekarek, R. S., Wannemacker, R. W., Jr., and Beisel, W. R. The effect of leucocyte endogenous mediator (LEM) on the tissue distribution of zinc and iron. *Proc. Soc. Exper. Biol. Med.* 140:685, 1972.
186. Pfeiffer, C. C., and Bacchi, D. Copper, zinc, manganese, niacin and pyridoxine in the schizophrenias. *J. Appl. Nutr.* 27:9, 1975.
187. Pinsent, J. The need for selenite and molybdate in the formation of formic dehydrogenase by members of the coli-aerogenes group of bacteria. *Biochem. J.* 57:10, 1954.
188. Polson, C. J., and Tattersall, R. N. *Clinical Toxicology.* London: Pitman, 1969.
189. Pomerantz, S. H. Separation, purification and properties of two tyrosinases from hamster melanoma. *J. Biol. Chem.* 238:2351, 1963.
190. Pories, W. J., and Strain, W. H. Zinc and wound healing. In A. S. Prasad (Ed.), *Zinc Metabolism.* Springfield, IL: Charles C Thomas, 1966. P. 378.
191. Prasad, A. S. Deficiency of Zinc in Man and its Toxicity. In A. S. Prasad (Ed.), *Trace Elements in Human Health and Disease.* New York: Academic, 1976. Vol. 1, p. 1.
192. Prasad, A. S. Zinc in human nutrition. *CRC Crit. Rev. Clin. Lab. Sci.* 8:1–80, 1977.
193. Prasad, A. S., Halsted, J. A., and Nadimi, M. Syndrome of iron deficiency, dwarfism and geophagia. *Am. J. Med.* 31:532, 1961.
194. Prasad, A. S., and Oberleas, D. Binding of zinc to amino acids and serum proteins in vitro. *J. Lab. Clin. Med.* 76:416, 1970.
195. Prasad, A. S., Schulert, A. R., Miale, A., Jr., Farad, Z., and Sandstead, H. H. Zinc and iron deficiency in male subjects with dwarfism and hypogonadism but without ancyclostomiasis, schistosomiasis, or severe anaemia. *Am. J. Clin. Nutr.* 12:437, 1963.
196. Prask, J. A., and Plocke, D. J. A role for zinc in the structural integrity of the cytoplasmic ribosomes of *Euglena gracilis. Physiology* 48:150, 1971.
197. Prieto, J., Barry, M., and Sherlock, S. Serum function in patients with iron overload and with acute and chronic liver disease. *Gastroenterology* 68:525, 1975.
198. Rahmat, A., Norman, J. N., and Smith, G. The effect of zinc deficiency on wound healing. *Br. J. Surg.* 61:271, 1974.
199. Raulin, J. Etudes cliniques sur la végétation. *Ann. Sci. Botan. Biol. Végétale* 11:93, 1869.
200. Raskin, N. H., Sligar, K. P., and Steinberg, R. H. Dark adaptation slowed by inhibitors of alcohol dehydrogenase in the albino rat. *Brain Res.* 50:496, 1973.
201. Reinhold, J. G., Faradji, B., Abadi, P., and Ismail-Beigi, F. Binding of Zinc to Fiber and other Solids of Wholemeal Bread. In A. S. Prasad (Ed.), *Trace Elements in Human Health and Disease.* New York: Academic, 1976. Vol. 1, p. 163.
202. Richards, M. P., and Cousins, R. J. Isolation of intestinal zinc: Proposed function in zinc absorption. *Fed. Proc.* 36:1106, 1977.
203. Riordan, J. F. Biochemistry of zinc. *Med. Clin. North Am.* 60:661, 1976.
204. Riordan, J. F., and Vallee, B. L. Structure and Function of Zinc Metalloenzymes. In A. S. Prasad and D. Oberleas (Eds.), *Trace Elements in Human Health and Disease.* New York: Academic, 1976.Vol. 1, p. 227.
205. Robertson, B. T., and Burns, M. J. Zinc metabolism and zinc deficiency syndrome in the dog. *Am. J. Vet. Res.* 24:997, 1963.
206. Robinson, W. O. J. *Assoc. Off. Agr. Chem.* 16:423, 1933.
207. Robinson, W. O., Edgington, G., and Byers, H. C. Chemical studies of infertile soils derived from rocks high in magnesium and generally high in chromium and nickel. *U.S. Department of Agriculture Technical Bulletin.* No. 471, 1935.
208. Rosenbusch, J. P., and Weber, K. Localisation of the zinc binding site of aspartate transcarbamoylase in the regulatory subunit. *Proc. Nat. Acad. Sci. US* 68:1019, 1971.
209. Rotruck, J. T., Hoekstra, W. G., Pope, A. L., Ganther, H., Swanson, A., and Hafeman, D. Relationship of selenium to GSH peroxidase. *Fed. Proc.* 31:691, 1972.

210. Rucker, R. B., Parker, H. E., and Rogler, J. C. Effect of copper deficiency on chick bone collagen and selected bone enzymes. *J. Nutr.* 98:57, 1969.
211. Sandstead, H. H. Zinc nutrition in the United States. *Am. J. Clin. Nutr.* 26:1251, 1973.
212. Sandstead, H. H., and Shephard, G. H. The effect of zinc deficiency on the tensile strength of healing surgical incisions in the integument of the rat. *Proc. Soc. Exper. Biol. Med.* 128:687, 1968.
213. Scheinberg, I. H. The effect of heredity and environment on copper metabolism. *Med. Clin. North Am.* 60:705, 1976.
214. Scheinberg, I. H., and Sternlieb, I. Metabolism of Trace Metals. In P. K. Bondy (Ed.), *Duncan's Diseases of Metabolism,* (6th ed.), Vol. II, 1969.
215. Schroeder, H. A. Losses of vitamins and trace elements resulting from processing and preservation of foods. *Am. J. Clin. Nutr.* 24:562, 1971.
216. Schroeder, H. A. The role of chromium in mammalian nutrition. *Am. J. Clin. Nutr.* 21:230, 1968.
217. Schroeder, H. A. Balassa, J. J., and Tipton, I. H. Abnormal trace elements in man: Chromium. *J. Chron. Dis.* 15:941, 1962.
218. Schubert, J. R., Muth, O. H., Oldfield, J. E., and Remmert, L. F. Experimental results with selenium in white muscle disease of lambs and calves. *Fed. Proc.* 20:689, 1961.
219. Schwarz, K. Dietary Necrotic Liver Degeneration: An Approach to the Concept of the Biochemical Lesion. In R. W. Brauer (Ed.), *Liver Function.* Washington, DC: American Institute of Biological Sciences, 1958. P. 509.
220. Schwarz, K. Essentiality and metabolic functions of selenium. *Med. Clin. North Am.* 60:745, 1976.
221. Schwarz, K., Bieri, J. B., Briggs, G. M., and Scott, M. L. Prevention of exudative diathesis in chicks by Factor 3 and selenium. *Proc. Soc. Exper. Biol. Med.* 95:621, 1957.
222. Schwarz, K., and Foltz, C. M. Factor 3 activity of selenium compounds. *J. Biol. Chem.* 233: 245, 1958.
223. Schwarz, K., and Foltz, C. M. Selenium as an integral part of Factor 3 against dietary necrotic liver degeneration. *J. Am. Chem. Soc.* 791:3292, 1957.
224. Schwarz, K., and McDade, M. Liver catalase levels in dietary necrotic liver degeneration. Quoted in K. Schwarz, *Med. Clin. North Am.* 60:745, 1976.
225. Scrutton, M. C., Reed, G. H., and Mildvan, A. S. Pyruvate carboxylase: VI. The presence of tightly bound manganese. *J. Biol. Chem.* 241: 3480, 1966.
226. Seeling, W., Dolp, R., Ahnefeld, F. W., Dick, W., and Hohage, R. Untersuchungen zum Verhalten des Chroms in Serum und Urin polytraumatisierter Patienten sowie der Chromkonzentration verschiedener Infusionslösungen. *Infusionstherapie* 2:144, 1975.
227. Shields, G. S., Coulson, W. F., and Kimball, D. A. Studies on copper metabolism: XXXII. Cardiovascular lesions in copper deficient swine. *Am. J. Pathol.* 41:603, 1962.
228. Shin, Y. A., and Eichhorn, G. L. Interaction of metal ions with polynucleotides and related compounds: XII. The related effect of various metal ions on DNA helicity. *J. Am. Chem. Soc.* 90: 7323, 1968.
229. Shokeir, M. H. K. Is ceruloplasmin a physiological ferroxidase? *Clin. Biochem.* 5:115, 1972.
230. Smith, J. C., Jr., Brown, E. D., and Cassidy, W. A. *Zinc and vitamin A: Interrelationships. Zinc Metabolism: Current aspects in Health and Disease.* New York: Liss, 1977. P. 29.
231. Smith, J. C., Jr., McDaniel, E. G., Fan, F. F., and Halstead, J. A. Zinc: A trace element essential in vitamin A metabolism. *Science* 131:954, 1973.
232. Solomons, N. W., Layden, T. J., and Rosenberg, I. H. Plasma trace metals during total parenteral alimentation. *Gastroenterology* 70:1022, 1976.
233. Sondergaard, E. Selenium and Vitamin E Interrelationships. In O. H. Muth, J. E. Oldfield, and P. H. Weswig (Eds.), *Selenium in Biomedicine.* Westport, CT: Avi, 1967. P. 365.
234. Spears, A. B., Kaufman, B. M., Mattock, M. B., Saharia, S. S., and Sachdeva, H S. Serum-zinc as an index of zinc status. *Lancet* 2:526, 1976.
235. Spencer, H., Osis, D., Kramer, L., and Norris, C. Intake, Excretion and Retention of Zinc in Man. In A. S. Prasad (Ed.), *Trace Elements in Human Health and Disease.* New York: Academic, 1976. Vol. 1, p. 345.
236. Spencer, H., Rosoff, B., Feldstein, A., Cohn, S. H., and Gusmano, E. Metabolism of zinc-65 in man. *Radiat. Res.* 24:432, 1965.
237. Sprinker, L. H., Harr, J. R., Newberne, P. M., Whanger, P. D., and Weswig, P. H. Selenium deficiency lesions in rats fed vitamin E supplemented rations. *Nutr. Rep. Int.* 4:335, 1971.
238. Stadtman, T. C. Biological function of selenium. *Nutr. Rev.* 35:161, 1977.
239. Steele, T. H. Dissociation of zinc excretion from other cations in man. *J. Lab. Clin. Med.* 81:205, 1973.

240. Stephan, J. K., and Hsu, J. M. Effect of zinc deficiency and wounding on DNA synthesis in rat skin. *J. Nutr.* 103:548, 1973.
241. Sternlieb, I., van den Hamer, C. J. A., Morell, A. G., Alpert, S., Gregoriadis, G., and Scheinberg, I. H. Lysosomal defect of hepatic copper excretion in Wilson's disease (hepatolenticular degeneration). *Gastroenterology* 64:99, 1973.
242. Stewart, R. D. H., Griffiths, N. M., Thomson, C. D., and Robinson, M. F. Quantitative selenium metabolism in normal New Zealand women. *Br. J. Nutr.* 40:45, 1978.
243. Sullivan, J. F., and Lankford, H. G. Zinc metabolism and chronic alcoholism. *Am. J. Clin. Nutr.* 17:57, 1965.
244. Summers, M., Worwood, M., and Jacobs, A. Ferritin in normal erythrocytes, lymphocytes, polymorphs and monocytes. *Br. J. Haematol.* 28:19, 1974.
245. Tasman-Jones, C., Kay, R. G., and Sum, P. L. Zinc and Copper Deficiency, with Particular Reference to Parenteral Nutrition. In Lloyd M. Nyhus (Ed.), *Surgery Annual.* New York: Appleton-Century-Crofts, 1978. Vol. 10, p. 23.
246. Tasman-Jones, C., and Kay, R. G. Zinc deficiency and skin lesions. *N. Engl. J. Med.* 283: 830, 1975.
247. Thompson, J. N., and Scott, M. L. Role of selenium in the nutrition of the chick. *J. Nutr.* 97:335, 1969.
248. Tipton, I. H., and Cook, M. J. Trace elements in human tissue: Part II. Adult subjects from the United States. *Health Phys.* 9:103, 1963.
249. Tipton, I. H., Schroeder, H. A., Perry, H. M., Jr., and Cook, M. J. Trace Elements in Human Tissue: Part III. Subjects from Africa, the Near and Far East and Europe. *Health Phys.* 11:403, 1965.
250. Toepfer, E. W., Mertz, W., Polansky, M. M., Roginski, E. E., and Wolf, W. R. Preparation of chromium-containing material of glucose tolerance factor activity from brewer's yeast extracts and by synthesis. *J. Agric. Food Chem.* 21:69, 1977.
251. Toepfer, W. W., Mertz, W., Roginski, E. E., and Polansky, M. M. Chromium in foods in relation to biological activity. *J. Agric. Food Chem.* 21:69, 1973.
252. Todd, W. R., Elvehjem, C. A., and Hart, E. G. Zinc in the nutrition of the rat. *Am. J. Physiol.* 107:146, 1934.
253. Topham, R. W., Sung, C. S., Morgan, F. G., Prince, D., and Jones, S. H. Functional significance of the copper and lipid components of human ferroxidase II. *Arch. Biochem. Biophys.* 167:129, 1975.
254. Truman, R. W., and Doisey, R. J. Studies in the Genetically Diabetic Mouse: Effect of Glucose Tolerance Factor (G.T.F.) and Clofibrate (C.P.I.B.) on the Diabetic Syndrome. *Proceedings of the Second International Symposium on Trace Element Metabolism in Animals.* Baltimore: University Park Press, 1974. P. 678.
255. Tucker, H. F., and Salmon, W. D. Parakeratosis or zinc deficiency disease in pigs. *Proc. Soc. Exper. Biol. Med.* 88:613, 1955.
256. Tucker, S. B., Schroeter, A. L., Brown, P. W., and McCall, J. T. Acquired zinc deficiency. Cutaneous manifestations typical of acrodermatitis enteropathica. *J.A.M.A.* 235:2399, 1976.
257. Underwood, E. J. *Trace Elements in Human and Animal Nutrition* (2nd ed.). New York: Academic, 1962.
258. Utter, M. F. The biochemistry of manganese. *Med. Clin. North Am.* 60:713, 1976.
259. Vaisrub, S. At the mercy of the elements. Editorial. *J.A.M.A.* 235:2422, 1976.
260. Vallee, B. L., and Neurath, H. Carboxypeptidase, a zinc metalloprotein. *J. Am. Chem. Soc.* 76:5006, 1954.
261. Vallee, B. L., Stein, E. A., Sumerwell, W. N., and Fischer, E. H. Metal content of α amylases of various origins. *J. Biol. Chem.* 234:2901, 1959.
262. Vallee, B. L., and Wacker, W. E. C. Metalloproteins. In H. Neurath (Ed.), *The Proteins, Composition, Structure and Function.* New York: Academic, 1970.
263. Van Caillie, M., Degenehart, H., Luijendijk, I., and Fernandes, J. Zinc content of intravenous solutions. *Lancet* 2:200, 1978.
264. Van Rij, A. M., McKenzie, J. M., and Dunckley, J. V. Excessive urinary zinc losses and aminoaciduria during intravenous alimentation. *Proc. Univ. Otago Med. Sch.* 53:77, 1975.
265. Van Vleet, J. F., Hall, B. V., and Simon, J. Vitamin E deficiency. A sequential light and electron microscopic study of skeletal muscle degeneration in weanling rabbits. *Am. J. Pathol.* 52:1067, 1968.
266. Van Vleet, J. F., Ferrans, V. J., and Ruth, G. R. Ultrastructural alterations in nutritional cardiomyopathy of selenium-vitamin E deficient swine: I. Fiber lesions. *Lab. Invest.* 37:188, 1977.
267. Van Vleet, J. F., Ferrans, V. J., and Ruth, G. R. Ultrastructural alterations in nutritional cardiomyopathy of selenium-vitamin E deficient swine: II. Vascular lesions. *Lab. Invest.* 37:201, 1977.

268. Van Vleet, J. F., Ruth, G. R., and Ferrans, V. J. Ultrastructural alterations in skeletal muscle of pigs with selenium-vitamin E deficiency. *Am. J. Vet. Res.* 37:911, 1976.
269. Versieck, J., Cornelis, R., Lemey, G., and DeRudder, J. Determination of manganese, in whole blood and serum. *Clin. Chem.* 26:531, 1980.
270. Vilter, R. W., Bozian, R. C., Hess, E. V., Zellner, D. C., and Petering, H. G. Manifestations of copper deficiency in a patient with systemic sclerosis on intravenous hyperalimentation. *N. Engl. J. Med.* 291:188, 1974.
271. Visek, W. J., Whitney, I. B., Kuhn, U. S. G., III, and Comar, C. L. Metabolism of Cr^{51} by animals as influenced by the chemical state. *Proc. Soc. Exp. Biol. Med.* 84:610, 1953.
272. Vittorio, P. V., Wright, E. W., and Sinnott, B. E. The distribution of $chromium^{51}$ in mice after intraperitoneal injection. *Can. J. Biochem. Physiol.* 40:1677, 1962.
273. Walshe, J. M. Disturbance of amino acid metabolism following liver injury. *Quart. J. Med.* 22:483, 1953.
274. Weismann, K. Lines of Beau: Possible markers of zinc deficiency. *Acta Dermatovener* 57:88, 1977.
275. Wells, N. Total Selenium in Top Soils. *N.Z. Soil Bureau Atlas,* Maps 89 and 90. Wellington: Govt. Printer, 1967.
276. Whanger, P. D., Weswig, P. H., Oldfield, J. E., Cheeke, P. R., and Muth, O. H. Factors influencing selenium and white muscle disease: Forage types, salts, amino acids and dimethyl sulphoxide. *Nutr. Rep. Int.* 6:21, 1972.
277. Whanger, P. D., Weswig, P. H., Schmitz, J. A., and Oldfield, J. E. Effects of selenium and vitamin E deficiencies on reproduction, growth, blood components and tissue lesions in sheep fed purified diets. *J. Nutr.* 107:1288, 1977.
278. Wiberg, J. S., and Newman, W. F. The binding of bivalent metals by deoxyribonucleic and ribonucleic acids. *Arch. Biochem. Biophys.* 72:66, 1957.
279. Widnell, C. C., and Tata, J. R. Studies on the stimulation by ammonium sulphate of the DNA-dependent RNA polymerase of isolated rat liver nuclei. *Biochem. Biophys. Acta* 123:478, 1966.
280. Wilgus, H. S., Norris, L. C., and Heuser, C. F. The role of certain inorganic elements in the cause and prevention of perosis. *Science* 84: 151, 1936.
281. Williams, D. M., Christensen, D. D., Lee, G. R., and Cartwright, G. E. Serum azide-resistant ferroxidase activity. *Biochem. Biophys. Acta* 350:129, 1974.
282. Willson, R. L. Iron Metabolism. In *Ciba Foundation Symposium 51.* Amsterdam, 1977.
283. World Health Organization. *Trace Elements in Human Nutrition.* Geneva: Technical Report Series No. 532, 1973.
284. Worwood, M., Summers, M., Miller, F., Jacobs, A., and Whittaker, J. A. Ferritin in blood cells from normal subjects and patients with leukemia. *Br. J. Haematol.* 28:27, 1974.
285. Wretlind, A. Complete intravenous nutrition. Theoretical and experimental background. *Nutr. Metabol. Suppl.* 14:1, 1972.
286. Wretlind, A. Future trends in parenteral nutrition. *Bibl. Nutr. Dieta* 21:177, 1975.
287. Wright, P. L., and Bell, M. C. Comparative metabolism of selenium and tellurium in sheep and swine. *Am. J. Physiol.* 211:6, 1966.
288. Zidar, B. L., Shadduck, R. K., Zeigler, Z., and Winkelstein, A. Observations on the anaemia and neutropenia of human copper deficiency. *Am. J. Hematol.* 3:177, 1977.
289. *Zinc in Human Nutrition: Summary of Proceedings of a Workshop.* Food and Nutrition Board, National Academy of Science. Washington, DC, 1970. Quoted in *Lancet* 1:229, 1973.

10

Two Dozen Syndromes: Pattern Recognition in Diagnosis and Treatment of Fluid and Electrolyte Disorders

Francis D. Moore

BACK TO NORMAL CELLULAR FUNCTION

Cellular metabolism, the process of life, is conducted in a salty, protein-rich body fluid. One component of this fluid lies within the cells themselves. Another portion circulates freely, is pumped through the blood vessels and capillaries, appears in the interstitial fluid, lymphatics, and gut, is rapidly replenished by oral intake, and serves as the secretory and excretory pathway of kidneys, lungs, liver, and bowel.

Whatever disorders arise in these intracellular and extracellular fluids, the ultimate message of damage or benefit is to be found in cellular function itself.

Homeostasis is the sum of bodily activities and inborn regulators by which these solute concentrations and solvent volumes are maintained to support normal cellular function. The inborn regulators—physiologic feedback systems—are the central issue in patient care: one must understand what the patient is doing for himself before effective assistance can be provided. Autoregulation and feedback loop regulators operate throughout this system. Their function or malfunction may be as important as the disease state or the external cause of the disorder. Fluid and electrolyte concentrations, pools, and volumes are interrelated and cross-connected through membrane boundaries: each acts directly on the other. The physician encounters these complex disorders in repetitive "patterns" or "syndromes." It is easier to understand and treat them if we learn to identify and recognize them by their distinct patterns. Pattern-recognition is the basis of effective fluid and electrolyte management.*

Complicated descriptions of the total system have been erected, often multivariate structures

**Author's Note:* The value of pattern-recognition and the use of identified patterns of fluid/electrolyte change as the basis for patient care was first explored in an article entitled "Common patterns of water and electrolyte change in injury, surgery, and disease" (Moore, F. D. *N. Engl. J. Med.* 258:277, 325, 377, 427, 1958). This concept was then applied to certain aspects of burn treatment (Moore, F. D. Burns. An annotated outline for practical treatment. *Med. Clin. North. Am.* 36:1201, 1962), and in a textbook of surgical management (*Metabolic Care of the Surgical Patient.* Philadelphia: Saunders, 1959). This pattern-chemistry was updated and the method further expanded in the Rhoads-Hardy text (Lippincott, 1975), and is here again brought up to date with several additional patterns observed in patients receiving parenteral nutrition.

involving exponential and logarithmic functions. Such mathematical models have their appeal, providing chemical and teleologic insight, but they are a poor guide for the clinician. The sailor lost at sea searches for a few buoys or lighthouses to guide him home safely, even though he may be intellectually fascinated by the total interaction of forces that determine wind, ocean currents, and the formation of beaches, reefs, and shoals.

It is the purpose of this chapter to identify and describe 24 syndromes of disorder in body fluids: the volume of body water, body composition, electrolyte concentration, and acid-base change.

"TWENTY-FOUR SYNDROMES"— A GUIDE TO CHAPTER 10

Introductory Tables

Useful Expressions and First Approximations	Table 10-1
Equations for Compositional Relationships	Table 10-2
Useful Expressions and First Approximations in Acid-Base Homeostasis	Table 10-3
Normal Values	Table 10-4

Fifteen Syndromes of Disordered Body Water, Salts, and Protein: Fluid Volumes and Tonicity

Syndrome 1	Hypovolemia	Table 10-5
Syndrome 2	Plasma Loss Hypovolemia	Table 10-6
Syndrome 3	Hypoproteinemia	
Syndrome 4	Hypervolemia	Table 10-7
Syndrome 5	Polycythemia	Table 10-8
Syndrome 6	Desalting Water Loss	Table 10-9
Syndrome 7	Oversalting: Extracellular Fluid Excess	Table 10-10
Syndrome 8	Desiccation-Dehydration	Table 10-11
Syndrome 9	Overhydration-Hypotonicity	Table 10-12
Syndrome 10	Solute-Loading Hypertonicity	Table 10-13
Syndrome 11	Hypokalemia	Table 10-14
Syndrome 12	Hyperkalemia	Table 10-15
Syndrome 13	Hypochloremia	
Syndrome 14	Hyperchloremia	Table 10-16
Syndrome 15	The Normal Post-operative Patient	Table 10-17

Three Syndromes Related to Starvation and Intravenous Feeding

Syndrome 16	Cellular Steal	
Syndrome 17	Parenteral Nutrition Overload	
	17-I	Fluid Overload
	17-II	Hyperosmolar Coma (Table 10-18)
	17-III	Hyperphosphatemia
	17-IV	Hypercalcemia
	17-V	Satiety
	17-VI	Amino Acid Overload
	17-VII	Acid-Base Distortion and Surgical Procrastination
Syndrome 18	Insulin Anomalies in Total Parenteral Nutrition	
	18-I	Weaning and Digestive Inhibition
	18-II	Flask Insulin Hypoglycemia
	18-III	Latent Diabetes and Post-Traumatic Pseudo-Diabetes

Six Syndromes of Disordered Acid-Base Homeostasis

Syndrome 19	Acute Hypercapnia	Table 10-19
Syndrome 20	Chronic Hypercapnia	Table 10-19
Syndrome 21	Acute Hypocapnia	Table 10-20
Syndrome 22	Post-Traumatic Alkalosis	Table 10-21
Syndrome 23	Base Loss Acidosis	Table 10-22
Syndrome 24	Low Flow Acidosis	Table 10-23

Body Composition

In normal body fluid composition, concentration is held constant while size is variable. The total mass of a solute is, in turn, the product of the volume of the solution multiplied by the concentration of the solute. Many clinical problems in the understanding of body fluid disorders and their treatment arise from confusion between total volume and total mass, and from the failure to appreciate the tremendous compositional differences among various patients, even though their ideal concentration parameters are identical.

The term "body composition" has been given to the study of these phenomena, relating mass and concentration in the body, and identifying the total of body cells, fluids, and salts in a meaningful way. Body composition is the study of the total mass and volume of body components in relation to body size, body configuration, age, sex, disease, and concentration changes.

An understanding of the patterns of disordered body fluid chemistry, as presented here, requires an adequate systematic knowledge of physiologic chemistry and body composition. This chapter does not provide such background introductory knowledge, but assumes it in the reader. In the bibliography at the close is presented a list of several volumes or summaries that provide a useful background review.

Addition or Subtraction?

Is the patient suffering from loss or gain? From deficit or plethora? Often obvious, this question should always be asked. Subtraction disorders include desalting water loss, various forms of dehydration, plasma volume deficit, and selective deficit of certain ions. But even here the balance between loss and gain is extremely important. A low hematocrit may mean the loss of red cells, but it also means an absolute increase in plasma volume.

Addition disorders, excesses in body fluid components, sometimes arise from disease, as in liver failure, heart failure, or renal failure. Quite frequently, in an age of intravenous therapy, excesses result from overzealous treatment. An overabundance of body fluid and salt can embarrass the circulation and become lethal; overtransfusion of blood and plasma can produce all the chamber-pressure alterations of congestive heart failure.

The balance of loss and gain will determine the most rational treatment. A low serum sodium concentration, for example, should often be treated by withholding water or by a water diuresis, rather than by the careless administration of huge amounts of sodium salts, which can overload the circulation, producing cerebral and pulmonary edema. What appears superficially to be a deficit of salt may, in such instances, actually be an overload of water. The question of whether the disorder is *addition* or *subtraction* is thus seemingly obvious, always important, and sometimes subtle.

Homeostatic Feedback Regulators

Land-dwelling vertebrates spend their lives fighting off acidosis and dehydration. The excretion of acid and conservation of body water are, in a sense, the most primitive life-maintaining systems of those organisms that have removed themselves from the watery buffers of the ocean.

In the last 50 years it has become evident that the human body contains an elaborate system of interlocking regulators that, sensing a disorder, then guide the body back to normal in a cybernetic fashion, a feedback loop.

When the body senses a disorder, for example, desalting water loss, there is an elaborate homeostatic regulator system that within moments, or hours at the most, results in the conservation of water and salt. These feedback loops regularly involve three components: a sensor (often vascular muscle walls or special sense organs in them), a central arc (usually neuroendocrine), and an effector arm (respiratory, excretory, or circulatory).

The physician should perceive the state of these homeostatic regulators, and determine by appropriate tests whether they are providing a feedback that is normal and corrective. If the inborn regulators are operating normally, it is a good portent that indicates a favorable outcome by simple treatment. If, owing to disease, the feedback regulator loop cannot operate normally, treatment becomes more complicated. Guides to progress must involve measures of the homeostatic regulators as well as the disorder itself. Examples to follow will make this point more clear.

In some cases, the disorder itself results from a primary malfunction of the homeostatic feedback mechanism. The simplest example is the unlimited diuresis seen in certain forms of kidney disease. A huge and unregulated loss of urine results in severe dehydration through the very organ whose normal function is to conserve water.

Four homeostatic regulatory mechanisms or feedback loops are pre-eminent in regulation of fluid and electrolyte, body water, salt, and acid.

Osmolar Regulation

Total osmolality is not to be confused with colloid osmotic pressure, the latter being a biologic property exhibited when any system of membranes is facing a solute to which the membranes are poorly permeable. Total osmotic pressure is a colligative property of all solutions based on the number of molecules dissolved. Colloid osmotic pressure is a biologic property regulated, in human plasma, by the concentration of albumin. Total osmotic pressure is approximately linear with sodium concentration in plasma water. Depressed osmolality of extracellular fluid (hypotonicity) has as its normal response a brisk free water clearance. Upward departure from the normal of 300 ± 10 mOsm/L is referred to as hypertonicity and is associated, in normal renal function, with a urine of increased osmolality and negative free water clearance.

Sodium Homeostasis

By the law of electroneutrality, the sum of cations (e.g., sodium and potassium) is balanced by an equal charge of anions in the plasma, chiefly chloride and bicarbonate. The sum of electrolytes present determines the normal water-holding property of the body, and for the extracellular fluid, the predominant and determining ion is sodium. It is, therefore, also water-volume determining. The sodium concentration is regulated by water clearance, aldosterone secretion, and reciprocal relationship with the plasma potassium concentration. Abnormalities in function of the adrenal glands, the pituitary, the central nervous system, and the kidneys may rob the body of its normal tendency to conserve water and/or sodium and maintain a normal sodium mass and concentration. In hypertension, heart disease, and chronic vascular disease, body sodium is chronically elevated owing to a distortion in the balance of sodium homeostatic regulators.

Volume Regulation

By a variety of subtle mechanisms, the body perceives the total volume of certain fluid components. When blood volume is expanded, diuresis ensues; when the blood volume is low, there is conservation of fluid and salt and an increased rate of synthesis of albumin. The total volume of extracellular fluid is closely guarded by the body, involving sensing mechanisms in the heart, mediastinum, great vessels, renal juxtaglomerular apparatus, and macula densa. Overfilling of the "capacitance-sensitive sensors" produces a water diuresis and a salt diuresis, while volume underfilling, often indicated by the decreased chamber pressures (i.e., lowered central venous pressure, diastolic pressure of the two ventricles, and a low mean pulmonary artery pressure) is associated with water and salt conservation. The term *chamber pressures* will be used throughout this chapter to indicate either left atrial pressure, pulmonary wedge pressure, pulmonary artery diastolic pressure, right ventricular and diastolic pressure, or central venous pressure. These pressures are all related and are measured by various methods. With a few very special exceptions pertaining to localized vascular disease in the lung, the pressures are all interrelated, especially in disorders of body fluid volume regulation.

When these volume sensing mechanisms are disordered or chronically stressed, as in chronic congestive heart failure, the body metabolism of water and salt is markedly altered, and the normal responses are no longer reliable, but blunted or totally distorted. The perception of this loss of normal feedback loop autoregulation is a vital element in rational treatment.

Acid Base Regulation

Cellular processes always result in the accumulation of acid wastes; stress, trauma, and the endocrinology of injury paradoxically favor the development of mild alkalosis. Balance between renal excretion of inorganic acids and protons, and the pulmonary excretion of CO_2 are responsible for normal acid base regulation. When either of these mechanisms is diseased, acid base regulation is lost, even though no external stress is introduced into the system.

In summary, then, disorders of body fluid and electrolyte may bear one of three relationships to the homeostatic regulators that would ordinarily compensate:

1. Feedback regulators *normal*:the body assists the therapist in restoration to normal.
2. Feedback regulators *abnormal*: the body fails to sense or to activate homeostatic responses.
3. Feedback regulators *at fault*: the disorder is due, per se, to an abnormality in the regulatory mechanism.

In the description of each syndrome, identification of normal and abnormal homeostatic responses will be included.

Tables 10-1 through 10-4 list helpful terms that are used in some of the mathematical expressions and derivations for the syndromes, as well as normal values and some conversion data for pH readings.

Table 10-1. *Useful Expressions and First Approximations*

Terms	
BV	Blood volume
PV	Plasma volume
RV	Red cell volume
LVH	Large vessel hematocrit
BWt	Body weight
Δ BWt	Change in body weight
TBW	Total body water
TBCl	Total body chloride
Total cation	Total "active" cation (i.e., exchangeable sodium + potassium)
Cation per kg	Total cation divided by body weight
ECF	Extracellular fluid
IF	Interstitial fluid
IF/PV	Ratio of interstitial fluid to plasma volume
ECF/PV	Ratio of extracellular fluid to plasma volume
Notations	
Subscript 1	Starting or normal value for term shown (e.g., LVH_1)
Subscript 2	Value observed during disease prior to treatment (e.g., PV_2)
Subscript 3	Value observed later on, or after treatment (e.g., PV_3)
Subscript def	Deficit of the term shown (e.g., PV_{def})
Subscript exc	Excess of the term shown (e.g., TBW_{exc})
(Delta) Δ	Change in the term shown (e.g., ΔPCO_2)
Subscript $(\ )_p$	Plasma concentration
Subscript $(\ )_u$	Urine concentration

Table 10-1 (Continued)

Blood Volume by Habitus in Health

Habitus	% BWt Males	% BWt Females
Normal	7.0	6.5
Obese	6.0	5.5
Thin	6.5	6.0
Muscular	7.5	7.0

LVH at Sea Level
  Males: 40–43% cells (0.40–0.43)
  Females: 38–41% cells (0.38–0.41)

Total Body Water by Habitus in Health

Habitus	% BWt Males	% BWt Females
Normal	55	48
Obese	48	40
Thin	50	44
Muscular	58	50

Cation per kg by Habitus in Health

Habitus	mEq/kg Males	mEq/kg Females
Normal	90	78
Obese	78	65
Thin	82	72
Muscular	95	82

Extracellular Fluid by Habitus in Health (Males: 42% of TBW; Females: 43% of TBW)

Habitus	% BWt Males	% BWt Females
Normal	0.23	0.21
Obese	0.21	0.17
Thin	0.22	0.20
Muscular	0.24	0.22

Extracellular Fluid Relationships

$$\text{ECF} = \text{Sum of plasma volume (PV)} + \text{interstitial fluid (IF)}$$

$$\text{ECF/PV} = 6.0 \pm 0.5$$

$$\frac{\text{IF}}{\text{PV}} = 5.0 \pm 0.4$$

$$\text{PV} = \text{BV} - (\text{LVH} \times \text{BV})$$

Table 10-2. *Equations for Compositional Relationships*

Blood Volume	Example (Normal 65 kg Male)
$BV = (\% \text{ BWt}) \times \text{BWt}$	$BV = 0.7 \times 6.5 = 4550$ ml
$LVH = 0.40 = \frac{BV}{RV}$	$LVH = \frac{1820}{4550} = 0.40$
$RV = BV \times LVH$	$RV = 4550 \times 0.4 = 1820$ ml
$PV = BV - (BV \times LVH)$	$PV = 4550 - 1820 = 2730$ ml
$BV = RV + PV$	$BV = 1820 + 2730 = 4550$ ml

Total Body Water and Total Cation	Example (Obese 60 kg Female)
$TBW = \frac{\text{BWt} \times \text{cation per kg}}{[(Na)_p + (K)_p + 15]}$	$\frac{60 \times 65}{163} = \frac{3900}{163} = 23.9$ L
$\text{TBW as \% BWt} = \frac{TBW}{BWt} \times 100$	$\frac{23.9}{60} \times 100 = 39.8\%$

Total cation = BWt × cation per kg = 60 × 65 = 3900 mEq

$$\text{Cation per kg} = \frac{[(Na)_p + (K)_p + 15] \times TBW}{BWt} = \frac{163 \times 23.9}{60} = 65 \text{ mEq/kg}$$

$$\text{Cation per kg} = \frac{163 \times (\text{TBW as \% BWt})}{100} = \frac{163 \times 29.8}{100} = 65 \text{ mEq/kg}$$

Total Body Chloride	Example (Muscular 80 kg Male)
$TBCl = BWt \times ECF/kg \times (Cl)_p$	$80 \times 0.24 \times 103 = 1978$ mEq

Cation ratio (Na_e/K_e where subscript "e" = total active or exchangeable ion)

Normal habitus male: $Na_e/K_e = \frac{40 \text{ mEq/kg}}{50 \text{ mEq/kg}} = 0.80$

Normal habitus female: $Na_e/K_e = \frac{39 \text{ mEq/kg}}{39 \text{ mEq/kg}} = 1.00$

Plasma Tonicity

Total tonicity = Electrolyte tonicity + Crystalloid tonicity

Electrolyte tonicity = $(Na)_p + (K)_p \times 2 = (143 + 5) \times 2 = 296$ mOsm/L

Crystalloid tonicity = glucose + urea = 5.0 + 0.5 = 5.5 mOsm/L

Total tonicity = 296 + 5.5 = 301.5 ± 5.0 mOsm/L

Crystalloid Tonicity

Glucose (mg/dl) ÷ 18 = glucose (mOsm/L)

Urea (mg/dl) ÷ 2 = urea N (mg dl)

Urea N (mg/dl) ÷ 30 = urea (mOsm/L)

"Unaccounted" Tonicity

"Unaccounted" tonicity = Total tonicity − (electrolyte tonicity) − (glucose + urea tonicity)

Table 10-3. *Useful Expressions and First Approximations in Acid-Base Homeostasis*

Conversion of pH to (H^+) in nM/L

pH (H^+)	pH (H^+)	pH (H^+)	ph (H^+)
7.10 = 79	7.32 = 49	7.38 = 42	7.44 = 37
7.15 = 71	7.34 = 48	7.39 = 41	7.46 = 36
7.20 = 63	7.35 = 46	**[7.40 = 40]**	7.48 = 34
7.25 = 58	7.36 = 44	7.41 = 39	7.50 = 32
7.30 = 50	7.37 = 43	7.42 = 38	7.60 = 25

Bedside Acid-Base Equation to Check Lab Work

$$(H^+) = \frac{24 \times PCO_2}{HCO_3} = \frac{24 \times 40}{24} = 40 \text{ nM/L} = \text{pH } 7.40$$

Quickie Conversions to Check Lab Work

Pure resp. acidosis: $\Delta(H^+) = 0.8\ \Delta PCO_2$
Comp resp. acidosis: $\Delta(H^+) = 0.3\ \Delta PCO_2$
Acute resp. alkalosis: $\Delta(H^+) = 0.8\ \Delta PCO_2$
Metabolic acidosis (addition): $PCO_2 = 1.1\ \Delta HCO_3^-$

Anion Gap

Anion gap = $(Na)_p - (Cl)_p = 143 - 103 = 40$ mEq/L

Anion gap ÷ 1.6 = predicted std. bicarb; $\frac{40}{1.6} = 25$ mEq/L

"Unaccounted" Anion

"Unaccounted" anion = $\left[\frac{\text{anion gap}}{1.6}\right]$ − std. bicarb.

Example: $(Na)_p = 145$ mEq/L; $(Cl)_p = 90$ mEq/L; std. bicarb. = 15 mEq/L

Then, $\frac{55}{1.6} - 15 = 19$ mEq/L "unaccounted" anion (Ketones? Lactate? Inorganic acids?)

Table 10-4. *Normal Values*

Datum	Units	Normal	Comments
Body weight	kg change		Reliable weight very difficult to measure in critically ill
Hematocrit	% cells	Males 40–43 Females 38–41	Spun large vessel venous hematocrit; centrifuge to constant meniscus
Plasma			
Protein	gm/dl	6.0–6.5	Marked method variance between hospitals
Tonicity	mOsm/L	290–300	Freezing point methods yield osmolality, not osmolarity
Nonelectrolyte tonicity	mOsm/L	5–10	See Table 10-2
Sodium	mEq/L	141–144	May be measured on either plasma or serum
Chloride	mEq/L	101–104	May be measured on either plasma or serum
Potassium	mEq/L	4.2–4.6	May be measured on either plasma or serum
Whole Blood			
Std. bicarbonate	mEq/L	24–27	CO_2 content of whole blood corrected to standard conditions
Urea N	mg/dl	10–18	
Blood pH_{art}	units	7.41–7.42	Must be measured on fresh chilled arterial blood
pH_{ven}	units	7.35–7.38	Varies somewhat with sampling site
$PCO_{2\ art}$	mm Hg	40	
$PCO_{2\ ven}$	mm Hg	43	Depends on sampling site
$PaO_{2\ art}$	mm Hg	70–90	Depends on inhaled gas mixture and shunting
$PVO_{2\ ven}$	mm Hg	30–50	Depends on sampling site
Urine			
Tonicity	mOsm/L	200–1400	Normal widest range of tonicity in man
		300–400	Characteristic tonicity in renal failure
Sodium	mEq/L	0.1–75	The low value shows good tubular function
Potassium	mEq/L	10–100	High potassium values accompany aldosterone effects and metabolic alkalosis (require good tubular function)
pH	units	4.5–6.5	Urine acidification below pH 5.5 not seen in renal failure
Volume	ml/hr	25–100	3 consecutive hours below 15 or over 150 requires explanation

Table 10-5. *Hypovolemia (Syndrome 1)*

		Major Findings	
	Unit	Typical	Extreme
Hematocrit	% cells	40 → 30	40 → 15
Plasma protein	gm/dl	6.5 → 6.0	6.5 → 5.0
Blood urea nitrogen	mg/dl	Normal	15 → 30
Blood volume	% BWt	7.0 → 6.0	7.0 → 4.0
Central venous pressure	cm H_2O	12 → 5	12 → 0

FIFTEEN DISORDERS OF BODY WATER, SALTS, AND PROTEIN; FLUID VOLUMES AND TONICITY

Syndrome 1. Hypovolemia (Table 10-5)

DEFINITION, TERMINOLOGY, AND RELATED TERMS

Hypovolemia is a blood volume that is lower than normal, without reference to hematocrit. Related or confusing terms include *oligemia* (synonymous), *hypotension* (refers to a low blood pressure without respect to cause), *shock* (a clinical picture), *low flow state* (generalized hypoprofusion without respect to cause), and *anemia* (usually used as meaning a low peripheral concentration of red blood cells).

The hematocrit, or fractional volume of cells in a blood sample centrifuged to constant meniscus, is a measure of the peripheral concentration of erythrocytes. It is used throughout this account, although the hemoglobin concentration and red cell count are linear functions, save in the presence of disordered red cell synthesis. The *large vessel hematocrit* is the hematocrit as measured on a sample of blood taken from a major vessel, usually a large vein of the arm. The *whole body hematocrit* is a conceptual term, to mean the ratio of the entire red blood cell volume to the entire blood volume (i.e., sum of measured PV + RV). Because of axial streaming of red cells in small blood vessels and capillaries, the whole body hematocrit is somewhat lower (0.85×–0.92×) than the large vessel hematocrit. Relationships between the two indicated by the WBH/LVH ratio are interesting and important in some very severe disorders of blood volume (late shock, severe polycythemia), but they do not appear in everyday blood volume measurement and therapy.

CLINICAL SETTING

1. Whole blood loss
2. Plasma loss
3. Desalting water loss
4. Desiccation, dehydration

The symptoms are weakness and faintness, particularly on assuming the erect posture. These mild symptoms progress to those of a severe low flow state, with hypotension, oliguria, and dangerous hypoperfusion of critical organs (brain, heart, and lungs) if the volume loss is severe and continuing.

ADDITION OR SUBTRACTION

Hypovolemia is always a subtraction disorder.

BODY COMPOSITION AND BODY WEIGHT

The normal blood volume is about 7 percent of body weight in males and 6.5 percent of body weight in females. The term *hypovolemia* refers to a blood volume approximately 1.0 percent of body weight lower than normal, approximately 10 to 15 percent reduced. In the chronic form, plasma volume gradually rises, owing to transcapillary refill, resulting in a "stabilized posthemorrhagic anemia" with a red cell volume lower than normal, plasma volume restored to values higher than normal, normal blood volume, and low hematocrit. Red cell synthesis is much slower.

Abnormalities of Autoregulation

The normal homeostatic regulation of blood volume in hypovolemia is by the inflow of interstitial fluid at the distal end of the capillary, occasioned by lowered venous pressure at the venular end of the capillary. Simple hydrostatic filling, resulting in an increase in the plasma volume, is the normal transcapillary refill of the blood volume. This results in the restoration of the blood volume to, or near, normal by the influx of a plasma-like fluid (interstitial fluid and lymph) with a low protein concentration. At the close of this period of refill there is a low red cell mass, a plasma volume much higher than normal, a blood volume close to or near normal (with the exceptions indicated), and a slightly low protein concentration. There is a low hematocrit.

An additional homeostatic regulator in hypovolemia is the secretion of antidiuretic hormone (stimulated by a volume receptor mechanism) and of aldosterone (stimulated by the juxtaglomerulus-renin-angiotensin-adrenal cortex effector arc). The firing off of these two homeostatic regulators after simple hemorrhage is a classic example of isotonic volume reduction as a stimulator of endocrine change. The result of this combination of hormone effectors is to save water and salt for the body so that the transcapillary refill may arise from an interstitial fluid of normal volume and tonicity. The principal abnormalities of this regulator, whose normal function is to conserve interstitial volume for transcapillary refill, occur in (1) *renal* disease, in which the response is abnormal or absent, (2) *adrenal cortical* disease, in which the aldosterone mechanism fails, (3) *central nervous system* disease, in which antidiuretic hormone production is abnormal, and (4) *low flow state,* wherein the loss has been more massive than these regulators can compensate and circulatory anoxia becomes a governing deterioration.

Treatment

The ideal infusion fluid for hypovolemia is fully compatible normal fresh human blood. However, if blood transfusion is to be less than 1,000 ml, one should exercise restraint in the use of bloodbank blood with its attendant problems. Hepatitis-virus-free plasma or one of its derivatives, or isotonic salt solutions free of both protein and cells, can be used. If a protein-free, cell-free electrolyte solution is used, approximately three times the volume of blood lost must be replaced to allow for equilibration throughout the extracellular volume.

Guides to Progress

Restoration of urine volume to normal is the most reliable sign of restoration of blood volume and tissue perfusion to normal. If hypotension has resulted from acute hypovolemia, the restoration of normal systolic blood pressure is an important sign, often confused by the administration of drugs. There are other, more subtle signs of volume restoration, such as the cessation of the transcapillary refill. If blood volume is restored by the use of cell-free solutions, the fall in the hematocrit is even more pronounced; this anemia is due to an expanded plasma volume and persists until red cell resynthesis restores the red cell volume to normal. The primary cellular signs of hypovolemia are to be seen in the kidney; if low flow is severe, all body cells suffer, finally the brain. Almost any index of cellular function demonstrates improvement when severe hypovolemia is returned toward normal. In elderly people, or those with cerebrovascular diseases, abnormalities of mental function and of the electrocardiogram indicate cerebral and myocardial responses to the hypoperfusion, and later to the restoration of normal blood volume and tissue perfusion.

One of the chamber pressures, such as central venous pressure, right atrial pressure, pulmonary artery pressure, pulmonary artery wedge pressure, or left atrial pressure, may profitably be measured in monitoring a patient who has suffered hypovolemia or hypervolemia from any cause. These pressures all tend to be lower than normal in hypovolemia; since the pressures are normally quite low, the initial reading is not as significant as the increase toward normal on restoration of volume to normal.

There is a further important precaution about blood transfusion in late hypovolemia when transcapillary refill has been complete. If at that point the volume of lost blood is transfused, acute hypervolemia will be produced. In the elderly patient or those with congestive heart failure this can be dangerous. Such an error results from a misreading of the low hematocrit in a stabilized post hemorrhagic patient: the low hematocrit indicates a high plasma volume, not a low blood volume.

Relevant Mathematical Expression

Mathematical expressions serve only as a guide to the appropriate general magnitude of treatment.

In Syndrome 1, *Hypovolemia,* the Red Cell Volume deficit after stabilization of transcapillary refill in a chronic bleed is given by:

$$RV_{def} = RV_1 - RV_2$$

BV_1 and RV_1 from Table 10-1

$$RV_2 = LVH_2 \times 0.9\ BV_1$$

This assumes refill to 90 percent of normal BV. For complete refill (bleed has stopped; hematocrit stable):

$$RV_2 = LVH_2 \times BV_1$$

Example: Obese woman, 50 kg, menorrhagia, continuing; hematocrit 18.

$$RV_2 = 0.18 \times 0.9\ (0.055 \times 50) = 445 \text{ ml}$$

$$RV_1 = (0.4 \times 0.055 \times 50) = 1{,}100 \text{ ml}$$

$$RV_{def} = 1{,}100 - 445 = 655 \text{ ml red cells}$$

$$RV_{def} = \text{about 3 units of cells}$$

This will restore deficit of oxygen transport capacity, but makes no allowance for further bleeding.

Syndrome 2. Plasma Loss Hypovolemia (Table 10-6)

Definition, Terminology, and Related Terms

Plasma loss hypovolemia refers to a lowering of the blood volume, owing to the loss of plasma or a plasma-like transudate. In this condition the plasma loss so predominates that the loss of red cells is trivial or negligible. A rising hematocrit is therefore inevitable. Plasma loss hypovolemia may progress to hypotension in a severe low flow state, resulting in death. The elevated hematocrit produces an increase in blood viscosity, which further slows tissue perfusion. Related terms include "third space effect," a term coined to signify the accumulation of plasma-like fluid in an area of traumatic edema. The same thing can be observed in peritonitis or in venous thrombosis.

Clinical Setting

1. Thermal burn
2. Acute peritonitis
3. Acute pancreatitis
4. Retroperitoneal edema
5. Mesenteric venous thrombosis
6. Portal thrombosis
7. Peripheral venous obstruction
8. Large surgical dissections

Addition or Subtraction

This is always a subtraction disorder, as fluid is moved out of the circulation into a peripheral injured or edematous area; nonetheless, if treat-

Table 10-6. *Plasma Loss Hypovolemia (Syndrome 2)*

		Major Findings	
	Unit	Typical	Extreme
Hematocrit	% cells	50 → 55	60 → 70
Plasma protein	gm/dl	6.5 → 6.0	6.5 → 5.0
Blood urea nitrogen	mg/dl	Normal	15 → 30
Blood volume	% BWt	7.0 → 6.0	7.0 → 4.0
Central venous pressure	cm H_2O	12 → 5	12 → 0

ment is instituted to restore the plasma volume to normal, the body gains weight. The increment of total body water and salt produced by treatment renders the net effect that of an addition disorder superimposed on an initial loss of plasma volume.

Body Composition and Body Weight

The normal plasma volume is approximately 4 percent of body weight in men and 3.6 percent of body weight in women. Loss of approximately one liter of plasma produces the typical rapidly rising concentration of erythrocytes as measured by hematocrit, red cell count, or hemoglobin concentration. Lesser amounts of plasma loss produce the same change, but it is less readily evident. If the plasma is lost within the body, weight is unchanged thereby. Since therapy consists of infusion of plasma and other fluids into the bloodstream in order to maintain an effective plasma volume, the situation in treated plasma-losing hypovolemia is one of a rapid gain in weight. From this gain of weight or from the high hematocrit, knowing the patient's starting body weight and predicted normal red cell volume, it is possible to calculate rather accurately either the amount of plasma required or the net water increment from treatment.

Abnormalities of Autoregulation

The body has no endogenous corrective mechanism for a severe generalized plasma-losing state, since the transcapillary refill of the plasma that would ordinarily compensate for hypovolemia is, by the very nature of the pathologic state, impaired or reversed. If the plasma loss occurs in one focal area (a small burn would be an example), transcapillary refill may occur from other undamaged areas of the capillary bed. This is the "parasite" effect of a burn.

The homeostatic regulators readily observed are those of the renal response to hypovolemia: antidiuresis and sodium conservation, with a low urine volume and very low sodium concentration. Some of the lowest urine sodium concentrations—as low as 0.1 mEq/L—are observed in plasma-losing states. The principal abnormality of this renal sodium and water conservation is seen in the diuretic phase of acute nephrosis or in renal or adrenal disease, in which a normal water-sodium conserving renal response cannot occur.

Laboratory Findings

A rising concentration of red cells in the plasma, usually measured as a rising hematocrit, is the most characteristic finding in plasma-losing states. The magnitude of elevation of the hematocrit is a linear function of the volume of plasma lost. It is therefore possible to formulate a simple mathematical expression to indicate the static deficit, i.e., the amount of plasma that must be infused over a short time to restore blood volume to normal. To this amount of rapid infusion must be added the amounts needed to compensate for concomitant losses. Urinary findings have been mentioned previously.

Chamber pressures are reduced, as in any other form of hypovolemia; their rise toward normal is a significant monitor of treatment. Their rise above normal is a sign of overtreatment.

TREATMENT

Infusion of plasma, various plasma fractions, albumin, and dextran are all effective. In plasma loss the infusion of ionic solutions without protein (for example, saline or Ringer's lactate) lowers the hematocrit and refills the plasma volume if rather large amounts are used, approximately three times the amount of plasma that has been lost. In such a case there is considerable dilution of plasma protein. A few days later, after diuresis of this water and salt, the plasma protein concentration usually returns to normal.

GUIDES TO PROGRESS

As is evident from the foregoing discussion, acute changes in the concentration of red cells (usually measured by hematocrit) are the most sensitive and direct guides to progress, with appropriate changes in renal function and in tissue perfusion. In most acute plasma-losing states—such as burns, pancreatitis, and peritonitis—the pathologic condition itself is limited by treatment or becomes self-limited; the only alternative is death if the loss continues unabated. Severe loss of body water of any variety can produce plasma loss secondarily, for example those described under Syndrome 6, Desalting Water Loss.

RELEVANT MATHEMATICAL EXPRESSION

In Syndrome 2, *Plasma Loss Hypovolemia,* the Plasma Volume Deficit is given by:

$PV_{def} = BV_1 - BV_2$ (assuming RV constant)

PV_1, RV_1, and BV_1 from Table 10-1

$$BV_2 = \frac{RV_1}{LVH_2}$$

Example: Muscular man, 80 kg, burn, hematocrit 65

$$BV_1 = 0.075 \times 80 = 6{,}000 \text{ ml}$$

$$RV_1 = 0.43 \times 6{,}000 = 2{,}580 \text{ ml}$$

$$BV_2 = \frac{2{,}580}{0.65} = 3{,}970$$

Then: $PV_{def} = 6{,}000 - 3{,}970 \text{ ml} = 2{,}030 \text{ ml}$

If plasma alone is used (or similar substitute), about 2,000 ml or 8 units will bring the hematocrit down to 40 to 45. If balanced salt is used, about 8,000 ml will be needed for the PV requirement alone; neither ration is in any sense a complete burn budget for skin, respiratory, and urinary losses. This is for the plasma volume deficit alone; continuing losses must be compensated.

Syndrome 3. Hypoproteinemia

DEFINITION, TERMINOLOGY, AND RELATED TERMS

Hypoproteinemia is a low concentration of proteins in the plasma, without reference to the volume of blood plasma, interstitial fluid, or total body water; it connotes a low colloid osmotic pressure. *Hypoalbuminemia* is essentially synonymous. *Lowered plasma oncotic* (or *colloid osmotic*) *pressure* is essentially synonymous. *Dilutional hypoproteinemia* refers to one of the common causes of hypoproteinemia.

CLINICAL SETTING

1. Overadministration of water and salt
2. Loss of whole protein from the body
3. Liver cell disease with failure of protein synthesis
4. Late starvation especially with overadministration of salt and/or water

ADDITION OR SUBTRACTION

Hypoproteinemia is due to addition of water and salt, masquerading as a subtraction syndrome (lack of albumin) in most cases. Only in advanced liver disease is the net albumin synthesis deficit the primary difficulty. In other instances some plasma or albumin loss has been overbalanced by water and salt administration and/or retention.

Body Composition and Body Weight

Because of the exogenous dilutional component in most cases of hypoproteinemia, body weight gain is a regular feature. As colloid osmotic pressure falls, edema readily forms in subcutaneous tissues and as ascites and hydrothorax. Body weight gain is therefore sometimes its most prominent feature. Diuretic treatment often results in a subsequent weight loss, with restoration of serum protein to normal.

Approximately one-half of the albumin in the body is outside the plasma volume, circulating in the much larger interstitial fluid volume (including lymph), but at a low concentration. Certain stimuli produce an increased flow of albumin up the thoracic duct from the liver to the great veins of the mediastinum, a sort of internal plasma infusion. One of the stimuli to this albumin influx is hemorrhage.

Abnormalities of Autoregulation

As mentioned, normal urinary excretion of water and salt and normal hepatic synthesis of albumin are the normal homeostatic regulators. Anything interfering with either tends to produce hypoproteinemia.

Serum albumin concentration is measured by a great many different methods, and one must know the hospital norms to ascertain the degree of abnormality. If the laboratory norm is a serum albumin concentration of 5 gm/day, values below 3.5 constitute significant hypoalbuminemia or hypoproteinemia. In the hypoalbuminemia of liver disease, there is characteristically an excess of globulins, both relative and absolute, with a reversal of the normal albumin/globulin ratio.

Treatment

Because the syndrome is often dilutional in part, the use of diuretics that increase the excretion of water and salt is sometimes effective. The administration either of concentrated human albumin or of plasma in a hepatitis-free form is rational. Concentrated salt-poor albumin should be reserved for patients in whom additional salt loads will embarrass cardiac function.

Guides to Progress

Rise of serum protein and albumin concentrations to normal are cardinal signs, with diuresis and weight loss where dilution has been prominent.

Syndrome 4. Hypervolemia (Table 10-7)

Definition, Terminology, and Related Terms

Hypervolemia is a blood volume larger than normal, without reference to the hematocrit. The term *plethora* has been used to indicate a high blood volume, but it connotes any elevated concentration of red cells. *Polycythemia* denotes a hematocrit that is higher than normal. Polycythemia and plethora often coexist with hypervolemia. Terms such as *congestive heart failure* should not be used interchangeably with *hypervolemia,* even though the two may coexist and chamber pressure elevation may develop in both.

Clinical Setting

1. Overinfusion of blood or other parenteral fluids
2. Chronic visceral failure (heart, kidneys, or lungs)

Addition or Subtraction

Hypervolemia is always an addition disorder; the source may be endogenous (as in visceral failure with ordinary oral intake) or exogenous, arising from infusions.

Table 10-7. *Hypervolemia (Overtransfusion) (Syndrome 4)*

		Major Findings	
	Unit	Typical	Extreme
Hematocrit	% cells	40 → 50	40 → 65
Protein	gm/dl	6.5 → 6.8	6.5 → 7.5
Blood volume	% BWt	7.0 → 8.0	7.0 → 10.0

Body Composition and Body Weight

The term *hypervolemia* denotes a blood volume that is more than 15 percent elevated. That is, it is elevated approximately 1.0 percent of body weight, or more. Body weight is usually elevated by an appropriate amount; if chronic visceral failure (heart, liver, lungs, kidneys) plays a role, the extent of weight elevation may be quite remarkable as all body water is expanded.

Abnormalities of Autoregulation

If produced acutely by overtransfusion of blood, hypervolemia results in a prompt plasma dispersal and disposal. This is the exact physiologic reverse of the transcapillary refill observed in hypovolemia. Plasma dispersal and disposal is effected by the selective loss of plasma by ultrafiltration from the capillary, the degradation of excess protein through its normal half-life, with the excretion of the extra water and salt. The result is a slowly rising plasma protein that then returns to normal, a rising hematocrit that remains high, appropriate to the half-life of the healthy red cells infused, as they live out their span. The abnormalities of these homeostatic regulators clearly reside in disease of those viscera concerned with plasma dispersal and disposal: the heart, the liver, and the kidneys. All are essential for the metabolism of excessive blood volume; when they are abnormal, plasma dispersal and disposal are impaired. When there is acute or chronic pulmonary disease or direct injury to the lungs, modest degrees of hypervolemia are much more likely to produce pulmonary edema.

In its acute phase the major *laboratory finding* is elevation of cardiac chamber pressures. Then, as plasma dispersal and disposal proceed, there is a rising concentration of red cells and protein. Of greatest significance are the laboratory findings relative to visceral function. If liver failure is present, hypervolemia is ill-tolerated. In the presence of oliguric renal failure, the renal mechanism for disposal is cut off and hypervolemia is dangerous. In heart failure, even modest degrees of exogenous hypervolemia added to the endogenous overexpansion of body water and salt rapidly produce pulmonary edema. If pulmonary function is embarrassed (particularly likely in primary pulmonary disease as in burns or crush, or chronic congestive heart failure), failing oxygenation and/or carbon dioxide accumulation are laboratory evidence of an uncorrected hypervolemia. Measurements of function of heart, lungs, liver, and kidneys are therefore essential in the management of hypervolemia.

Treatment

When hypervolemia results from overenthusiastic infusion of blood or other fluids, a most important step is often somewhat difficult: stop those infusions! Phlebotomy or direct bleeding is an effective emergency measure. The application of limb tourniquets is, at best, a weak substitute for phlebotomy. When renal failure also exists, hypervolemia (associated with a high volume of intracellular fluid and body water) can be managed, though with difficulty, by pressure filtration dialysis.

Guides to Progress

In most instances of hypervolemia, a reduction of chamber pressures to normal is the primary indicator of a response to treatment. Renal functional changes are an inconstant guide to progress. The chest x-ray film may be valuable if pulmonary edema has been a feature. Phlebotomy and diuretics have very different effects on volume, since diuretics act on all components of body water, particularly the extracellular phase, whereas bleeding operates initially on blood volume alone and, in the presence of chronic disease of liver, kidney, or heart, may be followed by transcapillary refill that is "inappropriate," as if the body intended to maintain a high volume. In some cases the body has become so "accustomed" to a high blood volume that some degree of hypotension and hypoperfusion may be observed if volume is restored to normal. For this reason, phlebotomy and/or diuretics must always be accompanied by careful measure of perfusion of organs, particularly brain and kidneys. Most cases of overtransfusion result from the sudden infusion of large amounts of blood bank blood to meet an unexpected emergency; in banked blood, the red blood cells are frequently approaching their expiration date, and hemolysis may be very prominent. In such a case, the hemolytic component adds greatly to the elevation of bilirubin that so frequently appears in low flow states.

Syndrome 5. Polycythemia (Table 10-8)

Definition, Terminology, and Related Terms

The term *polycythemia* should be reserved for those states in which there is elevation in hematocrit, regardless of the blood volume; just as *anemia* signifies a low hematocrit without reference to volume. The term *hypervolemia* is not strictly synonymous, because the hematocrit may not be elevated, at least in the early stages. The term *polycythemia vera* denotes an excessive volume of red cells associated with primary disease of the bone marrow. *Secondary polycythemia* denotes the compensatory elevation of red cell mass that occurs in response to a deficit of oxygen transport capacity. "Oxygen transport capacity" (OTC) is a product of cardiac output times effective oxygen carrying capacity, including total hemoglobin, the state of the hemoglobin, and location of the oxyhemoglobin association curve. Barring unusual variations in hemoglobin chemistry, it is a simple product of cardiac output times whole blood oxygen-carrying capacity. A term little used in the conventional cardiac or cardiovascular literature, it is of great importance in the management of acutely ill or injured patients.

Clinical Setting

The idiopathic form of polycythemia vera will not be discussed further. With a hematocrit over 55, there is a severe viscosity increase, threatening thrombosis of the mesenteric circulation, the brain, or the limbs.

Secondary polycythemia occurs most commonly in response to congenital heart disease and chronic obstructive pulmonary disease. The former, by left-to-right shunting, deprives the periphery of oxygenated red cells. The latter interferes with oxygenation by loss of ventilation. In both cases there is a reduction in OTC modified in turn by the ability of the hemoglobin present to unload oxygen in the tissues. The symptoms of polycythemia are initially those of the underlying disease, the polycythemic component responsible for the cyanotic appearance, increased blood viscosity, and susceptibility to thrombosis.

Addition or Subtraction

This is an addition disorder due to overproduction of erythrocytes by the marrow, in response to a deficit in OTC.

Table 10-8. *Polycythemia (Secondary) (Syndrome 5)*

		Major Findings	
	Unit	Typical	Extreme
Hematocrit	% cells	55	80
Protein	gm/dl	6.5	7.0
Uric acid	mg/dl	8.5	10.0
Blood volume	% BWt	7.5	12.0
Plasma volume	% BWt	2.0	1.0
Red cell volume	% BWt	5.5	11.0
Arterial oxygen saturation	% sat.	90	75
Reticulocytes	%	5.0	15.0
Central venous pressure	cm H_2O	5–10	20–30

Body Composition and Body Weight

In mild polycythemia due to chronic obstructive lung disease, the blood volume is normal. In the more severe forms of the disorder, due either to heart or lung disease, the blood volume is elevated. In congenital heart disease (such as tetralogy of Fallot), the blood volume may be as high as 12 percent of body weight, with a hematocrit of 75 to 80 percent. Uric acid concentrations in plasma tend to be elevated in the presence of any sort of polycythemia, probably a manifestation of an increased turnover rate of red cells. In hyperparathyroidism there is a low plasma phosphate concentration; for this reason, there is a very low value for red cell diphosphoglycerate (2,3-DPG). This produces a left shift of the oxyhemoglobin association curve with a resultant slight but very chronic anoxia of perishable tissues, including bone marrow. This, in turn, leads to reticular cytosis and a high red cell production rate. The combination of hyperparathyroidism, polycythemia, and hyperuricemia is, therefore, a rare but interesting syndrome, demonstrating some of these interrelationships.

Abnormalities of Autoregulation

As volume rises with polycythemia, plasma disposal and dispersal are hastened. The plasma volume is therefore low. In extreme cases, with hematocrits as high as 75 percent and blood volume as high as 10 to 12 percent of body weight (in congenital heart disease), the plasma volume is diminished to become a small component of the total blood volume. This dispersal of plasma is merely a chronic homeostatic response to the excessive volume of red cells. This increases viscosity and further reduces tissue perfusion. Under ordinary circumstances, an excess of total oxygen transport capacity (red cell concentration multiplied by cardiac output) results in bone marrow inhibition. This is frequently observed following surgical repair of congenital heart disease. There will be a gradual downward restitution of red cell volume to normal by inhibition of marrow erythropoiesis, as cardiac output is restored. In polycythemia secondary to chronic obstructive disease, the chronic desaturation constitutes a continuous stimulus to the marrow, and most treatment (other than the fringe benefits from decreased smoking, for example) is unavailing. In cases of chronically depressed inorganic phosphate concentration in the plasma (in hyperparathyroidism and in certain types of hyperalimentation), a left-shifted oxyhemoglobin dissociation curve may be severe enough to constitute a stimulus to increased erythropoiesis, with resultant polycythemia.

Table 10-9. *Desalting Water Loss (Syndrome 6)*

		Major Findings	
	Unit	Typical	Extreme
Body weight	Change	Fall 1–5 kg	Fall 4–7 kg
Hematocrit	% cells	40 → 45	45 → 55
Protein	gm/dl	6.5 → 6.8	6.5 → 8.0
Plasma tonicity	mOsm/L	295 → 270	295 → 250
Plasma sodium	mEq/L	143 → 125	143 → 115
Plasma chloride	mEq/L	103 → 95	103 → 80
Plasma potassium	mEq/L	4.2 → 4.5	4.2 → 6.5
Std. bicarbonate	mEq/L	24 → 20	24 → 15
Blood pH		7.42 → 7.30	7.42 → 7.22

Treatment

It may be advisable to carry out preoperative phlebotomy (with or without replacement of the shed blood with plasma) to carry the patient through operation with a lower hematocrit. In such instances, high oxygen concentration in the airway should be used to compensate for the sudden apparent deficit in OTC. If the basic cause of secondary polycythemia remains uncorrected, the polycythemia with its attendant problems of hypervolemia, blood viscosity, hypercoagulability, chronic desaturation, and cyanosis will remain.

Guides to Progress

These are primarily based on hematocrit and viscosity; in some cases of polycythemia vera the platelets are also elevated, contributing further to the hypercoagulable state.

Syndrome 6. Desalting Water Loss (Table 10-9)

Definition, Terminology, and Related Terms

Desalting water loss is the loss of water and salt from the body at concentrations close to isotonic, regardless of the final concentration of sodium or other salts in the plasma. The term *extracellular fluid deficit* refers to the result. *Third space effect* refers to one of the causes. *Dehydration* is carelessly used to include this syndrome, failing to differentiate it from desiccation-dehydration (see below). *Hyponatremia* and *hypotonicity* refer to a frequent late result of desalting water loss.

Clinical Setting

Extrarenal causes: loss from the gastrointestinal tract as in fistula, obstruction, vomiting, short bowel syndrome, typhoid fever, colitis.

Renal desalting: unregulated diuresis in the diuretic phase of recovering acute tubular necrosis; profound osmotic diuresis in diabetes mellitus.

Addition or Subtraction

In all instances this is a subtraction disorder.

Body Composition and Body Weight

The normal extracellular fluid volume is approximately 20 percent of body weight or 12 to 14 liters in 60- to 70-kg adults. Approximately one liter of volume, or 8 percent of the normal extracellular fluid volume, may be considered as tolerable variation in either direction. Losses of more than this produce the symptomatology referred to here. Extracellular fluid deficit is usually partitioned throughout the extracellular fluid and ultimately throughout total body water; the initial reduction is in the entire extracellular fluid; plasma and interstitial fluid are in hydrostatic and ionic equilibrium. Losses of extracellular fluid are therefore represented to the extent of approximately 25 to 30 percent of the total as plasma volume reduction. The normal ratio of plasma volume to interstitial fluid (PV/IF) is 0.25, and of plasma volume to total extracellular fluid 0.20.

Abnormalities of Autoregulation

Desalting water losses initially produce an isotonic volume reduction, the characteristic renal responses being decreased urine volume with increased urine osmolality and decreased sodium concentration. The principal abnormality of this homeostatic regulator is renal—a failure to implement the feedback loop. In adrenal disease (or in diseases of the central nervous system involving the area above the pituitary), there may be an accentuation of borderline renal insufficiency, or diabetes insipidus, impeding the homeostatic regulation. With impaired homeostatic regulation, the task of replacement becomes much more formidable, and much larger volumes are required.

In response to lower tissue pressure (and aldosterone secretion) sodium-free water enters (and is retained in) the bloodstream, largely from cells; this is a weak compensation toward volume restoration, but at the expense of sodium concentration, which falls. There is an increased excretion of potassium.

Initially with desalting water loss, the principal *laboratory findings* are in the urinary responses already described. In some instances, abnormalities of renal response are noteworthy (with unregulated diuresis or adrenal impairment): anomalous natriuresis indicates this failure of normal homeostasis.

Approximately one-quarter to one-third of the volume lost (depending on rate) may be considered as emanating from the plasma. There is, therefore, a gradual rise in hematocrit, somewhat slower than that seen in loss of plasma alone. Associated changes in blood viscosity are seen when the hematocrit rises above 50 or 55.

Any addition of sodium-free water adds further to the hyponatremia observed in desalting water loss. The ingress of sodium-free water into the extracellular fluid, diluting the sodium concentration, occurs by three principal routes: mobilization of cell water, oxidation of fat, and the administration of salt-free water by vein. The fall in sodium concentration with desalting water loss is thus primarily dilutional, resulting from the addition of sodium-free water to the system. Only in rare circumstances, such as pancreatic fistulas, is sodium lost from the body in actually hypertonic concentrations, leading immediately to hyponatremia.

The circulatory effects of decreased effective extracellular fluid volume are hypovolemia, low cardiac output, oliguria, and a low flow state. These are accentuated by hyponatremia. The low sodium concentration in plasma contributes to decreased cardiovascular responsiveness; if the loss from the gastrointestinal tract is primarily alkaline, severe acidosis results (see below). This combination is particularly unfriendly to normal cardiac function, rendering the heart insensitive to digitalis alkaloids, and in elderly patients, it may prove fatal.

Treatment

The treatment consists of replacement by intravenous infusion of saline liquids. If the disease is long-standing, some protein should be added. If hematocrit is markedly elevated, the early replacement components should be largely plasma,* to rectify the circulatory disorder first. In young people with normal renal function, the use of isotonic sodium chloride solutions is

*This can be whole plasma, or a plasma protein preparation.

acceptable. In elderly people, this results in hyperchloremia, and it is wiser to infuse some sort of a balanced salt solution, such as Ringer's lactate. If sodium concentration is low, a portion of the replacement fluid may consist of hypertonic salt solutions.

Guides to Progress

These consist of restoration of renal function and plasma electrolyte concentrations to normal; reduction of hematocrit; restoration of normal tissue perfusion and of consciousness.

Relevant Mathematical Expression

In Syndrome 6, *Desalting Water Loss,* with rehydration (not including salt administration) back to normal body weight but with severe dilution, the total cation deficit is given by:

$\text{Cation}_{def} = \text{Total cation}_1 - \text{Total cation}_2$

$\text{Total cation}_1 = \text{BWt} \times (\text{cat. per kg})_1$

$\text{Total cation}_2 = \text{TBW}_1 \times [(\text{Na})_p + (\text{K})_p + 15]_2$

$(\text{Cation per kg})_1$ and TBW_1 from Table 10-1

Example: Muscular male, 65 kg; intestinal obstruction, treated without salt. Plasma sodium 115 mEq/L; potassium 5 mEq/L

$\text{Total cation}_1 = 65 \times 95 = 6175$ mEq

$\text{Total cation}_2 = (0.58 \times 65) \times (115 + 5 + 15) = 37.7 \times 135 = 5089$ mEq

$\text{Cation}_{def} = 6175 - 5089 = 1086$ mEq

Note: Although both sodium and potassium are lost in this situation, the primary deficit is in the extracellular phase; some guess as to the proportionality may be gained from the associated hematocrit changes. In any event, a reasonable starting ration would be 750 mEq of sodium, given as concentrated salt solution; extreme caution is necessary because of the tendency of this therapy to lower the potassium concentration. KCl (totaling at least 400 mEq) will have to be used once resalting has begun.

Syndrome 7. Oversalting: Extracellular Fluid Excess (Table 10-10)

Definition, Terminology, and Related Terms

Oversalting with extracellular fluid excess is isotonic expansion of the extracellular fluid volume regardless of the sodium concentration. *Fluid overload* is a common term more or less synonymous, but less specific. *Hypertonicity* is one occasional result of oversalting. *Congestive heart failure* is one visceral cause of extracellular fluid excess.

Clinical Setting

1. Overadministration of saline fluids
2. Visceral disease of heart, kidneys, or liver

Addition or Subtraction

Oversalting with extracellular fluid excess is an addition disorder; as in the case of hypervolemia, however, the superimposition of visceral failure adds an important endogenous component. When this is present and severe, extracellular fluid oversalting can occur spontaneously on the basis of ordinary oral intake with no specific "fluid overload."

Body Composition and Body Weight

Elevated extracellular fluid volumes, approximating 30 percent of body weight or more, are seen in this disorder. Total body water is elevated, but cell water expansion is rarely, if ever, proportional to the extracellular expansion, particularly in chronic congestive heart failure. In mitral stenosis, for example, extreme cellular wasting accompanies the extracellular excess. Very characteristic disjunctions are therefore seen, with extreme constriction of the total body potassium as a manifestation of the diminished cell

Table 10-10. *Oversalting: Extracellular Fluid Excess (Syndrome 7)*

		Major Findings	
	Unit	Typical	Extreme
Body weight	Change	Gain 3–4 kg	Gain 5–10 kg
Hematocrit	% cells	32–36	28–32
Plasma protein	gm/dl	5.5–6.0	4.5–5.0
Plasma sodium	mEq/L	140–150	140–155
Plasma chloride	mEq/L	103–110	103–115
Plasma potassium	mEq/L	4.5–4.0	4.5–3.5
Std. bicarbonate	mEq/L	24–26	24–26
Central venous pressure	cm H_2O	5–20	29–60

mass, on the one hand, together with overexpansion of total body sodium as a manifestation of extracellular components, on the other. The ratio of total exchangeable sodium to potassium therefore becomes a very meaningful index. In the normal male the Na_e/K_e ratio is slightly below 1.0 and in the female slightly more than 1. In disorders of this category, Na_e/K_e ratio is markedly elevated and may be as high as 2.5. The curious reciprocal relationships that exist with these two cations are nowhere better epitomized than in congestive heart failure with a very high Na_e/K_e ratio, when the plasma concentration of sodium is characteristically low and of potassium characteristically high; concentration and body content are inversely related.

Abnormalities of Autoregulation

When extracellular fluid expansion is due simply to overtreatment with such solutions as Ringer's lactate (e.g., in treating hemorrhage with huge amounts of isotonic salt solution), a homeostatic regulation in the form of greatly increased urinary output is present and normal. There is a sharp cutoff of secretion of aldosterone and, under most circumstances, of antidiuretic hormone. Experiments in man have demonstrated that, given a choice between maintaining volume and tonicity, the body will sacrifice tonicity. Thus, in some overexpanded body water syndromes, there is an anomalous and continuing high renal excretion of sodium, leading to dangerous degrees of hypotonicity.

If renal function is normal, and there has been overadministration of saline fluids, huge urine volumes (5,000 to 7,000 ml per day) are seen. In the visceral forms of extracellular fluid expansion, particularly when due to disease of the heart, liver, or kidney, the disorder itself is due in part to an abnormality of this homeostatic regulator; there is a pathologic failure of diuresis with retention of fluid and salt. With extracellular fluid overexpansion and a restricted urine sodium concentration (i.e., less than 15 mEq/day), one has clear evidence of this abnormality of homeostasis. Frequent measurements of total urine volume are useful in the critically ill patient; the normal oliguric response to volume reduction has been mentioned several times in the foregoing. Here, normal renal response results in urine volumes over 100 ml per hour for three hours or more; such large urine volumes should indicate to the therapist that intravenous infusion rates should be sharply reduced, as long as the rest of the picture indicates good renal function.

In simple isotonic overexpansion of the extracellular fluid, *concentrations* are often normal save for the protein concentration, which is low by dilution. The hematocrit is also low by dilution. In more chronic forms, particularly in diseases of heart, lungs, liver, and kidneys, hypotonicity accompanies the volume overexpansion. Plasma sodium concentration and osmolality are therefore depressed. The ingestion or injection of large amounts of water adds to this depression of serum sodium and osmolality. Central venous pressure is usually high.

Treatment

When overadministration of fluids is the cause of the condition, fluid administration must be stopped promptly; this may require very strong steps because of the heavy-handed habits of those in attendance. If renal function shows a normal diuretic response, no other treatment is usually needed. In other instances, if some degree of pulmonary edema has resulted, the use of concentrated human albumin, with sodium-losing diuretic agents such as furosemide (Lasix), is effective. In the more difficult forms of extracellular fluid overload seen in diseases of heart, liver, and kidney, however, such simple measures will not suffice. The use of digitalis and diuretics in heart disease is beyond the scope of this chapter. The use of diuretics plus concentrated albumin in diseases of liver and lung may be quite effective to combat fluid overload. Such steps are an important aspect of preoperative management.

Guides to Progress

Lowering of central venous pressure (and other chamber pressures) to normal; gradual tapering off of diuresis if overadministration has been the cause; or the establishment of diuresis in chronic visceral disease—all of these are important guides to progress. A fall in body weight should occur.

Syndrome 8. Desiccation-Dehydration (Table 10-11)

Definition, Terminology, and Related Terms

Desiccation-dehydration is loss of water from the body, essentially as pure water. The term *dehydration* alone is more appropriately used here than for desalting water loss. Here we are dealing with a global body water deficit distributed throughout all compartments of the body; the term is therefore not synonymous with desalting water loss, which always involves the extracellular fluid first. *Hypernatremia* is a result of desiccation-dehydration, as is *hypertonicity,* yet neither of them is synonymous nor specific. The term *intracellular dehydration* was often used to refer to the results of desiccation-dehydration, implying thereby that there must be an increase in intracellular tonicity to match the increase in extracellular tonicity indicated by the hypernatremia. Although this is true, the term is unnecessarily limiting.

Clinical Setting

1. Loss of pure water from the respiratory tract (intubation, dry gas ventilation).
2. Evaporative loss from normal, burned, or injured skin or tissue.
3. Castaways in hot, dry atmosphere, desert or ocean.
4. Renal desiccation: diabetes insipidus or diseases of distal renal tubular water reabsorption.

Addition or Subtraction

Desiccation-dehydration is always a subtraction disorder. One may think of it as the loss of distilled water as vapor or "steam" from the body.

Body Composition and Body Weight

Total body water comprises approximately 50 to 55 percent of the body weight. Body fat, being anhydrous, constitutes a component of body composition that is not included in body water; the fraction of body weight occupied by water is inversely proportional to the degree of obesity. For this reason, very fat people have very low values for total body water and its various divisions. Approximately 10 percent of normal body

Table 10-11. *Desiccation-Dehydration (Syndrome 8)*

		Major Findings	
	Unit	Typical	Extreme
Hematocrit	% cells	50	60
Plasma protein	gm/dl	6.5–7.0	7.5–8.0
Plasma tonicity	mOsm/L	320–340	350–370
Plasma nonelectrolyte tonicity	mOsm/L	5	10–20
Plasma sodium	mEq/L	155	175
Plasma chloride	mEq/L	110	120
Std. bicarbonate	mEq/L	25–27	15–20
Plasma potassium	mEq/L	3.5–4.0	5.0–7.0
Blood urea nitrogen	mg/dl	15–20	40–70

water, or approximately 5 percent of normal body weight (2,500 to 4,000 ml in a normal individual), is the magnitude of loss required to produce significant hypertonicity and severe thirst. The loss of body weight is appropriate and exactly equal to the degree of water loss. The body weight change should be followed during rehydration.

Abnormalities of Autoregulation

The principal symptom of desiccation-dehydration is severe thirst. If the individual is conscious, hypertonicity produces an overpowering thirst; the slaking of this thirst by the oral intake of water is the primary homeostatic response. If the individual is unconscious, the complaint of thirst is neither felt nor made, and it is up to the physician to sense it and provide the water.

Desiccation-dehydration produces hypertonicity, the primal stimulus to antidiuretic hormone production and distal renal tubular reabsorption of water. Secretion of small volumes of urine of high osmolality is therefore the principal manifestation of a normal homeostatic response. If this is lacking, as in diabetes insipidus, and in water-losing nephritis, it is evident that the lack of this homeostatic regulator is, per se, largely responsible for the disorder itself.

A gradual increase in serum osmolality and sodium concentration is the characteristic *laboratory finding*. The concentration of potassium may not rise at an equal rate; that of chloride usually rises; the bicarbonate is variable. Urinary findings have been mentioned in the foregoing discussion. In general, serum sodium concentrations over 160 mEq/L are very dangerous and values over 175 mEq/L are rarely compatible with survival. These values would correspond to osmolality of 325 to 375 mOsm/L, depending to some extent on the quantity of nonelectrolyte osmolar solute present. With oliguria, blood urea rises, and therefore in acute, severe dehydration-desiccation (sometimes seen in heat stroke or in poorly conditioned athletes suddenly exercising in hot weather), the accumulated urea makes a real contribution to the elevated osmolality, as does the sugar concentration in diabetic dehydration.

Treatment

The primary treatment of desiccation-dehydration is the administration of water. This can be done by mouth, by gastric tube, or by vein (using 5 percent dextrose in water). The actual amounts of water required are almost always more than one might expect, particularly since the pathologic condition producing the water loss usually continues for at least a day or two. Body weight, osmolality, and renal function should all be followed with care. It is particularly important to be assured that one is not dealing with some element of solute loading (see Syndrome 10), in which case simple massive rehydration can be very dangerous.

Guides to Progress

Urinary output changes with beginning diuresis are the key occurrence. If the osmolality is elevated over 310 mOsm/L and serum sodium is over 150 to 155 mEq/L, sudden restoration of body water to normal will result in acute cerebral overhydration, with cerebral edema. This is due to the fact that the brain is more permeable to water than it is to salt. With sudden rehydration, therefore, the brain gains water before it loses salt. Cerebral edema can therefore be the result of too rapid restoration of desiccation-dehydration to normal. Pulmonary edema is likewise a threat if cardiopulmonary function is impaired. Body weight should be followed during rehydration.

Relevant Mathematical Expression

In Syndrome 8, *Desiccation-Dehydration,* the Total Body Water deficit is given by:

$$TBW_{def} = TBW_1 - TBW_2$$

$$TBW_1 = \frac{\text{body wt}_1 \times \text{cation per kg}_1}{[(Na)_p + (K)_p + 15]_1}$$

$$TBW_2 = \frac{\text{body wt}_1 \times \text{cation per kg}_1}{[(Na)_p + (K)_p + 15]_2}$$

(Cation per kg)$_1$ from Table 10-1, or use (TBW)$_1$ directly from Table 10-1.

Example: Muscular 85-kg male, 1 week after burn, with massive losses from skin and lungs. Sodium 162 mEq/L; Potassium 6.8 mEq/L.

$$TBW_1 = \frac{85 \times 95}{163} = \frac{8075}{163} = 49.5$$

$$TBW_2 = \frac{8075}{(162 + 6.8 + 15)} = \frac{8075}{183.8} = 43.9 \text{ liters}$$

$$TBW_{def} = 49.5 - 43.9 = 5.6 \text{ liters}$$

Note: This TBW_{def} (5.6 liters) needs to be given *and retained* in order to lower tonicity to normal. With large continuing losses, frequent estimates of intake and output and body weight must be done to document an actual weight gain achieved with rehydration. The figure of 5.6 liters is the *net water gain* required for rehydration; an amount much larger than that must be given. This assumes constant total cation (i.e., no salt loss).

Syndrome 9. Overhydration-Hypotonicity (Table 10-12)

Definition, Terminology, and Related Terms

Overhydration-hypotonicity is an abnormally large body water unaccompanied by a proportional increase in body salt or solute. It is the hypotonic analogue of extracellular fluid excess described in Syndrome 7; it is the hypotonic converse of dehydration-desiccation with hypertonicity as described in Syndrome 8. *Hyponatremia* is a related term; although hyponatremia is a result of overhydration with hypotonicity, it is also observed in late desalting water loss. *Water intoxication* is an analogous term for the severe form of overhydration hypotonicity.

Clinical Setting

1. *Overadministration* of water by mouth or vein.
2. *Postoperative* patients, particularly sensitive to overadministration of free water or hypotonic fluids.
3. Patients with *chronic visceral disease,* particularly that of the heart, who have been on a salt-free diet and taking large amounts of water by mouth.

Table 10-12. *Overhydration-Hypotonicity (Syndrome 9)*

		Major Findings	
	Unit	Typical	Extreme (water intoxication)
Body weight		gain 1–5 kg	gain 4–10 kg
Hematocrit	% cells	30–35	25–30
Plasma protein	gm/dl	4.0–5.0	3.0–4.0
Plasma tonicity	mOsm/L	260	220
Plasma sodium	mEq/L	120	105
Plasma chloride	mEq/L	80	70
Std. bicarbonate	mEq/L	25	20
Plasma potassium	mEq/L	4.0	3.5
Blood urea nitrogen	mg/dl	8–10	5–8

Addition or Subtraction

Overhydration-hypotonicity is usually an addition disorder, and there is associated weight gain. If compounded by concomitant loss of salt (renal or extrarenal), the disorder is a combined one, and with severe degrees of hypotonicity the body weight increase may be much less.

Body Composition and Body Weight

In the pure state of overhydration-hypotonicity, total body salt content is normal, but total body water is markedly elevated. The normal elasticity of total body water volume would permit the addition of 2000 to 3000 ml with little symptomatic change. Amounts larger than this produce significant hypotonicity. An appropriate weight gain will therefore have occurred. Weight measurement usually can begin only at the time of the diagnosis. Weight loss is to be expected during repair.

Abnormalities of Autoregulation

Free water clearance due to complete cessation ("ADH cutoff") of antidiuretic hormone secretion is the normal homeostatic response to the overadministration or overaccumulation of water. In the presence of visceral disease, this homeostatic feedback loop is impaired on either the sensor or the effector side, and one may therefore see this disorder develop because of restricted water excretion. After operations, or when there has been any prior injury or volume reduction, water excretion is impaired by a variety of mechanisms. The postoperative or post-traumatic state is therefore one in which water retention regularly occurs. Overhydration-hypotonicity so severe as to justify the term *water intoxication* is readily produced by overzealous administration of salt-free fluid in the post-operative or post-traumatic state. Anomalous increase in sodium excretion due to volume expansion ("aldosterone cutoff") may further complicate the hypotonicity.

A fall in the serum sodium concentration linear with the fall in serum osmolality is the characteristic *laboratory finding*. In this disorder, the sum of sodium and potassium concentrations (mEq/L) multiplied by 2 is almost always exactly equivalent to the serum osmolality (mEq/L). If water loading has been severe, there may be elevation of chamber pressures. Urinary findings are discussed earlier in this section.

Treatment

Cessation of water administration is mandatory. The establishment of a water diuresis is, in some cases, attainable by the use of a solute diuretic such as mannitol. When total body solute is elevated (Syndrome 10), its sudden hydration by the administration of large amounts of water is dangerous because of the production of cerebral or pulmonary edema. We have the exact analogue when total body water is elevated in hypotonicity: restoration to normal solute concentration by the careless administration of huge amounts of salt solutions is dangerous because of the threat of cerebral and pulmonary edema. For this reason, in overhydration-hypotonicity, the loss of water should be the objective, with loss of weight, rather than mere restoration of salt concentration.

Guides to Progress

Weight loss with restoration of tonicity to normal are the objectives. Serum sodium concentrations above 130 mEq/L are rarely symptomatic, but when they fall to 115 to 120 mEq/L, weakness, lassitude, drowsiness, and hypotension occur. Serum sodium concentrations below 115 mEq/L are dangerous (hypotension, coma) and below 100 mEq/L are rarely compatible with survival.

Relevant Mathematical Expression

In Syndrome 9, *Overhydration-Hypotonicity,* the body water excess is given by:

$$TBW_{exc} = TBW_2 - TBW_1$$

TBW_1 from Table 10-1

$$TBW_2 = \frac{(\text{total cation})_1}{[(Na)_p + (K)_p + 15]_2}$$

Example: 65 kg, normally built male, stressed by continued infection, given large extra amounts of water to carry antibiotics. Found to have gained weight, with a plasma sodium concentration of 110 mEq/L and potassium 3.5 mEq/L.

$TBW_1 = 35.7$ liters (from Table 10-1).

$$TBW_2 = \frac{65 \times 90}{128} = 45.7$$

$$TBW_{exc} = 45.7 - 35.7 = 10 \text{ liters}$$

Note: The 10 liters of excess body water is represented by 10 kg overweight. Using whatever therapy is employed, including water restriction and possibly diuretics, about 10 kg must be lost to bring salt concentrations up to normal. There will be some continuing electrolyte loss in the urine, particularly if an anomalous sodium excretion has occurred. For this reason urine electrolytes must be measured, with close monitoring throughout the period of water restriction and weight loss.*

Syndrome 10. Solute-Loading Hypertonicity (Table 10-13)

Definition, Terminology, and Related Terms

The term *solute-loading hypertonicity* refers to an elevated plasma osmolality due to the combined action of two pathogenic factors: ingestion of a large amount of osmotically active solute, accompanied by a continued profuse solute diuresis. Although other solutes are important, sodium concentration is always elevated, so that the term *hypernatremia* is sometimes used, though it is nonspecific as to cause. *Tube feeding syndrome* refers to the initial description of this disorder as a complication of tube feeding of

Editor's Note: Dr. Moore's caution is appropriate. My experience is that a total deficit should not be replaced immediately or rapidly and indeed is not often required. During the first 24 hours after discovery of one of these syndromes described, to replace or correct approximately one-third the deficit in a patient with reasonable renal function will allow a patient to participate in and complete the correction. Too rapid a correction of hypotonicity may be damaging to the brain, as pointed out repeatedly in this section.

Table 10-13. *Solute Loading Hypertonicity (Syndrome 10)*

		Major Findings	
	Unit	Typical	Extreme
Hematocrit	% cells	50	55
Plasma protein	gm/dl	6.0–6.5	6.0–6.5
Plasma tonicity	mOsm/L	320	370
Plasma nonelectrolyte tonicity	mOsm/L	40	60
Plasma sodium	mEq/L	160	170
Plasma chloride	mEq/L	110	115
Std. bicarbonate	mEq/L	25	15
Plasma potassium	mEq/L	4.5	6.5
Blood urea nitrogen	mg/dl	20–40	60–80
Sugar	mg/dl	120	1000
Central venous pressure	cm H_2O	5–15	20–40

a mix rich in solute, with inadequate water provision, in unconscious patients. *Hyperosmotic nonketotic hyperglycemic coma,* or some variant of that term, is used to describe an extreme form of this disorder accompanied by high blood sugar elevations and anomalously low plasma insulin concentrations; this is usually associated with prolonged enteral or parenteral feeding in unconscious patients. This variant is described separately (Syndromes 10 and 17-II).

Clinical Setting

1. *Solutes forced* by mouth or vein for nutrition, with too little water, particularly prone to occur in patients who are semicomatose.
2. *Insulin lack* (pancreatectomy, untreated diabetes).
3. *Borderline renal failure* (inadequate distal tubular water reabsorption, or water-losing nephritis).
4. *Coma or head injury,* and in some cases CNS injury salt retention.

Addition or Subtraction

Solute loading hypertonicity is due to the addition of large amounts of low-molecular-weight solutes to the body fluids, with inadequate water, together with the inability to excrete them in a concentrated urine. It is usually a mixture of addition of solutes and subtraction of water.

Body Composition and Body Weight

In desiccation-dehydration with hypertonicity, the total body sodium is normal, water has been subtracted, and sodium concentration is elevated. In solute-loading hypertonicity, there is a large increase in total body solute, including sodium. In some cases total body water may also be high. Body water and salt are therefore at extremely high levels, and weight has been gained. If the body solute is rapidly rehydrated by careless administration of large amounts of water, generalized edema occurs, with cerebral and pulmonary edema that are life-endangering. Sudden massive rehydration of solute-loading hypertonicity is one of the dangerous and immediately lethal errors that can be made in body fluid therapy.

Abnormalities of Autoregulation

In *desiccation-dehydration* with hypertonicity, a normal renal response is extreme oliguria with production of a scanty, highly concentrated urine. A key diagnostic signal that *solute-loading hypertonicity* is developing is the continued production of a high volume of urine (solute diuresis) at a fixed osmolality around 750 mOsm/L. High urine volumes with a rising plasma tonicity are the first clue.

Any diabetic trend worsens this syndrome. If a patient is on tube feedings or prolonged intravenous alimentation, and has undergone pancreatic surgery or has had pancreatitis or borderline diabetes in the past, or is on long-continued cortisone administration, this syndrome should be suspected if hypertonicity is found.* The diagnosis is established by finding a large amount of nonelectrolyte solute in the plasma, as indicated by the difference between the observed plasma osmolality and the sum of sodium and potassium multiplied by 2. This "osmolar gap," normally trivial, may rise to 20 to 40 mOsm/L in this disorder (see Table 10-2).

A high serum sodium concentration with proportionally higher osmolality, as mentioned, is the cardinal *laboratory finding*. The rise in hematocrit is slow to occur, since overwatering and oversalting rather than true water loss are the pathogenic factors. The urinary findings have been mentioned. Calculation of the "osmolar gap" is helpful.

Treatment

In this syndrome, a rapidly lethal outcome is produced if an attempt is made to rehydrate body solutes suddenly by the administration of large amounts of water. Because total body solute is high, the result of such an effort is merely a massive overhydration and oversalting, with rapid elevation of cardiac chamber pressures and the production of pulmonary and cerebral edema. It is for this reason that treatment should consist in cessation of solute loading, the administration of insulin in some cases (if blood glucose is high), and the cautious administration of water. The key to success is the excretion of solute, as well as the rehydration of residual body salt. If renal failure is present, dialysis is essential to success. If diuretics are used, the urine must be analyzed to be certain that solute is being excreted, rather than a urine of low osmolality, which would only accentuate the defect.

*The patient with severe bleeding from the upper gastrointestinal tract (e.g., duodenal ulcer) is frequently treated with large amounts of milky and salty substances by mouth (antacid therapy) with inadequate water. He is frequently in and out of coma. He cannot complain of thirst. He fails to move his bowels. Hypertonicity with severe fecal impaction is a serious complication seen in this circumstance.

Guides to Progress

Monitoring of body weight, blood and urine chemical values, electrocardiogram, cerebral function, and chamber pressures is essential to safety during rehydration.

Syndrome 11. Hypokalemia (Table 10-14)

Definition, Terminology, and Related Terms

Hypokalemia signifies a low plasma potassium concentration without reference to total body potassium content. *Hypokalemic alkalosis* and *hypokalemic hypochloremic alkalosis* refer to the frequently accompanying alkalosis and depressed chloride concentration. They are terms that include many cases of hypokalemia. *Potassium deficiency* is a misnomer, since hypokalemia may occur with little or no potassium deficit. By the same token, huge losses of body potassium with cellular wasting may be accompanied by a perfectly normal or high plasma potassium concentration.

Clinical Setting

1. *Loss of acid gastric juice* in duodenal or pyloric obstruction.
2. *Loss of acid gastric juice* in the presence of small bowel obstruction; rare cases of bowel foreshortening.

Table 10-14. *Hypokalemia (with Hypochloremia and Alkalosis) (Syndrome 11)*

		Major Findings	
	Unit	Typical	Extreme
Body weight	Change	None	Loss 1–2 kg
Hematocrit	% cells	40	38
Plasma protein	gm/dl	6.0–6.5	5.5–6.0
Plasma tonicity	mOsm/L	300–310	280–300
Plasma sodium	mEq/L	143	150
Plasma chloride	mEq/L	80	60
Std. bicarbonate	mEq/L	35	50
Plasma potassium	mEq/L	2.0–2.5	1.2–1.5
Blood urea nitrogen	mg/dl	30	70
Blood pH	Units	7.52	7.55
Blood PCO_2	mm Hg	35	45
Blood PaO_2	mm Hg	80–90	75–80

3. *Loss of acid gastric juice* in the Zollinger-Ellison syndrome.
4. *Hyperaldosteronism* due to adrenocortical disease or tumor.
5. *Hyperaldosteronism* due to renal artery stenosis or with other stimuli to excessive renin-angiotensin-aldosterone administration.
6. Chronic administration of *ACTH, cortisone,* or *aldosterone,* particularly if the patient is traumatized or operated on.

Addition or Subtraction

Hypokalemia is another combination syndrome due both to addition and subtraction. Loss of potassium plays a role, but is not critical; losses as small as 100 mEq may be sufficient. Loss of hydrogen ion, with production of a subtraction alkalosis, is very important. Then, if sodium salts are given by mouth or vein, the syndrome becomes much worse.

Body Composition and Body Weight

Body compositional changes may be negligible; possibly the most important is the reduction in extracellular volume that stimulates aldosterone production; body weight changes are then appropriate to this rather mild extracellular fluid loss.

Potassium exists within body cells in a rather fixed ratio to protein (approximately 3 mEq of potassium per gram of nitrogen). Balanced cellular loss, as in starvation, does not produce noticeable disorders of plasma potassium regulation. In a stressful situation, or with marked secretion of aldosterone or cortisone, potassium is lost from the cell at a high K:N ratio (as high as 15 mEq/gm). This *"differential potassium loss"* is the setting for hypokalemia, and as mentioned, it need not be large in magnitude. It is characteristic of this syndrome that the plasma sodium concentration is normal or slightly elevated. Again, note the tendency of these two ion concentrations to move in opposite directions.

Abnormalities of Autoregulation

"Alkalosis begets hypokalemia, hypokalemia begets alkalosis, alkalosis is difficult to repair in the presence of potassium deficiency, and hypokalemia is almost impossible to repair in the presence of a continuing alkalosis." This disorder is a disorder of the complex neuro-endocrine-renal feedback loop betwen potassium metabolism and acid base homeostasis. This is a complex homeostatic arrangement regulating cation distribution across cellular membranes, and the retention or excretion of hydrogen ion. The disorder is imposed from without, in the excessive loss of protons as in vomiting of highly acid gastric juice, but this engenders an inner disorder of one of the body's most delicate homeostatic arrangements. The intracellular potassium concentration is around 150 mEq/L. If extracellular potassium concentration is allowed to approach even one-twentieth of this value, death results. It is thus clear that the regulation of potassium concentration in the plasma is of extreme importance.

The loss of acid gastric juice, threatening extracellular alkalosis, would ordinarily be accompanied by an alkaline urine designed, as it were, to correct the disorder. With the slight volume reduction, aldosterone is instead secreted. Sodium bicarbonate is reabsorbed, and the "paradoxical aciduria" so characteristic of hypokalemia and alkalosis is produced. This tendency to secrete an acid urine is greatly intensified by operative stress or by anything that increases ACTH or cortisone production, as well as aldosterone. The alkalosis therefore becomes suddenly much worse. Loss of acid gastric juice may occur without any warning, simply through an indwelling gastric tube, by suction. The alkalosis itself causes a sharp reduction in plasma potassium concentration, and thus an "inappropriate positive feedback" is initiated, in which the alkalosis produces loss of acid and potassium in the urine, lowering plasma potassium concentration in a self-perpetuating cycle. As one might predict, this disorder is virtually never observed in oliguric renal failure. Its development requires a normal kidney, responding normally to endocrine influences activated by volume reduction and loss of hydrogen ion.

Plasma potassium concentrations in the region of 2.5 to 3.5 mEq/L are regular *laboratory findings* in this syndrome; levels below 1.5 mEq/L are very dangerous. The plasma sodium concentration is usually normal or slightly elevated. One would expect to find the plasma sodium concentration at about 135 mEq/L; in hypokalemic alkalosis the value is quite regularly approximately 143 to 145 mEq/L. The degree of metabolic alkalosis is indicated by the bicarbonate concentration, which is virtually always over 30 mEq and may approximate 40 to 60 mEq/L. The loss of acid gastric juice results in loss of chloride and, therefore, hypochloremia, with plasma chloride concentrations below 90 mEq/L.

The urinary findings are of key importance. Early in the syndrome there is secretion of an acid urine with large amounts of potassium. This is typically the aldosterone-induced urinary change. At the height of this syndrome, renal tubular reabsorption of sodium bicarbonate is almost 100 percent.

Electrocardiographic changes are characteristic: the heart becomes very sensitive to digitalis effects, and if the patient has previously been digitalized, the occurrence of this syndrome produces digitalis toxicity without alterations in digitalis dosage. Cardiac chamber pressures are normal or low, unless heart failure develops. In any case, arrhythmias are commonplace.

Treatment

Treatment is the administration of potassium with a proton equivalent. The administration of chloride ion has an acidifying effect on the extracellular fluid. For this reason the administration of KCl is standard therapy. The administration of ammonium chloride is another way of adding large amounts of hydrogen ion to the extracellular fluid and, in certain cases, actually brings the plasma potassium concentration toward normal without administration of any potassium. Mixtures of the two are usually administered. When there is volume reduction as indicated by oliguria, some sodium can be administered after the first or second day of treatment. In some instances, the alkalosis is remarkably resistant to therapy; the intravenous administration of 0.1 N HCl is rational and effective.

Table 10-15. *Hyperkalemia (with Renal Failure) (Syndrome 12)*

	Major Findings		
	Unit	Typical	Extreme
Body weight	Change	Gain	Gain
Hematocrit	% cells	Variable	Variable
Plasma protein	gm/dl	Variable	5.5–6.0
Plasma tonicity	mOsm/L	290	320
Plasma nonelectrolyte tonicity	mOsm/L	40	70
Plasma sodium	mEq/L	120	110
Plasma chloride	mEq/L	105	105
Std. bicarbonate	mEq/L	10	5
Plasma potassium	mEq/L	7.5	9.0
Blood urea nitrogen	mg/dl	70–100	100–200
Blood pH	Units	7.25	7.15

GUIDES TO PROGRESS

The electrocardiographic changes are quite remarkable and were for some time thought to be a function of the plasma potassium concentration, but alkalosis itself produces similar changes. Nonetheless, electrocardiographic changes are helpful. This is a metabolic alkalosis, and blood pH is rarely elevated much above 7.5; restoration to normal occurs with treatment. Restoration of plasma potassium concentration to normal is the principal index of rectification.

Renal artery stenosis, with high values for renin, angiotensin, and aldosterone, produces mild hypokalemic alkalosis along with hypertension. Here, the aldosterone effect has, alone and without any loss of gastric juice or other chemical stimuli, produced hypokalemic alkalosis. As accounted in Syndrome 15 (The Normal Postoperative Patient), hemorrhage, stress, and trauma tend to move the patient in the direction of hypokalemic alkalosis.

Syndrome 12. Hyperkalemia (Table 10-15)

DEFINITION, TERMINOLOGY, AND RELATED TERMS

Hyperkalemia is an elevation of plasma potassium concentration without reference to total body potassium content. The term is appropriate regardless of any other concomitant changes that may be occurring, the most common being acidosis. Few other terms are used for this disorder. As mentioned, renal acidosis is a regular accompaniment, but it is not synonymous. *Potassium toxicity* refers to a hazard of hyperkalemia, but it is not a synonymous physiologic term. *Chloride acidosis* refers to a metabolic acidosis with an elevated chloride concentration; potassium concentration does not always follow, and therefore the term is not a synonym.

CLINICAL SETTING

1. *Renal failure.*
2. Overadministration of *potassium salts* with borderline renal function.
3. *Very severe injury* (with loss of intracellular potassium) greatly accentuates the rate of potassium rise when renal failure coexists.

ADDITION OR SUBTRACTION

This is an addition syndrome, but the addition to extracellular potassium arises within the body, owing to redistribution of potassium; the disorder is greatly accentuated by the administration of exogenous potassium.

BODY COMPOSITION AND BODY WEIGHT

The body compositional change can be quite trivial. A redistribution of potassium sufficient to cause death by hyperkalemia and potassium toxicity can occur with no change in total body potassium. Body weight usually rises, owing to the accumulation of fluid (in renal failure).

ABNORMALITIES OF AUTOREGULATION

Potassium is a strong diuretic, excreted both by filtration and by tubular secretion. The absence of normal renal function therefore obliterates the normal homeostatic regulator of serum potassium concentration. Potassium administered to a normal person is distributed largely (98 percent) within cells, particularly if there is protein synthesis and cellular growth. It is the absence of this normal intracellular potassium-holding aspect of the body cell mass, in stress or after injury, that makes the potassium distribution so abnormal; if renal function were normal, the stress-induced cellular potassium loss would be reflected by increased renal potassium excretion. When a large meat meal is eaten in the course of a normal diet, more potassium is ingested by mouth than is required to cause severe hyperkalemia, were it all to remain in the extracellular phase. The rapid distribution, partition, and excretion of potassium is markedly inhibited by severe injury or in renal failure.

Just as *alkalosis* usually accompanies *hypokalemia* and/or potassium deficiency, so also *acidosis* characteristically accompanies *hyperkalemia* and/or potassium excess. Acidosis is also an end-result of renal failure because of the loss of the normal renal functional capacity for excretion of metabolic acids. If acidosis is corrected by dialysis, hyperkalemia tends to be more tractable. If large amounts of protons are removed from the body, for example, by gastric acid aspiration, hyperkalemia is much less notable even though the amounts of potassium so removed are trivial. Plasma potassium concentrations over 5.5 mEq/L are dangerous; with concentrations over 7.5 mEq/L, severe cardiac arrhythmias and death may suddenly occur. The degree of acidosis is quite impressive in these cases, with pH values around 7.15 to 7.25 in typical renal acidosis with hyperkalemia.

TREATMENT

The treatment consists in removal of potassium from the extracellular fluid, either by hemodialysis or peritoneal dialysis, or by the use of exchange resins in the gastrointestinal tract; the removal of gastric acid by suction is a mildly effective treatment and is helpful if prolonged.

GUIDES TO PROGRESS

The restoration of potassium concentration downward or toward normal may require dialysis daily. If urine volumes are in the range of 500 to 1500 ml per day, dialysis is less important and other measures may be more effective. Since acidosis is an important component, the restoration of pH toward normal is a sign of progress. Attempts to rectify this acidosis by the administration of large amounts of alkali salts is dangerous. The treatment of renal failure by any sort of infusion of sodium salt rapidly produces pulmonary edema, hypertension, and congestive heart failure.

Electrocardiogram must be monitored closely. A sudden fall in potassium concentration will accentuate digitalis effects.

Syndrome 13. Hypochloremia

DEFINITION, TERMINOLOGY, AND RELATED TERMS

Hypochloremia is a lowering of the plasma chloride concentration regardless of other findings. *Hypochloremic alkalosis* describes the frequent accompaniment of extracellular alkalosis, with hypochloremia. *Gastric juice loss hypo-*

chloremia describes the most common cause of hypochloremia in surgical patients. *Metabolic alkalosis* refers to an acid-base disorder that may or may not coexist with hypochloremia.

Clinical Setting

1. Chloride loss through *gastric juice;* vomiting and obstruction.
2. Treatment of *gastric obstruction* without chloride.
3. *Gastric hypersecretion* (Zollinger-Ellison syndrome or other causes), particularly with outlet obstruction or gastric fistula.

Addition or Subtraction

Hypochloremia is always a subtraction disorder.

Body Composition and Body Weight

The total chloride of the body is markedly reduced in hypochloremia, the reduction being linear with the reduction of concentration. This is one situation in body composition and chemistry wherein the plasma concentration changes occur *pari passu* with changes in total body content. As mentioned earlier, hypokalemia regularly accompanies hypochloremia, but the latter may be extremely marked with only minor degrees of hypokalemia if operative stress has been absent.

Abnormalities of Autoregulation

As the body is depleted of chloride, gastric secretion of hydrochloric acid is diminished. When gastric secretion of hydrochloric acid is maintained at a very high level (e.g., with duodenal ulcer, or in disorders such as the Zollinger-Ellison syndrome), the losses become massive. Severe and dangerous degrees of alkalosis can be produced. Hypergastrinemia from any cause, with obstruction, greatly accentuates hypochloremia and alkalosis. One occasionally observes situations in which the bicarbonate concentration (at 60 or 70 mEq/L) is actually higher than the chloride concentration, which has fallen to similar or lower values. In the more typical case, bicarbonate is in the region of 35 mEq/L and chloride approximately 75 to 85 mEq/L.

Renal conservation of chloride does not follow the renin-aldosterone cycle, but instead bears on renal acid-base regulation. Since the kidney expends energy to secrete an acid urine, one ordinarily finds only minor amounts of chloride present in the urine during gastric juice loss hypochloremia.

In any case of hypochloremia, the plasma potassium concentration should be watched closely as it will fall rapidly to low levels, given the addition either of a corticosteroid stimulus, of operative stress, or acute volume reduction. The sodium concentration in plasma is normally 135 to 140 mEq/L in hypochloremia.

Treatment

Treatment with sodium bicarbonate or other sodium salts low in chloride such as lactate makes the disorder much worse by further diluting the chloride ion. The best treatment is the use of KCl with sodium chloride, the latter in modest amounts. Only by close monitoring of chloride and bicarbonate concentrations, as well as plasma potassium concentrations and the electrocardiogram, can such patients be brought back to normal. With close attention, however, essentially normal extracellular chemical values can be produced in 36 hours if it should be necessary to operate on a patient with obstructive duodenal ulcer and severe hypochloremia. If gastric juice loss by nasogastric suction is playing a role, one might inquire as to whether such suction must be continued; if the amount of gastric juice is large, one should question the presence of either some gastric secretogogue in the drug mix or the Zollinger-Ellison syndrome. On several occasions the diagnosis of the Zollinger-Ellison syndrome has been rightly suspected on the basis of a severe and intractable hypochloremia.

Guides to Progress

All plasma chemical values are important here. Either arterial or venous pH may be followed. The pH values are normally not very high (7.52 for example). Close monitoring of all components is essential, including chamber pressures (if there is any evidence of cardiopulmonary disease).

As indicated under Syndrome 11, Hypokalemia, alkalosis renders the heart very sensitive to digitalis alkaloids, and produces cardiac arrhythmias in elderly patients with myocardial ischemia. In the patient with heart disease, particularly if digitalized, close monitoring of cardiovascular function is therefore essential in hypochloremia and alkalosis.

Nasogastric suction has become such a regular part of the surgical armamentarium that it has been easy to forget that in most patients the purpose of such suction is only the removal of swallowed air. Swallowed air constitutes the gas of the gastrointestinal tract; the body can neither absorb nor solubilize the gas, which is mostly nitrogen, and it leads to distention if not expelled as flatus. Most of the fluid removed in routine nasogastric suction can be reinfused into the stomach for absorption lower down, as long as the swallowed air is vented.

Any sort of alkalosis exerts a weak inhibitory effect on the respiratory center; a mild inhibition of ventilation, with a very mild elevation of the carbon dioxide tension in whole blood (PCO_2 42 to 45 mm Hg), is often seen.

Relevant Mathematical Expression

In Syndrome 13, *Hypochloremia,* Chloride deficit is given by:

$$TBCl_{def} = TBCl_1 - TBCl_2$$

$TBCl_1$ = from Table 10-1 (extracellular fluid volume × normal plasma chloride concentration)

$$TBCl_2 = ECF_1 \times Cl_2$$

Example: Thin male, 70 kg, vomiting from obstructing duodenal ulcer. Plasma chloride 70 mEq/L; Plasma sodium 143 mEq/L.

$$TBCl_1 = 70 \times 0.23 \times 103 = 1658 \text{ mEq}$$

$$TBCl_2 = 70 \times 0.23 \times 70 = 1127 \text{ mEq}$$

$$Cl_{def} = 1658 - 1127 = 531 \text{ mEq}$$

Note: Because of the marked tendency to depression of potassium concentration in this type of subtraction alkalosis, the chloride deficit can be made up using potassium chloride, ammonium chloride, and sodium chloride, the last in less abundance because of the tendency toward normal sodium in this disorder.

Syndrome 14. Hyperchloremia (Table 10-16)

Definition, Terminology, and Related Terms

Hyperchloremia is elevation of plasma chloride concentration regardless of other considerations. *Hyperchloremic acidosis* refers to the fact that hyperchloremia is usually accompanied by acidosis. *Renal acidosis* is another term that is sometimes used interchangeably, although renal acidosis can be quite severe without hyperchloremia. *Metabolic acidosis* is not synonymous, since it refers to any increase in hydrogen ion concentration that is due to metabolic rather than respiratory factors.

Clinical Setting

1. Administration of *large amounts of chloride* by mouth or by vein, particularly where renal function is poor and an acid urine cannot be excreted.
2. Chronic *obstructive uropathy* as with prostate diseases.
3. *Acute tubular necrosis in diuresis* may show this change.

Addition or Subtraction

Hyperchloremia is an addition syndrome. It is due to the addition of chloride ion when renal

Table 10-16. *Hyperchloremia (Syndrome 14)*

		Major Findings	
	Unit	Typical	Extreme
Body weight	Change	No change	Slight gain
Hematocrit	% cells	40–43	38–40
Plasma protein	gm/dl	6.0–6.5	6.0–6.5
Plasma sodium	mEq/L	140	130
Plasma chloride	mEq/L	115	125
Plasma potassium	mEq/L	5.2	6.0
Std. bicarbonate	mEq/L	12	8
Blood pH	Units	7.30	7.18
Blood PCO_2	mm Hg	35	25
Blood urea nitrogen	mg/dl	40	75–100

tubular function is abnormal and the kidney is unable to secrete an acid urine high in chloride.

Body Composition and Body Weight

Extracellular fluid volume is high and total body chloride elevated. Body weight rises because of the water and salt loading components.

Abnormalities of Autoregulation

As noted, some element of renal tubular disorder, with inability to excrete titratable acidity and a urine of low pH, is essential to the development of this syndrome. It is the lack of this normal homeostatic response to chloride administration that makes the syndrome most common in older people, particularly older men with prostatic disease. The overadministration of sodium chloride solutions is, in the normal individual, a stimulus to gastric secretion of hydrochloric acid. With hyperchloremia one may therefore find increased gastric secretion, and in patients with a history of duodenal ulcer this can be significant.

Chloride concentrations in the vicinity of 108 to 120 mEq/L are characteristic *laboratory findings*. The acidosis is usually severe, pH being approximately 7.2. Bicarbonate depression is usually a linear function of the chloride elevation. The "anion gap" is here reduced proportionally.

Treatment

The treatment consists of the cessation of chloride administration and the administration of sodium bicarbonate by mouth or by vein. In chronic renal tubular disease, the regular administration of sodium bicarbonate is advisable. Patients with ureterosigmoidostomies or other forms of ureteral diversion that result in abnormal reabsorption of ammonium chloride from the right colon should be given sodium bicarbonate by mouth to avoid hyperchloremic acidosis. Oversalting, hypoproteinemia, and edema result if too much sodium is given.

Guides to Progress

These are restoration of serum chloride, bicarbonate, and pH to normal, and downward adjustment of ventilation to normal, with rise of PCO_2 to normal levels.

Table 10-17. *Normal Postoperative Patient (Syndrome 15)*

		Major Findings	
	Unit	Typical	Overadministration of Fluid
Body weight	change	Loss 1–2 kg	Gain 1–2 kg
Hematocrit	% cells	35	30
Plasma protein	gm/dl	6.5	5.0
Plasma sodium	mEq/L	130	120
Plasma chloride	mEq/L	100	105
Plasma potassium	mEq/L	3.0	2.5
Std. bicarbonate	mEq/L	30	35
Blood pH	Units	7.52	7.62

Syndrome 15. The Normal Postoperative Patient (Table 10-17)

Definition, Terminology, and Related Terms

With unanesthetized trauma, or elective surgery of mid-grade severity or greater, there are stimuli to alterations in body fluid and electrolyte metabolism that justify consideration of this as a "syndrome"; if managed by even the simplest of means, no manifest disorder need result. *Post-traumatic alkalosis* is a very common disorder after severe injury and is described later, in Syndrome 19. *Low flow acidosis* is another acid-base disorder seen after injury, when a severe low flow state has supervened (see Syndrome 21). Neither of the foregoing terms is synonymous with the normal postoperative physiology.

Clinical Setting

1. Severe unanesthetized *traumatic injury.*
2. Major *operations.*
3. Either of the above with unwise *overadministration of alkalinizing fluids.*
4. Either of the above with *overadministration of hypotonic fluids* or excesses of salt.
5. Any one of the above with continued physiologic "*stress factors,*" particularly sepsis, undrained abscesses, severe immobilization, and pain.
6. Any of the above with added *cortisone* or *ACTH* administration.

Addition or Subtraction

If properly managed, the normal postoperative patient need show no abnormalities of either addition or subtraction.

Body Composition and Body Weight

The normal postoperative patient tends to lose body weight by the oxidation of fat and the catalytic destruction of protein, with the excretion of the end products of both (water, CO_2, and nitrogen). This is normal; if the patient is given so much fluid that no weight loss is experienced, he is being given too much fluid.

Abnormalities of Autoregulation

The normal postoperative patient is under the sway of a variety of endocrine influences, all of which are normal homeostatic regulators: conservation of salt, conservation of water, stimulation of fat oxidation, stimulation of gluconeogenesis from muscle protein, and maintenance of cardiovascular function by increased levels of catecholamines and corticosteroids.

If the patient is well managed, these normal post-traumatic influences quickly pass off (2 to 6 days, depending on the severity of the trauma), and the patient can return to normal intake as needed.

Treatment

For minor grades of trauma, no intravenous infusions need be given, and the patient can weather several hours or even a day with little fluid intake and with no challenge to his welfare. If the patient is elderly or has poor renal function, one should not hazard even that degree of dehydration, since it can be a setting for renal failure if there is a later complication such as sepsis or a mismatched blood transfusion. It has become customary to provide intravenous fluids to a large number of postoperative patients, in some of whom it is not a necessity.

If the patient has been the subject of injury of mid-grade or greater severity (e.g., ruptured spleen, fractured femur, bowel resection, closed cardiac surgery), intravenous infusion should be given to maintain normal hydration. Many of the disorders seen in the postoperative patient result from a wrongly prescribed intravenous regimen, usually excessive water and salt.

"Moderation in all things" seems to describe the management of the postoperative patient better than any other single aphorism. If large amounts of water or hypotonic fluids are administered, the antidiuretic hormone activity produces water retention with hypotonicity and, in severe cases, a rapid water intoxication. The same sort of analogous maladjustment results from too much salt, too much glucose, too much fat, too much transfusion, and too many amino acids.

If given nothing by mouth for several days and given infusions without potassium, the patient will show a typical hypokalemia after a few days; this is greatly accentuated by continued nasogastric suction or vomiting.

Therefore, the keynote should be administration of enough water to counterbalance skin and lung losses as well as the secretion of a slightly concentrated urine (in the volume of about 1,200 ml/24 hours). This amount of water will total about 1,500 to 2,000 ml in a normal-sized adult male, somewhat less in the female. He should be given an amount of salt required to fill up any "third space effect" from the operative trauma itself and to compensate for a urine sodium excretion of 10 to 50 mEq during the first day. This would correspond to approximately 500 ml of Ringer's lactate solution with added protein. Finally, if it is anticipated that he is to be without oral intake for a few days, he should be given 40 to 80 mM of KCl daily.

Moderation in transfusion has already been mentioned. If the patient is to receive only 500 to 1,000 ml of blood transfusion, it is advisable for him to be awake before it is given, so that he can complain of the early symptoms of a transfusion reaction (itching, restlessness, fever, pain in the back); it may be wise to omit such transfusion completely, realizing that the patient's own albumin synthesis and erythropoiesis will soon compensate for such minor losses. If more blood must be given, one must recall the readiness with which massive blood transfusion produces alkalosis after trauma, through the combination of an aldosterone effect and the oxidation of sodium citrate to sodium bicarbonate (see Syndrome 19).

The use of antibiotics and vitamins is beyond the scope of this chapter. The use of large volume infusions of fluid to maintain dosage of drugs is one of the common causes of overwatering and oversalting, as already mentioned. Frequently, to save the patient the discomfort of repeated venipuncture, a "keep open" intravenous is left in; if poorly guarded, this may also result in overinfusion of fluid. In such a situation the use of a heparin lock intravenous catheter may save the patient the venipunctures without challenging him with an overinfusion of fluid.

Guides to Progress

Repetitive laboratory determinations after injury have become a costly hospital habit. Prior to operation, or as soon as possible after injury, a simple laboratory profile should be undertaken to assess renal function, the presence or absence of diabetes, and the normal homeostatic relationship of ions and acids. Hematocrit, blood urea nitrogen, blood sugar, sodium potassium, chloride, bicarbonate—all analyzed on venous blood—should suffice.

On the first postoperative morning a repetition of these measurements is advisable in anyone with severe trauma. If convalescence is normal, such chemical determinations need not be repeated for 48 to 72 hours and, if normal at that time, can be discontinued.

If the patient's condition is more complicated—if he develops infection or has a large dissection area, burn or thrombosis, heart disease, diabetes, or an acid-base disorder—careful planning of the nature and frequency of chemical tests will effect not only an economy of funds but an economy of blood. It is not unusual for patients to lose 350 to 500 ml of blood in the first 10 days if overzealous blood sampling for repetitive chemical determinations is made a habit.

SYNDROMES RELATED TO STARVATION AND INTRAVENOUS FEEDING

Syndrome 16. Cellular Steal

Definition, Terminology, and Related Terms

This term is used to denote a monovalent deficiency, usually of a mineral, an electrolyte, or a vitamin, brought on in a starving patient by the initiation of cellular anabolism with intravenous macronutrients. As an example, the case of zinc deficiency is described here. *Zinc deficiency* is therefore an analogous term as are, under other circumstances, *potassium deficiency, phosphate deficiency, monovalent deficiency,* and various *vitamin deficiencies.*

Clinical Setting

Prolonged starvation, followed by macronutrient provision intravenously without one or more key anabolic elementary requirements.

Addition or Subtraction

This might be thought of as a subtraction syndrome, since it is the lack of a single element or compound that brings it on. Rather than simple lack, however, it is the *failure to provide the element during a period of cellular anabolism* that causes the disorder. It is therefore a syndrome of *addition failure.*

Body Composition and Body Weight

The characteristic situation compositionally is that of prior global weight loss (or "balanced starvation") through the loss of fat and muscle tissue. Then, with the addition of intravenous (or oral) feeding of a highly purified or unbalanced food mixture (an example would be amino acids plus glucose without additives of any sort), cellular anabolism and protein synthesis suddenly recommence. The occurrence of cellular protein synthesis without the trace substance lacking, "steals" this material from its available concentration in the extracellular fluid. Concentration in plasma abruptly falls, and the signs and symptoms of deficiency develop.

It is a platitude to suggest that deficiency syndromes (examples: zinc deficiency or potassium deficiency) are poorly correlated with the plasma concentration but are more a product of total body stores. Yet this is only partly true. The lowering of body stores renders the patient *vulnerable* to the acute fall in plasma concentration which, in turn, produces the acute peripheral symptoms and signs.

In the case of zinc, this element is required for the synthesis of a large number of zinc metalloenzymes. If protein anabolism commences without it, plasma concentration is "robbed" as the only available source of zinc. Thus, while chronic balanced starvation may produce little change in the plasma zinc concentration, and no skin changes of zinc deficiency, it falls drastically with beginning anabolism in its absence. The signs suddenly appear. In hospital care this is most noticeable in patients given hyperalimentation intravenously in which the single element is lacking.

Abnormalities of Autoregulation

Autoregulation of the body content of minerals such as zinc, magnesium, manganese, chromium, and cobalt is not well understood. There is a good deal of information on autoregulation of certain electrolytes, such as potassium, sodium, and phosphate. In the monovalent cellular steal syndromes of trace mineral deficiency, abnormalities of autoregulation involve both intracellular and plasma concentrations.

But far more important are the disorders of protein synthesis that result when general anabolism commences in the absence of these elements. In the case of zinc there is every reason to believe, as with iron, that when a complex organic molecule containing the element (a zinc metalloenzyme or hemoglobin, for example) is broken down, the heavy metal is recycled and can be incorporated into a new molecule being synthesized. It is only when there is a lack of that element in the extracellular fluid, and synthesis has begun, that the deficiency becomes manifest. In the case of zinc, this produces the symptoms of zinc deficiency, which, in the acute form, consist of a papular eruption around the mouth, lips and tongue, often with secondary staphylococcal infection; loss of hair; and dermatitis of the extremities (acrodermatitis). In growing children, protein synthesis occurring in the absence of zinc produces these manifestations, anabolism being the result of normal growth in the absence of the element, rather than macronutrient-induced growth, as is seen in the treatment of adult starvation.

In the case of the iron example already mentioned, an analogous situation prevails. When acute hemorrhage occurs (i.e., balanced loss of all the components of blood), the initial findings in the peripheral blood or marrow do not suggest deficiency of any element other than a gross reduction in the red cell volume. It is days, weeks, or months later—if red cell synthesis is again begun, but without provision of adequate iron—that the so-called "iron deficiency anemia" occurs. This is a classic example of the cellular steal syndrome and is accompanied by very low plasma iron concentrations with normal or elevated concentrations of the transport protein.

Treatment

The treatment consists of providing the missing element. The effects are often dramatic and virtually immediate. Of all the nutritional syndromes, monovalent deficiencies of this type are among the most rewarding for their consideration, recognition, and treatment.

Determination of the plasma zinc concentration is not always easy; the same goes for chromium, cobalt, manganese. Determination of plasma concentrations of iron, folate, and other elements or compounds notable for monovalent deficiency during intravenous feeding are more straightforward. There is not space here to review all the different treatment modalities that can be used depending on the element missing. In the case of zinc, if a patient has the clinical manifestations of zinc deficiency, zinc should be given intravenously in small doses. It might as well be given in a trace mineral solution containing other trace minerals.

Syndrome 17. Parenteral Nutrition Overload Syndromes

Definition, Terminology, and Related Terms

This is not one, but a series of several syndromes of fluid overload or overuse of parenteral nutrition solutions. These will be described briefly under several headings.

Syndrome 17-I. Parenteral Nutrition: Fluid Overload

This is to be compared with Syndrome 7, *Oversalting—Extracellular Fluid Excess,* and Syndrome 10, *Overhydration—Hypotonicity.* With

Table 10-18. *Hyperosmolar, Nonketotic, Hyperglycemic Coma (Syndrome 17-II)*

		Major Findings	
	Unit	Mild	Severe
Hematocrit	% cells	45	55
Plasma protein	gm/dl	6.0–6.5	6.5–7.0
Plasma tonicity	mOsm/L	320	390
Plasma nonelectrolyte tonicity	mOsm/L	10	20
Plasma sodium	mEq/L	155	185
Plasma chloride	mEq/L	140	170
Std. bicarbonate	mEq/L	27	22
Plasma potassium	mEq/L	4.5	6.5
Blood urea nitrogen	mg/dl	20–40	80–120
Blood sugar	mg/dl	175	1500
Central venous pressure	cm H_2O	5–15	20–40

TPN solutions,* the exact response of the patient to an overload depends to some extent on his prior condition and the nature of the fluids given. All intravenous nutrition is in a sense a race between provision of substrate and utilization; if the former prevails, utilization and excretion are unable to keep up and an overload syndrome of some type results.

Because of the high solute content, an acute overload readily produces pulmonary edema under almost any circumstance, and a high urine volume is a first warning. If a solution is given briskly, an overload will produce pulmonary edema without a marked increase in chamber pressures. The warning signals here are to be found, over the short-term, in a persistently high urine volume (assuming renal function to approximate the normal); consistent urine outputs of greater than 100 ml/hour for three hours or more strongly suggest that the patient is fighting off a fluid overload. Other indices constitute a warning: anomalous weight gain, fall in hematocrit or protein concentration, rise in plasma osmolality (see below). The ominous finding in all cases, however, is a finding of bubbly wet rales at the lung bases and, in many cases, a beginning rise in central venous pressure. If amino acids are given, disorders of mental and CNS function result from overload (see below).

*TPN refers to "total parenteral nutrition." Whether or not the nutrition is total is a side issue in this chapter. This refers to large amounts of parenteral nutritive substances given intravenously. The slang term "TPN" is used for brevity.

Syndrome 17-II. Hyperosmolar Nonketotic Hyperglycemic Coma in TPN (Table 10-18)

This is a highly specific syndrome that can be produced by overload of rich parenteral feeding solutions containing a large amount of low-molecular-weight solute, and particularly large amounts of glucose (as well as by tube feedings). See Table 10-13 for "solute loading hypertonicity," of which this is a remarkable exaggeration. A notable event here is the finding not only of high plasma tonicity (for example, 350 mOsm/L or higher), but excessively high glucose concentrations (as high as 1,500 mg/percent). From the first description of this syndrome, it was noted that this high blood glucose was not accompanied by an appropriate insulin concentration or degree of ketosis. Excessive urine volumes for several previous days are a characteristic sign of the persistent solute diuresis that underlies the dehydration.

Treatment consists in providing water at modest load rates to provide the kidneys with enough water to float out the excess solute. Beware overtreatment with water! As previously described, overwatering is a hazard in treatment of any form of hypertonicity, in which excretion of excess solute must be considered as well as rehydration.

The addition of insulin is essential. The plasma insulin concentration is found to be inappropriately low for the degree of hyperglycemia, and yet, there is no permanent damage to the pancreas. It was thought for a time that this indicated a sort of "pancreatic exhaustion" syndrome, analogous in this sense to pituitary-induced diabetes mellitus. This is an aspect of the syndrome that is still not well understood. After a few days of treatment with insulin, no more insulin is usually required.

If unrecognized, this situation is rapidly fatal. Its persistence, even for 24 hours (once the extreme hypertonicity and hyperglycemia have developed), may be considered to be life-threatening. Its avoidance is clearly a matter of awareness in monitoring, especially a check on the plasma osmolality, plasma sodium concentration, and plasma glucose. The calculation of "unaccounted or nonelectrolyte tonicity" shows extreme values in this syndrome. Sudden emergence of hyperglycemia in a patient who has previously tolerated TPN well is usually associated with sepsis.

Syndrome 17-III. Hyperphosphatemia in TPN

Hyperphosphatemia occurs in parenteral nutrition when large amounts of phosphorus-containing solutions are given, especially in the presence of borderline renal failure. The most common cause of this is the administration of large amounts of intravenous fat emulsion in the presence of poor renal function. Stabilizing phosphatides in the commercial fat emulsion known as "Intralipid" contain organic phosphorus. As this material is metabolized and hydrolyzed, inorganic phosphate is released to the extracellular fluid, and if renal function is not normal, it produces a rapidly rising phosphate. This can be accompanied by a falling calcium concentration and may be part of the pathogenesis of the pseudohyperparathyroidism mentioned below, since a chronic imbalance of this type should stimulate parathyroid function much as in long-standing uremia. A rising inorganic phosphate concentration far out of proportion to the rise in BUN or creatinine is the clue that this complication of parenteral nutrition is occurring. A high parathormone concentration confuses the diagnosis, but does not rule it out.

Syndrome 17-IV. Hypercalcemia in TPN

In the early days of total parenteral nutrition, many patients were reported to have a syndrome closely resembling hyperparathyroidism. In one or two instances, exploration of the parathyroid gland was undertaken or was imminent before the nature of the syndrome was recognized.

This is not necessarily due to the excessive infusion of calcium, but is a more subtle complication of total parenteral nutrition, not always well understood. An acutely threatened hyperphosphatemia might be one aspect. Contrariwise, the chronic infusion of a TPN mixture without any phosphorus in it at all would be associated with hypophosphatemia, and this might be accompanied by a high calcium concentration even in the absence of hyperparathormonemia. In some of these instances, elevated levels of parathormone in the blood have been reported, however.

In any patient receiving total parenteral nutrition who is considered to be suffering from hyperparathyroidism, it is absolutely essential to discontinue all parenteral feeding solutions for at least 7 to 10 days to determine whether or not the patient actually has hyperparathyroidism. There are few situations in human nutrition in which the lack of large amounts of macronutrients for 7 to 10 days is in any way threatening.

Syndrome 17-V. The Satiety Syndrome in TPN

About 25 years ago, when a fat emulsion known as "Lipomul" was available, some studies were carried out in normal human volunteers in whom normal dietary intake was continued by mouth and a superimposed large supply of calories in the form of fat emulsion was provided. Fever, right upper quadrant pain, and deterioration of liver function were reported. It was thought at that time that this was specific for fatty overload, was due to "Lipomul," and was pathognomonic of fatty liver.

More recently it has become evident that caloric super-supply far in excess of energy needs, whether as a result of the provision of fat or carbohydrate, can produce right upper quadrant pain and deterioration of liver function (as manifested by a rise in transaminase enzymes and, in some cases, in bilirubin). This can result from overloads of either carbohydrate or fat, but with fat it may well be more common. More recently a case report has suggested that overloads of carbohydrate that are excessive in relation to the provision of protein precursors, such as amino acids, can likewise produce liver functional changes. Unpublished data from our laboratory corroborate this.

The satiety syndrome is defined as that of a patient who is being given more caloric supply than required. This is usually manifested by a supracaloric intake of either carbohydrate or fat, or a feeding that is at an excessively high calorie: nitrogen ratio. Liver function deteriorates. If the patient is conscious, right upper quadrant pain is often a feature of this syndrome.

Patients with intravenous feeding for prolonged periods of time are subject to gallstones and the precipitation of sludge and mud in the biliary tract. Presumably part of the mechanism here is the lack of secretion of secretin and cholecystokinin in patients without any food intake by mouth. Right upper quadrant pain can therefore be confusing, signifying either the satiety syndrome or hepatobiliary disease.

It is important to understand that fatty liver is also produced by patients who lose their own body fat at excessively rapid rates of oxidation. An example would be excessive weight loss in small bowel shunt surgery. It has also been reported in ulcerative colitis with rapid weight loss. The mechanism is possibly the inability of the liver to adequately phosphorylate endogenous fat. It is conceivable that there is a kindred mechanism in the satiety syndrome in which fat may be appearing intravenously at a rate more rapid than hepatic metabolism can accommodate it.

Syndrome 17-VI. Amino Acid Overload in TPN

Early in our experience with intravenous feeding we encountered a few patients who, receiving central vein mixtures involving 2 to 4 liters of amino acid solution per day, showed some abnormalities of emotional or mental function. Often these patients were septic or had been acutely ill in the days preceding.

More recently it has become evident that patients may be especially sensitive to loading rates of the phenolic and polycyclic amino acids, particularly if sepsis and/or liver function impairment are present.

It is not clear at this time whether all these abnormalities have a single cause. Provision of carbohydrate alone lowers the plasma branched-chain amino acid concentration either in starvation or with the provision of amino acids intravenously. The provision of carbohydrate lowers the concentration of amino acids in patients who have been starving.

Summarizing these aspects, it appears that excessive amounts of amino acid, if not properly metabolized, can produce toxic manifestations, and that this syndrome is most marked in patients with sepsis or liver disease with respect to the phenolic amino acids (tyrosine and tryptophan, and possibly histidine and histamine). The clinical lesson is a simple one: if patients are receiving large amounts of amino acids and have any mental symptoms, sepsis, and/or liver disease, caution should be exercised. The determination of individual amino acids or an amino acid profile in the blood may at times be helpful.

A "balanced diet" is again emphasized as the surest guide to sound parenteral alimentation. Glucose assists not only in protein synthesis, but in the metabolism of amino acids; glucose likewise fosters normal metabolism of fat. If either glucose or fat is given in excess or alone, the situation is harmful. A balance not only in total amounts, but in relationship among constituents is essential. "Meat intoxication" can be produced by excess doses of amino acids by peripheral vein as well as by an Eck fistula or liver failure; hyperammonemia is not a feature in most of these cases.

Syndrome 17-VII. Acid-Base Distortion and Surgical Procrastination in TPN

Both alkalosis and acidosis (metabolic in both cases) can be made worse by large amounts of parenteral alimentation solutions, including amino acids, particularly when renal function is poor.

The pathogenesis is variable, depending on the clinical background of the patient.

When the loss of gastric juice is partly responsible for the alkalosis (gastric suction with an obstructed duodenal ulcer), the mechanism seems evident enough: with adequate energy and amino acids in good supply, gastric secretion is stimulated and supported at a high level. There may be some actual stimulation of gastrin by the amino acid mixture. The tube suction is actively maintained. Gastric losses are therefore high and continuing, and alkalosis becomes much worse. Large-scale infusions are also gastric secretogogue in effect. In a sense, this worsening of alkalosis is a byproduct of the "surgery of procrastination," all too common in total parenteral nutrition.

The worsening of metabolic acidosis with multiple amino acids is probably related to borderline renal function (especially in children with some evidence of renal tubular acidosis or in elderly adults who have had obstructive uropathy). In these situations, when global renal function is not reduced but the ability of the kidney to secrete a strongly acid urine has been compromised, the infusion of large amounts of amino acids, some of which are infused in the acidic form or as the amino acid hydrochloride, has a net acidifying effect on the extracellular phase, much as if it were an equal volume of dilute ammonium chloride.

These syndromes are mentioned briefly since, in our experience with parenteral alimentation patients, we have seen worsening of acidosis or of alkalosis on several occasions. Physicians are often mystified as to how a single form of intravenous nourishment can make either acidosis or alkalosis worse, seemingly direct opposites.

Related to this, in the general strategy of surgical care, is the prolonged and inadvisable procrastination regarding surgery itself, which sometimes occurs in patients on hyperalimentation, for whom almost indefinite postponement of needed surgery (e.g., for pancreatic abscess) is encouraged and tolerated because the patient appears to be maintaining "good nutrition." The worst example of alkalosis promoted by intravenous alimentation we have observed was a patient with high-grade outlet obstruction due to chronic duodenal ulcer, being treated on a Medical Department unit. He was kept in "good nutrition" for several weeks of total parenteral alimentation. His gastric juice outputs were gigantic. A severe gastric juice loss resulted, with typical hypochloremia and hypokalemia (Syndromes 11 and 13). He could be given additional potassium, and this helped somewhat, but the gastric juice volume persisted. The situation suggested that some element in the amino acid/glucose mixture acted as a strong gastric stimulus. This could either be the high load of sodium and chloride itself, which is a mild gastric secretogogue, or the presence of certain amino acids, which may stimulate gastrin production. This was a classic example of a case in which the best nutritional step for the patient was a surgical operation and the cessation of all efforts at intravenous feeding.

Syndrome 18. Insulin Anomalies in TPN

Syndrome 18-I. Weaning Syndrome: Lingering Hyperinsulinemia; Digestive Inhibition Prior to Weaning

The human pancreas has tremendous insulin production capacity. In individuals receiving glucose at concentrations around 5 percent, the blood sugar is maintained in a normal range and the plasma insulin rarely exceeds 8 mμ/ml. In high-dose glucose infusions (as in central vein alimentation), i.e., at glucose concentrations around 20 percent or higher (up to 80 mμ/ml) and total glucose loads of 500 gm/day or more, plasma insulin concentration ranges as high as 35 to 70 mμ/ml.

At these higher rates of glucose infusion with high plasma insulin concentration, the sudden cessation of glucose infusion will be followed by reactive hypoglycemia. In patients with heart disease this can be dangerous. In subjects undergoing surgical operations, it could lead to death if not recognized during anesthesia. The way to avoid this type of weaning syndrome is merely to reduce gradually the concentration of glucose by administering, after the hypoglycemic mixture, an infusion of 5 percent dextrose for 12 to 24 hours.

The provision of glucose intravenously inhibits gastric peristalsis and gastric secretions. This may be a part of the normal decline in gastric secretion that follows the intestinal phase of digestion and the normal postprandial hyperglycemia. Whatever its origin, the provision of high-calorie macronutrients by vein is inhibitory to gastric function.

Clinical evidence suggests that it is also inhibitory to small bowel motility, though this is less clearcut.

In any event, before the transition can be made from parenteral to oral nutrition, it is essential that the parenteral nutrition be stopped, even for several days or a week, to permit normal gastric responses, whether to the presence of food or to psychologic stimuli ("cephalic phase"), to manifest themselves. Although this is not a disorder of water and electrolyte metabolism, it is mentioned here because the undue prolonged continuation of parenteral alimentation may be due to this biofeedback mechanism, whereby the provision of the alimentation itself tends to inhibit its discontinuance.

Syndrome 18-II. Flask Insulin Hypoglycemia

Patients requiring insulin with hyperalimentation procedures (see below) are rare. It is most exceptional (less than 1 percent of instances) for ordinary hyperalimentation, even with concentrated central vein mixtures, to require concomitant insulin.

In patients with borderline diabetes, with overt diabetes following pancreatectomy, with pancreatitis, or with other diabetes-threatening situations, insulin must be used: Regular, or isophane insulin (NPH) should be given subcutaneously and the blood sugar and urine sugar used to monitor the insulin dose, just as in the treatment of a diabetic patient.

Under no circumstances should the insulin be added directly to the intravenous flask or bag, because of the danger of sudden, unintentional discontinuation of the infusion by displacement of the line, occlusion of the line if the patient lies on it, or interruption of the drip for anesthesia or some other purpose, which should be forbidden in any case.

With sudden cessation of an infusion containing both glucose and insulin, the glucose is oxidized within moments, whereas the insulin has a half-life of 6 to 12 hours, depending on the patient and the nature of the insulin used. This will produce an insulin reaction much more certainly and much more severely than the weaning syndrome already mentioned. It is for this reason that insulin should be given subcutaneously and should not be added to the infusion mix.

Syndrome 18-III. Latent Diabetes and Post-Traumatic Pseudo-Diabetes in TPN

This situation is recognized readily and is far less hazardous than the two syndromes of excessive insulin mentioned previously. The simplest forms of monitoring of parenteral nutrition will uncover hyperglycemia, glycosuria, or polyuria. Any high urine volume should of course be accompanied by studies of urine sugar. In post-traumatic diabetes, for instance after burns ("burn pseudo-diabetes"), after certain types of pancreatic resection, even though some pancreas is left behind, in pancreatitis, and in certain forms of trauma, one sees a tendency toward diabetes that mandates the temporary administration of insulin to normalize blood sugar. With a normal pancreas, infusions of high glucose loads produce blood sugars of 110 to 120 mg/dl fairly regularly. This mild hyperglycemia is harmless and is accompanied by an appropriate high level of insulin. If the blood sugar exceeds 150 mg/dl, the patient should be given insulin subcutaneously, with blood and urine sugars monitored as with any mild diabetic. We have seen insulin requirements as high as 40 units per day after severe burns, accentuated by the provision of large amounts of glucose intravenously. Upon recovery, the patient was totally free of any diabetic taint and carried a normal glucose tolerance curve.

SIX SYNDROMES OF DISORDERED ACID-BASE HOMEOSTASIS

In many of the foregoing syndromes of disordered body water and salt metabolism, there has been some reflection in acid-base distortion, sometimes a very important feature. In the following six syndromes, disorders of acid-base homeostasis predominate, and the disturbances of other ions or water distribution appear as secondary effects. In some instances, when repetitious description would result, cross-reference is indicated.

Confusion regarding terminology and mathematical expressions for disordered acid-base balance have led to much misunderstanding. We believe it is important to emphasize the Bronsted schema, namely, that the only acid is hydrogen ion and that bases are substances, such as bicarbonate or hydroxyl ion, that will accept hydrogen ion in buffer linkage. Most of the ionic components of human plasma, in the Bronsted schema, are therefore referred to as cations and anions and they include sodium, potassium, chloride, certain trace minerals, calcium, phosphorus, and magnesium.

On the mathematical side, it is possible to construct elaborate curvilinear plots or logarithmic analyses of hydrogen ion relationships, traceable in part to the fact that the conventional terminology of pH has been used for so many years and is based on the negative logarithm of the hydrogen ion concentration. We have preferred to continue to use the pH mode of expression rather than the H^+ concentration in most cases, since it is so widely adopted and so readily adapted to a wide variety of acid-base disorders. For graphic representation of acid-base disorders, we believe that the simple linear plot of pH against bicarbonate (the pH-bicarbonate diagram), as illustrated in Davenport's book [1], is by far the simplest and most useful. Using this, it is possible to discern at a glance the mixture of metabolic and respiratory components and to understand significant departures from expectation. By converting pH to direct hydrogen ion concentration, it is possible also to make simple linear expressions for "pure" respiratory and metabolic acid-base disturbances. Some of these formulations are shown in Table 10-3.

One other preliminary note concerns the "standard bicarbonate." Since there is no direct

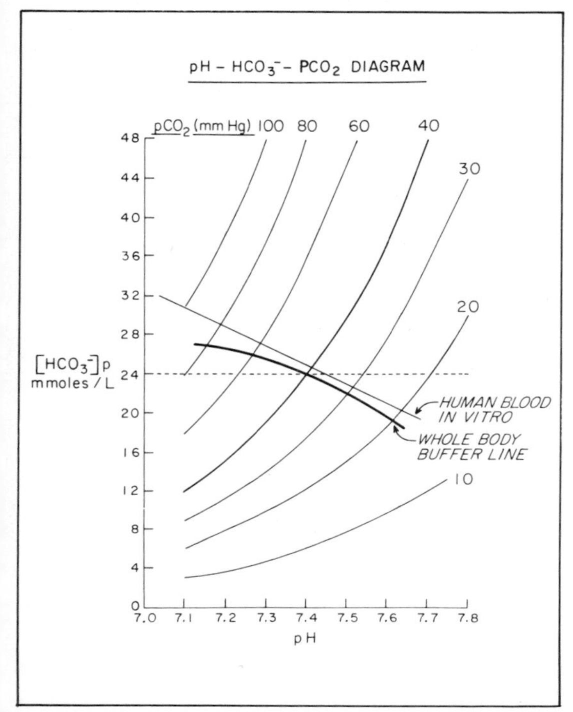

Figure 10-1. *Shown at right, a pH bicarbonate diagram as first developed by Davenport. It is the simplest way to analyze acid base disturbances. Every student should be able to draw one reasonably accurately on a free-hand basis. The in vitro blood buffer line shows what the change in bicarbonate and pH would be with a progressive change in carbon dioxide tension if there were no other metabolic, renal, or compensatory mechanisms and if one were dealing with whole blood in a test tube. Actually, the in vivo whole body buffer line is much less steep and is shown as such because blood in the body is in contact with extracellular and cellular buffers, which modulate the change in bicarbonate with alteration in PCO_2. Each student should take one or two clinical examples of acid-base disturbance encountered in the hospital and locate them on this pH bicarbonate diagram. Enter the bicarbonate (sometimes given as the "plasma CO_2") as best estimated from your lab, and the PCO_2 and calculate the pH. Check it. More complicated curvilinear diagrams are adapted for the use of certain commercial acid-base analytic machinery and are far more difficult to visualize graphically. The terms* base deficit *or* base excess *add little conceptual clarity to the simple expression of pH, bicarbonate, and PCO_2.*

analytic method for bicarbonate, it must always be estimated from a direct analysis of the arterial CO_2 content, with appropriate corrections for carbon dioxide tension and pH. The result is a figure for bicarbonate referred to as the "standard bicarbonate." The corrected venous CO_2 content can be thus used if performed on whole blood. It is this simple form of expression that we use for bicarbonate, namely the pH and PCO_2 of whole blood measured at two separated pH levels, and appropiately corrected to normal carbon dioxide tension. This sort of correction is evident from the pH-bicarbonate diagram previously mentioned. To depart from this simple terminology by introducing the phrases "base excess," and "negative base excess" (to signify a base deficit), appears to us to be an elaborate and scholastic nicety that only confuses the clinician. Better, by far, to stick with the simple "standard bicarbonate," understanding its derivation and meaning (Figure 10-1).

Syndrome 19. Acute Hypercapnia (Table 10-19)

Definition, Terminology, and Related Terms

Acute hypercapnia is an acute elevation of the partial pressure of carbon dioxide in the blood. *Acute hypoventilation* refers to the usual mechanism; *acute respiratory acidosis* is synonymous. *Hypoventilation acidosis* is synonymous.

Clinical Setting

Acute Hypoventilation

1. *Central*—drug or brain tumor.
2. *Nerve conduction or mechanical*—injury in the neck or phrenic nerve areas and/or diaphragm, chest wall, pleural space (pneumo- or hemothorax).
3. *Pulmonary*—acute failure of ventilation due to tracheal stenosis, tracheal impingement, tracheobronchial disease, chronic bronchopulmonary disease with an acute exacerbation, pneumothorax.

Table 10-19. *Hypercapnia (Syndromes 19 and 20)*

		Major Findings	
	Unit	Acute	Chronic
Body weight	Change	None	Gain in CHF
Hematocrit	% cells	38–42	45–50
Plasma proteins	gm/dl	6.0–6.5	7.0
Plasma tonicity	mOsm/L	295–300	295–300
Plasma nonelectrolyte tonicity	mOsm/L	5	5
Plasma sodium	mEq/L	143	150
Plasma chloride	mEq/L	103	80
Std. bicarbonate	mEq/L	29–30	45
Blood urea nitrogen	mg/dl	15	50
Blood PCO_2	mm Hg	85	60
Blood PaO_2	mm Hg	85	70
Blood pH	Units	7.05	7.25
Blood oxy Hgb D.C.		Right shift	Left shift

Addition or Subtraction

This is an addition disorder of endogenous source, the CO_2 arising from the normal metabolism.

Body Composition and Body Weight

There is no acute change in body composition, save for slight increase in total body carbon dioxide. There is no acute change in body weight.

Abnormalities of Autoregulation

This is clearly a disorder due to an abnormality of the prime homeostatic regulator of carbon dioxide partial pressures: pulmonary alveolar ventilation. There is no compensation for this save for the excretion of an acid urine and bicarbonate generation. This is such a slow and ineffective regulator that it is of little short-term significance. Acute hypercapnia can result from rebreathing or from acute upper respiratory tract obstruction, and progress to virtually lethal proportions within minutes.

Elevation of the partial pressure of carbon dioxide in the blood (PCO_2) is the most common and the characteristic *laboratory finding* in this disorder. This is best measured on arterial blood, freshly sampled. However, in acute respiratory acidosis, one should not stand on ceremony for arterial puncture, since the venous PCO_2 also is markedly elevated. There is an immediate slight increase in bicarbonate, as shown by the whole body buffer line, but this has little or no significance in acute hypoventilation.

The concomitant arterial oxygen tension is almost always low, but may not be threatening, depending on the balance between ventilation and perfusion in the pulmonary circulation.

Arterial pH values may fall below 6.95 within 20 to 30 minutes of the onset of rebreathing or acute hypoventilation, with PCO_2 approaching 100 mm Hg. When the onset is less acute, as in pneumothorax, hydrothorax, or early pulmonary edema, the fall in pH is much more gradual, and the arterial oxygen desaturation is due largely to shunting of blood through nonventilated portions of the lung rather than hypoventilation as such.

TREATMENT

Adequate ventilation. There is no substitute or alternative treatment. It is beyond the scope of this chapter to deal with the various respiratory steps taken to restore ventilation to normal.

No other form of acidosis lowers the whole blood pH as rapidly or to such profound levels. The principal laboratory guides to progress are therefore a reduction of the partial pressure of carbon dioxide and restoration of pH to normal.

Acute trauma or wounds to the upper airway, bleeding directly into the bronchus, rupture of the bronchus, mediastinal emphysema, and bilateral pneumothorax are all acute traumatic events that demand immediate clearing of the airway by surgical steps, usually including endotracheal intubation or tracheotomy. Details are beyond the scope of this chapter. Very aggressive surgical steps are often required for the correction of this respiratory disorder.

Syndrome 20. Chronic Hypercapnia (Table 10-19)

DEFINITION, TERMINOLOGY, AND RELATED TERMS

Chronic hypercapnia is underventilation, with hypercapnia that is long-standing enough to permit a compensatory metabolic change to occur. *Chronic respiratory acidosis* is synonymous. *Compensated respiratory acidosis* is, in a sense, a misnomer, since the compensation is never complete. *Respiratory acidosis with metabolic alkalosis* is a confusing mixture of terminologies. As long as the hydrogen ion concentration is elevated and the pH lower than normal, this must be referred to as acidosis, even though the metabolic changes that occur are "in the direction of" metabolic alkalosis. *Chronic obstructive pulmonary disease (COPD)* refers to the disease usually at fault.

CLINICAL SETTING

1. Chronic heavy *smoking* habit.
2. *Asthma, emphysema,* bronchiectasis on the basis of intrinsic infection.
3. Asthma and emphysema on the basis of *allergic* disease.
4. Chronic *dust diseases* and other chronic inhalation disorders producing emphysema and respiratory insufficiency.

ADDITION OR SUBTRACTION

This is an addition disorder due to the accumulation of carbon dioxide of endogenous sources, when pulmonary excretion is inadequate; it is in part compensated by the renal excretion of metabolic acid, a subtraction component. This accounts for the characteristic elevation of bicarbonate concentration and lowering of plasma chloride concentration.

BODY COMPOSITION AND BODY WEIGHT

There is no essential change in body weight through chronic obstructive pulmonary disease, per se. As the disease progresses, the sufferer becomes thin and wasted, possibly owing to the sheer effort and energy cost of respiration. Finally, if right heart failure is produced, there is weight gain with edema.

ABNORMALITIES OF AUTOREGULATION

As noted under Syndrome 18 (Acute Hypercapnia), the homeostatic regulator, pulmonary excretion of carbon dioxide, is itself impaired, accounting for the disorder. In the more chronic form, another homeostatic regulator consists in the renal excretion of urine of low pH and high titratable acidity, and containing large amounts of chloride. Thus, the change in the direction of "metabolic alkalosis" may actually lower the hydrogen ion concentration and raise the pH so that there is a restoration toward normal, if not fully to normal; the characteristic chemical signs of this are the low plasma chloride concentration and elevated bicarbonate, and a urine of pH as low as 4.5 if renal tubular function is good.

Once chronic congestive heart failure (cor pulmonale) becomes manifest, the renal excretion of acid becomes less efficient and the acidosis becomes more severe. Any supervening infection, such as bronchopneumonia, or transient respiratory infection of the epidemic virus variety, makes the condition much worse and may be fatal.

In acute hypercapnia the PCO_2 may rise to levels of 70 to 120 mm Hg. This is the characteristic *laboratory finding*. In chronic hypercapnia the PCO_2 values rarely exceed 50 or 60 mm Hg. Even those levels are harbingers of extreme illness if some pneumonic infection is superimposed. Bicarbonate values, usually normal in acute hypercapnia, may now exceed 35 to 50 mEq/L. Chloride concentration is usually depressed to the region of 75 to 90 mEq/L. Urine pH is acid.

Treatment

Normalization of ventilation is the ideal. In chronic obstructive lung disease it may be difficult or impossible to achieve. If, in chronic lung disease, superimposed infection or pulmonary edema develops, treatment of the infection may ameliorate the situation, at least temporarily. Anything that interferes with the excretion of an acid urine, such as abnormalities of renal tubular function or renal failure, inhibits the metabolic compensation of chronic hypercapnia and makes the disease much more difficult to treat, and much more apt to become lethal. The lethal mechanism is usually cardiac failure or acute arrhythmia.

Syndrome 21. Acute Hypocapnia (Table 10-20)

Definition, Terminology, and Related Terms

Acute hypocapnia is acute hyperventilation, with depression of the carbon dioxide tension in the blood. *Hyperventilation tetany* refers to one occasional end result. *Respiratory alkalosis* is a synonymous term.

Clinical Setting

1. *Anxiety* or emotional excitement with hyperventilation.
2. *Induced* hyperventilation due to an erroneous setting of machine-assisted ventilation.
3. With pulmonary *shunting,* a persistent hyperventilation of the perfused segment as seen in post-traumatic pulmonary insufficiency.

Addition or Subtraction

This is a subtraction disorder due to excessive removal of carbon dioxide from the blood.

Body Composition and Body Weight

There is no gross change in body composition and no essential change in body weight.

Abnormalities of Autoregulation

With chronic respiratory alkalosis, one would predict some compensatory metabolic changes. There is a decreased renal secretion of acid and a tendency toward a compensatory metabolic acidosis, with depression of bicarbonate. This is a weak response, and it is of more theoretic than clinical interest. Acute hypocapnia can progress to severe degrees of alkalosis with tetany and/or cardiac arrhythmias in short order (minutes or hours).

The blood carbon dioxide tension may fall below 30 mm Hg with great rapidity, this being the characteristic *laboratory finding* of the disease. Levels around 30 to 35 mm Hg are characteristic of most acutely ill patients, particularly those on assisted ventilation. If the PCO_2 falls below 15 mm Hg, alkalosis can become extremely severe (pH over 7.70), and there is a threat of sudden death due to cardiac arrhythmias. Characteristically, potassium is depressed—again an association of the hypokalemia with

Table 10-20. *Acute Hypocapnia (Syndrome 21)*

		Major Findings	
	Unit	Typical	Extreme
Body weight	Change	No change	No change
Hematocrit	% cells	38–42	43–46
Plasma protein	gm/dl	6.0–6.5	6.5–7.0
Plasma sodium	mEq/L	140	140
Plasma chloride	mEq/L	100	100
Plasma potassium	mEq/L	3.5–4.0	2.5–3.0
Std. bicarbonate	mEq/L	24	15
Blood pH	Units	7.65	7.75
Blood PCO_2	mm Hg	25	10
Blood PaO_2	mm Hg	80–90	80–90

alkalosis. In acute hypercapnia, whole blood pH falls directly to low levels with great rapidity. Here, conversely, in hypocapnia, whole blood pH rises to levels higher than in any other situation and is characteristically highly refractory to treatment; pH values as high as 7.75 have been recorded. If the patient is digitalized, digitalis toxicity can occur without any change in dose or blood level.

TREATMENT

Normalization of ventilation is the only treatment for this disorder. There are many ways of doing this in patients on respiratory assistance. In acute hypocapnia, an essentially respiratory situation, treatment by the infusion of metabolic acids is both unavailing and dangerous.

Alkalosis shifts the oxyhemoglobin dissociation curve to the left without any acute change in synthesis of diphosphoglycerate. This produces an anomalous failure to oxygenate the tissues, even though the hyperventilation would appear to be a sort of "super oxygenation." There is, therefore, a rising concentration of lactate which, in this disorder, may reach levels around 3.0 mM/L, a lesser elevation of lactate than is associated with low-flow acidosis. The anomalous association of lactate accumulation with alkalosis should be noted. If carbon monoxide poisoning is suspected, if the patient has been a heavy smoker or has been in a closed space with a conflagration, or if the patient has been exposed to drugs or industrial toxins, the oxyhemoglobin dissociation curve should be measured. A markedly left shifted oxyhemoglobin dissociation curve may also be associated with hypophosphatemia, and an anomalous increase in lactate owing to failure of tissue oxygenation. A mild hypocapnia is the tip-off to the compensatory hyperventilation.

Syndrome 22. Post-Traumatic Alkalosis (Table 10-21)

DEFINITION, TERMINOLOGY, AND RELATED TERMS

Post-traumatic alkalosis is the alkalosis characteristically observed in the severely injured patient, the result of multifactorial pathogenesis, as will be described. *Transfusion alkalosis* refers to one very important component of post-traumatic alkalosis without reference to the remainder of the picture. *Post-traumatic pulmonary insufficiency with hyperventilation* refers to a component, likewise. *Acute post-traumatic*

Table 10-21. *Post-Traumatic Alkalosis (Syndrome 22)*

		Major Findings	
	Unit	Typical	Extreme
Body weight	Change	Gain 1 kg	Gain 3–4 kg
Hematocrit	% cells	37	37
Plasma protein	gm/dl	6.0	5.0
Plasma sodium	mEq/L	135	130
Plasma chloride	mEq/L	90	70
Plasma potassium	mEq/L	3.5–4.0	2.5–3.0
Std. bicarbonate	mEq/L	28	32
Blood pH	Unit	7.55	7.70
Blood PCO_2	mm Hg	30	25
Blood PaO_2	mm Hg	70	60
Blood lactate	mM/L	2.0	4.0

hyperaldosteronism refers to a third component. None of these terms is synonymous with the total picture as described here.

Clinical Setting

1. *Severe injury* with adequate resuscitation.
2. *Severe injury,* particularly if associated with:
   a. Prolonged *nasogastric suction* with removal of gastric juice.
   b. Multiple *transfusions* with transfusion alkalosis.
   c. A prior volume-reduction with a prolonged *aldosterone* effect on the kidney.
   d. Some pulmonary shunting with hyperventilation of perfused segments.

Addition or Subtraction

As evidenced from the above, this is a combined syndrome. The addition of sodium citrate in transfusion obviously contributes to the alkalosis, while renal excretion of acid, hyperventilation, and gastric juice loss are all subtraction components in a multifactorial disorder whose net vector is in the alkalotic direction.

Body Composition and Body Weight

As noted in the section on the normal post-operative patient, severe trauma brings in its wake a transiently elevated level of catecholamines in the blood, followed by a gradually rising level of blood glucagon. There is gluconeogenesis at the expense of muscle protein. Fat oxidation is hastened. This net combination produces weight loss, and that is the typical situation during post-traumatic alkalosis. Nonetheless, overinfusion of sodium-rich fluid greatly accentuates the disorder and may obliterate the normal weight loss. After severe trauma patients should be expected to lose some weight; the net deficit in body composition is negligible through the oxidation of this small amount of fat and protein. If the weight loss is obliterated by infusions, it usually means that too much fluid has been given.

Abnormalities of Autoregulation

As is evident from the foregoing, this disorder, like several other syndromes described herein, is a mixture of pathogenic factors, some of which are the result of the exaggerated operation of normal homeostatic regulators. Post-traumatic hyperaldosteronism is an obvious example here. In general, any stress that tends to produce hypokalemia and alkalosis (e.g., liver disease with hemorrhage and transfusion) is made much worse by the superimposition of the surgical operation because of its greatly increased stimulus to adrenocortical production of aldosterone. Clearly, this should be taken into consideration by the surgeon in the administration of potassium-enriched acidifying solutions such as KCl.

The typical combination of *laboratory findings* in post-traumatic alkalosis on the second or third day is a pH mildly elevated at 7.55; a chloride mildly depressed at 85 mEq/L; and potassium depressed at 2.5 to 3.0 mEq/L. Serum sodium concentration is usually 135 to 138 mEq/L. Oxygenation may be borderline, as indicated by an arterial oxygen tension of 80 mm Hg on room air. There are rapid respiration and hyperventilation of portions of lung normally perfused. The carbon dioxide tension is in the region of 28 to 34 mm Hg, and the urine is acid, containing large amounts of potassium and almost no sodium.

Treatment

The best treatment of post-traumatic alkalosis is merely the continued energetic management of the patient to maintain good tissue perfusion, bearing in mind the factors that will make the alkalosis worse. Gastrointestinal suction should be discontinued as soon as possible. As already mentioned, some of the fluid removed by aspiration can be replaced, as long as the gastrointestinal tract is prevented from accumulating swallowed air. The administration of acidifying solutions such as KCl should be liberal (e.g., 120 to 160 mM per day). If hyperventilation is a persistent component and the patient is on assisted ventilation, it is possible to normalize the carbon dioxide tension. In extreme cases with continued obstinate inability to excrete sodium in an acid potassium-rich urine, the use of aldosterone antagonists is rational, but should be done with great care in cardiac patients who have been digitalized. Treatment with HCl is rational, if carried out with caution and close monitoring.

Post-traumatic alkalosis in mild form is both common and harmless.

The principal hazard of post-traumatic alkalosis when it is severe lies in the production of cardiac arrhythmias and increased sensitivity to digitalis, arrhythmias that may be sudden and fatal and often come without warning. In addition, there is a tendency to narcosis, sleepiness, and lack of normal cerebral function.

Reduction of bicarbonate and pH to normal with the opening up of urinary excretion of sodium are signs that the post-traumatic alkalosis is abating. Post-traumatic alkalosis of very severe grades can occur after open heart surgery; as noted several times in the preceding, hypokalemia and alkalosis are especially hazardous in cardiac patients.

Syndrome 23. Base Loss Acidosis (Table 10-22)

Definition, Terminology, and Related Terms

Base loss acidosis is a metabolic acidosis due to a desalting water loss in which the fluid lost from the body has an alkaline pH. There are several other types of metabolic acidosis, including renal acidosis and diabetic acidosis, that will not be discussed here. Base loss acidosis is the most common form of subtraction acidosis found in surgical patients.

Clinical Setting

1. *Diarrheal disease* in the infant or adult, including salmonella, typhoid, cholera, ulcerative colitis, Crohn's disease.
2. *Pancreatic fistula.*
3. *Small bowel fistula.*

Addition or Subtraction

This is a subtraction acidosis, pure and simple.

Table 10-22. *Base Loss Acidosis (Syndrome 23)*

(See Table 10-9. Desalting Water Loss, for general setting)
The acid-base changes depend on the extent of the loss of sodium bicarbonate in gastrointestinal secretions (such as diarrhea), the extent of the ventilatory-respiratory compensation (hypocapnia), and the ability of the kidney to secrete an acid urine. Three groups are discernible:

		Acute	Chronic	
	Unit	Severe Acute	Poorly Compensated (Pulmonary and Renal Disease)	Well Compensated
Std. bicarbonate	mEq/L	15	10	10
Blood pH	Units	7.25	7.16	7.35
Blood PCO_2	mm Hg	35	30	20
Blood PaO_2	mm Hg	80	80	90
Urine pH	Units	5.0	6.0	4.5
Urine titratable acidity		Low	Low	Very high

Body Composition and Body Weight

Body composition shows a marked reduction in the total exchangeable sodium; there is loss of weight corresponding to the desalting water loss.

Abnormalities of Autoregulation

The homeostatic regulator called into play here is renal conservation of sodium by both of the mechanisms that stimulate aldosterone—the renin-angiotensin mechanism on the one hand, and the ACTH on the other. This conservation mechanism may become chronically active in patients with ileostomies who are constantly in a mild state of hyperaldosteronism.

Though this homeostatic regulator tends to conserve sodium and favor loss of potassium in the urine, it is not particularly effective when the loss of alkaline juices from the body exceeds 1500 ml per day, a common occurrence in diarrheal diseases, intestinal fistulas, pancreatic fistulas, and the like.

The deep respirations so often seen in diabetic acidosis (an addition metabolic acidosis), compensating to some extent for addition of acid by ventilatory loss of carbon dioxide, are rarely seen here and would be of little effectiveness in any event.

In this type of metabolic acidosis, the typical *laboratory finding* is a pH that rarely falls below 7.25. In pure metabolic acidosis this is a dangerously low pH. Bicarbonate falls commensurately to the region of 15 mEq/L. Plasma sodium concentration usually drops and potassium concentration rises. The "anion gap" or difference between sodium and chloride concentrations will be narrowed to an extent usually proportionate to the fall in bicarbonate.

Treatment

As already indicated, desalting water loss is the ideal setting for the infusion of sodium-rich fluids. In this syndrome, in which acidosis is a complication, the infusion of sodium bicarbonate is uniquely appropriate; sodium lactate also can be used, the lactate being rapidly oxidized to bicarbonate.

It should be noted in passing that metabolic acidosis of the addition type (examples are renal acidosis and diabetic acidosis) should not be treated with sodium bicarbonate save with the

Table 10-23. *Low Flow Acidosis (Syndrome 24)*

		Major Findings	
	Unit	Typical	Extreme
Body weight	kg change	Falling	Falling rapidly
Hematocrit	% cells	37	30
Plasma protein	gm/dl	5.0	4.5
Plasma tonicity	mOsm/L	280	270
Plasma nonelectrolyte tonicity	mOsm/L	5–10	5–10
Plasma sodium	mEq/L	130	120
Plasma chloride	mEq/L	100	100
Std. bicarbonate	mEq/L	12	8
Blood lactate	mM/L	5	15
Blood urea nitrogen	mg/dl	15–30	70–90
Blood PCO_2	mm Hg	30	25
Blood PaO_2	mm Hg	70	60
Blood pH	Units	7.25	7.15
Blood oxy Hgb D.C.		Left shift	Right shift

most extreme caution, because of the danger of oversalting and cardiac failure. In the pure base loss acidosis, sodium bicarbonate infusion is most appropriate.

Syndrome 24. Low Flow Acidosis (Table 10-23)

Definition, Terminology, and Related Terms

Low flow acidosis is the lactic acidosis of the low flow state. *Lactic acidosis* refers to a chemical state, but without reference to the cause. *Hypoxic acidosis* is a misnomer, since ventilatory hypoxia is a weak stimulus to lactate generation. *Hypoperfusion acidosis* and *ischemic acidosis* are synonymous terms. *Shock acidosis* is synonymous; *washout acidosis* refers to an analogous situation arising from the reperfusion of localized ischemic tissue.

Clinical Setting

1. *Hypoperfusion of tissues due to shock,* and low flow states resulting from trauma.
2. *Hypoperfusion of tissues resulting from cardiac damage,* as in myocardial infarction with shock.
3. *Other low flow states* associated with trauma to the mediastinum or hemopericardium, and pericardial tamponade.
4. *Occlusion of the aorta* or other arteries, sometimes large enough in mass to produce a generalized acidosis, particularly when circulation is restored as a "washout effect."

Addition or Subtraction

This is an addition acidosis due to the accumulation of lactic acid within cells. In this regard it is unique, since the acidosis arises within the cells rather than within the extracellular fluid; the changes in blood are therefore but a dim reflection of the primary disorder within the cell.

Body Composition and Body Weight

Changes are not marked in most cases and, in any event, depend on the underlying cause and the rest of the clinical setting. Low flow states are usually associated with such severe stressful disease that rapid loss of body weight is the rule.

Abnormalities of Autoregulation

It is the intracellular acidosis, dimly perceived as an extracellular pH change and lactate accumulation, that is fundamentally at fault in low flow acidosis. Lactate is itself a harmless anionic intermediary in carbohydrate oxidation. It can be injected in large amounts without harm and is quickly oxidized in most situations. In the lactic acidosis of low flow state, the accumulation of extracellular lactate is a barometer of the extent of hydrogen ion accumulation within cells. The homeostatic regulator is therefore lactate oxidation, and in low flow state this cannot occur. If flow is returned to normal, lactate oxidation rapidly occurs, but it is noteworthy that patients that have been in a low flow state for a relatively long time may show residual lactate elevations for several days after recovery. Both hydrogen ion and lactate can be excreted by the kidney; in a low flow state renal function is essentially nil, and this pathway is unavailable. Upon return to normal, lactate can be burned in many tissues, notably heart and liver; it disappears rapidly. Treatment of patients in a low flow state by infusions of lactate-containing solutions, such as Ringer's lactate, does not make the disorder worse, because the lactate ion is merely a harmless bystander; it is the hydrogen ion that has been at fault. Ringer's lactate solution is buffered to a pH above that of normal blood in the pharmacy before it is used; while providing lactate, it does not present the threat of increasing the acidosis. If its infusion helps the circulation it may assist in cleaning the lactate.

Depression of plasma bicarbonate as a linear function of the lactate accumulation is the typical *laboratory finding* in almost all cases. The lactate accumulates at a more rapid rate than pyruvate, with an elevated lactate:pyruvate ratio, otherwise expressed as an accumulation of excess lactate. These various measurements of lactate and pyruvate are not clinically essential, but they may be helpful and instructive. The pH typically is in the region of 7.15 to 7.25. It must be emphasized again that pH values in this range are dangerous when they are of metabolic origin, whereas they are quickly produced and rectified when the cause is purely respiratory. The patient who has been in a low flow state and is observed to have a low plasma bicarbonate level with an arterial pH of 7.15 is in severe and dangerous low flow acidosis.

Treatment

The treatment of low flow acidosis is the restoration of tissue perfusion to normal. There can be no better example of the importance of viewing the patient in his entire perspective than the treatment of this particular form of metabolic acidosis by blood transfusion. Whatever steps are taken to restore flow to normal—and they include many details not covered in this section—the result should be an improvement in perfusion, with diffuse oxidation of lactate. In many instances, syndromes have been described in this chapter wherein surgical steps themselves are essential to the treatment of metabolic disorders. Low flow acidosis is the prototypic example. If this is due to hemorrhage, for example, or undrained sepsis, aggressive surgical steps, including major operation, may be necessary for its rectification. The infusion of sodium bicarbonate must be considered as both dangerous and temporizing. If large amounts are given, pulmonary edema and death will almost surely ensue. In the appropriate dosage, it may tide the patient through a difficult phase of low flow acidosis. Most important, however, is the realization that low flow acidosis is rather quickly rectified if tissue perfusion is returned to normal, and it is this, rather than the mere buffering of acid, that should be the objective of treatment.

Restoration of blood flow, urine volume, and tissue perfusion to normal is essential. The pH and plasma bicarbonate concentration are important guides to progress. If lactate itself has been measured, its gradual disappearance and oxidation is a demonstration that the metabolic products of the low flow state have been oxidized.

BIBLIOGRAPHY

Davenport, H. C. *The ABC of Acid Base Chemistry* (6th ed.). Chicago: University of Chicago Press, 1974.

Gamble, J. L. *Chemical Anatomy, Physiology and Pathology of Extracellular Fluid: A lecture syllabus* (6th ed.). Cambridge, MA: Harvard University Press, 1967.

Harper, H. A. *Review of Physiologic Chemistry* (14th ed.). Los Altos, CA: Lange, 1974.

Moore, F. D. *Metabolic Care of the Surgical Patient: III. Body Fluid and Electrolyte.* Philadelphia: Saunders, 1958.

Moore, F. D., et al. *The Body Cell Mass and Its Supporting Environment.* Philadelphia: Saunders, 1963.

Rose, B. D. *Clinical Physiology of Acid Base and Electrolyte Disorders.* New York: McGraw-Hill, 1977.

Wilmore, D. W. *The Metabolic Management of the Critically Ill.* New York: Plenum, 1977.

Patient Evaluation

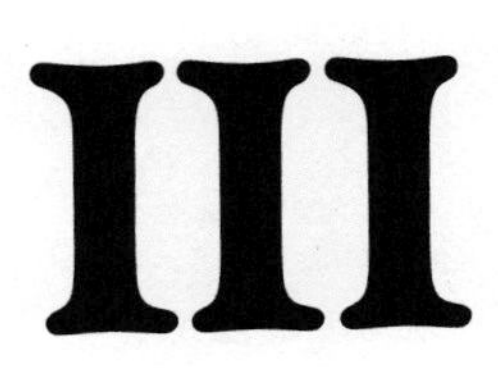

Evaluation of Efficacy

Sheldon Margen

11

The efficacious nutritional management of pre- and postoperative patients would appear to require only a relatively simple determination of whether protein and energy catabolism have been halted. Unfortunately, over the short term this is often quite difficult, since the evaluation process can vary from a simple clinical observation to the most complex research methodology.

BODY STORES AND BODY COMPOSITION

Changes in body composition take place when macronutrients (protein, carbohydrate, fat) are lost from the body (catabolism), are maintained in a state of equilibrium (homeostasis), or are built up during a reparative period (anabolism) [23]. In order for these energy sources to be available when needed, a storage mechanism must exist. Storage of carbohydrate in humans is essentially negligible and can be ignored when considering body composition. The only exception to this is that certain tissues such as central nervous system tissues and red blood cells require carbohydrate even after adaptation to a low intake has taken place. However, this amount is insignificant. Fat is stored in the adipose organ, and protein, in the form of nitrogen, is stored in all tissues (including fat), but primarily in adult muscle mass.

Body composition remains homeostatic when at least two essential conditions are met. First, *adequate protein must be available to replace mandatory (exogenous) losses.* In normal individuals, these relatively small losses amount to only 3 to 3.5 gm of nitrogen (20 ± 3 gm protein) per day [15]. This represents approximately 10 percent of the total protein turned over per day, as measured by radioactive or ^{15}N-labeled amino acids. The turnover values reported in the literature range from approximately 3.0 to 4.6 gm of protein per kg body weight per day, with a rather wide standard deviation [43]. The primary source of initial protein breakdown is thought to be a pool known as the "labile stores." Although this has never really been identified as to source or distribution, it constitutes a relatively small proportion of the total protein that is lost.

The major protein store is muscle, and during prolonged protein deprivation, after small initial losses from active organs such as the liver, kidney, and spleen, muscle becomes the primary source of protein. The minimum amount of protein necessary to sustain an individual varies with the rate of catabolism and turnover, but primarily depends on the total energy supplied [15]. If the amount of energy intake matches or exceeds the catabolic process, then some unspecified minimum amount of protein will suffice. In normal individuals, the evidence suggests that the mean "requirement" for high quality orally administered protein, such as egg, is less than 70 mg nitrogen per kg body weight if energy is optimum. There is some question whether this protein requirement can be reduced slightly in the presence of excessive quantities of energy, but this seems unlikely. Excess energy would be stored as body fat, thus increasing the size of the adipose organ which would then result in a slight *increase* in protein "requirements." However, this would be quite minor and not measurable by existing techniques. (2) *In addition to protein, adequate energy must also be available.* It is not known whether energy requirements can be totally met from either carbohydrates or fats alone. Some recent work on parenteral nutrition indicates that it *may* be possible to maintain the organism in energy balance in the total absence of fat as long as essential fatty acids are provided. However, the reverse question has never been answered, namely, whether it is possible to maintain an individual in energy balance utilizing only pure protein and fatty acids. (This experiment has not been attempted in either humans or animals. Although a small amount of carbohydrate may be obtained from some 3-carbon skeleton fragments, this might theoretically come from certain amino acid precursors and hence would require increased quantities of protein.) However, when a fat-carbohydrate mixture is used, more calories are required to maintain lean body mass than when only carbohydrate is used [31].

It is important to remember that during catabolism, virtually all other nutrients (in addition to protein, fat, and glycogen) are also depleted. This can lead to seriously impaired functioning in other areas. Therefore, although we will be primarily emphasizing body composition in terms of protein and fat, the clinician must always be alert to the possibility that single or multiple nutrient deficiencies may impair treatment.

MEASUREMENT OF BODY COMPOSITION

In order to be certain that anabolism has begun, a clinician must understand how to evaluate both short- and long-term alterations in body composition that occur as a result of the disease process and/or surgical intervention. Over the years many investigators have developed techniques to evaluate body composition and/or nutritional status. Among these we should particularly mention the contributions of Pace [28, 29], Behnke [4, 5], Brozek [10, 11], Moore [24], and Anderson [3]. Almost all their techniques are indirect and based on either principles of differential tissue density or measurements of administered or normally contained isotopes and extrapolation to their content in tissues. Unfortunately, these techniques are fraught with complex assumptions, which become subject to more error as the individual deviates from normal. Even under ideal conditions the reliability, accuracy, and replicability of these methods are frequently so poor that they are virtually worthless for following an individual who is ill and whose condition is changing rapidly. They are, therefore, generally reserved for careful, detailed research techniques.

Balance Technique

One of the simplest and most widely used techniques is the measurement of nitrogen and energy balance. Using this technique, an individual is given a known quantity of substance X, and if the same amount of the substance (or its metabolites) is excreted, the individual is said to be in equilibrium. If, however, an individual excretes less, and thus retains some portion of the substance, she or he is in positive balance (anabolic state). Likewise, if an individual excretes more of the compound or metabolite, a negative, or catabolic, state exists. Balance can be expressed as $B = I - (U + F + O)$.* Various authors [1, 24] have suggested that by applying equivalent factors to the amount of nitrogen, either excreted or retained, one can determine alterations in lean body mass. Likewise, by knowing alterations in weight and correcting these for rapid changes in water retention (which may or may not be possible), one can theoretically predict overall alterations in energy by extrapolating to changes in the size of the adipose organ.

Because this technique is used so extensively, it must be critically examined in order to determine its usefulness, particularly for short-term measurements, and under conditions of severe stress.

Nitrogen Balance and Requirements

The human requirement for nitrogen is partially met by ingesting certain highly specific amino acids that the organism is unable to synthesize (essential amino acids). In addition, humans also require a certain amount of nonspecific nitrogen ("nonessential amino acids"), which can be derived from other nitrogenous compounds that have, or are capable of forming, amino groups by various biochemical mechanisms. Certain microorganisms can convert urea to ammonia, which then reacts with certain ketoácids to form amino acids.

From the middle nineteenth to the early twentieth century, investigators attempted to quantify human nitrogen requirements first in adults and then in children. These early efforts were primarily epidemiologic and involved approximations of the quantity of protein (or nitrogenous substances) consumed. As a result, however, it became clear that the protein intake varied considerably in different population groups, all with the same general degree of health. It was also shown that in adults protein intake could be experimentally decreased below the level generally consumed without adversely affecting health. Since most investigators conceded that actual consumption might not bear any direct relationship to the "minimum" requirements, other avenues were explored. Ultimately, the balance technique emerged as the best way to define nitrogen requirements for individuals who had ceased growing. Under highly controlled conditions, it could also be used during states of disequilibrium (growth, disease states, and the like).

The history of the techniques, as well as some critical appraisals, have recently been published [2, 20]. During the last 25 to 50 years, many studies have been carried out under different environmental conditions to determine the protein and amino acid requirements of various populations. Unfortunately, the lack of standardized techniques makes it difficult, if not impossible, to interpret and compare these results. All of the classic studies on nitrogen balance have been carried out with orally administered protein or amino acids. By this route, the amino acids, or possibly small peptides, are absorbed by the intestinal tract, traverse the portal system, and are filtered by the liver, which serves as a regulator for the remaining body pools of amino acids. In the case of parenteral nutrition, this route is bypassed, and although the liver is very active and helpful in regulating amino acid levels, the fact that amino acids frequently reach the peripheral tissues before being regulated by the liver, complicates the situation and makes interpretation of the data very difficult.

In order to understand the mechanisms inherent in this system, we have devised a simple 2-compartment (pool) model, which could easily be expanded to incorporate a third compartment (Figure 11-1). Although the 3-pool model may, in some ways, more closely approximate reality, it does not help to understand the construct, and the data available can generally be explained by means of the 2-pool model.

Pool 1 ("labile") changes rapidly with alterations in dietary intake. This relatively small pool is probably composed of enzymes for protein

*B = balance; I = intake; U = urine; F = feces; O = other (skin, menstrual blood, saliva, etc.).

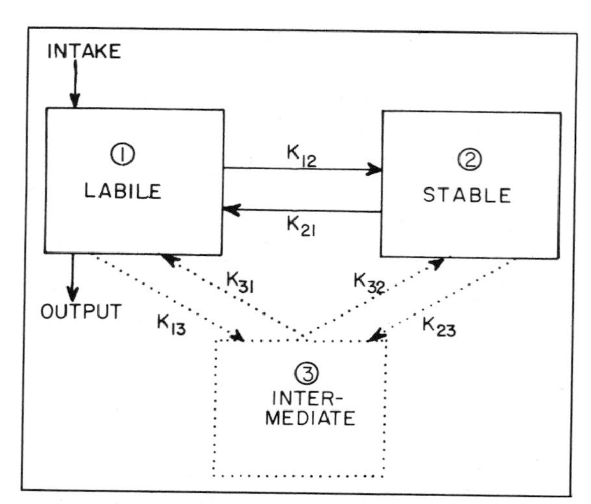

Figure 11-1. *Model of protein pools in the body.*

degradation, total body urea, total free amino acids, and other nitrogenous compounds. The second compartment is the major pool of the body and is represented principally by the muscle, which is, of course, the primary protein-containing organ system. In a sense, this is the protein storage pool, even though we do not ordinarily think of protein as a substance that is "stored." Pool 3, which is intermediate, can be introduced for those interested in thinking more anatomically or physiologically and may be of importance in disease states. However, this pool is not pertinent to our discussion.

At any given moment in time, pools 1 and 2 are in dynamic equilibrium. Pool 1 may constantly change in size and dynamic turnover because dietary protein (and thus nitrogen) varies from day to day (and during a given day). Pool 1 may also vary markedly during parenteral nutrition because of the large increase in amino acid pools and the synthesis and degradation of protein. There is also a large individual variation of loss that we do not believe is entirely random. In fact, this nonrandom variability in protein balance is the major drawback to using nitrogen or protein equilibrium for defining protein requirements [39]. However, in healthy people, the control mechanisms generally tend to keep the size and dynamics of the pools relatively constant, and this is reflected largely in autocorrelations of individuals maintained on dietary intakes within the so-called normal range [39]. During the diminished intake, this equilibrium or homeostatic mechanism is stressed. Interestingly enough, the same equilibrium appears to occur in normal individuals who consume protein at levels two to three times above the requirements but at higher levels it disappears.

For our purposes we might define requirements as "that amount of protein necessary to maintain total body nitrogen levels unchanged." This allows us to consider requirements not only in the static phase of unchanged protein levels, but also in terms of the periodicity of protein excretion and degradation products, even on a fixed nitrogen intake. This definition essentially implies no significant changes in the size of pool 1 or 2, but allows for a regulated, systematic variation in these pools on a day-to-day basis. Using this definition, it would be impossible to ascertain actual requirements, since at time zero (T_0), the moment at which we make the observation, the individual would be in equilibrium between the pools in Figure 11-1. Obviously, we would have to know ahead of time precisely what the intake and output were, as well as any change in output as a result of the regulatory mechanism just described. If we knew this, requirements could be defined by intake, but the possibility of accurately estimating intake by any means now available is very small. The exception to this, of course, is in the controlled environment of a metabolic ward, or in hospital patients receiving enteral or parenteral nutrition. Although this definition might be statistically useful, it is operationally untenable, since it does not define requirements for maintaining health, physiologically normal changes in pool size, or alterations as a result of disease states.

An alternative definition might be "that amount of protein necessary to maintain a regulated state called homeostasis in terms of individual nitrogen equilibrium." This has previously been interpreted as keeping the individual in nitrogen balance; our concept is that nitrogen balance is not a specific, but rather a changing, point which is part of an autoregulated process. This is borne out by the nitrogen balance of individuals maintained on constant nitrogen intake. If one knows the nature of the autoregulation and the day on which the nitrogen balance is calculated, the balance on the following day can be predicted. In normal individuals, the range over which nitrogen balance fluctuates is clearly evident by oscillations of regular amplitude and frequency. By this reasoning, individuals can (within limits) adapt to different nitrogen intakes over a period of time by changes in lean body mass. Obviously, these effects are more significant in long-term than in short-term changes in nitrogen balance. In dealing with short-term changes, it is useful to consider that the reason for protein administration is to alter the stable body protein pool when catabolism begins or, if the individual is normal, to maintain this. By using this definition we imply that changes could occur in pool 1, but not in pool 2, when the individual is in nitrogen equilibrium. However, in disequilibrium, the size of pool 2 is decreased (catabolism) or increased (anabolism).

In order to understand this model better, we must examine the experimental approaches that have been utilized to determine protein requirements in terms of nitrogen balance.

Factorial Method. Using the factorial method in adults, one assumes that when protein intake is zero and all other nutrients (particularly energy) are supplied in adequate quantities, the total output of nitrogen (or output plus the increment for true growth) at some observation time will define nitrogen requirements. One further assumes that if an "ideal protein" is supplied in quantities equal to output, nitrogen equilibrium will be obtained. The weakness of this theory, in its unrefined state, is that it takes no account of less than 100 percent efficient conversion of dietary to body protein.

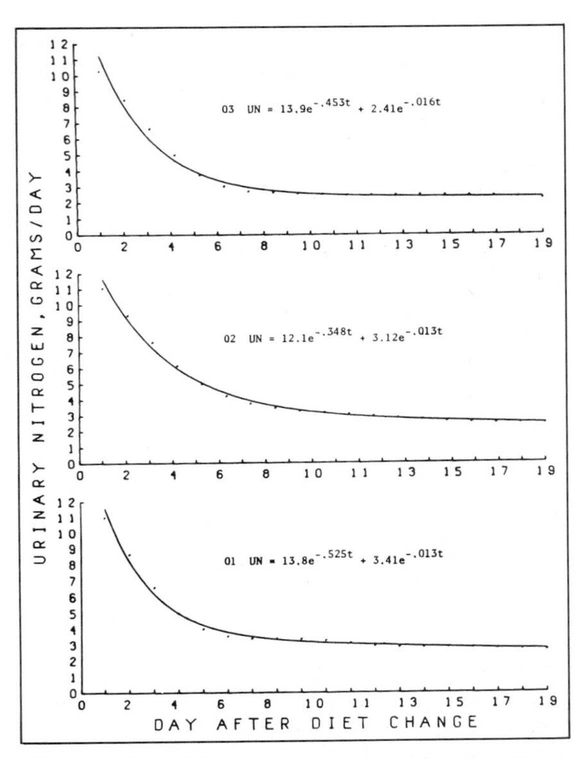

Figure 11-2. *Nitrogen excretion in three subjects on 0- to 3-gm nitrogen intake. Data have been smoothed using a cubic spline technique.*

When nitrogen input is dropped to zero, there is an almost immediate alteration of both urinary nitrogen and nitrogen balance (Figure 11-2) [15]. As can be seen, there is a rapid drop in nitrogen excretion and/or a rapid increase in negative nitrogen flux, which appears to be relatively constant after 6 to 9 days. It was originally thought that this minimal protein loss would be the individual protein requirement. However, experimental work suggests that at least 30 percent more high-quality protein (egg) was necessary to re-establish equilibrium [15]. Recent long-term experiments in our laboratory have shown that both nitrogen balance and autoregulation can be established in 17 to 31 days on as little as 57 mg nitrogen per kg per day [13].

The apparent constancy of urinary nitrogen output and/or nitrogen balance after approximately 9 days at zero protein intake is deceptive, and it is reasonable to question whether methodologic intervention itself alters the model and makes it impossible to determine output by this method. Because of the inherent biologic variations in the autoregulatory process, it is impossible to see changes that might occur in urinary excretion or balance. Even if we ignore the normal oscillations that have been attributed to intra-individual variability and we assume that there is no methodologic error, a simple calculation will show us the problem. The total body protein of an adult male equals about 10 kg (1.6 kg of nitrogen). Daily endogenous excretion equals approximately 3.5 gm of nitrogen or approximately 0.2 percent of total body protein per day. Since the maximal observations made at zero protein intake are about 18 days long, a constant state has not been observed for periods of more than about 10 days. The total loss of lean body mass over these 10 days would therefore be approximately 2 percent, and we have no techniques available to detect such a small degree of change.

However, if we use the proper statistical methods, a gradual decline in nitrogen excretion over time can be noted (Figure 11-2). In fact, according to our model, after a period of time at decreased protein and/or energy intake resulting in a marked decrease in the size of pool 2, the individual could be at a new stage of equilibrium, where survival will probably be possible at a lower level of nitrogen input.

Balance Methods. If we go back to our second definition of protein requirements, i.e., "that amount of protein which will keep the individual in a regulated state" and add to this "without change in stable body protein" (pool 2), we find that it is fraught with problems because the size of the stable pool may vary downward as a result of prior protein deprivation, surgery, and/or decreased food intake after surgery. As physicians, we are not so much concerned with individual requirements at any given time as with the requirements when pool 2 is at its "optimal" state for a given individual. Our objective is always to restore the individual to his or her optimal state as rapidly as possible, which means repletion of pool 2 when it has been depleted because of stress or disease. In most animals (including man), there is a certain relatively stable pool that can achieve a maximal size in healthy individuals. Man's ability to change his stable pool and/or body composition points out the importance, and frequently the difficulty, of ascertaining individual status by means of the balance technique.

As we have noted, individuals who are stable and eating at levels close to their requirements vary between positive and negative balance [39]. However, there are methodologic and conceptual problems with protein balance for which we still have no explanation. The usual method for determining minimal protein requirements, while attempting to keep pool 2 constant, is referred to as the slope intercept ratio and involves a series of 10- to 14-day metabolic studies. The mean balance of the last 4 to 6 days of each study represents the balance achieved at the dietary protein level administered, and the points thus obtained will be both above and below balance, and sometimes points at or above balance are not even noted. Thus, any interpretation of positive balance on days 10 to 14 and beyond is baffling. In part this can now be explained by the fact that equilibrium is not achieved in such a short period of time [13].

Theoretically, the model states that at any level above minimum, although pool 1 may expand, I(t) should be equal to O(t) in a relatively short time. Therefore, a prolonged positive balance should only mean an expansion of pool 2. In a 60-day metabolic study of individuals receiving 36 gm protein [26], a consistently positive balance of approximately 1.4 gm nitrogen per day was noted. This was associated with some weight gain, and possibly some increase in lean body mass. However, the actual degree of expansion could not be reasonably detected with methods

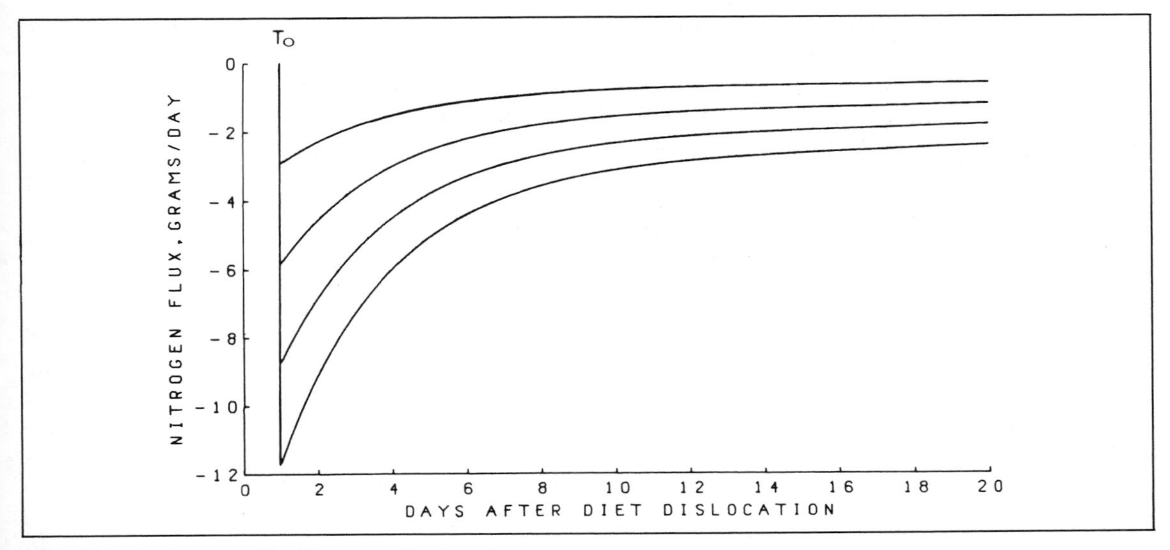

Figure 11-3. *Relationship between dietary nitrogen dislocation and nitrogen flux.*

currently at our disposal. This appears to be a consistent finding in all nitrogen balance studies; that is, with increasing nitrogen intake there is increasing positive balance. This disquieting phenomenon brings into question definitions of requirements in terms of balance, particularly as regards the anabolic status of individuals exhibiting positive nitrogen balance in short-term experiments.

After the series of points has been determined, it is plotted and a linear regression is drawn. The point of intercept at nitrogen equilibrium is taken to indicate the quantity of protein necessary to achieve nitrogen balance, and this is defined as the protein requirement. It is clear from examining the model and the technique employed that at each level of nitrogen administration a series of changes in pool sizes and turnover rates has occurred. These changes in balance at varying protein intakes can best be described by a series of curves, the exact nature of which is unknown. Nevertheless, analogies to certain physical processes and mathematical considerations suggest that the curves are most likely of the general configuration shown in Figure 11-3. The curves have been taken from a normal individual participating in one of our metabolic experiments. It can be seen from these smoothed curves that the greater the dislocation or translocation of nitrogen intake, the longer it takes to reestablish equilibrium, even though equilibrium is not necessarily at the zero point. This means that the greater the repletion and/or depletion (translocation), the greater the apparent change in nitrogen balance will be, the less likely it is that any significant interpretation can be made, and the longer it will be necessary to follow the patient to be assured that what we are observing is really the result of an anabolic process.

Young et al. [41] demonstrated that when the dislocation is above nitrogen balance levels, positive balance apparently ensues, although regression is not linear. Likewise, there is no linear fit when dislocation is extreme in the direction of protein restriction. For this reason alone one must question the significance and validity of the balance method for evaluating protein needs and the degree of anabolic/catabolic changes from nitrogen balance per se. The complexities of using balance techniques are even better exemplified in a recent paper by Garza, Scrimshaw, and Young [17]. Here, in long-term studies, marked intra-individual variations are obvious, and the use of simple statistical procedures to evaluate or ignore these leads to dangerous conclusions. In this paper, the observed values for nitrogen balance, with predicted changes from total body potassium measurements, do not correlate and tend to substantiate our misgivings about the use of nitrogen balance and other methodologies for determining requirements. In another paper, Young et al. [40] question the autocorrelations of intra-individual variation, but unfortunately the data as presented do not lend themselves to time series analysis.

Energy Balance and Requirements

We know there is a close relationship between energy and protein requirements; the latter tend to increase when inadequate energy is available for maintenance. Undoubtedly, this is because protein will be used as energy when energy balance is negative. In addition, the hypercatabolic state itself probably increases the turnover rate so that more protein is lost even when sufficient energy can be supplied. The nature of the protein-energy interaction is still uncertain, but recent experimental work suggests that protein requirements, as determined by excretion and balance, are extremely sensitive to energy change, particularly when energy balance is negative. However, the quantification of this interaction is extremely difficult and has not yet been clearly determined. One of the principal difficulties in determining energy balance is measuring the degree of energy output. The criterion generally used is weight equilibrium, but even under the most carefully controlled conditions, the variability is at least 0.5 kg/day. When one adds to this the marked changes in fluid balance seen in ill patients, body weight is obviously of little value. Furthermore, recent analyses from our long-term experiments may change. Although the degree of change has not yet been ascertained, in view of the marked hypercatabolic state that often characterizes severe medical and surgical illnesses, it is not significant. In order to minimize the effect of protein loss, it is simply necessary to supply sufficient energy and hope that the organism possesses all the other essential nutrients and the mechanisms for energy utilization.

Efficacy of the Balance Technique

All of the above criticisms are obviously leveled at long-term balance studies, and the essential question that is asked in this chapter is whether short-term observations of nitrogen balance, particularly nitrogen retention, can be used as a measure of anabolic response. The evidence to date indicates that short-term (2- to 4-day) demonstrations of positive nitrogen balance do not necessarily indicate that an anabolic effect for protein has been achieved. If a positive balance of more than 2 to 3 gm is maintained over 6 to 7 days in the presence of ideal caloric intake, if urinary functions remain adequate, and if skin losses can be accounted for, then it may be significant. This assumes that the total amount of protein fed contains no more than 24 to 30 gm of nitrogen per day, since normal individuals may exhibit this same degree of positive nitrogen balance for as long as 60 days, and retention would have to be greater than this in order to be significant. Thus, increasing the protein level and noting an increase in protein retention does not assure us that we have accelerated the anabolic process.

Another unanswerable question concerns the maximum rate at which protein can be laid down after depletion and thus the maximum rate of protein anabolism. After moderate surgical trauma, whole body protein synthesis appears to fall, but we do not know whether this can be modified, and whether it is possible to visualize a self-regulating system of protein turnover in which the rate of breakdown is related to and governed by the rate of synthesis.

The only conclusion that can be drawn from all this is that although at present the simplest method for measuring alterations is protein balance—as a short-term indicator of anabolism or catabolism—in some instances, it may lead to entirely erroneous conclusions. It is therefore necessary to continue to seek other techniques to better measure protein catabolism or anabolism.

3-Methylhistidine Excretion

The most complete review of the present status of 3-methylhistidine and its relation to protein muscle turnover is a review by Young and Munro [40]. They point out that there are various methylated amino acids in muscle, and for the most part, we do not understand their functions. However, there appears to be some evidence that they may be regulators of DNA synthesis and chromatin activity. It was hoped that their primary usefulness would be as indicators of muscle breakdown, since they fulfill certain criteria for such a substance. These criteria are: (1) the substance must be modified only after being incorporated into the muscle protein; (2) once it is in the protein, it must not be further metabolized; (3) its composition in muscle must remain relatively constant, related at least to the protein of the muscle; (4) it must not be present to significant degrees in other tissues; (5) when other amino acids are released during metabolism, it should be released in the same proportion as general muscle breakdown; (6) there should be no reutilization of this compound; (7) the compound itself should be known—not further metabolized; (8) the compound or its metabolites should have a low renal threshold; and (9) it must be virtually 100 percent excreted. Much like creatinine, 3-methylhistidine tends to fulfill these criteria. However, there are certain difficulties with interpretation in 3-methylhistidine. In humans this material is excreted almost entirely in its preformed state, although in rats almost half is acetylated. In humans less than 5 percent of the material is excreted as N-acetyl-3-methylhistidine. Fortunately, 3-methylhistidine appears to be attached to actin and myosin, which are the myofibrillar proteins most actively degraded and resynthesized (turned over).

3-Methylhistidine appears only in slight amounts elsewhere. About 88 percent is in the skeletal muscle (about 10 percent is found in smooth muscle of skin and intestinal tract). Yet, in terms of turnover, as much as 17 percent of the turnover may be accounted for in smooth muscle of skin and intestinal tract.

Probably the most significant problem associated with 3-methylhistidine has to do with the rate of excretion in response to dietary alterations. It is well known that dietary changes in protein and energy lead to changes in muscle protein turnover rates. However, the actions of protein and energy are not totally independent, and their interaction can lead to complex problems. Although we may discuss turnover as such, in the nonsteady state, which is what we are dealing with in disease, the pool size does not remain the same. The alteration may result from either change of synthesis or degradation or both. Therefore, both with diet as well as with disease states, the interpretation of change must be made with caution.

In both rats and humans, protein restriction leads to a reduction of 3-methylhistidine expressed on a per-unit body-weight basis. On refeeding, the excretion rates tend to rise [19, 27]. In rats on severely restricted energy intake, the output of 3-methylhistidine per unit body weight rose to higher values than in controls. It is interesting to note that the most significant decrease occurred when protein was withheld, more so than when energy was withheld. Although the adaptive response of muscle to prolonged fasting appears to be a decrease in the rate of protein turnover, this is probably not the case during surgical trauma and hypercatabolism [22]. This suggests that trauma may be associated with impaired synthesis rather than degradation of muscle [7]. In a study of four patients undergoing surgery [22], two developed sepsis during the course of surgery and exhibited a marked increase in 3-methylhistidine excretion. This was accompanied by an increase in creatinine excretion. All the patients had been on total parenteral nutrition prior to surgery and for 32 days postoperatively. In the two patients who did not develop sepsis, although the 3-methylhistidine was below normal at onset, it continued to decrease markedly, suggesting decreased muscle breakdown. Immediately after surgery, all the patients showed a decrease in 3-methylhistidine excretion associated with an increase in nitrogen excretion, suggesting that this nitrogen was not being derived from muscle.

Ward et al. [42] and Schenkin et al. [30] clearly point out the difficulties in utilizing 3-methylhistidine in isolation as an indicator of alterations in muscle metabolism. It can increase because of increased metabolism and a good diet. It can also increase because of catabolism associated with an injury. Ward et al. [42] state that more work is necessary to determine whether this method is of more value than creatinine.

Creatinine Excretion

Creatinine excretion has been used for a long time to predict muscle mass. It fulfills most of the criteria mentioned by Young [40], but like 3-methylhistidine, it responds to exogenous ingestion of the material in foods. Therefore, experiments with this material must be conducted on a creatinine-free diet. Predicting lean body mass from creatinine excretion is of some value in a relatively normal individual. However, it assumes a constancy of excretion which is not seen under controlled metabolic conditions. The coefficient of variability of creatinine excretion is probably ± 8 percent. The usual values given for estimating muscle mass from creatinine excretion are as follows:

$$\text{Creatinine weight coefficient} = \frac{\text{actual creatinine excretion}}{\text{ideal creatinine excretion}}$$

$$\text{Creatinine coefficient (men)} = \text{IBW}^* \times 23 \text{ mg/kg}$$

$$\text{Creatinine coefficient (women)} = \text{IBW} \times 18 \text{ mg/kg [8]}$$

*IBW = intracellular body water.

Other Methods for Measuring Body Composition

Classic Techniques

Some other classic techniques for measuring body composition are inappropriate for ill people. Among these are underwater weighing [4], water displacement [4, 5], helium displacement [35], or other techniques for determining body volume, total body water measurements [42], and ^{40}K counting [11] for determining lean body mass. Obviously, ill people cannot be subjected to underwater weighing. Further, the measurement of total body and extracellular water to estimate the alteration in intracellular fluid is fraught with compounded errors, particularly because the rate of change is so rapid. The inherent accuracy of ^{40}K measurements is limited, and ^{40}K concentration in the cells can vary considerably in relation to protein,† making the use of ^{40}K questionable as a measure of protein anabolism.

None of these techniques can tell us whether a given therapy is of significant short-term benefit in terms of change in protein or in the fat stores.

Recent Advances

We will now look at some newer techniques to see whether they are potentially of greater use and applicability at the bedside. As a result of the work done by Moore and others [24], multiple isotope dilution techniques have been used to estimate body composition. However, most of these are much too complex for routine use and have too great a magnitude of error to allow for repeated measurements. More recently, a simpler isotope dilution technique has been suggested by Shizgal and Spanier [33] and others [25]. Their work is based on an old postulated cellular phenomenon that the osmolarity between intra- and extracellular fluid must be constant, and that the cell membrane is therefore freely permeable to water. This was tested by Edelman et al. [14]

†This is particularly noticeable in diabetic acidosis, where the amount of potassium can fall markedly in a very short time without significant alteration in lean body mass.

and confirmed in 1958. Based upon this evidence, no osmotic gradient exists between the extra- and intracellular fluid compartments. Since sodium and potassium are the principal cations and sources of the osmotic pressure, techniques have been developed, utilizing this phenomenon, to simplify determination of intracellular fluid and hence lean body mass. This determination was first carried out in 1963 by Muldowney [25]. By taking muscle biopsies, he attempted to measure sodium and potassium in water and to estimate the normal exchangeable potassium (K_e) from the ratio of measured muscle to normal muscle potassium. This technique was useful, but required a minor surgical procedure and a rather sophisticated measurement. Although theoretically this is an excellent procedure, errors are always possible because the ratio of tissue K to K_e might change because of a loss of tissue K without an accompanying loss of muscle. In order for the procedure to work, we must assume that the potassium to muscle ratio is always constant. It is possible to measure K utilizing ^{40}K in the total body counter, but the difficulties with this method have already been described. Fortunately, 99 percent of the K_e is readily exchangeable, and this would suggest that measurement with potassium isotopes might be useful. However, ^{42}K has a half-life of 12.4 hours, and ^{43}K has a half-life of only 22.4 hours. This makes these materials, which are very expensive, logistically inconvenient to use.

Edelman et al. [14] postulated that the ratio (R) of the sum of sodium and potassium, divided by the water content, would be the same for all tissues of the body, namely,

$$R = \frac{Na + K}{H_2O}$$

A rearrangement of this equation shows that

$K_e = R(TBW - Na_e)$*

*K_e = exchangeable potassium; Na_e = exchangeable sodium; R = the ratio of sodium and potassium content in whole blood.

The remaining measurements that have to be made in order to determine K_e are exchangeable sodium and total body water. These can be accomplished by isotope dilution measurements made for 24 hours after injecting tritium-labeled water and ^{22}Na. The correlation between ^{42}K and the indirect measure of K_e gives the coefficient relationship of $R = 0.88$. However, as Shizgal points out, the standard error of the estimate is 70 percent of the mean. In order to improve this method even further and to estimate both the extracellular fluid and blood volume, Shizgal, and Spanier et al., have suggested the use of ^{22}Na-labeled water, ^{51}Cr-labeled red blood cells, and radioactive labeled serum albumin [34]. To help estimate the lean body mass, they use the Pace-Rathburn constant of fat-free tissue equal to 73 percent water [28]. In other words, total body water divided by 73 equals lean body mass. Using this technique, they [36] studied 20 patients after surgical bypass who were each followed for approximately 8½ months. Twenty-one percent of the patients showed a 17 percent decrease in body weight, supposedly due entirely to loss of body fat. Eight of the patients who were followed for 14 to 21 months showed a 27 percent decrease in body weight, of which 26.6 kg was a reduction in body fat and 13 kg was a reduction of lean body mass, the latter associated with an increase in extracellular mass. As they point out, this latter condition is characteristic of changes seen in malnutrition.

Shizgal et al. [32] attempted to apply this techique to studying the effects of parenteral nutrition on body composition in critically ill patients. They made 24 measurements on six severely catabolic patients receiving hyperalimentation. The patients suffered from sepsis, gastrointestinal fistulas, and gastroenteritis. They were each supposed to be treated with 3 liters of 25 percent glucose and 5 percent casein, but actually received only approximately 2.4 liters (about 50.4 ± 4.8 Kcal/kg). They also studied 18 patients who were ill but not receiving hyperalimentation and a group of 16 normals. All of the nonhyperalimented ill patients showed expanded extracellular fluid volume (52 percent compared with 40 percent). In addition, they all showed some increase in total exchangeable sodium, a decrease in body cell mass, and a decrease in exchangeable potassium. The intracellular mass showed a mean of 47.9 percent compared with 60.3 percent in the normals. The exchangeable sodium and potassium, over total body weight, was 49.2 for the ill patients who were not receiving hyperalimentation and over 80.2 in the controls.

The hyperalimented group were even more interesting. Their total exchangeable sodium over total body water was 87.4; intracellular water was 52.2. The mean K_e over total body water was 63.5, with many in the normal range. However, the Na_e/K_e ratio of the normals was 0.98, of the ill nonhyperalimented 2.07, and of the hyperalimented 1.46. Likewise, in the hyperalimented group the Na_e/TBW ratio was 96.9, whereas the ICW was 47.9. What was most interesting, however, was that a repeat carried out approximately 25 days later on the hyperalimented group showed no change in body composition. It appeared that the treatment allowed the individual to remain stable, but except for some increase in total exchangeable sodium, no true rehabilitation was noted. In addition, although the measurement error of K_e is approximately 8 percent, when all measurements are combined, the error undoubtedly adds up to a larger figure. This technique appears to be scientifically promising, but requires a great deal of isotope manipulation and a 24-hour equilibrium period. It is, therefore, not a simple routine procedure suitable for regular use.

Neutron activation is a fairly new technique which allows for measurement of total body composition (usually in segments) by using a neutron source and counting the specific element or spectra one wishes to examine. This technique can only be used in those places where there is a cyclotron and adjacent total body counting equipment.

Various isotope techniques have been developed for estimating the total body content of minerals, the first of which concentrated on calcium [38]. In the last several years, intensive efforts have been made to measure body nitrogen in this way [6, 18, 21, 37]. In this procedure, the individual is usually irradiated in segments. A specific isotope is measured after allowing several minutes for the short-term isotopes to decay. Because of the segmental distribution, the absolute total amount of nitrogen cannot be estimated, and attempts are now being made to either integrate these measurements or to irradiate the total individual.

Two methods for determining ^{15}N have been reported.

1. *^{14}N (n, ^{2}N) ^{13}N.* In this method the individual is irradiated with 14 mev neutrons and ^{13}N, which is a positron emitter with a 9.96 minute half-life, no γ-ray emission, and only 0.511 mev annihilation quanta produced. However, there are a number of nonspecificity problems. For example, approximately 29 percent of the counts are from the nitrogen alone. The major portion comes from a ^{16}O (p, α) ^{13}N reaction. Likewise, there is considerable spatial insensitivity, which can amount to as much as ± 81 percent. This means that great care must be taken when interpreting measures using this technique.
2. *^{14}N (n, p) ^{15}N.* This method has slightly more widespread use. Approximately 15 percent of the cited ^{15}N decays, emitting 10.8 mv γ rays. Since most other isotopes produced by this reaction are below 10 mv, this is more specific and thus more effective. This can be done at a total radiation dosage of 0.1 rem or less. Harvey et al. [18] conducted a study in which 65 patients were examined on 19 occasions, utilizing the body nitrogen analyses in sectors. Over a year they found that the coefficient of variation was only 2 percent, or approximately ± 2.5 percent, at $\pm$ one standard deviation. In studies of two patients, one who had had a laparotomy, another with liver disease and edema, both demonstrated changes that could be followed in terms of total body nitrogen. They also attempted to

estimate the nitrogen/potassium ratio utilizing ^{40}K counting, and found that the ^{40}K/nitrogen ratio had a correlation coefficient of 0.88. However, the problem does involve difficulties of careful positioning and geometry, and therefore changes in the size of the adipose organ can cause difficulties.

More recently, the ^{11}N (p, α) ^{11}C method has been investigated, but nothing has been published on this as yet.

Since severe malnutrition leads to serious impairment of the immune system, various measurements of this mechanism have been studied in an attempt to predict both degrees of malnutrition and rate of recovery. The difficulty, obviously, is that these techniques are complex, and it is difficult to know at what level of any specific nutrient a specific immunologic mechanism may be affected and at what level it may return to normal. Therefore, the problem is complicated both by the methodologies and the interpretations. It has also been noted that most of the changes seen earlier relate to tissue immunity rather than humoral immunity. The most common method of evaluation that has been suggested is to count total lymphocytes and the reactivity to intradermally administered antigens or sensitizing materials. Miller [23] points out many of the pitfalls in the immunologic assays as measurements of nutritional status. Each must be interpreted with great caution because they are quite nonspecific.

1. *Decrease in total lymphocytes.* It is often stated that a lymphocyte count under 1200 per cubic millimeter of blood is suggestive of malnutrition. However, this interpretation must be made carefully because a lowered level of lymphocytes is not a specific reaction and may be induced by many other factors, and the relationship of this to immune function is far from clear.

2. *Measurements of the T and B cells.* Unfortunately, this tells us very little about the A cells, which seem to be the ones most critically involved with the immune mechanism. So, the number of T and B cells may or may not be correlated with immune competence.

3. *Tests of mitogen-induced proliferation of T or B cells with phytohemagglutinin (PHA), concavalin A (CON A), pokeweed mitogen (PWM), and peanut agglutinin (PA).* These substances seem to stimulate carbohydrate receptors and cause the cells to divide. Great care is needed to perform and interpret these tests. If carefully done, they may give information on A-T or A-T-B cell interactions, and may detect some suppressive activity. Although there have been some enthusiastic reports suggesting TPN restores PHA or PWM responsiveness, data are really quite inconclusive.

4. *The mixed leucocyte response.* This test is supposedly more sensitive than the aforementioned. It is used to measure the ability to respond to a specific antigen challenge. It is also difficult to carry out and has been used very little in the study of malnutrition. Its usefulness is therefore quite unknown.

5. *Humoral mechanisms and antibody production.* These have been shown to be a poor predictor of malnutrition. It was hoped that the concentration of certain immunoglobulins would prove to be more specific, particularly immunoglobulin A (IgA). Unfortunately, most of these hopes have not been borne out.

6. *Complement.* Complement appears to be an interesting area to study. However, problems arise since there are so many portions to the complement system, and since the one that is usually measured (C3 complement) is subject to many factors aside from malnutrition, which can raise or lower its levels.

7. *Delayed cutaneous hypersensitivity (DCH) skin test.* This is probably mediated by the effector in the A cell. In this test a purified protein derivative or chemical material is administered subcutaneously. In severe malnutrition it is generally anticipated that the reaction will disappear and may reappear when good nutritional status is restored. However, the response of these purified protein derivatives is not specific and is generally due to a complex series of im-

mune reactions. A wide variety of metabolic defects, such as electrolyte imbalance, circulatory restriction, altered capillary permeability, and epidermal vascularity, can interfere. Likewise, the antigens themselves may be variable in strength. The most commonly used have been Candida, streptokinase-streptodornase, dinitrochlorobenzene (DNCB), coccidioidins, and mumps vaccine. In the case of DNCB, which is probably the most commonly used, only about 20 percent of normal individuals will react when this material is administered the first time. Most investigators attempt to use the recall to DNCB as a measure of protein depletion/repletion. However, it is still questionable whether any of these tests really measures defective immune systems in a hospitalized patient. Dr. Miller reports that the use of these tests, although widely reported, is "not impressive" in controlled work [23].

In clinical PEM, particularly in children, some plasma protein levels (especially albumin) are unusually low. Clinicians have been interested in the possibility of using such measurements to gauge recovery and with the advent of TPN, they hoped that the response to administration of some plasma proteins might serve as a convenient indicator of response to total body protein repletion. Fischer [16] has described the characteristics of such a usable protein. They include a small body pool, rapid rate of synthesis, specific and rapid catabolic response to protein and energy depletion, short biological half-life, high intravascular/extravascular ratio and relatively high specificity in response only to changes in protein or energy "balances." Unfortunately, no protein measured to date meets all of these requirements.

The most commonly measured plasma proteins are albumin and transferrin. Albumin has been used for the longest time. It has a slow rate of turnover and fair specificity. However, since there is a large extravascular pool in the body and since the fractional catabolic rate is related to the size of this pool and the ability of the organism to transfer albumin intravascularly, it is not totally satisfactory for measurement purposes. Likewise, there are factors other than protein or energy intake which may significantly influence synthesis rates. Therefore, albumin levels are not highly specific or rapid indicators of change in protein status.

Transferrin has been suggested as a better measure than albumin. Its half-life is shorter, but unfortunately, it is most responsive to changes in iron status. However, in the absence of significant iron fluctuation, it does reflect changes in protein and energy levels better and more rapidly than albumin.

Recently, attention has focused on prealbumin (thyroxine binding) and retinol binding protein (which also may be bound to prealbumin). Both of these have rapid turnover rates and are mainly intravascular. They also respond to changes in the "substrates" they carry. However, the specificity of responses of these proteins to energy and protein alterations needs more extensive investigation.

To date, it is difficult to measure short-term changes and determine the effectiveness of total parenteral nutrition or nutritional supplementation for the surgical patient. Each technique is fraught with difficulties in interpretation and we wish to recommend caution to both the investigator and the practicing clinician when utilizing any method, whether complex, or relatively simple as those advocated by Blackburn et al. [9]. Although we appear to be making progress, it is slow. There is no doubt that nutrition plays an important role in the rehabilitation of the surgical patient, and that rehabilitation and growth are possible utilizing enteral or parenteral means [12]. However, in spite of almost four decades of intensive investigation, the nature of the metabolic changes over the short term remains a mystery.

REFERENCES

1. Allison, J. B. Interpretation of nitrogen balance data. *Fed. Proc.* 10:676, 1957.
2. Allison, J. B., and Bird, W. C. Elimination of

Nitrogen from the Body. In H. Munro and J. B. Allison (Eds.), *Mammalian Protein Metabolism.* New York: Academic, 1964. Vol. I.

3. Anderson, E. C., and Langham, W. H. Average potassium concentration of the human body as a function of age. *Science* 130:173, 1959.
4. Behnke, A. R. Fat content and composition of the body. *Harvey Lect.* 37:198, 1941–1942.
5. Behnke, A. R. Anthropometric evaluation of body composition throughout life. *Ann. N. Y. Acad. Sci.* 110:450, 1963.
6. Biggin, H. C., Chen, N. S., Ettinger, K. V., Fremlin, J. H., Morgan, W. D., Novtony, R., and Chamberlain, M. J. Determination of nitrogen in living patients. *Nat. New. Biol.* 236:187, 1972.
7. Bilmazes, C., Vavy, R., Haverberg, L. N., Munro, H. N., and Young, V. R. Muscle protein breakdown rates in humans, based on Nτ-methylhistidine (3-methylhistidine) content of mixed proteins in skeletal muscle and urinary output of Nτ-methylhistidine. *Metabolism* 27:525, 1978.
8. Blackburn, G. L., Bistrian, B. R., Maini, B. S., Schlam, H. T., and Smith, M. F. Nutritional and metabolic assessment of the hospitalized patient. *J.P.E.N.* 1:11, 1977.
9. Blackburn, G. L., Flatt, J. P., and Cowles, G. H. A., Jr. Protein sparing therapy during periods of starvation with sepsis or trauma. *Ann. Surg.* 177: 588, 1973.
10. Brozek, J. (Ed.). *Body Measurements and Human Nutrition.* NRC Committee on Nutritional Anthropometry. Detroit: Wayne State University, 1956.
11. Brozek, J. (Ed.). Body composition. *Ann. N.Y. Acad. Sci.* 110. 1963.
12. Dudrick, S. J., Wilmore, D. W., Vars, H. M., and Rhoads, J. E. Long-term total parenteral nutrition with growth and development and positive nitrogen balance. *Surgery* 64:134, 1968.
13. Durkin, N., Ogar, D. A., Tilve, S. G., and Margen, S. Human protein requirements: Autocorrelation and adaptation to a low-protein diet containing .356 gm protein/kg or 57 mg N/kg body weight. Information Paper #7, FAO/WHO/UNV, Joint Expert Consultation on Energy and Protein Requirements, Sept., 1981.
14. Edelman, I. S., Leibman, J., O'Meara, M. P., and Birkenfeld, L. W. Interrelations between serum sodium concentration, serum osmolarity, and total exchangeable sodium, total exchangeable potassium and total body water. *J. Clin. Invest.* 37:1236, 1958.
15. *Energy and Protein Requirements. Report of a Joint FAO/WHO Ad Hoc Expert Committee.* Geneva: WHO/FAO, 1973.
16. Fischer, J. E. Plasma Proteins as Indicators of Nutritional Status. In *Nutritional Assessment-Present Status, Future Directions and Prospects. Report of the Second Ross Conference on Medical Research.* Columbus, OH: Ross Laboratories, 1981.
17. Garza, G., Scrimshaw, N. S., and Young, V. R. Human protein requirements: A long-term metabolic nitrogen balance study in young men to evaluate the 1973 FAO/WHO safe level of egg protein intake. *J. Nutr.* 107:335, 1977.
18. Harvey, T. C., Jain, S., Dykes, P. W., James, H., Chen, N. S., Chettle, D. R., Ettinger, K. V., Fremlin, J. H., and Thomas, B. J. Measurement of whole body nitrogen by neutron activation analysis. *Lancet* 2:395, 1973.
19. Haverberg, L. N., Deckelbaum, L., Bilmazes, C., Munro, H. N., and Young, V. R. Myofibrillar protein turnover and urinary methylhistidine output. Response to dietary supply of protein and energy. *Biochem. J.* 152:503, 1975.
20. Hegsted, D. M. Assessment of nitrogen requirements. *Am. J. Clin. Nutr.* 31:1669, 1978.
21. Leach, M. O., Thomas, B. J., and Vartsky, D. Total body nitrogen measured by the ^{14}N (n, ^{2}N) ^{13}N method. *Int. J. Appl. Radiat. Isotopes* 28:263, 1977.
22. Long, C. K., Schiller, W. R., Blackmore, W. S., Geiger, J. W., O'Dell, M., and Henderson, K. Muscle protein catabolism in the septic patient as measured at 3-methylhistidine excretion. *Am. J. Clin. Nutr.* 30:1349, 1977.
23. Miller, C. L. Immunological assays as measurements of nutritional status: A review. *J.P.E.N.* 2:554, 1978.
24. Moore, F. D., Olesen, K. H., McMurray, J. D., Parker, H. V., Ball, M. R., and Boyden, C. M. *The Body Cell Mass and Its Supporting Environment: Body Composition in Health and Diseases.* Philadelphia: Saunders, 1963.
25. Muldowney, F. P., and Williams, R. T. Clinical disturbances in serum sodium and potassium in relation to alteration in total exchangeable sodium, exchangeable potassium, and total body water. *Am. J. Med.* 35:768, 1963.
26. Oddoye, E. A., and Margen, S. Nitrogen balance studies in humans: Long-term effect of high nitrogen accretion. *J. Nutr.* 109:363, 1979.
27. Olmstedt, P. T., Kihlberg, R., Tinquall, P., and Shenkin, A. Effect of dietary protein on urinary excretion of 3-methylhistidine in rats. *J. Nutr.* 108:1877, 1978.
28. Pace, N., and Rathbun, E. N. Studies on body composition: III. The body water chemically com-

bined nitrogen content in relation to fat content. *J. Biol. Chem.* 158:685, 1945.

29. Rathbun, E. N., and Pace, N. Studies on body composition: I. The determination of total body fat by means of the body's specific gravity. *J. Biol. Chem.* 158:667, 1945.
30. Shenkin, A., and Steele, L. W. Clinical and laboratory assessment of nutritional status. *Proc. Nutr. Soc.* 37:95, 1978.
31. Shizgal, H. M. (Ed.). Symposium of nutritional requirements of surgical patients: I. Nutrition and body composition. *Can. J. Surg.* 21:483, 1978.
32. Shizgal, H. M., Milne, C. A., and Spanier, A. H. Effects of N-sparing intravenous administration of fluids on post-operative body composition. *Surgery* 85:496, 1979.
33. Shizgal, H. M., Spanier, A. H., Humes, J., and Wood, C. D. Indirect measurements of total exchangeable potassium. *Am. J. Physiol.* 233: F253, 1977.
34. Shizgal, H. M., Spanier, A. H., and Kurtz, R. S. The effect of parenteral nutrition on the body composition in the critically ill patient. *Am. J. Surg.* 131:156, 1976.
35. Siri, W. E. The gross composition of the body. *Adv. Biol. Med. Phys.* 4:239, 1956.
36. Spanier, A. H., Kurtz, R. S., and Shibata, H. R. Alterations in body composition following intestinal bypass for morbid obesity. *Surgery* 80:171, 1976.
37. Spinks, T. J. Measurement of body N by activation analysis. *Int. J. Appl. Radiat. Isotopes* 20:409, 1978. (Letter.)
38. Spinks, T. J., Bewley, D. K., Ranicar, A. S. O., and Joplin, G. F. Measurement of total body calcium in bone disease. *J. Radioanalyt. Chem.* 37: 345, 1977.
39. Sukhatme, P. V., and Margen, S. Models for protein deficiency. *Am. J. Clin. Nutr.* 31:1237, 1978.
40. Young, V. R., and Munro, H. N. N^{τ}methylhistidine (3-methylhistidine) and muscle protein turnover: An overview. *Fed. Proc.* 37:2291, 1978.
41. Young, V. R., Taylor, T. S. M., Rand, W. M., and Scrimshaw, N. S. Protein requirements of egg protein utilization at maintenance and submaintenance in young men. *J. Nutr.* 103:1164, 1974.
42. Ward, L. C., and Buttery, P. J. N^{τ}methylhistidine—an index of the true rate of myofibrillar degeneration? An appraisal. *Life Sci.* 23:1103, 1978.
43. Waterlow, J. E., Garlick, P. J., and Millward, D. J. *Protein Turnover in Mammalian Tissues and in the Whole Body.* Amsterdam: North-Holland, 1978.

Nutritional Assessment

Kenneth A. Kudsk
George F. Sheldon

12

Nutritional assessment in the broadest sense is applied clinical medicine. The experienced clinician usually identifies with ease the patient with severe protein-calorie malnutrition (PCM). Moreover, most physicians should be aware that the septic or injured patient is likely to develop pronounced wasting of body cell mass as illness evolves. An essential feature of nutritional assessment is identification of the patient's interaction with his illness, so that PCM can be prevented rather than treated.

Implicit in rational nutritional assessment are the concepts of static and dynamic methods for assessing the status of nutrition. Static nutritional assessment includes anthropometric measurements such as height, weight, ideal body weight, triceps skinfold, and arm muscle circumference, as well as albumin and other values that have been useful in the evaluation of third world populations with chronic malnutrition. Dynamic assessment includes measurements such as weight, nitrogen balance, and 3-methylhistidine measurement, which allow monitoring of the patient receiving nutritional support.

Many authors have used static nutritional assessment to evaluate the prevalence of malnutrition in the hospital setting. Bistrian and Blackburn found that 50 percent of surgical patients [4] and 44 percent of medical patients [5] surveyed met the World Health Organization's (WHO) criteria for PCM. Hypoalbuminemia, commonly associated with PCM, was reported to be present in 43 percent of medical patients (Butterworth) [10] and 26 percent of surgical patients (Hill) [24]. Mullen [31] and others have corroborated the prevalence of PCM in the hospital setting if the WHO criteria are used.

The current nutritional assessment methodology is simple and inexpensive, and makes possible a chart display of nutritional parameters which can be of value to the entire health care team. Moreover, these static nutritional assessment parameters document the diagnostic bases upon which sophisticated and expensive nutritional support is based.

Nutritional assessment using WHO parameters, however, has many deficiencies. It is questionable how applicable nutritional survey

Supported by US Army Grant #DADA 17-72-C-2020 and National Institutes of Health Grants #GMO-7032 and #NIGMO-18470.

methods are to the evaluation of hospitalized patients, in whom malnutrition is usually secondary to a disease. Moreover, sophisticated assessment of body composition by isotope methodology has demonstrated that tests such as triceps skinfold (fat layer) are quite inaccurate in predicting body composition [24]. In addition, dynamic alteration in body composition associated with acute illness is not usually identified by such methods. Finally, the predictive value of static nutritional assessment methods in identifying morbidity and mortality has not been established. Nevertheless, if one avoids over-interpretation, these tests have some value.

When nutritional intake contains inadequate calories and protein to equal metabolic expenditure and protein requirements for maintenance of body cell mass and growth, deterioration of body cell mass occurs. A patient who is starved, but not stressed, undergoes diminution of the basal metabolic rate [22], which is associated with transition from a glucose- to a fat-burning economy and gradual weight loss. Fat is usually the most abundant potential fuel, providing more calories per unit mass than any other tissue (Figure 12-1). Utilization of fat is associated with a metabolic conversion that is suppressed by elevated levels of catecholamines and glucocorticoids. Skeletal muscle is the largest single tissue in the body [32], containing protein, from which amino acids necessary for tissue repair, leukocyte production, and albumin synthesis derive. If other forms of energy, such as glucose or fat, are unavailable, the carbon skeletons of protein by gluconeogenesis become sources of energy. In the hypermetabolic, infected, or stressed patient [30], protein-sparing fails to occur in spite of an increased glucose space and rapid lipid turnover. Conceptually, the protein stores mobilized during stress provide an endogenous source of energy from amino acids, which represent an adaptive response to injury.

Although the metabolic response to injury is probably beneficial, if brief, body composition alteration secondary to stress, if severe and prolonged, contributes to weight loss [50], susceptibility to infection [16], muscle mass deterioration, and morbidity and mortality [47].

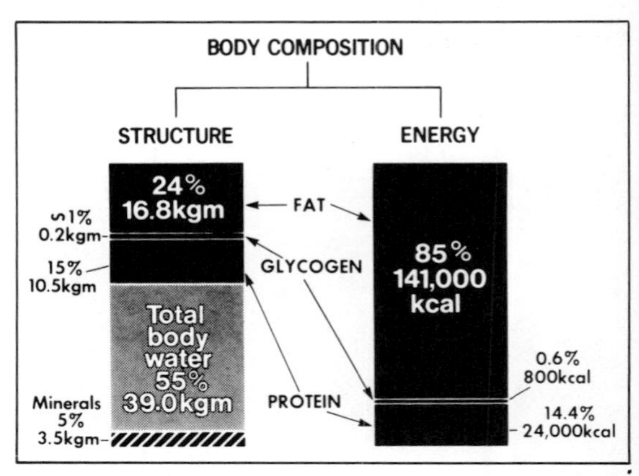

Figure 12-1. *Body composition is the basis of many nutritional assessment techniques. The idealized human has substrate-serving structure functions. The same compositional material has potential for conversion from structure into energy.*

Decreased intake and increased utilization of energy and protein are associated with dissolution of lean body mass. Decreased intake of foodstuffs occurs in anorexia associated with many disorders, and may accompany increasing tumor bulk, lesions of the gastrointestinal tract, and heart or liver failure. Different patterns of specific nutrient deficiencies occur with malabsorption due to bacterial overgrowth in an intestinal loop. Operative removal or disease of the terminal ileum common in granulomatous disease of the small intestine may cause failure of vitamin B_{12} absorption and resultant macrocytic anemia. Loss of bile salts from anatomic or functional loss of the terminal ileum can result in malabsorption of fat soluble vitamins (A, D, E, K). The most common identifiable defect with fat malabsorption is bleeding or prolonged prothrombin time from insufficient vitamin K.

Weight loss is a gross but useful index of the state of nutrition. Weight loss after medical therapy for ascites fluid in an alcoholic or cancer patient or in an extensively hydrated patient has different implications for body composition than does gradual weight loss. Rapid weight loss from vomiting and diarrhea may be largely reversible with hydration alone, with little alteration in body composition of fat, protein, or carbohydrate. A well-regulated dietary program can reduce body fat mass while preserving lean body mass. Clearly, clinical judgment and precise nutritional history are the cornerstones of nutritional assessment.

Measurement of body weight is often an inexact, infrequent, and underevaluated assessment tool. A careful history of weight, plus evaluation of its meaning, is a potentially useful tool. Interpretation of weight loss should take into consideration several known facts regarding weight loss. First, an otherwise normal individual who takes water, but no foodstuffs, will die of starvation in 60 to 70 days. Hypocaloric feeding will attenuate the effects of starvation and extend the period of time before death ensues. An acute loss of 10 percent of body weight (2 weeks or less) obviously has graver implications than a more gradual weight loss of the same magnitude. Weight loss of 25 percent of body weight is associated with comparable loss of weight of most of the body's functional organs (heart, lung, liver) and is the time period when severe complications of malnutrition such as pneumonia begin to occur. Body weight loss should be recorded by means of maximal monitoring. This is best done by using available tables of weights for age, height, and sex. It also is useful to obtain a history of weight change relative to ideal and usual body weight.

$$\%\ \text{Ideal body weight} = \frac{\text{actual weight} \times 100}{\text{ideal body weight}}$$

$$\%\ \text{Usual body weight} = \frac{\text{actual weight} \times 100}{\text{usual weight (history)}}$$

$$\%\ \text{Weight change} = \frac{\text{usual weight} - \text{weight} \times 100}{\text{usual weight}}$$

Obviously, frequent re-evaluation by daily, weekly, or monthly weight measurement is a readily available, noninvasive measurement tool that gives useful therapeutic and diagnostic information.

The physical examination is essential to the diagnosis of altered nutrition. Although gross cachexia, as seen in marasmus or severe PCM is diagnosed with ease, profound weight loss may not be obvious in a previously obese patient. Moreover, pronounced weight loss in a previously obese patient is often associated with profound loss of lean body mass and visceral protein (kwashiorkor).

Although the terminology derived from nutrition surveys in third world countries (marasmus, kwashiorkor) is not precisely applicable to most clinical states of malnutrition in the hospital setting, the terms are useful as broad categories. Marasmus is a state of protein and energy deficiency. Kwashiorkor is considered to be protein deficiency in the presence of adequate energy. Regardless of the applicability of specific terminology, all classification systems of disease include starvation and subgroups of starvation or malnutrition, e.g., adult marasmus (I.C.D.A. #268), kwashiorkor (I.C.D.A. #267). In most instances, malnutrition is secondary to another illness, such as cancer, burns, or pneumonia. A good practice is to code malnutrition on hospital discharge summaries, if it is a visible feature of the illness.

Some physical characteristics of malnutrition include dry, scaly, and atrophic skin, prone to decubitus ulcers because of loss of fat pads. Various specific nutrient deficiencies are occasionally seen, such as vitamin deficiencies (e.g., follicular dermatitis) of vitamin A, constipation or polyneuritis (thiamine), stomatitis and glossitis (niacin and riboflavin), macrocytic anemia (vitamin B_{12} and folic acid), increased capillary fragility and splinter hemorrhages (ascorbic acid), or intramuscular hemorrhages (vitamin K). Ascites and intra-abdominal organomegaly are usually associated with low serum albumin and may require additional diagnostic considerations. The overall result is a patient with functional and biochemical disturbances in association with significant somatic depletion.

Among the most important judgments required for nutritional assessment is metabolic rate. Although methodology exists for precise calculation of metabolic expenditure, assessment of metabolic expenditure is primarily a clinical judgment. In most instances, substrate requirements are predicated on estimated metabolic demand. Nitrogen balance is then used to adjust the prescribed solutions.

Although nitrogen excretion tends to parallel resting energy expenditure, the relationship is not predictable in individual patients [15]. A major operation causes minimal increase in metabolic expenditure. Serious injuries—such as burns, fractures, or sepsis—are accompanied by substantial increases in metabolic expenditure. The measurement of oxygen consumption ($\dot{V}O_2$) provides the most exact measurement of resting energy expenditure and is among the best methods available to correlate body composition with catabolism, as $\dot{V}O_2$ declines linearly with decreases in body weight [22]. In orally refed, malnourished children, feeding results in increased $\dot{V}O_2$. In starvation, $\dot{V}O_2$ is quite low. With refeeding, $\dot{V}O_2$ increases to high rates during rapid weight gain and then achieves a steady plateau between the nadir of starvation and the peak during immediate refeeding [8]. A different $\dot{V}O_2$ is characteristic of patients given parenteral nutrition if they are starved or stressed. Depleted patients whose treatment was changed from 5 percent dextrose infusion to higher carbohydrate load demonstrated little increase in $\dot{V}O_2$, but substantial (32 percent) increase in CO_2 production [15]. Injured and septic patients, unlike depleted patients, have substantial increases in both $\dot{V}O_2$ (29 percent increase) and CO_2 production (56 percent increase), when high concentrations of glucose are administered.

Nutritional assessment of the metabolic rate, coupled with judgment as to whether the patient is starvation adapted and depleted, or stressed and catabolic, provides the basis for rational selection of therapy. In the depleted patient, the therapeutic goal is restoration of body cell mass through provision of all nutrients. In the catabolic patient, the goal is to prevent body cell mass deterioration by providing sufficient energy, protein, and micronutrients.

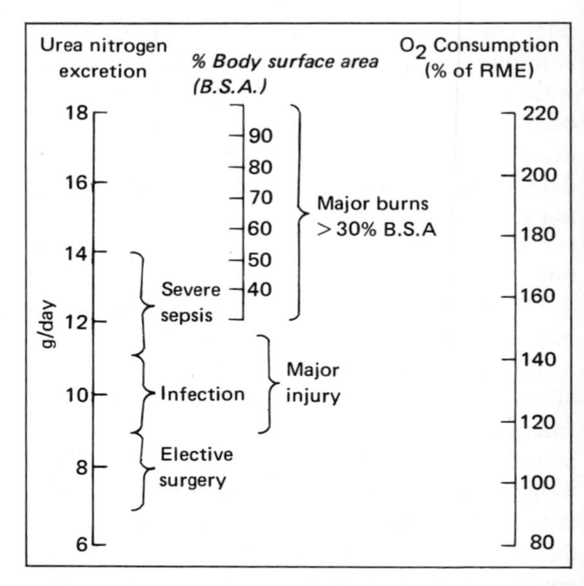

Figure 12-2. *Rates of hypermetabolism estimated from urinary urea nitrogen excretion. (From G. L. Blackburn et al. Nutritional and metabolic assessment of the hospitalized patient.* J.P.E.N. *1:11, 1977.)*

The disease process itself can increase the metabolic demands by 80 to 100 percent over normal basal metabolic demands [14] (Figure 12-2). The degree of hypermetabolism is a function of both the severity of injury and the presence of fever, infections, and/or sepsis.

If the gastrointestinal tract is functional, it is the optimal route to provide nutrition. Because most foodstuffs are absorbed in the proximal small intestine, its length and function require clinical evaluation if it is to be used as the source of nutrients. Even in the presence of normal intestinal mucosa, abnormalities in hepatic, pancreatic, and gastric function can affect digestion and absorption of nutrients. Moreover, malnutrition can create a vicious cycle in which malabsorption occurs and the malnutrition is worsened.

Table 12-1. *Standards for Anthropometric Measurements**

	Triceps Skinfold (mm)	Arm Circumference (cm)	Arm Muscle Circumference (cm)
Male	12.5	29.3	25.3
Female	16.5	28.5	23.2

*American standards have recently been developed (A. R. Frisancho. *Am. J. Clin. Nutr.* 27:1052, 1974).
Source: By permission of JPEN: G. L. Blackburn, et al. Nutritional and metabolic assessment of the hospitalized patient. *J.P.E.N.* 1:11, 1977.

STATIC NUTRITIONAL ASSESSMENT

Somatic Profile

Unless obesity is extensive, the skeletal muscle mass constitutes the greatest volume of tissue in the human body [32]. The greatest energy reserves, however, are contained within adipose tissue. Attempts to quantify the state of nutrition through indirect measurements of body compartments are popular, and include mid-arm circumference (AMC) and skinfold thickness (TSF) (Table 12-1) correlated with age, weight, height, and other measurements. Collectively referred to as anthropometric measurements, they are of perhaps greater value when used as intended, as survey material in underdeveloped countries. Anthropometric measurements have not proved reliable to assess body composition in individual patients, but are somewhat reliable when applied to groups of patients. In a study of 82 surgical patients and 10 volunteers [18], changes in arm circumference, arm muscle circumference, and weight/height ratio failed to correlate well enough with changes in total body nitrogen (as measured by neutron analysis techniques) to serve as biologic markers of total nitrogen. Skinfold thickness demonstrated no better correlation with lean body mass [24], and its value in monitoring fat stores is limited in populations with limited fat layers [14].

Creatinine-Height Index

Since creatinine is a by-product of muscle metabolism, correlations have been demonstrated between muscle mass and urinary excretion of creatinine. Muscle mass increases roughly in proportion to ideal body weight, resulting in a correlation between ideal body weight and creatinine. Marasmic malnutrition is considered moderate if creatinine-height index is 60 to 80 percent of normal, and severe if less than 60 percent of normal [7] (Table 12-2). Although creatinine-height index is a reasonable measure of muscle mass in patients with chronic nutritional deprivation, it is probably of less value in the stressed, septic, or injured patient.

Visceral Protein Status

Plasma proteins provide a more sensitive index of PCM than is reflected by anthropometric data [49]. Virtually all plasma proteins decrease as a consequence of PCM. The extent to which different plasma proteins decrease is largely a function of the half-life of the protein measured. Knowledge of the half-life of various plasma proteins allows interpretation of their absolute value to be usefully employed. Moreover, levels of protein are influenced by factors other than PCM. For example, many are diluted by resuscitation solutions and most function as acute phase proteins. In general, the rate of total body protein synthesis, breakdown, and turnover decreases in malnourished and stressed patients [19] and returns to normal in parallel with nutritional recovery. Visceral protein analysis includes measurement of serum albumin, transferrin, retinol-

Table 12-2. *Ideal Urinary Creatinine Values*

Men[a]		Women[b]	
Height (cm)	Ideal Creatinine (mg)	Height (cm)	Ideal Creatinine (mg)
157.5	1288	147.3	830
160.0	1325	149.9	851
162.6	1359	152.4	875
165.1	1386	154.9	900
167.6	1426	157.5	925
170.2	1467	160.0	949
172.7	1513	162.6	977
175.3	1555	165.1	1006
177.8	1596	167.6	1044
180.3	1642	170.2	1076
182.9	1691	172.7	1109
185.4	1739	175.3	1141
188.0	1785	177.8	1174
190.5	1831	180.3	1206
193.0	1891	182.9	1240

[a]Creatinine coefficient (men) = 23 mg/kg of ideal body weight.
[b]Creatinine coefficient (women) = 18 mg/kg of ideal body weight.
Source: By permission of JPEN: G. L. Blackburn, et al. Nutritional and metabolic assessment of the hospitalized patient. *J.P.E.N.* 1:11, 1977.

binding protein, and thyroxin-binding prealbumin.

Albumin

Albumin is a satisfactory index of subtle, progressive PCM if one excludes causes other than malnutrition of hypoalbuminemia [25, 42]. Albumin is the major protein produced by the liver during health, and the exchangeable albumin pool is about 4.0 gm/kg in women and 10 to 20 percent greater in men [37]. Normally, only about one-third of the total exchangeable albumin resides in the intravascular space; the remainder is distributed through the extravascular space [39] in the skin, muscle, and viscera. Fifteen grams of albumin are synthesized and catabolized daily, and newly produced albumin has a half-life of about 17 days.

Unfortunately, many extraneous factors besides protein and caloric intake influence albumin metabolism and distribution. In animals, deprivation of food produces a rapid decrease in albumin synthesis, but the extravascular compartment serves as a reservoir for the decreasing intravascular compartment, and serum albumin levels are thus maintained for prolonged periods [38]. Fractional catabolic rate (FCR) also slows as the extra-plasma compartment decreases [36]. Shifts in albumin occur in association with stress and hydration [46]. Investigators have also noted a greater decrease in extra-plasmic albumin mass than in the intravascular mass after a major operation such as gastric surgery [3]. Although not sensitive as a short-term indicator, albumin levels help to evaluate nutritional status in chronic PCM. If other causes, such as liver disease, are excluded, and the history is compatible with PCM, a low albumin is perhaps the most important single laboratory test that supports the diagnosis of PCM. In most series, recent and past, albumin values below 3.0 mg/100 ml correlate indirectly with morbidity and mortality.

Transferrin

Although transferrin is a more sensitive indicator of PCM than albumin [25], because of a half-life of 8 days, it is also a nonspecific indicator of PCM [2]. Metabolic studies done on obese women given various protein diets supplemented with high or low caloric intake showed decreasing levels of transferrin when protein intake was low. Significant decreases occurred, however, only when calories were also restricted, as severe energy deprivation, with adequate protein intake, may be accompanied by relatively normal transferrin values. In many primary disease states associated with coexisting iron deficiency, anemia may stimulate transferrin production, even in the presence of PCM, and may accentuate any putative correlation between PCM and transferrin values.

Retinol-binding Protein (RBP) and Thyroxin-binding Pre-albumin (TBPA)

Recently, many investigators have explored the usefulness of serum proteins with a shorter half-life and more biologic specificity than albumin, transferrin, or haptoglobin. Starvation diets in 12 healthy but obese patients showed much more acute changes in serum RBP and TBPA than in levels of transferrin and haptoglobin. Serum levels of RBP and TBPA appeared to develop a rapid decrease, levelling to a plateau at one week, whereas the albumin and transferrin gradually decreased [17]. Shelty [42] demonstrated that TBPA levels fell in response to energy restriction alone, although the early diminution of protein depletion could be blunted with adequate caloric intake [42]. RBP, however, decreased when deficits of either protein or calories were administered. Recovery rates of TBPA and RBP levels, assessed during repletion of 37 children with clinical PCM, were predictably more rapid than albumin values [25]. Rapid decrease and increase in TBPA and RBP probably reflect a brief half-life of 2 days and 12 hours, respectively, of TBPA and RBP [35]. Although both TBPA and RBA are proteins of relatively short half-life and have parallel values during CPM and repletion, they contain different biologic properties. Although the correlation between RBP and TBPA remains constant in healthy individuals, elevated levels of RBP and vitamin A occur with normal levels of TBPA in patients with chronic renal disease [21]. In addition, like albumin, both proteins are produced by the liver and are depressed with severe liver disease. Other chronic disorders, such as hyperthyroidism and vitamin A deficiency, may cause low serum levels of RBP and TBPA and reflect specific diseases, not just PCM [35].

Immunologic Profile

The immunologic profile provides an assessment of delayed cutaneous hypersensitivity (Candida, mumps, streptokinase-streptodornase, Trichomonas, Coccidioidin), total lymphocyte count, serum complement levels, and cellular immune function.

Protein-calorie malnutrition is known to be associated with decreased humoral and cellular immunity. Virulence of bacterial and viral infections is greater in patients with PCM than in normally nourished subjects [10, 16]. Only recently have assays become available which promise to unravel the problem of specificity of immunodeficiency associated with PCM. Considerable investigation is required in order to more clearly define the specifics of host defense alteration associated with PCM and catabolic illness. Prominent among known immunologic defects associated with PCM is the decreased ability of neutrophils to kill bacteria [40]. In addition, some diminution in opsonization function of the patient's serum occurs with injury and PCM [41]. Many complement components and immunoglobulins also decrease during both starvation and stress states. Alterations in leukocyte subpopulations, specifically the T-cell, appear to be altered following injury or PCM. Host defense, however, requires successful interaction of B, T, and Accessory (A) cells, as well as cooperative interactions through lymphokines and complement [29]. Protein synthesis is required for all of these responses to a lesser or greater degree. Unfortunately, the readily available tests of host defense provide the least information of actual immune function.

Delayed Cutaneous Hypersensitivity

Tests of delayed cutaneous hypersensitivity constitute the most practical manner available to analyze immunologic function of malnutrition. Intradermal injection of 0.1 ml of Candida, PPD, Trichophyton, Coccidioidin, streptokinase-streptodornase, or mumps antigen will cause induration and erythema in patients (1) sensitive to the antigens and (2) capable of generating a response. An additional, slightly different method of determining anergic recall, is to apply dinitrochlorobenzene (DNCB) on a small area of skin. Only 20 percent of normal patients responded to DNCB on first application, in one series, but most normal patients will respond to a second application [29]. In general, patients are considered anergic if they fail to develop induration and erythema to a second application of DNCB, or if one or none of the intradermal injections elicit the appropriate induration at 48 hours.

Numerous variables affect the interpretation of the response to skin tests. Peripheral edema is common in many acutely ill patients, and the inability to obtain erythema and induration may be due to insufficient cellular interaction, inflammation, or induration. Many extraneous factors, including uremia, hepatic failure, ongoing septic processes [26], and deficiencies of nutrients other than proteins can blunt or eliminate the response. In malnourished children administered bilateral skin tests, the application of zinc sulfate to one area reversed the local anergy response occurring simultaneously on the opposite arm [20]. In an investigation of DCH in cancer patients [13], 57.5 percent of DCH-negative patients and 28.5 percent of DCH-positive patients converted from negative to positive and positive to negative, respectively, after nutritional support. Even normal subjects may fail to respond as expected to skin tests [29]. Moreover, different preparations of antigen vary in strength and potency, a fact that adds to the difficulty of interpreting data from various reports [34].

Nevertheless, failure to achieve anergic recall to a battery of skin test antigens does seem to correlate with age and severity of illness. MacLean and Meakins reported a 34 percent incidence of sepsis and 212 percent mortality in anergic patients, which contrasted sharply with a 7 percent incidence of infection and 2 percent death rate in patients with normal skin test profiles. Skin test anergy will identify groups of sick patients. Lack of skin test anergy, however, is not necessarily caused by PCM, nor does it identify a specific defect in the immune system. Data from any individual patient must be considered in the context of the clinical state, with recognition of the shortcomings of skin test methodology.

Total Lymphocyte Count

Calculation of the total lymphocyte count (TLC) from the equation

$$TLC = \% \text{ of lymphocytes} \times \text{total white count}$$

has been used to assess mass of the peripheral blood lymphocytes, which is considered abnormal if less than 1500/ml. These data must be used, as before, in the context of the overall patient status, recognizing that lymphopenia may result from various primary disease states, such as cardiac failure, uremia, or Hodgkin's disease [48]. Administration of some immunosuppressive drugs, in particular, adrenocorticosteroids, also cause lymphopenia. Total lymphocyte counts are nonspecific for PCM and correlate poorly with outcome.

Complement Levels

Serum complement levels have been evaluated in children suffering from protein and caloric deficits. The simultaneous presence of chronic infection with PCM probably explains the inconsistent data reported. In general, malnutrition is associated with low values of C3 in uninfected individuals without stress [33]. If stress, infection, or injury occur, C3 behaves as an acute phase protein and is usually normal or elevated.

Specialized techniques to evaluate individual components of cellular immunity and inflammatory response have provided insights into the diverse effects of PCM on the immunologic systems. Effects on immunoglobulin profiles [1], and opsonins [41] have been described, and defects in neutrophil bacteriocidal ability have been noted [40] to accompany PCM. Further investigations are necessary to determine whether defects in components of the host defense mechanism can be identified and treated.

PROGNOSTIC NUTRITIONAL ASSESSMENT

The goal of nutritional assessment is to identify patients at risk for morbidity or mortality from malnutrition. The ability to provide nutrient support and potentially minimize or avoid morbidity and mortality from PCM has stimulated efforts to identify, by a variety of methods, patients at risk. Implicit in the identification of criteria for increased risk from malnutrition is the expectation that normalization by nutritional support of abnormal findings will positively benefit patients. The limitations and advantages of the various test methods have been discussed. An attempt to refine the interpretation of some of the tests has been developed, by Mullen, into a "prognostic nutritional assessment."

If a battery of biochemical, immunologic, and anthropometric measures are administered to any patient group, most patients will have at least one abnormal value. Moreover, a single abnormal value has little clinical significance. Because no single test is available that can quantitate nutritional status and predict an increased likelihood of postoperative problems, Mullen and associates have been successful in defining a population of patients with an increased morbidity and mortality using 4 parameters, i.e., albumin, triceps-skinfold, transferrin, and delayed cutaneous hypersensitivity (DCH). Mathematical modeling is used to improve predictive value:

Prognostic nutritional index (PNI)—(%) = 158 − 16.6 (Alb) − 0.78 (TSF) − 0.2 (transferrin) − 5.8 (DCH) was graded as:

0 = nonreactive

1 = less than 5 mm reactivity

2 = greater than 5 mm reactivity to mumps, Candida or streptokinase-streptodornase

The authors noted a significant increase in mortality, complications, and sepsis as PNI increased. Twelve other commonly cited nutritional assessment variables failed to improve the reliability of the test. Complications appear to increase in linear relation to PNI. Patients identified to be at risk suffered a 6- to 12-fold increase in complications and mortality, with most of the complications related to infection. In one study, the PNI defined 89 percent of patients developing complications and over 90 percent of all patients that became septic [11, 31]. The correlations described by Mullen represent a thoughtful, analytic approach which attempts to be more specific in terms of nutritional assessment. Preliminary results from this method suggest that it is more specific in predicting complications, particularly septic ones, than mortality. It remains unclear whether this methodology will truly predict potential morbidity more precisely than clinical judgment.*

DYNAMIC NUTRITIONAL ASSESSMENT

Nitrogen Excretion and Balance

Both the severity of the catabolic response to injury and inadequate nutrient intake, separately

**Editor's Note:* It is worth noting that the prognostic nutritional index is in large part made up of albumin as a major component. It is not clear that greater accuracy is introduced by taking the other components (TSF, transferrin, and DCH) into account. These and other studies by Mullen and his group, while interesting, unfortunately have all the defects of retrospective analysis.

or in concert, may result in PCM. Because protein is the limiting factor in determining survival, most assessments of nutrition focus on protein-derived functions. Because no single biochemical test is available to identify or quantitate malnutrition, or to follow progress during repletion, nitrogen balance is a useful though gross measure of protein breakdown and intake. Moreover, nitrogen balance provides a dynamic, as opposed to a static, measure of protein and energy balance.

Less than 5 gm/day of nitrogen as urea is excreted in the unstressed, starvation-adapted state, because fat serves as the major source of energy. Following injury or during infection, excretion of 10 to 30 gm daily of urea nitrogen commonly occurs. If nitrogen loss of this magnitude is prolonged, over 25 percent of lean body mass may be lost in less than one month.

Collection and analysis of a 24-hour urine for urea nitrogen can help to quantify the magnitude of protein breakdown. Since nitrogen excretion roughly parallels metabolic rate, measurements of nitrogen excretion are a crude index of catabolism. When nitrogen intake (+) is added to nitrogen excretion (−), it becomes possible to calculate nitrogen balance. Because protein is the only tissue and food containing nitrogen (6.25 × nitrogen gm = protein gm), nitrogen balance measurement reflects protein balance. In calculating nitrogen balance, 4 gm of nitrogen are commonly added to the measure of urine urea nitrogen, to account for nitrogen losses through the skin, feces, and unmeasured end-products of protein breakdown, such as ammonia. Obviously, abnormal protein loss through the skin in burns or the gastrointestinal tract in fistulas detract from the accuracy of the measurement. Nitrogen balance techniques have been justly criticized as inaccurate because of underestimation of losses through the skin, nails, and hair, which result in overestimation of the positive nitrogen balance [23]. Because nitrogen balance data by themselves do not reflect the rate of catabolism [6], a catabolic index, calculated as follows:

$$\text{CI} = \left(1 - \frac{\text{net protein utilization}}{100\%}\right) \text{(dietary nitrogen intake)}$$

aids in interpretation because energy intake and utilization are included in the equation.

In spite of the limitations of nitrogen balance, it remains the best quantitative and dynamic measure of ongoing nutritional therapy. Daily weight in patients receiving therapeutic nutrition fails to differentiate weight alteration due to fat and water. Biochemical tests, such as albumin, require a prolonged period of protein adequacy to restore values to normal. Nitrogen balance allows quantitation of therapy, so that excess or deficient therapy can be adjusted, based on the most significant structural component, protein.

3-Methylhistidine

As a product of actin and myosin metabolism, 3-methylhistidine is occasionally employed as an index of skeletal muscle breakdown. 3-Methylhistidine, when liberated from actin and myosin, is excreted without being recycled for energy or protein synthesis and therefore has the potential for quantitating catabolism. However, 3-methylhistidine increases during refeeding of starved patients and is not as specific for catabolism as originally thought. 3-Methylhistidine is a dynamic measure of protein status, but provides little practical information that cannot be obtained by nitrogen balance. Moreover, the measurement of 3-methylhistidine is complex and not a clinically practical test.

EXPERIMENTAL METHODS FOR NUTRITIONAL ASSESSMENT

Multiple Isotope Dilution

The metabolically active tissues of the body are enclosed in an intracellular environment in which lie 99 percent of the total exchangeable potassium (K) [43]. Skeletal muscle constitutes about 60 percent of this mass, with an additional 20 percent accounted for by the viscera. The remainder is made up of red blood cells, connective tissue, etc. Assuming that no osmolar discrepancies are present, the osmotic forces in the intracellular compartment are counterbalanced by the exchangeable sodium (Na_e) in the extracellular compartment. Only water distributes itself freely across the intracellular and extracellular compartments, roughly in a 2:1 ratio. A constant ratio (R) can be defined by the equation:

$$R = \frac{Na_e + K_e}{TBW}$$

and determined through the analysis of peripheral blood. The compartment defined by K_e provides the most useful information of lean body mass, but measurements using K isotopes are restrictive. Plasma volume, red cell mass, extracellular water, and total body water can be characterized by ^{125}I human serum albumin, ^{51}Cr red blood cells, ^{22}Na, and $^{3}H_2O$, so that K_e can be calculated indirectly with excellent correlation between calculated K and total body K [43]. The evaluation with this technique in postoperative patients [45] and in morbidly obese patients [44] undergoing intestinal bypass has defined changes in body composition through the derivation of the Na_3/K_3 ratio, i.e., extracellular mass as a function of body cell mass. Protein calorie malnutrition (PCM) is defined in terms of an Na_e/K_e ratio greater than 1:22. The technique may underestimate skeletal muscle protein in certain states; TBW, usually increased in PCM, may be excreted as nutritional support evolves and increases in total body nitrogen occur. As a result, skeletal muscle mass may remain unchanged even though an increase in nitrogen composition occurs. The technique has been useful in the quantitation of degrees of malnutrition. It has also confirmed the suspected magnitude of deterioration of different body compartments during injury and refeeding. Multiple isotope studies have demonstrated that body composition based on anthropometric measurements are estimates.*

**Editor's Note:* As pointed out in Chapter 11, while Na_e and other determinations are reasonable, attempts to derive further information from calculated ratios are likely to yield information which is only approximate at best. The reason is that while each estimate has approximately a 10% error, multiplying such errors yields enormous variations which may be almost without value.

Neutron Activation

Body composition can also be measured by a gamma neutron activation technique. The method allows analysis of absolute levels of calcium, phosphorus, sodium, and chloride by delayed neutron activation analysis. Body composition analysis of protein can be determined from total body nitrogen and potassium. Total body water and total bone calcium can be measured by these methods. Multi-element analysis provides the potential of supplementing or replacing balance techniques, as they provide the potential of determining body compartment size as well as distribution. Neutron activation, however, is not precise enough to measure visceral protein—a measurement that is essential to nutritional assessment.

NUTRITIONAL ASSESSMENT—IN PERSPECTIVE

Current methods for performing nutritional assessment have many limitations. The simple, noninvasive methods have the disadvantages of (1) lack of specificity; (2) minimal monitoring usefulness; and (3) limited predictive value. The more precise methods have the disadvantages of being primarily research tools which (1) are expensive; (2) often employ ionizing radiation; and (3) have limited predictive value. Advantages of the simple noninvasive methods are (1) simplicity; (2) awareness identification; and (3) potential for repletion. The research tools have provided information about body compositional changes in various states of malnutrition and during nutritional repletion. Both simple and complex assessment modalities have a role in patient care if overinterpretation is avoided.

Although it is known that malnutrition adversely affects a variety of illnesses, and may be a primary disease, the degree to which PCM influences morbidity and mortality is unclear. Moreover, it is quite likely that specific protein-dependent systems—such as host defense—may be more important in some illnesses than in others. It is quite possible that in terms of morbidity, body composition studies may contribute less information of value in terms of morbidity than is provided by evaluation of enzyme systems. Lacking a clearly defined defect to treat, and an end-point to strive for, it is not surprising that current nutritional assessment tools fall short of critical expectations.

The following approaches, however, can complement currently available assessment methodology after the history, dietary evaluation, and other methods are completed. They include the "5-day rule," which imparts an urgency to the clinician to have performed an estimation of the patient's metabolic and nutritional status within 5 days and project his ability to eat within one week. If it is clear that anatomic or physiologic loss of gastrointestinal function has occurred and will continue, nutritional support should be implemented. Obviously, if the patient is clinically malnourished on initial evaluation, nutritional support may need to be initiated immediately. The next consideration is whether the patient is starting from a state of relatively normal body composition or is cachectic or obese. Therapeutic nutrition designed to preserve or restore body cell mass will then be implemented.

The next decision involves a judgment as to the metabolic rate, using the following estimates:

Basal energy	25 kcal/kg/day
Trauma	5–60 kcal/kg/day
Protein	500–800 gm amino acid nitrogen or 1–3 gm protein/kg/day

The accuracy of these estimates is then evaluated by daily nitrogen balance until the patient is stable, and then twice a week. Finally, a knowledge of the pathophysiology of the underlying disease often is enough indication for therapeutic nutrition. A hypermetabolic patient with a third-degree thermal burn extensive enough to require hospitalization should receive aggressive nutritional support. A patient with an enterocutaneous fistula usually has insufficient gastrointestinal function to maintain body cell mass and requires nutritional support to survive. In all instances, the therapeutic goal should be prevention of malnutrition rather than correction after nutritional assessment parameters have identified the problem.*

REFERENCES

1. Alexander, J. W., et al. A comparison of immunologic profiles and their influence on bacteremia in surgical patients with a high risk of infection. *Surgery* 86:94, 1979.
2. Awai, M., and Brown, E. B. Studies of the metabolism of I^{131} labelled human transferrin. *J. Lab. Clin. Med.* 61:363, 1963.
3. Beno, I., and Cirven, A. Albumin metabolism and gastric surgery. *Nutr. Metab.* 22:44, 1978.
4. Bistrian, B. R., et al. Protein states of general surgical patients. *J.A.M.A.* 230:858, 1974.
5. Bistrian, B. R., et al. Prevalence of malnutrition in general medical patients. *J.A.M.A.* 235:1567, 1976.
6. Bistrian, B. R. A simple technique to estimate severity of stress. *Surg. Gynecol. Obstet.* 148:675, 1979.
7. Blackburn, G. L., et al. Nutritional and metabolic assessment of the hospitalized patient. *J.P.E.N.* 1:11, 1977.
8. Brooke, O. G., and Ashworthe, A. The influence of malnutrition on the postprandial metabolic rate and respiratory quotient. *Br. J. Nutr.* 27:407, 1972.
9. Burkinshaw, L., Morgan, D. B., and Hill, G. L. Loss of protein from muscle and other tissues in patients with pre-operative weight loss. *Br. J. Surg.* 65:816, 1978.
10. Butterworth, C. E. The skeleton in the hospital closet. *Nutr. Today.* Mar-Apr, 1974. Pp. 4–8.
11. Buzby, G. P., et al. Prognostic nutritional index in gastrointestinal surgery. *Am. J. Surg.* 139:160, 1980.
12. Collins, J. P., McCarthy, I. D., and Hill, G. L. Assessment of protein nutrition in surgical patients—the value of anthropometrics. *Am. J. Clin. Nutr.* 32:1530, 1979.
13. Copeland, E. M., MacFayden, B. V., and Dudrick, S. J. Effect of intravenous hyperalimentation on established delayed hypersensitivity in the cancer patient. *Ann. Surg.* 184:60, 1976.

******Editor's Note:* **This prognostic approach has much to recommend it. Our primary goal should be to prevent malnutrition rather than attempt to replete patients after the damage has been done.**

14. Duke, J. H., et al. Contribution of protein to caloric expenditure following injury. *Surgery* 68:168, 1970.
15. Elwyn, D. Nutritional requirements of adult surgical patients. *Crit. Care Med.* 8:9, 1980.
16. Faulk, D. W. P., Demaeyer, E. M., and Davies, A. J. Some effects of malnutrition on the immune response in man. *Am. J. Clin. Nutr.* 27:638, 1974.
17. Frey, B. M., et al. Dysproteinaemia during total fasting. *Metabolism* 28:363, 1979.
18. Frisancho, A. R. Triceps skinfold and upper arm muscle size norms for assessment of nutritional status. *Am. J. Clin. Nutr.* 27:1052, 1974.
19. Golden, M. H. N., Waterlow, J. C., and Picon, D. Protein turnover, synthesis and breakdown before and after recovery from protein-energy malnutrition. *Clin. Sci. Mol. Med.* 53:473, 1977.
20. Golden, M. H., Harland, P. S., Golden, B. E., and Jackson, A. A. Zinc and immunocompetence in protein-energy malnutrition. *Lancet* 1:1226, 1978.
21. Goodman, D. S. Retinol-Binding Protein, Prealbumin and Vitamin A Transport. In G. A. Jamieson and T. J. Greenwalt (Eds.), *Trace Components of Plasma: Isolation and Clinical Significance.* New York: Liss, 1976. P. 313.
22. Grande, F., Anderson, J. T., and Keys, A. Changes of basal metabolic rate in man in semistarvation and refeeding. *J. Appl. Physiol.* 12:230, 1958.
23. Hegsted, D. M. Balance studies. *J. Nutr.* 106:307, 1976.
24. Hill, G. L., et al. Fat-free body mass from skinfold thickness: A close relationship with total body nitrogen. *Br. J. Nutr.* 39:403, 1978.
25. Ingenbleck, Y., et al. Albumin, transferrin and the thyroxine-binding prealbumin/retinol -binding protein (TBPA-RBP) complex in assessment of malnutrition. *Clin. Chim. Acta* 673:61, 1975.
26. Johnson, M. W., Maibach, H. I., and Salmon, S. E. Skin reactivity in patients with cancer—impaired delayed hypersensitivity or faulty inflammatory response? *N. Engl. J. Med.* 284:1255, 1971.
27. Kaminski, M. V., Ruggiero, R. P., and Mills, C. B. Nutritional assessment. A guide to diagnosis and treatment of the hypermetabolic patient. *J. Florida Med. Assoc.* 66:390, 1979.
28. King, J. C., Calloway, D. H., and Morgan, S. Nitrogen retention, total body 40K and weight gain in teenage pregnant girls. *J. Nutr.* 103:772, 1973.
29. Miller, C. L. Immunological assays as measurements of nutritional status: A review. *J.P.E.N.* 2:554, 1978.
30. Moore, F. D., and Brennan, M. F. Surgical Injury: Body Composition, Protein Metabolism and Neuroendocrinology. In *Manual of Surgical Nutrition.* Committee on Pre- and Postoperative Care, American College of Surgeons. Philadelphia: Saunders, 1975.
31. Mullen, J. L., et al. Prediction of operative morbidity and mortality by preoperative nutritional assessment. *Surg. Forum* 30:80, 1979.
32. Munro, H. N. Nutrition and muscle protein metabolism: Introduction. *Fed. Proc.* 37:2281, 1978.
33. Palmbold, J., et al. Acute energy deprivation in man: Effect on serum immunoglobulins antibody response, complement factors 3 and 4, acute phase reactants and interferon-producing capacity of blood lymphocytes. *Clin. Exp. Immunol.* 30:50, 1977.
34. Palmer, D. L., and Reed, W. P. Delayed hypersensitivity testing: I. Response rates in a hospitalized population. *J. Int. Dis.* 130:132, 1974.
35. Robbins, J., et al. Thyroxine transport proteins of plasma. Molecular properties and biosynthesis. *Rec. Prog. Horm. Res.* 34:477, 1978.
36. Rossing, N., Parving, H. H., and Lassen, N. A. Albumin Transcapillary Escape Rate as an Approach to Microvascular Physiology in Health and Disease. In R. Bianchi, G. Mariani, and A. S. MacFarlane (Eds.), *Plasma Protein Turnover.* London: 1976. Pp. 357–370.
37. Rothschild, M. A., Oratz, M., and Schreiber, S. S. Albumin synthesis. *N. Engl. J. Med.* 286:748, and 286:816, 1972.
38. Rothschild, M. A., Oratz, M., and Schreiber, S. S. Albumin metabolism. *Gastroenterology* 64:326, 1973.
39. Rothschild, M. A., Oratz, M., and Schreiber, S. S. Extravascular albumin. *N. Engl. J. Med.* 301:497, 1979.
40. Selvaraj, R. J., and Bhat, K. S. Metabolic and bactericidal activities of leukocytes in protein-calorie malnutrition. *Am. J. Clin. Nutr.* 25:166, 1972.
41. Setl, V., and Chandra, R. K. Opsonic activity, phagocytosis and bactericidal capacity of polymorphs in undernutrition. *Arch. Dis. Child.* 47:282, 1972.
42. Shetty, P. S., et al. Rapid turnover transport proteins: An index of subclinical protein-energy malnutrition. *Lancet* 2:230, 1979.
43. Shizgal, H. M., et al. Indirect measurement of total exchangeable potassium. *Am. J. Physiol.* 233:253, 1977.
44. Shizgal, H. M., et al. Protein malnutrition following intestinal bypass for morbid obesity. *Surgery* 86:60, 1979.

45. Shizgal, H. M., Milne, C. A., and Spanier, A. H. The effect of nitrogen sparing, intravenously administered fluids on postoperative body composition. *Surgery* 85:496, 1979.
46. Smith, P. C., et al. Albumin uptake by skin, skeletal muscle and lung in living and dying patients. *Ann. Surg.* 187:31, 1978.
47. Studley, H. O. Percent of weight loss; a basic indicator of surgical risk. *J.A.M.A.* 106:458, 1936.
48. Wintrobe, M. M. *Clinical Hematology*. Philadelphia: Lea & Febiger, 1974.
49. Young, G. A., and Hill, G. L. Assessment of protein-calorie malnutrition in surgical patients from plasma proteins and anthropometric measurements. *Am. J. Clin. Nutr.* 31:424, 1978.
50. Young, V. R., and Munro, H. N. N^{τ}-methylhistidine (3-methylhistidine) and muscle protein turnover: An overview. *Fed. Proc.* 37:229, 1978.

Physiologic Alterations in Disease

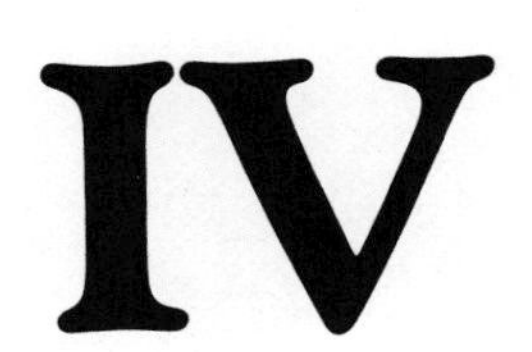

Starvation: Metabolic and Physiologic Responses

Stanley M. Levenson
Eli Seifter

13

Physicians have been aware for at least 2,500 years of the effects of diet and nutritional status on health and on the body's response to injury and disease (Hippocrates [84]). A large number of clinical and experimental studies during the past 70 years, beginning with the classic studies of Dubois [38], Benedict [10], Cuthbertson [33] and their associates, have confirmed and extended this understanding. This chapter deals with some of the metabolic and physiologic responses to food deprivation per se to lay the basis for later discussions in this volume of the metabolic and physiologic responses to injury and disease and how these are affected by food intake, for it is clear that the latter plays a critical modulating role. We will be concerned primarily with effects of inadequate food intake in the presence of adequate water intake. The reader is referred to the book by Wolf entitled *Thirst* [220]. Vitamin, unsaturated fatty acid, and trace mineral deficiencies per se will not be discussed, except to point out that the appearance of such deficiencies is slowed during starvation [67]. Nor will we discuss the psychologic changes possibly associated with (caused by?) starvation. This complicated subject is beyond the scope of this book; some relevant references are cited in the reference list for this chapter [100, 118].

Food deprivation can occur as a primary event in previously healthy individuals, as in famine, or it may come about as a secondary result of injury or disease. Also, in recent years, purposeful fasting of obese patients has become an increasingly popular therapeutic regimen. The metabolic responses to food deprivation are quantitatively and often qualitatively different in these various circumstances, and one of our efforts will be to point out some of the major differences in the metabolic responses to starvation by otherwise healthy individuals and by seriously ill and injured patients.

HISTORICAL SURVEY

Never in history has there been enough food for all people. Throughout evolution, man's exis-

Supported in part by the U.S. Army Research and Development Command, Contract #DADA 17-70-C, and a Research Career Award (S.M.L.) #5KO6 GM14,208 from the National Institutes of Health to the Albert Einstein College of Medicine, Yeshiva University, Bronx, New York.

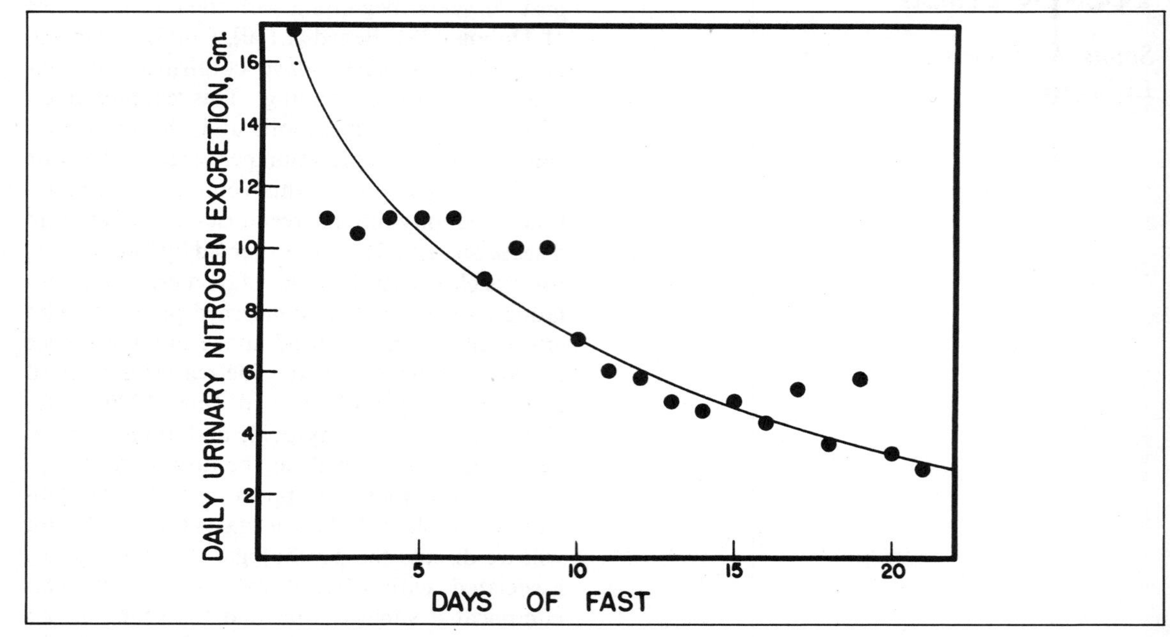

Figure 13-1. *Daily urinary nitrogen excretion during one of Succi's prolonged fasts. (From E. Freund and O. Freund,* Beiträge zum Stoffwechsel im Hungerzustande. Weiner Klin. Rundschau *15:91, 1901).*

tence has been facilitated by his ability to survive long periods of enforced fasting. It is a sad commentary on our civilization that severe hunger is rampant throughout much of the world, even in developed countries. Paradoxically, in some of these same countries, obesity is a major health problem. A discussion of the complex social, economic, political, and cultural causes for this situation is beyond the scope of this chapter, but the primacy of their solution is self-evident.

Descriptions of some of the overall physical, functional, and psychologic effects of severe food deprivation can be found in the earliest writings, but it was not until the late nineteenth century that prospective studies of experimental animals (Voit) and of men who subjected themselves to voluntary food deprivation began (Succi, in Italy; Tanner, in the United States; and Merlotti, in France).

Early studies established the relative rates of weight loss during starvation and demonstrated that after several days 10 to 15 percent of the calories expended during fasting were the result of protein metabolism, whereas 85 to 90 percent were supplied by fat. Liver and muscle glycogen fell rapidly, but some glycogen was present even after 3 weeks. These early investigations showed also that (1) urinary nonprotein nitrogen and sulfur fell during the first weeks of starvation of men (Figure 13-1) and (2) the proportion of urea in urinary nonprotein nitrogen fell from about 85 to 55 percent within 3 weeks, while urinary ammonium increased substantially, paralleling the developing metabolic acidosis reflected by the appearance of large quantities of β-hydroxybutyric acid and acetone in the urine. It was noted that gluconeogenesis declined during fasting in parallel with the decreased rate of body protein loss, as evidenced by a gradual decline in urinary nitrogen. There followed a prolonged period in which urinary nitrogen plateaued at a level of about 3 gm daily.

Table 13-1. *Calculation of Amounts of Carbohydrate, Protein, and Fat Metabolized by Benedict's Fasting Man*

		Food Metabolized		
Days of Fast	Nitrogen Excreted (gm)	Carbohydrate (gm)	Protein (gm)	Fat (gm)
1	7.1	69	43	135
2	8.4	42	50	142
3	11.3	39	68	130
4	11.9	4	71	136
5	10.4		63	133
6	10.2		61	133
7	9.8		59	134

Source: J. P. Peters and D. D. Van Slyke. *Quantitative Clinical Chemistry Interpretations.* Vol. 1. Baltimore: Williams & Wilkins, 1946.

These early investigators found that survival during starvation depended on the amount of fat present in the organism at the beginning of food deprivation. When the fat stores became markedly depleted, there was an increase in urinary nitrogen excretion, the so-called "pre-mortal rise." Body temperature and the normal diurnal variations in temperature were generally maintained close to normal until just a short time before death when there was a marked decline in temperature.

These early observations have been further elucidated during the past 80 years, owing to an increased understanding of mammalian biochemical and physiologic processes in general. Key advances were made between 1915 and 1920, when Dubois [38] began his classic studies of metabolic rates in healthy volunteers and in patients (especially those with infectious diseases). In the same period, Benedict [11] began his equally classic studies on the biochemical, physiologic, and psychologic responses of young men subsisting voluntarily on a modestly reduced diet that led to a weight loss of about 10 percent over many months. Their metabolic rates gradually declined about 12 to 18 percent per kilogram body weight (16 to 22 percent/m^2 body surface), demonstrating that the fall in metabolic rate was proportionately greater than the loss of total body mass.

Benedict [10] also studied (a tour de force) the effects of total nutrient deprivation (other than water) for 31 days in a male volunteer living in a whole-body calorimeter. His caloric expenditure dropped gradually from an average of 1650 calories per day during the first week to an average of 1290 calories per day during the third week, remaining at or near the latter level for the duration of the study. A calculation of the amounts of carbohydrate, protein, and fat metabolized during the first week was made some years later from Benedict's published data by Peters and Van Slyke [138] (Table 13-1). After a few days, the percentage of calories obtained from carbohydrate was minimal (less than 5 percent), whereas the proportions of calories derived from protein and fat were essentially constant for the next 3½ weeks, about 15 to 18 percent and 80 to 85 percent respectively. Gamble, Ross, and Tisdall [53] reported similar findings in fasting children; these children, like adults, showed a prompt decline in urinary nitrogen excretion in the first 10 days of fasting.

Wars have always accentuated the problems of supplying adequate nutrition to populations and have provided opportunities to study the effects of undernutrition on large numbers of people of all ages. Notable among the number of studies and publications describing the effects of undernutrition in Western Europe during and after World War II are those edited by McCance and Widdowson [118], by Burger, Drummond, and Sandstead [16], and by Winick [218]. In 1944, Keys, Brozek, Henschel, Mickelsen, and Taylor [95] began their remarkable study of semistarvation in 32 men, all healthy conscientious objectors to war. The reader is urged to read their excellent book, *The Biology of Human Starvation.*

The 1950s saw relatively few studies of starvation per se, but large numbers of studies dealing with the metabolic effects of injury and illness, in which reduction of food intake plays such an important role.

In 1959, there began a great resurgence of investigative interest in the effects of starvation per se when Bloom [13], and later Duncan [41], introduced prolonged total fasting with free access to water for weight reduction of obese people. This stimulated a great number of studies in the 1960s which have continued unabated through the 1970s; Cahill [18], Owen [135], Felig [43, 45], and their coworkers have been among the major contributors in this field.

CURRENT CONCEPTS OF THE EFFECTS OF STARVATION

At the basis for all the responses to starvation lies a common denominator: lack of exogenous energy substrates and of essential dietary nutrients, such as certain amino acids. Man's survival is based in large measure on his ability to produce and renew regulatory peptides and proteins. This, in turn, involves a wide range of other reactions involving all metabolites. In starvation, the range of metabolic activity is altered, sometimes drastically: some metabolic pathways that are active in the normal state are partially or completely turned off; others that normally are minimally active achieve major importance; and some pathways are newly developed and function only during prolonged starvation. The ability to respond adaptively to a variety of external stimuli becomes impaired during starvation, and at times a response will be elicited only when the stimulus poses a threat to survival. The organism faced with severe food deprivation channels all its metabolic activity to one goal: survival. Regulatory neuroendocrine mechanisms regulate the levels of certain major metabolic fuels. This is particularly important for organs like the brain, which have constant and high energy demands but minimal fuel depots.

METABOLIC RATE; ENERGY CONSERVATION

Paramount among the metabolic tasks is the need for the starving organism to regulate its energy expenditure and, therefore, energy requirement. Among the important adaptations to starvation are two that result in a lowering of caloric expenditure and a slowing of the rate of deterioration. One of these is voluntary, a reduction in physical work, while the other is involuntary, a reduction in basal metabolic rate proportionately greater than the loss of both body weight (Figure 13-2) and "lean-body mass" [10, 31, 95]. Body temperature decreases slightly at this time, but has little effect in lowering metabolic rate. A major difference, then, between the response to food deprivation per se and the response to injury or sepsis, with or without a concomitant reduction in food intake, is an increase in metabolic rate in the latter and a lowering in the former.

Much of an animal's (including human) resting energy expenditure is devoted to maintenance of ionic and other compartments against diffusion gradients and to a certain amount of mechanical work, e.g., respiration, cardiac contractility, and peristalsis. Resting energy expenditure is also involved in peptide and protein synthesis, particularly the synthesis of hormones and enzymes, which permit the body to respond to alterations in the internal or external environments. In the body's dynamic response to starvation, regula-

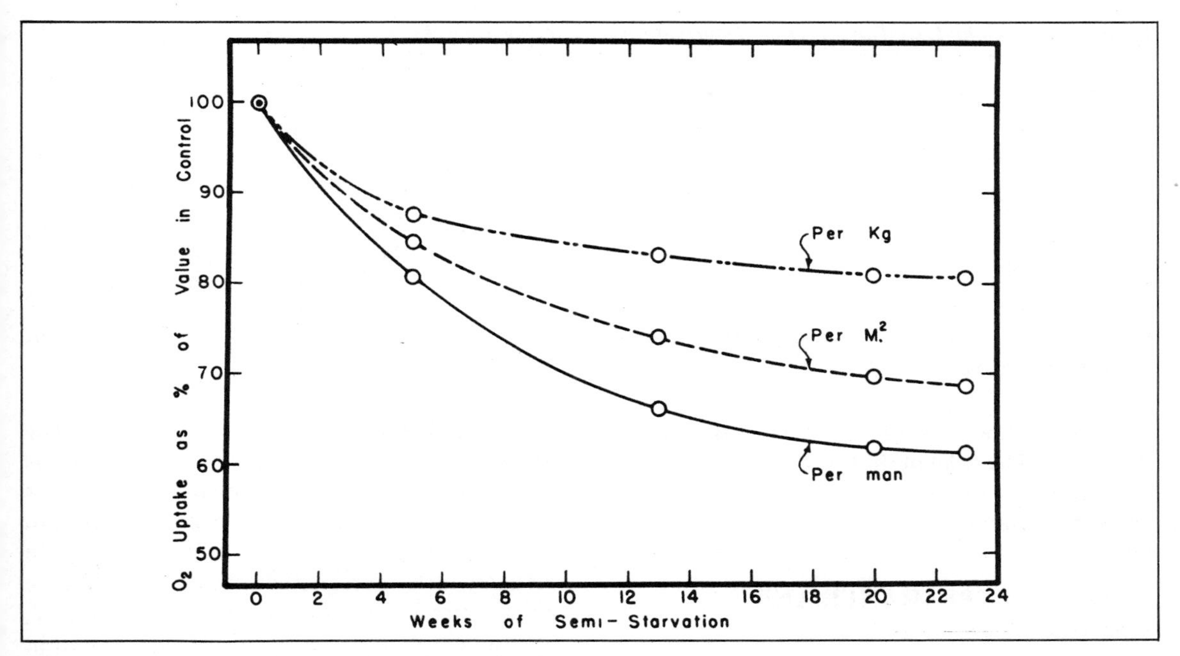

Figure 13-2. *Mean basal metabolism for 32 men before and during 24 weeks of semi-starvation. All values are expressed as percentage of the pre-starvation (control) values for the oxygen uptake per man, per square meter of body surface, and per kilogram of body weight (Minnesota experiment). (From A. Keys, J. Brožek, A. Henschel, O. Mickelson, and H. L. Taylor,* The Biology of Human Starvation. *Minneapolis: The University of Minnesota Press, 1970.)*

tory neuroendocrine and other metabolic mechanisms lower the metabolic rate to help safeguard survival, maintaining the blood levels of certain major metabolic fuels within relatively narrow limits. Concomitant with the reduced overall metabolic rate in starvation per se is the possible loss of cell mass by certain metabolically active tissues, such as the liver, pancreas, and gut. Kleiber [99] has shown that the changes in metabolic rate differ for various organs in starving rats, but no such comparable comprehensive measurements are available in humans.

Cardiac work is sharply reduced (bradycardia, decreased cardiac output) in starvation. The resting metabolic rate of skeletal muscle is likely to be lowered for the following reasons: (1) Maintenance of muscle mass is dependent on active (i.e., endergonic) reactions involving substrate uptake (glucose, amino acids) and the uptake of ions (K^+, Mg^{2+}, HPO_4^{2-}) against concentration gradients. Since muscle glycogen and certain protein syntheses are depressed in starvation, the energy required even in the basal state is lessened. (2) As muscle tone is decreased (characteristic of starved individuals), resting energy need is decreased. (3) There is a disproportionate loss of red muscle fibers compared to white muscle fibers; red muscle fibers contain myoglobin in the cell sap and numerous mitochondria and are metabolically more active than and contain more capillaries than white muscle. (4) There is a voluntary decrease in muscular activity of starving individuals.

With the decreased metabolic rate during starvation, there is a decrease in circulating T_3. However, during starvation the metabolic rate of thyroidectomized rats also falls, showing that some mechanism(s) in addition to (other than) decrease in circulating T_3 is responsible for the

Table 13-2. *Weight Loss During Food Deprivation of Varying Degrees*

Duration (mo.)	Caloric Intake as Percentage of Normal Balance							
	90	80	70	60	50	40	30	20
	Weight Loss (%)							
3	5	8	10	12	15	20	25	30
6	8	12	15	20	25	30	35	45
12 or more	10	15	20	25	30	35	40	

Source: A. Keys, J. Brožek, A. Henschel, O. Mickelson, and H. L. Taylor. *The Biology of Human Starvation.* Minneapolis: The University of Minnesota Press, 1970.

progressive lowering of metabolic rate during starvation. The roles of the thyroid hormones and the catecholamines in starvation are discussed in more detail later in this chapter (pp. 458–460).

GENERAL APPEARANCE AND WEIGHT LOSS

Progressive weight loss is an inevitable consequence of starvation. "Haggard-faced, lean, bony, chronically starved people are recognized at a glance, even by the layman" [92]. The skin is loose, flaccid, rough, and flaking. There are areas of overkeratinization and increased pigmentation. Plugs of hardened protein material distend the hair follicles and often project as spikes. Children are particularly affected by starvation because of their relatively greater nutrient requirement. The following was reported from Phnom Penh, Cambodia by a journalist:

> Waves of mothers carrying gravely ill children—swollen children [kwashiorkor], children with stick-like concentration camp bodies [marasmus], children with parchment skin hanging in flaccid folds, coughing children, weeping children, silent children too weak to respond anymore.... The child had been malnourished before. Now she is a skeletal horror, little more than bulging eyes and a protruding rib cage. Every few seconds she produces a wail that racks her body. In three hours she is dead [171].

The rate of weight loss, which is proportional to the reduction in food intake, generally is greatest at the beginning of food deprivation, reflecting a disproportionate loss of water. The rate then decreases gradually, leveling off as physical activity lessens and metabolic rate falls (Table 13-2). Most previously healthy adults can tolerate a weight loss of 5 to 10 percent with relatively little functional disorganization. At the other extreme, save for exceptional individuals, human beings and animals do not survive weight losses greater than 40 percent. Experimental studies have shown that early in starvation there is a rapid reduction in the weight of certain viscera, notably the liver, gastrointestinal tract, and pancreas. Autopsy studies [147] of people dead of prolonged starvation showed that the greatest organ weight losses were by the pancreas, spleen, kidney, liver, genitals, gut, and muscles, and least by the skeleton and eyes.

BODY COMPOSITION

The overall changes in body composition during semi-starvation are depicted in Figure 13-3 [20]; the increases in extracellular fluid, the disproportionate loss of fat, the lesser loss of lean body mass, and the maintenance of bone mineral are evident. The mechanisms underlying the relative increase in extracellular water, which is general in most tissues and may accumulate as gross edema in dependent areas, are not known fully.

> It is not yet clear if any local abnormality need be invoked to explain the edema, but it is natural to suppose that a reduction of muscle size and intercellular colloid, and a loss of elastic fibers from a skin now too

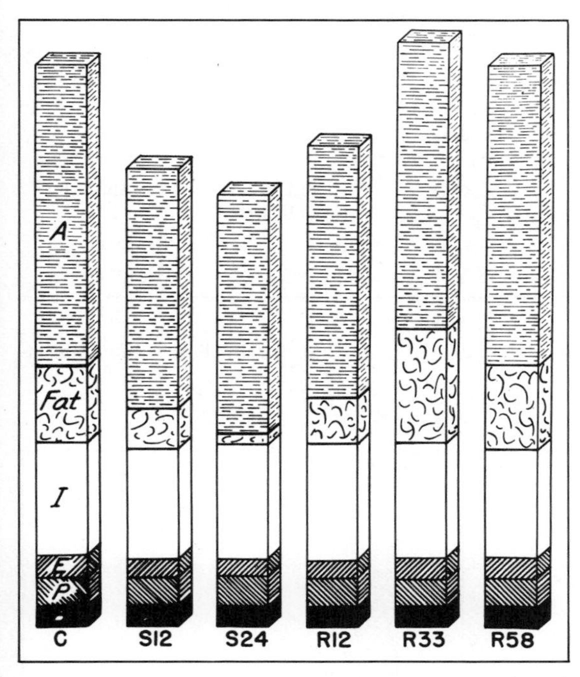

Figure 13-3. *The major compartments, as weight, of the bodies of young men in a normal state of nutrition, in semi-starvation, and in subsequent rehabilitation. Columns:* C = *control (pre-starvation): S12 and S24* = *12 and 24 weeks of semi-starvation; R12, R33, and R58* = *12, 33, and 58 weeks of rehabilitation. Compartments:* B = *bone;* P = *blood plasma;* E = *erythrocytes;* I = *interstitial fluid (thiocyanate space less plasma volume);* A = *active tissue (total body weight less the other indicated compartments). (From A. Keys, J. Brožek, A. Henschel, O. Mickelson, and H. L. Taylor,* The Biology of Human Starvation. *Minneapolis: The University of Minnesota Press, 1970.)*

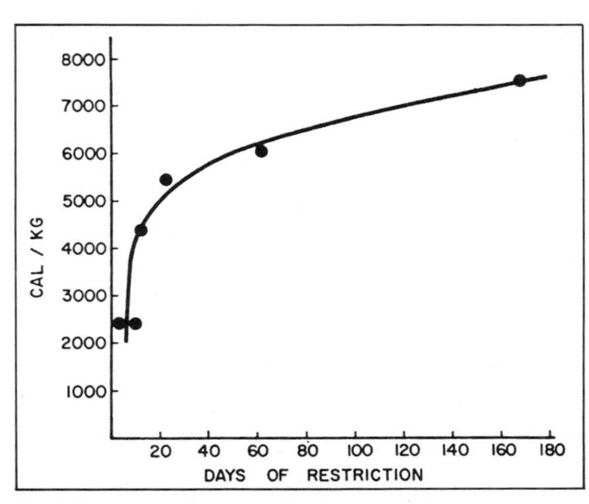

Figure 13-4. *Caloric equivalent of the weight loss and duration of the restriction period. (From F. Grande, Energetics and weight reduction.* Am. J. Clin. Nutr. *21:305, 1968.)*

large for the structures it was designed to enclose will all favour localized collection of fluid in the dependent parts... If and when there is a fall in the concentration of serum proteins, it is natural to suppose that this will also operate, and a large intake of salt must also help. Theories based on overactivity of the hormones of the suprarenal cortex, a deficiency of aneurin [vitamin B_1] and abnormalities of renal function must be regarded for the moment as not proven [118].

Others have suggested that abnormal amounts of ferritin are released from the liver and stimulate the production of antidiuretic hormone. Other aspects of sodium and water metabolism and renal function are discussed later in this chapter (see pp. 456, 462–465).

The caloric value of the tissue lost during semi-starvation is much greater later on than earlier, a reflection of the increasing utilization of body fat as starvation proceeds. During the early periods of semi-starvation, the body loses a mixture of fat, protein, and water; the caloric equivalent of the lost tissue may be about 2000 Cal/kg which does not correspond to the composition of any tissue of the body. Fat storage tissue is about 90 percent fat and one kilogram of storage fat would be expected to supply about 8100 Calories. A figure very close to the aforementioned (8000 Cal/kg tissue) was found by Grande as the caloric equivalent of the tissue lost late in semi-starvation [72] (Figure 13-4).

The reason why fat becomes the major fuel metabolized during starvation is evident from Table 13-3. The amount of stored carbohydrate is minimal, whereas the amount of potential calories in fat, especially in storage depots such as the subcutaneous tissue, is proportionately large. Most organs appear to lose fat in propor-

Table 13-3. *Normal Stores of Available Energy and Rates of Utilization in a Man Weighing 65 Kg*

	Total Body Content (gm)	Available Store (gm)	(mj)	(kcal)	Daily Utilization* (gm)	Exhaustion Time (days)
Carbohydrate	500	150	2.5	600	All used in first 24 hr.	Less than 1
Protein	11,000	2,400	40	9,600	60	About 40
Fat	9,000	6,500	235	58,500	150	About 40

*Assuming an energy expenditure of about 6.7 mj (1600 kcal)/day.
Source: R. Passmore and J. S. Robson. *A Companion to Medical Studies,* Vol. 3. Oxford: Blackwell Scientific Publications, 1974.

tion to their initial fat content. Exceptions are the brain and nervous tissues, and possibly the kidney. As fat is lost, the fat cells shrink until the cytoplasm becomes merely a limiting membrane. There is potentially a fairly large caloric source in protein, but there is little, if any, "storage" protein that can be "burned" to help meet the caloric expenditure without some loss of important cellular and enzymatic functions. Protein must be conserved if organ and body functions are to continue. The metabolic events and adaptations that occur during starvation and underlie the greater utilization of fat and relative preservation of protein are discussed in the following sections.

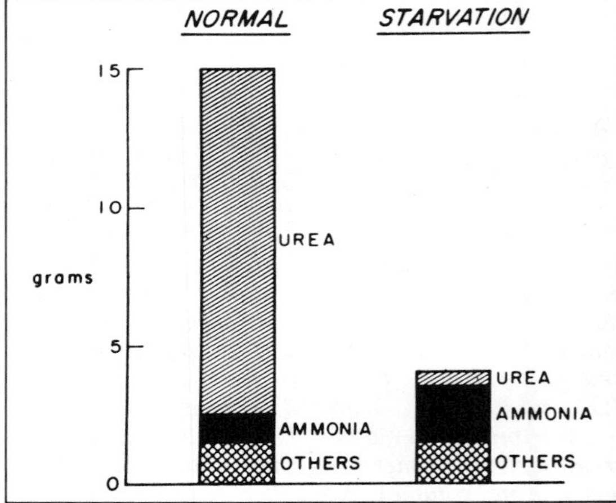

Figure 13-5. *Urinary nitrogen excretion in the post-absorptive state after a standard diet of 90 to 100 gm of protein and after five to six weeks of starvation, showing marked reduction in total nitrogen, the relative increase in ammonia, and the relatively unchanged excretion of the sum of uric acid, creatinine, and other nonprotein-nitrogen metabolites. (From G. J. Cahill, Jr., Starvation in man.* N. Engl. J. Med. *282:668, 1970. Reprinted by permission.)*

INTERMEDIARY METABOLISM

We have mentioned that during fasting the following occur: (1) a gradual drop in urinary nitrogen (chiefly urea), which begins within one or two days and plateaus in man after about 2 weeks, until shortly before death when it rises moderately; (2) a prompt but modest lowering of blood sugar, after which it plateaus until the end stages of the fast when it falls sharply; (3) a gradual increase in plasma fatty acids, keto acids, and ketones leading to metabolic acidosis and ketonuria; (4) a gradual increase in urinary NH_4^+ (Figure 13-5); and (5) an increase in urinary sodium and potassium excretions.

In normal men fasted for 10 days, the early loss includes a negative water balance (500 ml/day), nitrogen loss (8.5 gm/day), and mineral losses (1.85 gm sodium and 1.5 gm potassium) [31]. As starvation continues, nitrogen losses are reduced to 2 to 4 gm/day; some glucose-burning organs, e.g., the brain, are by this time utilizing ketones derived from the fat stores.

Urinary nitrogen losses are much greater following injury than during uncomplicated starva-

Table 13-4. *Relative Losses of Protein From Various Organs and Tissues of Albino Rats in a 7-Day Fast, as Percentages of Control Values*

Organ or Tissue	Percentage Loss	Organ or Tissue	Percentage Loss
Liver	40	Heart	18
Prostate	29	Muscle, skin, and skeleton	8
Seminal vesicles	29	Brain	5
Gastrointestinal tract	28	Eyes	0
Kidneys	20	Testicles	0
Drawn blood	20	Adrenals	0

Source: T. Addis, L. J. Poo, and W. Lew. The quantities of protein lost by the various organs and tissues of the body during a fast. *J. Biol. Chem.* 115:111, 1936.

tion. The data presented by Kinney [96, 97] suggest that the proportionate amounts of protein and fat lost after injury are not much different than in healthy, fed subjects; the disproportionate higher utilization of fat seen during starvation per se is not seen following injury. In addition, water and sodium conservation are immediate following injury, and although administration of carbohydrate to the starved individual has an immediate protein-sparing effect, this effect is less in the injured individual.

As noted, there is a disproportionately large reduction in the weight of certain viscera—notably the liver, gastrointestinal tract, and pancreas—during starvation. This reduction is rapid (a matter of days) in small mammals such as rats [2]. Significant amounts of protein are lost from these viscera (Table 13-4), and the activities of certain enzymes are altered. As a result of the selective loss of liver proteins in early starvation, those enzymes related directly to fatty acid oxidation and gluconeogenesis appear to be conserved best, whereas those enzymes concerned with urea synthesis are decreased. The early starvation period results also in a loss of intestinal mucosal digestive hydrolases. At the same time, the rate of regeneration of gut mucosal epithelial cells is slowed. During starvation, exocrine pancreatic function is lost because of decreased synthesis of pancreatic and gastrointestinal enzymes, and digestion of dietary protein, fat, and polysaccharides is inhibited. The gastrointestinal tract may become relatively intolerant of food, and the refeeding of starving patients becomes a challenge.

Amino acid and protein turnover and cell loss involve the breakdown of a portion of the protein, amino acid, and nucleic acid pools. This breakdown results in an obligatory loss of nitrogen, largely in the form of urea, but also as free amino acids, peptides, creatine, creatinine, uric acid, and ammonia. The amount of nitrogen lost is a function of the balance of energy intake and output and the size of the protein and amino acid pools, which in turn are affected by dietary intake of all nutrients and the physiologic state. Protein intake increases the size of the amino acid pool, as do exercise and other stimuli for gluconeogenesis and glycogenolysis, such as injury or glucocorticoid administration. The pool size can be increased by states in which both protein synthesis and breakdown are speeded up, but overall breakdown exceeds synthesis, as in hyperthyroidism. The mechanism of salvage or recycling of amino acids (e.g., hydrolysis of digestive enzymes and absorption and reutilization of the amino acids) conserves amino acids, but at a significant expenditure of energy. This salvage, however, makes possible many different metabolic and physiologic responses by various organs regardless of their size.

In prolonged starvation, the amino acid pool is decreased for three reasons: (1) amino acid intake is nil, (2) protein breakdown decreases gradually and reaches a near-plateau because metabolic rate falls and fat becomes the major fuel, and (3) turnover of certain proteins may be decreased. One consequence is that the starving animal may not synthesize certain enzymes in amounts adequate to respond appropriately to environmental stimuli. For example, as starvation proceeds, the liver urea cycle enzymes decrease. As a result, the starving individual cannot respond quickly to a load of ammonia by synthesizing more urea. The body may become less or nonresponsive in a variety of other ways. For example, the liver may not respond adequately to catecholamine stimuli for glucogenesis because (a) it has decreased numbers of catecholamine receptors or decreased levels of adenylate cyclase, or both (b) it has decreased amounts of glycogen, or (c) it has decreased amounts of enzymes and cofactors required for glycogenolysis and gluconeogenesis.

Normal adults can make metabolic adjustments to a wide variety of nutrient intakes. When caloric and protein intakes are adequate, the proportions of fat, carbohydrate, and protein may be varied within wide limits without upsetting the steady state, once a small amount of unsaturated fatty acids (about 2 to 4 percent of calories) and small amounts of glucose (75 to 100 gm daily) are included. Once the minimal intake requirement of protein (about 0.3 to 0.5 gm/kg body weight/day) for nitrogen equilibrium is met, "extra" amino acids absorbed as the result of a higher protein intake are deaminated, transaminated, and their nitrogen is converted to urea and excreted. Some of the carbon chain is oxidized and/or converted to carbohydrate and fat. A new steady state is again reached within three to four days. If less than adequate amounts of protein are ingested, there is a gradual depletion of body protein, with certain organs and tissues being more affected than others, as already described. The rate of protein depletion is hastened when dietary non-protein calories are low. When the protein intake is marginal or inadequate, the protein-sparing effect of carbohydrate is somewhat greater than that of fat, because carbohydrate may be used for the synthesis of non-essential amino acids.

Body protein losses by injured patients with limited food intakes are much larger than protein losses by uninjured people with comparable levels of decreased food intake. Also, as mentioned, the disproportionately high utilization of fat seen during prolonged food deprivation per se is not seen following injury. Whereas administration of small amounts of glucose (50 to 100 gm) to the starved but uninjured individual has an immediate protein-sparing effect, this effect is considerably less in the severely injured individual.

GLUCONEOGENESIS AND AMINO ACID METABOLISM IN STARVATION

When dietary intakes of fat, carbohydrate, and protein are all inadequate, glucose homeostasis and "sparing" of certain critical proteins and lipids (e.g., nervous system proteolipids, lipoproteins) are central factors. Stored fat is expendable. Glucose is normally the major or sole energy source for certain key organs, notably the central nervous system, peripheral nerves, red blood cells, white blood cells, active fibroblasts, and certain phagocytes. The brain normally oxidizes the glucose to CO_2 and water, and glycolysis goes on in the other tissues and cells and the lactic acid is recycled into glucose by the liver and kidney (the Cori cycle). Provision of glucose (gluconeogenesis) during starvation is thus essential [3].

The trigger that induces the initial metabolic adaptations during starvation is the arterial glucose level, which begins to fall in humans within 15 hours of fasting. This fall occurs because the peripheral organs continue to utilize glucose, while the supply of exogenous energy substrates is abolished. As the blood glucose level falls, the stimulus for insulin secretion diminishes and this is reflected by the falling serum insulin levels. The falling glucose and insulin levels are accompanied by rising glucagon and growth hormone levels (Figure 13-6). Only limited data are avail-

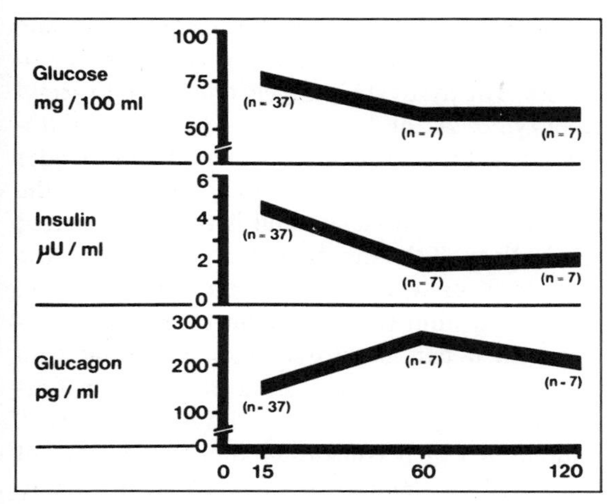

Figure 13-6. *Arterial glucose, insulin, and glucagon levels after 15, 60, and 120 hours of fasting. (From F. W. Ahnefeld, C. Burri, W. Dick, and M. Halmagyi,* Parenteral Nutrition. *New York: Springer-Verlag, 1976.)*

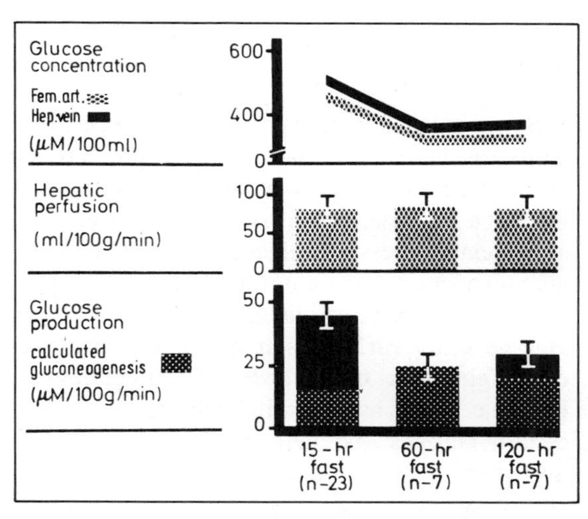

Figure 13-7. *Arterial and hepatic-venous glucose concentrations, liver perfusion, and contributions of gluconeogenesis and glycogenolysis to glucose production after 15, 60, and 120 hours of fasting. (From F. W. Ahnefeld, C. Burri, W. Dick, and M. Halmagyi,* Parenteral Nutrition. *New York: Springer-Verlag, 1976.)*

able regarding the catecholamines, and the findings are conflicting. (Hormonal changes are discussed in more detail later in this chapter.)

In the first 24 hours of starvation, hepatic glycogenolysis provides the necessary blood sugar, but at the end of this time hepatic glycogen is nearly exhausted and gluconeogenesis becomes the main route for the provision of glucose (Figure 13-7). The rate of gluconeogenesis then diminishes gradually, coincident with the overall decline in metabolic rate and an increase in ketone utilization by the central nervous system.

The brain does not metabolize fatty acids directly. Fatty acids generally do not cross the blood:brain barrier, but ketones and keto acids provided by the liver do. During starvation, adaptive changes occur in the transport system which result in an increase in the rate at which ketones cross the blood:brain barrier [61]. In addition, competitive inhibition for ketone transport by lactate and pyruvate is decreased because of their lower levels in starvation. The brain begins to metabolize ketones and keto acids increasingly in starvation as glucose availability decreases. Current evidence indicates that enzyme induction for this is not necessary; the brain is set to use ketones even when the individual is well fed, but under that circumstance the brain uses glucose preferentially [136]. However, starvation leads to derepression of β-hydroxybutyrate dehydrogenase and β-keto acid CoA transferase, thereby increasing the levels of these two enzymes, which are important for ketone oxidation. It should be noted that certain areas of the brain metabolize glucose preferentially (solely?), while other areas of the brain may metabolize either glucose or ketones depending on their relative availability. The metabolism of ketones by the brain seems to be limited to specific regions by their permeability characteristics—areas with no blood:brain barrier show the highest rate of utilization [80]. During starvation the brain's respiratory quotient (RQ) may be about 0.8. This indicates that either the ketones or the glucose, or both, are not completely oxidized to CO_2 and H_2O, because in that case the RQ would be significantly higher (1.0

for glucose and acetoacetic acid and 0.9 for β-hydroxybutyric acid) or that CO_2 fixation is taking place.

Some glucose is derived from the glycerol released as a result of fat mobilization, but the amount so provided is inadequate by itself to meet the starving individual's general need. The additional necessary glucose is provided by gluconeogenesis. The amount of gluconeogenesis required has been estimated to be about 60 gm glucose daily early in starvation; stored or recycled glucose is of the order of 120 gm daily at this time. Later, as the brain begins to metabolize certain ketones and keto acids, its glucose requirement falls substantially, about 70 percent, and the amount of gluconeogenesis required falls about 50 percent; at this time the amount of stored or recycled glucose falls to about 80 gm per day [18].

MUSCLE AS AN ENERGY STORE AND ITS METABOLIC ROLE IN STARVATION

In the starved state the skeletal muscle becomes a tissue necessary for the survival of the organism because it provides biochemical intermediates essential to the maintenance of vital metabolic activities, particularly of the brain and kidneys.

Skeletal muscle normally uses glucose and fatty acids as its main energy sources. The glucose is derived directly from the circulation or indirectly from muscle glycogen. Uptake of glucose by muscle from blood is dependent in part on the blood glucose concentration, but it is most strongly dependent on serum insulin levels. This insulin effect can be blocked by other hormones, notably growth hormone.

Once glucose enters the muscle cells, its fate depends largely on whether the muscle is resting or at work. If the latter, the glucose enters the glycolytic pathway and, depending on the amount of work, the pyruvate either enters the Krebs cycle or is converted to lactate, which goes to the liver where it is partially converted to glucose. Muscle glycogen is utilized in normal metabolism and work by conversion of glucose 1-phosphate to glucose 6-phosphate to pyruvate in the extramitochondrial portion of the cytoplasm. The pyruvate is largely converted to acetyl coenzyme A and metabolized in the mitochondria to carbon dioxide and water. Under these conditions only a small amount of the pyruvate goes to lactate and is then transported to the liver. If the muscle is at rest, glucose in the muscle is preferentially converted to glycogen. There is a limit to the amount of muscle glycogen which can be stored, namely, about 0.75 percent of muscle mass. Because of the proportionately large mass of skeletal muscle, however, muscle glycogen constitutes the largest store of carbohydrate calories in the body; it is three to four times as large as the store of liver glycogen. Very early in starvation (in rats), 60 percent of the glucose derived from glycogen comes from the liver and 40 percent from the muscle [196]. However, stored liver and muscle glycogen are of little quantitative significance in the fuel economy of the starving individual, since they could supply less than a day's energy during total starvation, even if totally metabolized. Fatty acids are key energy sources for muscle during starvation.

Additional Aspects of Skeletal Muscle Metabolism

A number of aspects of muscle metabolism are relevant to the metabolic responses and adaptations to starvation:

1. Uptake of glucose and the subsequent conversion to glycogen are largely under insulin control. In starvation, glucose uptake by muscle is affected mainly by the low levels of serum insulin. There is evidence that in starvation the insulin effect on glucose uptake by muscle is increased. The glucose uptake in vivo of starved animals is independent of the elevated fatty acid or ketone levels in the blood [159]. Ruderman et al. [158] have shown in studies of the isolated perfused rat hindquarter that after a 48-hour fast, glucose oxidation decreased 75 percent. The

decrease in lactate oxidation was in general paralleled by changes in the activity of the active form of pyruvate dehydrogenase, indicating that glucose metabolism was inhibited at the step of pyruvate oxidation.

2. Muscle cannot provide blood glucose from its own glycogen since it lacks the enzyme glucose-6-phosphatase.

3. Formation of creatine phosphate by muscle.

4. Muscle glycogenesis.

5. Gluconeogenesis from alanine via pyruvate does not occur in the muscle because muscle has very little pyruvate carboxylase, the enzyme that generates oxaloacetate, a precursor of phosphoenol pyruvate (PEP) needed for de novo hexose synthesis.

$$\text{Pyruvate} + \text{ATP} + CO_2 \xrightarrow[\text{almost absent in muscle}]{\text{pyruvate carboxylase}} \text{oxaloacetate} + \text{ADP} + \text{Pi}$$

$$\text{Oxaloacetate} + \text{GTP} \xrightarrow[\text{present in muscle}]{\text{phosphoenol pyruvate carboxykinase}} \text{PEP} + \text{GDP} + CO_2$$

Sum:

$$\text{Pyruvate} + \text{ATP} + \text{GTP} \longrightarrow \text{PEP} + \text{ADP} + \text{GDP} + \text{Pi}$$

6. Muscle provides amino acids to the liver and kidney for gluconeogenesis. (A detailed discussion of these points follows.)

Muscle Creatine Phosphate

As mentioned, skeletal muscle activity is diminished in starvation to a near basal amount of ATP-dependent muscle contraction. Under conditions of minimum ventilatory activity and decreased muscle perfusion, glycolysis in white muscle is favored. The PEP formed in glycolysis can go into various pathways. In cells that are at low energy levels and therefore have increased levels of ADP and AMP (starvation), the system is driven in the direction of making ATP, i.e.,

$$\text{ADP} + \text{PEP} \xrightarrow{\text{pyruvate kinase}} \text{ATP} + \text{Pyruvate}$$

The energetics of the reaction strongly favor ATP formation. The formation of this ATP acts to moderate (slow down) both glycolysis and the Krebs cycle, by the inhibitory allosteric effects of ATP on glycolytic enzymes and by the depletion of ADP, which is both a necessary substrate and a positive allosteric effector of some glycolytic enzymes. The relative lack of ATP is an appropriate response to starvation. High amounts of ATP could favor synthetic reactions (glycogen or fat synthesis) or could limit the amount of PEP that could phosphorylate ADP. These synthetic reactions would be inappropriate in the starving individual because they would be energy-consuming.

One factor that modulates the amounts of ATP and ADP in muscle cells is the amount of creatine present. The energetics of the reaction $\text{ATP} + \text{Creatine} \rightleftharpoons \text{Cr} \sim \text{P} + \text{ADP}$ favor ATP synthesis. This is a very good adaptive mechanism for energy storage when high levels of ATP are present since high levels of ATP (which would be generated by high levels of respiration or glycolysis) would favor the synthetic reaction $\rightarrow$ Creatine phosphate ($\text{Cr} \sim \text{P}$) at times when the cells can afford the energy expenditure. Thus, the potential energy of glucose or fatty acid oxidation would yield a high amount of immediately available $\sim$P. A reasonably small proportion of this ATP energy is spent to synthesize the high energy compound $\text{Cr} \sim \text{P}$, which represents a readily available store of $\sim$P. Thus, during oxidations, ADP + Pi stimulate respiration and ATP synthesis and stimulate the reaction $\text{ATP} + \text{Cr} \rightarrow \text{Cr} \sim \text{P} + \text{ADP}$.

Under the conditions of glycolysis and respiration the *net* synthesis of high energy bonds is limited by available inorganic phosphorus. Therefore, oxidation increases the amount of ATP, $\text{Cr} \sim \text{P}$ and decreases the amounts of Pi. As the ATP is used for muscle or other work, $\text{Cr} \sim \text{P}$ is converted to ATP until the $\text{Cr} \sim \text{P}$ is used up. This gives rise to increased levels of

ADP + Pi, which in turn stimulate glycolysis and respiration leading to ATP synthesis. Therefore, glycolysis and respiration are stimulated by ADP and inorganic P and tend to be inhibited by ATP. This is a useful adaptive phenomenon because low energy levels in the cell stimulate respiration and glycolysis, which then produce the energy (ATP) that slows glycolysis and respiration.

The presence of high concentrations of creatine permits the muscle to store five times as much readily available phosphate bond energy as would be the case if ATP and ADP were the only reservoirs of ~P energy. The creatine phosphate reservoir is a useful mechanism for the nourished active muscle. For starved, inactive muscle, it represents an unnecessary and perhaps useless or futile cycle. Certain events that occur in the starving muscle decrease the activity of the creatine kinase system and therefore have adaptive value in starvation. The muscle wasting that occurs in starvation involves the loss of the enzymatically active protein, creatine kinase, and the loss of small substrate molecules such as creatine. This means that Cr ~ P concentrations are lowered, decreasing the total ~P available for work. The loss of the Cr ~ P mechanism in starvation decreases the amount of work muscle can carry out, but it represents a way of conserving energy and muscle mass. It is clear that the decreased work in starvation has adaptive value. What may not be obvious is that the decrease in the amounts of ATP + Cr ~ P inhibits the ATP-dependent synthetic phases of wasteful "futile" metabolic cycles and the ATP-dependent phases of glucose assimilation, thus conserving body glucose mainly for nonmuscle uses, e.g., brain and blood cell metabolism.

Muscle Glycogenesis

Although muscle is the source of metabolites that provide energy for other tissues, it cannot provide this in the form of glucose from its own glycogen because muscle lacks the enzyme glucose-6-phosphatase. Thus, although muscle can synthesize glycogen from blood glucose and can degrade glycogen to glucose-6-phosphate, the glucose-6-phosphate so formed must be used within the muscle cell.

In addition to muscle's ability to synthesize glycogen from glucose, it has a *limited* ability to synthesize glycogen or glucose-6-phosphate from the carbon chains of some glucogenic amino acids, especially those that can be converted to oxaloacetate by either transamination or the Krebs cycle, but at a considerable energy cost.

CYTOSOL REACTIONS

$$\text{Aspartate} + \alpha\text{-ketoglutarate} \xrightarrow[\text{oxaloacetate transaminase}]{\text{glutamic acid}} \text{oxaloacetate (OAA)} + \text{glutamate} \quad (1)$$

$$\text{OAA} + \text{NADH} + \text{H}^+ \xrightarrow{\text{malic dehydrogenase}} \text{malate} \quad (2)$$

Malate shuttle (malate in cytosol $\longrightarrow$ malate in mitochondria) (3)

MITOCHONDRIAL REACTIONS

$$\text{NAD}^+ + \text{malate} \xrightarrow[\text{dehydrogenase}]{\text{malic}} \text{OAA} + \text{NADH} + \text{H}^+ \quad (4)$$

$$\text{OAA} + \text{GTP} \xrightarrow[\text{carboxykinase}]{\text{phosphoenol pyruvate}} \text{phosphoenol pyruvate (PEP)} + CO_2 + \text{GDP} \quad (5)$$

PEP transport (mitochondrial PEP $\longrightarrow$ cytosol PEP) (6)

The glutamate generated in reaction 1 is used to regenerate the α-ketoglutarate necessary for reaction 1 in the following way:

Glutamate transport (cytosol glutamate $\longrightarrow$ mitochondrial glutamate) (7)

$$\text{mitochondrial glutamate} + \text{NAD}^+ + H_2O \xrightarrow{\text{glutamic dehydrogenase}} \alpha\text{-ketoglutarate} + NH_4^+ + \text{NADH} \quad (8)$$

As is evident from the following summation of the foregoing reactions, the flow of carbon from aspartate to PEP and to glycogen requires the OAA-malate shuttle, while the flow of aspartate N requires the glutamate–α-ketoglutarate shuttle:

$$\text{Aspartate carbon} \xrightarrow{\text{OAA-malate shuttle}} \text{PEP} + CO_2$$

$$\text{Aspartate nitrogen} \xrightarrow{\text{glutamate–}\alpha\text{-ketoglutarate shuttle}} \text{N of other amino acids, amides, and } NH_4^+$$

The PEP produced from aspartate and some other glycogenic amino acids can be resynthesized into glycogen, but at a considerable energy cost. However, it is not only the energetics that limit muscle glycogen synthesis from amino acids, but in starvation there are mechanisms that limit the availability of amino acids for this purpose. The synthesis of muscle glycogen from glucogenic amino acids depends on a net synthesis of PEP. The shuttle mechanisms could give rise to a net formation of PEP and, therefore, a net synthesis of glucose from aspartate as illustrated.

PEP can be formed also from some other amino acids by similar types of reactions involving the various shuttles:

valine, methionine, isoleucine → succinyl COA → succinate → OAA → PEP → glycogen

and

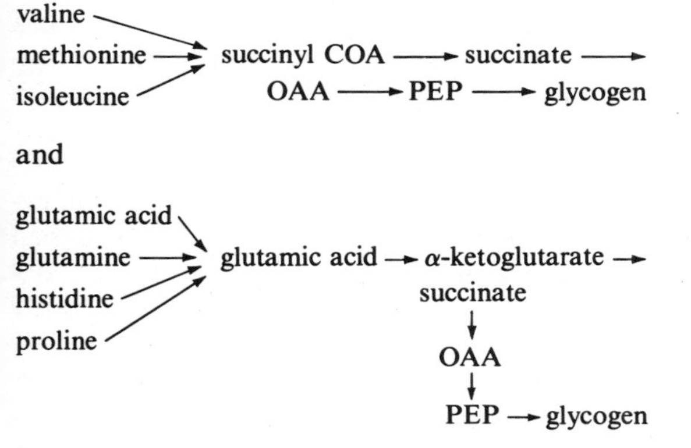

However, in order for gluconeogenesis to proceed from these amino acids in addition to a functional malate oxaloacetate shuttle, it is necessary that mitochondria carry out the oxidation of some substrates derived from the amino acids (e.g., α-ketoglutarate and succinate) at a more rapid rate than usual to provide PEP. Additionally, mitochondrial oxidation of the reduced cofactors (mainly NADH generated by substrate oxidation) by the electron transport chain would have to proceed at normal or greater-than-normal rates. In muscle, these conditions are *not* met during starvation when a reducing environment prevails as a result of decreased capillarity, decreased myoglobin, decreased red fibers with proportionate increase of white fibers, and decreased mitochondria. Aoki, Finley, and Cahill [6] have pointed out that in starvation, proteolysis of muscle is diminished because of the existence of large amounts of reduced nicotinamide coenzymes. Chua and associates [29] have pointed out that in the fed state both reduced blood flow of muscle and muscle hypoxia without ischemia favor proteolysis over protein synthesis. Thus the effect on proteolysis may be mediated by both the tissue O_2 levels and failure to remove metabolites, both of which lead to a reduced environment. In contrast to the fed state, muscle protein is conserved in starvation by mechanisms that inhibit proteolysis and gluconeogenesis. Cahill and his colleagues [19] suggest that control over muscle metabolism by thyroid hormone is important in conserving muscle mass and energy in starvation, since thyroid hormone creates an oxidizing environment in the cell. We have pointed out elsewhere in this chapter that circulating T_3 is low in starvation (see pp. 427, 428, 458–460).

How else may increased reducing power lessen mitochondrial PEP synthesis and glycogen synthesis? High NADH concentration in the cytosol favors the formation of malate from OAA, the first part of the shuttle. However, in the reducing environment of the mitochondria, malate would not readily be reoxidized. Therefore, PEP synthesis would be inhibited. In the reducing environment, malate participates in coupled reactions which result in lactate and alanine formation. Increased reducing power, then, favors cytosol reactions involving the formation of lactate, malate, glycerolphosphate, and alanine. Of these, only alanine and lactate leave the cell. Both may be synthesized into glycogen by the liver, or they may be oxidized by the heart. Additionally, reducing power favors the formation of amino acids from their more highly oxidized keto analogues. Thus glutamine synthesis is favored in muscle under starving conditions; as this glutamine can be exported, it influences the flow of carbon and nitrogen throughout the body.

GLUCONEOGENESIS

The cycle described by the Coris demonstrated that lactate produced by skeletal muscle could be converted to liver glycogen and glucose at high rates and suggested that (1) the mechanism involved a reversal by the liver of the glycolytic sequence, and (2) this was an important normal metabolic phenomenon by which two major organ systems (muscle and liver) interacted. At about the same time Krebs described the citric acid cycle as (1) a mechanism for the oxidation of pyruvate to carbon dioxide and water, and (2) a way of generating alanine and glutamic and aspartic acids by amination of the appropriate keto acids. Since the latter reactions are reversible, Krebs suggested that the metabolites of this cycle, including pyruvate, could be used as a way of coupling amino acid metabolism to carbohydrate metabolism. Later, he singled out alanine as key among the amino acids whose carbon skeleton is converted to glucose.

Corroboratory data concerning the close relationship between alanine and glucose metabolism were obtained from the study of amino acid metabolism in exercising healthy male subjects in postabsorptive states. During mild exercise, alanine release increased by 25 percent, whereas with more intense exercise, alanine release increased by 60 to 96 percent. Increases in arterial alanine concentrations were directly proportional to the rise in arterial pyruvate and to the intensity of the work; glutamine measurements were not obtained [46].

Some quantitation of the early skeletal muscle metabolic changes in starvation was achieved by measurements of arteriovenous differences of amino acids across the deep tissues (largely skeletal muscles) of the forearm and leg [48, 135]. When normal and obese subjects were fasted for a 12- to 14-hour overnight period, there was a consistently negative arteriovenous difference, indicating a net output of amino acids from the skeletal muscle. Alanine output exceeded that of all other amino acids, representing, together with glutamine, over 50 percent of the total α amino acid released (Figure 13-8). Similar results were obtained from measurements of the amino acid output from the myocardium [22] and gut [46].

Muscle alanine is produced from several sources including the transamination of pyruvate produced in glycolysis and the alanine liberated by proteolysis. Felig [43] proposed the following metabolic scheme, called the glucose-alanine cycle (Figure 13-9). In this reaction sequence, involving the liver and muscle, some blood glucose (derived from the liver) is taken up by muscle and converted to pyruvate via glycolysis. The pyruvate is then transaminated using, in particular, the amino groups of branched-chain amino acids to yield alanine and a keto acid capable of metabolism by the muscle. There is a linear correlation between circulating concentrations of alanine and pyruvate in humans in the basal state; no other amino acid has this relationship to pyruvate. Following exercise or fasting there is increased muscle pyruvate production and release of alanine. The alanine is then transported to the liver, where oxidative deamination of the substrate provides the energy for gluconeogenesis.

Although the glucose-alanine cycle accounts for some aspects of carbohydrate and protein metabolism, it does *not* account for a net flow of amino acid carbon to carbohydrate during starvation, since no carbon is lost in the glucose-alanine cycle. Several groups of workers (our-

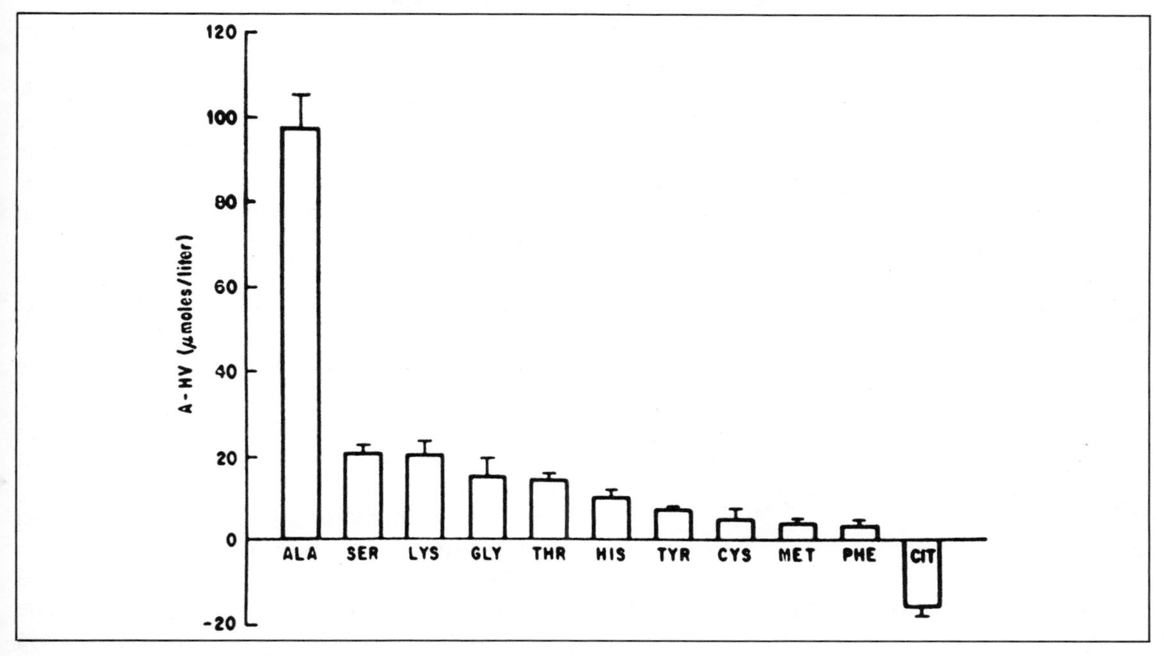

Figure 13-8. *Net balance of individual amino acids across the splanchnic bed (arterio-hepatic venous differences) in 12 subjects in the resting postabsorptive state. Only those amino acids whose mean A-HV differences were significantly different from zero are shown. (From P. Felig and J. Wahren, Amino acid metabolism in exercising man.* J. Clin. Invest. *50:2703, 1971. Reprinted by permission.)*

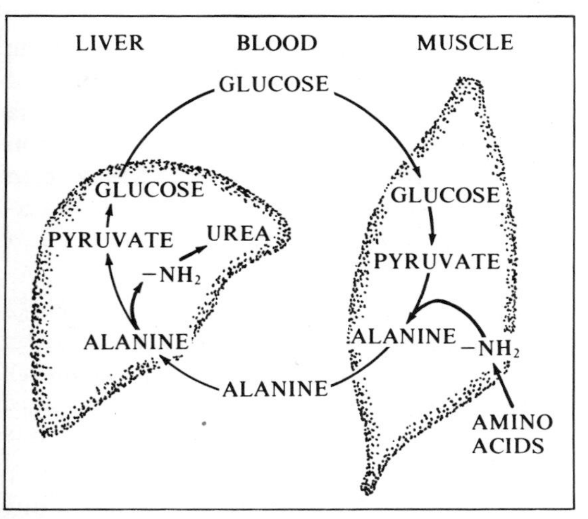

Figure 13-9. *The glucose-alanine cycle. (From P. Felig, The glucose-alanine cycle.* Metabolism *22:179, 1973.)*

selves included) have pointed out that the carbon of alanine released by muscle must have its origin in the amino acids released by proteolysis or in the carbon chain of one of the acids of the Krebs cycle [54, 107]. In the example cited below, Seifter speculated on the critical importance of malate, malic enzyme, and the Krebs cycle in such a scheme [107].

$$\text{Malate} + \text{NAD}^+ + \xrightarrow[\text{malic enzyme}]{Mn^{2+}} \text{pyruvate} + \text{NADH} + \text{HCO}_3^-$$

$$\text{Pyruvate} + \text{aspartate} \longrightarrow \text{alanine} + \text{oxaloacetate}$$

$$\text{Oxaloacetate} + \text{acetyl CoA} \longrightarrow \text{citrate}$$

$$\text{Citrate via Krebs cycle} \longrightarrow \text{malate}$$

Pertinent sum:

$$\text{Malate} + \text{aspartate} \longrightarrow \text{alanine} + \text{malate} + \text{HCO}_3^-$$

The following concepts advanced by Seifter derive from this scheme:

1. The synthesis of extra alanine (other than alanine derived from 3 carbon amino acids) by muscle is possible because of the presence of malic enzyme in the muscle.
2. Since malate is both a reactant and a product (Krebs cycle), the net carbon transfer involved in alanine biosynthesis comes from the degradation of muscle amino acids (e.g., aspartate, glutamate, and valine).
3. Most amino acids metabolized in the muscle according to this scheme would yield (a) some alanine, (b) carbon dioxide, (c) fatty acid derivatives in a partially oxidized state, and (d) energy.

Clarification of amino acid metabolism and transport in and out of muscle was brought by Garber, Karl, and Kipnis [55] in a series of in vitro experiments with rat epitrochlaris muscle. The pattern of amino acid release by this muscle preparation is remarkably similar to that observed in studies of arteriovenous differences across skeletal muscle in postabsorptive humans; alanine and glutamine account for more than 60 percent of the total amino acid release. Despite the disproportionately high release of alanine and glutamine, the tissue levels of these amino acids were found to be virtually unchanged. The following observations support the view that alanine carbon is not derived from glucose:

1. No correlation was found between glucose uptake and alanine release.
2. Muscle alanine and glutamine release were not changed by added insulin.
3. When glycolysis was blocked by iodoacetate, alanine and glutamine release were not decreased.
4. Using amino-oxyacetate, which inhibits alanine aminotransferase, a decrease in alanine release and a reciprocal increase in glutamine formation were noted, showing that an alanine transaminase rather than alanine dehydrogenase was involved in alanine synthesis.
5. Addition of amino acids such as aspartate, leucine, and valine increased the total carbon efflux from muscle, as measured by pyruvate + lactate + alanine + glutamate + glutamine release, by 70, 54, and 40 percent, respectively, in the presence of iodoacetate.
6. Addition of pyruvate did not increase the rate of alanine formation above that produced by aspartate, leucine, serine, and valine. These findings demonstrate that the increased carbon efflux from muscle is derived principally from metabolic transformation of amino acids to alanine and glutamine (Figures 13-10, 13-11).

Alanine formation from pyruvate and glutamate via transamination by alanine aminotransferase represents the final common pathway. Carbon derived from glycolysis and metabolic transformation of amino acids contributes to the intracellular pyruvate pool. The rate of glycolysis is not rate-limiting for alanine formation, whereas pyruvate formation from amino acids is reflected in corresponding changes in alanine synthesis and release.

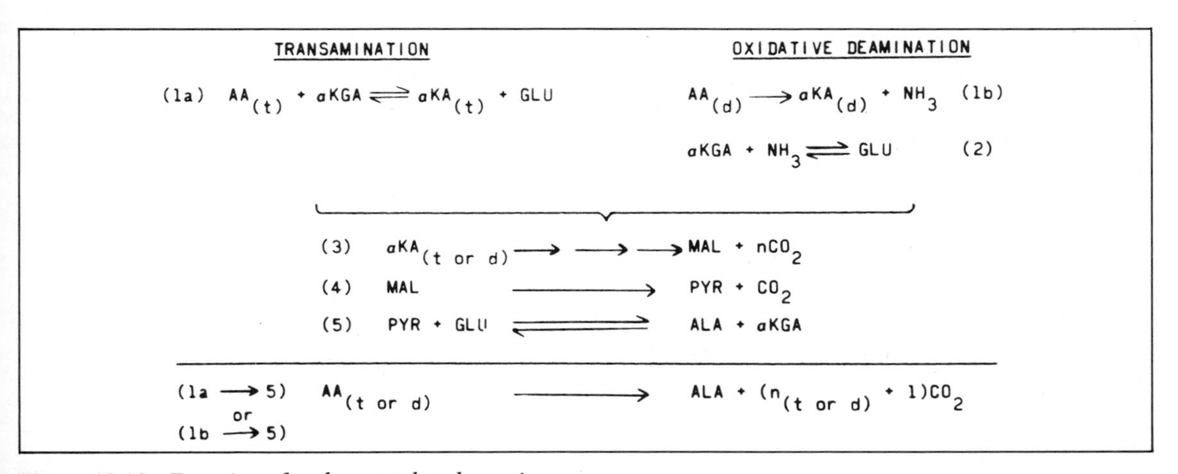

Figure 13-10. *Equations for the postulated reactions involved in synthesis of alanine (ALA) in skeletal muscle. Amino acid may transaminate ($AA_{(t)}$) with α-ketoglutarate (α-KGA) (1a) or may be oxidatively deaminated ($AA_{(d)}$) (1b) with subsequent glutamate (GLU) formation (2). For amino acids that form pyruvate directly, Equations 3 and 4 are to be omitted. Equation 3 represents the number of steps necessary to form malate (MAL) in the citric acid cycle, with the subsequent formation of pyruvate by $NADP^+$-malate dehydrogenase (4). Identical equations of summation (for carbon atoms) result regardless of the mechanism of glutamate formation (1a versus 1b and 2). (From A. J. Garber, I. E. Karl, and D. M. Kipnis, Alanine and glutamine synthesis and release from skeletal muscle.* J. Biol. Chem. *251:836, 1976.)*

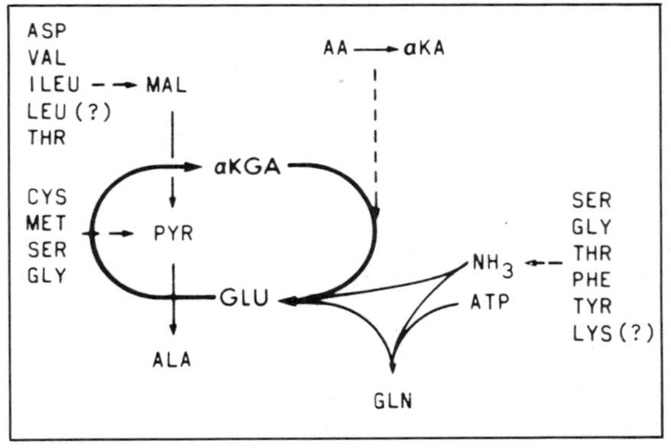

Figure 13-11. *Summary of the intracellular mechanisms leading to alanine and glutamine formation. AA = amino acid; KA = ketoacid. (From A. J. Garber, I. E. Karl, and D. M. Kipnis, Alanine and glutamine synthesis and release from skeletal muscle.* J. Biol. Chem. *251:836, 1976.)*

Net synthesis of alanine from cysteine, methionine, glycine, and serine can be accounted for, since they all lead ultimately to formation of pyruvate and glutamate. Methionine, isoleucine, and valine can lead to net alanine formation by generating succinyl CoA, which then becomes oxidized to malate via the Krebs cycle. The malic enzyme action is now known to possess sufficient activity in skeletal muscle to divert 4-carbon intermediates to pyruvate formation as suggested by Seifter [107].

Pozefsky et al. [149] found in normal men that the plasma concentrations of most amino acids in arterial blood had fallen after a 12-hour overnight fast, but those of the branched-chain amino acids (valine, leucine, and isoleucine) and α-aminobutyrate had risen. The arterial concentration of the branched chain amino acids rose even more at 60 hours of starvation. The glutamine-asparagine peak remained unchanged. The A-V difference (forearm) of several other amino acids (threonine, glycine, alanine, α-aminobutyrate, methionine, tyrosine, and lysine) became increasingly more negative with starvation (12 → 60 hours). The A-V difference for the branched-chain amino acids was somewhat more negative at 60 hours than at 12 hours, but not significantly so. Serine was actively taken up by muscle during the postabsorptive state, whereas it was released after the 60-hour fast. The 60-hour fast increased the rate of total amino acid (notably alanine) release from the forearm muscles by 69 percent over the postabsorptive levels.

Intracellular skeletal muscle amino acid concentrations were studied by Bergstrom et al. [12] in quadriceps muscle biopsies obtained from healthy subjects after an overnight fast. They found that eight dietary essential amino acids represent only 8.4 percent of the total pool of muscle free amino acids, whereas glutamine, glutamic acid, and alanine constitute about 79 percent. The intracellular concentrations of the branched-chain dietary essential amino acids (valine, leucine, and isoleucine) were greater than the plasma concentrations.

In many areas of nutrition and metabolism currently there is a good deal of interest in the branched-chain amino acids and their keto analogues. There are some special aspects of the metabolism of branched-chain amino acids that relate to starvation. Muscle, particularly red and heart muscle, is capable of utilizing leucine, isoleucine, and valine for energy to a greater extent than is the liver. It is this property that permits these compounds and their metabolites to act as regulators of muscle protein breakdown. Some of the intermediates of branched-chain amino acid can give rise to either muscle or liver glycogen.

Among factors that regulate muscle protein breakdown it has been found that the branched chain amino acids, their keto derivates, and their decarboxylated products inhibit muscle protein catabolism. For example: in muscle, valine, a branched chain amino acid, is converted to α-ketoisovaleric acid and then oxidized to isobutyric acid (as shown at the top of the next column). All of these compounds inhibit muscle protein breakdown. It is not known whether the subsequent metabolites of valine also share this property. It has been suggested that the partial oxidation of the

Valine

$(CH_3)_2CH{-}CH(NH_2){-}C(=O)OH$

↓

α-Ketoisovaleric acid

$(CH_3)_2CH{-}C(=O){-}C(=O)OH$

↓

Isobutyric acid

$(CH_3)_2CH{-}C(=O)OH + CO_2$

branched-chain amino acids and the partial oxidation of ketoacids by muscle contributes to the reducing environment of the muscle cell and that the inhibition of proteolysis is due to this reducing environment.

Insulin, in addition to promoting muscle protein synthesis, also inhibits protein breakdown. In starvation, insulin levels are low and therefore the control (inhibition) of protein breakdown derives in greater part from the branched chain amino acids and their metabolites. In an earlier discussion of this (1970, 1971), we had suggested an analogous approach using aromatic and branched-chain α-hydroxy and α-keto analogues of the amino acids; supportive evidence for the effectiveness of this approach using the α-keto analogues has since been reported by Sapir and colleagues [165–168].

The branched-chain amino acids (which by themselves inhibit protein breakdown) do not augment the inhibitory action of insulin on protein breakdown. Some workers [17], have speculated that leucine plays a special role in the inhibition of proteolysis. Since other branched-chain amino acids and some of their metabolites also are active in this regard [29], the existence of a special role for leucine has been questioned. We suggest that the latter view is probably correct for the fasted or starved animal. For the fed animal, though, it is likely that circulating leucine is an important regulator of insulin secretion. We think that it is not by accident that leucine, the one purely ketogenic amino acid, is a stimulus for hormonal changes that can abrogate the ketotic state.

Most studies directed toward evaluating the role of the liver and gut in amino acid exchange in normal humans have used measurements of arterial-hepatic venous differences, since the portal vein is not readily accessible for catheterization. Felig and Wahren [47] showed in normal, healthy volunteers that alanine predominates in the amino acid uptake across the splanchnic bed in the postabsorptive state. Studies of overnight fasted patients undergoing elective cholecystectomy and intraoperative portal vein sampling showed that the organs (principally the gastrointestinal tract) drained by the portal vein consistently released alanine, and that liver took up alanine, glycine, leucine, and isoleucine. The splanchnic bed (chiefly the gut) takes up glutamine and releases glutamate and alanine [47, 113]. The importance of the gut in glutamine metabolism is indicated by the observation that removal of the gastrointestinal tract, pancreas, and spleen, but not the liver, which was left in situ with its blood supply ligated, causes a greater rise in plasma glutamine than does nephrectomy [116].

Shulman et al. [181] have reported observations suggesting that the plasma glucose level can itself, independently of insulin or glucagon, modify the metabolism of the two main gluconeogenic precursors. They studied dogs that were fasted and given somatostatin and constant infusions of insulin and glucagon. They found that hyperglycemia leads to an elevation in the plasma lactate concentration primarily as a consequence of decreased lactate uptake by the liver. In addition, hyperglycemia causes the plasma alanine level to rise as a result of an increase in the production rate of the amino acid and a fall in its fractional extraction by the liver. Finally, hyperglycemia not only alters the net rate of entry of the aforementioned gluconeogenic precursors into the liver, but also decreases the efficiency with which they are converted to glucose.

IMPORTANCE OF OXALOACETATE IN MUSCLE AND LIVER METABOLISM

Muscle and liver oxaloacetate is a key metabolite in gluconeogenesis because it acts as a link between the carbon chain of some glucogenic amino acids and the carbon chain of glucose. For example, in muscle net oxaloacetate is generated from amino acids such as aspartate derived from protein:

Aspartate + keto glutarate ⟶ oxaloacetate + glutamate

Oxaloacetate ⟶ Krebs cycle ⟶ $CO_2 + H_2O$
Oxaloacetate ⟶ Krebs cycle ⟶ malate
Oxaloacetate ⟶ PEP ⟶ limited muscle gluconeogenesis

Muscle oxaloacetate also is critical because it provides the carbon chain for gluconeogenesis in liver and because it provides substrates for heart muscle metabolism.

In muscle:

$$\text{OAA} + \text{NADH} + \text{H}^+ \xrightarrow[\text{dehydrogenase}]{\text{malic (MDH)}} \text{malate} + \text{NAD}^+$$

$$\text{Malate} + \text{NAD}^+ \xrightarrow[\text{enzyme}]{\text{malic}} \text{pyruvate} + CO_2 + \text{NADH} + \text{H}^+$$

$$\text{Pyruvate} + \text{NADH} + \text{H}^+ \xrightarrow[\text{dehydrogenase}]{\text{lactic}} \text{lactate} + \text{NAD}^+$$

Sum:

$$\text{Muscle OAA} + \text{NADH} + \text{H}^+ \longrightarrow \text{muscle lactate} + CO_2 + \text{NAD}^+$$

Muscle lactate ⟶ liver lactate ⟶ glycogen
Muscle lactate ⟶ uptake and utilization by heart

Thus oxaloacetate serves to carry the carbon chain of amino acids (as lactate) to the liver for resynthesis into glycogen. It should be noted that lactate here also functions as part of an inter-organ transport of excess reducing power generated by muscle because the starving muscle carries out less complete oxidation than does well-nourished and perfused muscle.

In addition to providing lactate to liver for gluconeogenesis and to heart for further oxidation, OAA is the key in supplying muscle *alanine* to the liver for gluconeogenesis:

$$\text{Aspartic acid} + \alpha\text{-ketoglutarate} \xrightarrow[\text{transaminase (GOT)}]{\text{glutamic oxaloacetic}} \text{OAA} + \text{glutamate}$$

$$\text{OAA} + \text{NADH} + \text{H}^+ \xrightarrow{\text{malic dehydrogenase (MDH)}} \text{malate} + \text{NAD}^+$$

$$\text{Malate} + \text{NAD}^+ \xrightarrow[\text{enzyme}]{\text{malic}} \text{pyruvate} + \text{CO}_2 + \text{NADH} + \text{H}^+$$

$$\text{Pyruvate} + \text{glutamate} \xrightarrow[\text{transaminase (GPT)}]{\text{glutamic pyruvic}} \text{alanine} + \alpha\text{-ketoglutarate}$$

Sum:

$$\text{Aspartic} \xrightarrow[\text{NAD}^+\text{, NADH, pyruvate}]{\text{GOT, MDH, GPT, OAA, malate, } \alpha\text{-ketoglutarate, H}^+} \text{alanine} + \text{CO}_2$$

Thus muscle oxaloacetate provides some carbon for muscle gluconeogenesis or liver gluconeogenesis, or lactate for peripheral utilization. There exists a group of glucogenic amino acids that cannot provide OAA or PEP in muscle. Therefore, they are not glucogenic in muscle, but give rise to alanine and lactate, which can be converted to glycogen in liver and several other tissues:

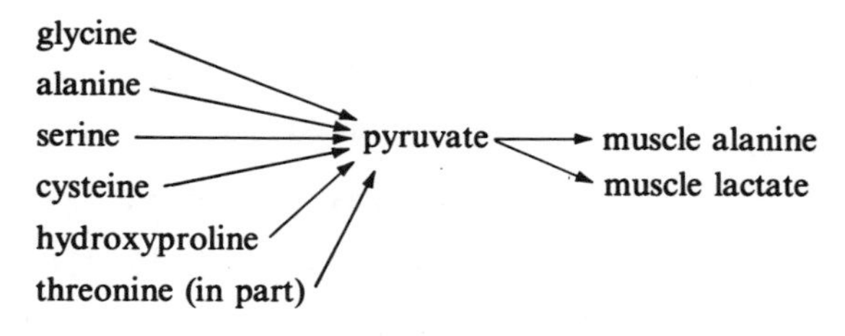

ROLE OF GLUTAMINE

Glutamine plays a major function in transporting some of the ammonia from muscle catabolism and a related function in providing a carbon skeleton which can be utilized for gluconeogenesis, although recent work of Goldberg [64] emphasizes this latter function. From the quantitative standpoint, about equal amounts of alanine and glutamine leave muscle under various metabolic states. Since the carbon of glutamine (as α-ketoglutarate) is convertible to the carbon of alanine (as pyruvate), either one can transport the carbon and nitrogen of other muscle amino acids to the liver or the kidney. In the muscle, glutamine is formed from glutamate which originates either from proteolysis or from transamination of α-ketoglutarate and then amidation. The α-ketoglutarate can be derived by a net synthesis from fatty acid oxidation and oxidation of the carbon skeleton of some amino acids, such as aspartic acid, via the Krebs cycle. Glutamine synthesis is an energy-dependent reaction requiring a glutamyl phosphate intermediate, which reacts with ammonia to yield the amino acid. Formation of glutamine by glutamine synthetase requires ammonia, glutamate, and ATP. The required glutamate is derived from either muscle protein glutamate, methionine, valine, or isoleucine. The latter three amino acids are precursors of succinyl CoA, therefore of α-ketoglutaric acid, and can contribute to a *net* synthesis of glutamine.

The preceding data are highly relevant to the glucogenic events in starvation. Alanine, the prime substrate for liver gluconeogenesis, and glutamine, the prime substrate for renal gluconeogenesis, are both derived from amino acid metabolism in muscle. Factors that regulate the rate of synthesis and release of these amino acids could directly affect the rate and importance of these two gluconeogenic pathways in different stages of starvation. Dependence on alanine as a gluconeogenic source poses problems to the body in terms of disposing of the ammonia formed in deamination. In the fed or postabsorption state, the ammonia is fed into the urea cycle in the liver and is synthesized into urea at the expense of considerable energy. In the prolonged starved state, urea is no longer the major nitrogen excretory product, but ammonium ion is; to a major extent this is because of the large amounts of ketones and ketoacids excreted at this time.

The adaptation of the kidneys to starvation becomes a major feature of the responses to food deprivation. Thus, early in starvation 90 percent of gluconeogenesis goes on in the liver and 10 percent in the kidney, but later in starvation 45 percent goes on in the kidney and 55 percent in the liver.

Kidney glutamine also contributes to the homeostasis of acid-base balance. By use of the enzyme glutaminase, glutamine becomes the immediate source of the ammonia, which accepts hydrogen ion and acts to neutralize some of the acidic products of metabolism. This reaction is quantitatively small in fed individuals, but in starvation becomes critical for survival for two reasons: (1) during starvation the body becomes depleted of sodium, potassium, and other fixed bases; and (2) the amounts of base required to neutralize the excreted keto acids (100 mEq/day) are large and require the production of a base by metabolism. The glutaminase reaction fulfills this requirement, permitting the excretion of ammonium and preserving the glutamate. The glutamate then acts as an acceptor of circulating ammonia and is converted to glutamine in the kidney, which can then give rise to urinary ammonium again. With a drop in circulating ammonia, some of the glutamate is cycled to the liver for glutamine or other syntheses and some of the glutamate is deaminated. Under similar conditions, α-ketoglutarate formed in the kidney is converted to kidney glycogen, and the ammonia handled by remaining glutamate as just described. Thus, deamination of glutamate is a major factor in the kidney's role as a glucose source during starvation. In acidosis (1) kidney glutamine arriving from the muscle is hydrolyzed by glutaminase to give NH_3, which picks up H^+ that is then excreted as NH_4^+; (2) the glutamate formed in this reaction is deaminated by glutamic dehydrogenase yielding a second molecule of ammonia, which combines with H^+ to be excreted as NH_4^+; (3) α-ketoglutaric acid in reaction 2 and under acidotic conditions tends to be used for renal gluconeogenesis. This means that the kidney can dispose of both the carbon and nitrogen of glutamine arriving from muscle (Figure 13-12).

The kidney also contains enzymes capable of carrying out a glutamate-based cycle, which converts glucogenic amino acids arriving from the circulation (muscle) into kidney glycogen and produces urinary ammonia.

(1) $\text{Glutamic acid} + NAD^+ \xrightarrow[H_2O]{\text{glutamic dehydrogenase (GDH)}} NADH + NH_4^+ + \alpha\text{-ketoglutaric acid}$

$NH_4^+ \xrightarrow{\text{excretion}} \text{urinary ammonium}$

(2) $\alpha\text{-Ketoglutaric acid} + \text{incoming glycogenic amino acid (e.g., alanine)} \xrightarrow{\text{glutamic pyruvic transaminase (GPT)}} \text{pyruvate} + \text{glutamate}$

(3) $\text{Pyruvate} \longrightarrow \text{glycogen}$

Sum:

$\text{Glycogenic amino acid} \xrightarrow{\text{glutamic acid, } NAD^+\text{, GDH, GPT}} \text{renal glycogen} + \text{urinary } NH_4^+$

ERYTHROCYTE AMINO ACIDS

Early equilibration studies of amino acids using red blood cells showed long equilibration times, and it was assumed that the plasma is the most important vehicle for amino acid transport. However, later studies indicate that large amounts of inter-organ and tissue amino acid exchange occur via the blood cellular elements, probably the erythrocytes, although a role for the leukocytes has not been ruled out [49]. Although the mechanism of the erythrocyte uptake and release of amino acids is not known, we think that the erythrocyte glutamyl transport system of Meister [122] could explain the transfer of amino acid into and out of the red blood cells. Moreover, this may provide the explanation for the

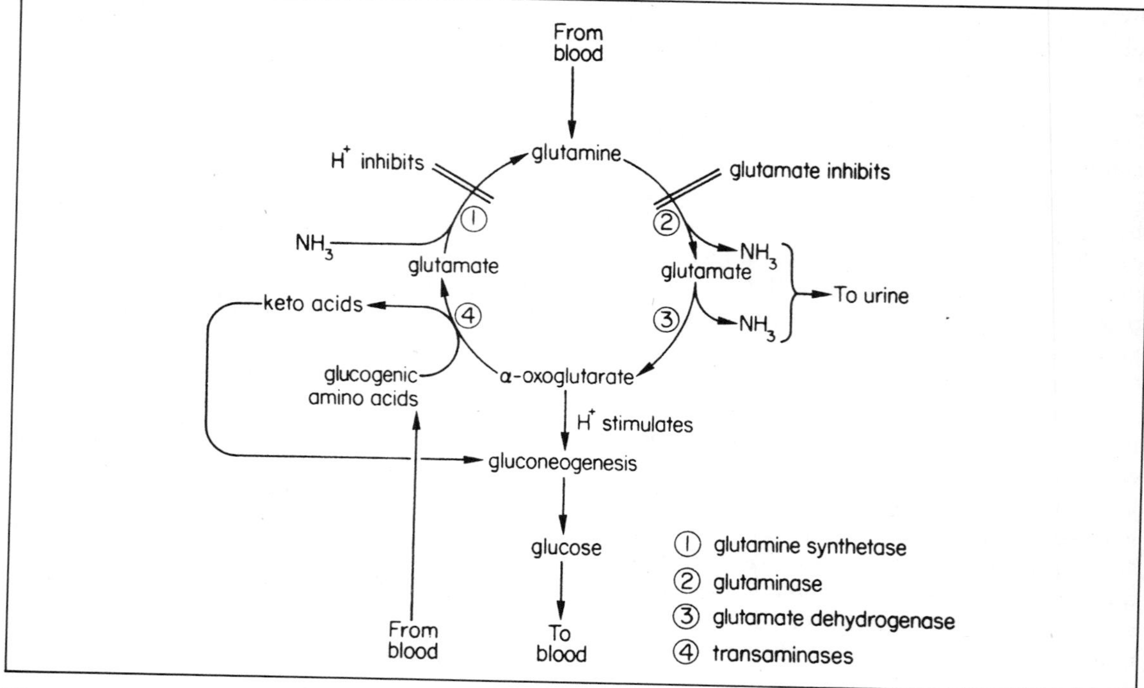

Figure 13-12. *Relationship between gluconeogenesis and ammonia production in the kidney. (From P. Banks, W. Bartley, and L. M. Birt,* The Biochemistry of the Tissues. *London: Wiley, 1976. Reprinted by permission.)*

existence of an amino acid transport system in cells that do not carry out protein synthesis. The situation parallels another function of red cells, i.e., oxygen transport by cells that utilize only minimal amounts of oxygen.

ERYTHROCYTE AND LEUKOCYTE GLUCOSE

In starvation, the brain and blood cells account for about 57 percent and 40 percent respectively of the glucose utilized [19]. Most brain glucose is oxidized to CO_2 and H_2O, but about 10 percent leaves the brain as lactate or pyruvate. Almost all the glucose used by blood cells is released as lactate. In starvation, the contribution of blood cell and brain lactate to the carbon of hepatic gluconeogenesis is as great as the carbon contribution from gluconeogenic amino acids and the glycerol from triglycerides.

FAT METABOLISM

One of the important adaptive changes of starvation is the increase in the absolute and relative amounts of fat consumed for energy purposes compared to the calories derived from protein. If the rate of protein breakdown and nitrogen excretion observed in the initial phases of starvation were to continue unchanged, the organism's protein stores would soon be depleted, resulting in dysfunction and death significantly sooner than, in fact, happens. Thus, after the initial phase of starvation, which is mainly concerned with gluconeogenesis, a second phase supervenes and is directed at minimizing protein breakdown by switching over from glucose to fat as the main source of energy, thereby decreasing gluconeogenesis. This changeover is accomplished by increasing the pool of free fatty acids by lipolysis, so that muscle increases its utilization of free fatty acids to a point at which 90 percent of its calories may be derived from their oxidation. Additionally, the liver increases its utilization of fatty acids. The main products of hepatic oxidation of fatty acids are the ketone bodies, acetoacetic acid, and β-hydroxybutyric acid, which are then transported to tissues (muscle, brain) that would otherwise require glucose. The accelerated hepatic ketogenesis during starvation is a result of both an enhanced activity of the enzymatic system(s) involved in ketone production and an increased FFA load, (enhanced activity of fatty acid synthesizing enzymes) [75, 103]. Once the early phase of starvation is over, the ketones are produced by the liver in greater amounts than glucose (130 gm versus 110 gm) [56]. During this phase, hepatic glucose output accounts for less than 30 percent of the total calories utilized by the body. As a result of these changes, in contrast to early starvation, in which the body uses about 4.8 calories derived from fat for every calorie derived from protein, the body in the adapted state uses about 17 calories from fat for each calorie derived from protein. It is this change in the relative amounts of protein catabolized during starvation, a drop from about 75 gm per day early in starvation to about 20 gm later in starvation, that makes longer survival possible.

Fatty acids are released from adipocytes following the hydrolysis of triglycerides by lipases [192]. Fatty acids are present in plasma in increased amounts under conditions of low circulating insulin, a characteristic of starvation; high insulin levels inhibit the lipolytic (lipase) activity of fat cells. Fatty acids are present in the serum in combination with either albumin or lipoproteins. In the former case, the linkage is a salt one with positively charged lysyl groups of albumin. In the latter case (lipoproteins), free fatty acids are taken up by the liver and secreted as part of macrostructures containing lipoprotein, triglyceride, phospholipid, cholesterol, and fatty acids. The binding of some of these structures involves noncovalent, hydrophobic associations. In advanced starvation the synthesis of lipoproteins declines, and fatty acid transport may become dependent on the albumin-bound complex.

Entrance of free fatty acids into muscle cells appears not to be directly under special hormonal regulation; rather, the concentration of serum fatty acids is critical in determining the rate of entry of fatty acids into the muscle cell. To the extent that insulin (or lack thereof) regulates release of free fatty acids from adipose tissue, it can be considered to regulate free fatty acid uptake by the muscle indirectly. Long-chain fatty acids cannot permeate the outer mitochondrial membrane, whereas some smaller-chain fatty acids are capable of permeating the outer, but not the inner, mitochondrial membranes. Fatty acids must be primed for utilization by mitochondria. The priming process consists of reactions occurring in the outer mitochondrial membrane and in some extramitochondrial organelles, which convert a fatty acid to its acyl coenzyme A derivative:

$$\text{Fatty acid} + \text{ATP} + \text{CoA} \rightarrow \text{fatty acid ester CoA} + \text{adenylic acid} + \text{PPi}$$

The acyl coenzyme A ester formed is now capable of crossing the outer membrane, but it is unable to permeate the inner mitochondrial membrane. This is made possible by a reaction carried out by an enzyme in the inner mitochondrial membrane:

$$\text{Acyl CoA} + \text{carnitine*} \rightarrow \text{Acyl carnitine} + \text{CoA}$$

It is the acyl carnitine that is able to cross the inner membrane. The coenzyme A diffuses back

$$* \; (CH_3)_3N^+{-}CH_2{-}CH(OH){-}CH_2{-}C(=O)OH$$

to the outer aspect of the outer membrane. On the inner aspect of the inner membrane, the reverse reaction occurs:

Acyl carnitine + CoA → Acyl CoA + carnitine

The acyl coenzyme A is now able to be oxidized inside the mitochondria, and the carnitine is free to diffuse out of the mitochondrial matrix, particularly back to the inner mitochondrial membrane.

These reactions can be summarized as follows:

Fatty acid + CoA + energy $\xrightarrow{\text{(outer membrane)}}$ Fatty acid CoA ester (Acyl CoA)

Acyl CoA + carnitine $\xrightarrow{\text{(inner membrane)}}$ Acyl carnitine + CoA

CoA + acyl carnitine $\xrightarrow{\text{(mitochondrial matrix)}}$ Acyl CoA + carnitine

Sum:

Fatty acid + CoA + energy $\longrightarrow$ Acyl CoA (inside mitochondrial matrix)

The system is of interest from two standpoints in starving individuals:

1. The synthesis of carnitine requires methyl groups from methonine and the carbon chain of lysine. Thus it is synthesized at the expense of a nutrient that cannot be synthesized in adequate amounts (methionine) or that cannot be synthesized (lysine) by the body. The biosynthesis of carnitine also involves ascorbic acid-dependent hydroxylations.
2. Carnitine levels in skeletal muscles of starved dogs and humans have been found to be higher than in samples from unstarved subjects [14]. Some workers have considered that elevations of carnitine are essential for the adaptation to starvation, suggesting that intracellular transport of fatty acids may be limiting for fatty acid oxidation during starvation. The maintenance of high carnitine levels during starvation may be accomplished by depleting some tissues of ascorbic acid.

Grey, Karl, and Kipnis [74] have shown that the accelerated hepatic ketogenesis during starvation is a result of increased free fatty acid load and an increase in the activity of the enzyme system(s) involved in ketone body production. As the supply of fatty acids to the liver rises, there is a parallel increase in the rate of hepatic extraction of these fatty acids. Concomitantly, ketone body production in the liver increases to 5 to 8 times the original value, and this leads to raised blood ketone levels. It has been calculated that after a 15-hour fast, 50 percent of the fatty acid uptake is converted to ketone bodies by the liver; this percentage increases to 80 percent after a 60-hour fast and to almost 100 percent after a 120-hour fast [36].

The increased hepatic ketogenesis is believed to result from inhibition of the citric acid cycle in the liver secondary to an accumulation of reduced coenzymes arising from increased fatty acid utilization and from substrate saturation of the citric acid cycle in the liver. Another, but quantitatively less important, source of ketone bodies is the deamination of some amino acids that are degraded via the acetyl CoA pathways. The increases in plasma ketones early in fasting reflect chiefly increased production and, to a lesser extent, some impairment of peripheral utilization, both processes being sensitive to insulin. Late in fasting, peripheral utilization of ketones is high.

Diabetes has been called "starvation in the midst of plenty." Starvation and uncontrolled diabetes both represent ketotic states, and these are compared in Figures 13-13 and 13-14. The key substance, in both the generation and utilization of ketone bodies, is acetyl CoA. In normal, fed animals, liver acetyl CoA derives from fatty acids released by adipocytes and from hepatic carbohydrate metabolism. Most of this acetyl CoA is oxidized via the Krebs cycle or resynthesized into fatty acids by the normal liver (see Figure 13-13). Only a minute amount (dotted

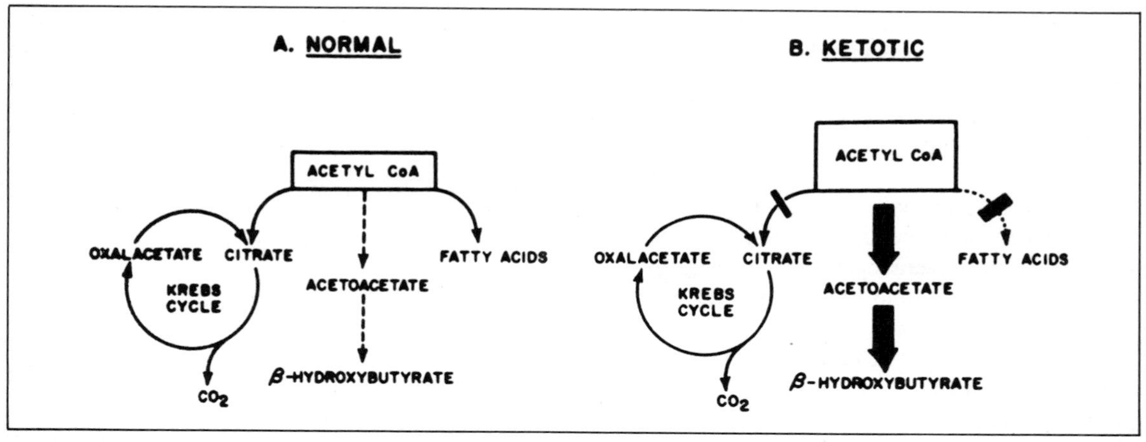

Figure 13-13. *Underutilization of acetyl-CoA in genesis of ketosis. In normal liver (A), acetyl-CoA is utilized primarily in Krebs cycle reactions or in fatty acid synthesis with minimal ketone formation. In ketotic states (B), fatty acid synthesis becomes negligible, hepatic acetyl CoA concentrations increase, and two-carbon flow to acetoacetate and β-hydroxybutyrate is enhanced. Krebs cycle activity is depressed only in severe ketosis. (From J. D. McGarry and D. W. Foster, Regulation of ketogenesis and clinical aspects of the ketotic state.* Metabolism *21: 471, 1972.)*

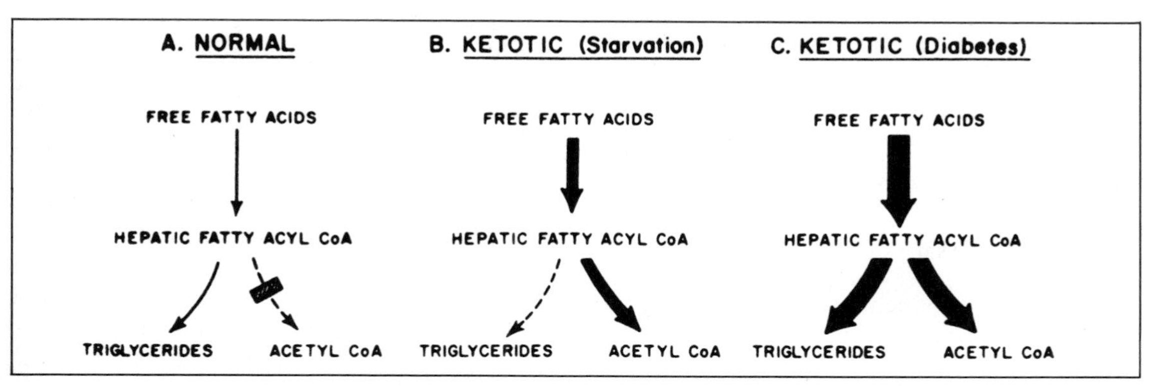

Figure 13-14. *Overproduction of acetyl-CoA in the genesis of ketosis. In the normal state (A), fatty acid oxidation is considered limited, probably at long chain fatty acyl CoA-carnitine transferase reaction with hepatic fatty acids utilized primarily for triglyceride synthesis. In starvation (B), entry of fatty acids into oxidative pathway is increased so that less substrate is available for triglyceride synthesis. In diabetes (C), fatty acid oxidation is maximally increased and free fatty acid delivery to liver is greater than in starvation, providing substrate sufficient for both accelerated ketogenesis and enhanced triglyceride synthesis. (From J. D. McGarry and D. W. Foster, Regulation of ketogenesis and clinical aspects of the ketotic state.* Metabolism *21:471, 1972.)*

line) goes to form ketones. In the liver of ketotic animals, the amount of acetyl CoA to be metabolized is greater. This is true for both the starved and diabetic state. The acetyl CoA levels rise because fatty acid synthesis becomes negligible and the amount of free fatty acids presented to the liver increases, probably owing to low plasma insulin levels or inadequate insulin activity. The activity of the Krebs cycle is only slightly decreased by ketosis, and most of the acetyl CoA goes into ketogenesis.

The liver has a mechanism for determining whether intermediates like acyl coenzyme A will go to ketone production or fatty acid synthesis. The mechanism explains why fatty acid breakdown in the liver does not usually occur at the same time as fatty acid synthesis, and how cessation of fatty acid synthesis stimulates fatty acid oxidation in the liver.

Normal State

High carbohydrate (CHO) ⟶ saturation of glycogen synthesis

then High CHO ⟶ high levels of AcCoA

High levels of AcCoA ⟶ high levels of citrate

High levels of citrate activate AcCoA carboxylase

(monomeric AcCoA carboxylase) (inactive) $\xrightarrow{+\text{ Citrate}}$ polymeric AcCoa carboxylase (active)

$$CO_2 + \text{AcCoa} \xrightarrow[\text{AcCoA carboxylase}]{\text{Polymeric}} \text{malonyl CoA}$$

$$\text{AcCoA} + 7 \text{ malonyl CoA} + 14 \text{ NAOPH} + 14H^+ \longrightarrow \text{palmitic acid} + 7\ CO_2 + 8\ \text{COA} + 14\ \text{NADP}^+ + 6\ H_2O \longrightarrow \text{palmitic acid} + 7\ CO_2 + 8\ \text{COA} + 14\ \text{NADP}^+ + 6\ H_2O$$

Fatty acid synthesis, then, is dependent (rate-limited) on malonyl CoA levels, which are in turn dependent on AcCoA carboxylase activity. In addition, malonyl CoA is an inhibitor of carnitine Acyl transferase (CAT), and as a consequence, fatty acid CoA derivatives that are formed in fatty acid biosynthesis are prevented from being oxidized:

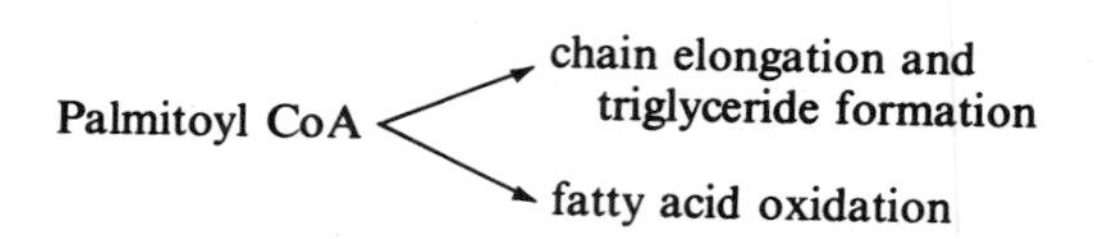

Malonyl CoA inhibits the mitochondrial transport of palmitoyl CoA by blocking the reaction

$$\text{Palmitoyl CoA} + \text{carnitine} \xrightarrow{\text{CAT}} \text{palmitoyl carnitine}$$

and therefore blocks fatty acid oxidation. As a result, fatty acid synthesis and oxidation do not occur simultaneously [119, 120].

Starvation

In starvation, there is a decrease in malonyl CoA levels in the liver (less glucose arriving to the liver), and at the same time, high levels of free fatty acids arrive from adipocytes. The fatty acids are activated by ATP + CoA, and the acyl CoA compounds formed are able to react with carnitine to form acyl carnitine, since there is little malonyl CoA to inhibit the process. As we have already noted, carnitine, a co-substrate for these reactions, is elevated in tissues of starved animals. These elevated carnitine levels further favor intracellular fatty acid transport and partial oxidation to ketone bodies.

In diabetes, levels of malonyl CoA and activity of AcCoA carboxylase are modified for different reasons than they are in starvation. A relative citrate deficit (and therefore deactivation of AcCoA carboxylase) exists owing to the shunting of oxaloacetate (citrate precursor) to gluconeogenesis. The end results (ketogenesis, decreased fat synthesis), however, are similar in starvation and diabetes.

Under-utilization of hepatic acetyl CoA for fatty acid synthesis, therefore, underlies ketone formation in both starved and diabetic animals. Whether the increased ketogenesis leads to ketonemia depends on the level of ketogenesis and the degree of peripheral utilization of the ketones.

Diabetic ketosis differs from starvation ketosis in several important ways:

1. Peripheral utilization of ketones is low in diabetes and in early starvation, but it is high in advanced starvation. However, because of the high production of ketones in starvation, ketonemia persists.
2. Although the liver in starvation decreases its ketone production following the infusion of antiketogenic substances (lactate, pyruvate, alanine), which are converted to glucose, the diabetic liver is nonreactive and ketone formation continues high.
3. The liver of diabetics produces large amounts of triglycerides even while producing large amounts of ketones, but this is not the case in starvation.

Influence of Fat Metabolism on Gluconeogenesis and Protein Catabolism

In the periphery, the ketone bodies block complete oxidation of glucose by inhibiting the activity of pyruvate dehydrogenase [120], and it is likely that this block plays a regulatory role in the switch-over in energy substrate from glucose to fatty acids and ketones that occurs in starvation.

Since ketogenesis reduces the need for glucose and therefore gluconeogenesis, ketonemia appears to provide a regulatory mechanism over the gluconeogenic pathway by inhibiting the release of glucogenic amino acids, especially alanine, by muscle and inhibiting alanine extraction from the plasma by the liver.

Sherwin, Hendler, and Felig [177] have shown, after prolonged starvation in obese subjects, that plasma alanine decreases to a greater extent than any other amino acid, whereas peripheral release and splanchnic uptake of alanine are reduced to less than 50 percent of the levels observed in postabsorptive states. They found also that during prolonged fasting, venous alanine concentration, which had already fallen by 40 percent below prefast levels, fell an additional 30 percent in response to the ketone infusion. In parallel with this decrease of plasma alanine, urinary nitrogen excretion fell in fasted subjects given prolonged infusions of ketones. The urinary nitrogen excretion returned to basal levels after the cessation of the infusions.

In summary, it seems clear that ketones play a major regulatory role in the second phase of starvation in addition to their role as energy sources. Whereas in the first phase, the drop in insulin and increase in glucagon are at the basis of the metabolic adaptations that occur, in the second phase, the ketone bodies play a dual role: on one hand, they represent a major energy substrate; on the other hand, they also play the major regulatory role in the metabolic adaptation, particularly in depressing gluconeogenesis.

WHOLE BODY PROTEIN TURNOVER

Golden and his associates [65, 66] found that whole body protein synthesis and breakdown were each reduced about 40 percent in seriously malnourished children. These values increased above normal during the period of rapid weight gain during refeeding (70 percent higher for synthesis, 50 percent higher for degradation) and then returned to normal when the children had recovered (Figure 13-15).

There are limited data in humans as to changes in protein turnover of individual organs and tissues. Interpretation of changes in whole body protein turnover during starvation poses problems similar to those we have already mentioned regarding interpretation of the changes in whole body metabolic rate during starvation. Millward [125] has pointed out that the average protein turnover rate of the lean tissue present in the malnourished children may not have been markedly depressed, but no measurements of lean body mass were made by Golden and his colleagues.

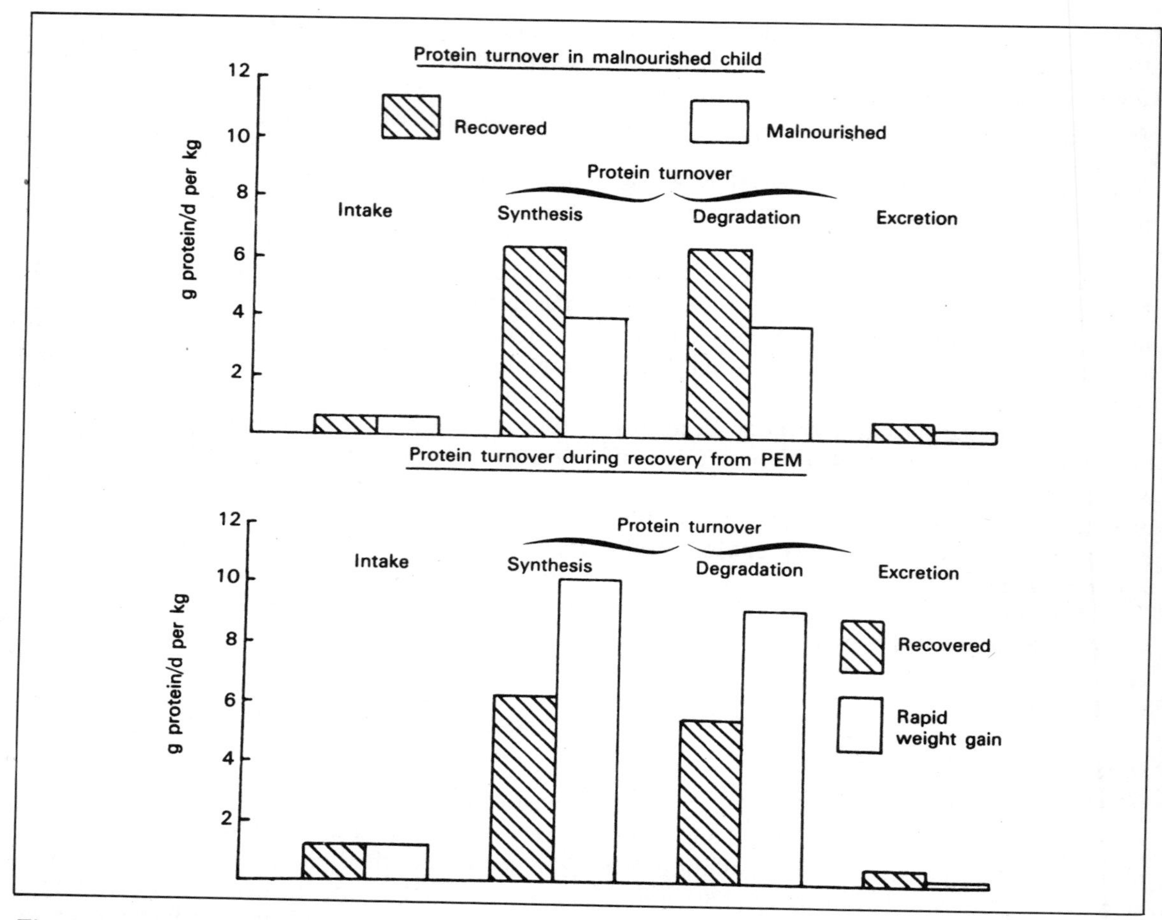

Figure 13-15. *Whole body protein turnover in malnourished, recovering, and recovered children. (From D. J. Millward, Protein deficiency, starvation and protein metabolism.* Proc. Nutr. Soc. *38:77, 1979.)*

LIVER AND MUSCLE PROTEIN TURNOVER

When rats are fed diets free of protein but adequate in calories, the liver loses protein immediately, without an apparent change in the fractional rate of protein synthesis [59]. During the next 3 weeks, the liver continues to lose protein, but more slowly, despite an increase in the fractional rate of hepatic protein synthesis. In contrast, when rats are starved, liver protein synthesis falls about 30 percent within 2 days [121], and liver protein falls rapidly. The decrease in liver protein synthesis correlates with a decrease of liver ribosomal RNA [82], but liver DNA is not altered.

Millward has pointed out that the rapid loss of liver protein by the rat early in starvation is almost exactly equal to the rate of export protein synthesis that is maintained at the expense of liver cytoplasmic protein [127]. He has stated that the liver's role in exporting protein may explain why the regulation of liver protein balance is achieved principally through regulation of protein degradation (increased in starvation)

[130] rather than protein synthesis [58], since a regulatory mechanism affecting principally protein synthesis would likely affect export protein synthesis, and this would be undesirable, at least as far as acute changes are concerned.

A decrease in skeletal muscle protein of starved rats occurs much more slowly. During the feeding of protein-free diets adequate in calories, a net loss of muscle protein occurs after 8 to 9 days, a result principally of a reduced rate of muscle protein synthesis. Protein degradation falls also, but not to the same extent as synthesis [59]. In contrast, starvation depresses synthesis and increases degradation of muscle protein in rats [126, 133, 193, 208]. The skeletal muscle (but not cardiac muscle) of starved rats (2 to 4 days) shows increased levels of ribosomal subunits along with a reduced rate of protein synthesis in vitro, demonstrating a starvation-induced inhibition of peptide chain initiation [152].

The changes in muscle protein synthesis during starvation may depend in part on the changes in insulin. Insulin not only stimulates amino acid transport into muscle, but also regulates muscle protein synthesis at the level of initiation of translation; in addition, insulin suppresses muscle protein breakdown [89]. Jenkins, Whittaker, and Schofield [90] have reported that the starvation-induced increase in muscle protein degradation is nonlysosomal in origin.

Of the amino acids liberated from muscle protein during fasting, two-thirds leave directly while the rest are deaminated, the nitrogen and carbon leaving as glutamine and alanine, and some of the carbon as CO_2 or branched-chain α-keto acids.

Amino acid deamination and oxidation in muscle are important because the essential amino acids involved (the branched-chain amino acids, particularly leucine) can be rate-limiting for tissue protein synthesis: the amount of leucine in proteins is high, whereas the amount in the free amino acid pool is relatively low. The amino acids effluxing from muscle tend to be relatively low in branched-chain amino acids, and Millward has pointed out that this may prejudice the ability of the liver to maintain normal export protein synthesis.

The aforementioned findings regarding protein turnover in muscle and liver are confirmatory of earlier findings by Waterlow and Stephen [209], who showed that the uptake of ^{14}C lysine by skeletal muscle of protein-deficient animals is reduced, indicating a substantially slowed rate of protein synthesis, while liver protein synthesis is reduced only moderately. Waterlow and Stephen [210] have shown in humans and animals that this latter finding is reflected by an increase in liver amino acid activating enzymes in protein depletion and a fall with refeeding, whereas the activity of argininosuccinase (a urea cycle enzyme) falls with protein depletion and rises with refeeding. In contrast, the amino acid activating enzymes of muscle fall rapidly with protein depletion and rise with refeeding.

Dice, Walker, Byrne, and Cardel [35] found that the enhanced protein degradation in starvation is fundamentally different from normal protein catabolism, i.e., correlations among molecular size, acidity, and nature (e.g., glycoproteins vs nonglycoproteins), which are present normally, are absent in starvation (liver and muscle) and diabetes, suggesting that starvation and diabetes alter the general characteristics of intracellular protein degradation in target tissues affected by insulin.

Wannemacher and Dinterman [207] have reported a gradual loss during starvation of the day:night differential in the rate of protein catabolism (normally greater at night). The differential in the normally fed rat may be related to the differential food intake (principally at night) as well as the diurnal variations in secretion of various hormones.

In obese men fasting for 20 days, excretion of urinary 3-methylhistidine was found to be decreased (34 percent), whereas the decrease in creatinine excretion and calculated loss of muscle mass was much less (15 percent), suggesting a decrease in skeletal muscle protein degradation

[222]. No reports are available of normal non-obese adults starving for long periods of time.

ALBUMIN SYNTHESIS AND CATABOLISM

A consistent change during starvation is a lowering of the serum albumin level. This change reflects a decreased rate of albumin synthesis, which occurs early (1 to 2 days) in starved rats and continues to fall, but at a slowed rate, dropping to about 20 percent of normal. This decrease is paralleled by a decreased ability of liver microsomes (ribosomes) from fasted rats to incorporate amino acids into protein [157]. The isolated perfused livers of starved rats also show lower rates of synthesis of fibrinogen, α-1 acid glycoprotein, α-2 acute phase globulin, and haptoglobulin. Albumin catabolism of rats slows late in starvation, but not proportionately to the slowing of its synthesis, as a result of which serum albumin falls.

In humans, a decrease in albumin synthesis occurs slowly during food deprivation; Keys et al. [95] found little change in serum albumin in volunteer men semi-starved for as long as 6 months.

ENDOCRINE SYSTEM

The thesis that starvation causes significant metabolic and physiologic changes, which enable the organism to better withstand food deprivation, is exemplified by the endocrinologic adaptations that occur in starvation. Hormonal adaptations occur hand in hand with other metabolic adaptations to starvation, e.g., the activities of certain enzymes. The degree to which the metabolic changes initiate and influence the hormonal modifications and the degree to which the hormonal changes initiate and influence the metabolic modifications have not been fully clarified. What is clear, however, is that the hormonal adaptations facilitate the organism's adaptation to food deprivation.

Some of the Major Endocrinologic Changes in Starvation

Almost all hormones are involved in the responses to food deprivation. Major changes in insulin, glucagon, growth hormone, catecholamines, thyroid hormones, glucocorticoids, and antidiuretic hormone occur, and these are reflected in alterations in carbohydrate, protein, fat, water, and electrolyte metabolism.

INSULIN

A key metabolic initiator of the hormonal changes is the early fall in blood sugar, which is followed by a variety of responses to maintain glucose homeostasis. Insulin secretion is decreased promptly, while glucagon, growth hormone, and possibly catecholamine secretions are increased and liver glycogenolysis is accelerated. At this early time, there is a beginning decrease in circulating T_3 with an increase in rT_3 and free cortisol.

As a result of the early hormonal responses, glucose production is increased, but as starvation goes on, the rate of glucose utilization outstrips its production. Blood sugar drops somewhat further and serum insulin continues diminished. The lowered serum insulin reduces glucose uptake by muscle and adipose tissue, promotes amino acid mobilization from muscle, and increases hepatic gluconeogenesis. The production of glucose is thereby enhanced, providing the glucose required by the brain and other glucose-using cells and tissues. Among the potential gluconeogenic precursors, only amino acids are hormonally dependent with regard to hepatic influx.

Lipolysis increases in starvation. It proceeds under the control of a number of lipases, one or more of which are under hormonal control. The functions of insulin in the inhibition, and of the catecholamines, growth hormone, and glucagon in the stimulation, of lipolysis play the major physiologic regulatory roles.

Insulin plays a major role in amino acid metabolism. It has long been known that insulin lowers plasma amino acid concentration and that the muscle is the main site of the insulin-mediated increased tissue amino acid uptake [129]. The in vitro sensitivity of skeletal muscle of rats to physiologic concentrations of insulin is enhanced during starvation (glucose uptake, glucose utilization, transport of α-aminoisobutyric acid) [68, 69]. Splanchnic uptake of alanine and other gluconeogenic amino acids is increased by glucagon, cortisol, and growth hormone by mechanisms yet undefined. Notable is the finding that insulin does not affect plasma levels of alanine in the peripheral blood or its release by muscle, but it does decrease the splanchnic uptake of alanine by 30 to 75 percent [47] and inhibits the incorporation of C^{14} alanine into glucose in the perfused liver [160]. Thus, amino acid gluconeogenesis, occurring in the initial phases of food deprivation, is facilitated by the decreased plasma insulin levels.

In humans, the plasma immunoreactive insulin levels after oral and intravenous glucose administration are subnormal in prolonged starvation and in protein-calorie malnutrition (starvation diabetes). In the earliest phases of food deprivation, the lowered plasma insulin levels are believed to be a response to the moderate decrease in plasma glucose, and at this early time the release of insulin in response to a glucose load may be normal. In prolonged malnutrition, at least in experimental animals subjected to protein malnutrition, the diminished islet cell volume may explain the persistently low insulin levels and poor responses to glucose administration [211]; no direct damage could be observed to either α or β cells, although the β cells contained unusually pale granules [212], and there may be a reduction in islet size [213]. Evidence regarding the responsiveness of the islet β cells in starvation to glucose as assessed in vitro is unsettled [81, 151, 224].

Improved tolerance with closely spaced successive glucose loads is known as the Staub-Traugott effect. Abraira and Lawrence [1] have found that while a clear Staub-Traugott effect was shown in the fed state, this effect was conspicuously absent after long-term caloric deprivation of obese humans. Compared to the findings before fasting, insulin levels after prolonged caloric deficit were similar during the initial intravenous glucose challenge, but successive glucose loads failed to elicit incremental insulin rises, in keeping with earlier suggestions from their laboratory that distinct mechanisms mediate the insulin-initiating and potentiating actions of glucose. After starvation there was greater suppression of plasma free fatty acids and immunoreactive glucagon levels. Absence of the Staub-Traugott effect after fasting would, in their view, appear to reflect a failure of nutrient induction of improved glucose metabolism, as alterations in glucoregulatory hormones and free fatty acids do not consistently explain the presence or absence of this phenomenon in the different metabolic states so far studied by them.

A close correlation has been noted between the lowered levels of serum potassium and serum insulin in protein-calorie malnutrition. The insulin response to oral or intravenous loading of glucose is markedly improved by giving large amounts of potassium during refeeding [5, 112].

Histologic studies of the pancreas in humans dead of starvation are hampered by the rapid postmortem autolysis that this organ undergoes. No specific abnormality in the islets has been reported, but pancreatic acinar atrophy and fibrosis have been found. These latter lesions are common in rats following prolonged calorie: protein deficiency.

Glucagon

The role of glucagon in the early and late phases of starvation is still not fully understood. Plasma glucagon levels rise in the early phases of starvation [195]. This increase appears to be secondary to a decreased rate of glucagon clearance rather than to a pancreatic hypersecretion [50]. During prolonged fasting (3 to 4 weeks), plasma glucagon values fall to pre-fast levels as a consequence of reduced pancreatic secretion despite a progressive decline in glucagon clearance.

Glucagon is a glucogenic hormone, and in the phase of maximal gluconeogenesis, it can lead to increased glucose levels by facilitating amino acid release from muscle and uptake by liver. Injected in pharmacologic doses, glucagon decreases the circulating levels of most amino acids, but its strongest effect is on alanine [45]. This decrease of the plasma amino acids occurs in parallel with an increased amino acid uptake by the splanchnic bed, especially for alanine [104, 179]. Glucagon's glucogenic action is also demonstrated by the fact that it increases the negative nitrogen balance in fasted subjects [114].

In the perfused liver, glucagon increases the conversion of alanine to glucose [110]. A stimulatory effect on cellular uptake and utilization of glucogenic amino acids, particularly alanine, also has been demonstrated. Karl, Garber, and Kipnis [93], using the in vivo epitrochlaris muscle preparation, found that 10^{-6} and 10^{-8} M concentrations of glucagon had no effect on the amino acid release from the muscle. Others have shown increased amino acid output from isolated muscle in response to glucagon at a concentration of 5×10^{-6} M [139].

When hepatic glycogen stores are intact, glucagon leads to a rise in plasma glucose by activating the adenylate cyclase system, which leads to increased phosphorylase activity and glycogen degradation. In fasting obese subjects, infusion of glucagon raises plasma glucose even after long-term fasting, by which time hepatic glycogen stores are depleted, and therefore some other mechanism(s) underlies its hyperglycemic effect [7]. Glucagon favors hepatic proteolysis, and this may provide substrates for glucogenesis and glycogenolysis.

Increased serum alanine and arginine stimulate glucagon secretion. Glucagon stimulates gluconeogenesis by stimulating the conversion of pyruvate to phosphoenol-pyruvate and increases the transport of alanine into hepatic cells. This results in a lesser fall in blood glucose and, thereby, lesser inhibition of insulin secretion. Increase in serum insulin in turn diminishes the breakdown of muscle protein and synthesis of alanine and slows gluconeogenesis. Thus, glucagon and insulin play essential roles in the cyclic interrelationships between alanine and glucose. The glucocorticoids appear to play a "permissive" role. During the period of maximal gluconeogenesis in starvation, glucagon appears to inhibit insulin secretion directly.

Glucagon also leads to increased lipolysis [195]. The major influence of glucagon on hepatic FFA metabolism appears to be the diversion of circulating FFA into the pathways of oxidation (ketone body and CO_2 formation) and away from esterification products. This indicates a special role for glucagon in the metabolic switchover to ketone bodies as starvation proceeds.

There are relatively few data regarding glucagon metabolism in prolonged starvation. Low levels have been reported in malnourished children with severe fasting hypoglycemia [76], and in these children glucagon administration causes a prompt rise in blood sugar levels [4]. Thus, hypoglycemia, a late occurrence in protein-calorie malnutrition, may be caused in part by decreased levels of circulating glucagon.

Walter, Dudl, Palmer, and Ensink [206] have reported studies in human volunteers, results of which suggest that the augmented glucagon release in man during starvation or after hypoglycemia is not significantly regulated by signals from the adrenergic nervous system.

The relationship between glucagon levels and the natriuresis that occurs at the beginning of starvation in obese subjects has been studied by Saudek, Boulter, and Arky [169]. Both the rise in glucagon levels and the natriuresis reach their maxima on the fourth day of starvation. Both are suppressed by glucose and both start to decline by the fifth day. By the seventh day, a time when sodium balance is achieved, plasma glucagon levels have fallen to normal baseline levels. A direct action of glucagon on the kidney has been demonstrated [150].

Pituitary Gland; Growth Hormone (GH)

Half a century ago it was observed that the acidophils of the anterior pituitary were atrophied and degranulated in starved rats [88]. Findings in malnourished patients have been variable, and are perhaps age dependent. For example, one study showed no changes in the pituitaries of infants dying from marasmus or kwashiorkor, or both [200], whereas another study of 101 malnourished patients (adults?) showed pituitary atrophy to be present in 49 of them. Degenerative lesions of the anterior lobe were present, including vacuolization, pycnosis, cellular atrophy, and calcification. The posterior lobe showed basophilic invasion [225].

Campbell et al. [20] have shown that severe reduction in food intake by rats decreases the release of at least five anterior pituitary hormones (GH, TSH, FSH, LH, prolactin). They suggest that this is due primarily to reduced hypothalamic stimulation rather than a reduced ability of the pituitary to secrete hormones.

Prior to the availability of radioimmunoassay techniques, growth hormone (GH) secretion was thought to be diminished in malnutrition, but recent studies in starving obese subjects have shown that the circulating GH levels increased between the third and tenth day of fasting; later, between days 10 and 38, there was a steady decline in circulating GH levels to well below 50 percent of the starting values [135]. In normal men subjected to fasting, serum GH levels also increased (three- to fivefold) during days 3 to 5; the values returned to prefast values by the ninth day of fasting [137]. In normal women, the early increases in serum GH during the first few days were more modest (one- to three-fold) [123, 124]. The elevated growth hormone levels early in starvation may have a diabetogenic effect.

In prolonged protein-calorie malnutrition, Smith et al. [189] found plasma GH levels elevated (fivefold). Despite this elevation, arginine infusion led to significant rises in plasma GH; glucose infusion caused rapid and significant falls in the plasma GH levels. Plasma GH levels are elevated also in children with kwashiorkor or marasmus; marasmic children generally have lower GH levels than those suffering from kwashiorkor [164]. Marasmic children in general showed no increases in GH secretion in response to arginine [9], or to insulin hypoglycemia, and the elevated plasma GH levels in marasmus and kwashiorkor were not suppressed by intravenous or oral glucose [143, 144], but did drop following the oral administration of a mixture of the dietary essential amino acids [128]. Tannenbaum and colleagues [198] found that circulating SRIF is a physiologic regulator of starvation-induced GH suppression in rats, but is not involved in mediating the inhibition of insulin.

Inverse correlations between (1) plasma GH and plasma albumin levels and (2) plasma GH and plasma alanine and valine levels have been observed in children with marasmus and kwashiorkor [108]. The strong relationship betwen the degree of body protein depletion and plasma GH levels is demonstrated further by the finding that high-protein refeeding produces a marked drop in plasma GH levels in malnourished children [164].

Administration of human GH on alternate days, for 12 days, to fasting obese women led to increases in the sodium and potassium urinary excretion, with no increase in ketoacidosis [174]. In contrast, Felig, Marliss, and Cahill [44] showed that administration of GH to obese males and females fasting for 5 to 6 weeks led to rises in serum free fatty acids, glycerol, and β-hydroxybutyrate plus acetoacetate. This was accompanied by a two- to threefold increase in plasma insulin. Urinary potassium and ketone excretion also increased significantly. There was no reduction in urinary total nonprotein nitrogen excretion. However, urinary urea excretion decreased, probably secondary to a reduction of protein catabolic processes, whereas urinary ammonia excretion increased, probably as a compensatory renal mechanism to the increased ketonemia.

Growth hormone secretion is stimulated by stress or injury. It stimulates free fatty acid release by increasing lipolysis. Moreover, Wilmore et al. [216] have shown that human GH administration to critically burned patients, together with a fixed intake of protein and amino acids and calories designed to meet projected metabolic needs, decreased nitrogen excretion (20 percent) during the net "catabolic" phase of injury.

Low serum somatomedin levels have been found in children with kwashiorkor, most of whom had high serum GH levels [73]. Work with rats had already shown that serum somatomedin levels are reduced in starvation [34, 142]. These findings suggest the possibility of a block in somatomedin formation in starvation. Although the somatomedins were thought initially to be dependent only on growth hormone, it now seems likely that they are regulated by insulin as well [140, 141].

Plasma heat-labile inhibitors of somatomedin activity have been found in starvation, both in experimental animals and in humans [83, 163, 203]. If such inhibitors have specific effects, it raises the possibility that selective control over certain aspects of GH activity with survival benefit may exist in starvation; thus, as a compensatory mechanism, GH might influence some metabolic events, e.g., lipolysis, in preference to others, e.g., growth, when protein stores are being depleted.

Somatomedins and somatomedin inhibitors may be produced largely by the liver, though the kidney may also produce somatomedins.

Thyroid

As noted earlier, the basal metabolic rate falls during starvation in contrast to the rise following injury, and the decrease in metabolic rate as starvation progresses is proportionately greater than the loss of weight. These observations have prompted many studies of the thyroid and thyroid hormones in both conditions.

Plasma TSH levels have been variously reported as low, normal, or high in malnourished children [63, 77, 145]. These varying results may be due to demographic factors related to nutritional and socioeconomic backgrounds or to differences in the radioimmunoassay techniques used. Diminutions of protein-bound iodine in the blood, butanol extractable iodine, and total thyroxine have been reported in infantile malnutrition. These decreases are parallel to, and may be related to, a reduction in the plasma levels of thyroxine-binding protein and pre-albumin [63]. Free plasma T_4 levels were found normal or elevated in kwashiorkor and normal or low in marasmus [71]. Thyroid involution occurs during prolonged protein-calorie malnutrition, and thyroid fibrosis has been noted in severely malnourished children [62]. In adults, prolonged protein-calorie malnutrition led to serum TSH levels that are high when compared to normal American standards, but did not change with refeeding [27].

In normal fasting adults, serum TSH levels were unchanged after a 60-hour fast [124], but significantly decreased after 10 days of fasting [137]. The secretion of TSH remains sensitive to changes in serum thyroid hormone concentrations [57, 78]. Short-term (2 days) starvation of rats did not alter the hypothalamic content of TRH, but did decrease pituitary TSH content and serum TSH concentration [79].

In healthy adults fasted for 60 hours, mildly elevated serum levels of free T_4 were found [124], whereas at 5 and 10 days, in normal males, serum T_4 was significantly decreased as were the serum total and free T_3 concentrations [78, 79, 137]. In obese humans, modest increases in serum free T_4 were found after 4 weeks of starvation [148]. Chopra and Smith [27] studied adult males with protein-calorie malnutrition and found that plasma-bound T_4 levels were normal, but free T_4 levels were elevated; total plasma T_3 levels were low. Although plasma albumin and thyroxine binding pre-albumin levels were decreased, the decrease in plasma T_3 was proportionately greater. The decrease in serum T_3 (total and free) has been confirmed in short-term starvation studies, both in normal and in obese humans [27, 137, 191, 214]. The decrease in serum T_3 levels is associated with a reciprocal rise in reverse (r) T_3 [27, 57, 137, 189] (Figure 13-16).

The high serum T_4 and low T_3 levels may reflect low peripheral conversion of T_4 to T_3 [199, 202], but studies on the degradation rates of either hormone have not been carried out. The decreased hepatic T_3 generation by the starved rat is associated with decreased NPSH (non-

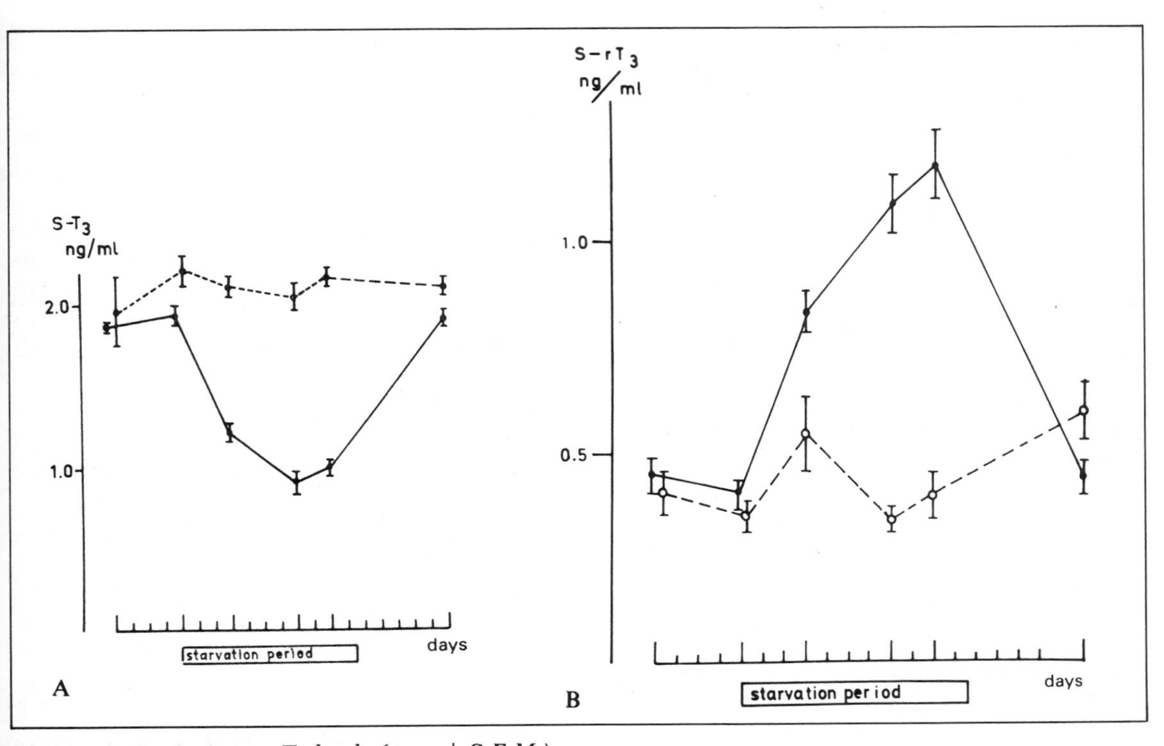

Figure 13-16. *A, Serum T_3 levels (mean ± S.E.M.). B, Serum rT_3 levels (mean ± S.E.M.).* •- - - - -• *Non-starved;* •———• *starved. (From J. Palmblad, et al., Effects of total energy withdrawal (fasting) on the levels of growth hormone, thyrotropin, cortisol, adrenaline, noradrenaline, T_4, T_3, and r-T_3 in healthy males.* Acta Med. Scand. *201:16, 1977.)*

protein sulfhydryl groups), but not with a decrease in the absolute quantity of the enzyme 5[1]-deiodinase; provision of sulfhydryl groups restored hepatic T_3 generation to normal in vitro [78, 79, 189]. There is a decrease in hepatic nuclear T_3 receptors in starved rats, and the induction of the cytosolic enzyme, malic dehydrogenase, known to be inducible by thyroid hormones, is blocked in starvation. The mechanism by which T_4 is converted to the poorly calorigenic rT_3 is not known. The increase of serum rT_3 concentrations during starvation appears to be due to both an increase in the rate of production of rT_3 and a decrease in the rate of degradation of rT_3 [197]. It is known that administration of corticoids to hypothyroid and hyperthyroid patients leads to increased production of rT_3 [28], thus implicating the raised levels of corticoids during starvation as responsible, in part, for the rise of rT_3 production.

It has been suggested that the decrease in serum T_3 during starvation spares muscle protein. Karl, Garber, and Kipnis [93], using an in vitro epitrochlaris muscle preparation, found that added thyroxine increased by 200 percent the amount of alanine released by the muscle, a fact that may be relevant to the early gluconeogenic events during starvation. Administration of T_3 to humans fasted for 3 days enhances protein catabolism, as indicated by a doubling of urinary urea excretion [23, 57], and increased fat catabolism, as demonstrated by increases in the free fatty acid and ketone levels [23].

Returning to the question of whether the decrease in serum T_3 may be one of the mechanisms underlying the lowered metabolic rate in starvation, it should be noted that Wimpfheimer, Saville, Voirol, and Danforth [217] have found that the decrease in resting oxygen consumption induced by starvation occurs not only in euthyroid rats, but also in hyperthyroid and hypothyroid rats treated with triiodothyronine. The effectiveness of triiodothyronine in raising metabolic rate was decreased when given to hypothyroid starved rats. It is clear that some factor(s) other than the plasma levels of the thyroid hormones influenced the changes in metabolic rate following starvation in these experiments.

L-Dopa, a substrate for catecholamine synthesis, given to obese patients ingesting a hypocaloric, normal protein diet, prevented the usual decline in metabolic rate, increased plasma norepinephrine to normal, and increased plasma epinephrine to levels slightly above normal. The low serum T_3 levels did not change with the administration of L-dopa, but the usual increase of plasma rT_3 was largely prevented. These data indicate that the changes in metabolic rate and T_3 can be dissociated by giving a precursor of the catecholamines. The mechanisms for the metabolic adaptation to semi-starvation may relate to an interplay of catecholamines and the thyroid hormones [91, 178] (see pp. 432 and 461 for additional discussion of catecholamines).

Adrenal Cortex; Glucocorticoids

Data regarding histologic changes in the adrenals during starvation are conflicting. Thus, the adrenal gland has alternately been described as atrophic in infants with protein-calorie malnutrition [25] or as hyperplastic in pigs subjected to experimental protein deficiency for about 1 to 3 months [146].

Studies by Galvao-Teles et al. of fasting obese humans show that rises in plasma-free cortisol and diminution of the day-night variation of these plasma levels occur [51]. Fasting of humans of normal weight also led to increases in plasma cortisol levels; the highest levels were reached on the tenth day, the last day of the fast [137].

There is a marked inverse correlation between plasma cortisol and albumin levels in children with protein-calorie malnutrition [108]. Thus, cortisol changed in the same direction as growth hormone in relation to serum albumin, i.e., it increased as the albumin level fell.

Plasma cortisol is also elevated significantly in adults suffering from protein-calorie malnutrition; there were no significant changes in plasma ACTH [188]. Urinary free cortisol excretion was normal, but when corrections were carried out for the reduction in the creatinine clearance that occurs in starvation, free urinary cortisol excretion was elevated in protein-calorie malnutrition. Urinary 17-hydroxysteroids and 17-ketosteroids were markedly reduced.

It appears that the metabolism of cortisol is impaired in starved patients, resulting in low urinary excretion of its metabolites in the face of high circulating and high urinary excretion of free cortisol. Also, the pituitary-adrenal axis appears to be defective in its feedback control, since normal response of the adrenal to ACTH persists while dexamethasone does not suppress cortisol plasma levels. In addition, normal secretion of ACTH continues despite raised plasma cortisol levels. By contrast, lower response to ACTH, as measured by plasma cortisol levels, has been found in children with kwashiorkor [154]. Circulating cortisol binding protein is also reported to be low in children with protein-calorie malnutrition.

In prolonged starvation, a pseudo-Cushingoid syndrome exists; in these subjects, ACTH and plasma cortisol levels are elevated simultaneously. Some of the immunologic abnormalities of starvation have been attributed to this, although during refeeding there is no correlation between the time of return to normal of the cortisol plasma binding protein levels and, for example, the reversal of the decrease in complement levels.

As to how the changes in cortisol metabolism may effect the metabolic response to starvation, glucocorticoids generally have a glucogenic function. Glucocorticoids given to experimental animals decrease protein synthesis by skeletal muscle and lead to augmented hepatic uptake and utilization of amino acids by increasing gluconeogenesis [111]. In the eviscerated rat, cortisol administration leads to increased levels of plasma amino acids, implicating the muscle as their source [187]. An in vitro study by Karl, Garber and Kipnis [93] of muscle obtained from rats given cortisone for 3 days showed an increased alanine release (145 percent) and decreased glutamine release (37 percent); tissue alanine level remained unchanged whereas that of glutamine decreased by 30 to 60 percent. Administration of dexamethasone to obese and nonobese fasting humans leads to a rise in plasma alanine, whereas the plasma levels of the other amino acids remain unchanged [219]. In line with this are experimental in vivo studies showing that administration of hydrocortisone leads to increases in intracellular hepatic and skeletal muscle alanine, exceeding that of all other amino acids.

The crossing over of gluconeogenic intermediates between pyruvate and phosphoenolpyruvate (PEP) observed in intact starved rats was not seen in adrenalectomized rats with constant serum insulin levels. This supports the concept that during starvation glucocorticoids enhance the rate of glucose production by the liver by permitting hepatic CAMP to stimulate the yet undefined mechanism that controls the substrate flow between pyruvate and PEP [175].

Of interest is the observation that glucocorticoid administration increases glucagon secretion, indicating a multifactorial hormonal drive for the gluconeogenesis of starvation. Owen and Cahill [134] showed in obese subjects that the proteolytic effect of glucocorticoids disappears in long-term starvation. This supports the strong correlation between the tissue protein changes and the hormonal adaptations that occur in starvation.

Adrenal Medulla, Sympathetic Ganglia, Catecholamines

The roles of the catecholamines (epinephrine, norepinephrine) in the early and, especially, the late phases of starvation unaccompanied by stress are still largely unknown. The plasma norepinephrine level has been reported to fall early during starvation, whereas the plasma epinephrine level does not change.

A recent study of healthy fasting men showed that the urinary levels of adrenaline (epinephrine) levels decreased, but not significantly [137]. The epinephrine released early in fasting can induce liver glycogenolysis and also can activate muscle phosphorylase via a cyclic AMP mechanism. This would lead to enhancement of glycolysis and, if intense enough, to the point where pyruvate and lactate become main end-products and contribute to acidosis and an oxygen debt. The pyruvate and lactate secreted into the blood enter liver pathways for gluconeogenesis, as already noted.

Fasting is associated with decreased rates of norepinephrine turnover in the heart, as demonstrated recently by Young and Landsberg [223] in rats fasted for 2 days. The fast-related suppression of norepinephrine turnover in the heart was found to also occur in the liver, pancreas, and spleen. These investigators interpret their data as indicating decreased catecholamine activity during early fasting. We have already mentioned the possible role of the decreased catecholamines in the lowered metabolic rate of starving people (p. 460).

In later stages of food deprivation (but not total starvation), Shoemaker and Wurtman [180] found reduced brain tissue levels of norepinephrine and dopamine in protein-malnourished rats. In a small number of marasmic children, low urinary levels of metanephrines have been reported [15], whereas in those with kwashiorkor, elevated epinephrine and low dopamine urinary excretion have been reported [85].

Much more work is needed in the area of catecholamine function in starvation, since their calorigenic function and their role in the release of polypeptide hormones and in the control of various metabolic substrates are of major importance.

Sex Hormones

There is a paucity of studies regarding the behavior of the sex hormones during starvation, particularly in humans. A few short-term studies have been carried out in animals. In terms of the hypothalamic control mechanism, total starvation for 7 days of normal and castrated male rats did not affect the hypothalamic content of LH-releasing hormone [156]. Starvation in male hamsters did not affect pituitary weight or pituitary LH content, but serum LH levels fell significantly, as did seminal vesicle and testicular weights; in female hamsters, starvation decreased pituitary weight, while pituitary LH content increased and serum LH content remained unchanged; female hamsters also demonstrated decreased uterine weight, but no change in ovarian weight [87]. Serum LH levels fell after 10 days, while pituitary LH levels increased after 20 days in female rats subjected to 50 percent food restriction. In male rats similarly semistarved, serum testosterone decreased at 20 days, but serum and pituitary FSH levels were not affected [86].

Fasting of prepubertal heifers led to a significant decrease in serum prolactin levels, without blunting the prolactin response to arginine [117]. Decreased serum prolactin levels were also observed in starving rats [183].

RENAL FUNCTION; SODIUM, POTASSIUM, MAGNESIUM, CALCIUM, PHOSPHORUS, AND URIC ACID URINARY EXCRETIONS

Increased urinary excretion of *sodium, potassium,* and *magnesium* begins promptly *during fasting* and continues elevated, although at lower levels. In contrast to the changes in starvation per se, *sodium* excretion *decreases* promptly *after injury,* while *potassium* excretion *increases.*

The basis for the early changes in sodium, potassium, and magnesium excretion in starvation is not known completely, although catabolism of tissue proteins with concomitant loss of intracellular cations has been implicated. Early studies by Gamble and his colleagues [52] showed that feeding small amounts of *glucose* (50 to 100 gm daily) early in starvation led promptly to *decreased* excretion of sodium and potassium (Figure 13-17). Feeding a calorically equivalent amunt of *fat* may *increase* the natriuresis and kaliuresis. Later investigators showed that plasma aldosterone and renin concentrations increase early in starvation [26, 60, 101, 102]. Feeding carbohydrates led to decreased urinary sodium excretion, but to no change in plasma renin activity or aldosterone levels. Aldosterone infusion had only 40 percent of the antinatriuretic effect it achieved before the fast, indicating a state of aldosterone resistance at the nephron. These observations are complemented by earlier studies by Schloeder and Stinebaugh [173], which demonstrated that fasting leads to increases in V/GFR and C_{H_2O}/V, but to decreases in C_{H_2O}/GFR, all of these changes being reversible by carbohydrate feeding. These changes reflect both maximal and distal nephron dysfunction and may be responsible in part for the natriuresis and aldosterone resistance of fasting. We have already pointed out (p. 456) the relationship between sodium excretion and plasma glucagon levels during fasting [169].

In the later phases of fasting, it has been suggested that the increased urinary excretions of sodium and potassium are to buffer the increased urinary ketones. Studies conducted by Sigler [182] of fasting obese women maintained on a fixed sodium intake showed a close correlation among urinary $Na^+ + K^+ + NH_4^+$ and urinary organic acid anions and $H_2PO_4^-$. Ammonium excretion rose and Na^+ excretion fell as the fast proceeded. Urinary excretion of Na^+ was greater than that of Cl^-. Glucose feeding led to the expected decrease in Na^+ excretion, and this correlated with a decrease in urinary organic acid anions. These data were interpreted by Sigler as indicating that obligatory cation coverage of the metabolically generated anions is a major mechanism responsible for the fasting natriuresis.

The mechanism of the carbohydrate action on urinary Na^+ and K^+ excretion is not completely understood, but may be related to its roughly parallel effects in lessening protein catabolism; it does not appear to be due to secondary effects on certain hormones (aldosterone, renin, insulin, glucagon, glucocorticoids, and catecholamines).

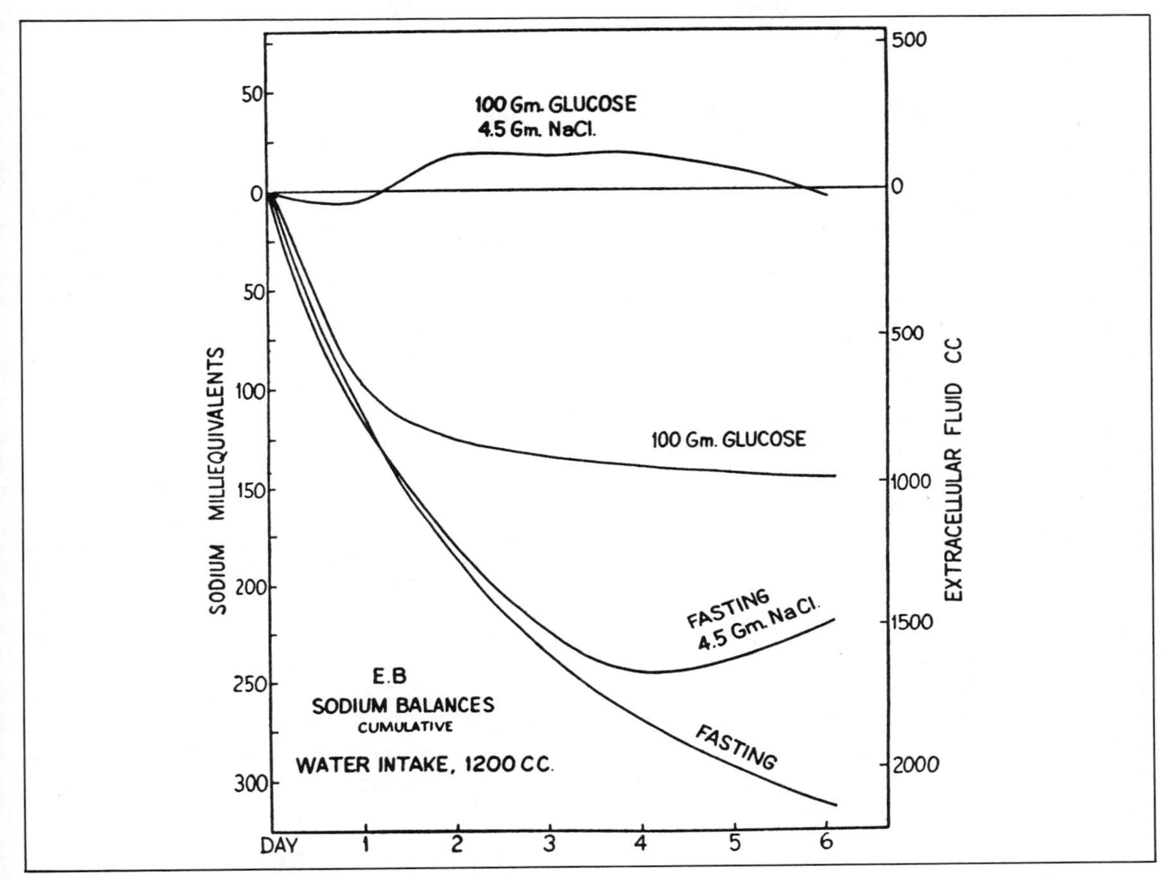

Figure 13-17. *Cumulative sodium balances and water intake. (From J. L. Gamble, Physiological information gained from studies on life raft ration.* Harvey Lecture *42:269, 1947.)*

Sodium plasma levels remain fairly stable for a long time, despite the high urinary losses, while plasma potassium levels fall [194]. In prolonged starvation, intracellular K^+ and Mg^+ fall. A relationship between K^+ and Mg^+ is evidenced by the following: Erythrocyte K^+ levels were 5 to 9 percent below normal in patients demonstrating decreased plasma Mg^{2+} levels; administration of Mg^{2+} corrected the low erythrocyte K^+ levels. These observations are interpreted as showing an effect of extracellular Mg^{2+} on the ATP-ase system associated with the cell membrane Na^+-K^+ transfer mechanism in prolonged starvation.

Administration of KCl, 0.5 mmol/kg/day, to obese subjects undergoing prolonged starvation reduced daily urinary ammonium and β-hydroxybutyrate excretion by one-third, improved potassium balance, and increased chloride excretion [165]. Administration of $KHCO_3$, 0.5 mmol/kg/day, rather than KCl, led to a similar fall in ammonium excretion, but ketone body and bicarbonate excretion remained unchanged; potassium balance improved.

Urine pH fell significantly in both groups as the rate of excretion of urinary buffer (ammonium) decreased. The mechanism of the decrease in β-hydroxybutyrate excretion after potassium chloride administration is not apparent; however, because it was associated with increased chloride excretion, anion competition may be involved. When the $KHCO_3$ was increased to 1.5 to 2.0 mmol/kg/day, the urine was alkalinized, and ammonium excretion fell to negligible levels, resulting in nitrogen sparing of 2.0 gm/day. Sapir, Chambers, and Ryan [165] interpret these findings as indicating that one-half of the increase in ammonium excretion observed in prolonged starvation is due to potassium deficiency. In their view, it is likely that nitrogen wastage caused by losses of urinary ammonium during starvation can be virtually eliminated by potassium supplementation and urinary alkalinization.

In the section of this chapter dealing with endocrine function, we have pointed out that potassium administration to fasting obese and nonobese subjects improves the glucose tolerance in these patients and leads to improved insulin secretion [5].

Sapir and Owen [166], in studies of fasting obese humans, found that there was no tubular maximal transport rate (reabsorption) for acetoacetate or β-hydroxybutyrate during the starvation ketonemia. They concluded that the reabsorption of ketones minimizes N loss (NH_4^+) and aids in maintaining ketonemia. More recently, Reichard and his colleagues [155] have demonstrated a significant loss of acetone via expired air in starvation. This results in a significant saving of fixed base and NH^{4+}.

Calcium and Phosphorus: Bone, Hydroxyproline

Serum calcium levels fall gradually during starvation, reflecting a reduction in serum albumin and magnesium deficiency. The effect appears to be mediated by way of parathormone (secretion and/or tissue responsiveness). Fecal calcium is low, since the amount of feces excreted is small (except late, when diarrhea may occur). Urinary calcium continues fairly high during starvation. The greatest urinary calcium excretion occurs when metabolic acidosis is well established. Significant loss of phosphate also occurs; the decrease in the ability of the kidney in starvation to excrete titratable acids is due in large measure to phosphate deficiency, since administration of phosphate corrects this dysfunction.

Bone is the major source of the excreted calcium and phosphorus, but the relative loss of bone mass is less than that of many organs and tissues in starvation; significant osteomalacia is not seen except after prolonged severe starvation. Urinary hydroxyproline excretion increases during starvation, presumably reflecting collagenolysis of bone collagen and collagenolysis of subcutaneous supporting tissue as storage fat is catabolized.

Uric Acid

One of the characteristic biochemical changes in starvation is a rise in serum uric acid consequent to a decreased urinary excretion of uric acid. This latter is due primarily to a "blocking" effect (competitive inhibition) of uric acid tubular secretion by the increased serum and urinary levels of β-hydroxybutyrate, acetoacetate, and other keto or hydroxy acids. We speculate that it may also be due to the low levels of urea in the glomerular filtrate.

SOME ORGAN CHANGES IN STARVATION

Kidneys

The kidneys maintain function for a long time during starvation, despite their high metabolic requirement. Their continued function is possible because of their high blood supply (about 20 percent of cardiac output) and their ability to metabolize amino acids, lactate, pyruvate, glycerol, fatty acids, and β-hydroxybutyrate efficiently. As starvation goes on, as noted, gluconeogenesis by the kidney increases, so that after a while it is producing almost half the glucose, the rest being produced by the liver. There is a net uptake of glycine, alanine, and proline by the kidney, and a net release of serine.

Polyuria, hyposthenuria, and proteinuria are common late in starvation. The decreased concentrative ability of the kidney is due in part to the decreased amounts of urea in the medulla, and thus lowering the medullary osmolar gradient. Infusions of urea to such subjects lead to the excretion of concentrated urine (see also pp. 456, 462–465).

The kidneys of individuals dying of "uncomplicated" starvation show little in the way of morphologic changes, either grossly or histologically (light microscopy).

Liver

We have already discussed some of the metabolic adaptations that occur in the liver during starvation and mentioned that the liver loses glycogen rapidly and gains fat. As starvation proceeds, liver fat decreases and liver protein is lost, but the number of hepatocytes seems unchanged for a long time. Liver biopsies were found to be generally normal histologically in undernourished people who had lost 2 to 55 kg weight, although the liver cells sometimes contained considerable amounts of iron and chromolipoid pigment. Liver function, as judged by clinical liver function tests, is maintained for a considerable period of time.

Pancreas

Pancreatic acinar atrophy and fibrosis are commonly seen in people dying of starvation. The islets generally are not involved morphologically; we have already mentioned the possible altered responsiveness of the β cells to glucose.

Gastrointestinal Tract

The gut is one of the more active organs metabolically, and so it is not surprising that it (especially the small intestine) decreases substantially in mass during starvation. Gastric emptying and intestinal transit times are prolonged. Digestion is impaired, reflecting a diminution in the production of pancreatic enzymes, but not bile. Intestinal absorption of amino acids may not be impaired for long periods of starvation. The rates of renewal and migration of the intestinal mucosal cells are slowed, but the composition of the cells seems unchanged (protein and RNA per unit DNA). Eventually there is a flattening of the villi and a reduction in absorptive surface area. The atrophic mucosa often has a lowered disaccharidase (especially lactase) activity. Absorption, particularly of fat and carbohydrate, may be impaired as a result of disturbance of small bowel mucosal cell functions and enzyme activity [42]. Terminally, there is generally severe diarrhea; postmortem examination has shown that the wall of the small intestine is so thin that it is almost transparent.

Little is known about the effects of starvation on the gut bacteria in humans. These bacteria influence mammalian metabolism and nutrition in important ways in health and disease [106], e.g., the presence of the indigenous gut bacteria (the facultative anaerobes) increase metabolic rate by 15 to 20 percent, without inducing an infectious disease. Body fat is greater in conventional rats than in germfree rats; associated with this is a longer survival for conventional rats than for germfree rats following starvation.

Respiratory and Cardiovascular Systems

Starvation of rats leads to decreased capacity of the lungs to synthesize protein, but the efficiency of synthesis is not reduced [153] and surface elastic forces are increased (decreased tissue elasticity?), leading to air-space enlargement [162]. These latter observations may be related to the decrease in lung lysyl oxidase activity, which falls dramatically in starved rats to 25 percent of control values after only 48 to 72 hours of starvation [109].

Doekel et al. [37] found that feeding a 500-calorie carbohydrate diet to normal humans for 10 days led to a significant diminution in the hypoxic ventilatory response (42 percent of control); the hypercapnea ventilatory response was not significantly altered. The reason for the decreased hypoxic ventilatory response has not been determined. After 5 days of refeeding with a normal diet, the hypoxic ventilatory response returned to normal.

One normally thinks of the lungs and the kidneys as exerting the primary regulatory influences on acid-base metabolism. The immediate and huge accumulation of organic acids that occurs with cardiac arrest serves to demonstrate the critical role the heart normally plays in maintaining acid-base homeostasis. The major part of this role is related to the muscular activity of the heart, which results in perfusion of tissues; maintenance of oxygen delivery and removal of acids resulting from tissue metabolism; delivery of lactate to the liver and kidney, which may recycle it to glucose; and delivery of hydroxybutyrate and acetoacetate to brain and muscles (including the heart), where they are metabolized to $CO_2 + H_2O$, or to the lungs where, in addition to being metabolized to these latter compounds, the hydroxybutyrate and acetoacetate may be oxidized or provide the hydrogen ions that serve to drive the reaction:

$$HCO_3^- + H^+ \longrightarrow CO_2 + H_2O$$

and thus participate in the respiratory compensation to metabolic acidosis. This respiratory mechanism, which serves to conserve fixed base and ammonia, may be one way in which keto acid oxidation spares nitrogen loss in starvation. The mechanism ultimately depends on the muscular work of the heart. The heart, in addition to its *muscular* work, carries out *metabolic* activities that regulate acid-base balance in the body.

The heart is a major consumer of acetoacetic acid in both well-nourished and starved states. The brain is the main consumer of ketoacids in starvation; depending on the rate of hepatic ketogenesis, the heart can use the ketones not used by the brain. Because of the relatively high concentration of mitochondria in both of these organs, they are able to generate high levels of succinyl CoA. The brain and heart are thus able to activate acetoacetic acid (as shown at the top of the next column).

$$\text{Acetoacetic acid} + \text{succinyl CoA} \longrightarrow \text{acetoacetyl CoA} + \text{succinate} \longrightarrow CO_2 + ATP + H_2O$$

Additionally, the heart has a unique metabolic action that influences acid-base balance. Consider the A-V differences in lactate for the heart and skeletal muscle:

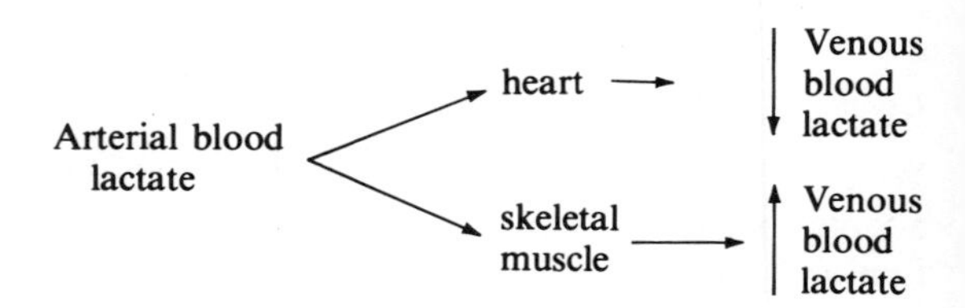

The *heart* is a *consumer* of lactate, which is normally oxidized completely by this tissue; it is the only organ that uses lactate as a direct energy source. *Skeletal muscle* is a *producer* of lactate. Liver and kidney use lactate, but mainly for glucose synthesis.

In the fed or fed-exercised state the heart reduces acidosis by oxidizing lactate, and permits maximal glucose utilization by skeletal muscle. In the postprandial state, glucose uptake by muscle is regulated by the blood levels of sugar and insulin. During exercise, muscle takes up additional glucose because of the increased circulation and metabolism. This is not true in the fasted state, in which blood insulin and glucose levels are both low. In the fasted state, muscle lactic dehydrogenase (LDH, M_4) activity decreases.

$NADH + H^+ + \text{pyruvate} \rightleftharpoons \text{lactate} + NAD^+$ is a reversible reaction. However, because the K_m for pyruvate is low and its V_{max} (pyruvate → lactate) high, muscle lactic dehydrogenase isoenzyme (LDH, M_4) is adapted to convert pyruvate to lactate at high rates. Rarely would it have occasion to work in the opposite direction since skeletal muscles import less lactate than they export. Additionally, in conditions in which glucose is completely oxidized by muscle, the LDH, M_4 would be nonfunctional because pyruvate would be converted to acetyl CoA and not to lactate. The LDH system in muscle is geared to provide lactate for export to the liver and kidneys for glucogenesis and to the heart for fuel, particularly during oxygen debt.

On the other hand, the lactic dehydrogenase isoenzyme in the heart (LDH, H) exerts an entirely different physiologic function. Whereas skeletal muscle is an exporter of lactate and its LDH, M_4 is adapted for this, the heart is an importer of lactate and its LDH, H isoenzyme is adapted for lactate oxidation. It has a high K_m for pyruvate, and a low V_{max} for pyruvate reduction. As a result, pyruvate reduction is slower in the heart than in the muscle, but oxidation of lactate is much faster in the heart. When the fed individual exercises, the excess lactate produced by skeletal muscle can be used by the heart, thus sparing the liver the work of converting all the lactate to glucose, and decreasing the glucose requirement of the exercising heart. In contrast, in the starved resting individual, lactate production by skeletal muscle is minimal. Even in starvation the blood cells and brain release about 50 gm of lactate/day, which is converted by the liver and kidney to glucose for use again by the blood cells and brain. Concomitant with decreased lactate production by muscle in starvation are decreased levels of heart LDH, H, and other heart enzymes connected with lactate and pyruvate metabolism. There is also a coincident loss of cofactors (magnesium, thiamine, potassium) for these enzymatic reactions; therefore, lactate utilization by the heart is decreased in starvation. It is not surprising, then, that cardiac function is impaired in starvation and cardiac failure is common. Losses of intracellular and extracellular electrolytes not only affect heart muscle tone and contractility, but influence its excitability as well.

Prolonged caloric deficiency induces significant alterations in cardiac morphology [185] and in several cardiac lysosomal enzymes, particularly cathepsin. D. Wildenthal and associates [215] speculate, from some studies of fetal mouse heart in culture, that this may be related to the prolonged low serum insulin and high concentrations of ketones and fatty acids in starvation. They had advanced the view that the altered cathepsin D activity might contribute to the net protein catabolism and cardiac atrophy of starvation. However, in a recent study, Crie, Sanford, and Wildenthal [32] showed that protein degradation of the hearts of starved rats was decreased as assessed in vitro, opposite in direction from what was predicted from the simultaneous changes in cathepsin D activity. Starvation has been reported to cause only a small decrease in the rate of protein synthesis by the heart, but since there is a progressive decrease in intrinsic cardiac proteolytic activity during starvation, the cardiac atrophy that occurs in starvation appears to result chiefly from the decrease in protein synthesis. Crie, Sanford, and Wildenthal [32] found cardiac alanine release to be significantly increased by starvation. Inhibition of pyruvate oxidation and consequent increased conversion of pyruvate to alanine seem to be an important components of the process. The branched-chain amino acids were released to a lesser extent from the hearts of starved animals than would be explained on the basis of decreased protein degradation alone. They believe that increased oxidation of these compounds during starvation is the probable explanation for this finding.

Consolazio and associates [31] found changes in cardiac function of previously healthy men as early as 10 days after total nutrient deprivation other than water. When such men carried out submaximal work on the treadmill, their electrocardiograms promptly became abnormal (AVF and GRS axis changes), reflecting, in their view, "severe stress." In the study of semistarvation conducted by Keys and his associates [95], there were electrocardiographic changes in response to moderate exercise that were maximal at 12 weeks. These consisted of an increase of the Q-T interval, a continuous decrease in amplitudes at all deflections, and marked shifts to the right of the QRS and T axes.

As starvation goes on, the heart decreases progressively in size and function. Bradycardia, hypotension, decreased cardiac output, elevated central venous pressure, and diminished ability to handle a fluid load all are characteristic. Digoxin may show little inotropic effect at this time. Some of the psychologic changes that may occur in starvation (decreased desire for muscular activity) may function indirectly to protect the heart.

Frank congestive failure consequent to the cardiac dysfunction, accentuated by anemia and excessive extracellular volume, may be a terminal event. In humans dying from starvation, the heart is often atrophied to half its normal size.

HEMATOLOGIC CHANGES

Progressive anemia (decreased erythrocyte formation and increased hemolysis) is common late in starvation. Early in starvation (10 days) there may be a relative increase in the circulating neutrophils, with a concomitant decrease in circulating lymphocytes, but later (after 1 to 2 months) neutropenia is characteristic. The neutrophils appear normal morphologically, and there is generally an increase in neutrophils in response to infection, even late in starvation. There are, however, abnormalities in neutrophil function, including impaired intracellular bactericidal and mobility defects, late in starvation [94].

STARVATION AND RESISTANCE TO INFECTION

Clinicians have known for many years that malnutrition is associated often with a decreased resistance to certain infections, and considerable experimental evidence confirming and extending this has been obtained during the last fifty years. The period of food deprivation need not be long. Smith and Dubos [186] showed that when mice were starved for as short a time as 36 hours, their resistance to staphylococcal infections was markedly decreased. This was shown also to be true for tuberculous infection in mice starved for 30 hours or made protein-deficient by dietary restriction [40]. Elsewhere, Dubos [41] states:

> Through a number of different mechanisms arrived at by evolutionary adaptation, man has achieved some sort of ecological equilibrium with the microorganisms that are ubiquitous in his environment. Indeed these microorganisms may be harbored in the body without causing disease, and establish relationships with the tissues—covering the whole gamut from the commensalism and symbiosis represented by the flora of the gut, to the various types of arrested or latent infections. The factors which determine whether the microbial agents are thus held in check, or undergo unrestrained multiplication, are, of course, highly complex... I have presented the view that natural and acquired resistance depends more often upon the ability of the inflammatory response to create in and around the lesion a micro-environment inimical to the infectious agent.
>
> It is likely that disturbances in the general state of health often bring about qualitative and quantitative changes in the biochemical characteristics of the inflammatory area. These, in turn, may interfere with the processes which control the activities of microorganisms within the lesion. As a result, the response of the body to infection and consequently the microenvironment in which the infectious process follows its course, are under the control of factors which may be metabolic or psychic in origin. This concept accounts in part for the fact that susceptibility to infection can change independently of the immunological state of the infected individual. Since changes in susceptibility can occur rapidly, and be extremely transient, the intensity of exposure to an infectious agent may be less decisive than the physiological state of the exposed individual, in determining whether infection fails to take hold, becomes established, runs an abortive course, or evolves into overt disease.

In recent studies of mice subjected to short-term starvation (1 to 3 days), Martinez, Cox, Lukassewycz, and Murphy [115] found a disproportionate depletion of lymphoid tissue, and a decrease in peripheral WBC, but no change in the peripheral differential count. Adoptive cell transfer experiments showed that immunocompetence of individual spleen immunocytes was *not* reduced by starvation.

Najjar, Stephen, and Asfour [131] reported elevated IgM levels in marasmic children; others have shown reduced levels of IgG globulin in such children [24]. In children with kwashiorkor, low, normal, and high levels of the immunoglobulins have been reported, but generally the levels have been found normal or elevated. Kwashiorkor complicated by overt infection led to a threefold increase in overall immunoglobulin synthesis. In fact, the initial high levels of immunoglobulins in kwashiorkor may reflect the subclinical infections common in such patients.

Law, Dudrick, and Abdou [105] found no significant decrease in the levels of IgG, IgM, and IgA in adult patients who had undergone severe food deprivation, had suffered weight losses of at least 20 pounds, and had serum albumin levels below 3.2 g/100 ml. The patients were a mixed group with regard to diagnosis—dementia, heart disease, including some in congestive failure, and cerebrovascular accidents; none had malignant, hepatic, or primary immunologic diseases.

In contrast to the immunoglobulins, the serum levels of all complement proteins, except C_4, were markedly decreased in children with protein-calorie malnutrition; this may result in abnormal opsonification [132, 184]. There was a rapid reversal of these changes following nutritional rehabilitation.

Although the levels of immunoglobulins are not reduced in starvation, the ability to synthesize antibodies is likely to be impaired. Cannon, Chase, and Wissler [21] demonstrated 39 years ago that rabbits made hypoproteinemic by food protein deprivation had decreased antibody responses to *Escherichia typhosa* and *Salmonella paratyphi* vaccines. There is also clinical evidence that humans suffering from malnutrition or starvation may be unable to make circulating antibodies and interferon adequately in response to certain bacterial or viral antigens [172]. Thus, Coovadia et al. [30] showed that although the numbers of β lymphocytes isolated from the blood of children with marasmus or kwashiorkor were not significantly different from normal, the ability of these cells to produce antibodies 10 days after TAB (typhoid) vaccination was depressed.

Cellular aspects of the immune response have also been studied in starvation. It has long been known that malnutrition is frequently associated with atrophy of the lymphoid tissues and depression of cellular immunity. Thymic and lymph node atrophy, low total lymphocyte counts, diminished or absent delayed hypersensitivity responses, and abnormal in vitro lymphocytic function have all been described [24, 70, 132, 161, 190, 204, 211].

There is evidence that the inflammatory response is depressed in starvation. Guggenheim and Buechler [75] showed that peritoneal granulocytes obtained from rats subjected to protein and/or calorie malnutrition have decreased bactericidal activity. Yoshida and colleagues [221] showed that leukocytes from patients with protein-calorie malnutrition had depressed glycolytic activity; it is well known that normal phagocytic function depends upon an intact glycolytic pathway. Subsequently, it was shown that malnutrition leads to motility defects in the granulocytes and an abnormality in intracellular bacterial activity [176]. Kendall and Nolan [94] found a highly significant difference in the function of the polymorphonuclear cells of children below the third weight percentile and those of heavier children as assessed by nitro-blue tetrazolim staining and latex particles phagocytosis. Correlated with the depression of function of the inflammatory cells were changes in the histology of the bone marrow [199]. Bone marrow biopsies obtained from humans who had starved for prolonged periods showed fat atrophy, hypoplasia of hematopoietic cells, and gelatinous changes in the ground substance. The gelatinous changes could also be reproduced in rabbits that had been undernourished for 4 months. In both humans and experimental animals, these changes were reversible with refeeding.

It is clear that part of the reduced capability of response of the starved organism to a variety of stimuli is reflected in its inability to mount adequate responses to challenges by various infectious agents. This is reflected both in the humoral and cellular components of the immune response and in nonimmune defense mechanisms. Nutritional rehabilitation reverses many of these alterations, although it is not known whether long-term malnutrition and starvation may leave some permanent insufficiencies in the immune responses and other defense reactions.

In recent years there has been increasing interest in possible adverse effects of malnutrition, primary and/or secondary, on the resistance of surgical patients to infection (chiefly bacterial and fungal). These matters are discussed at length elsewhere in this volume.*

A wide variety of metabolic changes and adaptations occur during starvation, all of which help animals and humans to survive a lack of exogenous nutrient supply in the face of continuing nutrient utilization for essential metabolic and physiologic processes.

These responses to food deprivation per se are different in many significant ways from the metabolic responses to severe injury and illness, although these latter are influenced in major ways by the nutrient intakes of the patients. As a result, the net physiologic and clinical consequences of injury and illness are conditioned importantly by the nutrient intakes of the patients. The nature of these effects, which are complex, additive, and at times synergistic; ways in which they are brought about; and methods of treating them are dealt with in other chapters of this volume.

The chapter has been concerned mainly with the ways in which the body adapts to conserve life in the absence of food intake. If the process has a purpose or subserves an important function in nature, it is not primarily to lengthen the period between the onset of starvation and death. The process is carried out in a singularly remarkable way, so that at almost any time, recovery, though not always complete, is possible, and fertility reestablished. This is possible because the integrity of some cells is maintained throughout starvation and because, even in those cells that are stripped of many structural and metabolically active features, the genetic material remains intact, as does the apparatus for expressing that material. Thanks to this fact, the remnants of starvation in Auschwitz, in Pnom Penh, and elsewhere, and their descendants survive.

**Editor's Note:* The interested reader is referred to the Third Ross Conference on Medical Research: Nutrition and Sepsis, Josef E. Fischer (Ed.) 1982, which is available from Ross Laboratories, Columbus, Ohio.

REFERENCES

1. Abraira, C., and Lawrence, A. M. The Staub-Traugott phenomenon: III. Effects of starvation. *Am. J. Clin. Nutr.* 31:213, 1978.
2. Addis, T., Poo, L. J., and Lew, W. The quantities of protein lost by the various organs and tissues of the body during a fast. *J. Biol. Chem.* 1115:111, 1936.
3. Adibi, S. A. Metabolism of branched-chain amino acids in altered nutrition. *Metabolism* 25:1287, 1976.
4. Alleyne, G. A. O., and Scullard, G. H. Alterations in carbohydrate metabolism in Jamaican children with severe malnutrition. *Clin. Sci.* 37:631, 1969.
5. Anderson, J. W., Herman, R. H., and Newcomb, K. L. Improvement in glucose tolerance of fasting obese patients given oral potassium. *Am. J. Clin. Nutr.* 22:1589, 1969.
6. Aoki, T. T., Finley, R. J., and Cahill, R. J., Jr. The Redox State and Regulation of Amino Acid Metabolism in Man. In P. B. Garland and C. N. Hales (Eds.), *Substrate Mobilization and Energy Provision in Man.* Biochem. Soc. Symposia, No. 43, July, 1977. London: The Biochemical Society, 1978. Pp. 17–30.
7. Arky, R. A., Finger, M. Veverbrants, E., et al. Glucose and insulin response to intravenous glucagon during starvation. *Am. J. Clin. Nutr.* 23:691, 1970.
8. Balsam, A., and Ingbar, S. H. Observations on the factors that control the generation of triiodothyronine from thyroxine in rat liver and the nature of the defect induced by fasting. *J. Clin. Invest.* 63:1145, 1979.
9. Beas, F., Contreras, I., Maccioni, A., et al. Growth hormone in infant malnutrition: The arginine test in marasmus and kwashiorkor. *Br. J. Nutr.* 26:169, 1971.
10. Benedict, F. G. A Study of Prolonged Fasting. Washington, DC: Carnegie Institute of Washington, 1915. Publication No. 280.
11. Benedict, F. G., Miles, W. R., Roth, P., and Smith, H. M. Human Vitality and Efficiency under Prolonged Restrictions. Washington, DC: Carnegie Institute of Washington, 1919. Publication No. 701.

12. Bergstrom, Y., Furst, P., Noree, L. O., et al. Intracellular free amino acid concentration in human muscle tissue. *J. Appl. Physiol.* 36:693, 1974.
13. Bloom, W. L. Fasting as an introduction to the treatment of obesity. *Metabolism* 8:214, 1959.
14. Border, J. R., Metabolic response to short-term starvation, sepsis and trauma. *Surg. Annu.* 2:11, 1970.
15. Bourgeois, B., Schmidt, B. J., and Bourgeois, R. Some Aspects of Catecholamines in Undernutrition. In L. Gardner and P. Amacher (Eds.), *Endocrine Aspects of Malnutrition.* Proceedings of a Symposium Sponsored by the Kroc Foundation, 1973. Pp. 163–179.
16. Burger, G. C. E., Drummond, J. C., and Sandstead, H. R. *Malnutrition and Starvation in Western Netherlands. September 1944–July 1945.* The Hague: General State Printing Office, 1948.
17. Buse, M. G., and Reid, S. S. Leucine: A possible regulator of protein turnover in muscle. *J. Clin. Invest.* 56:1250, 1975.
18. Cahill, G. F., Jr. Starvation in man. *N. Engl. J. Med.* 282:668, 1970.
19. Cahill, G. F., Herrera, M. G., Morgan, A. P., et al. Hormone-fuel interrelationships during fasting. *J. Clin. Invest.* 45:1751, 1966.
20. Campbell, G. A., Kurcz, M., Marshall, S., and Meites, J. Effects of starvation in rats on serum levels of follicle-stimulating hormone, LH, thyrotropin, GH, and prolactin; response to LH-releasing hormone and thyrotropin-releasing hormone. *Endocrinology* 100:580, 1977.
21. Cannon, P. R., Chase, W. E., and Wissler, R. W. The relationships of the protein reserves to antibody production: I. The effects of a low-protein diet and of plasmapheresis upon the formation of agglutinins. *J. Immunol.* 47:133, 1943.
22. Carlsten, A., Hallgren, B., Jagenburg, R., et al. Myocardial metabolism of glucose, lactic acid, amino acids and fatty acids in healthy human individuals at rest and at different work loads. *Scand. J. Clin. Lab. Invest.* 13:418, 1961.
23. Carter, W. J., Shakir, K. M., Hodges, S., et al. Effect of thyroid hormone on metabolic adaptation to fasting. *Metabolism* 24:1177, 1975.
24. Chandra, R. K. Immunocompetence in undernutrition. *J. Pediatr.* 81:1194, 1972.
25. Chatterji, A., and Sen Gupta, P. C. Adrenals in malnourished infants. *Indian J. Pathol.* 27:353, 1960.
26. Chinn, R. H., Brown, J. J., Fraser, R., et al. The natriuresis of fasting: Relationship to changes in plasma renin and plasma aldosterone concentrations. *Clin. Sci.* 39:437, 1970.
27. Chopra, I. J., and Smith, S. R. Circulating thyroid hormones and thyrotropin in adult patients with protein calorie malnutrition. *J. Clin. Endocrinol. Metab.* 40:221, 1975.
28. Chopra, I. J., Williams, D. E., Orgiazzi, J., et al. Opposite effects of dexamethasone on serum concentrations of 3,3′,5′-triiodothyronine (reverse T_3) and 3,3′,5-triiodothyronine (T_3). *J. Clin. Endocrinol. Metab.* 41:911, 1975A.
29. Chua, B., Kao, R., Rannels, D. E., and Morgan, H. E. Hormonal and Metabolic Control of Proteolysis. In P. B. Garland and C. N. Hales (Eds.), *Substrate Mobilization and Energy Provision in Man.* Symposia 43, July 1977. London: The Biochemical Society, 1978. Pp. 1–15.
30. Coovadia, H. M., Parent, M. A., Loenig, W. E. K., et al. An evaluation of factors associated with the depression of immunity in malnutrition and in measles. *Am. J. Clin. Nutr.* 27:665, 1974.
31. Consolazio, C. F., Matoush, L. O., Johnson, H. L., Nelson, R. A., and Krzywicki, H. J. Metabolic aspects of acute starvation in normal humans (10 days). *Am. J. Clin. Nutr.* 20:672, 1967.
32. Crie, J. S., Sanford, C. F., and Wildenthal, K. Influence of starvation and refeeding on cardiac protein degradation in rats. *J. Nutr.* 110:22, 1980.
33. Cuthbertson, D. P. The disturbance of metabolism produced by bony and non-bony injury with notes on certain abnormal conditions of bone. *Biochem. J.* 24:1244, 1930.
34. Daughaday, W. H., and Kipnis, D. M. The growth-promoting and anti-insulin actions of somatotropin. *Rec. Prog. Horm. Res.* 22:49, 1966.
35. Dice, J. F., Walker, C. D., Byrne, B., and Cardiel, A. General characteristics of protein degradation in diabetes and starvation. *Proc. Nat. Acad. Sci. USA* 75:2093, 1978.
36. Dietze, G., Wicklmayer, M., and Mehnert, H. Physiology of Metabolism During Starvation. In F. W. Ahnefeld, C. Burri, W. Dick, M. Halmagyi (Eds.), *Parenteral Nutrition.* Berlin: Springer, 1976. Pp. 17–30.
37. Doekel, R. C., Jr., Zwillich, C. W., Scoggin, C. H., Kryger, M., and Weil, J. V. Clinical semistarvation: Depression of hypoxic ventilatory response. *N. Engl. J. Med.* 295:358, 1976.
38. Dubois, E. F. Metabolism in Fever and in Certain Infections. In L. F. Barker (Ed.), *Endocrinology and Metabolism.* New York: Appleton, 1922. Vol. IV, pp. 94–151.
39. Dubos, R. J. Effect of metabolic factors on the susceptibility of albino mice to experimental tuberculosis. *J. Exper. Med.* 101:59, 1955.
40. Dubos, R. J. The micro-environment of inflam-

mation or Metchnikoff revisited. *Lancet* 2:1, 1955A.

41. Duncan, G. G., Jenson, W. K., Fraser, R. I., and Cristofori, F. C. Correction and control of intractable obesity. Practical applications of intermittent periods of total fasting. *J.A.M.A.* 181:309, 1962.
42. Ecknauer, R., and Raffler, H. Effect of starvation on small intestinal enzyme activity in germfree rats. *Digestion* 18:45, 1978.
43. Felig, P. The glucose-alanine cycle. *Metabolism* 22:179, 1973.
44. Felig, P., Marliss, E. B., and Cahill, G. F., Jr. Metabolic response to human growth hormone during prolonged starvation. *J. Clin. Invest.* 50:411, 1971.
45. Felig, P., Owen, O. E., Wahren, J., et al. Amino acid metabolism during prolonged starvation. *J. Clin. Invest.* 48:584, 1969.
46. Felig, P., and Wahren, J. Amino acid metabolism in exercising man. *J. Clin. Invest.* 50:2703, 1971.
47. Felig, P., and Wahren, J. Influence of endogenous insulin secretion on splanchnic glucose and amino acid metabolism in man. *J. Clin. Invest.* 50:1702, 1971A.
48. Felig, P., and Wahren, J. Protein turnover and amino acid metabolism in the regulation of gluconeogenesis. *Fed. Proc.* 33:1092, 1974.
49. Felig, P., Wahren, J., and Raf, L. Evidence of inter-organ aminoacid transport by blood cells in humans. *Proc. Nat. Acad. Sci. USA.* 70: 1775, 1973.
50. Fisher, M., Sherwin, R. S., Hendler, R., et al. Kinetics of glucagon in man: Effects of starvation. *Proc. Nat. Acad. Sci. USA.* 73:1735, 1976.
51. Galvao-Teles, A., Graves, L., Burke, C. W., et al. Free cortisol in obesity: Effect of fasting. *Acta Endocrinol.* 81:321, 1976.
52. Gamble, J. L. Physiological information gained from studies on the life raft ration. *Harvey Lect.* 42:247, 1947.
53. Gamble, J. L., Ross, G. S., and Tisdall, J. Metabolism of fixed base during fasting. *J. Biol. Chem.* 57:633, 1923.
54. Garber, A. J., Karl, I. E., and Kipnis, D. M. Carbon sources of alanine and glutamine released by skeletal muscle. *J. Clin. Invest.* 52:31A, 1973.
55. Garber, A. J., Karl, I. E., and Kipnis, D. M. Alanine and glutamine synthesis and release from skeletal muscle. *J. Biol. Chem.* 251:826, 1976.
56. Garber, A. J., Menzel, P. H., Boden, G., et al. Hepatic ketogenesis and gluconeogenesis in humans. *J. Clin. Invest.* 54:981, 1974.
57. Gardner, D. F., Kaplan, M. M., Stanley, C. A., and Utiger, R. D. Effect of triiodothyronine replacement on the metabolic and pituitary responses to starvation. *N. Engl. J. Med.* 300: 579, 1979.
58. Garlick, P. J., Millward, D. J., and James W. P. The diurnal response of muscle and liver protein synthesis in vivo in meal-fed rats. *Biochem. J.* 136:935, 1973.
59. Garlick, P. J., Millward, D. J., James, W. P., et al. The effect of protein deprivation and starvation on the rate of protein synthesis in tissues of the rat. *Biochem. Biophys. Acta* 414:71, 1975.
60. Garnett, E. S., Cohen, H., Nahmias, C., et al. The roles of carbohydrate, renin and aldosterone in sodium retention during and after total starvation. *Metabolism* 22:867, 1973.
61. Gjedde, A., and Crone, C. Induction processes in blood-brain transfer of ketone bodies during starvation. *Am. J. Physiol.* 229:1165, 1975.
62. Godard, C. The endocrine glands in infantile malnutrition. *Helv. Paediat. Acta* 29:5, 1974.
63. Godard, C., and Lemarchand-Beraud, T. Plasma thyrotropin levels in severe infantile malnutrition. *Horm. Res.* 4:43, 1973.
64. Goldberg, A. L., and St. John, A. C. Intracellular protein degradation in mammalian and bacterial cells. Part 2. *Annu. Rev. Biochem.* 45:747, 1976.
65. Golden, M. H. N., Waterlow, J. C., and Picou, D. Protein turnover, synthesis and breakdown before and after recovery from protein-energy malnutrition. *Clin. Sci. Mol. Med.* 53:473, 1977A.
66. Golden, M., Waterlow, J. C., and Picou, D. The relationship between dietary intake, weight change, nitrogen balance, and protein turnover in man. *Am. J. Clin. Nutr.* 30:1345, 1977B.
67. Goodhard, R. S., and Shils, M. *Modern Nutrition in Health and Disease,* (5th ed.). Philadelphia: Lea & Febiger, 1973.
68. Goodman, M. N., Berger, M., and Ruderman, N. B. Glucose metabolism in rat skeletal muscle at rest. Effect of starvation, diabetes, ketone bodies and free fatty acids. *Diabetes* 23:881, 1974.
69. Goodman, M. N., and Ruderman, N. B. Insulin sensitivity of rat skeletal muscle: Effects of starvation and aging. *Am. J. Physiol.* 236: E519, 1979.
70. Grace, H. J., and Armstrong, D. Reduced lymphocyte transformation in protein-calorie malnutrition. *South Afr. Med. J.* 46:402, 1972.
71. Graham, G. G., Baertl, J. M., Claeyssen, G., et al. Thyroid hormonal studies in normal and

severely malnourished infants and small children. *J. Pediatr.* 83:321, 1973.

72. Grande, F. Energetics and weight reduction. *Am. J. Clin. Nutr.* 21:305, 1968.
73. Grant, D. B., Hambley, J., Becker, D., et al. Reduced sulphation factor in undernourished children. *Arch. Dis. Childh.* 48:596, 1973.
74. Grey, N. J., Karl, I., and Kipnis, D. M. Physiologic mechanisms in the development of starvation ketosis in man. *Diabetes* 24:10, 1975.
75. Guggenheim, K., and Buechler, E. Nutrition and resistance to infection. *J. Immunol.* 54:349, 1946.
76. Hansen, J. D. L., cited by Pimstone, B. Endocrine function in protein-calorie malnutrition. *Clin. Endocrinol.* 5:79, 1976.
77. Harland, P. S. E. G., and Parkin, J. M. TSH levels in severe malnutrition. *Lancet* 2:1145, 1972.
78. Harris, A. R. C., Fang, S. L., Azizi, F., Lipworth, L., Vagenakis, A. G., and Braverman, L. E. Effect of starvation on hypothalamic-pituitary-thyroid function in the rat. *Metabolism* 27:1074, 1978.
79. Harris, A. R. C., Fang, S. L., Hinerfeld, L., and Braverman, L. E. The role of sulfhydryl groups on the impaired hepatic 3′,3,5-triiodothyronine generation from thyroxine in the hypothyroid, starved, fetal, and neonatal rodent. *J. Clin. Invest.* 63:516, 1979.
80. Hawkins, R. A., and Biebuyck, J. F. Ketone bodies are selectively used by individual brain regions. *Science* 205:325, 1979.
81. Hedeskov, C. J., and Capito, K. The pentose cycle and insulin release in isolated mouse pancreatic islets during starvation. *Biochem. J.* 152:571, 1975.
82. Henshaw, E. C., Hirsch, C. A., Morton, B. E., et al. Control of protein synthesis in mammalian tissues through changes in ribosome activity. *J. Biol. Chem.* 246:436, 1971.
83. Hintz, R. L., Suskind, R., Amatayakul, K., Thanangkul, O., and Olson, R. Plasma somatomedin and growth hormone values in children with protein-calorie malnutrition. *J. Pediat.* 92:153, 1978.
84. Hippocrates. *The Genuine Works of Hippocrates, translated from Greek by Francis Adams.* Baltimore: Williams & Wilkins, 1939.
85. Hoeldtke, R. D., and Wurtman, R. J. Excretion of catecholamines and catecholamine metabolites in kwashiorkor. *Am. J. Clin. Nutr.* 26:205, 1973.
86. Howland, B. E. The influence of feed restriction and subsequent refeeding on gonadotrophin secretion and serum testosterone levels in male rats. *J. Reprod. Fertil.* 44:429, 1975.
87. Howland, B. E., and Skinner, K. R. Effect of starvation on LH levels in male and female hamsters. *J. Reprod. Fertil.* 32:505, 1973.
88. Jackson, C. M. The Effects of Inanition and Malnutrition Upon Growth and Structure. Cited by Platt, B. S., Heard, C. R. C., and Stewart, R. J. C. (1925). In H. N. Munro and J. B. Allison (Eds.), *Mammalian Protein Metabolism.* New York: Academic, 1964. Vol. 2, p. 445.
89. Jefferson, L. S., Li, J. B., and Rannels, S. R. Regulation by insulin of amino acid release and protein turnover in the perfused rat hemicorpus. *J. Biol. Chem.* 252:1476, 1977.
90. Jenkins, A. B., Whittaker, M., and Schofield, P. J. The starvation induced increase in muscle protein degradation is non-lysosomal in origin. *Biochem. Biophys. Res. Commun.* 86:1014, 1979.
91. Jung, R. T., Shetty, P. S., Barrand, M., Callingham, B. A., and James, W. P. The role of catecholamines and thyroid hormones in the metabolic response to semistarvation. *Proc. Nutr. Soc.* 38:17A, 1979.
92. Kark, R. M. Food hunger in a world of turmoil. *World Rev. Nutr. Diet.* 6:1, 1966.
93. Karl, I. E., Garber, A. J., and Kipnis, D. M. Alanine and glutamine synthesis and release from skeletal muscle: III. Dietary and hormonal regulation. *J. Biol. Chem.* 251:844, 1976.
94. Kendall, A. C., and Nolan, R. Polymorphonuclear leukocytic activity in malnourished children. *Central Afr. J. Med.* 18:73, 1972.
95. Keys, A., Brozek, J., Henschel, A., Mickelsen, O., and Taylor, H. L. *The Biology of Human Starvation.* Minneapolis: University of Minnesota Press, 1950.
96. Kinney, J. M., Duke, J. H., Long, C. L., and Gump F. E. Carbohydrate and nitrogen metabolism after injury. *J. Clin. Pathol.* (Suppl.) 4:65, 1970.
97. Kinney, J. M., Long, C. L., and Duke, J. H., Jr. Carbohydrate Metabolism After Injury. In R. Porter and J. Knight (Eds.), *Energy Metabolism in Trauma.* London: Churchill, 1970. Pp. 103–126.
98. Kinney, J. M., Gump, F. E., and Long, C. L. Energy and tissue fuel in human injury and sepsis. *Adv. Exp. Med. Biol.* 33:401, 1972.
99. Kleiber, M. *The Fire of Life. An Introduction to Animal Energetics.* New York: Wiley, 1961.
100. Klein, P. S., Forbes, G. B., and Nader, P. R. Effects of starvation in infancy on subsequent learning disabilities. *J. Pediatr.* 87:8, 1975.
101. Kolanowski, J. Influence of glucose, insulin, and glucagon on sodium balance in fasting obese subjects. *Persp. Biol. Med.* Spring:366, 1979.

102. Kolanowski, J., Desmecht, P., and Crabbe, J. Sodium balance and renal tubular sensitivity to aldosterone during total fast and carbohydrate refeeding in the obese. *Eur. J. Clin. Invest.* 6:75, 1976.
103. Korchak, H. M., and Masoro, E. J. Changes in the level of the fatty acid synthesizing enzymes during starvation. *Biochim. Biophys. Acta* 58: 354, 1962.
104. Lacy, W. W., Lewis, S. B., Liljenquist, J. E., et al. Control of plasma amino acids by glucagon and insulin. *Diabetes* 21:340, 1972.
105. Law, D. K., Dudrick, S. J., and Abdou, N. I. Immunocompetence of patients with protein-calorie malnutrition. *Ann. Intern. Med.* 79:545, 1973.
106. Levenson, S. M. The influence of the indigenous microflora on mammalian metabolism and nutrition. *J. Parent. Enter. Nutr.* 2:75, 1978.
107. Levenson, S. M., Crowley, L. V., and Seifter, E. Starvation. In W. Ballinger, S. A. Collins, W. R. Drucker, S. J. Dudrick, and R. Zeppa (Eds.), *Manual of Surgical Nutrition.* Philadelphia: Saunders, 1975. Pp. 236–264.
108. Lunn, P. G., Whitehead, R. G., Hay, R. W., et al. Progressive changes in serum cortisol, insulin and growth hormone concentrations and their relationship to the distorted amino acid pattern during the development of kwashiorkor. *Br. J. Nutr.* 29:399, 1973.
109. Madia, A. M., Rozovski, S. J., and Kagan, H. M. Changes in lung lysyl oxidase activity in streptozotocin-diabetes and in starvation. *Biochim. Biophys. Acta* 585:481, 1979.
110. Mallette, L. E., Exton, J. H., and Park, C. R. Control of gluconeogenesis from amino acids in the perfused rat liver. *J. Biol. Chem.* 244:5713, 1969.
111. Manchester, K. L. Site of Hormonal Regulation of Protein Metabolism. In H. N. Munro (Ed.), *Mammalian Protein Metabolism.* New York: Academic, 1970. Vol. IV, p. 229.
112. Mann, M. D., Becker, D. J., Pimstone, B. L., et al. Potassium supplementation, serum immunoreactive insulin concentration and glucose tolerance in protein-energy malnutrition. *Br. J. Nutr.* 33:55, 1975.
113. Marliss, E. B., Aoki, T. T., Pozefsky, T., et al. Muscle and splanchnic glutamine and glutamate metabolism in postabsorptive and starved man. *J. Clin. Invest.* 50:814, 1971.
114. Marliss, E. B., Aoki, T. T., Unger, R. H., et al. Glucagon levels and metabolic effects in fasting man. *J. Clin. Invest.* 49:2256, 1970.
115. Martinez, D., Cox, S., Lukasewycz, O. A., and Murphy, W. H. Immune mechanisms in leukemia: Suppression of cellular immunity by starvation. *J. Nat. Cancer Inst.* 55:935, 1975.
116. Matsutaka, H., Aikawa, T., Yamamoto, H., et al. Gluconeogenesis and amino acid metabolism: III. Uptake of glutamine and output of alanine and ammonia by non-hepatic splanchnic organs of fasted rats and their metabolic significance. *J. Biochem.* 74:1019, 1973.
117. McAtee, J. W., and Trenkle, A. Effects of feeding, fasting, glucose and arginine on plasma prolactin levels in the bovine. *Endocrinology* 89: 730, 1971.
118. McCance, R. A., and Widdowson, E. M. *The German Background. Studies of Undernutrition, Wuppertal 1946-1949.* London: Spec. Rep. Ser. Med. Res. Coun., No. 275, 1951.
119. McGarry, J. D., and Foster, D. W. In support of the roles of malonyl-CoA and carnitine acyltransferase in the regulation of hepatic fatty acid oxidation and ketogenesis. *J. Biol. Chem.* 254: 8163, 1979.
120. McGarry, J. D., and Foster, D. W. Regulation of ketogenesis and clinical aspects of the ketotic state. *Metabolism* 21:471, 1972.
121. McNurlan, M. A., Tomkins, A. M., and Garlick, P. J. The effect of starvation on the rate of protein synthesis in rat liver and small intestine. *Biochem. J.* 178:373, 1979.
122. Meister, A. On the enzymology of amino acid transport. *Science* 180:33, 1973.
123. Merimée, J. J., and Fineberg, S. E. Growth hormone secretion in starvation: A reassessment. *J. Clin. Endocrinol. Metab.* 39:385, 1974.
124. Merimée, J. J., Pulkkinen, A. J., and Burton, C. E. Diet-induced alterations of hGH secretion in man. *J. Clin. Endocrinol. Metab.* 42:931, 1976.
125. Millward, D. J. Protein deficiency, starvation, and protein metabolism. *Proc. Nutr. Soc.* 38:77, 1979.
126. Millward, D. J., Garlick, P. J., James, W. P. T., Nnanyelugo, D. O., and Ryatt, J. S. Relationship between protein synthesis and RNA content in skeletal muscle. *Nature* 241:204, 1973.
127. Millward, D. J., Garlick, P. J., James, W. P. T., Sender, P., and Waterlow, J. C. Protein Turnover. In *Protein Metabolism and Nutrition* (EAAP Publication 16). London: University of London Press, 1976. Pp. 49–69.
128. Milner, R. D. G. Metabolic and hormonal responses to oral amino acids in infantile malnutrition. *Arch. Dis. Childh.* 46:301, 1971.
129. Mirsky, I. A. The influence of insulin on the protein metabolism of nephrectomized dogs. *Am. J. Physiol.* 124:569, 1938.
130. Mortimore, G. E., and Ward, W. F. Behavior of

the lysosomal system during organ perfusion. An inquiry into the mechanism of hepatic proteolysis. *Front. Biol.* 45:157, 1976.
131. Najjar, S. S., Stephan, M., and Asfour, R. J. Serum levels of immunoglobulins in marasmic infants. *Arch. Dis. Childh.* 44:120, 1969.
132. Neuman, C. G., Lawlor, G. J., Jr., Stiehm, E. R., et al. Immunologic responses in malnourished children. *Am. J. Clin. Nutr.* 28:89, 1975.
133. Ogata, E. S., Foung, S. K., and Holliday, M. A. The effects of starvation and refeeding on muscle protein synthesis and catabolism in the young rat. *J. Nutr.* 108:759, 1978.
134. Owen, O. E., and Cahill, G. F., Jr. Metabolic effects of exogenous glucocorticoids in fasted man. *J. Clin. Invest.* 52:2596, 1973.
135. Owens, O. E., Felig, P., Morgan, A. P., et al. Liver and kidney metabolism during prolonged starvation. *J. Clin. Invest.* 48:574, 1969.
136. Owen, O. E., Reichard, G. A., Jr., Patel, M., and Boden, G. Energy metabolism in feasting and fasting. *Adv. Exp. Med. Biol.* 111:169, 1979.
137. Palmblad, J., Levi, L., Burger, A., Melander, U., et al. Effect of total energy withdrawal (fasting) on the levels of growth hormone, thyrotropin, cortisol, adrenaline, noradrenaline, T_4, T_3, and rT_3 in healthy males. *Acta Med. Scand.* 201:15, 1977.
138. Peters, J. P., and Van Slyke, D. D. *Quantitative Clinical Chemistry Interpretations.* Baltimore: Williams & Wilkins, 1946. Vol. 1.
139. Peterson, R. D., Beatty, C. H., and Bocek, R. M. Effects of insulin and glucagon on carbohydrate and protein metabolism of adductor muscle and diaphragm. *Endocrinology* 72:71, 1963.
140. Phillips, L. S., and Vassilopoulou-Sellin, R. Nutritional regulation of somatomedin. *Am. J. Clin. Nutr.* 32:1082, 1979.
141. Phillips, L. S., and Vassilopoulou-Sellin, R. Somatomedins. *N. Engl. J. Med.* 302:371, 1980.
142. Phillips, L. S., and Young, H. S. Nutrition and somatomedin: I. Effect of fasting and refeeding on serum somatomedin activity and cartilage growth activity in rats. *Endocrinology* 99:304–314, 1976.
143. Pimstone, B., Barbezat, G., Hansen, J. D. L., et al. Growth hormone and protein-calorie malnutrition. Impaired suppression during induced hyperglycemia. *Lancet* 2:1333, 1967.
144. Pimstone, B., Barbezat, G., Hansen, J. D. L., et al. Studies in growth hormone secretion in protein-calorie malnutrition. *Am. J. Clin. Nutr.* 21:482, 1968.
145. Pimstone, B., Becker, D., and Hendricks, S. TSH response to synthetic thyrotropin-releasing hormone in human protein-calorie malnutrition. *J. Clin. Endocrinol. Metab.* 36:779, 1973.
146. Platt, B. S., and Stewart, R. J. C. Experimental protein deficiency: Histopathological changes in the endocrine glands of pigs. *J. Endocrinol.* 38:121, 1967.
147. Porter, A. *The Disease of the Madras Famine of 1877–1878.* Madras, India: Government Press, 1889.
148. Portnay, G. I., O'Briand, J. T., Bush, J., et al. The effect of starvation on the concentration and binding of thyroxine and triiodothyronine in serum and on the response to TRH. *J. Clin. Endocrinol. Metab.* 39:191, 1974.
149. Pozefsky, T., Tancredi, R. G., Moxley, R. T., et al. Effect of brief starvation on muscle amino acid metabolism in non-obese man. *J. Clin. Invest.* 57:444, 1976.
150. Pullman, T. N., Lavender, A. R., and Aho, I. Direct effect of glucagon on renal hemodynamics and excretion of inorganic ions. *Metabolism* 16:358, 1967.
151. Rabinovitch, A., Grill, V., Renold, A. E., and Cerasi, E. Insulin release and cyclic AMP accumulation in response to glucose in pancreatic islets of fed and starved rats. *J. Clin. Invest.* 58:1209, 1976.
152. Rannels, D. E., Pegg, A. E., Rannels, S. R., and Jefferson, L. S. Effect of starvation on initiation of protein synthesis in skeletal muscle and heart. *Am. J. Physiol.* 235:E126, 1978.
153. Rannels, D. E., Sahms, R. H., and Watkins, C. A. Effects of starvation and diabetes on protein synthesis in lung. *Am. J. Physiol.* 236: E421, 1979.
154. Rao, K. S. J., Spikantia, S. G., and Gopalan, C. Plasma cortisol levels in protein-calorie malnutrition. *Arch. Dis. Childh.* 43:365, 1968.
155. Reichard, G. A., Jr., Haff, A. C., Skutches, C. L., Paul, P., and Holroyde, C. P. Plasma acetone metabolism in the fasting human. *J. Clin. Invest.* 63:619, 1979.
156. Root, A. W., Reiter, E. O., Duckett, G. E., and Sweetland, M. L. Effect of short-term castration and starvation upon hypothalamic content of luteinizing hormone-releasing hormone in adult male rats. *Proc. Soc. Exp. Biol. Med.* 150:602, 1975.
157. Rothschild, M. A., Oratz, M., and Mongelli, J., et al. Effects of a short-term fast on albumin synthesis studies in vivo, in the perfused liver, and on amino acid incorporation by hepatic microsomes. *J. Clin. Invest.* 47:2591, 1968.
158. Ruderman, N. B., Goodman, M. N., Berger, M., and Hagg, S. Effect of starvation on muscle glu-

cose metabolism: Studies with the isolated perfused rat hindquarter. *Fed. Proc.* 36:171, 1977.

159. Ruderman, N. B., Schmahl, F. W., and Goodman, M. N. Regulation of alanine formation and release in rat muscle in vivo: Effect of starvation and diabetes. *Am. J. Physiol.* 233:E109, 1977.
160. Rudorff, K. H., Albrecht, G., and Staib, W. Effect of insulin and proinsulin on the metabolism of alanine in the rat liver. *Horm. Metab. Res.* 2:49, 1970.
161. Saha, K., Mehta, R., Misra, R. C., Chaudhury, D. S., and Ray, S. N. Undernutrition and immunity: Smallpox vaccination in chronically starved, undernourished subjects and its immunologic evaluation. *Scand. J. Immunol.* 6:581, 1977.
162. Sahebjami, H., and Vassallo, C. L. Effects of starvation and refeeding on lung mechanics and morphometry. *Am. Rev. Respir. Dis.* 119:443, 1979.
163. Salmon, W. D., Jr. Interaction of somatomedin and a peptide inhibitor in serum of hypophysectomized and starved, pituitary-intact rats. *Adv. Metabol. Disord.* 8:183, 1975.
164. Samuel, A. M., and Deshpande, U. R. Growth hormone levels in protein calorie malnutrition. *J. Clin. Endocrinol. Metab.* 35:863, 1972.
165. Sapir, D. G., Chambers, N. E., and Ryan, J. W. The role of potassium in the control of ammonium excretion during starvation. *Metabolism* 25:211, 1976.
166. Sapir, D. G., and Owen, O. E. Renal conservation of ketone bodies during starvation. *Metabolism* 24:23, 1975.
167. Sapir, D. G., Owen, O. E., Pozefsky, T., and Walser, M. Nitrogen sparing induced by a mixture of essential amino acids given chiefly as their keto-analogues during prolonged starvation in obese subjects. *J. Clin. Invest.* 54:974, 1974.
168. Sapir, D. G., and Walser, M. Nitrogen sparing induced early in starvation by infusion of branched-chain ketoacids. *Metabolism* 26:301, 1977.
169. Saudek, C. D., Boulter, P. R., and Arky, R. A. The natriuretic effect of glucagon and its role in starvation. *J. Clin. Endocrinol. Metab.* 36: 761, 1973.
170. Saudek, C. D., and Felig, P. The metabolic events of starvation. *Am. J. Med.* 60:117, 1976.
171. Schanberg, S. The New York Times. February, 1975.
172. Schlesinger, L., Ohlbaum, A., Grez, L., et al. Decreased interferon production by leukocytes in marasmus. *Am. J. Clin. Nutr.* 29:758, 1976.
173. Schloeder, F. X., and Stinebaugh, B. J. Renal tubular sites of natriuresis of fasting and glucose-induced sodium conservation. *Metabolism* 19: 1119, 1970.
174. Schwarz, F., der Kinderen, P. J., van Reit, H. G., et al. Influence of exogenous human growth hormone on the metabolism of fasting obese patients. *Metabolism* 21:297, 1972.
175. Seitz, H. J., Kaiser, M., Krone, W., and Tarnowski, W. Physiologic significance of glucocorticoids and insulin in the regulation of hepatic gluconeogenesis during starvation in rats. *Metabolism* 25:1545, 1976.
176. Selvaraj, R. J., and Bhat, K. S. Phagocytosis and leukocyte enzymes in protein-calorie malnutrition. *Biochem. J.* 127:255, 1972.
177. Sherwin, R. S., Hendler, R. G., and Felig, P. Effect of ketone infusions on amino acid and nitrogen metabolism in man. *J. Clin. Invest.* 55:1382, 1975.
178. Shetty, P. S., Jung, R. T., Barrand, M., Callingham, B. A., and James, W. P. The effect of catecholamine replacement on the metabolic response to semistarvation. *Proc. Nutr. Soc.* 38: 18A, 1979.
179. Shoemaker, W. C., and VanItallie, T. B. The hepatic response to glucagon in the unanesthetized dog. *Endocrinology* 66:260, 1960.
180. Shoemaker, W. J., and Wortman, R. J. Perinatal undernutrition: Accumulation of catecholamines in rat brain. *Science* 171:1017, 1971.
181. Shulman, G., Williams, P., Lacy, W. W., and Cherrington, A. D. Adaptation of glucose production to a physiologic increment in glucagon. *Diabetes* 26 (Suppl. 1):383, 1977.
182. Sigler, M. H. The mechanism of the natriuresis of fasting. *J. Clin. Invest.* 55:377, 1975.
183. Sirek, A. M., Horvath, E., Ezrin, C., and Kovacs, K. Effect of starvation on pituitary growth hormone cells and blood growth hormone and prolactin levels in the rat. *Nutr. Metab.* 20:67, 1976.
184. Sirisinha, S., Suskind, R., Edelman, R., et al. Complement and C_3-proactivator levels in children with protein-calorie malnutrition and effect of dietary treatment. *Lancet* 1:1016, 1973.
185. Smith, A. L. Effects of starvation on vacuolar apparatus of cardiac muscle tissue determined by electron microscopy, marker-enzyme assays and electrolyte studies. *Cytobios* 18:111, 1977.
186. Smith, J. M., and Dubos, R. J. The effect of nutritional disturbances on the susceptibility of mice to staphylococcal infections. *J. Exper. Med.* 103:109, 1956.
187. Smith, O. K., and Long, C. N. H. Effect of corti-

sol on the plasma amino nitrogen of eviscerated adrenalectomized diabetic rats. *Endocrinology* 80:561, 1967.

188. Smith, S. R., Bledsoe, T., and Chhetri, M. K. Cortisol metabolism and the pituitary-adrenal axis in adults with protein-calorie malnutrition. *J. Clin. Endocrinol. Metab.* 40:43, 1975.
189. Smith, S. R., Edgar, P. J., Pozefsky, T., et al. Growth hormone in adults with protein-calorie malnutrition. *J. Clin. Endocrinol. Metab.* 39:53, 1974.
190. Smythe, P. M., Schonland, M., Brereton-Stiles, M. M., et al. Thymolymphatic deficiency and depression of cell mediated immunity in protein-calorie malnutrition. *Lancet* 2:939, 1971.
191. Spaulding, S. W., Chopra, I. J., Sherwin, R. S., et al. Effect of caloric restriction and dietary composition on serum T_3 in man. *J. Clin. Endocrinol. Metab.* 42:197, 1976.
192. Spencer, I. M., Hutchinson, A., and Robinson, D. S. The effect of nutritional sate on the lipoprotein lipase activity of isolated fat cells. *Biochim. Biophys. Acta* 530:375, 1978.
193. Stein, T. P., Oram-Smith, J. C., Leskiw, J., et al. Effect of nitrogen and calorie restriction on protein synthesis in the rat. *Am. J. Physiol.* 230:1321, 1976.
194. Stewart, W. K., and Fleming, L. W. Relationship between plasma and erythrocyte magnesium and potassium concentrations in fasting obese subjects. *Metabolism* 22:535, 1973.
195. Stout, R. W., Henry, R. W., and Buchanan, K. D. Triglyceride metabolism in acute starvation: The role of secretion and glucagon. *Eur. J. Clin. Invest.* 6:179, 1976.
196. Sugden, M. C., Sharples, S. C., and Randle, P. J. Carcass glycogen as a potential source of glucose during short-term starvation. *Biochem. J.* 160:817, 1976.
197. Takagi, A., Isozaki, Y., Kurata, K., and Nagataki, S. Serum concentrations, metabolic clearance rates, and production rates of reverse triiodothyronine, triiodothyronine, and thyroxine in starved rabbits. *Endocrinology* 103:1434, 1978.
198. Tannenbaum, G. S., Epelbaum, J., Colle, E., Brazeau, P., and Martin, J. B. Antiserum to somatostatin reverses starvation-induced inhibition of growth hormone but not insulin secretion. *Endocrinology* 102:1909, 1978.
199. Tavassoli, M., Eastlund, D. T., Yam, L. T., Neiman, R. S., and Finkel, H. Gelatinous transformation of bone marrow in prolonged self-induced starvation. *Scand. J. Haematol.* 16:311, 1976.
200. Tejada, C., and Russfield, A. B. A preliminary report on the pathology of the pituitary gland in children with malnutrition. *Arch. Dis. Childh.* 32:343, 1957.
201. Vagenakis, A. G. Thyroid Hormone Metabolism in Prolonged Experimental Starvation in Man. In R. A. Vigersky (Ed.), *Anorexia Nervosa.* New York: Raven Press, 1977. Pp. 243–253.
202. Vagenakis, A. G., Portnay, G. I., O'Brian, J. T., Rudolph, M., Arky, R. A., Ingbar, S. H., and Braverman, L. E. Effect of starvation on the production and metabolism of thyroxine and triiodothyronine in euthyroid obese patients. *J. Clin. Endocrinol. Metab.* 45:1305, 1977.
203. Van den Brande, J. L., and DuCaju, M. V. L. Plasma somatomedin activity in children with growth disturbances. Cited in Pimstone, B., Endocrine function in protein-calorie malnutrition, *Clin. Endocrinol.* 5:79, 1976.
204. Vint, F. W. Post-mortem findings in natives of Kenya. *East African Med. J.* 13:332, 1937.
205. Walser, M., Sapir, D. G., Mitch, W. E., Batshaw, M., Brusilow, S., and Maddrey, W. C. Evidence for an anabolic action of essential amino acid analogues in uremia and starvation. *Z. Ernaehrung Swiss* (Suppl.) 19:5, 1976.
206. Walter, R. M., Dudl, R. J., Palmer, J. P., and Ensinck, J. W. The effect of adrenergic blockade on the glucagon responses to starvation and hypoglycemia in man. *J. Clin. Invest.* 54:1214, 1974.
207. Wannemacher, R. W., Jr., and Dinterman, R. E. Total body protein catabolism in starved and infected rats. *Am. J. Clin. Nutr.* 30:1510, 1977.
208. Wassner, S. J., Orloff, S., and Holliday, M. A. Protein degradation in muscle: Response to feeding and fasting in growing rats. *Am. J. Physiol.* 233:E119, 1977.
209. Waterlow, J. C., and Stephen, J. M. L. Adaptation of the rat to a low-protein diet: The effect of a reduced protein intake on the pattern of incorporation of L-^{14}C lysine. *Br. J. Nutr.* 20:461, 1966.
210. Waterlow, J. C., and Stephen, J. M. L. Use of carbon-14-labelled arginine to measure the catabolic rate of serum and liver proteins and the extent of amino-acid recycling. *Nature* 211:978, 1966A.
211. Watts, T. Thymus weights in malnourished children. *J. Trop. Pediatr.* 15:155, 1969.
212. Weinkove, C. Insulin release and glucose tolerance in malnourished rats. Ph.D. Thesis, University of Cape Town. Cited by Pimstone,

B. in Endocrine function in protein-calorie malnutrition. *Clin. Endocrinol.* 5:79, 1976.
213. Weinkove, C., Weinkove, E. A., and Pimstone, B. L. Glucose tolerance and insulin release in malnourished rats. *Clin. Sci. Mol. Med.* 50:153, 1976.
214. Weissel, M., Stummvoll, H. K., and Kolbe, H. T_3 metabolism in starvation. *N. Engl. J. Med.* 301:163, 1979. (Letter)
215. Wildenthal, K., Poole, A. R., Glauert, A. M., and Dingle, J. T. Dietary control of cardiac lysosomal enzyme activities. *Rec. Adv. Stud. Cardiac Struc. Metab.* 8:519, 1975.
216. Wilmore, D. W., Moylan, J. A., Bristow, B. F., et al. Anabolic effects of human growth hormone and high caloric feedings following thermal injury. *Surg. Gynecol. Obstet.* 138:875, 1974.
217. Wimpfheimer, C., Saville, E., Voirol, M. J., Danforth, E., Jr., and Burger, A. B. Starvation-induced decreased sensitivity of resting metabolic rate to triiodothyronine. *Science* 205: 1272, 1979.
218. Winick, M. (Ed.) *Nutrition, Pre- and Postnatal Development.* New York: Plenum, 1979.
219. Wise, J. K., Hendler, R., and Felig, P. Influence of glucocorticoids on glucagon secretion and plasma amino acid concentrations in man. *J. Clin. Invest.* 52:2774, 1973.
220. Wolf, A. V. *Thirst.* Springfield, IL: Thomas, 1958.
221. Yoshida, T., Metcoff, J., and Frenk, S. Reduced pyruvic kinase activity, altered growth patterns of ATP in leukocytes and protein-calorie malnutrition. *Am. J. Clin. Nutr.* 21:162, 1968.
222. Young, V. R., Haverberg, L. N., Bilmazes, C., and Munro, H. M. Potential use of 3-methylhistidine excretion as an index of progressive reduction in muscle protein catabolism during starvation. *Metabolism* 22:1429, 1973.
223. Young, J. B., and Landsberg, L. Suppression of sympathetic nervous system during fasting. *Science* 196:1473, 1977.
224. Zawalich, W. S., Dye, E. S., Pagliara, A. S., Rognstad, R., and Matschinsky, F. M. Starvation diabetes in the rat: Onset, recovery, and specificity of reduced responsiveness of pancreatic beta-cells. *Endocrinology* 104:1344, 1979.
225. Zubiran, S., and Gomez-Mont, F. Endocrine disturbances in chronic human malnutrition. *Vitamins and Hormones* 11:97, 1953.

14 Metabolic Response to Trauma and Infection

Martin B. Popp
Murray F. Brennan

Trauma is an injury to a living body caused by the application of some external force and may range from minor elective surgery to a massive insult, such as a severe burn or multiple system injury. The influence of the traumatic insult may be conveniently divided into the local effect and the systemic response. With successful treatment, the local effect usually is resolved, results in loss of function depending on the tissue injured, and dictates specific local therapy. The systemic effects are highly dependent on the nature and magnitude of the local injury, represent a somewhat stereotyped response, may jeopardize survival, dictate systemic therapy, and are the physiologic alterations of sepsis and trauma.

These physiologic alterations are mediated by four basic effects of the local injury: the neuroendocrine response; the cardiovascular response; a toxic response secondary to necrotic tissue resorption and invasive infection; and a starvation response, which occurs if adequate nutrient intake cannot be rapidly reestablished. These mediators affect total body fluid and electrolyte balance, and carbohydrate, protein, and fat metabolism. If these systemic effects are prolonged, severe, or untreated, body energy supplies become depleted, the body's protein "machinery" is damaged, and an unfavorable clinical result occurs.

The development of a major physiologic response is dependent on the local injury, the treatment, and the degree to which each of the aforementioned effector pathways is activated. A herniorrhaphy performed with good anesthesia, little blood loss or edema formation, no infection, and rapid reinstitution of enteral feeding provokes little systemic response. A 60 percent full-thickness burn causes a maximal neuroendocrine response, lethal hypovolemia if not treated properly, certain toxicity from infection, and nutritional problems from inadequate food intake and hypermetabolism. This thermal injury is currently lethal in an average adult in 50 percent of cases, and the outcome is highly dependent on the skill of the physician in managing the systemic and local problems [44]. The influence of the four mediating factors is synergistic, and the net result of the injury is dependent on the severity of each component.

Recent research has clarified much of the neuroendocrine response and its influence on protein, carbohydrate, and fat metabolism. Hemodynamic changes, invasive infection, and starvation basically modify the overall neuroendocrine response to injury. This review considers the basic neuroendocrine response; its effect on protein, carbohydrate, and fat metabolism; and the special effects of altered circulation, infection, and starvation.

NEUROENDOCRINE RESPONSE

The initial stimulus of the wounding agent sets in motion a basic neuroendocrine response. This is a neurophysiologic reflex with an afferent limb composed primarily of the neural pain pathways, integration at higher central nervous system (CNS) levels, and both neurologic and endocrine efferent paths. Selye [152], when he described a "general adaptation syndrome," first suggested that this reflex response is a stereotype common to many different stressful stimuli (i.e., surgical operation, trauma, burn injury, cold, or psychic stress). Albright [1], in 1943, noted the similarities between this stereotyped response to stress and Cushing's syndrome and suggested the importance of adrenal cortical function in the overall response. Cannon [37] noted the inability of sympathectomized animals to withstand various stresses and emphasized the importance of the sympathetic nervous system and the adrenal medulla in this response. Other investigators have suggested that severe stress may provoke a maximal neurophysiologic stress response and that inadequate reserve in this response is associated with death [74, 181]. A detailed analysis of this reflex response, with consideration of the extent to which it is graded to the strength of the stimulus, can be of significant importance in patient care.

Neurologic Afferent Pathway

Strong evidence exists to suggest that neurologic mechanisms are the primary afferent limb and transmit information from the peripheral area of injury to high CNS centers for integration. Hume and Egdahl [91], in a classic series of experiments, studied the corticosteroid response to thermal injury in the leg of an anesthetized dog. They demonstrated that this response could be blocked by section of either peripheral nerve, cervical spinal cord, or medulla oblongata. Egdahl [58], in a further group of experiments, removed the cortex, the cortex and thalamus, the entire brain down to the hypothalamus, or the entire brain including the hypothalamus. The adrenocortical response to trauma remained intact in all groups, except in those animals with hypothalamus removed. Further, these animals all had elevated basal adrenocortical steroid output, suggesting that an inhibitory cortical center had been removed [57].

Support for the concept of neural transmission of afferent impulses through the peripheral nervous system and spinal cord in man can be found in studies of the response of paraplegics and patients under spinal anesthesia to operative trauma. Hume [90] directly measured adrenal vein secretion during abdominal operation and over the first 24 hours postoperatively in a series of patients including two paraplegics. Neither paraplegic demonstrated an adrenocorticotropic response similar to that of patients with intact nervous systems. Newsome and Rose [128] noted that the response of both adrenocorticotropic hormone (ACTH) and growth hormone (GH) in male patients undergoing herniorrhaphy was abolished by spinal anesthesia, but was present in those patients placed under general anesthesia. In contrast to Hume's work, Bromage [28], in studying response to surgical operation, found the plasma hydroxycortisone elevation preserved in a series of patients having prolonged epidural blockade and light general anesthesia, although the hyperglycemic response was abolished. These authors suggested that afferent vagal fibers transmitted information to the CNS, and that the efferent sympathetic response mediating the hyperglycemia through the adrenal medulla was blocked.

The foregoing clinical phenomena suggest the importance of the CNS in integrating the response to various forms of stress. The anatomic pathways most likely to mediate this response (Figures 14-1 and 14-2) have been described in basic neuroanatomic and neurophysiologic studies and give some

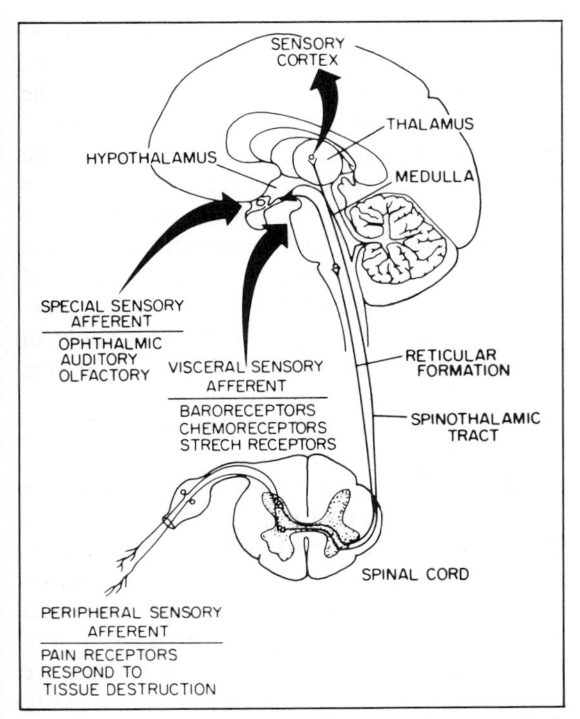

Figure 14-1. *Afferent neurologic pathways, which transmit sensory perceptions of traumatic injury or infection to higher central nervous system centers.*

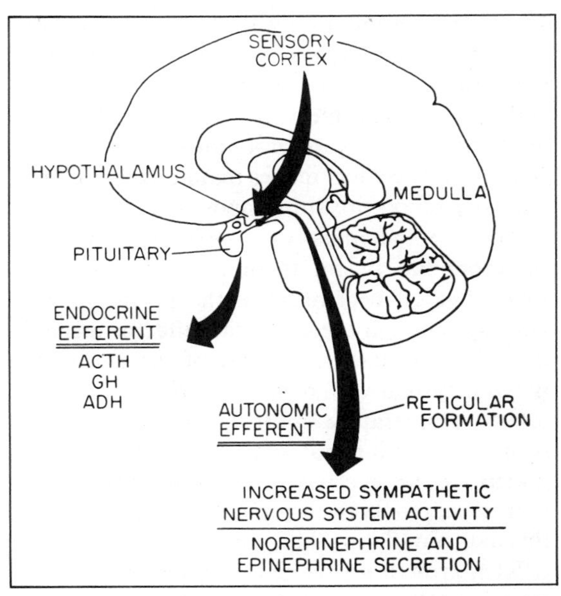

Figure 14-2. *Efferent neurologic pathways, which mediate the autonomic and endocrine components of the central nervous system response to trauma to the periphery.*

understanding as to why the responses occur as they do [127].

The initial and most direct effect of injury is on the afferent nociceptive mechanism. This system responds to local tissue damage, the local production of proteolytic enzymes, and production of other chemical mediators to excite afferent peripheral myelinated delta and C nerve fibers [120]. These fibers synapse in both the dorsal horn and the lateral horn gray matter. The dorsal horn cells give rise to axons, which carry information to the thalamic relay nuclei via the lateral spinothalamic tracts. Direct fibers from the thalamus are projected to the somatesthetic cortex, and this system is thought to mediate short latency, sharply localized pain sensation [46]. A multisynaptic system that accompanies this direct system is thought to mediate a much more poorly localized, highly disagreeable pain sensation, which can be perceived at thalamic levels. The spinothalamic tracts give off many fibers to reticular gray matter throughout their course, and these fibers allow integration of information to occur at many different brain levels [46].

The neurologic response to painful stimulus also occurs at many levels. The direct synapses of afferent peripheral nerve fibers with lateral horn cells give rise to afferent fibers and cause a "spinal reflex," which is integrated entirely at the spinal level. The efferent response usually extends only one segment above and one segment below the segment that received the sensory input [101]. The short latency and segmental distribution of this response is well demonstrated in electrophysiologic studies, as is the much longer latency supraspinal response, which can be eliminated by cord section [146]. The medulla is also a major autonomic regulating center. At this level, more complex reflexes—blood pressure, blood sugar, and respiratory regulation—occur (see Figure

14-1). Integration of responses involving both sympathetic and parasympathetic components of the autonomic nervous system occurs. The spinal and medullary centers contribute sympathetic discharge necessary for vasomotor tone. Destruction of these centers makes maintenance of a satisfactory blood pressure impossible [82].

The hypothalamus is the next important level of autonomic control. It controls both the neurologic effector mechanism of the autonomic nervous system and the endocrine effector mechanism of the pituitary. Activity of the autonomic nervous system with regard to food intake, water intake, temperature control, and the stress response are all integrated at this level. Also integrated are the levels of the anterior pituitary hormones: adrenocorticotropic hormone (ACTH), thyroid stimulating hormone (TSH), prolactin (PRL), growth hormone (GH), luteotropic hormone (LH), and follicle stimulating hormone (FSH), and the important posterior pituitary hormone: antidiuretic hormone (ADH). The importance of the hypothalamus is emphasized by the observation that most autonomic functions are relatively normal when brain structures superior to the hypothalamus are removed [101]. For most practical purposes, the hypothalamus is the highest level of integration of the stress response. The major efferent paths of the hypothalamus are the endocrine via the pituitary and the efferent sympathetic and parasympathetic systems.

Information transmission from peripheral pain sensors via the spinothalamic paths is the major CNS information source during anesthesia and surgical procedures. This concept is supported by the diminished or absent response to surgical trauma in paraplegics and denervated animal preparations [28, 90, 128]. Under the less-controlled circumstances of most major trauma and with neurologically intact individuals, other paths can also stimulate the response. One secondary path is the psychic impact of traumatic situations in which information may be transmitted via the visual and auditory paths independent of information from the site of injury. Examples of pure psychic stimulation of the stress response include rises in urinary corticosteroids documented in Korean War soldiers, which fluctuated with the level of hostilities being encountered [88]. The development of ulcers in "executive monkeys" given responsibility for determining the feeding patterns of "subordinate monkeys" has also been attributed to chronic stimulation of a stress response [25]. Hume [89] has demonstrated a marked increase in both catecholamine and corticosteroid levels by an untrained, highly agitated dog exposed to a controlled bleed compared to either an anesthetized dog or a trained, calm, resting dog exposed to the same procedure.

Many of the physiologic systems that usually monitor bodily function and serve as feedback control systems also transmit information to the CNS during periods of trauma. If the injury produces hypovolemia, atrial stretch receptors transmit information that is integrated at the medullary and hypothalamic levels [130]. Hypotension is registered by the baroreceptors of the aortic arch and carotid areas. Declines in blood pressure are immediately perceived at medullary levels [150]. The rapidity and efficiency of these two systems in compensating for acute hemorrhage or hypovolemia is demonstrated by experimental bleeding and transfusion studies in normal man, in whom neither the pain afferent nor the emotional input would be operative. Studies by Skillman [158] and by Frye [67] demonstrate short latency compensation to bleeds or transfusion of 1,000 to 1,500 ml in normal man and relatively little physiologic dysfunction. This compensation occurs initially by shifts of blood from splanchnic areas, and the short latency of the response that preserves blood pressure suggests that it is mediated entirely via the autonomic nervous system. The ability of resting, normal man to readily compensate to large losses of red cell mass (down to a hematocrit of 20 percent) by minimal change in pulse and no change in blood pressure, emphasizes the importance of rate as well as volume of blood loss as neurogenic stimuli [173].

Other receptor systems capable of relaying information to the CNS during trauma and sepsis include the chemoreceptors of the carotid bodies and the oxygen receptors of the medulla. These systems can provoke one of the strongest short-term blood pressure responses known during periods of hypoxia [83]. Glucose receptors in the hypothalamus have also been demonstrated, and thus abnormalities in glucose concentration produced peripherally in traumatic situations may be perceived directly by the CNS as part of the afferent limb of a neurophysiologic response [145]. Similarly, the CNS may directly perceive many different amino acid levels, and the concentrations of these substances may provide afferent information [51].

Another possible afferent in the CNS response to trauma is the production, from the areas of wounds, of specific toxins that interact with CNS receptors. One example of a specific chemical afferent is endogenous pyrogen (EP), which is released in response to stimuli such as infectious agents, bacterial products, fungal products, immune processes, and a variety of other exogenous pyrogens [53]. Cell sources of EP include neutrophils, monocytes, eosinophils, and both circulating and fixed tissue macrophages. The principal site of action of EP appears to be the preoptic anterior hypothalamic area of the brain, and it functions by elevating the physiologic set point for body temperature [119]. This is a normal response to EP. All the physiologic mechanisms that maintain temperature function normally to maintain this new temperature.

Data suggesting CNS input from direct wound toxins are sparse and the existence of such toxins is questionable. Allgower [3] has isolated, from thermally injured mouse skin, a lipid-protein complex that kills 100 percent of normal mice when 0.3 mg/gm body weight is injected intraperitoneally. A similar material isolated from normal skin by the same biochemical procedure causes no mortality. Allgower postulates that the toxin is a polymer of a normally occurring membrane component that is produced by direct heating of skin. Similarly, Holder [87] has demonstrated enhanced survival in burned mice protected with antisera to burned skin, and Baxter [15] has demonstrated a myocardial depressant factor that is produced in thermally injured dogs. All of these studies suggest that "toxins" can be produced by injury and adversely affect the injured organism. Whether these toxins are abnormal molecular species produced by the injury, as suggested by Allgower [3], or are normal intercellular constituents that only become toxic when they enter the circulation, as suggested by Holder [87], is unknown. The mode of action of these substances, and particularly any effect on the CNS and the stress reflex, is similarly unknown.

Efferent Neurologic Reflex Paths

After integration of the vast array of afferent input in higher CNS centers, the efferent discharge is channelled to the periphery through the hypothalamus. Outflow from the hypothalamus is through either the autonomic nervous system or the pituitary. Both paths are important and contribute to the overall response (see Figure 14-2).

Autonomic Nervous System

It has been widely accepted, since the work of Cannon [37] and previous investigators, that the autonomic nervous system exerts CNS control over internal homeostasis. The autonomic nervous system consists of two major divisions: the craniocaudad or parasympathetic and thoracolumbar or sympathetic. All organs of the body and all smooth muscle, including that of the vasculature, is innervated by one or both of these divisions of the autonomic nervous system. Under conditions of normal activity, much bodily function—heart rate, vasomotor tone, and gastrointestinal motility—and much endocrine function are under the tonic influence of one or both branches of this system [101].

It has also long been suspected that the sympathetic branch of the autonomic nervous system is a chief effector of the response to stress. Cannon [37] noted that the thoracolumbar ganglion chain is a diffuse multiplying system in which a few preganglionic fibers synapse with a large number of axons to the periphery. Early investigators ob-

Table 14-1. *Hypersecretion of Catecholamines in Trauma and Sepsis (% Increase in Blood Levels or 24-hr Urinary Excretion Over Control Values)*

Condition	Epinephrine (%)	Norepinephrine (%)
Normal		
Blood	100	100
Urine	100	100
Myocardial infarction		
Blood	189	158
Elective surgical operation		
Urine	136	289
Burn injury		
Blood	386	248
Urine	421	205
Severe infection		
Blood	950	868

Table compiled from data in references 42, 64, 79, and 136.

served that many of the clinical features of stress—such as piloerection, hyperhydrosis, increased pulse rate, peripheral vasoconstriction, and decreased gastrointestinal motility—can be abolished by ablation of parts of the sympathetic nervous system. Early investigators were also aware of many of the details of epinephrine secretion from the adrenal medulla which effectively distributes the effect of sympathetic discharge throughout the entire body via the circulation. They were aware that metabolic effects, particularly hyperglycemia following stressful stimulation, are mediated by this path [37].

More recent studies confirm these previous concepts and have indicated a primary role for the sympathetic nervous system as the primary mediator of the stress response. Strong evidence (Table 14-1) to support this has come from the measurement of blood catecholamine levels and urinary catecholamine excretion in traumatic conditions including operation [64], trauma [64], burns [75, 85, 136, 181], infection [79], and myocardial infarction [42]. These studies indicate that both epinephrine and norepinephrine are elevated, and that their levels may fluctuate independently of each other. The other striking finding is that the levels correlate with the severity of the stress, and the duration of their elevation correlates with the duration of the stress (see Table 14-1). A major surgical operation, with good anesthesia and without blood loss, provokes little response from either catecholamine [64]. Operations followed by complications, trauma, and burns cause greater levels of response, and these persist as long as the stress continues [64, 75, 181].

As epinephrine is secreted only by the adrenal medulla and norepinephrine is thought to come only from "leaks" at sympathetic nerve endings, norepinephrine levels are an indicator of overall sympathetic activity, whereas the epinephrine activity indicates action of the adrenal medulla. The relative proportions of the two catecholamines are of some importance as norepinephrine selectively stimulates the alpha receptors, whereas the epinephrine selectively stimulates beta receptors [68]. A variable physiologic response is possible, dependent on the ratio of the two agents. In most situations, however, similar elevations of both catecholamines are observed (see Table 14-1).

It is also worth noting that circulating and urinary norepinephrine levels are only a crude index of sympathetic activity. Most norepinephrine is released at adrenergic nerve endings, and only a small portion escapes into the bloodstream [86]. Reliable assays have only recently become available for measurement of the small amounts of this transmitter in blood. After escape into the bloodstream and transport to the liver, or in either the postsynaptic neuron or the effector cells, both epinephrine and norepinephrine are methylated by catechol-O-methyl transferase, oxidized by monoamine oxidase, and excreted in the urine primarily as metanephrine, normetanephrine, and VMA [101]. Therefore, measurements of either blood or urinary epinephrine and norepinephrine are only crude estimates of basic sympathetic activity. An improved estimation of sympathetic activity has been suggested by Maas on the basis of isotope tracer studies. This work indicates that measurement of urinary norepinephrine and normetanephrine is an accurate index of overall sympathetic activity [111].

The foregoing evidence of excessive sympathetic activity in severe trauma raises the question: what is its effect? The most prominent effects are the immediate cardiovascular, gastrointestinal, and CNS alerting effects: the so-called "fight or flight" response of Cannon [37]. These effects are quite useful in preventing trauma and provide powerful mechanisms to protect vital structures. The cardiovascular response includes increased pulse rate and cardiac output and shunting of blood from storage areas (spleen, splanchnic bed, and deep leg veins) into the more central areas, where it can support circulation to the brain, heart, and somatic masculature [77]. Thus sympathetic activity is the ideal initial defense in most traumatic circumstances, in which blood and fluid loss is the immediate problem. Peripheral skin vasoconstriction is important in preventing hemorrhage in traumatic situations and gives rise to the cold, clammy feeling of peripheral skin in hypovolemic patients. This protective sympathetic effect is well demonstrated in experimental bleeding studies, which show that normal man can lose 30 percent of his blood volume and show little physiologic defect [157, 158, 173].

The other major effect of sympathetic stimulation is the metabolic response. The primary effect of both epinephrine and norepinephrine is best demonstrated by experiments involving infusion of these substances into normal man. Porte has demonstrated that the metabolic response to epinephrine infusion at 6 μg/min includes a prompt increase in glucose and free-fatty acid (FFA) levels and a suppression of the expected rise in insulin levels, which would usually accompany this rise in glucose [139]. The response to infusion of norepinephrine at 6 μg/min in normal adults is a more moderate rise in glucose and FFA levels, but a similar flattening of the insulin response, which is observed when similar rises in blood sugar are created by glucose infusion [138]. This response could not be elicited by rapid removal of 15 percent of the blood volume of a normal individual [84]. In similar infusion studies, the insulin response to both glucose and tolbutamide can be shown to be blocked by either catecholamine [138, 139].

The mechanism underlying the effect of the catecholamines on insulin secretion has been related to the occurrence of both alpha and beta receptors on the islet cell [94]. Stimulation of the alpha receptors causes inhibition of insulin secretion, whereas stimulation of beta receptors causes increased secretion of insulin. The exquisite sensitivity of the alpha receptors and the demonstration of rich sympathetic nerve innervation of the endocrine pancreas suggest that sympathetic discharge to the pancreas under conditions of stress is of importance in suppressing insulin. The suppression of insulin by epinephrine infusions, which produce blood levels similar to those frequently found in stress, likewise suggests that circulating epinephrine levels can suppress insulin.

Another basic metabolic effect of circulating catecholamines may be the stimulation of glucagon. Glucagon elevation has been well demonstrated in trauma [105, 117], blood loss [105], burns [185], and infection [142] (see Figure 14-2). This rise seems to be most prominent during the period of initial trauma and returns to normal as the stressful insult abates. There is evidence accumulating which suggests that the combined influence of elevated glucagon levels and suppressed

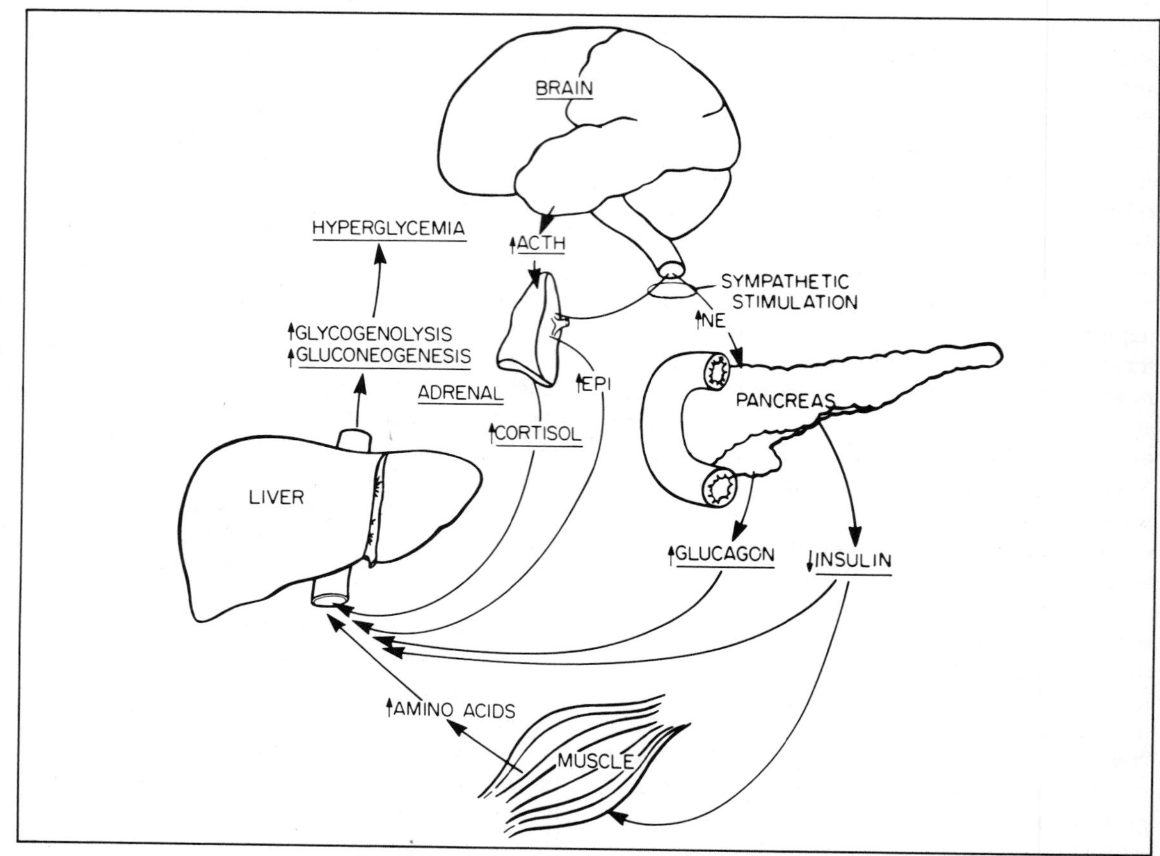

Figure 14-3. *Neuroendocrine response to trauma, which results in increased gluconeogenesis and hyperglycemia.*

insulin levels is of major importance in controlling hepatic gluconeogenesis (Figure 14-3). This influence may be expressed as the molar insulin: glucagon ratio, and as this ratio falls, hepatic gluconeogenesis is favored [168]. This ratio is decreased in all trauma states. The mechanism that produces hyperglucagonemia during alpha cell stimulation has not been determined. The work of Iversen would suggest that alpha cells are stimulated by beta adrenergic agents, and thus the hyperglucagonemia could result from circulating catecholamines or direct neural stimulation [94].

Pituitary Efferent Pathway

The second major efferent pathway from the hypothalamus is via the pituitary. This path includes the hypothalamico-hypophyseal portal system, which consists of a capillary bed starting in the hypothalamus and extending into the anterior lobe of the pituitary. Blood had been noted to flow from the hypothalamus to the pituitary as early as 1936, and during the past 30 years it has become clear that the secretory activities of the anterior pituitary lobe are largely controlled by substances formed in the hypothalamus. These are transported humorally to the hypophysis via this portal system [50]. The substances carried in this portal system may be termed releasing factors, and nine such substances are now known to either stimulate or inhibit anterior pituitary hormones [149]. These releasing factors are small polypeptides, and they are produced in central neurons, travel down their axons, and are released into the CNS end of the portal system. They are then carried by this system to the cells of the anterior pituitary gland, where they regulate hormone secretion.

Pituitary Adrenal Axis and Growth Hormone. There are six anterior pituitary hormones: ACTH, GH, TSH, PRL, FSH, and LH. Of these, only ACTH and its effect on the adrenal cortex during traumatic and stressful situations has been well studied. Initially, Albright [1] noted the similarity between Cushing's syndrome and stressful situations. Subsequently, the development of assays for urinary steroid concentrations and the fractionation of the ketosteroids from the hydroxysteroids have allowed further description of the pituitary-adrenal hyperactivity found in traumatic situations. The only known control of adrenal glucocorticoid activity is ACTH secreted from the pituitary. Therefore, evidence of hypersecretion of adrenal glucocorticoid is good evidence for excessive activity of both pituitary ACTH and of hypothalamic corticotropin-releasing factor.

Evidence for increased pituitary and adrenal-cortical activity in post-traumatic states is abundant. Elevated glucocorticoids have been found in patients after severe trauma [38, 90, 117], burns [137, 187], operation [162], and infection [19]. These elevations persist throughout the period of stress in burn patients and correlate directly with the magnitude of the injury [137, 187]. Moderate hemorrhage in normal man, however, does not produce an elevation in serum cortisol [157]. In situations of moderate surgical trauma (e.g., cholecystectomy) the degree of corticosteroid response can be markedly altered by the degree of pre- and perioperative hydration [72].

The functional significance of elevated levels of circulating glucocorticoids in stressful situations is unclear. It has been long noted that the elevation in glucocorticoid activity does not correlate well with the obligate loss of urinary nitrogen that occurs with trauma as first described by Cuthbertson [48]. Ingle [93] has demonstrated and Campbell [36] has confirmed this lack of correlation by demonstrating that adrenalectomized rats on a fixed maintenance dose of glucocorticoid have a urinary nitrogen loss after femur fracture that is similar to the loss experienced by normal animals after similar fracture. On the basis of these experiments, it appears that the excessive nitrogen wasting occurs as long as adequate corticoids are available, but little function can be attributed to increased hormone levels. The glucocorticoid response has thus been termed "permissive" in that glucocorticoids are necessary for the stress response, but do not appear to mediate it [92].

Growth hormone has also been intensively studied as a possible mediator of the metabolic response to trauma. Striking elevations in circulating GH levels have been observed as part of the initial response to severe trauma [38], shock [38], operation [41, 128, 129], and exercise [129]. This response appears to be brief, however, as normal GH levels are observed in 1 to 2 days after trauma and throughout the first month after burn injury [38, 41, 137]. The origin of this early GH response is unclear at this time. Primary CNS stimulation of growth hormone-releasing factor by the arcuate nucleus of the hypothalamus seems most likely [113]. A response to peripherally released amino acids has also been proposed and, if operative, would also have to act through the hypothalamus, as both the ACTH and GH response to stress can be blocked by pituitary stalk section [29]. The significance of this response may be questioned. Its limitation to the very early period makes it an unlikely contributor to the metabolic derangement that follows severe trauma or a large thermal burn. An interesting finding, however, is that exogenously administered GH can enhance positive nitrogen balance in burn patients by elevating circulating insulin levels [183].

TSH and Thyroid Function. Another potential CNS effector mechanism is the hypothalamic production of thyrotropin-releasing factor (TRF), causing pituitary production of TSH and altering thyroid hormonal function. Early investigations of metabolic changes in trauma and sepsis indicated increased oxygen consumption and metabolic rate [43]. The influence of thyroid hormones on these functions encouraged much investigation into this area, but this investigation produced little evidence of altered function. However, the recent development of direct assays for thyroid hormones is producing a clearer picture of both the pituitary and the thyroid components of this system. Studies of TSH activity have revealed little evidence of abnormality in either the acute response to illness or the prolonged course of thermal trauma [30, 41, 137, 151]. Measurement of the thyroid hormones T_3, T_4, and reverse T_3 in the postoperative period [32] and after acute illness [30] has demonstrated a characteristic picture of normal T_4, depressed T_3, and elevated reverse T_3. This depression in T_3 has also been demonstrated in long-term stress in burn patients [137], and appears to be characteristic of most stress states [151]. These changes cannot be explained by changes in either prealbumin or thyroid-binding globulin [151]. However, in spite of evidence that T_3 is the active thyroid hormone in the periphery, this depression of circulating T_3 in acute stress states does not appear to cause hypothyroid symptoms [161].

New evidence is emerging to suggest a strong inverse correlation of circulating T_3 levels with both circulating epinephrine and norepinephrine levels in burn patients [17]. In this study, burn patients treated with metabolically active T_3 had higher circulating T_3 levels, lower catecholamine levels, and similar metabolic rates when compared with untreated burn patients. Thus, although depressed levels of T_3 are common after stress and injury, and may be related to sympathetic nervous system function, the significance of these findings is unknown. TSH and T_4 levels remain the best index of thyroid function after injury and are normal.

Pituitary-Gonadal Axis and Prolactin. The other three hormonal secretions of the anterior pituitary are LH, FSH, and PRL. Of these, LH is theoretically most important, as its level of activity controls the interstitial cells of both the ovaries and the testes. It thus controls the circulating levels of estrogen and testosterone. Of these gonadal hormones, testosterone is of particular interest because of its anabolic effects on skeletal muscle [192]. FSH is of some interest as a controller of the amenorrhea often mentioned as part of the response to trauma. PRL is of little potential influence in the trauma response.

The response of LH and testosterone to operative trauma has been examined. Both Aono [7] and Carstensen [39] have reported decreased testosterone levels for periods of one to two weeks following major operation. LH levels appear depressed during the first two days after operation and then return to normal levels [7, 41]. Over the first four weeks following severe thermal injury in young males, little depression in LH values was noted [137]. These studies suggest that the anabolic effect of testosterone may be diminished during the post-traumatic period. Diminished circulating testosterone may be mediated by the pituitary, or by some direct effect on the testis. FSH has also been studied in the operative and postoperative period, and little change in activity has been noted [7, 41]. FSH levels are, however, depressed in young males over the four weeks after thermal trauma [137].

Posterior Pituitary Response, Renin-Angiotensin Aldosterone Axis, and Control of Fluid and Electrolyte Balance. The posterior pituitary is distinct from the anterior pituitary in that (1) it has only one hormone active in the metabolic response to trauma and (2) it does not share the hypothalamaco-hypophyseal-portal system. Antidiuretic hormone is synthesized by neurons in the supraoptic nucleus of the hypothalamus, travels down axons through the pituitary stalk into the posterior lobe of the pituitary, and is secreted directly into the general systemic circulation [114]. It acts on the collecting system of the nephron to increase its permeability to water and thereby has a strong antidiuretic effect, decreasing free water clearance and decreasing urine output. Under normal circumstances this system responds primarily to osmotic stimuli and, along with CNS thirst mechanisms, maintains osmotic homeostasis [114].

It has been well demonstrated that operative trauma is a strong stimulus to ADH release and that the release lasts as long as the operation [125]. Further, the very short response time and the fact that regional anesthesia completely blocks the ADH response is evidence for a strictly neural transmission [125]. ADH is also known to be released by a variety of nonspecific stress stimuli including trauma and hypoglycemia [16, 18]. The practical significance of this system is that it prevents traumatized patients from excreting a free water load and is responsible for the hyponatremia that results when excessive free water is given to oliguric post-traumatic patients. This response to trauma is strong enough to totally over-ride the usual volume and osmotic feedback system [125]. This pathologic response can be treated with simple fluid intake restriction. Clinically, this situation is indicated by secretion of a hyperosmolar urine in the presence of a hypo-osmolar serum and is called the syndrome of inappropriate ADH secretion.

The renin-angiotensin aldosterone system is the second major endocrine system that may be under primary control of the autonomic nervous system in the post-traumatic state. Under normal circumstances, this system primarily responds to intravascular pressure and can be considered to be jointly controlled by the sympathetic nervous system, by the perfusion pressure of the arteriole in the area of the juxtaglomerular apparatus of the kidney, and by sodium flux at the macula densa of the kidney [134]. However, recent experience with burned children has demonstrated ninefold elevations of plasma renin activity (PRA) and fivefold elevations of serum aldosterone in children who are normotensive or hypertensive, normovolemic or hypervolemic, and with high levels of urinary sodium excretion [13, 136]. This evidence suggests that this system is highly active in the post-traumatic state and that it is not responsive to the usual feedback controls of blood pressure, vascular volume, and sodium balance. Experience with the beta blocking agent propranolol is providing further evidence of the importance of sympathetic control of this system [52]. The effect of this hyperactive system is to strongly influence the kidney to conserve sodium and excrete potassium. The combined effect of both the posterior pituitary response and the renin-aldosterone response is to make post-traumatic patients oliguric, hyponatremic, edematous, hypervolemic, and alkalotic (Figure 14-4).

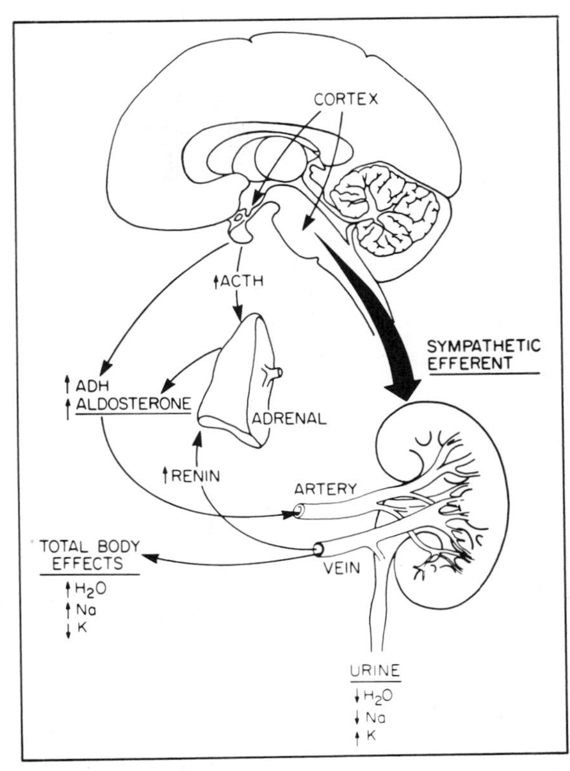

Figure 14-4. *Influence of neuroendocrine response to trauma on fluid and electrolyte balance.*

EFFECT OF STRESS AND INJURY ON BODY COMPOSITION

All of the alterations in neuroendocrine control mechanisms resulting from trauma profoundly affect total body composition and organ function. The most obvious change in body composition is change in total body weight. Body weight may increase if excess fluids are accumulated or de-

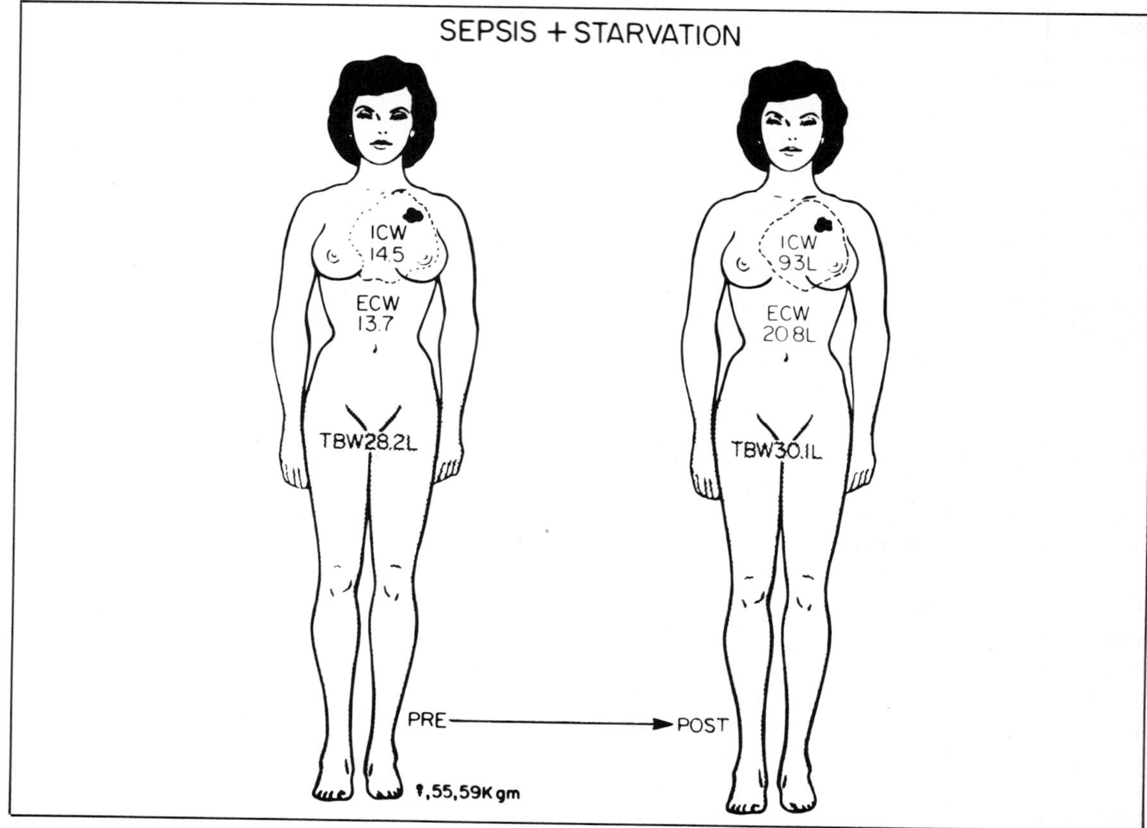

Figure 14-5. *Minimal change in total body water (TBW) associated with severe sepsis, starvation, and estimated change of body cell mass from 18.7 kg to 11.8 kg. Note decrease in intracellular water (ICW) and increase in extracellular water (ECW). (Adapted from F. D. Moore et al.* The Body Cell Mass and Its Supporting Environment. *Philadelphia: Saunders, 1963.)*

crease if some combination of fluid, fat, and lean body mass (muscle, viscera, and skeleton) is lost. Because of the tendency of fluid accumulation to mask decreases in lean body mass and fat, total body weight is a poor indicator of general nutritional and metabolic condition (Figure 14-5). Attention must therefore be focused on the individual components of body composition (Table 14-2). Changes in these components can be divided into two broad categories with regard to their responses to trauma: (1) changes in fluid and electrolyte components, and (2) changes in body tissue components. Changes in body tissue components are intimately related to changes in whole body energy exchange.

Fluid and Electrolytes in Response to Injury

Acute injury, whether it is an elective surgical procedure, local trauma, a burn, or hemorrhage, is accompanied by characteristic fluid and electrolyte changes that act to preserve intravascular fluid volume and maintain perfusion. There is an obligatory sodium retention, which is inevitably accompanied by fluid retention and mediated by the release of ADH and aldosterone. This fluid retention is accompanied by transcapillary refill and maintains blood volume (see Figure 14-4) [122, 156]. Tissue anoxia is prevented initially by

Table 14-2. *Normal Body Fluid and Tissue Components in Adult Men and Women*

	70-Kg Male		60-Kg Female	
	Total Wt. (kg)	% of Total Body Wt. (%)	Total Wt. (kg)	% of Total Body Wt. (%)
Total body water	42.0	60	31.2	52
Cellular tissue components				
Carbohydrate	0.5	1	0.5	1
Protein	9.8	14	6.5	11
Fat	12.5	18	17.4	29
Extracellular solids*	5.2	7	4.4	7
Total	70.0	100	60.0	100

*Primarily skeleton and supporting structures.

increased oxygen extraction so that the venous PO_2 falls [173]. This increased oxygen extraction allows compensation for quite large defects in red cell mass with little change in hemodynamics. Unfortunately, red cell mass loss frequently exceeds this compensatory mechanism, and major changes in cardiac function occur. These changes consist of selective organ perfusion and blood volume redistribution from peripheral venous reservoirs to the central circulation. When these adaptive mechanisms are overwhelmed by rapid or prolonged hemorrhage, hypovolemic shock characterized by low cardiac output and poor tissue perfusion results.

In addition to the aforementioned fluid shifts, a variety of acid-base balance changes and electrolyte changes frequently occur. Specific disorders are dependent on the magnitude of the injury, forms of treatment, and previous health of the patient. These disorders have been reviewed recently, and a full description of them is beyond the scope of this discussion [153]. The most common change is a mild alkalosis caused by hyperventilation, nasogastric tube loss of acid, increased aldosterone production, and administration of blood. This is frequently accompanied by potassium loss. The alkalosis may convert to acidosis if problems with oxygen exchange or tissue perfusion, or both, arise.

Mild changes in fluid retention and fluid redistribution are quickly overcome if the insult is removed or corrected. In situations of severe and profound sepsis, ongoing trauma, or massive body injury, a low flow state occurs, and one changes from compensated volume loss to a nonreversed low flow state. This latter is accompanied by cellular anoxia and death, with loss of organ function and content. This process is life-threatening and pre-empts any attempts at the preservation of the patient's surgical nutrition.

Energy Balance

Energy Requirements

A fundamental requirement in the postinjury state is the need for adequate energy to continue normal body function, to respond to pathologic energy demands, and to fuel the reparative process. Sources of this energy are either the exogenous (enteral or parenteral nutrition) or the endogenous utilization of body fuel stores.

Energy needs are normal or increased in traumatized man (Table 14-3). There is little or no increased need in uncomplicated postoperative patients [99]. Multiple fractures and sepsis cause moderate increases of 120 to 140 percent of normal resting needs. Major burns cause marked hy-

Table 14-3. *Energy Expenditures Measured in Different Clinical Conditions*

Condition	Resting Energy Expenditure	
	Calories (kcal/24 hrs)*	% of Normal*
Normal man	1800	100
Simple starvation (20 days)	1080	60
Postoperative	1800	100
Multiple fractures	2160	120
Major sepsis	2520	140
60% Burn:		
In 21°C environment	3600	200
In 25°C environment	3819	212
In 33°C environment	3342	185

*All values calculated assuming normal resting energy expenditure is 1800 kcal/24 hr.
Data from references 99, 103, and 181.

permetabolism, with increases in energy requirements of 180 to 200 percent [98, 99, 181]. Wilmore has further demonstrated that the degree of elevation of metabolic rate in burn patients is directly related to the size of the burn [181]. These elevations in metabolic rate observed in injured patients are in marked contrast to starving man, in whom a decreased metabolic rate is a prominent adaptive mechanism (see Table 14-3) [103].

Well-studied possible mediators of this hypermetabolic response to trauma include thyroid function and sympathetic nervous function. The data previously reviewed indicate that thyroid function is normal or depressed and should result in a hypometabolic state [137, 151]. A likely mediator of the hypermetabolic response is the sympathetic nervous system. Catecholamine secretion, which indicates sympathetic nervous system activity, is elevated in the traumatized patient [42, 64, 79, 136]. Further, both Wilmore [181] and Harrison [85] have demonstrated in burn patients that the degree of hypermetabolism can be related to total catecholamine excretion. Alpha and beta adrenergic blockade significantly decreases the metabolic rate of burn patients, and epinephrine infusions in normal man increase metabolic rate [181].

Two additional defects in energy metabolism in burned patients with bacteremia and with extensive injury have been demonstrated [181]. Patients studied during bacteremia had markedly decreased metabolic rates compared to their predicted rates or rates measured during nonseptic intervals. They also had excessively high catecholamine excretion rates during bacteremia; these were inappropriately high for the metabolic response measured. Patients with extensive injury also could not respond to a cool ambient temperature (21°C) with an increase in catecholamine excretion and metabolic rate elevation. The failure to increase metabolic rate in response to both increased levels of circulating catecholamines and cool ambient temperature is abnormal. These data all suggest that increased energy expenditure of up to 200 percent of normal is a fundamental component of the metabolic response to trauma, and that this response is mediated by the sympathetic nervous system. Bacteremia and extensive injury impair this response. These considerations indicate the increased need of injured patients for energy sources. Kinney [99] has estimated that an excess of 50 percent over resting metabolic energy expenditure is necessary for anabolism.

Effects on Body Composition

Recovery from severe injury, with or without sepsis, requires that the energy needs be met and that

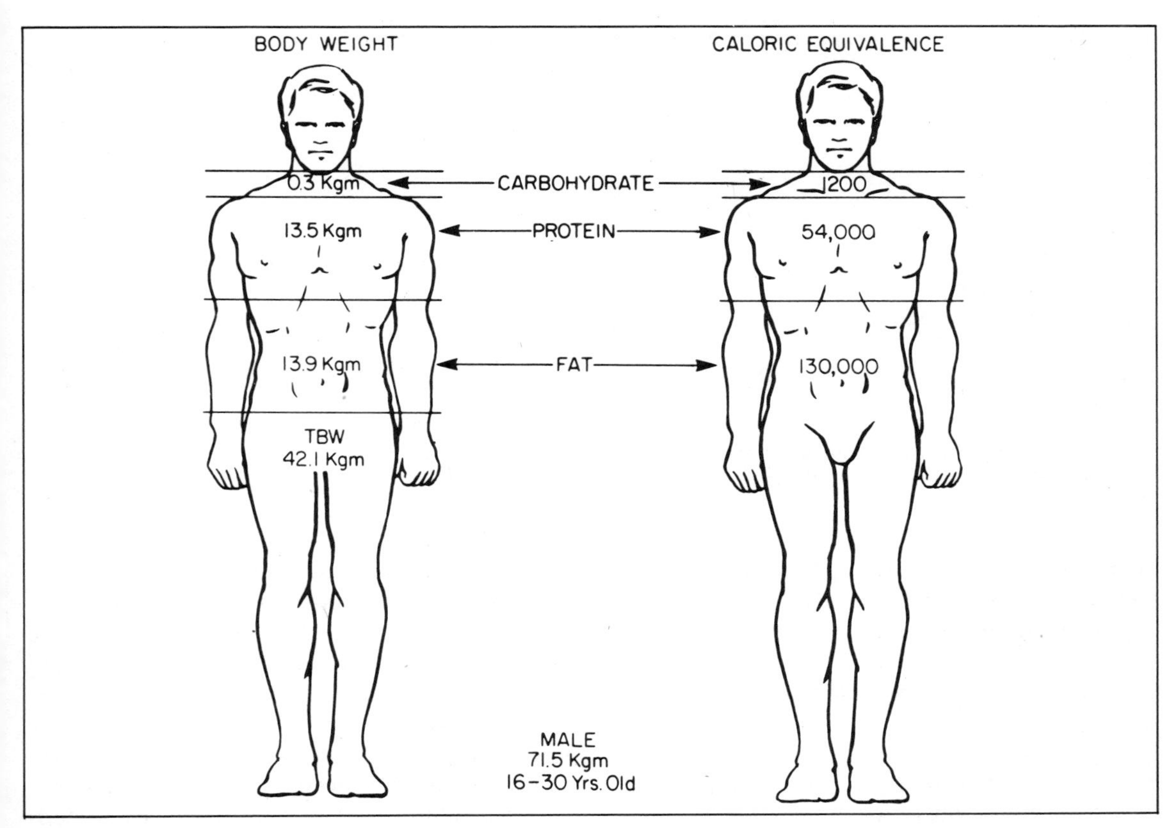

Figure 14-6. *Caloric equivalence of body mass in a healthy adult. (Adapted from M. F. Brennan, Metabolic response to surgery in the cancer patient: Consequences of aggressive multimodality therapy.* Cancer *43:2053, 1979.)*

biologic materials necessary for tissue repair be available [160]. An estimate of the normal body reserves of fuel has been derived from radioisotope dilution studies of the different body compartments [124, 155]. These estimates indicate that there is almost no reserve energy stored as carbohydrate, that the majority of energy is stored as fat, and that considerable energy can be mobilized from protein stores (Figure 14-6). In traumatized man, fat stores supply 80 to 85 percent of body energy needs [55].

Mobilization from protein reserves also occurs to a considerable extent. This is well demonstrated in the work of both Moore [124] and Shizgal [155], in which losses of 20 to 30 percent of the body cell mass have been observed during recovery from severe injury. This loss of body cell mass from catabolism of protein is also quite evident from studies of nitrogen balance. Losses of 20 gm of nitrogen daily are common in traumatized patients [23, 141]. As each gram of nitrogen is equivalent to approximately 30 gm of lean tissue, losses of 500 to 600 gm of lean body mass daily can occur in the severely injured, septic patient.

The effect of this catabolism frequently is loss of body weight. Both the composition of this weight loss and its effect on survival have been studied. Studies by Kinney [98] have suggested that, regardless of the total quantity of weight loss, protein makes up 10 percent of the total and fat 20 percent. Studies by Studley suggest that a 30 percent total body weight loss is usually fatal and that only occasional patients may sustain greater

Table 14-4. *Depletion of Components of Body Composition During Different Levels of Stress*

	Chronic Starvation	Postoperative State (Acute Starvation)	Major Injury/Burn
Caloric expenditure (kcal/24 hrs)	1200	1500	3500
30-Day weight loss (kg)[a]	6.3	12.6	23.0
Nitrogen loss (gm N/24 hrs)	3.0	10.0	20.0
Lean tissue loss (gm/24 hrs)	90	300	600
Days to lose 50% of total muscle mass[b]	128	38	19
Days to lose 50% of body cell mass[b]	217	65	33

[a]Often obscured by increases in total body water and electrolytes.
[b]Usually fatal.

losses [166]. The influence of the effect of various metabolic rates on the rate of weight loss is evident in Table 14-4.

Changes in Body Tissue Components

Protein Metabolism

Following an acute injury without a low flow state such as a major operation or burn, lean tissue mass is first mobilized and then lost. The loss is one of cellular content rather than cellular number, and the body protein reservoir is diminished. The major reservoir in man is skeletal muscle. These protein losses are manifested by mobilization of amino acids for the central (visceral) synthesis of energy substrate or protein. This loss of protein is accompanied by increased urinary nitrogen excretion with the major component of nitrogen excreted as urea. The increased urea excretion reflects increased gluconeogenesis. In the acute situation, these losses have little long-term effect, provided the injury is rapidly reversed.

Changes in Synthesis and Catabolism. The manner in which this net protein catabolism takes place is a subject of great debate. Recently attempts have been made to determine whether these events are the consequence of increased muscle protein catabolism or decreased protein synthesis. Available data indicate that changes in both protein synthesis and catabolism may depend on the severity of the injury (Table 14-5) [23, 97]. Severe burns [97], skeletal trauma [23], and sepsis [106] appear to cause marked increases in both synthesis and catabolism. Mild burns [97] and elective operation [45, 133] cause only minimal changes and may result in decreased synthesis and unchanged catabolism (see Table 14-5). These studies, unfortunately, have not been corrected for nutrient intake, which is a major factor influencing protein synthesis [76]. The effects of immobilization have also not been taken into account.

The foregoing data assume the validity of the methods used to measure protein synthesis and catabolism. These methodologies have recently been reviewed in depth, and several important concepts concerning available methodologies are emerging [172]. The use of constant infusion of ^{14}C-tyrosine probably underestimates whole body protein synthesis as plasma-specific activity of tyrosine underestimates the size of the precursor pool. However, this is balanced by an overestimation as constant infusions do not measure any oxidation of the labeled tracer. If perhaps 20 percent of the turnover could be accounted for by this oxidation, then an overestimation of turnover of 20 percent is possible. In man and in the rat, 12 to 15 percent of the turnover on a normal

Table 14-5. *Whole Body Protein Synthesis and Catabolism as Measured by Isotopic Tracer Methods in Various Clinical Conditions*

Author	Clinical Condition	Nutrient Intake of Subjects Relative to Control	% Normal Protein Synthesis	% Normal Protein Catabolism
Kien [97]	Severe burn	Variable	203	203
	Mild burn	Variable	114	106
Birkhahn [23]	Skeletal trauma	Same	150	179
Crane [45]	Elective operation	Same	77	94
O'Keefe [133]	Elective operation	Decreased	88	101
Long [106]	Sepsis	Same	121	121

diet can be accounted for by amino acid oxidation [172].

The variable response of protein synthesis and breakdown, depending on the severity of the injury, is also suggested by studies of urinary 3-methylhistidine (3-MEH) excretion. 3-MEH is formed by methylation of histidine in the peptide chains of actin and myosin only after protein synthesis [193]. 3-MEH is totally excreted in the urine after muscle breakdown without either reutilization or oxidation [193]. As 3-MEH is found in only skeletal muscle and platelets in significant quantities, measurement of urinary excretion of 3-MEH predicts skeletal muscle breakdown. 3-MEH has been measured sequentially during starvation in obese subjects and demonstrates a progressive decline similar to the decline in total nitrogen excretion classically observed during adaptation to starvation [193].

3-MEH has also been measured during injury and sepsis. Measurements in patients with large burns [22] and patients with normoketonuric trauma [176] both indicate marked increase in muscle catabolism after severe injury. Similar marked increases in 3-MEH excretion have been observed during severe septic events [108]. Patients after minor operative procedures and with hyperketonuria after trauma had normal rates of 3-MEH excretion [176]. These studies suggest that the catabolic response of skeletal muscle, as measured with 3-MEH excretion, is similar to total body protein catabolism, as measured with isotopic tracers. In severe injury there is a marked increase in muscle and total body catabolism, whereas in minor or moderate trauma, both skeletal muscle and total body protein breakdown are little changed. In the studies of Bilmazes [22], in which patients with large burns were studied with both 3-MEH excretion and isotopic tracers, the percentage contribution of muscle breakdown to whole body protein breakdown (19.1 ± 7.6%, mean ± SD) was similar to that of unburned children, even though both muscle and total body protein catabolism were markedly elevated.

The response of nitrogen balance and 3-MEH excretion to exogenously administered amino acids in traumatized patients is also of interest. Addition of adequate levels of amino acids with adequate energy substrate markedly improves nitrogen balance compared to administration of energy substrate alone [171]. Measurement of 3-MEH under each of these conditions, however, indicates no difference in skeletal muscle catabolic rates [171]. These data suggest that exogenous nutritional support is effective in increasing protein synthesis in the presence of increased protein catabolism, and that increased protein synthesis results in improved nitrogen balance.

Plasma and Muscle Amino Acid Changes in Response to Injury. Much recent interest has focused on plasma and muscle amino acid changes in trauma and sepsis as a means of understanding changes in protein metabolism and of devising optimal nutritional therapy. Plasma amino acids are not influenced by general anesthesia [49]. Elective operations of moderate severity (cholecystectomy or vagotomy and pyloroplasty) cause a slight decrease in nonessential amino acids and a mild rise in the essential amino acids (valine, leucine, isoleucine, phenylalanine, lysine, and tyrosine) [49]. Operations of greater severity (abdominal aortic bifurcation graft) cause changes identical to those of moderate operative trauma [49]. Severe trauma causes a twofold rise in the branched chain amino acids (valine, leucine, isoleucine), which is maximal 4 to 7 days after the trauma and is much more pronounced in patients who remain normoketonuric than in those developing a hyperketonuria [174]. Severe sepsis causes marked elevations of phenylalanine and methionine, with few changes in the branched-chain amino acids [65, 189].

Studies of intracellular muscle-free amino acids have been performed on specimens of quadraceps muscle obtained from percutaneous needle biopsy before and 4 days after total hip replacement [10]. These studies reveal increases in branched-chain amino acids, phenylalanine, tyrosine, and methionine, which were accompanied by parallel changes in plasma amino acids. There was a marked decrease in intracellular-free glutamine, which was not accompanied by a similar plasma change. These changes were not affected by isotonic infusions of dextrose or amino acids, or both.

These studies all suggest that there is a specific plasma and intracellular pattern of amino acid concentration change in response to trauma. The interpretation of these changes is obscure at this time. The elevations in branched-chain amino acids are of interest because they are thought to be the main source of energy derived from proteolysis in muscle and to participate in a branched-chain amino acid-alanine shunt, which shuttles amino and gluconeogenic precursors to the liver [132]. It has also been reported that infusions of branched-chain amino acids may be as effective in promoting positive nitrogen balance as are balanced mixtures containing all essential and nonessential amino acids [66]. Increased branched-chain amino acids may either reflect increased muscle catabolism or be a necessary stimulus to increased protein synthesis. The finding that 3-methylhistidine excretion shows postoperative muscle protein breakdown that parallels the increased total body nitrogen loss, and that exogenous amino acid administration improves nitrogen balance in spite of increased protein turnover, implies that amino acids act by stimulating protein synthesis. Therefore, the observed increases in plasma and muscle branched-chain amino acids would be expected to stimulate protein synthesis and limit rather than reflect the post-traumatic protein catabolism.

The finding of high levels of aromatic (phenylalanine and tyrosine) and sulfur-containing (methionine and cysteine) amino acids in sepsis and trauma suggests impaired liver function in clearance. The aromatic amino acids have also been implicated as adversely influencing neurotransmission and perhaps causing the metabolic encephalopathy sometimes observed in severe sepsis [65]. Attempts have been made to treat both postoperative trauma and metabolic encephalopathy with intravenous administration of solutions high in branched-chain amino acids and low in aromatic amino acids [65, 66]. The decreased intracellular glutamine concentrations are prominent and enigmatic. They are probably important, as glutamine comprises more than 50 percent of the free intracellular amino acid pool and decreased levels may limit protein synthesis [10].

Effects of Amino Acid Infusions. Isotonic amino acids have been administered to man as the sole nutritional substrate under a variety of clinical conditions. Interest in these infusions was stimulated by reports indicating that positive nitrogen balance could be achieved by quantities of these infusions that were insufficient to meet the patient's caloric needs [24]. It was further suggested that isotonic amino acids alone were more beneficial than amino acids and glucose or glucose alone, because the glucose stimulated insulin secretion, which suppressed lipolysis and interfered with the utilization of endogenous fat as energy substrate [24]. The "protein sparing" effect of isotonic amino acids then resulted, because endogenous fat became the primary energy source rather than the utilization of endogenous protein for gluconeogenesis.

This proposed beneficial effect of isotonic amino acids has been vigorously investigated. Tweedle [167] infused isotonic amino acids in fasting normal man and was unable to demonstrate positive nitrogen balance. Wolfe [188] compared amino acids alone with glucose alone, lipid alone, and combinations of amino acids, glucose, and lipid in fasting normal man. These studies suggest that nitrogen balance is most dependent on calorie intake, but that provision of amino acids and energy substrate is better than provision of energy substrate alone [188]. All of these studies in fasting normal man indicate that large quantities of infused amino acids are utilized as energy substrate with increased production of urea when amino acids are infused without adequate energy substrate.

Similar, although less extensive, studies of isotonic amino acid infusions with and without energy substrate have been conducted in postoperative patients [78] and in burned patients [116]. Studies in postoperative patients demonstrated a protein sparing effect of amino acid infusion, but this could not be related to the degree of endogenous fat mobilization [78]. The study in burn patients indicates a similar effect of isocaloric infusions of amino acids or glucose in patients with or without bacteremia [116]. The effects of both infusions were additive and nitrogen balance was most dependent on caloric intake [116].

Changes in Carbohydrate Metabolism

Glucose Kinetics. Hyperglycemia has long been recognized as a principal biochemical abnormality in traumatized and septic patients [81, 177]. This finding can result from either increased production of glucose or decreased utilization, or both. Only recently have the mechanisms involved been clarified.

Early studies documented increased blood glucose levels and glucose tolerance curves resembling those seen in diabetic patients [81, 177]. These data give rise to the concept of "stress diabetes" and suggested an insulin deficiency and decreased peripheral glucose utilization. However, recent data, summarized in Table 14-6, suggest that glucose production and utilization are increased in hypermetabolic traumatized patients. Wilmore has demonstrated markedly increased glucose flow in burn patients by mathematical analysis of glucose tolerance curves [182] and by measuring blood flow and arteriovenous glucose differences across the splanchnic circulation [179]. Long [109] administered U-^{14}C-glucose to normal subjects, postoperative patients, and patients with severe trauma and sepsis. Analysis of disappearance of the labeled glucose and appearance of labeled CO_2 suggested little change in glucose turnover in postoperative patients, but a doubling of both glucose pool size and glucose turnover in the traumatized patients [109]. Gump [80] used arterial, peripheral venous, and hepatic venous catheters with infusion of indocyanine green to measure hepatic glucose production and peripheral glocuse utilization in septic and traumatized patients. These studies demonstrated increased hepatic production of glucose and impaired hepatic uptake of an administered glucose load. Insulin was released from the splanchnic bed during glucose infusion, but did not decrease hepatic glucose production. All these studies indicate two- to threefold increases in hepatic glucose production in injured and septic patients.

The destination of the increased glucose produced in injured patients has recently been clarified. Studies of glucose utilization in fasting postabsorptive man have suggested that approximately 225 gm/day of glucose is utilized by brain, red cells, white cells, marrow, and cardiac muscle [61]. Measurements of glucose production in burned and traumatized patients suggest glucose production from 278 gm/day in trauma patients [80] to 1016 gm/day in patients with 40 percent burns [182]. Wilmore [178] has studied leg blood flow and substrate utilization in patients with 40 percent burns who either had burns involving legs or did not. Patients in both groups had similar

Table 14-6. *Glucose Production Rates in Man (% of Postabsorptive Control)*

	Rate of Gluconeogenesis (%)	Glucose Pool Size (%)
Postabsorptive man	100	100
Resuscitated burn	155	230
Hypermetabolic burn	255	116
Septic burn	141	145
Elective operation	109	125
Major injury and sepsis	213	201

Data from references 109 and 177.

sized burns and similar elevations in cardiac output and oxygen consumption. Patients with leg burns, however, demonstrated increased blood flow, glucose utilization, and lactate production in the burned legs. Oxygen consumption was not increased in burned legs. This study and in vitro studies of energy requirements of reparative tissues (fibroblasts, macrophages, leukocytes) suggest that the wound is highly dependent on anaerobic energy production from glucose.

Substrate for Gluconeogenesis. The primary question raised by the high levels of gluconeogenesis just demonstrated is: What is the metabolic substrate utilized for production of glucose? It is well known that fat cannot be converted to glucose, although the glycerol released by hydrolysis of triglyceride would be readily converted to glucose [175]. Quantitative estimates of glycerol release in trauma patients are not, however, currently available to permit estimation of the utilization of this source.

Another gluconeogenic substrate available in large quantities in traumatized patients is lactate. The studies of burn wounds already discussed have suggested that 80 percent of glucose consumed by an injured extremity is converted to lactate [178]. These studies can be used to estimate lactate production from the entire burn wound, and these estimates of peripheral lactate production have been found to be comparable to recent measurements of hepatic lactate uptake [178, 179]. In the same studies, measurements of glucose flow across the kidney indicated a net uptake of glucose by the kidney, thus suggesting the liver as the sole source of glucose production in injured man [179]. All these data can be used in calculations that suggest that lactate provides approximately 30 percent of the gluconeogenic substrate for the liver in patients with major burns under most circumstances and can provide up to 45 percent of the substrate in patients with severe complications [179].

The marked negative nitrogen balance, muscle wasting, weakness, and decrease in lean body mass demonstrated by body composition studies in traumatized patients suggest that amino acids stored in skeletal muscle would also be a likely source of gluconeogenic substrate. Previous discussion of amino acid metabolism in skeletal muscle suggests that oxidation of branched-chain amino acids occurs preferentially in the muscle of trauma patients. There are also extensive data from postabsorptive man (subjects after an overnight fast), man after prolonged starvation, and exercising man to suggest that alanine is synthesized de novo in muscle and accounts for as much as 33 percent of the substrate utilized by the liver for gluconeogenesis under these circumstances [61-63]. This evidence is primarily derived from arterial and venous sampling of glucose and substrate, and of blood flow measurements across the liver and muscle beds.

Similar studies have been accomplished in patients with major burns. Aulick [12] has measured

Table 14-7. *Amino Acid Release by Skeletal Muscle and Uptake by Liver in Postabsorptive Man and Man After Thermal Injury (% of Total Molar Quantity of Amino Acids)*

	Skeletal Muscle Release		Liver Uptake	
	Postabsorptive	Burn	Postabsorptive	Burn
Alanine	−39	−26	+45	+35
Glycine	−13	−18	+8	+18
Lysine	−11		+9	+10
Proline	−10	−11		+3
Threonine	−7	−8	+8	+14
Histidine	−6		+7	−2
Leucine	−6	−11		+1
Valine	−5	−7		−5
Arginine	−4			−3
Phenylalanine	−3	−5	+2	+9
Tyrosine	−2		+5	+5
Methionine	−2	−1	+3	+4
Isoleucine	−2	−5		+1
Taurine	+1			−2
Ornithine	+1			+8
Cysteine	+4		+4	+2
Serine	+4	−8	+9	+4
Total μmol/min	−135	−655	+253	+619

Data from references 61 and 179.

amino acid release by skeletal muscle in burn patients. These studies indicate that 26 percent of released amino acid is alanine and 18 percent is glycine (Table 14-7). As the composition of skeletal muscle contains far less alanine and glycine than is being released by muscle, it is evident that alanine and glycine are being synthesized de novo from the nitrogen and portions of the carbon skeletons of other amino acids. A recent study of splanchnic uptake of amino acids in burn patients indicates that alanine and glycine are preferentially taken up by the liver [179]. Hepatic glucose production was also measured in this study of burn patients and combined with the amino acid uptake data in calculations that indicate that 22 to 34 percent of substrate for gluconeogenesis is provided by amino acids [179].

These data suggest that an alanine "shunt" for the movement of three carbon fragments and ammonia from skeletal muscle to the liver for production of glucose and urea is functional in traumatized patients (Figure 14-7). The production of radioactive tracer-labeled glucose from infusions of labeled alanine in traumatized man is further evidence that alanine is a functional substrate under these conditions [61, 107].

One problem with the foregoing data is that all measurements have been performed on plasma and that glutamine and glutamate have not been measured. The dynamic relationship between amino acids in the red cell, plasma, and tissue has been demonstrated [4, 60]. Aoki has provided data that suggest that the red cell compartment may contribute quantities of amino acid substrate to tissue equal to that contributed by the plasma compartment [5, 6]. Studies of glutamine and glutamate levels in forearm arterial and venous blood indicate that these amino acids are quantitatively

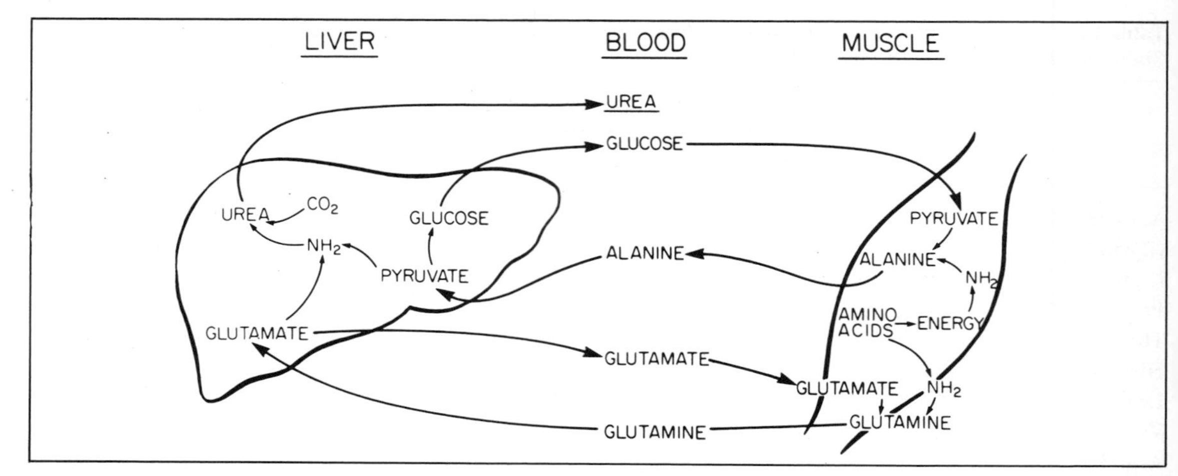

Figure 14-7. *Glucose-alanine shunt and glutamine-glutamate shunt, which result in transfer of ammonia from muscle to liver for production of urea. Alanine also transfers 3-carbon units, which serve as substitute for hepatic gluconeogenesis.*

important substrates and that glutamine release by muscle and glutamate uptake by the liver can shunt amino groups to the liver in a manner similar to the alanine shunt [4]. Therefore, the aforementioned measurements of amino acid uptake by the liver as gluconeogenic substrate in burned patients may be underestimated [179].

Effect of Glucose Infusions. Studies of glucose infusions in starving man and in depleted man demonstrate that exogenous glucose markedly decreases urinary nitrogen excretion [70, 131]. Similar studies in injured man have demonstrated this effect, but glucose is not nearly so effective in hypermetabolic injured patients as in hypometabolic starving subjects [8]. Measurements of gluconeogenic rates from tracer infusions of labeled amino acids similarly suggest that glucose will suppress gluconeogenesis in injured man, but that much higher rates of glucose infusion are necessary than in starving man [31, 59, 107].

The mechanisms involved in this exaggerated gluconeogenic response are most likely the altered hormonal environment of the traumatized patient. The elevations in circulating catecholamines, glucagon, and cortisol, and the relative deficiency of insulin have been described. The importance of the relative insulin deficiency in promoting gluconeogenesis is evident from recent studies of infusion of glucose and insulin. In these studies, insulin markedly enhances the nitrogen sparing of glucose [190]. An interesting recent finding is evidence that epinephrine secretion correlates with the rate of glucose infusion [8, 59]. The significance of this later finding is unclear at this time.

Another area currently being studied is the effect of glucose infusion rates that are in excess of energy expenditure. This area of study is important because of the ease with which this can be accomplished with current total parenteral nutrition techniques. These studies suggest that glucose oxidation increases with increases in glucose infusion up to about 5 mg/kg/min (504 gm/70 kg/day) in injured patients, but that little additional glucose is oxidized at rates beyond this [31, 59]. The fate of glucose that is not oxidized is currently being examined. Studies by Askanazi [8] suggest that an RQ above 1.0, indicating fat synthesis, is rarely observed in hypermetabolic patients. Excess glucose given to these patients appears to be stored primarily as glycogen [8]. However, these authors have not studied patients receiving more than 5 mg/kg/min or past the fifth day of TPN. Burke [31] has studied rates of infusion almost twice this high in burned patients. He has noted definite increases in nonprotein RQ above 1.0, has documented extensive fat deposits in the liver in patients dying after intravenous glucose infusions of 9.3 to 17 mg/kg/min, and has stressed the disadvantages of the high glucose load [31]. Askanazi has also demonstrated the increased ventilation necessary to increase oxygen uptake and CO_2 excretion at high levels of glucose infusion [9, 11]. Both studies suggest that glucose loads in TPN should not greatly exceed metabolic expenditures.

Changes in Fat Metabolism

Fat Utilization and Kinetics. A primary question regarding fat metabolism in traumatized patients is: To what extent is fat utilized? The relatively large store of energy in body fat is readily apparent from body composition studies (see Figure 14-7). There is little question that fat is used extensively during starvation and that the body adapts to starvation by decreasing the metabolic rate and increasing the quantity of fat used to supply energy [34, 103]. The meager supplies of carbohydrate stored as glycogen are utilized during the first two days of starvation, and the decline of protein used to low levels is evident from the decrease in urinary nitrogen excretion [103].

In traumatized and septic patients, however, metabolic rate increases and high levels of urinary nitrogen excretion persist. This had led some investigators to postulate that protein is the primary fuel following injury [35]. Detailed calorimetry studies by Duke [55], however, demonstrate little difference in the percent of protein contribution to the resting metabolic rate in patients studied preoperatively (16.5 percent) and during postoperative days 1 to 4 (15.6 percent). Groups of patients studied late in the postoperative period (18 to 21 days) with sepsis, with trauma, and with burns had percentages of protein contribution ranging from 9.4 to 20.4 percent. These results differ from those of Moore [124], who used sequential body composition studies in the postoperative period and concluded that 50 percent of tissue loss was fat and 50 percent protein. However, most studies indicate that the predominant fuel in traumatized man is fat.

Evidence supporting fat utilization in traumatized patients is also found in the descriptions of elevated levels of circulating free fatty acids and glycerol [117, 181]. The kinetics of fatty acid metabolism have not been studied in this clinical setting, and in the absence of data suggesting decreased peripheral utilization of fat, it can only be presumed that high levels of circulating free fatty acids indicate net lipolysis of adipose tissue. The hormonal milieu of traumatized patients, which includes increased levels of catecholamines and levels of insulin inappropriately low for glucose levels, would strongly favor lipolysis. Catecholamines stimulate lipolysis by cyclic AMP-mediated increases in lipase activity [163]. Insulin is the chief storage hormone, and low levels of insulin favor free fatty acid release [33].

Effects of Exogenous Fat Infusion. The recent availability of fat emulsions that can be infused as a caloric source has allowed study of the metabolic effects of exogenous lipid infusions. The aqueous solution most commonly used consists of an emulsion of 10 percent soybean oil, 2.25 percent glycerol, and 1.2 percent egg yolk phospholipids. Fifty-four percent of the soybean oil is essential linoleic acid. These solutions can be given as a caloric source and/or to prevent essential fatty acid deficiency.

The major questions arising when fat solutions are given as caloric sources are: Are they utilized and are they as effective as glucose in preventing proteolysis? Evidence suggesting utilization rests primarily on the findings that fat is cleared from plasma and stabilizes patient weight when given in relatively large quantities over prolonged periods of time to traumatized patients [170, 184]. No suggestion of toxicity has developed during this administration [184]. ^{14}C-labeled triglycerides have been given to postoperative patients as part of a 10 percent lipid solution and suggest approximately 30 percent of the infused lipid is metabolized to carbon dioxide during the first 24 hours [56].

The protein sparing ability of infused fat has been debated. Jeejeebhoy [95] compared parenteral nutrition solutions containing either all glucose or predominantly lipid as the energy source for a group of nutritionally depleted patients. In this well-designed crossover study, no difference in protein sparing was noted between either the lipid or the glucose systems. Long [110] administered a series of solutions with varying proportions of fat and glucose to patients with severe burns. This study showed that urea nitrogen excretion was inversely related to carbohydrate intake and directly related to metabolic rate. Fat infusions exerted no nitrogen sparing effect. Maximal nitrogen sparing was achieved when carbohydrate calories were given in quantities approximating the resting metabolic rate. These later findings are supported by studies in normal fasting man, in which all protein sparing from lipid infusions is demonstrated to be secondary to the glycerol contained in the solutions [27].

OTHER MAJOR FACTORS INFLUENCING THE METABOLIC RESPONSE TO TRAUMA

The common sequelae of major trauma include invasive infection, shock and low-flow states, and inability to resume oral intake of nutrients. These factors can markedly enhance the neurophysiologic stress response, which has just been described, and can independently influence the metabolic response to trauma.

Trauma Complicated by Infection

Hypermetabolic Response

The development of invasive infection intensifies the metabolic response to trauma. Kinney [99] has demonstrated that the energy expenditure of patients after major uncomplicated elective operation rarely differs from preoperative values by more than 10 percent. In contrast, development of a serious complicating infection, such as peritonitis, is accompanied by an increase of 20 to 50 percent over the predicted resting energy expenditure [55, 99]. Similarly, uncomplicated gastrectomy has little effect on the body cell mass (95 to 99 percent of predicted), whereas the same operation complicated by peritonitis causes a major reduction in body cell mass (63 to 78 percent of predicted) [124]. Urinary nitrogen excretion is higher in postoperative patients with complicating infection than in those with uncomplicated postoperative courses [55]. Although the aforementioned trend toward greatly increased catabolism with infection is usually observed, it is of interest that Wilmore's studies [181, 182] of burned patients during periods of bacteremia have demonstrated a significant decrease in energy expenditure and in glucose turnover when compared to the extremely high rates (energy expenditure 50 to 120 percent higher than predicted) usually observed in hypermetabolic burn patients [181, 182].

Mediation of Response to Infection

Local Inflamation and Increased Tissue Destruction. The increase in catabolism caused by infection raises the question: How is it mediated? Experimental studies of infection have suggested three basic pathways (Figure 14-8). The first of these is the increase in local tissue destruction caused by the infecting organism and the resulting inflammatory response. This inflammatory reaction includes increased vascular permeability, leukocyte migration, and cell death. This reaction results in the release of lysosomal enzymes as well as specific chemical mediators including histamine, kinins, prostaglandins, and serotonin [186]. These substances are all capable of stimulating afferent nerve endings and thereby amplifying the entire neurophysiologic response to stress.

Effects of Fever. A second major effect of infection complicating a traumatic injury is the production of fever. The mechanism involving the release of endogenous pyrogen (EP) by phagocytic cells after the ingestion of bacteria, and the action of EP on the hypothalamus to increase

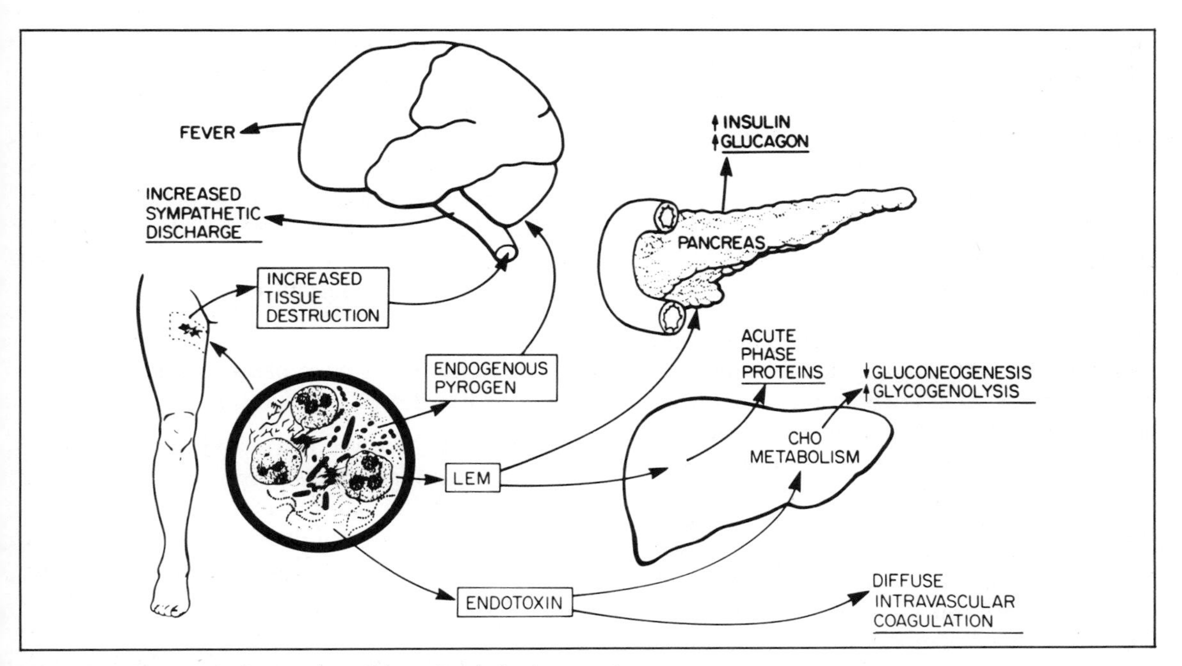

Figure 14-8. *Metabolic results of invasive infection mediated by increased tissue destruction, endogenous pyrogen, leukocyte endogenous mediator (LEM), and endotoxin.*

body temperature have been previously discussed. The effect of this elevation is to dramatically increase the catabolic response. DuBois [54] has demonstrated a 13 percent average increase in energy expenditure for each degree centigrade of temperature elevation. He also found a linear relationship between energy expenditure and body temperature for five different bacterial infections. Similarly, Beisel [20] has demonstrated that hyperthermia mechanically induced in normal human volunteers results in decreased nutrient intake and increased urinary excretion of nitrogen and resulting negative nitrogen balance. Both of these studies indicate that the production of fever markedly increases the catabolic response, probably by increasing the rate of all bodily biochemical reactions, as suggested by DuBois [54].

Effects of Other Chemical Mediators. The third effect of infection is the release of other chemical mediators, which may come either from phagocytosing cells or the bacteria themselves. Endogenous pyrogen is one example of a well-classified mediator released by phagocytes. Another recently described substance (or group of substances) is leukocyte endogenous mediator (LEM). LEM is a protein of molecular weight 10,000 to 30,000, which is chemically distinguishable from both pyrogen and endotoxin [112]. LEM appears to act directly on the liver to increase amino acid flux and cause production of acute phase globulin proteins [96, 140]. It also may act directly on the pancreas to increase insulin and glucagon secretion [71]. Endotoxin released by gram-negative bacteria is another chemical mediator capable of producing profound metabolic effects. It influences both the hormonal and cellular immune systems and the coagulation system. These influences can be extensive and have recently been reviewed [126]. Animal work by McCallum and Berry [115] also suggests that endotoxin can markedly influence carbohydrate metabolism. Effects include liver glycogen depletion and reduced gluconeogenesis from ^{14}C-labeled alanine and pyruvate. Animals poisoned with endotoxin also had markedly reduced circulating blood glucose. This experimental interference with glucose production by endotoxin is similar to the diminished glucose turnover in burned patients during gram-negative bacteremia [182].

Metabolic Effects of Infection in the Absence of Trauma

The effects of an infectious process in the absence of trauma are catabolic and similar to the response to trauma. Beisel has demonstrated negative balances of nitrogen and other intracellular minerals in response to experimentally induced intracellular infections in man [19, 21]. The negative nitrogen balances are the result of both decreased nutrient intake and enhanced urinary excretion of urea and ammonia. Hormonal changes are also similar to those seen in trauma and consist of elevations in catecholamines [79], cortisol [21], glucagon [142, 194], aldosterone [21], and insulin [21]. The elevations in insulin that have been reported are not elevated appropriately to the elevations in glucose that are concomitantly observed. Elevations of glucagon are high, and the molar ratio of insulin to glucagon is usually depressed into the range observed in trauma [105, 117], hemorrhagic shock [117], early starvation [168, 169], and severe exercise [169]. All of these are energy-requiring catabolic situations, and the low insulin:glucagon ratio indicates the predominance of the catabolic and gluconeogenic hormone glucagon over the anabolic hormone insulin. In addition to the inappropriately low levels of insulin observed in infection, there is evidence to suggest that there is diminished peripheral sensitivity to its anabolic action [144]. All of the foregoing data suggest that the response to infection is similar to the response to trauma. The effect of infection when it complicates trauma is to both increase the intensity and prolong the activity of the catabolic response.

Effects of Shock and Low-Flow States

Another mechanism that mediates the systemic response of trauma or sepsis is shock and poor tissue perfusion. This may be brought on by loss of bodily fluids into the traumatized area (i.e., burn wound edema or gastrointestinal losses with intestinal obstruction), or by the effects of toxins on either the vasculature or the myocardium (endotoxin or myocardial depressant factor). The net effect of all these mechanisms is to deprive normal tissues distant from the wound of their required oxygen substrate and nutrient requirements.

Enhancement of Neuroendocrine Stress Response

Blood and fluid loss is a strong stimulus to the neurophysiologic stress response. The afferent receptors are the baroreceptors of the aortic arch, the chemoreceptors of the carotid body, the atrial volume receptors, and the juxtaglomerular apparatus of the kidney. Stimulation of these by diminished circulating volumes and perfusion pressures cause a massive sympathetic response, which includes the outpouring of catecholamines, sympathetic nervous discharge, glucagon, cortisol, renin, aldosterone, and ADH. All these mechanisms tend to shunt blood from storage areas (spleen, splanchnic, and extremity veins) to provide increased flow to vital structures (brain, heart, and wound). This response can be quite effective in compensating for moderate degrees of fluid loss (1500 ml blood in normal man) or for more severe losses for short periods of time [157, 158]. During this time, this response induces severe bodily catabolism, and therefore compensated marginal perfusion situations should be corrected as soon as they are recognized.

Cellular Damage from Low-Flow States

Blood or fluid losses significant enough to cause major impairment of tissue perfusion, usually indicated by low blood pressures, oliguria, cyanosis, and mental confusion can also markedly influence the systemic response to trauma by causing distant tissue damage. Haldane clearly recognized this situation when he remarked that "anoxia not only stops the machine, but wrecks the machinery" [14]. The effect is well demonstrated in the laboratory by the "taking up" phenomenon in animal shock models. This occurs when the systemic pressure is reduced to shock levels (usually 40 to 50 mm Hg) by bleeding into a reservoir kept in continuity with the animal's arterial system and maintained at that pressure level. The animal's cardiovascular system initially adjusts to this low perfusion pressure. For a limited time period, the animal can be completely resuscitated by simply reinfusing the shed blood. After a period of several hours, however, the arterial system dilates and increased quantities of blood (130 to 150 percent) must be reinfused to continue the same low level of perfusion pressure. Following this point, most investigators term the shock "irreversible," since most animals will die regardless of treatment [73]. This laboratory model clearly illustrates the systemic damage inflicted by blood loss and prolonged low-flow states. The same phenomenon is readily observed in the clinical sequelae following shock resuscitation. Brain death can occur after as little as four minutes of cardiac arrest [165]. Acute renal failure and acute pulmonary insufficiency are frequently observed after episodes of circulatory insufficiency and poor tissue perfusion [104, 123]. Hepatic impairment secondary to poor tissue perfusion during periods of shock has also been described [40].

Cell Membrane Effects. Recent research utilizing shock animal models is detailing many of the events that occur at the cellular level (see Figure 14-5). The work of Shires [154] and that of Sayeed [148] suggest that the initial insult to the cell interferes with the sodium pump located in the cell membrane. This causes loss of the normal cell membrane potential difference, allows sodium and water to enter the cell, and allows potassium to escape. If resuscitation is performed, these abnormalities disappear. Sayeed [148] also tested the sodium pump capability in liver slices from shocked animals by cooling them to stop the Na-K pump, measuring the major shifts of sodium into and potassium out of the cooled cells, and then measuring cation changes that occur with warming. Liver tissue slices from control animals were able to decrease intracellular sodium and increase intracellular potassium upon warming to a much greater extent than were liver slices from shocked animals. Further, if liver slices are incubated with ouabain and oxygen consumption is measured, liver slices from control animals demonstrate a 30 percent decrease in respiration, whereas liver slices from shocked animals exhibit no change. As ouabain is considered to selectively inhibit respiration coupled to the Na-K transport process, these data suggest that the low-flow state has selectively damaged the ion pump mechanism [148].

Effects on Mitochondria. The effects of low-flow state on mitochondrion have also been studied. The work of Sayeed [147] and that of Mela [118] demonstrate marked impairment in mitochondrial function and the production of ATP as the low-flow state progresses. This biochemical impairment correlates with the swelling and bursting of the mitochondria that are observed in electron microscopic preparations of mitochondria taken from animals at various times after the onset of shock [14]. Baue [14] has also measured concentration of glucose-6-phosphate, ATP, ADP, AMP, and inorganic phosphate levels in liver, muscle, and kidney from animals in early and in late shock and compared them with tissue from control animals. This determination indicated that concentrations of glucose and the adenosine phosphates fell markedly in shocked animals, while levels of inorganic phosphates increased. These data are interpreted as demonstrating a progressive fall in intracellular energy from deficient mitochondrial activity.

Insulin Insensitivity. One further area of cellular abnormality, as demonstrated in hemorrhagic shock models, is insulin insensitivity. Ryan [144], working with adipose tissue and muscle from rabbits exposed to circulating pressures of 30 mm Hg for 30 minutes and then resuscitated, showed decreased oxidation of glucose to CO_2 and decreased incorporation of glucose into both glycogen and neutral lipid in the presence of insulin. Insulin stimulation of amino acid incorporation of leucine into muscle protein was also diminished in shocked animals. However, the capacity of muscle to oxidize leucine in the presence of insulin was enhanced by shock. These studies were continued at intervals up to 30 days in surviving animals, and insulin resistance was noted to persist for 7 to 10 days in animals that made complete recoveries.

Baue [14] has found that there was no change in insulin-stimulated uptake of glucose in muscle from shocked rats compared to a twofold increase in uptake observed in muscle from normal animals. Wright and Henderson [191] have demonstrated a marked decrease in glucose utilization in shocked pigs which was accompanied by a large increase in both portal and systemic insulin levels. They also demonstrated that cellular free glucose rose in both red blood cells and muscle cells in response to a glucose load, but fell in liver cells. They interpreted these data to indicate that transport of glucose across cell walls in response to insulin was intact, but that a defect in phosphorylation existed. All of these studies of response to insulin of tissues exposed to periods of decreased tissue perfusion indicate derangement of several important metabolic activities.

From these data, it has been suggested that cell death occurs when the energy processes are damaged to the extent that they no longer will support the sodium pumping activity of the cell membrane. Excess sodium and water then enter the cell, causing swelling of intracellular organelles including mitochondria and lysosomes. Lysosomes rupture, releasing proteolytic enzymes, and the cell dies [14].

Whatever the final mechanism, all these studies demonstrate severe derangement at the cellular level, which is caused by the low-flow states that result from either trauma or sepsis.

Effects of Starvation

The usual course of major injury includes cessation of normal oral intake. This results from either direct injury to the gastrointestinal tract, from toxicity secondary to infection or tissue destruction, or from interference with feeding caused by various treatment modalities (i.e., endotracheal tubes, medications). The duration of this period of starvation depends on how quickly the clinical situation can be brought under control, so that oral feeding can be resumed or the decision to institute TPN can be made, if early resumption of oral feeding is not anticipated.

The response to starvation by the traumatized or septic patient is considerably different from the response of the normal fasting individual. The normal response to fasting has been extensively studied and has been reviewed in another chapter. It can, however, briefly be summarized as consisting of a series of adaptations, which include a 30 to 40 percent decline in metabolic rate and a shift by brain and heart from utilization of glucose as primary energy substrate to the use of ketone bodies as primary substrate. This later adaptation indicates that the body has markedly less need for gluconeogenesis from protein stores. The major energy store, fat, is then consumed and vital protein is conserved [34, 103]. These adaptations mean that a normal 65-kg fasting individual has approximately 40 days of survival until both fat and protein stores are exhausted [135]. The hypermetabolic response of the injured patient overrides these normal adaptations to starvation and considerably shortens the time an injured patient can be expected to live without nutritional support.

EFFECT OF NUTRITIONAL SUPPORT IN TRAUMA AND INFECTION

The negative nitrogen balance and negative energy balance in trauma and infection make nutritional supplementation theoretically appealing. Given the practical experience of the severely cachectic intensive-care patient, most actively practicing physicians have experienced situations in which survival has appeared to be related to a major degree to the ability to nutritionally replete patients during times of hypercatabolism. Many problems, however, were experienced in early attempts to get these patients into positive energy and nitrogen balance. The recent development of intravenous and better enteral techniques for administration of calories and nitrogen have to a large extent overcome these problems.

The critical information that, in fact, nutritional support can actually reverse some of the complications of injury and infection is rather minimal. Infection does occur much more frequently in the undernourished [19]. Given this observation, many clinicians have assumed that nutritional supplementation will prevent or help to resolve infection in the severely ill. Certainly patients in whom body compositional changes can be identified are more likely to have immune defects that reverse along with reversal of the defects in body composition [160]. Unfortunately, the observation that low-dose exogenous glucose rather poorly suppresses the obligatory gluconeogenesis of trauma and injury [59, 107] causes concern that the nutritional support may be ineffective. Other attempts to characterize demonstrable improvement in response to nutrition have been minimal. One group was able to demonstrate restoration of intracellular electrolyte concentrations in major trauma following nutritional supplementation [47]. Alexander has recently presented data indicating that survival and immune function can be improved by increasing the quantity and quality of the amino acid used to nutritionally supplement burned children [2].

Much of these data supporting aggressive nutritional supplementation of the injured and traumatized patient have been based on changes in rather crude immunologic parameters, such as skin testing for cellular immunity and total lymphocyte counts [102, 160]. It remains unquestionable that complications and mortality are more frequent in the anergic patient. Anergic patients can be shown to have major deficits in body composition, and reversal of the body compositional changes will be reflected in changes in immunologic reactivity [160]. It is important not to assume that, if nutritional support can reverse some aspects of immunologic incompetence, and if immunologic incompetence is associated with increased complications, then nutritional support increases survival, and any patient with impaired immunity should be nutritionally supported by whatever method is available. Unfortunately, the over-riding problem is that the agent that rendered the sick, septic, traumatized patient anergic will inevitably receive appropriate aggressive care at the same time nutritional support is administered. There is therefore little chance to dissect whether or not the patient's anergy reverse is because of nutritional response, or because of the reversal of the underlying defect, which was as important in the development of the anergic state as the nutritional deficiency. It would currently seem prudent to aggressively support hypercatabolic patients with either parenteral or enteral nutrition, while continuing to investigate the extent to which this support is being utilized to improve organ system function.

The stereotyped neuroendocrine response; disordered metabolism of protein, carbohydrate, and fat; and devastating effects of infection, shock, and starvation on the injured patient have been described. There is little question that effective efforts to minimize this systemic response to trauma will be rewarded with improved patient survival. The complexity of this response is evident. Because of this complexity, the effectiveness of attempts to manipulate this response must be clearly demonstrated before therapeutic efforts are widely accepted and applied. Design of these manipulations will be aided by better understanding of the pathophysiology involved. Improved understanding and more effective manipulation of this metabolic response to trauma and infection present a challenge to future researchers in this area.

REFERENCES

1. Albright, F. Cushing's syndrome. *Harvey Lect.* 38:123, 1943.
2. Alexander, J. W., et al. Beneficial effects of aggressive protein feeding in severely burned children. *Ann. Surg.* 192:505, 1980.
3. Allgower, M., et al. Burn toxin in mouse skin. *J. Trauma* 13:95, 1973.
4. Aoki, T. T., Brennan, M. F., Muller, W. A., Moore, F. D., and Cahill, G. F. Effect of insulin on muscle glutamate uptake: Whole blood versus plasma glutamate analysis. *J. Clin. Invest.* 51: 2889, 1972.
5. Aoki, T. T., Brennan, M. F., Muller, W. A., Soeldner, J. S., Alpert, J. S., Saltz, S. R., Kaufmann, R. I., Tang, M. T., and Cahill, G. F. Amino acid levels across normal forearm muscle and splanchnic bed after a protein meal. *Am. J. Clin. Nutr.* 29: 340, 1976.
6. Aoki, T. T., Muller, W. A., Brennan, M. F., and

Cahill, G. F. Blood cell and plasma amino acid levels across forearm muscle during a protein meal. *Diabetes* 22:768, 1973.
7. Aono, T., et al. Influence of surgical stress under general anesthesia on serum gonadotropin levels. *J. Clin. Endocrinol. Metab.* 42:144, 1976.
8. Askanazi, J., Carpentier, Y. A., Elwyn, D. H., Nordenstrom, J., Jeevanandam, M., Rosenbaum, S. H., Gump, F. E., and Kinney, J. M. Influence of total parenteral nutrition on fuel utilization in injury and sepsis. *Ann. Surg.* 191:40, 1980.
9. Askanazi, J., Elwyn, D. H., Silverberg, P. A., Rosenbaum, S. H., and Kinney, J. M. Respiratory distress secondary to a high carbohydrate load. *Surgery* 87:596, 1980.
10. Askanazi, J., Furst, P., Michelsen, C. B., Elwyn, D. H., Vinnars, E., Gump, F. E., and Kinney, J. M. Muscle and plasma amino acids after injury: Hypocaloric versus amino acid infusion. *Ann. Surg.* 191:465, 1980.
11. Askanazi, J., Rosenbaum, S. H., Hyman, A. I., Silverberg, P. A., Milic-Emili, J., and Kinney, J. M. Respiratory changes induced by large glucose loads of total parenteral nutrition. *J.A.M.A.* 243: 1444, 1980.
12. Aulick, L. H., and Wilmore, D. W. Increased peripheral amino acid release following burn injury. *Surgery* 85:560, 1979.
13. Bane, J. W., et al. The pattern of aldosterone and cortisone blood levels in thermal burn patients. *J. Trauma* 14:605, 1974.
14. Baue, A. E., et al. Cellular alterations with shock and ischemia. *Angiology* 25:31, 1974.
15. Baxter, C. R., Cook, W. A., and Shires, G. T. Serum myocardial depressant factor of burn shock. *Surg. Forum* 17:1, 1966.
16. Baylis, P. H., and Heath, D. A. Plasma-arginine-vasopressin response to insulin-induced hypoglycemia. *Lancet* 2:428, 1977.
17. Becker, R. A., et al. Plasma norepinephrine, epinephrine, and thyroid hormone interactions in severely burned patients. *Arch. Surg.* 115:439, 1980.
18. Becker, R. M., and Daniel, R. K. Increased antidiuretic hormone production after trauma to the craniofacial complex. *J. Trauma* 13:112, 1973.
19. Beisel, W. R. Magnitude of the host nutritional responses to infection. *Am. J. Clin. Nutr.* 30:1236, 1977.
20. Beisel, W. R., Goldman, R. F., and Joy, J. T. Metabolic balance studies during induced hyperthermia in man. *J. Appl. Physiol.* 24:1, 1968.
21. Beisel, W. R., et al. Metabolic effects of intracellular infections in man. *Ann. Intern. Med.* 67:744, 1967.
22. Bilmazes, C., et al. Quantitative contribution by skeletal muscle to elevated rates of whole-body protein breakdown in burned children as measured by 3-methylhistidine output. *Metabolism* 27:671, 1978.
23. Birkhahn, R. H., et al. Effects of major skeletal trauma on whole body protein turnover in man measured by L-[1, ^{14}C]-leucine. *Surgery* 88:294, 1980.
24. Blackburn, G. L., et al. Peripheral intravenous feeding with isotonic amino acid solutions. *Am. J. Surg.* 125:447, 1973.
25. Brady, J. V. Ulcers in "executive" monkeys. *Sci. Am.* 199:95, 1958.
26. Brennan, M. F. Metabolic response to surgery in the cancer patient: Consequences of aggressive multimodality therapy. *Cancer* 43:2053, 1979.
27. Brennan, M. F., et al. Glycerol: Major contributor to the short-term protein sparing effect of fat emulsions in normal man. *Ann. Surg.* 182:386, 1975.
28. Bromage, P. R., Shibata, H. R., and Willoughby, H. W. Influence of prolonged epidural blockade on blood sugar and cortisol responses to operations upon the upper part of the abdomen and the thorax. *Surg. Gynecol. Obstet.* 132:1051, 1971.
29. Broun, G. M., Schalch, D. S., and Reichlin, S. Hypothalamic mediation of growth hormone and adrenal stress response in the squirrel monkey. *Endocrinology* 89:694, 1975.
30. Burger, A., et al. Reduced active thyroid hormone levels in acute illness. *Lancet* 1:653, 1976.
31. Burke, J. F., et al. Glucose requirements following burn injury. *Ann. Surg.* 190:274, 1979.
32. Burr, W. A., et al. Serum tri-iodothyronine and reverse tri-iodothyronine concentrations after surgical operations. *Lancet* 2:1277, 1975.
33. Cahill, G. F., Jr. Physiology of insulin in man. *Diabetes* 20:785, 1971.
34. Cahill, G. F., Jr. Starvation in man. *N. Engl. J. Med.* 282:668, 1970.
35. Cairnie, A. B., et al. The heat production consequent to injury. *Br. J. Exp. Pathol.* 38:504, 1957.
36. Campbell, R. M., et al. Cortisone and the metabolic response to injury. *Br. J. Exp. Pathol.* 35: 566, 1954.
37. Cannon, W. B. *The Wisdom of the Body.* New York: Norton, 1939.
38. Carey, L. C., Cloutier, C. T., and Lowery, B. D. Growth hormone and adrenal cortical response to shock and trauma in the human. *Ann. Surg.* 174:451, 1971.
39. Carstenson, H., et al. Testosterone, luteinizing hormone and growth hormone in blood follow-

ing surgical trauma. *Acta Chir. Scand.* 138:1, 1972.

40. Champion, H. R., et al. A clinicopathologic study of hepatic dysfunction following shock. *Surg. Gynecol. Obstet.* 142:657, 1976.
41. Charters, A. C., Odell, W. D., and Thompson, J. C. Anterior pituitary function during surgical stress and convalescence radioimmunoassay measurement of blood TSH, LH, FSH, and growth hormone. *J. Clin. Endocrinol. Metab.* 29:63, 1969.
42. Christensen, N. J., and Jorgeon, V. Plasma catecholamines and carbohydrate metabolism in patients with acute myocardial infarction. *J. Clin. Invest.* 54:278, 1974.
43. Cope, O., et al. Metabolic rate and thyroid function following acute thermal trauma in man. *Ann. Surg.* 137:165, 1953.
44. Cornell, R. G., and Feller, I. Evaluation of emergency medical services with a national burn registry. Dept. of Biostatics, School of Public Health, University of Michigan, Ann Arbor, MI, 1979. P. 20.
45. Crane, C. W., et al. Protein turnover in patients before and after elective orthopedic operations. *Br. J. Surg.* 64:129, 1977.
46. Crosby, E. C., Humphrey, T., and Lauer, E. W. *Correlative Anatomy of the Nervous System.* New York: Macmillan, 1962. P. 288.
47. Curreri, P. W., et al. Inhibition of active sodium transport in erythrocytes from burned patients. *Surg. Gynecol. Obstet.* 139:538, 1974.
48. Cuthbertson, D. P. Observations on the disturbance of metabolism by injury to the limbs. *Q. J. Med.* 1:233, 1932.
49. Dale, G., et al. The effect of surgical operation on venous plasma free amino acids. *Surgery* 81:295, 1977.
50. Daniel, P. M. The blood supply of the hypothalamus and pituitary gland. *Br. Med. Bull.* 22:202, 1966.
51. Danksepp, J. Hypothalamic regulation of energy balance and feeding behavior. *Fed. Proc.* 33: 1150, 1974.
52. Davies, R., and Slater, J. D. H. Is the adrenergic control of renin release dominant in man. *Lancet* 2:594, 1976.
53. Dinarello, C. Production of endogenous pyrogen. *Fed. Proc.* 38:52, 1979.
54. DuBois, E. F. The Mechanism of Heat Loss and Temperature Regulation. In *Lane Medical Lectures.* Stanford, CA: Stanford University Press, 1937.
55. Duke, J. H., Jr., et al. Contribution of protein to calorie expenditure following injury. *Surgery* 68:168, 1970.
56. Eckart, J., et al. Metabolism of radioactive-labelled fat emulsions in the postoperative and post-traumatic period. *Am. J. Clin. Nutr.* 26:578, 1973.
57. Egdahl, R. H. Cerebral cortical inhibition of pituitary adrenal secretion. *Endocrinology* 68:574, 1961.
58. Egdahl, R. H., Story, J. L., and Melby, J. C. Effect of progressive removal of the brain on adrenal cortical hypersecretion due to operative trauma. *Fed. Proc.* 17:435, 1958.
59. Elwyn, D. H., Kinney, J. M., Malayappa, J., Gump, F. E., and Broell, J. R. Influence of increasing carbohydrate intake on glucose kinetics in injured patients. *Ann. Surg.* 190:117, 1979.
60. Elwyn, D. H., Launder, W. J., Parikh, H. C., and Wise, E. M., Jr. Roles of plasma and erythrocytes in interorgan transport of amino acids in dogs. *Am. J. Physiol.* 222:1333, 1972.
61. Felig, P. The glucose-alanine cycle. *Metabolism* 22:179, 1973.
62. Felig, P., and Wahren, J. Amino acid metabolism in exercising man. *J. Clin. Invest.* 50:2703, 1971.
63. Felig, P., et al. Alanine: Key role in gluconeogenesis. *Science* 167:1003, 1970.
64. Franksson, C., Gemzell, C. A., and von Euler, U. S. Cortical and medullary adrenal activity in surgical and allied conditions. *J. Clin. Endocrinol. Metab.* 14:608, 1954.
65. Freund, H. R., Ryan, J. A., and Fischer, J. E. Amino acid derangements in patients with sepsis: Treatment with branched chain amino acid rich infusions. *Ann. Surg.* 188:423, 1978.
66. Freund, H., Yoshimura, N., and Fischer, J. E. The effect of branched chain amino acids and hypertonic glucose infusions on postinjury catabolism in the rat. *Surgery* 87:401, 1980.
67. Frye, R., Braunwald, E., and Cohen, E. Studies on Starling's law of the heart: I. The circulatory response to acute hypervolemia and its modification by ganglionic blockade. *J. Clin. Invest.* 39: 1043, 1960.
68. Furchgott, R. I. The receptors for epinephrine and norepinephrine (adrenergic receptors). *Pharmacol. Rev.* 11:429, 1959.
69. Furst, P., et al. Influence of amino acid supply on nitrogen and amino acid metabolism in severe trauma. *Acta Chir. Scand. Suppl.* 494:136, 1978.
70. Gamble, J. L. Physiological information gained from studies on the life-raft ration. *Harvey Lect.* 42:247, 1947.
71. George, D. T., Abeles, F. B., and Powanda, M. C. Alterations in plasma glucose, insulin, and gluca-

gon induced by a leukocyte derived factor. *Clin. Res.* 23:320, 1975.
72. Gibbs, J. M., et al. Alterations of plasma 11-hydroxy corticosteroid response to surgery by a fluid load. *J. Endocrinol.* 58:517, 1972.
73. Glasser, O., and Page, I. Experimental hemorrhagic shock: A study of its production and treatment. *Am. J. Physiol.* 154:297, 1948.
74. Goodall, McC., and Moncrief, J. A. Sympathetic nerve depletion in severe thermal injury. *Ann. Surg.* 162:893, 1965.
75. Goodall, McC., Stone, C., and Haynes, B. W. Urinary output of adrenaline and noradrenaline in severe thermal burns. *Ann. Surg.* 145:479, 1957.
76. Golden, M., Waterlou, J. C., and Picou, D. The relationship between dietary intake weight change, nitrogen balance, and protein turnover in man. *Am. J. Clin. Nutr.* 30:1345, 1977.
77. Goldenberg, M., et al. The hemodynamic response of man to norepinephrine and epinephrine and its relation to the problem of hypertension. *Am. J. Med.* 5:792, 1948.
78. Greenberg, G. R., et al. Protein-sparing therapy in postoperative patients. *N. Engl. J. Med.* 294: 1411, 1976.
79. Groves, A. C., et al. Plasma catecholamines in patients with serious postoperative infection. *Ann. Surg.* 178:102, 1973.
80. Gump, F. E., Long, C. L., Geiger, J. W., and Kinney, J. M. The significance of altered gluconeogenesis in surgical catabolism. *J. Trauma* 15:704, 1975.
81. Gump, F. E., Long, C., Killian, P., and Kinney, J. M. Studies of glucose tolerance in septic injured patients. *J. Trauma* 14:378, 1974.
82. Guyton, A. C., Harris, J. G., and Coleman, T. G. Autoregulation of the total systemic circulation and its relation to control of cardiac output and arterial pressure. *Circ. Res.* 28:1, 1971.
83. Guyton, A. C., et al. Arterial pressure regulation: Over-riding dominance of the kidneys in long-term regulation and in hypertension. *Am. J. Med.* 52:584, 1972.
84. Hanson, E. I., et al. Response of glucose, insulin, free fatty acid, and human growth hormone to norepinephrine and hemorrhage in normal man. *Ann. Surg.* 177:453, 1973.
85. Harrison, T. S., Seton, J. F., and Feller I. Relationship of increased oxygen consumption to catecholamine excretion in thermal burns. *Ann. Surg.* 165:169, 1967.
86. Hertling, G., Potter, L. T., and Axelrod, J. Effect of decentralization and ganglionic blocking agents on the spontaneous release of ^{3}H-norepinephrine. *J. Pharmacol. Exp. Ther.* 136:289, 1962.
87. Holder, I. A., and Jogan, M. Enhanced survival in burned mice treated with antiserum prepared against normal and burned skin. *J. Trauma* 11: 1041, 1971.
88. Howard, J., et al. Studies of adrenal function in combat and wounded soldiers. *Ann. Surg.* 141: 314, 1955.
89. Hume, D. M. Endocrine and Metabolic Responses to Injury. In S. I. Schwartz (Ed.), *Principles of Surgery*. New York: McGraw-Hill, 1969. Pp. 3–46.
90. Hume, D. M., Bell, C. C., and Bartter, F. Direct measurement of adrenal secretion during operative trauma and convalescence. *Surgery* 52:174, 1962.
91. Hume, D. M., and Egdahl, R. H. The importance of the brain in the endocrine response to injury. *Ann. Surg.* 150:697, 1959.
92. Ingle, D. J. Permissive action of hormones. *J. Clin. Endocrinol. Metab.* 14:1272, 1954.
93. Ingle, D. J., Ward, E. O., and Kuizenga, M. H. The relationship of the adrenal glands to changes in urinary non-protein nitrogen following multiple fractures in the force-fed rat. *Am. J. Physiol.* 149:510, 1947.
94. Iversen, J. Adrenergic receptors and the secretion of glucagon and insulin from the isolated, perfused canine pancreas. *J. Clin. Invest.* 52:2102, 1973.
95. Jeejeebhoy, K. N., et al. Metabolic studies in total parenteral nutrition with lipid in man: Comparison with glucose. *J. Clin. Invest.* 57:125, 1976.
96. Kampschmidt, R. F., et al. Multiple biological activities of a partially purified leukocytic endogenous mediator. *Am. J. Physiol.* 224:530, 1973.
97. Kien, C. L., et al. Increased rates of whole body protein synthesis and breakdown in children recovering from burns. *Ann. Surg.* 187:383, 1978.
98. Kinney, J. M. Energy requirements in injury and sepsis. *Acta Anaesthesiol. Scand.* (Suppl.) 55:15, 1974.
99. Kinney, J. M. Energy Requirements of the Surgical Patient. In Committee on Pre- and Postoperative Care, American College of Surgeons (Eds.), *Manual of Surgical Nutrition*. Philadelphia: Saunders, 1975. Pp. 223–235.
100. Kinney, J. M., et al. Carbohydrate and nitrogen metabolism after injury. *J. Clin. Pathol.* 23:65, 1970.
101. Koizumi, K., and McBrooks, C. The Autonomic Nervous System and Its Role in Controlling Visceral Activities. In V. B. Mountcastle (Ed.), *Medical Physiology* (13th ed.). St. Louis: Mosby, 1974. P. 783.
102. Law, D. K., Dudrick, S. J., and Abdou, N. I. Immunocompetence of patients with protein-calorie

malnutrition: The effects of nutritional repletion. *Ann. Intern. Med.* 79:545, 1973.

103. Levenson, S. M., Crowley, B. S., and Seifter, E. Starvation. In Committee on Pre- and Postoperative Care, American College of Surgeons (Eds.), *Manual of Surgical Nutrition.* Philadelphia: Saunders, 1975. P. 236.
104. Levinsky, N. Pathophysiology of acute renal failure. *N. Engl. J. Med.* 296:1453, 1977.
105. Lindsey, A. F., et al. Pancreatic alpha-cell function in trauma. *J.A.M.A.* 227:775, 1974.
106. Long, C. L., Jeevanandam, M., Kim, B. M., and Kinney, J. M. Whole body protein synthesis and catabolism in septic man. *Am. J. Clin. Nutr.* 30: 1340, 1977.
107. Long, C. L., Kinney, J. M., and Geiger, J. M. Nonsuppressibility of gluconeogenesis by glucose in septic patients. *Metabolism* 25:193, 1976.
108. Long, C. L., Schilller, W. R., Blakemore, W. S., Geiger, J. W., O'Dell, M., and Henderson, K. Muscle protein catabolism in the septic patient as measured by 3-methylhistidine excretion. *Am. J. Clin. Nutr.* 30:1349, 1977.
109. Long, C. L., Spencer, J. L., Kinney, J. M., and Geiger, J. W. Carbohydrate metabolism in man: Effect of elective operations and major injury. *J. Appl. Physiol.* 31:110, 1971.
110. Long, J. M., III, et al. Effect of carbohydrate and fat on nitrogen excretion during total intravenous feeding. *Ann. Surg.* 185:417, 1977.
111. Maas, J. W., and Landis, H. The metabolism of circulating norepinephrine by human subjects. *J. Pharmacol. Exp. Ther.* 177:600, 1971.
112. Mapes, C. A., and Sobocinski, P. Z. Differentiation between endogenous pyrogen and leukocytic endogenous mediator. *Am. J. Physiol.* 232:C15, 1977.
113. Martin, J. B. Neural regulation of growth hormone secretion. *N. Engl. J. Med.* 288:1384, 1973.
114. McBrooks, C., and Koizumi, K. The Hypothalamus and Control of Integrative Processes. In V. B. Mountcastle (Ed.), *Medical Physiology* (13th ed.). St. Louis: Mosby, 1974. P. 813.
115. McCallum, R. E., and Berry, J. Effects of endotoxin on gluconeogenesis, glycogen synthesis, and liver glycogen synthetase in mice. *Infect. Immunol.* 7:642, 1973.
116. McDougal, W. S., Wilmore, D. W., and Pruitt, B. A., Jr. Effect of intravenous near isosmotic nutrient infusions on nitrogen balance in critically ill injured patients. *Surg. Gynecol. Obstet.* 145:408, 1977.
117. Meguid, M. M., et al. Hormone substrate relationships following trauma. *Arch. Surg.* 109:776, 1974.
118. Mela, L., Bucalzo, L. V., and Miller, L. D. Defective oxidative metabolism of rat liver mitochondria in hemorrhagic and endotoxin shock. *Am. J. Physiol.* 200:571, 1971.
119. Milton, A. S., and Wendlant, S. Effects of body temperature of prostaglandins of the A, E, and F series on injection into the third ventricle of unanesthetized cats and rabbits. *J. Physiol. (Lond.)* 218:325, 1971.
120. Monnier, M. *Functions of the Nervous System.* Amsterdam: Elsevier, 1975. Vol. 3, P. 85.
121. Moore, F. D. Bodily changes in surgical convalescence. *Ann. Surg.* 137:289, 1953.
122. Moore, F. D. The effect of hemorrhage on body composition. *N. Engl. J. Med.* 273:567, 1965.
123. Moore, F. D., Lyons, J. H., Pierce, E. C., Morgan, A. P., Drinker, P. A., MacArthur, J. D., and Dammin, G. J. *Post-Traumatic Pulmonary Insufficiency.* Philadelphia: Saunders, 1969.
124. Moore, F. D., Olesen, K., McMurrey, J. D., Parker, H. V., Ball, M. R., and Boyden, C. M. *The Body Cell Mass and Its Supporting Environment.* Philadelphia: Saunders, 1963. Pp. 224–278.
125. Moran, W. H., et al. The relationship of antidiuretic hormone secretion to surgical stress. *Surgery* 56:99, 1964.
126. Morrison, D. C., and Ulevitch, R. J. The effects of bacterial endotoxins on host mediation systems. *Am. J. Pathol.* 93:525, 1978.
127. Mountcastle, V. B. Pain and Temperature Sensibilities. In V. B. Mountcastle (Ed.), *Medical Physiology* (13th ed.). St. Louis: Mosby, 1974. P. 348.
128. Newsome, H. H., and Rose, J. C. The response of human adrenocorticotrophic hormone and growth hormone to surgical stress. *J. Clin. Endocrinol. Metab.* 33:481, 1971.
129. Noel, G. L., et al. Human prolactin and growth hormone release during surgery and other conditions of stress. *J. Clin. Endocrinol. Metab.* 35:840, 1972.
130. Oberg, B., and White, S. Circulatory effects of interruption and stimulation of cardiac vagal afferents. *Acta Physiol. Scand.* 80:383, 1970.
131. O'Connell, R. C., et al. Nitrogen conservation in starvation: Graded response to intravenous glucose. *J. Clin. Endocrinol. Metab.* 39:555, 1974.
132. Odessey, R., Khairallah, E. A., and Goldberg, A. I. Origin and possible significance of alanine production by skeletal muscle. *J. Biol. Chem.* 249: 7623, 1974.
133. O'Keefe, S. J. D., Sender, P. M., and James, W. P. T. Catabolic loss of body nitrogen in response to surgery. *Lancet* 2:1035, 1974.
134. Oparil, S., and Haber, E. The renin-angiotensin system. *N. Engl. J. Med.* 291:389, 1974.

135. Passmore, R., and Robson, J. S. *A Companion to Medical Studies,* Vol. 3. Oxford: Blackwell, 1974.
136. Popp, M. B., Silberstein, E. B., Srivastava, L. S., Loggie, J. M. H., Knowles, H. C., Jr., and MacMillan, B. G. A pathophysiologic study of the hypertension associated with burn injury in children. *Ann. Surg.* 181:817, 1981.
137. Popp, M. B., Srivastava, L. S., Knowles, H. C., and MacMillan, B. G. Anterior pituitary function in thermally injured male children and young adults. *Surg. Gynecol. Obstet.* 145:517, 1977.
138. Porte, D., Jr., and Williamson, R. H. Inhibition of insulin release by norepinephrine in man. *Science* 152:1249, 1966.
139. Porte, D., Jr., et al. The effect of epinephrine on immunoreactive insulin levels in man. *J. Clin. Invest.* 45:228, 1966.
140. Powanda, M. C. Changes in body balances of nitrogen and other key nutrients: Description and underlying mechanisms. *Am. J. Clin. Nutr.* 30: 1254, 1977.
141. Reiss, E., et al. The metabolic response to burns. *J. Clin. Invest.* 35:62, 1956.
142. Rocha, D. M., et al. Abnormal pancreatic alpha cell function in bacterial infections. *N. Engl. J. Med.* 288:700, 1973.
143. Ryan, N. T., Blackburn, G. L., and Clowes, G. Differential tissue sensitivity to elevated endogenous insulin levels during experimental peritonitis in rats. *Metabolism* 23:1081, 1974.
144. Ryan, N. T., et al. Chronic tissue insulin resistance following hemorrhagic shock. *Ann. Surg.* 180: 402, 1974.
145. Sakata, K. S., Hayano, S., and Sloviter, H. A. Effect on blood glucose concentrations of changes in availability of glucose to the brain. *Am. J. Physiol.* 204:1127, 1963.
146. Sato, A., and Schmidt, R. Spinal and supraspinal components of the reflex discharges into lumbar and thoracic white rami. *J. Physiol.* 212:839, 1971.
147. Sayeed, M. M., and Baue, A. E. Mitochrondrial metabolism of succinate, β-hydroxybutyrate, and α-ketoglutarate in hemorrhagic shock. *Am. J. Physiol.* 220:1275, 1971.
148. Sayeed, M. M., and Baue, A. E. Na-K transport in rat liver slices in hemorrhagic shock. *Am. J. Physiol.* 224:1265, 1973.
149. Schally, A. V., Arimura, A., and Kastin, A. J. Hypothalamic regulatory hormones. *Science* 179: 341, 1973.
150. Scher, A. M. Carotid and aortic regulation of arterial blood pressure. *Circulation* 56:521, 1977.
151. Schimmel, M., and Utiger, R. D. Thyroidal and peripheral production of thyroid hormones: Review of recent findings and their clinical implications. *Ann. Intern. Med.* 87:760, 1977.
152. Selye, H. A syndrome produced by diverse noxious agents. *Nature* 138:32, 1936.
153. Shires, G. T., and Canizaro, P. C. Fluid and Electrolyte Management of the Surgical Patient. In D. C. Sabiston, Jr. (Ed.), *Textbook of Surgery: The Biological Basis of Modern Surgical Practice.* Philadelphia: Saunders, 1977. Pp. 95–118.
154. Shires, G. T., et al. Alterations in cellular membrane function during hemorrhagic shock in primates. *Ann. Surg.* 176:288, 1972.
155. Shizgal, H. M., Spanier, A. H., and Kurtz, R. S. Effect of parenteral nutrition on body composition in the critically ill patient. *Am. J. Surg.* 131: 156, 1976.
156. Skillman, J. J., Awwad, H. K., and Moore, F. D. Plasma protein kinetics of the early transcapillary refill after hemorrhages in man. *Surg. Gynecol. Obstet.* 125:983, 1967.
157. Skillman, J. J., Lauler, D. D., Hickler, R. B., Lyons, J. H., Olson, J. E., Ball, M. R., and Moore, F. D. Hemorrhage in normal man: Effect on renin cortisol, aldosterone, and urine composition. *Ann. Surg.* 166:865, 1967.
158. Skillman, J. J., Olson, J. E., Lyons, J. H., and Moore, F. D. The hemodynamic effect of acute blood loss in normal man, with observations on the effect of the valsalva maneuver and breath holding. *Ann. Surg.* 166:713, 1967.
159. Spanier, A. H., and Shizgal, H. M. Caloric requirements of the critically ill patient receiving intravenous hyperalimentation. *Am. J. Surg.* 133: 99, 1977.
160. Spanier, A. H., et al. The relationship between immune competence and nutrition. *Surg. Forum* 27:332, 1976.
161. Spector, D. A., et al. Thyroid function and metabolic state in chronic renal failure. *Ann. Intern. Med.* 85:724, 1976.
162. Steenberg, R. W., Lennihan, R., and Moore, F. D. Studies in surgical endocrinology: II. The free blood 17-hydroxycorticoids in surgical patients; their relation to urine steroids, metabolism and convalescence. *Ann. Surg.* 143:180, 1956.
163. Steinberg, D., et al. Hormonal regulation of lipase, phosphorylase and glycogen synthetase in adipose tissue. *Adv. Cyclic Nucleotide Res.* 5:549, 1975.
164. Stephens, R. V., and Randall, H. T. Use of a concentrated, balanced, liquid elemental diet for nutritional management of catabolic states. *Ann. Surg.* 170:642, 1969.
165. Stephenson, H. E. *Cardiac Arrest and Resuscitation* (3rd ed.). St. Louis: Mosby, 1969. P. 520.

166. Studley, H. O. Percentage of weight loss, a basic indicator of surgical risk. *J.A.M.A.* 106:458, 1936.
167. Tweedle, D. E. F., et al. Intravenous amino acids as the sole nutritional substrate. *Ann. Surg.* 186: 60, 1977.
168. Unger, R. H. Glucagon and the insulin:glucagon ratio in diabetes and other catabolic illnesses. *Diabetes* 30:834, 1971.
169. Unger, R. H., and Orci, L. The essential role of glucagon in the pathogenesis of diabetes mellitus. *Lancet* 1:14, 1974.
170. Van Itallie, T. B., et al. Will fat emulsions given intravenously promote protein synthesis? Metabolic studies on normal subjects and surgical patients. *Surgery* 36:720, 1954.
171. Vinnars, E., et al. The effect of intravenous nutrition on nitrogen and amino acid metabolism in postoperative trauma. *Acta Chir. Scand.* (Suppl.) 494:133, 1978.
172. Waterlow, J. C., Garlick, P. J., and Millward, D. J. *Protein Turnover in Mammalian Tissues and in the Whole Body*. Amsterdam: North-Holland, 1978.
173. Watkins, G. M., et al. Bodily changes in repeated hemorrhage. *Surg. Gynecol. Obstet.* 139:161, 1974.
174. Wedge, J. H., et al. Branched-chain amino acids, nitrogen excretion and injury in man. *Clin. Sci. Mol. Med.* 50:393, 1976.
175. White, A., et al. Carbohydrate Metabolism I. In *Principles of Biochemistry* (5th ed.). New York: McGraw-Hill, 1978. P. 431.
176. Williamson, D. H., et al. Muscle-protein catabolism after injury in man, as measured by urinary excretion of 3-methylhistidine. *Clin. Sci. Mol. Med.* 52:527, 1977.
177. Wilmore, D. W. Carbohydrate metabolism in trauma. *J. Clin. Endocrinol. Metab.* 5:731, 1976.
178. Wilmore, D. W., Aulick, L. H., Mason, A. D., and Pruitt, B. A. Influence of the burn wound on local and systemic responses to injury. *Ann. Surg.* 186:444, 1977.
179. Wilmore, D. W., Goodwin, C. W., Aulick, L. H., Powanda, M. C., Mason, A. D., and Pruitt, B. A. Effect of injury and infection on visceral metabolism and circulation. *Ann. Surg.* 192:491, 1980.
180. Wilmore, D. W., Long, J. M., Mason, A. D., and Pruitt, B. A. Stress in surgical patients as a neurophysiologic reflex response. *Surg. Gynecol. Obstet.* 142:257, 1976.
181. Wilmore, D. W., Long, J. M., Mason, A. D., Skreen, R. W., and Pruitt, B. A., Jr. Catecholamines: Mediator of the hypermetabolic response to thermal injury. *Ann. Surg.* 180:653, 1974.
182. Wilmore, D. W., Mason, A. D., and Pruitt, B. A. Insulin response to glucose in hypermetabolic burn patients. *Ann. Surg.* 183:314, 1976.
183. Wilmore, D. W., Moylan, J. A., Jr., Bristow, B. F., Mason, A. D., Jr., and Pruitt, B. A., Jr. Anabolic effects of human growth hormone and high caloric feedings following thermal injury. *Surg. Gynecol. Obstet.* 138:875, 1974.
184. Wilmore, D. W., Moylan, J. A., Helmkamp, G. M., and Pruitt, B. A., Jr. Clinical evaluation of a 10% intravenous fat emulsion for parenteral nutrition in thermally injured patients. *Ann. Surg.* 178:503, 1973.
185. Wilmore, D. W., Moylan, J. A., Pruitt, B. A., Lindsey, C. A., Faloona, G. R., and Unger, R. H. Hyperglucagonemia after burns. *Lancet* 1:73, 1974.
186. Winkelmann, R. K. Molecular inflammation of the skin. *J. Invest. Dermatol.* 57:197, 1971.
187. Wise, L., Margraf, H. W., and Ballinger, W. F. Adrenalcortical function in severe burns. *Arch. Surg.* 105:213, 1972.
188. Wolfe, B. M., Celebras, J. M., Sim, A. J. W., Ball, M. R., and Moore, F. D. Substrate interaction in intravenous feeding. *Ann. Surg.* 186:518, 1977.
189. Woolfe, L. I., et al. Arterial plasma amino acids in patients with serious postoperative infection and in patients with major fractures. *Surgery* 79:283, 1976.
190. Woolfson, A. M., Heathy, R. V., and Allison, S. P. Insulin to inhibit protein catabolism after injury. *N. Engl. J. Med.* 300:14, 1979.
191. Wright, P. D., and Henderson, K. Cellular utilization during hemmorhagic shock in the pig. *Surgery* 78:322, 1975.
192. Young, V. R. The Role of Skeletal and Cardiac Muscle in the Regulation of Protein Metabolism. In H. N. Munro (Ed.), *Mammalian Protein Metabolism*. New York: Academic, 1969. Vol. IV, pp. 585–674.
193. Young, V. R., et al. Potential use of 3-methylhistidine excretion as an index of progressive reduction in muscle protein catabolism during starvation. *Metabolism* 22:1429, 1973.
194. Zenser, T., et al. Infection induced hyperglucagonemia and altered hepatic response to glucagon in the rat. *Am. J. Physiol.* 227:1299, 1974.

Nutritional Changes in Neoplasia

Edward M. Copeland III
Stanley J. Dudrick
John M. Daly
David M. Ota

15

Often malnutrition is the common denominator of the multiple complications ultimately causing the death of patients with cancer. At some point during treatment of most malignant diseases, particularly when metastases have occurred, malnutrition becomes a problem because the antineoplastic treatment modalities result in tissue injury and consequent need for repair. Surgery, chemotherapy, and radiotherapy each have the potential to limit calorie intake for extended periods of time, and if the primary treatment fails to eradicate the disease, subsequent antineoplastic therapy may be compromised by malnutrition. Cancer cachexia should no longer be a contraindication to appropriate oncologic therapy. Adequate nutritional replenishment should be undertaken prior to the indicated antineoplastic therapy because the malnourished patient has a much narrower safe therapeutic margin for most antineoplastic therapy, and because the tumoricidal doses of these agents may be much closer to the lethal doses for normal tissues in malnourished patients than in well-nourished ones. Physicians must be alert to the complications resulting from the treatment of a patient with an inadequate nutritional status and should be prepared to individualize nutritional therapy for each patient.

Absorption of nutrients via a functional gastrointestinal tract is the best means of maintaining adequate nutrition; however, delivery of nutrients to the gut does not always result in nutritional restoration of the starving patient because the syndrome of malnutrition may include malabsorption. In some patients, such as those with malignant disease of the head and neck region, restoration of good nutritional status may be possible by nasogastric intubation with a small feeding tube. Gastrostomy and jejunostomy feeding tubes may be used in patients with obstructing carcinomas of the esophagus, stomach, or pancreas. Unfortunately, nutritional supplementation via the gastrointestinal tract can be time consuming, or the gastrointestinal tract may be unavailable for nutrient administration. Under these circumstances, the use of intravenous hyperalimentation (IVH) has been indicated.

The anorexia and cachexia associated with cancer often can be explained by the anatomic location of the malignant disease, the anxiety associated with it, and the consequent decrease in total daily caloric intake. Weight loss occurs when energy expended by an individual is not balanced by equal energy or caloric sources gained. As Holland and her group [44] have indicated, much of the depression and hopelessness encountered in cancer patients can be a reactive state associated with the diagnosis of cancer, the effects of treatment, or the stage of the disease. Even more important to the early diagnosis of anorexia and weight loss in the cancer patient is the observation that depression can occur in response to the anticipated threat of a symptom or sign that the individual perceives as evidence of a potential malignant process. Since symptoms of malignant disease often antedate diagnosis by as long as six months, it is not unusual to find that patients have lost 5 percent of their usual body weight prior to diagnosis. Nevertheless, patients with certain cancers, such as oat cell carcinoma of the lung, can have extreme weight loss prior to diagnosis, and when diagnosed, the volume of tumor is relatively small. It has been proposed that anorexia and weight loss are secondary to certain peptides, oligonucleotides, and other metabolites produced by the cancer. Theologides [64] believes that the cancer itself initiates and contributes most to the genesis of the syndrome of cancer cachexia. Others, including the authors, believe that much of the malnutrition seen in cancer patients is iatrogenic and the result of inadequate nutritional intake during and after treatment with antineoplastic agents.

Nutritional manipulation of cancer cells as a therapeutic tool has been discussed for many years, but results of such therapy remain either anecdotal or speculative. Recently, the enzymatic approach to selective amino acid depletion of rapidly growing malignant lymphocytes in acute lymphocytic leukemia has been promising [6]. Asparaginase blocks the metabolism of asparagine in the malignant T or null lymphocyte, whereas normal cells are affected very little. Methotrexate and 5-FU, both antimetabolites, are most effective when vitamin and nutritional deficiencies do *not* coexist. Both drugs give suboptimal results in folate-deficient patients, and Moertel et al. [36] demonstrated a significantly better response to 5-FU in patients who were nutritionally intact and active compared to those who had limited performance status.

In animal tumor models, starvation inhibits transmissibility of transplantable tumors and impedes the growth of these tumors once established in the host animal. Nutritional repletion of the host results in renewed growth of the transplanted neoplasm. These observations have been made by most investigators working with experimental tumors and has lead to speculation that nutritional repletion might result in tumor growth stimulation in man. Minimal evidence for such an occurrence has been published. Terepka and Waterhouse [63] enterally force-fed eight patients with terminal cancer and found that three patients "from clinical impression" appeared to have accelerated tumor growth during the 24- to 63-day period of forced feeding. These three patients died one to 16 days after the end of the forced feeding period, making interpretation of the results difficult. In adult and pediatric cancer patients, Copeland [9], Solassol [57], Filler [24], and their colleagues have reported large series of patients nutritionally replenished with intravenous hyperalimentation, and no evidence of growth stimulation has been noted. These reports are criticized because the analyses were retrospective; nevertheless, they represent data from almost 3,000 patients who have received IVH, with no indication that tumor growth was increased by the use of the nutritional solutions.

This chapter will outline current attitudes on anorexia and cachexia of malignancy, the use of intravenous hyperalimentation as a supportive technique in nutritional maintenance and rehabilitation of the cancer patient, and the possible use of nutritional manipulation as a therapeutic modality in the treatment of cancer.

ANOREXIA AND CACHEXIA

DeWys [22] has made important contributions in the study of the pathophysiology of anorexia in cancer patients. This process is poorly understood and difficult to investigate because of the multiple variables that influence the experimental data.

There is no evidence that hypothalamic centers stimulate or depress feeding behavior. DeWys has identified abnormalities of taste sensation, particularly elevation of the recognition threshold for sweet and lowering of the recognition threshold for bitter. Symptoms of meat aversion were associated with an altered taste sensation for urea, a bitter taste. Changes in taste sensation could be correlated with changes in disease status and in response to antineoplastic therapy. In his series, nine patients responded to antineoplastic therapy with a reduction in tumor size, and in four of these patients, low thresholds for urea returned to near-normal levels. Similarly, patients responding to antineoplastic therapy regained a normal threshold for the recognition of sucrose. DeWys [49] has also demonstrated that there are abnormalities in taste sensation associated with malnutrition, and these abnormalities may be reversed by nutritional repletion with IVH. Thus interpretation of the data on taste sensation collected by DeWys and his coworkers must be evaluated relative to the nutritional status of the patient at the time the studies were done.

Several investigators have demonstrated that cancer patients as a group have abnormal or diabetic glucose tolerance curves. Schein and his colleagues [53] compared the results of standard oral glucose tolerance tests for cachectic cancer patients and for control subjects. Blood glucose levels for the malnourished patients were statistically higher than those for controls for the one- to four-hour period after ingestion of glucose. Plasma insulin levels rose at a slightly lower rate in the cachectic patients, but similar concentrations were achieved in both groups two hours after glucose ingestion. Malnourished patients and controls were given 15 gm of oral glucose every 15 minutes for four hours, and the cachectic patients maintained a steady state of blood glucose concentration 30 to 40 mg/dl higher than that of the control subjects. Also, the glucose response to an exogenous insulin infusion was markedly impaired in the group of cachectic patients. The authors were unable to demonstrate a quantitative or qualitative alteration in insulin receptors to explain the observed differences. An explanation offered was that the increase in gluconeogenesis in cachectic cancer patients might serve as a contributory mechanism for the elevation in blood glucose.

In our laboratory, Solomon et al. [58] also demonstrated diabetic glucose tolerance curves and depressed serum insulin levels, as well as increased levels of serum growth hormone, in malnourished patients with metastatic cancer. Nutritional replenishment for ten days with IVH resulted in normalization of glucose tolerance curves, a return toward normal of serum insulin levels, and a reduction in serum growth hormone concentration. Possibly, the normalization of values for these indicators after nutritional replenishment indicates that the previous abnormalities were secondary to malnutrition rather than to the malignant disease process, and that the abnormalities can be corrected by intravenous hyperalimentation.

A characteristic of normal mammalian species in the presence of adequate food supplies is to alter nutrient intake to meet changes in nutritional needs. Morrison [38] believes there is a relative and an absolute hypophagia in tumor-bearing patients. The capacity of the cancer patient to increase food intake on the basis of need appears to be limited. Experimentally, he found that the feeding response of normal rats to dilution of food with non-nutritive bulk was to progressively increase intake in accordance with the percent of dilution. Thereby, if nutritive density of the administered food was reduced by one-half, the animal would ingest twice as much food. This control mechanism was altered in rats with transplanted tumors. As the animals began to lose weight and cachexia became apparent, the feeding response to food dilution was abolished. Excision or regression of the tumor resulted in increased nutrient intake and a reversal of the cachetic process.

It is clear that the tumor requires energy substrates to grow and that these substrates are exacted from the host. As tumor bulk increases, nutritive demands are greater and host intake may be less. The result of this process may be extreme weight loss and malnutrition. Moreschi [37] initially developed the concept that malnutrition in the cancer patient might be a result of competition for nutrients between the host and the cancer. As Costa [15] points out, however, the great majority of patients who die from cancer and are examined at autopsy seldom have more than a total of 500 gm of cancer; it is difficult to imagine that such tumor volume in a 70 kilogram man can actively compete for nutrients to the extent that the host becomes malnourished. Nevertheless, cancer cells are thought to concentrate and incorporate amino acids and glucose better than do normal cells. Christiansen et al. [7] demonstrated that Erlich ascites tumor cells were more active in accumulating amino acids than were hepatic or muscle cells from the same animal. Pimpstone's group [43] demonstrated that malnourished patients had elevated levels of serum growth hormone, and we postulated that this increased growth hormone level might cause preferential uptake of amino acids by some human tumor cells [10]. If growth hormone increases incorporation of amino acids within neoplastic cells and normal cells, the former with intrinsically better concentrating power, the balance of nutrient flow in the malnourished patient might favor the tumor; consequently, the malnourished cancer patient should benefit from nutritional repletion, thereby lowering serum growth hormone levels. Moreover, Lundholm et al. [33] observed that protein synthesis in muscle from cancer patients was depressed, but could be stimulated by the addition of high levels of amino acids. This observation suggested that, in cancer patients, there was a reduced efficiency of amino acid utilization for muscle protein synthesis during periods of normal levels of amino acid supply, but that this decreased synthesis could be overcome by raising the supply of amino acids to muscle.

Although gluconeogenesis occurs within a cancer cell, apparently any nitrogen released is reutilized by the cancer cell for the production of tumor protein. Thus, once amino acids are within the cancer cell, they are not available for participation in the turnover of the amino acid pool of the host [35]. Protein-calorie malnutrition has been identified in some rat tumor models, even though the animals remained in postive nitrogen balance [56]. A proposed theory to explain this observation was that energy for tumor metabolism was derived from host protein stores through gluconeogenesis within the host, and that the nitrogen liberated from gluconeogenesis was utilized by the tumor for protein synthesis and was not available for use or elimination by the host's body.

The energy for tumor metabolism is derived from both aerobic and anaerobic metabolism of glucose. Anaerobic glycolysis is thought to predominate in malignant cells because of their limited oxygen supply and resultant enzymatic makeup. The partial pressure of oxygen in some human cancers is reduced by as much as 50 percent when compared with normal tissues [55]. Also, the administration of dextrose to rats bearing transplanted tumors has resulted in a decrease in tumor pH, whereas the pH of normal tissues did not change. The end product of anaerobic glycolysis is lactic acid, which is thought to cause the decrease in pH within the tumor environment. Waterhouse [67] demonstrated an increased recycling of lactic acid and pyruvate to glucose in human beings with cancer. The amount of recycling correlated directly with the total volume of malignant tissue. Holroyde et al. [26] demonstrated an increase in Cori cycle activity in patients with metastatic cancer and progressive weight loss when compared to similar patients without weight loss. Total glucose turnover, glucose oxidation, and total caloric expenditure were higher in the former group, and caloric expenditure was highest in those patients with a marked increase in Cori cycle activity. Reichard and coworkers [45] demonstrated that almost all lactic acid generated from anaerobic glucose metabolism by cancer cells enters the blood stream to be resynthesized into glucose by the liver. Only two moles of adenosine triphosphate (ATP) are generated by glycolysis, and six moles of ATP are required by the liver to resynthesize glucose from lactic acid. Therefore, the metabolism of one mole of glucose by the tumor is accomplished at the expense of eight moles of ATP from the host since the two moles of ATP generated by tumor metabolism are not available for host use, and the six moles of ATP required by the host for lactic acid metabolism are lost for other uses. Moreover, for each mole of glucose metabolized by the cancer, one mole of glucose is lost to the host for energy metabolism via the Krebs cycle, a process that can result in the production of 36 moles of ATP for host energy purposes. These concepts of recycling of lactate by the host and trapping of nitrogen by the tumor are used by some investigators to explain the syndrome of cancer cachexia; it is difficult, however, for many investigators to reconcile the small volume of malignant disease seen in most cachectic cancer patients as primarily responsible for the syndrome of cancer cachexia via these postulated mechanisms. Young [71] has published a review on energy metabolism and requirements in the cancer patient and notes that basal metabolic rate among cancer patients has considerable variation, and no consistent change in resting metabolism can be identified.

Theologides [64] remains a proponent of the theory that cancers produce peptides and other small molecules responsible for modification of activity of host enzymes that modulate the metabolism of many compounds potentially responsible for maintenance of host nutritional homeostasis. Our group continues to believe that malnutrition in cancer patients generally is secondary to a decrease in nutritional intake related to the anatomic location of the neoplasm or to the adverse gastrointestinal or general systemic effects of radiation therapy, chemotherapy, and surgery.

Brennan postulates that cancer patients are less well adapted to respond to the added insult of starvation than are noncancer patients [3]. Normal homeostatic mechanisms exist to conserve lean tissue mass and to conserve total body protein. The cancer patient seems less able to utilize these lean tissue-conserving mechanisms and to decrease gluconeogenesis from protein stores in the presence of host starvation. Thus, the loss of lean tissue mass continues unabated in the malnourished cancer patient. Brennan does agree, however, that these observations in a tumor-bearing host are inevitably compounded by decreases in intake and a decrease in the efficient utilization of ingested nutrients.

NUTRITIONAL MANIPULATION AS A THERAPEUTIC TOOL

Although cancer cells have the enzymatic machinery for the tricarboxylic acid cycle reactions, there is evidence that this cycle in the cancer cell functions poorly at a pH below 7.4. Warburg [66] has shown that in vitro glycolysis is inhibited progressively by a decreasing pH and is inhibited completely at a pH of 6. Thus, in the metabolism of glucose, a vicious cycle might occur within the cancer cell: As more glucose is metabolized, more lactic acid is generated via anaerobic glycolysis, causing a decrease in interstitial and cellular pH; the tricarboxylic acid cycle ceases to function and more dependence on anaerobic glycolysis ensues, thereby producing more lactic acid and a further fall in pH. If the pH reaches 6 within the cancer cell, conceivably tumor metabolism might be severely restricted because both anaerobic and aerobic glycolysis would cease. Such a situation would be unusual, however, in the dynamic, homeostatic state within the host, since an adequate blood supply to the tumor tissue would constantly "wash out" the lactic acid produced within the tumor, thus preventing tumor pH from reaching such low levels. Nevertheless, the possibility of a progressively decreasing pH within the tumor environment secondary to an increase in glucose infusion is intriguing and deserves further evaluation.

Meyer [34] developed the concept that certain chemotherapeutic agents, especially methotrexate, enjoy an increased penetration into the cancer cell in an acid environment, another benefit that a lower pH might have within the tumor cell. He tested his hypothesis in rats with transplanted Walker carcinosarcoma-256 and found that those animals maintained on a high-glucose oral diet had better tumor regression when treated with methotrexate than did animals maintained on normal rat chow. Intravenous hyperalimentation contains 250 gm of glucose per 1,000 ml along with amino acids, minerals, and vitamins to provide host anabolism. Properly managed, 750 to 1,000 gm of glucose can be administered to man daily with maintenance of a normal blood sugar and a negative urine sugar. Consequently, both normal and malignant cells are exposed to an excess of glucose. If the biochemical reactions described by Warburg, Meyer, and others occur, IVH might act synergistically with certain chemotherapeutic agents and simultaneously result in nutritional rehabilitation of the host.

In vitro data derived from studies of glucose absorption and transport across small bowel gut sacs from hyperalimented rats suggest that there is a four-fold increase in the ratio of glucose transported to that metabolized within the mucosal cell during bowel rest and nutritional maintenance with IVH [52]. An explanation of this increased efficiency of glucose utilization could be that glucose metabolism within the mucosal cell is predominantly aerobic during hyperalimentation. Those tissues most affected by chemotherapy are the cancer cell, white blood cell, and mucosal cell. Hyperalimentation might disassociate the metabolism of glucose in these cells, resulting in anaerobic glycolysis in the cancer cell and aerobic glucose metabolism in the normal cell. This differential in glucose metabolism may partially explain why certain chemotherapeutic drugs, such as F-FU [54], are better tolerated in the patient treated with IVH without resulting in a decrease in tumor responsiveness to the antimetabolite. Patients receiving IVH do appear to have less anorexia, nausea, vomiting, and diarrhea in response to some chemotherapeutic protocols and consequently may tolerate a larger dose of antitumor drug.

The treatment of cancer by selectively inducing an amino acid deficiency lethal to the neoplasm, but tolerated by the host, is not a new concept. The experimental difficulty lies in finding a good method of long-term administration of diets lacking in one or more amino acids while otherwise maintaining nutritional equilibrium. That this approach has some therapeutic promise is suggested from several reported experiments. Holt and Albanese [27] first reported the dependence of normal spermatogenesis on the amino acid arginine. Schachter et al. [51] treated male patients with oligospermia with arginine and noted a 100 percent increase in sperm count in 23.6 percent of patients. Withholding arginine from patients with normal spermatogenesis would severely depress the sperm count. If arginine had such an effect on rapidly multiplying sperm cells, one might postulate that it or another amino acid might have a similar effect on rapidly multiplying cancer cells. Jose and Good [29] fed tumor-bearing mice restricted casein diets in order to render them deficient in cystine, methionine, and tryptophan. The effect of a deficiency of a single amino acid was tested by feeding a series of diets in which the selected amino acid was reduced to 50, 25, or 10 percent of its composition in a standard amino acid diet. A selected depression in tumor growth was noted in the mice fed low casein diets. Specific dietary restriction of phenylalanine, tyrosine, valine, threonine, methionine, cystine, isoleucine, or tryptophan profoundly reduced serum blocking antibody without affecting cell-mediated immunity. Thus, by dietary manipulation, the immunologic balance of the animal was shifted toward the host. Moderate leucine restriction, however, resulted in depression of cell-mediated immunity and had no effect on serum blocking antibody. Theurer [65] showed that growth of a C57BL mouse adrenocarcinoma was inhibited by reducing dietary levels of phenylalanine, valine, or isoleucine without affecting host weight. Dietary levels of tryptophan, threonine, leucine, or methionine that significantly inhibited tumor growth also significantly depressed host weight. Moderate leucine restriction resulted in moderate stimulation (19 percent) of tumor growth. Allan and associates [1] added L-phenylalanine and L-tyrosine to the normal diet of five leukemic patients. Serum amino acid imbalance was documented, and regression of the leukemic process for a short period of time was identified in each patient. Demopoulous [21] restricted phenylalanine and tyrosine from the diet of patients with metastatic melanoma and noted tumor regression in four of five patients. He stated, however, that this diet was "cumbersome, complex, and unpalatable, making its application difficult."

Few studies are available on the serum, urine, and tissue amino acid profiles of patients with cancer, but available results suggest that free amino acids in the blood of cancer patients do not differ dramatically from those of normal patients [70]. Lorincz and associates [32] demonstrated widely varying patterns of tissue amino acids in various tumors, but in each individual, geographically separate metastases showed remarkable similarity in amino acid patterns. Thus, background information on free amino acid profiles from a variety of malignant neoplasms seems necessary to provide more speculative information as to which amino acids to manipulate.

Young and Richardson [72] recently have summarized the information available on minerals in the prevention of malignancies. They conclude that there is no evidence to suggest that manipulation or change in our usual trace element intake would have any important impact on the incidence of human cancers. However, they do recommend that trace element intake and balance studies receive clinical evaluation in order to determine whether they serve as cocarcinogens in the induction of malignant neoplasms in human beings. Several English investigators [42] have reported their experience with the effect of electrolyte depletion on cancer growth. They observed tumor regression in 11 of 13 patients when the serum magnesium was maintained below 1.0 mg/dl and serum potassium was maintained below 3 mEq/L. The investigators used hemodialysis to produce the desired electrolyte pattern and observed that the better nourished patients had a greater effect of potassium and magnesium depletion on tumor regression. Similar effects of magnesium and potassium depletion on tumor growth have been demonstrated in the rat model [50, 62]. The purpose of IVH is to reverse negative nitrogen balance, to produce anabolism, and to effect a net increase in new cells. Potassium and magnesium are major intracellular ions. As anabolism is stimulated by IVH, hypokalemia and hypomagnesemia will regularly result, unless potassium and magnesium are added to the IVH solutions. We have postulated that these electrolytes are utilized in forming the intracellular milieu of the new cells and, consequently, routinely have added them to the IVH solutions. In fact, the more severe the initial malnutrition or the more rapid anabolism becomes once IVH is begun, the greater is the need for exogenous magnesium and potassium. Since hypomagnesemia and hypokalemia can be produced by the induction of anabolism with IVH and patients can be carefully monitored during such intervals, depletion of potassium and magnesium while maintaining appropriate amino acid and calorie intake is an interesting avenue of research and deserves some consideration. Rudman and his associates [48] have confirmed that anabolism and nitrogen retention in the normal host will not proceed unless adequate quantities of nitrogen, sodium, potassium and phosphorus are provided; thus, the tumor and the host may be functioning similarly in that neither is capable of an anabolic response to proper caloric intake unless adequate minerals are available. In this light, the results obtained by the English investigators during hemodialysis of patients with metastatic cancer are difficult to interpret.*

NUTRITIONAL REPLETION: WHO PROFITS? HOST OR TUMOR

Adjunctive nutritional therapy in experimental animals initially identified host and tumor competition for nutrient substrates and caused concern over the potential for accelerated growth during nutritional repletion. Cameron et al. [5] and Steiger et al. [60] suggested that nutritional therapy in tumor-bearing, malnourished rats

**Editor's Note:* The experience with potassium and magnesium depletion [42] may be a reflection of differential sensitivities of tumor and host cells to the same disturbance—tumor cells being more sensitive due to the rapid growth rate.

stimulates tumor growth, and in studies from our laboratory, this possibility has also been identified. Controversy exists, at least in the rat, whether nutritional therapy preferentially benefits the malnourished host or increases tumor growth to the detriment of the host. Munro et al. [39] reported that total RNA content of a rat hepatoma did not vary with dietary intake of the host, whereas the total RNA content of the host liver was significantly higher in animals on a 25 percent protein diet compared with animals maintained on a protein-free diet. Ota et al. [40] made similar observations in rats with Morris hepatomas. His group studied the effects of protein depletion and subsequent repletion on host liver enzymes and protein content and compared these effects with those obtained from Morris hepatomas growing as a transplant in the flank of the host animal. The tumor-bearing, protein-depleted rats were assigned randomly to one of three feeding groups which: (1) continued to receive the protein-depleted diet; (2) resumed ingestion of a normal protein diet; or (3) received all nutrients parenterally as IVH. As anticipated, the protein content of the liver was reduced significantly during protein depletion. Ota hypothesized that the host liver was relinquishing its protein for use elsewhere in the organism by both the host and the tumor. In the hepatoma, protein content remained unchanged during variations of the quantity of protein in the diet. Apparently, the tumor had the ability to capture essential amino acid moieties to maintain the protein content of its malignant cells even when host protein intake was negligible. During dietary protein repletion, there was no measurable difference in tumor protein content, but host liver protein content was restored to predepletion levels. In terms of total RNA and protein content, hepatomas in the experiments of Munro and Ota appeared to be insensitive to dietary intake, whereas the host liver manifested wide fluctuations in RNA and protein content, depending on the protein level in the diet. These results suggested that nutritional repletion was advantageous to the host by restoring depleted cellular RNA and protein content, whereas tumor biosynthetic function did not appear to be altered.

Alterations in the biosynthesis of specific enzymes in tumors do appear to fluctuate with change in dietary intake of the host. Wu et al. [69] reported that Morris hepatomas increased their glutamine synthetase activity when host dietary intake of protein was reduced. In experiments of Ota et al. [40] similar observations were made. Host and tumor metabolism were evaluated by measuring fructose-1,6-diphosphatase (FDPase), an enzyme in the gluconeogenic pathway between pyruvate and glucose, and by measuring glutamate-pyruvate transaminase (GPT) and glutamate-oxaloacetate transaminase (GOT). These latter two enzymes degrade alanine and aspartic acid to pyruvate and oxaloacetate, respectively. In the protein-depleted host liver, FDPase activity was elevated significantly, whereas GPT and GOT activities were reduced significantly. The increase in FDPase activity suggested that liver protein was being utilized to provide amino acid moieties for gluconeogenesis, a compatible explanation since liver protein content was reduced in protein-depleted rats. The low transaminase activities in the livers of the protein-depleted rats suggested that the amino acid enzyme-degrading pathways were reduced in order to conserve the diminished hepatic protein stores. In the hepatoma, FDPase activity was unchanged by varying the protein in the diet, but GOT and GPT activities were increased significantly after a period of protein depletion. Possibly, the increase in tumor GOT and GPT activities represented a compensation by the tumor for the protein deficiency of the host. If so, the hepatoma might have been in a better condition than the host liver to compete actively for amino acids to utilize as energy substrates and nitrogen sources. Although protein repletion had no effect on tumor FDPase activity, GOT and GPT activities were lowered significantly. In host liver, nutritional repletion resulted in normalization of the activities of FDPase, GOT, and GPT. These data suggest that nutritional repletion of the malnourished host decreased tumor utilization of alanine and aspartic acid for energy production and allowed gluconeogenic activities within the host liver to function more normally. In these experiments, tumor growth was not stimulated out of proportion to nutritional repletion of the host. Thus, the study of enzyme changes in host liver and hepatoma indicated that nutritional repletion preferentially benefited the host.

The effect of dietary manipulation on tumor growth in rat-tumor models remains somewhat confusing because of the different experimental methods utilized. Most investigators have shown that malnourished rats have significantly smaller tumors than their well-nourished counterparts. Reilly et al. [46] made similar observations, but noted that during starvation, the tumor increased its specific DNA activity, whereas specific activity of DNA in the livers of both tumor- and non-tumorbearing animals decreased during starvation. These authors believed that such data suggested a failure of the tumor to recognize normal host controlling mechanisms and, in the presence of host starvation, the tumor maintained its specific activity of DNA at the expense of the host. These studies were done with tritiated thymidine, and in vivo tracer studies of protein, RNA, and DNA are dependent on: (1) pool size of the substrate, (2) tissue uptake of the substrate, (3) the distribution of the substrate within the host. Because these three parameters may vary widely with changes in host nutrition, it becomes difficult to compare data in protein-depleted or starved animals with information obtained from a well-nourished group. Possibly, monitoring the capacity of host and tumor tissues to synthesize messenger RNA and its specific translocation products can prevent problems encountered in interpreting data from radioactive substrate labeling experiments during dietary changes.

If nutritional repletion does stimulate tumor cell replication and metabolism, there may be an optimal time period during early nutritional repletion when tumor cell growth and division are maximal, and the tumor is most susceptible to antimetabolites such as methotrexate. Daly et al. [20] demonstrated that protein-calorie repletion of malnourished Sprague-Dawley rats with transplanted Walker-256 carcinosarcomas accelerated host and tumor growth within 48 hours and within six days resulted in growth patterns similar to those of well-nourished, tumor-bearing animals. Reynolds et al. [47], utilizing the same experimental protocol, gave animals methotrexate either two days or six days after protein repletion had begun. These times were chosen to correspond with the period of rapid tumor growth after nutritional repletion identified by Daly. Methotrexate administration had no effect on tumor or carcass weight if a protein-free diet was continued. The greatest inhibition of tumor growth occurred in rats fed a regular diet and treated with methotrexate two days after nutritional repletion had begun. The greatest reduction in tumor weight compared with the greatest gain in carcass weight also occurred in this group of rats. Since methotrexate inhibits DNA synthesis, Reynolds concluded that the good response to methotrexate after nutritional repletion had begun was secondary to an increase in tumor cell replication stimulated by feeding the regular diet. Conversely, the poor response to methotrexate in rats continued on the protein-free diet was secondary to depressed tumor cell metabolism and replication coincident with minimal carcass weight gain in these animals. If specific DNA activity in tumor had been increased during protein depletion, as might be expected from the results of Reilly et al. [46], an effect of methotrexate on tumor growth in those animals continued on the protein-free diet would have been expected also.

Although acceleration of tumor growth in human beings has not been observed during short intervals of nutritional repletion, the results from rat experiments suggest that this possibility exists in the mammalian species, and that appropriate antineoplastic therapy should be instituted early during nutritional rehabilitation. Data in rats, however, cannot be applied directly to malnourished cancer patients, since doubling times of human malignant tumors are measured in days or weeks, and the cancer may not kill the patient until several years after the initial clone of malignant cells has developed. Since the doubling times of animal tumors often can be measured in hours, the relatively rapid growth can result in death of the animal within five to seven weeks after initial tumor inoculation. Thus, dietary protein repletion or depletion can be expected to have a more obvious and measurable effect on a tumor such as a Walker-256 carcinosarcoma because of its rapid growth characteristics. As in rats, however, tumors in cachectic human beings have not been noted to be more responsive to DNA-specific chemotherapeutic agents, and to recommend a period of starvation as treatment for cancer in man is undesirable, but it has been suggested by others in the past.

Although Jose and Good [29] postulated a potential benefit from malnutrition in cancer patients because serum blocking antibodies appeared to be depressed out of proportion to any depression of cell-mediated immunity when tumor-bearing rats became moderately protein-calorie malnourished, severe restriction of the protein in the diet of their animals resulted in depression of both humoral and cellular immune responses. Using complete Freund's adjuvant to sensitize nontumor-bearing, young rats to purified protein derivative (PPD), our group demonstrated that protein depletion rapidly led to a loss of weight and of PPD reactivity [17]. Feeding an amino acid diet adequate in minerals and vitamins to these protein-malnourished rats maintained body weight at the lower levels, but did not result in restoration of PPD reactivity. Feeding a diet adequate in protein, minerals, vitamins, and nonprotein calories restored both body weight and PPD reactivity to normal. This study demonstrated that loss of PPD reactivity occurred when inadequate protein and/or nonprotein calories were fed to an immunocompetent rat, and that both adequate protein and calorie substrates were necessary to restore immune reactivity to normal in the malnourished rat. Although serum blocking antibody was not measured in this study, the deleterious effects on PPD reactivity secondary to protein and/or nonprotein calorie restrictions were obvious.

Cancer and malnutrition are both thought to be singularly immunosuppressive. To examine the interrelationships between cancer and malnutrition in an animal-tumor model, Daly et al. [16] designed an experimental protocol to mimic the clinical situation often seen in human beings with cancer, that is—malnourished, immune-incompetent animals with viable neoplasms. PPD reactive rats bearing transplanted Morris hepatomas were protein-depleted by feeding them a high-carbohydrate protein-free diet for two weeks. Next, the rats were randomized to receive either (1) continuation of the high-carbohydrate protein-free diet, (2) normal rat chow, or (3) IVH. After one week, none of the animals continuing the high-carbohydrate protein-free diet regimen regained PPD reactivity, whereas almost all animals receiving the regular diet or IVH became PPD reactive. Tumor weight to body weight ratios were not significantly different in all groups, although tumors in the nutritionally repleted animals were somewhat larger. Tumor growth had not been stimulated out of proportion to host nutritional repletion by either IVH or the normal diet, and nutritionally replenished animals were immunocompetent. Although certain malignant neoplasms might produce a substance that is directly immunosuppressive, in this experimental model, PPD reactivity could be correlated with dietary intake and was restored by proper nutritional repletion.

IVH: A HISTORICAL AND IMMUNOLOGIC EVALUATION

Prior to 1974, IVH had not been used widely to nutritionally replenish malnourished cancer patients. Physicians feared stimulation of tumor growth by the nutritional solutions and, from a more practical and realistic standpoint, feared potential septic complications from the indwelling superior vena cava feeding catheter in patients with depressed leukocyte counts secondary to chemotherapy or radiotherapy, and with depressed immunocompetence secondary to oncologic treatment, malnutrition, or tumor burden. Dudrick et al. [68] had shown previously that proper aseptic management of the indwelling catheter and the IVH delivery system and aseptic mixing of the IVH solutions by the pharmacist minimized septic complications secondary to IVH in a noncancer patient population, and our group speculated that similar results could be obtained in cancer patients if proper technique was utilized. At our institution in 1974, there was a group of cachectic cancer patients who were *not* considered candidates for oncologic therapy because of the fear of complications that would result from the use of antineoplastic agents in malnourished patients. These patients would have been denied adequate oncologic treatment had they not received nutritional repletion with IVH, since enteral repletion had failed already. Under these circumstances, stimulation of tumor growth by the nutritional solutions was moot, and any risk of infection secondary to the indwelling subclavian vein feeding catheters was acceptable. Intravenous hyperalimentation was initially used to treat 93 cachectic cancer patients with a wide variety of malignant diseases [12]. Half the patients in the study received chemotherapy and had leukocyte count depressions below 2,500 cells per cubic millimeter for an average duration of 7.2 days. The average period of IVH was 24.8 days. No organisms were grown from the catheters in place for less than ten days, and eight positive cultures (7.3 percent) were obtained from catheters in place longer than ten days. The catheter could be incriminated as a source of infection in only two patients (2.2 percent), both of whom had *Candida albicans* cultured from the catheter and the bloodstream. These patients subsequently tolerated a therapeutic course of chemotherapy, or radiation therapy, or a major surgical procedure, any of which could have been potentially fatal without nutritional rehabilitation with IVH. From these observations, the application of IVH as adjunctive nutritional therapy for cancer patients appeared to be safe and efficacious, and no stimulation of tumor growth was identified.

An additional factor in the low rate of observed catheter sepsis may have been a return to normal function of the immune mechanism. Cell-mediated immunity can be divided into two broad categories: (1) primary and initiated by contact with a new antigen and (2) established in the past, capable of immediate recall, and demonstrable by response to skin test antigens. Short-term chemotherapy suppresses primary cell-mediated immunity, but should have no effect on established immunity. Malnutrition suppresses established cell-mediated immunity. Both types of cell-mediated immunity are important in preventing sepsis during chemotherapy; therefore, if the patient becomes malnourished during chemotherapy or is malnourished at the outset of treatment, he may have minimal immunologic defense against infection, and susceptibility to sepsis may increase.

The relative extent to which malnutrition contributes to immune incompetency during oncologic therapy is unknown. Suppression of immune function after various forms of oncologic therapy is well documented. Anesthetic agents such as chloroform and halothane inhibit delayed hypersensitivity and phagocytic activity [4]. Jubert and coworkers [30] observed that major intraabdominal or intrathoracic procedures, or an intraoperative blood loss greater than 500 ml, were associated with marked suppression of in vitro lymphocyte transformation to mitogens and antigens. The nutritional status of these surgical patients, however, was not identified. The response of the immune system to the effects of chemotherapy is both dose- and time-related. Hersh and coworkers [25] noted the immunologic advantages of intensive, intermittent drug therapy over continuous chemotherapy and thought that these advantages were critical for patient survival and tumor response. The nutritional status of patients in these studies was not reported. Hersh and his group did suggest that recovery of the host immune response and regression of cancer might be related in a cause and effect manner, and that this relationship might be responsible for prolonged survival obtained in patients who were immunologically competent. Potentially, patients who received intermittent chemotherapy might have maintained a better nutritional status, and the improved nutritional status contributed to the competency of the immune system. Radiation therapy appears to result in a more permanent suppression of cell-mediated immunity than does either surgery or chemotherapy. Stjernsward et al. [61] reported that radiation therapy increased the ratio of B-cells to T-cells in the peripheral blood by specifically reducing the T-cell population. Several investigators [14] observed a persistent lymphopenia for more than ten years after radiation therapy had ended, and suggested that suppression of host immunity by radiation therapy was specific for the cell-mediated immune response. Patients described in these studies were well nourished, and any long-term suppression of cell-mediated immunity by radiation therapy probably could not be attributed to malnutrition.

In our attempts to define the contribution of malnutrition to the suppression of immunocompetence associated with oncologic therapy, 160 patients who were malnourished or whose treatment would ordinarily result in malnutrition were tested with a battery of five recall skin test antigens at seven- to ten-day intervals throughout antineoplastic therapy and nutritional rehabilitation with IVH [19]. Skin tests were read 48 hours after intradermal injection, and a reaction to any of the five antigens consisting of 10 × 10 mm of induration was considered to be a positive result. Originally negative tests were interpreted as having converted to positive if at least 10 mm of induration existed in one or more antigen sites and if a 100 percent increase in the diameter of induration was attained when compared with the pre-IVH reaction. Forty-five patients in the chemotherapy group were initially skin-test negative; 25 of these patients converted their skin tests to positive reactions in an average period of 18.8 days of IVH. Thirty-eight percent of the patients who manifested positive skin test reactions throughout nutritional therapy or converted results from negative to positive responded to chemotherapy, compared with only 20 percent of patients whose skin test reactions remained negative. In patients who converted skin test reactions from negative to positive and responded to chemotherapy, skin test conversion usually occurred prior to any measurable reduction in tumor size. In the group of 49 surgical patients, postoperative complications developed in 69 percent of patients whose skin test reactions remained negative throughout IVH or converted to negative despite IVH, whereas only 25 percent of surgical patients who maintained positive skin test reactivity or converted skin tests to positive preoperatively had postoperative complications. In the supportive care group, 56 percent of the negative reactors converted skin tests from negative to positive in an average period of 11.6 days of IVH and gained an average weight of 5.8 pounds during this time interval. For patients whose skin test responses remained positive or converted to positive during treatment with IVH, subsequent oncologic therapy was uncomplicated.

Of the 20 patients in the radiation therapy group, nine failed either to convert skin test reactions from negative to positive or to maintain positive skin test reactions during radiotherapy. These patients usually were receiving radiation therapy to T-cell bearing areas, such as the thymus or large areas of bone marrow, and possibly the number or efficacy of circulating T-lymphocytes that are responsible for delayed cutaneous hypersensitivity were reduced significantly. Although positive skin test reactivity was often difficult to achieve in this group, there were no complications secondary to radiotherapy, and nutritional rehabilitation was considered adequate.

Evaluation of these 160 patients represents an expansion of a study of 47 patients initially done to determine the effect of IVH on established cell-mediated immunity in the cancer patient [10]. Conclusions reached in the initial study remain justified and consistent with the additional patient information. Those conclusions were: (1) immune depression attributed to chemotheraphy, in part, may be secondary to malnutrition; (2) skin test reactivity, in general, was depressed during radiation therapy to the mediastinum and pelvis, even though nutrition was estimated to be adequate; and (3) surgical patients with negative skin tests either expired or had prolonged postoperative recovery periods, whereas patients with positive tests had an uncomplicated postoperative recovery. Intravenous hyperalimentation was responsible for nutritional repletion in each of these 160 patients and probably was responsible for, and at the very least associated with, return of the positive skin test reactivity in the majority of negative reactors. Radiotherapy, certain chemotherapeutic drugs, and the physiologic events associated with anesthesia and operative intervention may be immunosuppressive. Nevertheless, this study indicates that a portion of the immunodepression associated with antineoplastic therapy is secondary to malnutrition and not necessarily a result of a direct suppressor effect on the immune system by the oncologic treatment regimen or by a circulating substance liberated by the neoplasm. Because established cell-mediated immunity is effective against many microorganisms, nutritional repletion with IVH might have improved host defense mechanisms against many bacteria, fungi, and viruses, which could have imposed an additional infectious problem because of the indwelling central venous catheter. Mortality usually occurred in those patients with persistently negative skin tests, and most often the precipitating cause of death was sepsis. Current concepts in cancer treatment dictate that surgery should be utilized to remove the bulk of the malignant disease whenever possible and that chemotherapy and radiation therapy should be employed to eliminate remaining cancer cells. No doubt, the immune mechanism participates with the oncologic agents in destruction and elimination of these neoplastic cells. Thus, a return to function of the immune mechanisms via nutritional repletion would be important, particularly if specific tumor immunity had been established in the host throughout the life span of the cancerous process. Some support for this hypothesis is evident in this study, since response to chemotherapy occurred most frequently in patients with positive skin tests.

Not all of the 160 patients studied by our group demonstrated an improvement in skin test reactivity during intravenous nutritional support, possibly because of a more severe degree of malnutrition prior to the initiation of IVH. To evaluate this hypothesis, *pretreatment* immunologic and nutritional parameters were measured in 140 cancer patients who *were* to receive IVH [18]. Serum albumin concentration, the degree of recent weight loss, total lymphocyte count, and skin test reactivity were the parameters used to quantitate nutritional status. Fifty-seven patients had a positive reaction to at least one skin test, whereas 83 patients had negative reactions to the battery of five recall skin test antigens. Negative reactors compared with positive reactors had greater body weight loss and lower serum albumin levels and total lymphocyte counts, each of which correlated with the degree of malnutrition. The negative reactors had a decreased response to chemotherapy and an increase in postoperative morbidity and mortality. Possibly, a more prolonged course of IVH prior to oncologic treatment might have resulted in a better outcome for the negative reactors. Unfortunately, the physician does not always have the luxury of waiting until nutritional repletion is complete before beginning specific therapy for a malignant lesion, and the risk of waiting too long to initiate antineoplastic therapy may outweigh the benefits of prolonged attempts at nutritional rehabilitation. The importance of nutritional rehabilitation cannot be overemphasized, but must be integrated into the overall management of the cancer patient.

CLINICAL MATERIAL

Our team defines malnutrition as a recent, unintentional loss of 10 percent or more of body weight, a serum albumin concentration of less than 3.4 gm/100 ml, and/or a negative reaction to a battery of recall skin test antigens. Patients who satisfy two of these three criteria and who have a reasonable chance of responding to appropriate oncologic therapy are candidates for IVH. Also, patients who are incapable of adequate enteral nutrition because of malnutrition imposed by previous cancer therapy are candidates for nutritional rehabilitation with IVH. Nutritionally healthy patients whose treatment plan requires multiple courses of chemotherapy, possibly combined with surgery or radiation therapy, also should be considered candidates for IVH if maintenance of optimal nutrition during therapy is considered important to maximize the chance for response to treatment, to reduce complications of oncologic therapy, and to improve the quality of life. There are many important tests for evaluating nutritional status, but without the aid of an organized nutritional support service, the practicing physician cannot do all available tests. From a practical standpoint, we rely on percent weight loss, serum albumin concentration, and reactivity to skin test antigens.*

At our institutions, over 2,000 patients have received IVH as nutritional support for oncologic therapy during the last five years. Our group evaluated the results of IVH in the treatment of 406 consecutive cancer patients suffering from a wide variety of malignant diseases [8, 9]. Treatment categories were: chemotherapy—43 percent; general and thoracic surgery—24 percent; head and neck surgery—10 percent; radiation therapy—10 percent; fistulas—6 percent; and supportive care—7 percent. Hyperalimentation was utilized for an average time of 23.9 days, and the average weight gain in these 406 patients during IVH was five pounds. Response to chemotherapy or radiation therapy was defined as a 50 percent or greater reduction in measurable malignant tissue mass.

Chemotherapy

Two hundred and sixty courses of chemotherapy were given to 175 patients. Intravenous hyperalimentation was utilized for an average period of 22.8 days, and the average weight gain was 5.6 pounds. Depression of the leukocyte count below 2,500 cells per cubic millimeter occurred in 51.5 percent of patients and lasted for an average duration of 7.7 days; nevertheless, only four pathogenic organisms were grown on cultures from 212 consecutive subclavian vein catheters. Three patients had simultaneous positive blood and catheter cultures for an incidence of catheter-related sepsis of only 1.4 percent. Patients completed a planned course of chemotherapy, and tumor response was obtained in 27.8 percent of patients (range 11 percent to 31 percent). Such a response rate represents our ability to select patients for IVH and chemotherapy rather than an overall percentage response of a patient group to a particular drug protocol. Many patients had failed to respond to primary chemotherapy and were being treated with drugs known to result in a limited response, or they were patients who had relapsed after an initial response to chemotherapy and were being treated with a different drug regimen. When discharged from the hospital, the responding patients were able to maintain the weight gained during IVH and seldom required intravenous nutritional support for follow-up courses of chemotherapy. Gastrointestinal symptoms of nausea, vomiting, and diarrhea were reduced or better tolerated if IVH was used with chemotherapy. The beneficial effect of IVH depended, however, on the drug protocol employed. For example, IVH had minimal effect on the systemic symptoms produced by the administration of Bleomycin and Vinblastine, whereas the gastrointestinal side effects of 5-FU might be eliminated completely.

The concept of increased tolerance for 5-FU during "bowel rest" and nutritional maintenance with IVH was initially tested in animals [59]. Rats that nourished themselves ad libitum with ordinary rat chow were compared with animals nourished entirely by IVH. Both groups received a single intraperitoneal dose of 5-FU, 15 mg/kg per day, for seven days. Eighty percent of animals eating ad libitum died within ten days of beginning 5-FU injections, whereas only 30 percent of animals nourished by IVH died during the ten-day interval. This experience was extrapolated to human beings, and 16 patients with metastatic colon carcinoma who had lesions evaluable for chemotherapeutic response were placed on IVH

**Editor's Note:* The reduced serum albumin concentration has traditionally been viewed as a manifestation of decreased albumin synthesis secondary to malnutrition. Recent studies from our laboratory (Karlberg [30a]) have suggested that synthetic rates are well maintained and that hypoalbuminemia is a reflection of increased body water and increased pool size, in other words, a dilutional effect. Thus, if hypoalbuminemia is not a reflection of decreased hepatic synthesis of albumin, it is not likely to be useful in the definition of malnutrition. Karlberg's findings may explain why some investigators have had difficulty in establishing a relationship between hypoalbuminemia and postoperative morbidity and mortality.

for seven to ten days prior to beginning treatment with 5-FU (15 mg/kg per day diluted in 50 ml of 5 percent dextrose and water and delivered intravenously during a one hour period). Ten control patients had similar disease patterns and degrees of malnutrition, but did not receive IVH. In the IVH group, five patients (31 percent) responded with a greater than 50 percent reduction in measurable tumor volume and received a total dose of 7.4 gm of 5-FU over an average period of 8.6 days. Only one control patient (10 percent) responded to an average total dose of 3.8 gm of 5-FU given over an average time of only 4.4 days. The control group lost an average weight of 4.2 pounds during 5-FU administration. Although conclusions in this study must be guarded because the patient groups are small, the percent response rate in the IVH group was the same as that noted by Moertel et al. [36] in patients who were treated with 5-FU for gastrointestinal cancer and had an excellent performance status. In Moertel's series, patients with a poor performance status had only 10 percent response to 5-FU. Whether the increased response in nutritionally healthy patients was secondary to nutritional repletion or to tolerance of a larger dose of 5-FU remains to be evaluated. Another explanation for the poor results of chemotherapy with 5-FU in malnourished patients may be related to folate-deficient states commonly found in cachectic cancer patients [2].

Issell et al. [28] recently reported preliminary results of a prospective, randomized trial utilizing patients with non-oat cell carcinoma of the lung. Twenty-six patients underwent oncologic therapy with Adriamycin, Ifosfamide, and *Corynebacterium parvum*. Thirteen patients were chosen randomly to receive IVH for ten days prior to chemotherapy and to continue it for 31 days throughout the first course of chemotherapy. The other patients were supported nutritionally by standard techniques that did not include IVH. During the first course of chemotherapy, the IVH group experienced less nausea and vomiting and had a significant improvement in anthropometric measurements when compared to the non-IVH control group. A response to chemotherapy was identified in four patients in the IVH group and in only one patient in the non-IVH group. These results are preliminary, but do support retrospective data previously reported by Copeland [11], Lanzotti [31], and their coworkers. Studies currently sponsored by the Diet, Nutrition and Cancer Program of the National Cancer Institute are nearing completion and, at present, neither response rates nor survival has been improved in patients receiving IVH [23]. In many of these studies, patients with only marginal degrees of malnutrition were entered into the randomization process. Little if any documentation of differences in response rates would be expected unless patients with severe malnutrition were selected for study. From the ethical and moral standpoint, most investigators are hesitant to deny patients suffering from severe degrees of malnutrition access to nutritional rehabilitation either parenterally or enterally for the purpose of obtaining randomized, prospective data. At this moment, IVH should be used in cancer patients as a means of nutritional rehabilitation when such a goal is desirable to optimize response to chemotherapy and to minimize complications from the antineoplastic agents.

Surgery

One hundred patients received IVH as nutritional support for a general or thoracic surgical procedure. Fifty-two patients underwent curative resections, which included esophagectomies, gastrectomies, and abdominal-perineal resections. Without IVH, recovery from surgical procedures of this magnitude would have been questionable in each instance. The average age of the patients was 56.6 years; IVH was utilized for an average period of 24.2 days; and patients gained an average weight of 4.2 pounds. Only four patients expired postoperatively, and catheter-related sepsis occurred in only one patient. In 57 patients, IVH was utilized for an average period of 12.3 days preoperatively and for an average period of 13.9 days postoperatively. In 11 patients, IVH was used preoperatively only for an average period of 18.1 days, and in 32 patients, IVH was used postoperatively only for an average period of 18.9 days. In patients who received IVH pre- and post-operatively, weight gain and a rise in serum albumin concentration were attained almost entirely during the preoperative period. Weight and serum albumin concentration were maintained during the postoperative period, but did not increase significantly. Those individuals who received IVH only postoperatively usually had developed one of the complications of prolonged inanition—i.e., wound infection, paralytic ileus, decubitus ulcer, or wound dehiscence—before IVH was instituted. Weight gain in these patients was difficult to obtain, probably because of increased energy expenditure secondary to the surgical complications. In contrast, patients who received IVH preoperatively had virtually no postoperative complications and often were eating within five days after bowel resection. Consequently, we recommend that a malnourished patient be nutritionally replenished *preoperatively,* and not only after some catastrophic postoperative complication occurs.

Patients with malignant neoplasms of the oropharyngeal area present a special nutritional problem because of prior dietary indiscretions, heavy alcohol intake, and smoking. These patients often are undernourished and have vitamin deficiencies at the time an oropharyngeal malignancy develops, and malnutrition is potentiated by the cancer if it produces obstruction or pain on eating. Intravenous hyperalimentation was used in 39 such patients who would not tolerate or respond favorably to nasogastric tube feedings. Prompt nutritional replenishment and weight gain were achieved in each patient; nevertheless, four patients died postoperatively, probably because the magnitude of the operative procedure exceeded the capability of wound healing. Cancers of the head and neck region often grow to a large size before metastasizing. Although these lesions may be anatomically removed, wound healing cannot be accomplished even during nutritional replenishment with IVH because of the extent of the surgical resection. Overzealous surgery should not be attempted in older patients, even if weight gain and an increase in strength has been attained on IVH.

Three patients had pharyngeal incompetence after a head and neck surgical procedure, and the incompetence was thought to be secondary to muscle weakness and reversible muscle injury. Nutritional rehabilitation was accomplished with IVH, and deglutitory muscular rehabilitation was begun. Concomitant with return of general body muscle strength and tone, swallowing function returned after 18 to 48 days of IVH.

Catheter-related sepsis was the most common complication resulting from the use of IVH in patients with malignant tumors of the head and neck. Secretions from pharyngostomy or tracheostomy stomas frequently contaminated the catheter dressings and necessitated daily dressing changes. Sixteen percent of all catheters used in these patients were contaminated upon removal. Pathogenic organisms were cultured from feeding catheters from seven (17.9 percent) patients. Four (10.3 percent) patients had simultaneous positive blood cultures associated with sepsis. In two patients, subsequent causes of the positive blood cultures other than the catheter were identified, but in the remaining two patients, the elevated temperature resolved after catheter removal. No deaths or complications secondary to catheter-related sepsis occurred in head and neck patients, and without IVH, these patients would have been extremely poor surgical risks. Nevertheless, a constant vigil against catheter-related sepsis is necessary, and IVH should be utilized in patients requiring major head and neck surgical resections only when other forms of nutritional replenishment are impossible.

A recent addition to parenteral infusion equipment is the long silastic catheter, the tip of which can be directed percutaneously through a vein in the anticubital space to lie in the middle of the superior vena cava. Thus, the catheter skin entrance site is removed to an area distant from the head and neck region. Preliminary results with the use of this catheter for infusion of IVH solutions have been acceptable, and sepsis has been minimized by meticulous catheter care identical to that followed for catheters inserted through the infraclavicular area. At present, our group continues to use the standard infraclavicular, subclavian vein approach unless the potential for infection in this area dictates that an alternate site be selected.

Radiation Therapy

Mucositis secondary to radiation therapy can produce pain on deglutition, nausea, diarrhea, and crampy abdominal pain. Radiation to the gastrointestinal tract may cause edema of the bowel wall and obstruction of an already partially compromised gastrointestinal lumen. The net result of acute radiation enteritis is a decrease in food intake and a diminished capacity to digest and absorb those nutrients that do reach the small intestine.

Thirty-nine malnourished patients required IVH in order to complete a planned course of radiation therapy. Intravenous hyperalimentation was utilized for an average period of 37.6 days, and the average weight gained during IVH was 7.8 pounds. Ninety-five percent of the patients completed their planned courses of radiation therapy and symptomatically improved. Anorexia, nausea, and vomiting disappeared during IVH unless the patients attempted oral feeding, in which case all symptoms recurred. A response to radiation therapy was attained in 54 percent of the patients. Responding patients gained an average of 13.0 ± 6.4 pounds during IVH, whereas nonresponding patients gained only 4.9 ± 8.8 pounds during a similar time interval. In responding patients, serum albumin rose from 3.12 ± 0.49 gm/dl to 3.51 ± 0.68 gm/dl, whereas serum albumin did not rise significantly from an initial average value of 3.09 ± 0.48 gm/dl in nonresponding patients. Intravenous hyperalimentation allowed a planned course of radiation therapy to be delivered to a group of poor-risk, malnourished cancer patients; a correlation between tumor response and improvement in nutritional status was identified; and symptoms of radiation stomatitis and enteritis were reduced or eliminated as long as "bowel rest" was maintained.

Fistulas

Management of cancer patients with enterocutaneous fistulas was quite rewarding. Such fistulas present unique problems because there may be cancer cells within the fistulous tract, the fistula may involve an area of irradiated bowel or abdominal wall, or the patient's life expectancy may be so short that the physician does not think the time required to treat the fistula is justified unless the fistula is immediately life threatening. Each of 24 patients with fistulas was extremely cachectic at the initiation of IVH; nevertheless, 44 percent of the fistulas closed spontaneously, and 28 percent were successfully closed surgically. Patients in whom fistula closure was achieved were able to lead comfortable and productive lives for at least a short period of time. In contrast, results with spontaneous closure of enterocutaneous fistulas arising from areas of irradiated bowel were dismal uniformly [13]. Although spontaneous fistula closure was achieved in several such patients, fistulas eventually recurred, and the patient either required operative therapy or died. We currently recommend that malnourished patients who have radiation-related fistulas of the gastrointestinal tract receive IVH for two to three weeks to stimulate weight gain and a state of anabolism prior to definitive operative intervention to bypass, close, or resect the fistula.

Nutritional Supportive Care

Attempts at enteral nutritional repletion failed in 28 patients who required admission to the hospital specifically for IVH. Although the gastrointestinal tract was functional in over half these patients, they had little desire to eat and were often depressed. Seventeen patients had completed a course of chemotherapy or radiation therapy as outpatients and were unable to recover from the inanition that occurred during treatment. Seven patients had not recovered sufficiently from a major abdominal surgical procedure before their discharge from the hospital and could not regain their weight on outpatient dietary nutritional regimens. Each of these patients improved symptomatically during IVH and was released from the hospital ingesting a regular soft diet after an average period of 13.4 days on IVH. The vicious cycle of malnutrition, anorexia, and further malnutrition had been interrupted by nutritional replenishment with IVH, and psychologic support relieved much of the depression initially identified in these patients. Possibly, the gastrointestinal digestive and absorptive processes were improved concomitant with improvement in the nutritional state, and even more possibly, the patients were psychologically better motivated to eat because of improvement in strength and general well-being. DeWys [49] has correlated anorexia and taste abnormalities with malnutrition, and an improved appetite might have been a manifestation of an improvement in taste sensation. Nevertheless, anorexia disappeared, hunger returned, and the patients looked forward to meals.

THE TERMINAL PATIENT

Occasionally, our group has begun IVH only to find that the patient has a metastatic malignant process for which there is no remaining treatment. In such a situation, we attempt to nourish the patient by enteral means and discontinue IVH. Forced enteral nutritional replenishment of terminal cancer patients has been reported to improve the quality of remaining life [41], and our group has made similar observations utilizing IVH in terminal cancer patients. We continue, however, to recommend that IVH not be used for patients who have received all possible modalities of oncologic therapy and are dying of the combined effects of malnutrition and progressive cancer growth. These patients' nutritional state should be maintained as adequately as possible utilizing all available enteral diets, but with the current state of the art, IVH is not often indicated. Terminal patients may feel somewhat better during IVH infusion, but this effect ceases immediately upon discontinuing IVH. Prolongation of pain for the patient and anguish for the family do not seem justified as indications for the use of IVH in cancer patients.

REFERENCES

1. Allan, J. D., Ireland, J. T., Miller, J., and Moss, A. D. Treatment of leukemia by amino acid imbalance. *Lancet* 1:202, 1965.
2. Bertino, J. R. Nutrients, vitamins and minerals as therapy. *Cancer* 43:2137, 1979.
3. Brennan, M. F. Uncomplicated starvation versus cancer cachexia. *Cancer Res.* 37:2359, 1977.
4. Bruce, O. L., and Wingrad, D. W. Anesthesia and the immune response. *Anesthesiology* 34:271, 1971.
5. Cameron, I. L., and Pavlat, W. A. Stimulation of growth of a transplantable hepatoma in rats by parenteral nutrition. *J. Natl. Cancer Inst.* 56:597, 1976.
6. Capizzi, R. L., Bertino, J. R., and Handschumacher, R. E. L-asparaginase. *Annu. Rev. Med.* 21:433, 1970.
7. Christensen, H. N., and Henderson, M. E. Comparative uptake of free amino acids by mouse-ascites carcinoma cells and normal tissues. *Cancer Res.* 12:229, 1952.
8. Copeland, E. M., Daly, J. M., and Dudrick, S. J. Nutrition as an adjunct to cancer treatment in the adult. *Cancer Res.* 37:2451, 1977.
9. Copeland, E. M., and Dudrick, S. J. Nutritional Aspects of Cancer. In R. C. Hickey (Ed.), *Current Problems in Cancer.* Chicago: Year Book, 1976. Vol. I.
10. Copeland, E. M., MacFadyen, B. V., and Dudrick, S. J. Effect of intravenous hyperalimentation on established delayed hypersensitivity in the cancer patient. *Ann. Surg.* 184:60, 1976.
11. Copeland, E. M., MacFadyen, B. V., Lanzotti, V. C., and Dudrick, S. J. Intravenous hyperalimentation as an adjunct to cancer chemotherapy. *Am. J. Surg.* 129:167, 1975.
12. Copeland, E. M., MacFadyen, B. V., McGown, C., and Dudrick, S. J. The use of hyperalimentation in patients with potential sepsis. *Surg. Gynecol. Obstet.* 138:377, 1974.
13. Copeland, E. M., Souchon, E. A., MacFadyen, B. V., Rapp, M. A., and Dudrick, S. J. Intravenous hyperalimentation as an adjunct to radiation therapy. *Cancer* 39:609, 1977.
14. Cosimi, A. B., Brunstetter, F. H., Kemmerer, W. T., and Miller, B. N. Cellular immune competence of breast cancer patients receiving radiotherapy. *Arch. Surg.* 107:531, 1973.
15. Costa, G. Cachexia, the metabolic component of neoplastic diseases. *Cancer Res.* 37:2327, 1977.

16. Daly, J. M., Copeland, E. M., and Dudrick, S. J. Effects of intravenous nutrition on tumor growth and host immunocompetence in malnourished animals. *Surgery* 84:655, 1978.
17. Daly, J. M., Dudrick, S. J., and Copeland, E. M. Effects of protein depletion and repletion on cell-mediated immunity in experimental animals. *Ann. Surg.* 188:791, 1978.
18. Daly, J. M., Dudrick, S. J., and Copeland, E. M. Evaluation of nutritional indices as prognostic indicators in the cancer patient. *Cancer* 43:925, 1979.
19. Daly, J. M., Dudrick, S. J., and Copeland, E. M. Intravenous hyperalimentation: Effect on delayed cutaneous hypersensitivity in cancer patients. *Ann. Surg.* 192:587, 1980.
20. Daly, J. M., Reynolds, H. M., Rowlands, B. J., Baquero, G., Dudrick, S. J., and Copeland, E. M. Nutritional manipulation of tumor-bearing animals: Effects on body weight, serum protein levels and tumor growth. *Surg. Forum* 29:143, 1978.
21. Demopoulous, H. B. Effects of reducing the phenylalanine-tyrosine intake of patients with advanced malignant melanoma. *Cancer* 19:658, 1966.
22. DeWys, W. D. Anorexia as a general effect of cancer. *Cancer* 43:2013, 1979.
23. DeWys, W. D., and Kisner, D. Maintaining caloric needs in the cancer patient. *Contemp. Surg.* 15:25, 1979.
24. Filler, R. M., Jaffe, N., Cassady, J. R., Traggis, D. G., and Das, J. B. Parenteral nutritional support in children with cancer. *Cancer* 39:2665, 1977.
25. Hersh, E. M., Gutterman, J. U., Mavligit, G., McCredie, K. B., Bodey, G. P., Freireich, E. J., Rossen, R. D., and Buttler, W. T. Host defense, chemical immunosuppression and the transplant recipient. Relative effects of intermittent versus continuous immunosuppressive therapy with reference to the objectives of treatment. *Transplant Proc.* 5:1191, 1973.
26. Holroyde, C. P., Gabuzda, T. G., Putnam, R. C., Paul, P., and Reichard, G. A. Altered glucose metabolism in metastatic carcinoma. *Cancer Res.* 35:3710, 1975.
27. Holt, L. E., and Albanese, A. A. Observations on amino acid deficiencies in man. *Trans. Assoc. Am. Phys.* 58:143, 1944.
28. Issell, B. F., Valdivieso, M., Zaren, H. A., Dudrick, S. J., Freireich, E. J., Copeland, E. M., and Bodey, G. P. Protection against chemotherapy toxicity by IV hyperalimentation. *Cancer Treat. Rep.* 62:1139, 1978.
29. Jose, D. G., and Good, R. A. Quantitative effects of nutritional essential amino acid deficiency upon immune responses to tumors in mice. *J. Exp. Med.* 137:1, 1973.
30. Jubert, A. V., Lee, E. T., Hersh, E. M., and McBride, C. M. Effects of surgery, anesthesia and intraoperative blood loss on immunocompetence. *J. Surg. Res.* 15:399, 1973.
30a. Karlberg, I. Unpublished observations.
31. Lanzotti, V. C., Copeland, E. M., George, S. L., Dudrick, S. J., and Samuels, M. L. Cancer chemotherapeutic response and intravenous hyperalimentation. *Cancer Chemother. Rep.* 59:437, 1975.
32. Lorincz, A. B., and Kuttner, R. E. Responses of malignancy to phenylalanine restriction. *Neb. St. Med. J.* 50:609, 1965.
33. Lundholm, K., Bylund, A. C., Holm, J., and Schersten, T. Skeletal muscle metabolism in patients with malignant tumor. *Eur. J. Cancer* 12:465, 1976.
34. Meyer, J. A. Potentiation of solid-tumor chemotherapy by metabolic alteration. *Ann. Surg.* 179:88, 1974.
35. Mider, G. B., Tesluk, H., and Morton, J. J. Effect of Walker Carcinoma-256 on food intake, body weight and nitrogen metabolism of growing rat. *Acta de L'Unio. Inter. Contrel Cancrum* 6:409, 1948.
36. Moertel, C. G., Schutt, A. J., Hahn, R. G., and Reitemeier, R. J. Effects of patient selection on results of Phase II chemotherapy trials in gastrointestinal cancer. *Cancer Chemother. Rep.* 58:257, 1974.
37. Moreschi, C. Beziehungen zwishen Ernahrung and Tumorwachstum: 2. Immunitaetsforsch. *Exper. Therap.* 2:651, 1909.
38. Morrison, S. D. Control of food intake during growth of a Walker-256 carcinosarcoma. *Cancer Res.* 33:526, 1973.
39. Munro, H. N., and Clark, C. M. The influence of dietary protein on the metabolism of ribonucleic acid in rat hepatoma. *Br. J. Cancer* 13:324, 1959.
40. Ota, D. M., Copeland, E. M., Strobel, H. W., Daly, J. M., Gum, E. T., Guinn, E., and Dudrick, S. J. The effect of protein nutrition on host and tumor metabolism. *J. Surg. Res.* 22:181, 1977.
41. Pareira, M. D., Conrad, E. J., Hicks, W., and Elman, R. Clinical response and changes in nitrogen balance, body weight, plasma proteins, and hemoglobin following tube feeding in cancer cachexia. *Cancer* 8:803, 1955.
42. Parsons, F. M., Anderson, C. K., Clark, P. B., Edwards, G. F., Ahmad, S., Hetherington, C., and Young, G. A. Regression of malignant tumors in magnesium and potassium depletion induced by diet and haemodialysis. *Lancet* 1:243, 1974.
43. Pimpstone, B. L., Wittman, W., Hansen, J. D. L., and Murray, P. Growth hormone in kwashiorkor. *Lancet* 2:770, 1966.
44. Plumb, M. J., and Holland, J. Comparative studies of psychological function in patients with ad-

vanced cancer: I. Self-related depressive symptoms. *Psychosom. Med.* 39:264, 1977.
45. Reichard, G. A., Moury, N. J., Hochella, N. J., Patterson, A. L., and Weinhouse, S. Quantitative estimation of the Cori-cycle in the human. *J. Biol. Chem.* 238:495, 1963.
46. Reilly, J. J., Goodgame, J. T., Jones, D. C., and Brennan, M. F. DNA synthesis in rat sarcoma and liver: The effect of starvation. *J. Surg. Res.* 22:281, 1977.
47. Reynolds, H. M., Daly, J. M., Rowlands, B. J., Dudrick, S. J., and Copeland, E. M. Effects of nutritional repletion on host and tumor response to chemotherapy. *Cancer* 45:3069, 1980.
48. Rudman, D., Millikan, W. J., Richardson, T. J., Bixler, T. J., Stackhouse, W. J., and McGarrity, W. C. Elemental balances during intravenous hyperalimentation. *Arch. Intern. Med.* 138:799, 1977. *J. Clin. Invest.* 55:94, 1975.
49. Russ, J., and DeWys, W. D. Correction of taste abnormality of malignancy with intravenous hyperalimentation. *Arch. Intern. Med.* 138:799, 1977.
50. Ryan, M. P., Smyth, H., and Hingerty, D. Effect of magnesium and potassium deficiencies on composition and cell growth in ascites tumor cells in vivo. *Life Sci.* 8:485, 1969.
51. Schachter, A., Goldman, J. A., and Zuckerman, Z. Treatment of oligospermia with the amino acid arginine. *J. Urol.* 110:311, 1973.
52. Schanbacher, L. M., Johnson, L. R., Copeland, E. M., Dudrick, S. J., and Castro, G. A. Glucose transport across the small intestine of parenterally nourished rats. *J. Int. Res. Commun. System* (Research on Alimentary System, Metabolism and Nutrition; Physiology; Surgery and Transplantation) 2:1459, 1974.
53. Schein, P. S., Kisner, D., Haller, D., Blecher, M., and Hamosh, M. Cachexia of malignancy. *Cancer* 43:2070, 1979.
54. Schwartz, G. F., Green, H. L., Bendon, M. B., Graham, W. P., and Blakemore, W. S. Combined parenteral hyperalimentation and chemotherapy in the treatment of disseminated solid tumors. *Am. J. Surg.* 121:169, 1971.
55. Shapot, V. S. Some biochemical aspects of the relationship between the tumor and the host. *Adv. Cancer Res.* 15:253, 1972.
56. Sherman, C. D., Morton, J. J., and Mider, G. B. Potential sources of tumor nitrogen. *Cancer Res.* 10:374, 1950.
57. Solassol, C., and Joyeux, H. Artificial gut with complete nutritive mixtures as a major adjuvant therapy in cancer patient's treatment. Proc. Internat. Soc. Parenteral Nutrition, Rio De Janiero, Brazil, Aug. 28, 1979. *Acta Chir. Scand.* (Suppl.) 494:186, 1979.
58. Solomon, N., Copeland, E. M., MacFadyen, B. V., Dudrick, S. J., and Samaan, N. A. Intravenous hyperalimentation and growth hormone in cancer patients. *Surg. Forum* 25:59, 1974.
59. Souchon, E. A., Copeland, E. M., Watson, P., and Dudrick, S. J. Intravenous hyperalimentation as an adjunct to cancer chemotherapy with 5-fluorouracil. *J. Surg. Res.* 18:451, 1975.
60. Steiger, E., Oram-Smith, J., Miller, E., Kuo, L., and Voss, H. N. Effects of nutrition on tumor growth and tolerance to chemotherapy. *J. Surg. Res.* 18:455, 1975.
61. Stjernsward, J., Jardal, N., Vanky, F., Wigzell, H., and Sealy, R. Lymphopenia and change in distribution of human B- and T-lymphocytes in peripheral blood induced by irradiation for mammary carcinoma. *Lancet* 1:1352, 1972.
62. Sugiura, K., and Benedict, S. R. The influence of magnesium on the growth of carcinoma, sarcoma and melanoma in animals. *Am. J. Cancer* 23:300, 1935.
63. Terepka, A. R., and Waterhouse, C. Metabolic observations during the forced feeding of patients with cancer. *Am. J. Med.* 20:225, 1956.
64. Theologides, A. Cancer cachexia. *Cancer* 43:2004, 1979.
65. Theuer, R. C. Effect of essential amino-acid restriction on the growth of female C57BL mice and their implanted BW10232 adenocarcinomas. *J. Nutr.* 101:223, 1971.
66. Warburg, O., Posener, K., and Negelein, E. Uber den Stosffwechsel der Karzinomzelle. *Biochem. Zeitschr.* 152:309, 1924.
67. Waterhouse, C. Lactate metabolism in patients with cancer. *Cancer* 33:66, 1974.
68. Wilmore, D. W., and Dudrick, S. J. Safe long-term venous catheterization. *Arch. Surg.* 98:256, 1969.
69. Wu, C., and Morris, H. P. Responsiveness of glutamine metabolizing enzymes in Morris hepatoma to metabolic modulation. *Cancer Res.* 30:2675, 1970.
70. Young, S. E., Griffin, C. A., Milner, A. N., and Stehlin, J. S. Free amino acids and related compounds in the blood and the urine of patients with malignant melanoma. *Cancer Res.* 27:15, 1967.
71. Young, V. R. Energy metabolism and requirements in the cancer patient. *Cancer Res.* 37:2336, 1977.
72. Young, V. R., and Richardson, D. P. Nutrients, vitamins and minerals in cancer prevention. *Cancer* 43:2125, 1979.

Changes in Immunologic Function

J. Wesley Alexander
J. Dwight Stinnett

16

Perhaps the most important advance in the control of surgical infection during the last decade has been a better understanding of the effects of nutrition on immunologic function and infection. It is somewhat surprising that the importance of this complex relationship has taken so long to be appreciated in surgical practice, since the association between famine and infectious disease has been known for centuries. In fact, the interaction of nutrition and infection has shaped the development of civilization from the very beginning.

McNeill recently reviewed the influence of infection on both population and power in human development [49]. Before the time of Christ, disease transmission among peoples of the world was limited because restricted transportation made it difficult for intermingling of distant communities. With the development of trade routes between the East and the Mediterranean countries, epidemics of disease ravaged both populations. As an example, in 165 A.D., 25 to 30 percent of all persons in the Mediterranean populations died of the plague. Later, in Rome alone, as many as 5,000 persons died per day during an epidemic from 251 to 266 A.D., which was probably caused by measles. In China during the period of 310 to 312 A.D., another pestilence, which was probably smallpox, was preceded by locusts and famine, leaving only one or two of every hundred persons alive in the northwest provinces. Another outbreak of disease started in China in 610 A.D., this time plague, which killed as much as one-half of the population in local areas. Thus, the population dropped sharply in both China and the Mediterranean areas during the first thousand years A.D.

After 1000 A.D., sea transportation developed progressively. By the time the Americas were discovered by Columbus in 1492, there were approximately 30,000,000 Aztec Indians living in Mexico, and an approximately equal number of Incans in Peru. It sometimes seems difficult to appreciate how the small armies of Cortez and Pizarro conquered these populations until it is realized that the peoples of the Americas had never been exposed to many of the infectious diseases that had previously decimated populations in the Old World. When Cortez invaded Mexico, so did smallpox, effectively destroying the Aztec army. Fifty years after Cortez came to Mexico,

Supported in part by USPHS Grant #AI-12936.

the population had dropped from 30 million to 3 million. The low point came in 1620, when the population dipped even further, to 1.6 million. After Cortez's invasion of Mexico, smallpox spread through Guatemala (1520), to the Incan Empire (1525), where most of the population died. It was then as easy a conquest for Pizarro as Mexico had been for Cortez. Both the Indians and the Spaniards believed that the diseases were the result of God's will, making mass conversion of the Indians to Christianity relatively easy for the Spaniards to accomplish. Measles followed the smallpox in Mexico and Peru in 1530-1531, killing one-third of the population. Typhus came in 1546, and influenza caused the death of 20 percent of the remaining population in 1558. Numerous other examples of the influence of infection on human civilization can be found.

In more recent history, of course, better documentation of disease processes has been preserved. In the American Revolution, Duncan [23] documents that in the Revolutionary forces, there was a death rate of 200 per 1,000 troops per year. Only twenty of these were a result of battle, but ten times as many died from infection. Intestinal diseases were apparently present at all times. Dysentery, typhus, and smallpox were the leading killers, followed by diarrhea, typhoid, measles, pneumonia, and malaria. During this conflict, 70,000 persons died, only 7,000 from battle and the rest from diseases that were nearly always of infectious origin. Virtually every able-bodied man served, and approximately half died. It was adequately documented that the army was poorly fed, but the degree of malnutrition, of course, was not as easy to determine.

During the Civil War, almost a hundred years later, the death rate from infectious disease was clearly reduced [13]. Thirty-three of every thousand troops died each year from battle in the Union army, and only sixty-five per thousand per year died from disease. There were a total of 620,000 deaths and 10,000,000 cases of sickness. Diarrhea was the most common disease, with an attack rate of 543 per thousand soldiers per year in the Union army and 987 per thousand per year for the Confederate troops. In the Union army, 60,000 soldiers died from diarrhea alone. Poor nutrition and bad food were the rule, since most of the men cooked for themselves. Brooks notes that at Vicksburg, the army ate fried dogs, boiled cats, and roasted wharf rats [13]. In most places, conditions were not quite that bad, but there was a general shortage of food, and sickness was often linked to the "scorbutic" diets.

In the recent wars, death from infectious or parasitic disease among troops has almost been eliminated. Reister documents that only 28 of every thousand troops per year died of infection or parasitic disease in the Korean War [62].

Although the impact of nutrition on the development of these diseases in the past is difficult to assess, it is now clear that virtually all infections aggravate malnutrition, especially when associated with diarrhea, and it is equally clear that malnutrition predisposes to infection. Thus, the vicious cycle of malnutrition and infection contributed to the death of major segments of the world's population prior to the last century.

Malnutrition remains a problem today. In a recent study conducted among Nigerian children of preschool age in a rural area, 95 percent had Ascaris, 60 percent *Plasmodium falciparium,* 30 percent *Strongyloides,* and 12 percent *Entamoeba histolytica* [48]. In 1973, Suskind et al. [78] reported that 90 percent of children between the ages of one and five who had marasmus or kwashiorkor were suffering from infections. Twenty-nine percent had hepatitis-associated antigen.

The effects of malnutrition were recognized as having an adverse effect on recovery from surgical therapy as early as 1936, when Studley emphasized that postoperative fatality rates correlated well with the extent of preoperative weight loss [77]. Cannon and his coworkers emphasized that protein malnutrition had an adverse effect on the outcome of surgical therapy in 1944 [15], and in 1946 Guggenheim and Buechler showed that protein and calorie malnutrition inhibited the bactericidal power and phagocytic properties of peritoneal fluids in rats [31]. Scrimshaw et al. reviewed the effects of multiple nutritional deficiency in 1968 and clearly documented a regular association with increased susceptibility to infection [69]. Malnourished individuals seem to be particularly susceptible to gram-negative septicemia, tuberculosis, herpes simplex infections, and candidiasis [18]. Even in developed societies, it has recently been estimated that 50 percent of patients in large, charity-type hospitals and 50 percent of surgical patients hospitalized for longer than one week have demonstrable malnutrition [9, 32].

Some of the effects of malnutrition may be long-lasting. In a long-term follow-up of World War II and Korean War prisoners, Beebe found a significantly higher rate of hospital admissions for infective and parasitic diseases after the time of discharge in patients who previously had been prisoners of war [6]. Similar findings were reported by Thygesen et al. for Danish survivors of concentration camps [80]. Not only was infection the leading cause of death in the concentration camps, but pulmonary tuberculosis, pneumonia, recurring cutaneous infections, and influenza occurred at a higher rate in a long-term follow-up of released prisoners.

It must be emphasized, however, that the relationship between malnutrition and infection is extremely complex. Indeed, undernutrition does not increase the incidence of infection in all instances. As a historic example, the English sweat swept recurrently through sixteenth century Europe, selecting primarily the well-to-do in preference to the poor [49, 52]. Murray and Murray have observed that falciparum malaria in eastern Niger was suppressed by famine, but was reactivated within five days after vigorous refeeding [52]. Cerebral malaria was restricted to undernourished children after they were re-fed with grain. These authors present further evidence to show that undernutrition often results in an increased resistance to viral and malarial infections at the same time that there is an increased susceptibility to most bacterial infections.

EFFECT OF CHRONIC UNDERNUTRITION ON IMMUNOLOGIC FUNCTION

The term "protein energy malnutrition" (PEM) is frequently used to describe undernutrition. For the most part, however, patients with PEM also have multiple and varied deficiencies of vitamins and minerals. Marasmus is a term used to describe severe, chronic undernutrition in which caloric deficiency predominates, whereas kwashiorkor is chronic undernutrition in which protein deficiency predominates, usually associated with ascites and peripheral edema. Most studies on immunologic changes associated with PEM have been performed in children, usually in underdeveloped countries.

T-Cell Immunity

Smythe and his colleagues [74] emphasized that the features of infection in children with PEM include a tendency to gram-negative septicemia, disseminated herpes infections, and gangrene rather than suppuration. Their studies also showed marked depression of cell-mediated immunity in such patients, and 70 percent of the malnourished children failed to respond to DNCB. Analysis of autopsy material from children who died with PEM revealed marked atrophy of the thymus and peripheral lymphoid tissues with depletion of both paracortical areas and germinal centers, predominately affecting the T-dependent areas. Schlesinger and Stekel [64] also showed a lack of responsiveness to DNCB in kwashiorkor and marasmus, but found that their lymphocytes stimulated with PHA had normal blastoid transformation. Schopfer and Douglas [65] studied individual lymphocyte functions in children with kwashiorkor and found that peripheral blood counts were normal, although atypical mononuclear cells were frequently seen on the peripheral blood smear. They found the in vitro response to phytohemagglutinin to be significantly depressed, whereas pokeweed mitogen caused a supranormal response. Rosette-forming lymphocytes of both T- and B-cell lineage were reduced in the peripheral blood. Similar reports have been made by Chandra [17] and by Law et al. [41]. Defined studies were done in marasmic pigs by Lopez et al. [44]. They also found marked thymic atrophy, decreased DNCB sensitivity, reduced reactivity to delayed hypersensitivity antigens (anergy), and delayed rejection of skin grafts. However, lymphocyte transformation to PHA was not altered. On the contrary, Rafii et al. [60] found that T-dependent immune function was normal when assessed by either cutaneous hypersensitivity reactions or in vitro response to PHA. Other T-lymphocyte functions are also in dispute—Schlesinger et al. [63] described reduced interferon production by lymphocytes from marasmic patients, whereas Palmblad et al. [58] failed to show any effect of experimental starvation on interferon production in normal volunteers.

B-Cell Function

Despite the frequent observation of atrophic germinal centers and decreased numbers of peripheral B-cells, immunoglobulin levels in children with PEM are usually normal and sometimes even elevated. However, there may be depressed reactivity to certain antigens. Chandra [19] has postulated that the recurrent infections in such individuals may provide a constant immunologic stimulus, resulting in hyperimmunoglobulinemia. In young infants, particularly those with low birth weights and chronic postnatal undernutrition, there may be a profound and prolonged hypoimmunoglobulinemia. Aref et al. [1] found that Egyptian children with kwashiorkor appearing before the age of seven months regularly had a delayed and deficient development of serum immunoglobulins, whereas children in whom the disease is noted at 18 to 48 months had elevated levels of IgG. Antibody responses to specific antigens are variable and may depend somewhat on the stage and severity of the disease [26]. In well-controlled rat experiments, Olusi and McFarlane [55] showed that intrauterine and early postnatal malnutrition produced severe changes in the thymus and spleen, which could be corrected by refeeding. Primary immune responses to sheep red blood cells, as measured by the number of plaque-forming cells in the spleen, could be corrected by refeeding for four months, but the secondary response could not, indicating that early postnatal malnutrition may result in prolonged impairment. On the other hand, Narayanan et al. [53] found similar antibody titers to typhoid-paratyphoid vaccine in animals either starved or fed ad libitum. They concluded that undernutrition depresses cell-mediated responses, but not humoral responses. In Lopez' study in marasmic pigs, antibody responses to erythrocyte A antigen were considerably depressed [44]. However, antibody response to tetanus toxoid, sheep erythrocytes, and bacteriophage 0X174 were similar to control animals. Chandra [19] has demonstrated a reduced synthesis of IgA and fewer IgA plasma cells in the submucosa of individuals with PEM.

Neutrophil Function

Incisive studies by Selveraj and Bhat [70], Seth and Chandra [71], and Schopfer and Douglas [66] have shown a deficiency of the capacity of neutrophils from children with PEM to kill bacteria. In general, phagocytic activity was not impaired compared to healthy controls, but there was a significant decrease in the intracellular killing of bacteria. Decreased chemotactic responses have been a regular accompaniment. A number of studies have reported reduced enzyme activity in neutrophils in malnutrition [50]. Gotch and his colleagues demonstrated similar findings of reduced granulocyte bactericidal capacity for *Staphylococcus aureus* and *E. coli* in patients with malnutrition secondary to anorexia nervosa [29]. The numbers of circulating neutrophils in all these studies have been normal, and the defects in neutrophil function are reversible following recovery from malnutrition. Our own early studies with marasmic guinea pigs showed a defect in the antibacterial capacity of neutrophils, but we have more recently been unable to reproduce the model [90]. In our studies with rats, we were never able to demonstrate a deficiency of neutrophil antibacterial activity in several kinds of malnutrition, and Lopez et al. [44] were unable to find a leukocyte bactericidal abnormality in marasmic pigs. Therefore, human neutrophils appear to be particularly susceptible to the effects of malnutrition, or some subtle alteration in nutrition has not been adequately reproduced in the animal models.

Serum Opsonic Proteins

Sirisinha et al. [72], Chandra [16], and Olusi et al. [56] have shown that nearly all serum complement components except C4 and C5 are low in patients with PEM. There appears to be an increased consumption of C3, as evidenced by the presence of C3 degradation products in the serum. Wunder et al. have shown significant reduction in C3 levels in marasmic guinea pigs [90]. Similarly, Palmblad et al. have shown that 10 days of total energy deprivation in humans could cause decreased levels of C3 in the serum, which were restored with refeeding [58]. Dionigi and his colleagues earlier reported similar findings in marasmic dogs [22].

Bacterial Clearance

Kwashiorkor is associated with a high incidence of septicemia, which has a high mortality rate. Infection, indeed, is the most important cause of death [67]. LaForce and Huber [40] investigated the effect of extrapulmonary infection on the antibacterial clearance of inhaled bacteria in mice. They noted that the infected mice had markedly decreased clearance when compared to controls, but also noted that they had marked weight loss because of decreased food intake. Noninfected mice fed amounts equivalent to those given the infected mice also showed impaired pulmonary clearance of bacteria, indicating that starvation alone can be responsible for impaired antibacterial defense.

EFFECT OF INDIVIDUAL NUTRITIONAL DEFICIENCIES ON IMMUNOLOGIC FUNCTION AND INFECTION

Protein Deficiency

Experiments of strict protein deficiency have been achieved only in animal models, and there are somewhat conflicting results. However, protein deficiency has been shown to alter almost all important immunologic functions (Table 16-1). Acute deprivation of protein can increase antibody synthesis, but moderate degrees of chronic protein restriction (4 to 10 percent of the caloric intake) with normal caloric intake have resulted in a depressed B-cell function, enhanced T-cell function, and increased resistance to the growth of transplantable tumor cells [35]. The effect on tumor cells has been found to result in part from the restricted synthesis of blocking antibody. Suppressor T-cells appear to be more sensitive than helper cells to moderate degrees of protein restriction.

Malave and Layrisse studied antibody responses in protein-deficient mice [45]. Such animals had a decrease in the total number of spleen cells, but direct plaque-forming cells were proportionately increased in the protein-deficient animals compared to normal controls. Titers of serum hemagglutinins were similar or higher in protein-deficient mice than in normal mice during the primary response, but markedly depressed during the secondary response. IgG hemagglutinins were depressed in protein-deficient mice during both primary and secondary responses. The results suggested that IgM synthesis was not affected by protein deficiency, whereas synthesis of IgG was markedly depressed. Kenney and her coworkers demonstrated that manipulation of dietary amino acids in protein-deficient animals could influence hemolysin titers after immunization [37, 38]. Tryptophan increased the hemolysin titers, whereas methionine did not. Furthermore, these investigators found that titers of antibody fell during protein depletion, and that the numbers of specific antibody-forming cells were about one-third

Table 16-1. *Immunologic Effects of Severe Protein Deficiency*

Function	Effects of Severe Protein Deficiency
Neutrophil function	Depressed oxidative pathway activity Depressed chemotaxis Impaired ability to kill bacteria
T-Lymphocyte	Decreased numbers in circulation Atrophy of thymus and T-cell dependent areas Impaired antibody response to T-cell dependent antigens Depressed response in vitro to T-cell mitogens Depressed cutaneous hypersensitivity
B-Lymphocyte	Circulating immunoglobulin variable Specific antibody responses usually impaired
Complement	Both classic and alternative pathway components and activity depressed
Inflammatory response	Decreased cell migration to both specific and nonspecific stimuli

of normal. However, antibody production on a per cell basis was not diminished in protein-depleted animals, suggesting that reduced antibody titers were due to fewer cells producing antibody. Subsequent studies by Mathur et al. [46] found that the addition of normal syngeneic thymocytes would restore the immune response, implying that depressed immunity might be due to a disturbance in thymic function. Law et al. [42] have verified the depressed antibody response of protein-depleted rats, and also demonstrated depressed cutaneous hypersensitivity and in vitro lymphocyte transformation responses.

Ratnakar et al. measured the clearance of both live and killed *E. coli* in protein-deficient Rhesus monkeys and found a marked depression of clearance compared to normal controls [61]. Bhuyan and Ramalingaswami report similar findings in protein-deficient rabbits [8]. *Staphylococcus aureus* injected intravenously had delayed clearance with persistence and multiplication of bacteria in the blood. This resulted in an increased mortality, and the findings in the protein-deficient animals were characterized by focal necrotizing lesions rather than well-formed abscesses. Wolf et al. [88] have used protein-deficient monkeys to study the intestinal clearance of a mildly enteropathic *E. coli.* The organisms were excreted for a longer time in the protein-restricted animals compared to normal animals, suggesting that clearance mechanisms were impaired. In our experiments, moderate protein restriction did not influence the antibacterial function of neutrophils, and even severe protein restriction did so irregularly, a finding supported by Bhuyan et al. [7]. Our own studies [75a] have shown that immunologic defects caused by protein-deficient diets in guinea pigs can be prevented by essential amino acids, but not by nonessential amino acids.

Carbohydrates

To our knowledge, no systematic study has been made of the effect of dietary deficiency of carbohydrates on immunologic functions. However, such deficiencies do not appear to be of practical consideration, since they are rarely, if ever, encountered clinically. It is well known, however, that carbohydrates supply the necessary energy for protein metabolism and may be a preferred fuel source in stress and sepsis, since fats are not as efficiently utilized in these conditions.

Fats

Essential fatty acid deficiency is occasionally encountered in patients during long-term periods of

Table 16-2. *Immunologic Effects of Vitamin Deficiency*

Vitamin	Effects of Deficiency
Vitamin A	Impairment of epithelial barriers Depressed function of phagocytic cells Reduced antibody response Increased susceptibility to infection
Pyridoxine (B_6)	Depressed antibody responses Depressed cutaneous hypersensitivity Delayed rejection of allografts Decreased lymphocytes Defective phagocytosis and killing of bacteria
Vitamin C	Depressed migration of phagocytes Increased predilection for infection
Pantothenic acid	Impaired antibody response
Thiamine and riboflavin	Depressed antibody response and increased susceptibility to infection

intravenous hyperalimentation, but such individuals have no obvious increase in their susceptibility to infection. Some studies would suggest that the administration of lipids during the course of acute infection may actually be harmful by blockading phagocytic cells [24, 57]. Because of this possible harmful effect, the lack of evidence that lipid deficiency has an adverse effect on immunologic resistance against infection, and the observation that lipids are not used efficiently as a fuel source during sepsis, we do not recommend that lipids be given in large quantities for nutritional support of the hypermetabolic or septic patient. Administration of a lipid emulsion once or twice a week should be sufficient to prevent essential fatty acid deficiency.

Vitamins

Vitamin deficiencies have a varied effect on immunologic responses (Table 16-2). Fortunately, in modern clinical practice, isolated vitamin deficiencies are almost never encountered, and the relative safety of vitamin preparations to prevent vitamin deficiency allows their routine use in most clinical settings. Numerous problems can be encountered, however, but these are difficult to separate from the effects of generalized undernutrition.

Vitamin A

Scrimshaw and his colleagues [69] have emphasized that deficiency of vitamin A is consistently synergistic with infectious disease. Indeed, an increased susceptibility to infection was one of the first recognized features of avitaminosis A. Studies in experimental animals have been designed largely to investigate antibody responses to a variety of antigens. Most of these have shown that vitamin A deficiency does not affect antibody formation, although others show mild to moderate inhibition [89]. Bang et al. [5] showed vitamin A deficiency would cause a marked atrophy and depletion of plasma cells of gut-associated lymphoid tissues in chickens. In addition, Krishan et al. [39] found that the yield and functional capabilities of phagocytes from deficient animals were depressed. Certainly, one of the major contributions of vitamin A deficiency to susceptibility is the deterioration of mechanical barriers, since retinol is required for the maintenance of epithelial layers [34].

Pyridoxine (B_6)

Axelrod has shown that pyridoxine deficiency impairs nucleic acid synthesis, causing a deleterious effect on cell multiplication, protein synthesis, antibody formation, and delayed hypersensitivity responses [2–4]. Delayed rejection of allografts and defective phagocytosis in killing of bacteria have also been reported in some experimental animal models.

Some of these defects may be due to impaired T-lymphocyte differentiation, since B_6 deficiency has been shown to affect thymic epithelial cell function [87]. Defects in antibacterial function of phagocytes appears to correlate with decreased myeloperoxidase content [82, 83]. Nonetheless, the effect of pyridoxine deficiency on the development and severity of infections in experimental animals has been variable.

Pantothenic Acid

Pantothenic acid deficiency somewhat resembles pyridoxine deficiency in that it may be antagonistic or synergistic to acquired infections. It is frequently antagonistic to viral or protozoal infections, but more often synergistic to bacterial infections. Deficiency in pantothenic acid causes a reduction in thymus weight, and inhibition of secretion of antibody to the extracellular compartment [2].

Vitamin C

Deficiency of vitamin C results in scurvy, which is associated with an increased predilection for infections. However, this may partly result from impaired wound healing and inhibition of reparative processes. In the guinea pig [28], there may be a severe depression of delayed hypersensitivity skin reactions, and depressed migration of phagocytes to inflammatory foci has been found in other animals. Normal antibody responses have been observed after vaccination of scorbutic humans with influenza virus, and the ability of neutrophils to kill bacteria is not impaired nor are other specific immunologic responses. Therefore, the primary adverse effect of vitamin C deficiency appears to be upon the development of nonspecific inflammatory responses.

Vitamin D

Deficiency of vitamin D is associated with clinical rickets. Responses to antigenic substances are usually normal, even in the face of rather severe growth retardation in experimental animals. There is no documented effect on phagocytic function associated with vitamin D deficiency, but opsonic activity can be impaired [76].

Vitamin B_{12} and Folic Acid

Pernicious anemia is believed to be an immunologically mediated disease, usually associated with chronic atrophic gastritis and autoantibodies to parietal cells and/or intrinsic factor. Horton and Burman [33] have demonstrated that such patients have reduced levels of C3 but not C4. After specific therapy with correction of the pernicious anemia, C3 levels rose to normal values, suggesting disordered synthesis of C3 in the affected patients.

The megoblastic anemias of B_{12} and folic acid deficiencies are both associated with abnormalities of the neutrophil in both the bone marrow and peripheral circulation. Such neutrophils are usually macrocytic, and circulating neutrophils often have hypersegmentation of their nuclei.

Kaplan and Basford [36] have shown that the neutrophils of patients with B_{12} deficiency have diminished metabolic responsiveness on activation and a slightly decreased capacity for killing bacteria, neither of which was found with neutrophils from patients with folic acid deficiency. Patients with pernicious anemia do not have a recognized increase in the incidence of bacterial infections.

Vitamin E

Eckman, Eaton, and Jacob [25] have shown that vitamin E deficiency reduces parasitemia and death in mice infected with *Plasmodium berghei.* Also, repletion with the vitamin led to activation of the disease and increased mortality.

Thiamine, Riboflavin, and Niacin

The effects of deficiencies in these vitamins are variable. They usually demonstrate only moderate or mild reduction in antibody synthesis. However, there is associated increase in susceptibility to infections [89].

Minerals

With few exceptions, little is known about specific mineral deficiencies on either immunologic variables or infection.

Iron

Chandra [17] estimates that iron deficiency affects 28 percent of the population in industrialized countries and 60 percent of the population in developing nations. It is not surprising, therefore, that iron deficiency is associated with general malnutrition and that it is also associated with a variety of infections. Iron deficiency may in itself increase susceptibility to infections, as has been suggested by a variety of animal experiments. Iron-deficient animals may have decreased responsiveness to delayed hypersensitivity antigens and reduced numbers of circulating T-cells, but other reports have suggested that cell-mediated immune responses in iron-deficient subjects are normal [20]. Some investigators have shown an inhibition of the antibacterial function of neutrophils associated with iron deficiency. Again, such findings have not always been documented. Whatever the effect of iron deficiency on immunocompetence, it is relatively clear that iron should not be administered during the course of acute bacterial infection, since numerous studies have shown that infection can be worsened by increasing the concentration of iron, which acts as a nutrilite for bacteria [86]. The binding of free iron by plasma transferrin during acute infections may be an important antibacterial defense mechanism, since the bacteriostatic reactions of serum for many bacteria can clearly be reversed by the saturation of the iron-binding capacity of transferrin [14]. Hemoglobin and hematin also increase the lethality of challenges with standardized doses of bacteria in experimental animals. Since transferrin levels are usually low in chronic malnutrition, this could provide a mechanism for increasing the severity of infections.

Zinc

The role of zinc in infection is not clear. However, it is known to be involved in numerous enzymes, which might potentially be important in defense against infection. Acrodermatitis enteropathica is a disease associated with profound deficiency of T-cell function, which can be corrected by the administration of zinc. Even topical zinc has been shown to restore reactivity to cutaneous injection of delayed hypersensitivity antigens. However, there is no clear association with hypozincemia and susceptibility to infection. On the other hand, hypozincemia usually occurs during the course of acute bacterial infections [43]. Chvapil and his coworkers have demonstrated that there are optimal concentrations of zinc for macrophage function—too little zinc as well as too much zinc are both inhibitory [21].

Copper

Copper deficiency has been documented in patients with chronic intravenous alimentation, and the condition may result in a significant and sometimes profound neutropenia. Studies of the antibacterial functions of such neutrophils have not been reported to our knowledge, but neutropenia in itself may result in increased susceptibility to infection.

Magnesium

Guenounou et al. [30] demonstrated that magnesium deficiency caused a significant inhibition of both primary and secondary immune responses, as measured by the spleen antibody-forming cells. McCoy and Kenney [47] also demonstrated specific antibody response to be impaired in magnesium-deficient rats.

EFFECT OF INFECTION ON NUTRITIONAL REQUIREMENTS AND IMMUNOLOGIC FUNCTION

It has long been appreciated that kwashiorkor can be precipitated by even trivial infections in children with a marginal nutritional status. Because of the potential therapeutic implications, the effects of infection on nutritional requirements and altered metabolism have been studied rather intensively in the past few years.

Infections have many effects on nutrition, including a decreased dietary intake, decreased absorption from the intestine, increased losses, increased requirements, and alteration in metabolic pathways [79]. In patients with severe sepsis, the metabolic rate is characteristically increased and may be almost twice normal. Fever itself is important, since basal metabolism increases about 13 percent for each degree centigrade rise in temperature [59]. Endogenous fuel stores, primarily muscle protein, are utilized early and extensively; thus, protein depletion is an early consequence of the septic state, which may be accompanied by negative nitrogen balance as great as 50 gm per day. Nitrogen balance is regularly disturbed during acute infection, and even minor infections may result in increased urinary nitrogen excretion. Obviously, altered protein metabolism may play a significant role in cellular and humoral defenses, as discussed previously.

Wannemacher [85] has analyzed the alterations of serum amino acids in response to infection. Free amino acid pools of plasma were studied in tularemia, typhoid fever, attenuated Venezuelan equine encephalomyelitis virus, vaccinia infection, and sand fly fever, all in man. In general, these infections resulted in depression of total free plasma amino acids before the onset of fever or other clinical indications of illness. The largest decrease was seen in the branched-chain amino acids. All the studies indicated that the infectious processes stimulated a marked flux of amino acids into the liver and away from skeletal muscles. Phenylalanine typically rose during infection, and further studies showed that infections did not initiate inhibitory effects on phenylalanine hydroxylation, nor was there an increased rate of renal absorption. Incorporation into serum proteins was significantly increased, suggesting that there was not a decreased utilization. Therefore, the increased serum levels of phenylalanine appeared to occur primarily as a result of increased catabolism of skeletal muscle with breakdown of contractile proteins. Tryptophan was likewise elevated in the serum, apparently as the result of accelerated release from skeletal muscles. Alanine, the major amino acid utilized by the liver as a substrate for gluconeogenesis, had a markedly increased flux during acute infection. Gluconeogenesis from alanine was increased not only in the acute, but also in the agonal state of some infections, but there was decreased gluconeogenesis from alanine precursor in other agonal infections. The branched-chain amino acids—leucine, isoleucine, and valine—were more profoundly decreased during acute infections, primarily because they are incorporated at a markedly elevated rate into newly synthesized serum proteins. However, incorporation into skeletal muscle protein was significantly depressed. It may be of particular interest that Odessey [54] showed that the addition of branched-chain amino acids in physiologic concentrations increased production of glutamine and alanine by rat diaphragm, and they also increased protein synthesis [27]. Thus, as circulating glucose is decreased, skeletal muscle breakdown releases branched-chain amino acids, which can be used as a source of energy. Until the point of organ failure, synthetic rates of the proteins associated with protection from infection is generally increased during infection. In contrast to the patient with chronic malnutrition from starvation, in which lipolysis of adipose tissue can supply energy needs, patients with sepsis are unable to mobilize fat stores at a very rapid rate, resulting in a marked increase in gluconeogenesis from amino acids and an increased breakdown in skeletal muscle and skin proteins to supply substrates (Figure 16-1).

In another study, Vaidyanath et al. [81] studied plasma concentrations and tissue uptake of free amino acids in dogs having sepsis and starvation.

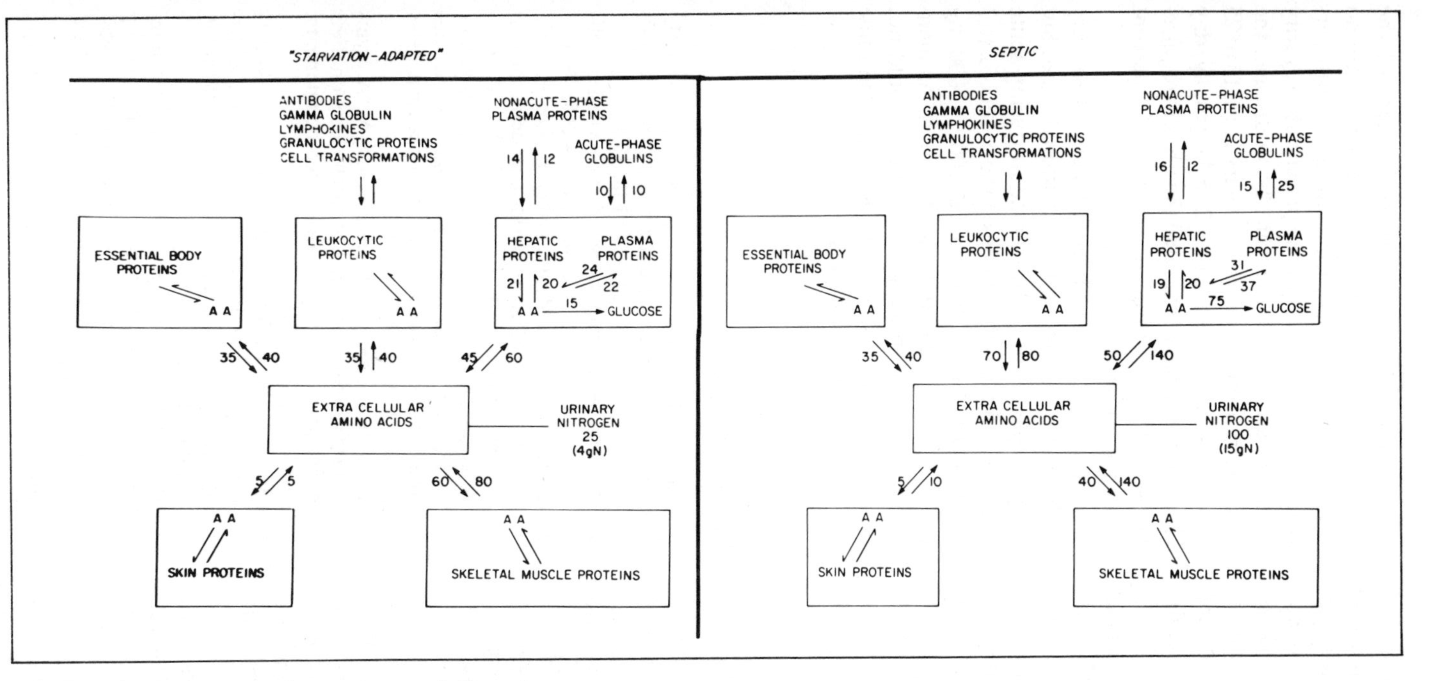

Figure 16-1. *Summary of protein metabolism in starvation-adapted and septic patient. Numbers next to arrows represent grams of protein per day. (From R. W. Wannemacher, Jr., Key role of various individual amino acids in host response to infection.* Am. J. Clin. Nutr. *30:1277, 1977. Published by The American Society for Clinical Nutrition, Inc.)*

During sepsis, there were high concentrations of threonine, glycine, tyrosine, lysine, histidine, and tryptophan. Asparagine, glutamine, leucine, isoleucine, α-aminobutyrate, and tyrosine were significantly depressed in severely ill septic dogs. The infusion of glucose increased the concentration of lactate and pyruvate and depressed the concentrations of most amino acids in both normal and septic dogs.

Various other studies have shown that clinical manifestations of vitamin A deficiency [73], thiamine deficiency (beriberi), folic acid deficiency, B_{12} deficiency, or vitamin C deficiency (scurvy) can be precipitated by acute infections in patients with marginal vitamin intakes [68, 79, 84]. Studies with labeled vitamin A have shown that this may result, in part, from decreased intestinal absorption[75].

NUTRITIONAL REPLETION IN INFECTION

Optimal nutritional support of an infected patient is not always an easy task since such therapy must be based not only upon the additional requirements caused by the infection (which may vary with different pathogens), but also upon the underlying nutritional status of each patient and the energy expenditure and requirements in excess of basal requirements associated with the patient's underlying disease(s) [11, 12, 51, 68].

Caloric support must reflect the needs for basal metabolism, excess energy requirements from disease and infection, internal losses, decreased utilization, and correction of previous deficits. In severely hypermetabolic patients, fats and lipids are not protein-sparing, and carbohydrates must be provided as the primary caloric source.

Disordered protein metabolism appears to be the most important nutritional cause of altered immunologic functions in both infected and noninfected patients. The quality of protein provided is of great importance, since all essential amino acids must be provided. Current evidence suggests that during acute infection, enrichment of the nutritional support with branched-chain amino acids may be beneficial. Depending on the underlying nutritional status of the patient, the severity of the infection, and the underlying disease, the amount of protein needed may vary from 15 to 25 percent of caloric intake or 1.2 to 2.0 gm/kg/day [10, 12]. Some have estimated the protein requirements during infection to be almost 50 percent greater than normal [68].

Vitamin and mineral requirements also vary with the disease and prior nutritional state, but daily supplementation for an adult during acute bacterial infection should be on the order of 2 to 3 times RDA for the B vitamins, 500 to 1000 mg vitamin C, and 25,000 units vitamin A. As mentioned before, iron supplementation should not be given, and vitamin E could be harmful in some infections but not in others.

REFERENCES

1. Aref, G. H., Badr El Din, M. K., Hassan, A. I., and Araby, I. I. Immunoglobulins in kwashiorkor. *J. Trop. Med. Hyg.* 73:186, 1970.
2. Axelrod, A. E. Immune processes in vitamin deficiency states. *Am. J. Clin. Nutr.* 24:265, 1971.
3. Axelrod, A. E., Fisher, B., Fisher, E., Lee, P. C. P., and Walsh, P. Effect of pyridoxine deficiency on skin grafts in the rat. *Science* 127:1388, 1958.
4. Axelrod, A. E., and Hojper, S. Effects of pantothenic acid, pyridoxine and thiamine deficiencies upon antibody formation to influenza virus PR-8 in rats. *J. Nutr.* 72:325, 1960.
5. Bang, B. G., Bang, F. B., and Foard, M. A. Lymphocyte depression induced in chickens on diets deficient in vitamin A and other components. *Am. J. Pathol.* 68:147, 1972.
6. Beebe, G. W. Follow-up studies of World War II and Korean War Prisoners: II. Morbidity, disability, and maladjustments. *Am. J. Epidemiol.* 101:400, 1975.
7. Bhuyan, U. N., Mohapatra, L. N., and Ramalingaswami, V. Phagocytosis, bactericidal activity and nitroblue tetrazolium reduction by the rabbit neutrophil in protein malnutrition. *Indian J. Med. Res.* 62:42, 1974.
8. Bhuyan, U. N., and Ramalingaswami, V. Re-

sponses of the protein-deficient rabbit to staphylococcal bacteremia. *Am. J. Pathol.* 69:359, 1972.
9. Bistrian, B. R., Blackburn, G. L., Hallowell, E., and Heddle, R. Protein status of general surgical patients. *J.A.M.A.* 230:858, 1974.
10. Bistrian, B. R., Blackburn, G. L., and Scrimshaw, N. S. Effect of mild infectious illness on nitrogen metabolism in patients on a modified fast. *Am. J. Clin. Nutr.* 28:1044, 1975.
11. Bistrian, B. R., Blackburn, G. L., Sherman, M., and Scrimshaw, N. S. Therapeutic index of nutritional depletion in hospitalized patients. *Surg. Gynecol. Obstet.* 141:512, 1975.
12. Blackburn, G. L., Flatt, J. P., Clowes, G. H. A., O'Donnell, T. F., and Hensle, T. E. Protein sparing therapy during periods of starvation with sepsis of trauma. *Ann. Surg.* 177:588, 1973.
13. Brooks, S. *Civil War Medicine*. Springfield, IL: Thomas, 1966.
14. Bullen, J. J., Rogers, H. J., and Griffiths, E. Annotation: Iron binding proteins and infection. *Br. J. Haematol.* 23:389, 1972.
15. Cannon, P. R., Wissler, R. W., Woolridge, R. L., and Benditt, E. P. The relationship of protein deficiency to surgical infection. *Ann. Surg.* 120:514, 1944.
16. Chandra, R. K. Serum complement and immunoconglutinin in malnutrition. *Arch. Dis. Child.* 50:225, 1975.
17. Chandra, R. K. Iron and immunocompetence. *Nutr. Rev.* 34:129, 1976.
18. Chandra, R. K. Nutrition as a critical determinant in susceptibility to infection. *World Rev. Nutr. Diet.* 25:166, 1976.
19. Chandra, R. K. Interactions of nutrition, infection and immune response. Immunocompetence in nutritional deficiency, methodological considerations and intervention strategies. *Acta Paediatr. Scand.* 68:137, 1979.
20. Chandra, R. K., Au, B., Woodford, G., and Hyam, P. Iron Status, Immunocompetence and Susceptibility to Infection. In A. Jacob (Ed.), *Ciba Foundation Symposium on Iron Metabolism*. Amsterdam: Elsevier, 1977. P. 249.
21. Chvapil, M., Stankova, L., Bernhard, D. S., Weldy, P. L., Carlson, E. C., and Campbell, J. B. Effect of zinc on peritoneal macrophages in vitro. *Infect. Immunol.* 16:367, 1977.
22. Dionigi, R., Zonta, A., Diminioni, L., Gres, F., and Ballabio, A. The effects of total parenteral nutrition on immunodepression due to malnutrition. *Ann. Surg.* 185:467, 1977.
23. Duncan, L. C. *Medical Men of the American Revolution*. New York: Kelley, 1970.
24. Du Toit, D. F., Villet, W. T., and Heydenrych, J. Fat-emulsion deposition in mononuclear phagocytic system. *Lancet* 2:898, 1978.
25. Eckman, J., Eaton, J. W., and Jacob, H. S. Role of vitamin E in regulating malaria expression. *Clin. Res.* 24:480A, 1976.
26. Faulk, W. P., Mata, L. J., and Edsall, G. Effects of malnutrition on the immune response in humans: A review. *Trop. Dis. Bull.* 72:89, 1975.
27. Fulks, R. M., Li, J. B., and Goldberg, A. L. Effects of insulin, glucose, and amino acids on protein turnover in rat diaphragm. *J. Biol. Chem.* 250:290, 1975.
28. Ganguly, R., Durieux, M. F., and Waldman, R. H. Macrophage function in vitamin C deficient guinea pigs. *Am. J. Clin. Nutr.* 29:762, 1976.
29. Gotch, F. M., Spry, C. J. F., Mowat, A. G., Beeson, P. B., and Maclennan, I. C. M. Reversible granulocyte killing defect in anorexia nervosa. *Clin. Exp. Immunol.* 21:244, 1975.
30. Guenounou, M., Armier, J., and Gaudin-Harding, F. Effect of magnesium deficiency and food restriction on the immune response in young mice. *Int. J. Vit. Nutr. Res.* 48:290, 1978.
31. Guggenheim, K., and Buechler, E. Nutrition and resistance to infection. The effect of quantitative and qualitative protein deficiency on the bactericidal properties and phagocytic activity of the peritoneal fluid of rats. *J. Immunol.* 55:133, 1947.
32. Hill, G. L., Pickford, I., Schorah, C. J., Blackett, R. L., Burkinshaw, L., Warren, J. V., and Morgan, D. B. Malnutrition in surgical patients: An unrecognized problem. *Lancet* 3:689, 1977.
33. Horton, M. A., and Burman, J. F. Reversible C3 hypocomplementaemia in megaloblastic anaemia due to vitamin B_{12} deficiency. *Br. J. Haematol.* 36:23, 1977.
34. Howell, J. M., Thompson, J. N., and Pitt, G. A. J. Changes in the tissues of guinea pigs fed on a diet free from vitamin A but containing methyl retinoate. *Br. J. Nutr.* 21:37, 1967.
35. Jose, D. G., and Good, R. A. Quantitative effects of nutritional protein and calorie deficiency upon immune responses to tumors in mice. *Cancer Res.* 33:807, 1973.
36. Kaplan, S. S., and Basford, R. E. Effect of vitamin B_{12} and folic acid deficiencies on neutrophil function. *Blood* 47:801, 1976.
37. Kenney, M. A., Arnrich, L., Mar, E., and Roderuck, C. E. Influence of dietary protein on complement, properdin and hemolysis in adult protein-depleted rats. *J. Nutr.* 85:213, 1965.
38. Kenney, M. A., Roderuck, C. E., Arnrich, L., and Piedad, F. Effect of protein deficiency on the

spleen and antibody formation in rats. *J. Nutr.* 95:173, 1968.
39. Krishan, S., Krishan, A. D., Mustafa, A. S., Talwar, G. P., and Ramalingaswami, V. Effect of vitamin A and undernutrition on the susceptibility of rodents to malarial parasite *Plasmodium berghei*. *J. Nutr.* 106:784, 1976.
40. LaForce, F. M., and Huber, G. L. Effect of a subacute extrapulmonary infection on antibacterial defense mechanisms of the lung. *Antimicrob. Agents Chemother.* 10:332, 1970.
41. Law, D. K., Dudrick, S. J., and Abdou, N. I. Immunocompetence of patients with protein-calorie malnutrition. The effects of nutritional repletion. *Ann. Intern. Med.* 79:545, 1973.
42. Law, D. K., Dudrick, S. J., and Abdou, N. I. The effect of dietary protein depletion on immunocompetence: The importance of nutritional repletion prior to immunologic induction. *Ann. Surg.* 179:168, 1974.
43. Lennard, E. A., Bjornson, A. B., Petering, H. G., and Alexander, J. W. An immunologic and nutritional evaluation of burn neutrophil function. *J. Surg. Res.* 16:286, 1974.
44. López, V., Davis, S. D., and Smith, N. J. Studies in infantile marasmus: IV. Impairment of immunologic responses in the marasmic pig. *Pediat. Res.* 6:779, 1972.
45. Malavé, I., and Layrisse, M. Immune response in malnutrition. Differential effect of dietary protein restriction on the IgM and IgG response to alloantigens. *Cell. Immunol.* 21:337, 1976.
46. Mathur, M., Ramalingaswami, V., and Deo, M. G. Influence of protein deficiency on 19S antibody-forming cells in rats and mice. *J. Nutr.* 102:841, 1974.
47. McCoy, J. H., and Kenney, M. A. Depressed immune response in the magnesium-deficient rat. *J. Nutr.* 105:791, 1975.
48. McFarlane, H. Malnutrition and impaired immune response to infection. *Proc. Nutr. Soc.* 35:263, 1976.
49. McNeill, W. H. *Plagues and Peoples.* Garden City, NY: Anchor, 1977.
50. Metabolic and enzyme activities of neutrophils in malnutrition. *Nutr. Rev.* 35:230, 1977.
51. Miller, J. D. B., Blackburn, G. L., Bistrian, B. R., Rienhoff, H. Y., and Trerice, M. Effect of deep surgical sepsis on protein-sparing therapies and nitrogen balance. *Am. J. Clin. Nutr.* 30: 1528, 1977.
52. Murray, J., and Murray, A. Suppression of infection by famine—A paradox? *Perspect. Biol. Med.* 20:471, 1977.
53. Narayanan, R. B., Nath, I., Bhuyan, U. N., and Talwar, G. P. The effect of undernutrition on immunological response to BCG and TAB vaccines in mice maintained on a natural diet. *Bull. WHO* 56:781, 1978.
54. Odessey, R., Khairallah, E. A., and Goldberg, A. L. Origin and possible significance of alanine production by skeletal muscle. *J. Biol. Chem.* 249:7623, 1974.
55. Olusi, S. O., and McFarlane, H. Effects of early protein-calorie malnutrition on the immune response. *Pediatr. Res.* 10:707, 1976.
56. Olusi, S. O., McFarlane, H., Ade-Serrano, M., Osunkoya, B. O., and Adesina, H. Complement components in children with protein-calorie malnutrition. *Trop. Geogr. Med.* 28:323, 1976.
57. Paape, M. J., and Guidry, A. J. Effect of fat and casein on intracellular killing of *Staphylococcus aureus* by milk leukocytes. *Proc. Soc. Exp. Biol. Med.* 155:588, 1977.
58. Palmblad, J., Cantell, K., Holm, G., Narberg, R., Strander, H., and Sunblad, L. Acute energy deprivation in man: Effect on serum immunoglobulins, antibody response, complement factors 3 and 4, acute phase reactants and interferon-producing capacity of blood lymphocytes. *Clin. Exp. Immunol.* 30:50, 1977.
59. Pollack, H. Disease as a factor in world food problems. *Am. J. Clin. Nutr.* 21:868, 1968.
60. Rafii, M., Hashemi, S., Nahani, J., and Mohagheghpour, H. Immune responses in malnourished children. *Clin. Immunol. Immunopathol.* 8:1, 1977.
61. Ratnakar, K. S., Mathur, M., Ramalingaswami, V., and Deo, M. G. Phagocytic function of reticuloendothelial system in protein deficiency—A study in Rhesus monkeys using ^{32}P-labeled *E. coli*. *J. Nutr.* 102:1233, 1972.
62. Reister, F. A. *Battle Casualties and Medical Statistics. US Army Experience in the Korean War.* Washington, DC: The Surgeon General, Department of the Army, 1973.
63. Schlesinger, L., Ohlbaum, A., Grey, L., and Stekel, A. Decreased interferon production by leukocytes in marasmus. *Am. J. Clin. Nutr.* 29: 758, 1976.
64. Schlesinger, L., and Stekel, A. Impaired cellular immunity in marasmic infants. *Am. J. Clin. Nutr.* 27:615, 1974.
65. Schopfer, K., and Douglas, S. D. *In vitro* studies of lymphocytes from children with kwashiorkor. *Clin. Immunol. Immunopathol.* 5:21, 1976.
66. Schopfer, K., and Douglas, S. D. Neutrophil function in children with kwashiorkor. *J. Lab. Clin. Med.* 88:450, 1976.
67. Scragg, J. N., and Appelbaum, P. C. Septicaemia

in kwashiorkor. *S. Afr. Med. J.* 53:358, 1978.
68. Scrimshaw, N. S. Effect of infection on nutrient requirements. *Am. J. Clin. Nutr.* 30:1536, 1977.
69. Scrimshaw, N. S., Taylor, C. E., and Gordon, J. E. *Interactions of Nutrition and Infection.* Monograph Series No. 57. Geneva: WHO, 1968.
70. Selvaraj, R. J., and Bhat, K. S. Metabolic and bactericidal activities of leukocytes in protein-calorie malnutrition. *Am. J. Clin. Nutr.* 25:166, 1972.
71. Seth, V., and Chandra, R. K. Opsonic activity, phagocytosis, and bactericidal capacity of polymorphs in undernutrition. *Arch. Dis. Child.* 47:282, 1972.
72. Sirisinha, S., Edelman, R., Suskind, R., Charupatana, C., and Olson, R. E. Complement and C3-proactivator levels in children with protein calorie malnutrition and effect of dietary treatment. *Lancet* 1:1016, 1976.
73. Sivakumar, B., and Reddy, V. Absorption of labelled vitamin A in children during infection. *Br. J. Nutr.* 27:299, 1972.
74. Smythe, P. M., Schonland, M., Brereton-Stiles, G. G., Coovadia, H. M., Grace, H. J., Loening, W. E. K., Mafoyane, A., Parent, M. A., and Vos, G. H. Thymolymphatic deficiency and depression of cell-mediated immunity in protein-calorie malnutrition. *Lancet* 2:939, 1971.
75. Srikantia, S. G. Human vitamin A deficiency. *World Rev. Nutr. Diet.* 20:184, 1975.
75a. Stinnett, J. D., Wunder, J. A., and Alexander, J. W. Alterations in complement metabolism during protein malnutrition and restoration by selected amino acids. *Fed. Proc.* 39:888, 1980 (abstract).
76. Ströder, J., and Kasal, P. Phagocytosis in vitamin D deficient rickets. *Klin. Wschr.* 48:383, 1970.
77. Studley, H. O. Percentage of weight loss. A basic indicator of surgical risk in patients with chronic peptic ulcer. *J.A.M.A.* 106:458, 1936.
78. Suskind, R. M., Olson, L. C., and Olson, R. E. Protein calorie malnutrition and infection with hepatitis-associated antigen. *Pediatrics* 51:525, 1973.
79. Taylor, C. E., and DeSweemer, C. Nutrition and infection. *World Rev. Nutr. Diet.* 16:203, 1973.
80. Thygesen, P., Hermann, K., and Willanger, R. Concentration camp survivors in Denmark persecution, disease, disability, compensation. A 23-year follow-up. A survey of the long-term effects of severe environmental stress. *Danish Med. Bull.* 17:66, 1970.
81. Vaidyanath, N., Birkhahn, R., Border, J. R., Oswald, G., Trietley, G., Yuan, T. F., Moritz, E., and McMenamy, R. H. Plasma concentrations and tissue uptake of free amino acids in dogs in sepsis and starvation: Effects of glucose infusion—some effects of low alimentation. *Metabolism* 27:641, 1978.
82. Van Bijsterveld, O. P. *In vitro* phagocytosis in pyridoxine deficiency. *J. Med. Microbiol.* 4:165, 1971.
83. Van Bijsterveld, O. P. The digestive capacity of pyridoxine-deficient phagocytes in vitro. *J. Med. Microbiol.* 4:337, 1971.
84. Vitale, J. J. The impact of infection on vitamin metabolism: An unexplored area. *Am. J. Clin. Nutr.* 30:1473, 1977.
85. Wannermacher, R. W., Dinterman, R. E., Pekarek, R. S., and Beisel, W. R. Urinary free amino acid excretion as a measure of alterations in protein metabolism during experimentally induced infections in man. *Fed. Proc.* 33:669, 1974.
86. Weinberg, E. D. Iron and susceptibility to infectious disease. *Science* 184:952, 1974.
87. Willis-Carr, H. F., and St. Pierre, R. L. Effects of vitamin B_6 deficiency in thymic epithelial cells and T lymphocyte differentiation. *J. Immunol.* 120:1153, 1978.
88. Wolf, R. H., Felsenfeld, O., Brannon, R. B., and Greer, W. E. Low protein intake and response to *Escherichia coli* 055 infection in Patas monkeys. *Am. J. Dig. Dis.* 15:819, 1970.
89. Worthington, B. S. Effect of nutritional status on immune phenomena. *J. Am. Diet. Assoc.* 65:123, 1974.
90. Wunder, J. A., Stinnett, J. D., and Alexander, J. W. The effects of malnutrition on variables of host defense in the guinea pig. *Surgery* 84:542, 1978.

Nutritional Support in Hepatic Failure

Craig A. Nachbauer
Josef E. Fischer

17

Among the most complex problems in patient management are those that involve failure of one of the metabolically active organs, such as the liver or kidney. The liver, which is the primary metabolic factory of the body, clears nutrients from the portal blood, processing and preparing them for distribution to the periphery. Management of hepatic failure is complicated by the myriad processes that normally take place in the liver, as well as by its central role in managing metabolism [25].

In general, the alternatives in management of organ failure are:

1. General supportive measures, allowing for recovery of organ function.
2. Employment of an extra- or intracorporeal device that assumes temporary or permanent function.
3. Organ transplantation.

Liver transplantation in patients with acute hepatic failure occasionally is successful, but long-term survival is rare, and will, in the future, rely heavily upon the development of an effective hepatic assist device. Thus, general supportive measures are likely to remain the major form of therapy for patients in hepatic failure.

Therapy in hepatic failure is thus a play for time until the powers of regeneration can resume normal function. Some of the many influences on hepatic failure and hepatic regeneration are known, such as insulin and glucagon (although the ideal stoichiometric relationship between the two is not clear); some are unknown, such as the ileal factor; others are permissive, such as steroids, growth hormone, and triiodothyronine. But few are as manageable as nutrition.

In discussing nutritional support in hepatic failure, it is reasonable to define the circumstances under which it may be useful. Hepatic failure can be defined as either acute or chronic failure, with some middle ground for mixed disease. Fulminant hepatic failure, usually occurring secondary to a viral or toxic hepatitis, involves a patient with previously normal nutrition and hepatic function. The course is progressive and acute, and the outcome is decided within two or three weeks. Nutri-

Supported in part by Lipid-Atherosclerosis-Nutrition Training Grant USPHS HL-07460, and PHS grant #AM-25347.

tional support may be useful in promoting hepatic regeneration or as an adjunct to catabolic forms of therapy, such as repeated polyacrylonitrile membrane hemodialysis [72].

In a chronic condition such as alcoholic hepatitis, elements of acute necrosis are usually superimposed on chronic liver damage. This often fatal condition, in our experience, requires prolonged nutritional support to improve survival [36]. In a group of patients with alcoholic hepatitis who were considerably less ill than those that we have seen, survival has been improved by an aggressive program of nutritional support [55].

Acute-on-chronic hepatic failure occurs in the patient with pre-existent liver disease, usually cirrhosis, who has sustained an acute insult secondary to gastrointestinal bleeding, infection, starvation, or surgical intervention. It is primarily these patients with whom this chapter deals and for whom nutritional support is most beneficial.

Finally, hepatic failure associated with sepsis is the cause of death in many surgical patients. One of the authors (JEF) has proposed that sustained gluconeogenesis at the expense of structural and functional protein in the liver itself, as well as in other essential organs, may be the etiology of this condition [28]. Our management of septic patients, therefore, does not differ markedly from our management of patients with acute-on-chronic hepatic failure.

PATHOPHYSIOLOGY OF ACUTE HEPATIC FAILURE

Normal Flow and Architecture

Under normal circumstances, the major source of blood supply to the liver is portal blood, containing both nutrient and toxic substances absorbed from the gut, and representing between 65 and 80 percent of total hepatic blood flow. It is nutrient-rich and relatively oxygen-poor, although the venous oxygen content of the afferent portal blood is not so low as other venous effluents from other parts of the body. Portal blood mixes at the level of the hepatic sinusoid with arterial blood, relatively nutrient-poor and oxygen-rich, which in turn comprises between 20 and 35 percent of normal hepatic flow.

Flow originates at the periphery of the hepatic lobule, at the portal triad, which contains the hepatic artery, portal vein, and bile cannuliculus surrounded by a small amount of fibrous tissue containing lymphocytes and macrophages. Mixed portal and arterial blood flows centripetally, perfusing single plates of hepatocytes in an orderly progression. Presumably, not all cells function simultaneously; as many as two-thirds may be "resting" at any given time. Possibly there exists a continuum of functional capacity that diminishes in a centripetal fashion; indeed those cells at the periphery of the lobule are relatively oxygen- and nutrient-rich, whereas those at the central portion may be marginal with respect to oxygen and nutrient supply.

Genesis of Portal Hypertension

The continued evolution of chronic liver disease with repeated insults to the liver, usually on the basis of alcohol and malnutrition, results in distortion of the lobular architecture—piecemeal necrosis, bridging necrosis, collapse of the fine reticular framework, and replacement by fibrous tissue. Nodules of regenerating hepatocytes derive their blood supply largely from the hepatic artery. The portal vein has little role in their perfusion, thus depriving them of a major source of nutrients. These hepatocytes are particularly vulnerable because hepatic artery flow is extremely responsive to sympathetic tone; dehydration, anesthesia, shock, or sepsis may rapidly compromise hepatic artery flow, resulting in acute deterioration. In addition, the cirrhotic architecture distorts the orderly access of single plates of hepatocytes to both arterial and portal flow [70].

Hepatocytes in regenerating nodules are of varying functional capacity. Depending upon the activity of the disease, they may manifest any degree of normal function, dysfunction, or necrosis. Intrahepatic shunts form in fibrous septa as a result of the regenerative process. These shunts, as well as compression of the hepatic venous radicles and sinusoids by regenerating nodules, result in increased resistance to portal flow. Portal pressure in turn rises, leading to the formation of extrahepatic portasystemic shunts. Initially, these low-resistance extrahepatic shunts reduce portal pressure toward normal; conceivably, some of the extrahepatic shunts may then close. With further disruption of hepatic architecture, intrahepatic shunting increases and portal pressure continues to rise, resulting in greater flow through extrahepatic shunts. This progresses toward hepatofugal flow. When the percentage of shunting is small, clearance of a particular portal substance (e.g., glucose, amino acids, insulin, glucagon, or endotoxin), is probably not significantly affected. The shunted substance, with subsequent circulation through the splanchnic circuit, may eventually be cleared; in addition, there would be prolonged exposure to peripheral tissues. Overall, concentration is likely to remain at or near normal. As the percentage of shunting progressively increases toward hepatofugal flow, a critical value is reached and systemic plasma concentrations of the substance rise to a new steady-state level.

It is wise to keep in mind that portal hypertension represents a homeostatic process; that is, an attempt on the part of the liver to maintain flow in the face of increased resistance. The associated plasma volume expansion, probably secondary to increased aldosterone and ADH, may be viewed teleologically as an attempt to increase perfusion pressure and thus flow. Consequently, though normalizing portal pressure may be advantageous or even life-saving in the instance of variceal bleeding, the concomitant decrease in hepatic flow may be ultimately deleterious and probably contributes to the longtime hepatic failure, which may follow shunting procedures. In addition, nutritional restriction secondary to encephalopathy results in further damage to the liver, as sufficient protein and calories for healing of the damaged parenchyma are no longer available [2, 27]. This in turn contributes to a vicious cycle of decreased hepatic function.

An important adaptive mechanism is hepatic vascular autoregulation: when portal flow is diminished, hepatic arterial flow increases. Following end-to-side portacaval shunt, patients who are capable of autoregulation seem to fare better [7, 63]. However, cause and effect are difficult to establish here. The ability to autoregulate may merely indicate the severity of liver disease; patients who compensate may simply have a less advanced form of the disease, and therefore tolerate shunting better. Our patients with central splenorenal shunts who, after a time, show diminished portal flow, also tend to manifest enormous hypertrophy of the hepatic artery and continue to do well [30].

ALTERATIONS IN VARIOUS METABOLIC PROCESSES

It is beyond the scope of this chapter to discuss the various derangements of metabolic function in hepatic failure. However, a brief review of the disorders in carbohydrate, fat, and protein metabolism is necessary to any discussion of nutritional support.

Alterations in Carbohydrate Metabolism

The hormonal milieu underlying carbohydrate metabolism involves the storage hormone insulin and the catabolic hormone glucagon. There is widespread evidence that diminished degradation of glucagon and insulin results in persistent elevation of both of these hormones in compromised hepatic function [71, 76, 77]. Hyperglucagonemia has been correlated with portasystemic shunting [71]. It is likely that hyperinsulinemia results by the same mechanism [76]. The net result, however, is an effectively decreased insulin:glucagon ratio due to glucagon predominance and/or cellular insensitivity to insulin. Thus, there exists in cirrhosis a tendency toward catabolism. In experimental animals, the decreased insulin:glucagon ratio becomes more prominent as the liver continues to fail [76]. Soon after portasystemic shunting, for example, insulin is mildly elevated and glucagon is elevated somewhat. As hepatic failure and hepatic coma supervene, glucagon increases precipitously, whereas insulin either remains the same or falls. More recently, similar data have been obtained in humans by Ziparo and associates [33]. In their studies, true alpha cell hyperfunction suppressable by somatostatin occurs in postshunt patients, especially those with hepatic encephalopathy.

The source of hyperglucagonemia is not entirely clear. Teleologically, one may argue that it is directed at increasing glucose production by a failing liver. Glucagon is responsive to a number of influences, including ammonia [78], and a number of amino acids, including the aromatic amino acids, which are present in excess concentration in the blood. The combination of hvperglucagonemia against the background of increased epinephrine and increased steroids (probably in turn due to decreased degradation) provokes a state of sustained gluconeogenesis as Sherwin and his coworkers have proposed [19].

The cirrhotic liver fails to store glucose; chronic hyperglucagonemia presumably results in depletion of glycogen. Despite this, fasting hypoglycemia is rare. Hepatic gluconeogenesis is active and, as in prolonged starvation, is probably assisted by renal gluconeogenesis. Other energy sources also lessen the requirement for glucose production. Lipolysis liberates glycerol (which contributes to gluconeogenesis) as well as fatty acids, which are utilized directly or oxidized to ketones, although this latter pathway may be impaired [5]. Skeletal muscle proteolysis liberates branched-chain amino acids; at least one carbon atom is oxidized locally while the amino groups and possibly some of the carbon skeleton [21] are contributed to pyruvate to form alanine (glucose-alanine cycle).

Postprandial hyperglycemia, however, is characteristic of cirrhosis. This glucose intolerance occurs after both intravenous and oral glucose, and is associated with an exaggerated insulin response. The latter is probably due to shunting; however, the hyperglycemia may be multifactorial. Shunting of glucose probably contributes little to this hyperglycemia. Peripheral cellular uptake of glucose is insulin-dependent and, although hepatocellular *uptake* of glucose is independent of insulin, hepatocellular *metabolism* of glucose is also insulin-dependent. The decreased insulin:glucagon ratio may therefore account for this hyperglycemia.

The primary hepatic responsibilities in carbohydrate metabolism are: (1) glucose storage, (2) glucose production, and (3) maintaining a steady fuel concentration, and therefore a steady plasma osmolarity. In summary, the cirrhotic liver fails only in the first of these, maintaining adequate capacity for the remaining functions. However, with superimposed acute deterioration, gluconeogenesis may ultimately fail, resulting in hypoglycemia. Hepatic uptake of substrates for this pathway ceases, resulting in gross hyperaminoacidemia and lactic acidemia.

Alterations in Lipid Metabolism

The abnormalities in metabolism extend to the treatment of fatty acids. Under normal circumstances, lipolysis is a major source of energy, accounting for approximately 75 to 85 percent of normal energy expenditure during resting starvation. The liver plays a central role in the metabolism of relatively long-chain fatty acids to ketone bodies, a major source of peripheral energy, as well as maintaining normal plasma concentrations of relatively short-chain fatty acids.

The issue with respect to metabolism of fatty acids is somewhat controversial. Although short-chain fatty acids together with ammonia and methane thiols occupy a relatively prominent place in one of the current hypotheses of hepatic encephalopathy [82], other investigators have given relatively large amounts of these substances without deleterious effects [53]. Thus, their role remains questionable. Morecver, in those conditions in which short-chain fatty acids have been implicated in the coma of congenital disorders or those involving hypoglycin A [6, 79], the concentrations of short-chain fatty acids are literally hundreds of times higher than those seen in patients with hepatic encephalopathy.

Nonesterified fatty acids circulate in the bloodstream at least partially bound to albumin. Their importance with respect to hepatic encephalopathy is their displacement of bound tryptophan from albumin [52]. With lipid mobilization and increased nonesterified fatty acids within the circulation, unbound tryptophan increases, thus becoming more available for absorption across the blood-brain barrier [13].

The overall effect of the failing liver on lipid metabolism is to deprive the body of a major source of energy, thus making the organism turn to gluconeogenesis as a primary source.

Alterations in Nitrogen Metabolism

The cirrhotic tendency toward gluconeogenesis requires an equal capacity for ureagenesis in order to prevent hyperammonemia. A wide range of hepatocellular dysfunction may be present in chronic cirrhotic failure; the reserve capacity for glucose production is adequate (at least initially), but the reserve capacity for ureagenesis may be less comparable.

It is difficult to distinguish the hyperammonemia resulting from a diminished ureagenic capacity from that resulting from shunting of ammonia of gut origin. Gut gluconeogenesis from glutamine is active; ammonia from this source, as well as from intraluminal deamination of amino acids, requires successful transport to the liver for urea synthesis. Shunting of a critical portion of portal blood would result in persistent elevation of plasma ammonia concentrations.

Of greater importance is the particular amino acid pattern that characterizes cirrhosis and acute-on-chronic failure. The branched-chain amino acids—leucine, isoleucine, and valine—are usually below normal, whereas phenylalanine, tyrosine, free tryptophan, methionine, glutamate, aspartate, and, to a lesser extent, histidine are usually elevated [34].

The branched-chain amino acids are unique in their partial utilization as an energy source by tissues other than the liver; relatively little oxidation occurs at the hepatic level. They represent between 60 and 100 percent of the splanchnic clearance of amino acids, as well as between 60 and 100 percent of peripheral nitrogen accumulation in patients in energy and nitrogen balance [22]. In circumstances in which the production or utilization of the usual energy substrates (glucose, fatty acids, ketones) is impaired, the branched-chain amino acids may be expected to contribute a greater percentage of energy needs, perhaps up to 30 or 40 percent. Enhanced peripheral consumption thus provides a reasonable explanation for the diminished plasma levels in acute-on-chronic failure.

In fulminant hepatic failure, the branched-chain levels remain relatively normal despite gross elevation of all other amino acids. Clearly their concentrations are maintained largely by the periphery with little effect by the liver [34, 67].

Tryptophan is unique in being albumin-bound. In acute-on-chronic failure, although the total concentration remains normal or diminished, the unbound fraction is elevated [11, 13, 52, 60]. Tryptophan appears to be displaced by nonesterified fatty acids or bilirubin [60], both of which are present in high concentration. Associated hypoalbuminemia may further compound this competitive process.

The elevations of phenylalanine, tyrosine, methionine, glutamate, aspartate, and histidine are not explained as easily. Why these particular amino acids are elevated, while others are relatively normal, is not immediately obvious. As mentioned earlier in regard to hyperammonemia, distinguishing the effects of hepatocellular dysfunction from those of shunting is often difficult.

The conversion of phenylalanine to tyrosine has been found to be impaired in cirrhosis; this seems to correlate well with the estimation of portal-systemic shunting [49].

It has been demonstrated that the hepatic uptake of each amino acid upon single circulatory passage through the liver varies quite dramatically [61]. Histidine, aspartate, glutamate, and the aromatics are at the upper end of this spectrum; that is, between 80 and 100 percent of these amino acids are cleared on initial passage through a normally functioning liver. Others such as alanine, lysine, proline, and arginine demonstrate only 20 to 40 percent clearance. This may shed some light on the selective elevations in cirrhosis and acute-on-chronic failure. The plasma concentrations of those amino acids with particularly high uptake indices on initial passage may be most seriously affected if shunting alone were to deny their direct access to the sinusoids. However, a particular problem at the hepatocellular membrane, impeding uptake, could conceivably account for these selective elevations as well.

Interestingly, phenylalanine, tyrosine, histidine, methionine, and tryptophan have recently been implicated perhaps in the control of flux of other amino acids through the hepatocyte membrane in vitro [46]. The liver serves as the principal site of catabolism of these amino acids, by enzymes that are inducible by and normally responsive to sharply increased concentrations in the circulation.

The common clinical setting of acute-on-chronic failure often involves a combination of starvation, surgical or traumatic insult, and sepsis resulting in extensive skeletal muscle proteolysis; amino acids from this source, as well as from the gastrointestinal tract (secondary to blood degradation), only tend to exacerbate the abnormal pattern that existed prior to the insult.

HYPOTHESES OF HEPATIC ENCEPHALOPATHY

From the foregoing discussion, it should be clear that the abnormalities in nitrogen metabolism, because of their dramatic impact, have proved to be a major handicap in providing nutritional support to patients with hepatic failure. Hepatic coma, with its intolerance to protein, imposes a most severe dietary restriction in these patients. Moreover, since protein is the essential component for protein synthesis and hepatic regeneration, as well as the metabolic substrate for immunologic host defense [1], it is clear that protein restriction, if carried out beyond a certain point, would be deleterious. Thus, the provision of adequate protein without provoking hepatic encephalopathy is critical in nutritional support.

The most long-lived villain in the etiology of hepatic encephalopathy is ammonia. Although a detailed description of the theories and hypotheses of hepatic encephalopathy is beyond the scope of this chapter (the interested reader is referred to reference 26), a few comments should suffice. The difficulties with ammonia as the principal etiologic agent in hepatic encephalopathy are well known. Hepatic encephalopathy in its various presentations is a subtle disease. Mood swings, subtle disturbances in judgment, day-night rhythm, and posture all bespeak a disorder which is not toxic but neurotransmissive in nature. The lack of correlation between ammonia and the grade of encephalopathy is well known. The excuses that ammonia cannot be measured accurately (after five decades!) begin to wear thin. In addition, it is relatively easy both in experimental animals and in man to dissociate blood levels of ammonia and symptomatology. Monoamine-oxidase inhibitors, for example, decrease blood ammonia, but patients become more symptomatic [15]. Glutamine synthetase inhibitors, such as methionine sulfoximine in experimental animals, increase brain ammonia, but decrease its toxicity [81]. Clearly, ammonia in and of itself does not explain hepatic encephalopathy.

Others have speculated that ammonia, mercaptans, methane thiols, and short-chain fatty acids in combination may be the source of symptomatology [82]. Aside from the fact that this is but another toxic hypothesis, it has been difficult for other laboratories to confirm these hypotheses because of difficulties in measurement. Furthermore, it is not clear how the failing liver allows the accumulation of these compounds. Short-chain fatty acids have been administered by some investigators to patients with a history of encephalopathy without provoking the symptom complex [53].

Unified Hypothesis of Hepatic Encephalopathy

Our present concept, which will henceforth be called the unified hypothesis, implies a multifactorial nature of hepatic encephalopathy in which ammonia is merely an indicator of disturbed nitrogen metabolism [45].

The clinical manifestation is conceptualized as being a disturbance in central and peripheral neurotransmitters, particularly in the aminergic system. This phylogenetically primitive midline system comprises less than 5 percent of the neurons in the central nervous system, but has tremendous ramifications and feedback circuits throughout. The locus ceruleus, for example, situated under the fourth ventricle, is largely noradrenergic in nature; although it consists of only 1,500 neurons, it has associations with the entire nervous system. Indeed, no central nervous system neuron seems to be a great distance from the ramifications of the aminergic system, suggesting a neuroregulatory function.

The anatomic relationship between aminergic neurons also suggests a regulatory function; the axons and dendrites tend to end free in the matrix instead of forming classic synapses [16].

The unified hypothesis points to the amino acid imbalance characteristic of cirrhosis and acute-on-chronic failure as the etiology of this aminergic disturbance. Phenylalanine, tyrosine, unbound tryptophan, methionine, and histidine, as well as the branched-chain amino acids, are all neutral pH. Blood-brain barrier transport of these neutral amino acids is via system-L [59, 62]. Presumably a common carrier is involved which each amino acid competitively employs. Increased brain concentrations of phenylalanine, tyrosine, unbound tryptophan, methionine, and histidine result directly from their high plasma concentrations, as well as indirectly, from diminished competition from low plasma branched-chain concentrations. An intrinsic alteration involving the velocity of transport across system-L may also be involved [44].

Phenylalanine, tyrosine, tryptophan, methionine, and histidine are all precursors of aminergic neutrotransmitters. The crux of the hypothesis is the imbalance of aminergic products that results from excessive brain concentrations of these amino acids. Studies in both experimental animals and humans suggest that decreased norepinephrine and dopamine [17, 20], as well as increased serotonin [3, 13, 14, 24, 60] and the phenylethylamines (tyramine, octopamine, and phenylethanolamine) [20, 29, 48, 51, 56, 68], correlate very well with the presence of hepatic encephalopathy. The presence of 5-hydroxyindoleacetic acid and homovanillic acid in CSF of patients with hepatic encephalopathy also supports this concept of aminergic derangement this concept of aminergic derangement [47, 60].

According to this hypothesis, where does ammonia fit in? As mentioned earlier, hyperammonemia stimulates the release of glucagon [78], thereby further promoting gluconeogenesis and the requirement for comparable ureagenesis. In the brain, however, ammonia is represented as glutamine, the product of a small, rapidly turning over pool of glutamate [4]. It has been known for some time that CSF glutamine in patients correlates very well with the level of hepatic encephalopathy [43]. In experimental animals, we have provided evidence that there is an excellent correlation between CSF glutamine and the concentrations of phenylalanine, tyrosine, and tryptophan [74]. Glutamine, being neutral pH, also traverses the blood-brain barrier via system-L. If the brain were to export glutamine in blood-brain fashion, the L-system carrier would then be free to exchange at an increased rate for the neutral amino acids [45]. This concept is supported by a series of experiments carried out both in experimental animals and in isolated brain capillaries from shunted and normal animals [10]. This concept also satisfactorily explains why the toxicity of ammonia is decreased when methionine sulfoximine, an inhibitor of glutamine synthetase, is given to experimental animals [81]; methionine sulfoximine inhibits the transport of neutral amino acids, possibly because of decreased glutamine synthesis within the brain [69].

The relationship between amino acid concentrations in plasma and brain in animals following portacaval shunt also lends support to this hypothesis. Simultaneous determination of plasma and brain neutral amino acids suggests that the brain accumulates neutral amino acids against a gradient. If the penetration of neutral amino acids across the blood-brain barrier is by facilitated diffusion, the brain concentrations of amino acids should not be higher than plasma unless another factor is at work.

One can predict the brain concentrations of various neutral amino acids from plasma competition ratios as calculated from the equations of Fernstrom and Faller [23]. The concentrations of neutral amino acids in brains of animals with liver disease are in considerable excess of predicted concentrations, but seem to follow linear correlations as if subjected to another influence.

If, however, glutamine is exchanged across the blood-brain barrier for other neutral amino acids, the excess of observed over predicted might be correlated with brain glutamine. In fact, the correlation is excellent; only animals with normal brain glutamine have normal brain neutral amino acids [10, 69]. Moreover, isolated brain capillaries preloaded with glutamine and incubated with ammonia, or capillaries from shunted animals manifest similar increases in capillary neutral amino acid uptake. Blocking synthesis of glutamine with methionine sulfoximine inhibits the increased in vitro uptake of neutral amino acids stimulated by ammonia. For further details, which are beyond the scope of this chapter, the interested reader is referred to the bibliography [10, 69].

Thus, if one examines the current unified concept of hepatic encephalopathy, there is provision for ammonia, the disturbed hormonal balance of insulin and glucagon, increased plasma concentrations of phenylalanine, tyrosine, unbound tryptophan, methionine, and histidine, as well as decreased plasma concentrations of their blood-brain barrier competitors, the branched-chain amino acids. Furthermore, this hypothesis explains the apparent beneficial clinical effects of such diverse compounds as L-dopa [32, 64], bromcryptine [54], and the branched-chain amino acids, as well as neomycin and lactulose.

NUTRITIONAL SUPPORT IN HEPATIC ENCEPHALOPATHY

Most of the following discussion will concern patients with acute decompensation. They are not likely to tolerate large amounts of oral nutrition and therefore the discussion will center around intravenous support.

In the event that patients with hepatic insufficiency present the necessity for nutritional support, one should remember that intravenous protein, especially synthetic solutions consisting of individual amino acids, is likely to be better tolerated than oral protein in equal amounts. In our clinical experience, even patients with grade I encephalopathy will sufficiently normalize their plasma amino acid patterns due to decreased catabolism and increased protein synthesis, so that approximately 50 to 60 percent will tolerate a commercially available glucose/amino acid mixture. However, if one is seeking to replenish patients with increased amounts of protein, a special formulation is necessary.

Beneficial Effects of the Branched-Chain Amino Acids

The approach we have taken to nutritional support of patients with hepatic encephalopathy has been to administer increased amounts of the branched-chain amino acids. The rationale is based on several beneficial effects:

1. A peripheral energy deficiency exists in patients with hepatic failure as described. Under these circumstances, the branched-chain amino acids may provide an energy substrate, thereby sparing gluconeogenesis and decreasing the amino acids released by muscle.
2. Increased concentrations of plasma branched-chain amino acids decrease the efflux of other amino acids from muscle [8, 57]. Concurrently,

increased protein synthesis both in liver and muscle occurs, thereby incorporating amino acids [37, 38].

3. In addition to decreasing the plasma concentrations of phenylalanine, tyrosine, unbound tryptophan, methionine, and histidine [31, 34], the branched-chain amino acids decrease these amino acids' penetration of the blood-brain barrier by providing increased competition.

4. More recent experiments have shown that the central nervous system hyperaminoacidemia, provoked by ammonia infusions in normal animals, can be counteracted by infusions of the branched-chain amino acids, presumably by decreasing the penetration of aromatic amino acids and decreasing exchange for glutamine. Once central nervous system hyperaminoacidemia is established, clearance of aromatic amino acids from the brain is more rapid with, and is dose-related to, infusion of branched-chain amino acids.

5. Even in anhepatic experimental animals, infusion of branched-chain amino acids restores plasma amino acids toward normal [40], suggesting that even in fulminant hepatic failure, part of the hyperaminoacidemia is derived from peripheral catabolism.

Our experience has been with a single formulation, in which the branched-chain amino acids have been increased and phenylalanine, tyrosine, tryptophan, and methionine have been decreased [31, 34]. Other solutions with various concentrations of branched-chain amino acids are available, particularly in other countries.

Animal Experiments Utilizing High Branched-Chain Amino Acid Mixtures in the Treatment of Hepatic Encephalopathy

Prior to testing in man, F080, or Hepatamine, as it is likely to be called when commercially available, underwent extensive animal testing. The two large animal models used were dogs and monkeys, which, following end-to-side portacaval shunt (especially in the dog), offer a severe if self-limited model of human hepatic encephalopathy, with a plasma amino acid pattern similar to that seen in man with acute-on-chronic failure. Conditioned animals had CSF cannulas [73] implanted, and after a two-week recovery period, baseline CSF and plasma samples were obtained. After two additional weeks, end-to-side portacaval shunts were performed under sterile conditions, and serial samples of both plasma and CSF were obtained as the animal was allowed to feed freely. When the animals developed grade III encephalopathy [31, 74], an internal jugular catheter was placed and 5 percent dextrose and saline was infused for three days. In general, no improvement in neurologic status was noted. Then either F080, a 35 percent branched-chain amino acid mixture in 24 percent dextrose, or another commercially available amino acid mixture in 24 percent dextrose was infused at a dose of 4 gm/kg body weight. The results clearly indicated that F080 was superior in that larger doses of amino acids were administered, and positive nitrogen balance and neurologic normality were achieved long-term. In those animals that had survived for 40 days on F080, a commercially available mixture was substituted, and hepatic encephalopathy once again supervened and the animals died in coma [31, 74]. Similar results were obtained in crossover fashion [75].

In monkeys, even more interesting results were obtained. Hepatic enchephalopathy occurred in some animals with normal plasma amino acids; however, there were markedly elevated aromatic amino acids within the CSF. When F080 was given, animals woke up simultaneous with or immediately following a return to normal of various CSF parameters. From these experiments, one can conclude that:

1. Hepatic coma occurs when CSF tryptophan, phenylalanine, tyrosine, octopamine, phenylethanolamine, and 5-hydroxyindoleacetic acid reach their highest concentrations.
2. Abnormalities in CSF precede and are more severe than those in plasma.

3. Awakening from hepatic encephalopathy occurs simultaneous with or immediately following return to normal of all these CSF parameters.
4. Most important, it is impossible to predict CSF and therefore brain amino acid concentrations from plasma alone, owing to the activity of the blood-brain barrier.

Use of Branched-Chain-Enriched Amino Acid Mixtures in Humans

Several groups, including our own, have had fairly extensive experience with a branched-chain-enriched amino acid mixture. There are two modes of employing branched-chain amino acids in the nutritional support of patients with hepatic encephalopathy. There are those who utilize a concentrated solution of branched-chain amino acids alone in dextrose principally as a drug directed toward treating the hepatic encephalopathy in rapid and effective fashion; then, after the patient is awake, a more complete amino acid mixture in hypertonic dextrose is administered specifically for nutritional support. The other alternative is to provide a more complete mixture from the start, accepting a slower resolution of encephalopathy because of a relatively lower dose of branched-chain amino acids, but providing complete nutritional support from the outset.

Criteria for Parenteral Nutrition in Hepatic Encephalopathy

The criteria that we have used in patients with hepatic encephalopathy for treatment with special amino acid mixtures include the following:

1. Lack of oral intake for 48 to 72 hours with no expectation of resuming adequate oral intake for an additional 48 to 72 hours.
2. Grade II to grade III hepatic encephalopathy.
3. A need for parenteral nutrition with intolerance to greater than 40 to 50 gm of a commercially available amino acid mixture. As previously stated, approximately half of the patients requiring parenteral nutrition will tolerate a commercially available amino acid mixture. However, 40 to 50 gm is insufficient for long-term nutritional support, and if additional dosages are not tolerated, changing to a branched-chain-enriched amino acid solution is indicated.

Administration of Branched-Chain Amino Acid Mixtures

We have begun at an amino acid dose of 0.75 gm/kg of body weight/24 hours, given with 24 percent dextrose according to the techniques of central parenteral nutrition. This rate is increased by 0.25 to 0.50 gm of amino acids/kg/24 hrs until a maximum of 120 gm of amino acids/24 hrs is reached. In general, at a rate of 75 to 80 gm of amino acids/24 hrs, nitrogen equilibrium is achieved, and in most patients with acute-on-chronic failure, normalization of the plasma amino acids occurs.

The results obtained in a group of approximately 80 patients with hepatic encephalopathy associated with different disease states suggests that the response to amino acid infusion is predicated in part on the disease process that is being treated. Patients with acute-on-chronic failure can be expected to have a more rapid and complete normalization of their plasma amino acid patterns, since the amino acids are primarily derived from muscle breakdown. Thus, the branched-chain amino acids are better able to supply the energy deficit, improve protein synthesis, and control efflux of other amino acids through the myocyte membrane. Resolution of encephalopathy has been relatively rapid; approximately 85 percent of the patients experience an improvement in one full grade within 72 hours. Over this period, approximately 60 percent of the patients can be expected to have a sustained improvement despite persistence of the precipitating insult. Such improvement is also manifested by improved Reitan trail test times and improvement in the electroencephalogram, which appears to follow rather than precede the clinical grade. Survival in the anectotal group of patients has been approximately 50 percent, which is quite reasonable, considering that the group had a mean bilirubin of

13, had been in coma for five days despite standard therapy, and had been hospitalized for two weeks prior to treatment.

A more interesting group of patients were those treated fortuitously, and then by design, with the branched-chain amino acid mixture while all other forms of therapy were discontinued. In this group, the resolution of encephalopathy remained about 60 percent over 48 to 72 hours, confirming the efficacy of this form of therapy.

Of greater interest is a recently completed randomized prospective trial involving a group of patients with acute-on-chronic hepatic encephalopathy treated with the three branched-chain amino acids alone either in hypertonic dextrose or in hypertonic dextrose and lactulose. These investigators, working in four centers in Rome, Italy, showed that branched-chain amino acids given in somewhat larger doses than we have used (up to 60 gm/24 hours) woke patients faster and to a greater extent than did lactulose and an isocaloric amount of hypertonic dextrose [9]. Though the differences were not statistically significant, it may be concluded that branched-chain amino acids are equally as efficacious as lactulose in arousing patients from hepatic encephalopathy. We, as well as others, have demonstrated some nutritional benefit from the branched-chain amino acids alone given with a hypocaloric or hypercaloric dextrose solution [37], but continue to prefer a complete nutritional support mixture. Several other randomized prospective trials involving either intravenous or oral use of branched-chain-enriched amino acid mixtures have recently been completed. Horst et al. [42] showed that Hepatic-Aid, a 35 percent branched-chain amino acid enriched elemental diet with glucose as a caloric source, was superior to protein in a group of cirrhotics with protein intolerance. When F080 was randomized against neomycin and isocaloric dextrose, more rapid recovery was seen both in the United States and in Brazilian multicenter trials [4a, 12], and survival was improved in the group receiving F080 in 23 percent dextrose. Several other trials, in which the randomization is suspect, also appear to show efficacy for branched-chain-enriched amino acid solutions [18, 41, 58, 66].

Only two trials have failed to show efficacy when branched-chain amino acids are used in hepatic coma [65, 80]. It is of interest that in both studies intravenous fat was the caloric source. It is not clear that intravenous fat can be utilized in hepatic failure. As if to confirm this suggestion, in one study [65] plasma aromatic amino acids did not change, thus suggesting that intracellular disposition of aromatic amino acids and protein synthesis did not take place. In the other study [80], most patients were dead within a month; whether nutritional support can help such patients in extremis is not clear.

It should also be stressed that the use of intravenous fat in patients with hepatic encephalopathy may be deleterious, as fat may displace tryptophan from albumin, increasing unbound tryptophan and making it more available for transport to the brain.

Results in Fulminant Hepatic Failure

The infusion of branched-chain-enriched amino acid solutions in fulminant hepatic failure does not return plasma amino acids to normal. However, at least in the anecdotal series, aromatic amino acid levels are reduced, and encephalopathy is improved. The gross amino acid elevations characteristic of this severe form of failure are only in part due to massive skeletal muscle proteolysis in the face of diminished gluconeogenic capacity; presumably the necrotizing liver itself contributes significantly to this hyperaminoacidemia [34]. Whether nutritional support will avert the myopathy seen after repeated polyacrylonitrile membrane dialysis, or improve the possibility for regeneration, is not clear at present.

LONG-TERM THERAPY FOR CHRONIC HEPATIC ENCEPHALOPATHY

In patients with chronic hepatic encephalopathy, occurring either spontaneously or following portasystemic shunting, a number of different approaches have been taken. Since such stable patients are rare, experience with any single group is necessarily limited. Maddrey, Walser, and coworkers have employed a mixture of ornithine salts of keto-analogues of the branched-chain amino acids [50]. They have modified their previous proposal of a more complete mixture, since the keto-analogues of phenylalanine and methionine appear to be present in abundance. In a crossover trial with nine chronic cases, they were able to show that results with these ornithine salts were superior to the results achieved with a rather low dose (10 gm per day) of branched-chain amino acids [50].

Our group has concentrated on the amino acids themselves, using a more complete mixture. Our longest-term patient has been treated for 4½ years with reversal of encephalopathy, improvement in hepatic function, reversal of seemingly irreversible features including grimacing, explosive speech, and hemiballismus, and perhaps some improvement in a spinal paralysis secondary to demyelination. In other patients, now totaling five, we have generally used large oral doses (24 to 30 gm) of the three branched-chain amino acids in equimolar concentrations. A more complete mixture, Hepatic Aid, has not been utilized because most of these patients, as predicted by Ziparo [33], have severe diabetes; the glucose load of Hepatic Aid is too high for most patients with hyperglucagonemia and post-shunt diabetes.

LIVER FAILURE IN PATIENTS WITH SEPSIS

It is reasonable to include a section on the septic patient, in whom mortality is attributable largely to liver failure. In these patients, long-term sepsis, compounded by surgical insult and inadequate nutrition, evolves into a clinical picture that is indistinguishable from acute-on-chronic liver failure. Possibly this is secondary to donation of hepatic structural and functional protein to gluconeogenesis in order to maintain cerebral function, the final priority of survival. Thus, our nutritional support in sepsis is not unlike that of acute-on-chronic failure.

The plasma amino acid patterns are markedly similar. Sepsis is characterized by high levels of phenylalanine, tyrosine, taurine, cysteine, and methionine, as well as mild elevations of alanine, aspartate, glutamate, and proline. The branched-chain amino acids are within normal limits [39]. Furthermore, patients who do not survive sepsis have higher levels of the aromatic and sulfur-containing amino acids than do patients who survive; on the other hand, survivors have higher levels of branched-chain amino acids, alanine, and arginine [35, 39].

We have also been struck by the similarity between septic and hepatic encephalopathy. Recent studies from this laboratory suggest that the alterations at the blood-brain barrier in patients with septic encephalopathy seem to be similar to those described in animals with liver disease. We, as well as others, have applied the concept that since there appears to be an energy crisis in terminal sepsis, either secondary to or associated with hepatic failure, it seems appropriate that the administration of increased amounts of branched-chain amino acids may be beneficial in providing a peripheral substrate. In our studies, administration of a branched-chain-enriched amino acid mixture appeared to improve the septic encephalopathy as well.

At present, a 45 percent branched-chain solution is being evaluated in cases of overwhelming sepsis. It is hoped that this tailored approach to nutritional support, along with appropriate surgical drainage and antibiotic therapy, will improve the survival of these critically ill patients.

REFERENCES

1. Alexander, J. W., et al. Beneficial effects of aggressive protein feeding in severely burned children. *Ann. Surg.* 192:505, 1980.
2. Baldessarini, R. J., and Fischer, J. E. S-adenosylmethionine following portacaval anastomoses. *Surgery* 62:311, 1967.
3. Baldessarini, R. J., and Fischer, J. E. Serotonin metabolism in rat brain after surgical diversion of

the portal venous circulation. *Nature (New Biol.)* 254:25, 1973.

4. Berl, S., et al. Metabolic compartments in vivo: Ammonia and glutamine acid metabolism in brain and liver. *J. Biol. Chem.* 237:2562, 1962.

4a. Bernadini, P. Personal communication.

5. Biebuyck, J. F., et al. Neurochemistry of hepatic coma: Alterations in putative transmitter amino acids. In R. Williams and I. M. Murray-Lyons (Eds.), *Artificial Liver Support* (Proceedings of an International Symposium on Artificial Support Systems for Acute Hepatic Failure. London: Pittman, 1974. Pp. 51–60.

6. Budd, M. A., et al. Isovaleric acidemia: Clinical features of a new genetic defect of leucine metabolism. *N. Engl. J. Med.* 277:321, 1967.

7. Burchell, A. R., et al. Hepatic artery flow improvement after portacaval shunt: A single hemodynamic clinical correlate. *Ann. Surg.* 184: 289, 1976.

8. Buse, M. G., and Reid, M. Leucine, a possible regulation of protein turnover in muscle. *J. Clin. Invest.* 56:1250, 1975.

9. Capocaccia, L., and Rossi-Fanelli, F. A randomized prospective trial of lactulose versus branched-chain amino acids in the treatment of hepatic encephalopathy. *Dig. Dis. Sci.* 1982. In Press.

10. Cardelli-Cangiano, P., et al. Uptake of amino acids by brain microvessels isolated from rats after portacaval anastomosis. *J. Neurochem.* 36:627, 1981.

11. Cascino, A., et al. Plasma amino acid imbalance in patients with hepatic encephalopathy. *Am. J. Dig. Dis.* 23:591, 1978.

12. Cerra, F., Chung, R., Fischer, J. E., et al. Treatment of hepatic encephalopathy with F080: A randomized prospective trial. In preparation.

13. Cummings, M. G., et al. Regional brain study of indoleamine metabolism in the rat in acute hepatic failure. *J. Neurochem.* 27:741, 1976.

14. Curzon, G., et al. Effects of chronic portacaval anastomosis on brain tryptophan, tyrosine and 5-hydroxytryptamine. *J. Neurochem.* 24:1065, 1975.

15. Dawson, A. M., and Sherlock, S. Effect of an amine oxidase inhibitor in liver disease. *Lancet* 1:1332, 1957.

16. Dismukes, K. New look at the aminergic nervous system. *Nature* 269:557, 1977.

17. Dodsworth, J. M., et al. Depletion of brain norepinephrine in acute hepatic coma. *Surgery* 75: 811, 1974.

18. Egberts, E. H., Hamster, W., Jurgens, P., Schumaker, H., Fondalinski, G., Reinhard, V., and Schomerus, H. Effect of Branched-Chain Amino Acids on Latent Portal-Systemic Encephalopathy. In M. Walser and R. Williamson (Eds.), *Metabolism and Clinical Implications of Branched-chain Amino and Ketoacids.* New York: Elsevier/North Holland, 1981. Pp. 453–463.

19. Eigler, N., Sacca, L., and Sherwin, R. S. Synergistic interactions of physiologic investment of glucagon, epinephrine and cortisol in the dog. A model for stress induced hyperglycemia. *J. Clin. Invest.* 63:114, 1979.

20. Faraj, B. A., et al. Evidence for central hypertyraminemia in hepatic encephalopathy. *J. Clin. Invest.* 67:395, 1981.

21. Felig, P. The glucose alanine cycle. *Metabolism* 22:179, 1973.

22. Felig, P. Amino acid metabolism in man. *Annu. Rev. Biochem.* 44:936, 1975.

23. Fernstrom, J. D., and Faller, D. V. Neutral amino acids in brain: Changes in response to food ingestion. *J. Neurochem.* 30:1531, 1978.

24. Fischer, J. E. False neurotransmitters and hepatic coma. *Res. Publ. Assoc. Res. Nerv. Ment. Dis.* 53:53, 1974.

25. Fischer, J. E. What can we expect from the artificial liver? *Int. J. Artif. Organs* 1:187, 1978.

26. Fischer, J. E. Portasystemic Encephalopathy. In R. Wright, K. G. M. M. Alberti, S. Karran, and G. H. Millward-Sadler (Eds.), *Liver and Biliary Disease: Pathophysiology, Diagnosis, Management.* Philadelphia: Saunders, 1979. P. 983.

27. Fischer, J. E. Portal hypertension and bleeding esophageal varices. *Am. J. Surg.* 140:337, 1980. Editorial.

28. Fischer, J. E. Nutritional Support in the Seriously Ill Patient. In M. M. Ravitch and F. M. Steichen (Eds.), *Current Problems in Surgery.* Chicago: Year Book, 1980. Vol. 17, No. 9.

29. Fischer, J. E., and Baldessarini, R. J. False neurotransmitters and hepatic failure. *Lancet* 2:75, 1971.

30. Fischer, J. E., Bower, R., Atamian, S., and Welling, R. Comparison of distal and proximal splenorenal shunts: A randomized prospective trial. *Ann. Surg.* 194:531, 1981.

31. Fischer, J. E., Funovics, J. M., Aguirre, A., James, J. H., Keane, J. M., Wesdorp, R. I. C., Yoshimura, N., and Westman, T. The role of plasma amino acids in hepatic encephalopathy. *Surgery* 78:276, 1975.

32. Fischer, J. E., and James, J. H. Treatment of hepatic coma and hepatorenal syndrome. Mechanism of L-dopa and aramine. *Am. J. Surg.* 123: 222, 1972.

33. Fischer, J. E., Jeppsson, B., James, J. H., and Ziparo, V. A Unified Hypothesis of Hepatic En-

cephalopathy. In M. J. Orloff, S. Stipa, and V. Ziparo (Eds.), *Medical and Surgical Problems of Portal Hypertension*. London: Academic, 1980. Vol. 34.

34. Fischer, J. E., Yoshimura, N., James, J. H., Cummings, M. G., Abel, R. M., and Deindorfer, F. Plasma amino acids in patients with hepatic encephalopathy: Effects of amino acid infusions. *Am. J. Surg.* 127:40, 1974.
35. Freund, H., Atamian, S., Holroyde, J., and Fischer, J. E. Plasma amino acids as predictors of the severity and outcome of sepsis. *Ann. Surg.* 190:571, 1979.
36. Freund, H., Dienstag, J., Lehrich, J. M., et al. Infusion of branched-chain amino acid solution in patients with hepatic encephalopathy. *Ann. Surg.,* 1982. In press.
37. Freund, H., Hoover, H. C., Jr., Atamian, S., and Fischer, J. E. Infusion of the branched-chain amino acids in postoperative patients. Anti-catabolic properties. *Ann. Surg.* 190:18, 1979.
38. Freund, H., James, J. H., and Fischer, J. E. Nitrogen-sparing mechanisms of singly administered branched-chain amino acids in the injured rat. *Surgery* 90:237, 1981.
39. Freund, H., Ryan, J., and Fischer, J. E. Amino acid derangements in patients with sepsis. *Ann. Surg.* 188:423, 1978.
40. Herlin, P. M., et al. Total hepatectomy as a model for fulminant hepatic failure (FHF)—Effects of branched-chain amino acid (BCAA) infusion. Submitted for publication.
41. Holm, E., Streibel, J. P., Moller, P., and Hartman, M. Amino Acid Solutions for Parenteral Nutrition and for Adjuvant Treatment of Encephalopathy in Liver Cirrhosis, Studies Concerning 120 Patients. In M. Walser and R. Williamson (Eds.), *Metabolism and Clinical Implications of Branched Chain Amino and Keto Acids*. New York: Elsevier/North Holland, 1981. Pp. 513–518.
42. Horst, D., Grace, N., Conn, H. O., Schiff, E., Schenker, S., Viteri, A., Law, D., and Atterbury, C. E. A double-blind randomized comparison of dietary protein and an oral branched chain amino acid (BCAA) supplement in cirrhotic patients with chronic portal-systemic encephalopathy (PSE) (ABS) *Hepatology* 5:518, 1981.
43. Hourani, B. T., Hamlin, E. M., and Reynolds, T. B. Cerebrospinal fluid glutamine as a measure of hepatic encephalopathy. *Arch. Intern. Med.* 127: 1033, 1971.
44. James, J. H., Escourrou, J., and Fischer, J. E. Blood-brain neutral amino acid transport activity is increased after portacaval anastomosis. *Science* 200:1395, 1978.
45. James, et al. Hyperammonemia, plasma amino acid imbalance, and blood-brain amino acid transport: A unified theory of portalsystemic encephalopathy. *Lancet* 2:772, 1979.
46. Jeejeebhoy, K. N., and Phillip, R. J. Isolated mammalian hepatocytes in culture. *Gastroenterology* 71:1086, 1976.
47. Knell, A. J., et al. Dopamine and serotonin metabolism in hepatic encephalopathy. *Br. Med. J.* 1:549, 1974.
48. Lam, K. C., et al. Role of a false neurotransmitter, octopamine, in the pathogenesis of hepatic and renal encephalopathy. *Scand. J. Gastroenterol.* 8:465, 1973.
49. Levine, R. J., and Conn, H. O. Tyrosine metabolism in patients with liver disease. *J. Clin. Invest.* 46:2012, 1967.
50. Maddrey, W. C., Herlong, H. F., and Walser, M. Ornithine Salts of Branched Chain Ketoacids in Portal-Systemic Encephalopathy. In M. Walser and J. R. Williamson (Eds.), *Metabolism and Clinical Implications of Branched Chain Amino and Keto Acids,* New York: Elsevier/North Holland, 1981. Vol. 18, pp. 433–440.
51. Manghani, K. K., et al. Urinary and serum octopamine in patients with portalsystemic encephalopathy. *Lancet* 2:943, 1975.
52. McMenamy, R. H., and Oncley, J. L. The specific binding of L-tryptophan to serum albumin. *J. Biol. Chem.* 233:1436, 1958.
53. Morgan, M. Y., et al. Medium chain triglycerides and hepatic encephalopathy. *Gut* 15:180, 1974.
54. Morgan, M. Y., et al. Successful use of bromcryptine in the treatment of patients with chronic portasystemic encephalopathy. *N. Engl. J. Med.* 296:793, 1977.
55. Nasrallah, S. M., and Galambos, J. T. Amino acid therapy in alcoholic hepatitis. *Lancet* 2:1276, 1980.
56. Nespoli, A., et al. The role of false neurotransmitters in the pathogenesis of hepatic encephalopathy and hyperdynamic syndrome in cirrhosis. *Arch. Surg.* 116:1129, 1981.
57. Odessey, R., Khairallah, E. A., and Goldberg, A. L. Origin and possible significance of alanine production by skeletal muscle. *J. Biol. Chem.* 249:7623, 1974.
58. Okada, A., Kamata, S., Kim, C. W., and Kawashima, Y. Treatment of Hepatic Encephalopathy with BCAA-Rich Amino Acid Mixture. In M. Walser and R. Williamson (Eds.), *Metabolism and Clinical Implications of Branched-chain Amino and Ketoacids.* New York: Elsevier/North Holland, 1981. Pp. 447–452.
59. Oldendorf, W. H. Brain uptake of radiolabelled

amino acids, amines and hexoses after arterial injection. *Am. J. Physiol.* 221:1629, 1971.
60. Ono, J., et al. Tryptophan and hepatic coma. *Gastroenterology* 74:196, 1978.
61. Pardridge, W. M., and Jefferson, L. S. Liver uptake of amino acids and carbohydrates during a single circulatory passage. *Am. J. Physiol.* 228: 1155, 1975.
62. Pardridge, W. M., and Oldendorf, W. H. Kinetic analysis of blood-brain barrier transport of amino acids. *Biochim. Biophys. Acta* 401:128, 1975.
63. Parke, W. F., Rousselot, L. M., and Burchell, A. R. A sixteen year experience with end-to-side portacaval shunt for variceal hemmorhage. Analysis of data and comparison with other types of portosystemic anastomoses. *Ann. Surg.* 168:957, 1968.
64. Parkes, J. D., Sharpstone, P., and Williams, R. Levodopa in hepatic coma. *Lancet* 2:1341, 1970.
65. Pomier-Layrangues, G., Duhamel, O., Lacombe, B., Culleret, G., Bellet, H., and Michel, H. Treatment of hepatic encephalopathy by perfusions of normal or modified solutions of amino acids—controlled study of 32 patients. *Gastroenterologie Clinique et Biologique,* 1980. Vol. 4 (IBIS), A79.
66. Rakette, S., Fischer, M., Reimann, H. J., and Sommoggy, S. V. Effects of Special Amino Solutions in Patients with Liver Cirrhosis and Hepatic Encephalopathy. In M. Walser and R. Williamson (Eds.), *Metabolism and Clinical Implications of Branched-chain Amino and Ketoacids.* New York: Elsevier/North Holland, 1981. Pp. 419–427.
67. Rosen, H. M., Yoshimura, N., Hodgman, J. M., and Fischer, J. E. Plasma amino acid patterns in hepatic encephalopathy of differing etiology. *Gastroenterology* 72:483, 1977.
68. Rossi-Fanelli, F., et al. Phenylethanolamine and Octopamine in Hepatic Encephalopathy. In A. D. Mosnaim and M. E. Wolf (Eds.), *Noncatecholic Phenylethylamines.* New York: Dekker, 1980. Pp. 231–244.
69. Samuels, S., Fish, F., and Freedman, L. S. Effect of gammaglutamyl cycle inhibitors on brain amino acid transport and utilization. *Neurochem. Res.* 3:619, 1978.
70. Sherlock, S. *Diseases of the Liver and Biliary System.* Oxford: Blackwell, 1975. P. 427.
71. Sherwin, R., et al. Hyperglucagonemia in Laennec's cirrhosis: The role of portalsystemic shunting. *N. Engl. J. Med.* 290:239, 1974.
72. Silk, D. B. A., et al. Treatment of fulminant hepatic failure by polyacrylonitrile-membrane hemodialysis. *Lancet* 2:1, 1977.
73. Smith, A. R., Freund, H., Rossi-Fanelli, F., Berlatzky, Y., and Fischer, J. E. Long-term sampling of intraventricular CSF in the unanesthetized monkey and dog. *J. Surg. Res.* 26:69, 1979.
74. Smith, A. R., Rossi-Fanelli, F., Ziparo, V., James, J. H., Perelle, B. A., and Fischer, J. E. Alterations in plasma and CSF amino acids, amines and metabolites in hepatic coma. *Ann. Surg.* 187: 343, 1978.
75. Soeters, P. B., Ebeid, A. M., and Fischer, J. E. Evidence for superiority of a branched-chain enriched amino acid solution in hepatic coma in dogs. Submitted for publication.
76. Soeters, P. B., and Fischer, J. E. Insulin, glucagon, amino acid imbalance, and hepatic encephalopathy. *Lancet* 2:880, 1976.
77. Soeters, P. B., Weir, G. C., Ebeid, A. M., and Fischer, J. E. Insulin, glucagon, portalsystemic shunting, and hepatic failure in the dog. *J. Surg. Res.* 23:183, 1977.
78. Strombeck, D. R., Rogers, Q., and Stern, J. S. Effects of intravenous ammonia infusion on plasma levels of amino acids, glucagon, and insulin in dogs. *Gastroenterology* 74:1165, 1978. (Abstract)
79. Tanaka, K., Isselbacher, K. F., and Shih, V. Isovaleric and alphamethylbutyric acidemias induced by hypoglycin A: Mechanism of Jamaican vomiting sickness. *Science* 175:69, 1972.
80. Wahren, J. J., Deňis, J., Desurmount, P., Ericson, S., et al. Is IV administration of branched-chain amino acids effective in the treatment of hepatic encephalopathy, results of multicenter study. *Europ. Soc. Parent. Enter. Nutr.* FC47:61, 1981.
81. Warren, K. S., and Schenker, S. Effect of an inhibitor of glutamine synthesis (methionine sulfoximine) on ammonia toxicity and metabolism. *J. Lab. Clin. Med.* 64:442, 1964.
82. Zieve, F. J., et al. Synergism between ammonia and fatty acids in the production of coma: Implications for hepatic coma. *J. Pharmacol. Exp. Ther.* 191:10, 1974.

18

Nutritional Management of Acute Renal Failure

Joel D. Kopple
Bruno Cianciaruso

METABOLIC AND NUTRITIONAL STATUS OF THE PATIENT WITH ACUTE RENAL FAILURE

The metabolic and nutritional status of patients with acute renal failure can vary enormously. Some patients show no evidence of negative nitrogen balance, and they have normal water balance, plasma electrolyte concentrations, and acid-base status. In general, these patients have no severely catabolic underlying illnesses. They are usually not oliguric, and the cause of their acute renal failure is typically an isolated, noncatabolic event, such as administration of radiocontrast drugs. However, most patients with acute renal failure have some degree of net protein breakdown (synthesis minus degradation) and disturbances in fluid, electrolyte, or acid-base status. Often, there is water overload, hyperkalemia, hyperphosphatemia, hypocalcemia, azotemia, hyperuricemia, and metabolic acidosis with a large anion gap.

Net protein degradation in acute renal failure can be massive, with a net loss of 150 to 200 gm/day or more [31, 67]; by comparison, the total protein mass of a 70-kg man is about 6 kg [23]. Patients are more likely to be catabolic when the acute renal failure is caused by shock, sepsis, or rhabdomyolysis. In the study of Feinstein et al., mean urea nitrogen appearance (UNA, net urea nitrogen production) was 12.0 ± 7.9 (SD) gm/day in patients in whom acute renal failure was caused by hypotension, or sepsis, or both and 12.3 ± 7.9 gm/day in those with rhabdomyolysis [31]. These UNA rates were significantly greater ($p < 0.001$ and $p < 0.05$ respectively) than in patients with acute renal failure from other causes (3.8 ± 2.4 gm/day).

In patients with acute renal failure, marked net protein breakdown can enhance the rate of rise in plasma potassium, phosphorus, and nitrogenous metabolites and the fall in blood pH. Studies in nonuremic humans indicate that wasting and malnutrition can impair normal wound healing and immune function [20, 65] and enhance morbidity and mortality. It is therefore likely that the profound catabolic response of many patients with acute renal failure may increase the risk of delayed wound healing and infection, prolong convalescence, and increase mortality.

Causes of Wasting in Acute Renal Failure

There are clearly multiple causes of wasting in acute renal failure. Several studies in animals suggest that acute uremia itself may cause disorders in amino acid and protein metabolism and promote wasting. In liver from acutely uremic rats, Lacy observed an increased uptake of several amino acids and enhanced urea production [64]. Fröhlich et al. studied glucose and urea output in perfused liver from rats with bilateral nephrectomies and reported increased hepatic release of glucose, urea, and the branched-chain amino acids valine, leucine, and isoleucine, which are not well metabolized by the liver [35]. When a mixture of amino acids was added to the perfusate in concentrations that were approximately physiologic, the increment in glucose and urea formation in the acutely uremic rats was significantly greater than in control rats [35]. These observations suggest that in rats, acute uremia stimulates both gluconeogenesis and protein degradation in liver.

Protein synthesis and degradation may vary independently and according to the organ studied. McCormick, Shear, and Barry reported increased incorporation of ^{14}C-leucine into trichloroacetic acid precipitable material in liver homogenates from acutely uremic rats [72]. This suggests enhanced protein synthesis. Shear reported that in acutely uremic rats, protein synthesis was increased in liver and heart and decreased in skeletal muscle [95]. Flügel-Link et al. studied protein synthesis and degradation in perfused posterior hemicarcasses of rats made acutely uremic by bilateral nephrectomy and in sham-operated control rats [33]. There was increased UNA in the acutely uremic rats, indicating enhanced net protein degradation. Muscle protein synthesis was not different in the two groups of rats, but protein degradation was significantly increased in the acutely uremic animals.

The mechanisms for increased gluconeogenesis and net protein degradation in rats with acute renal failure are not well defined. In the liver of acutely uremic rats, Sapico and coworkers report that activity of glutamic oxaloacetic aminotransferase, which catalyzes the transamination of glutamate, is increased [92, 96]. Also, there appears to be increased activity of two enzymes involved with metabolism of urea cycle amino acids: ornithine transaminase, which catalyzes the conversion of glutamate to ornithine, and arginase, which catalyzes formation of urea and ornithine from arginine. In addition, Sapico and coworkers reported that in liver of acutely uremic rats, there is normal activity of phenylalanine hydroxylase and increased activity of tyrosine aminotransferase, key enzymes in the major degradative pathway of phenylalanine and tyrosine [93].

Glycogen metabolism may also be altered in acute uremia. Bergström and Hultman reported decreased muscle glycogen content in acutely uremic patients who are catabolic [11]. Hörl and Heidland observed reduced muscle glycogen in rats with bilateral nephrectomies as compared with sham-operated controls [50]. They also reported that in muscle from these rats there is increased activity of phosphorylase a, which catalyzes glycogenolysis, and decreased activity of glycogen synthetase I, which catalyzes glycogen synthesis. Whether or not these alterations may predispose to protein wasting in acute uremia is unknown. It is of interest that Hörl and Heidland found that supplementing a low-protein diet with serine increased glycogen synthetase I activity in these rats.

Whether these metabolic changes in acute uremia are due to altered endocrinologic function (see the following) or to retention of toxic metabolic products is not known. It is also possible that the surgical procedure for making rats uremic (e.g., bilateral nephrectomy) may itself constitute a greater catabolic stress to the animal than does the sham surgery. If so, the enhanced net protein catabolism in these animals might represent a response to the surgical stress rather than the influence of uremia. Nonetheless, since virtually every study indicates that acute uremia in rats is a catabolic stress, it seems likely that enhanced catabolism is due to uremia per se rather than solely to the methods of causing renal failure.

The catabolic effects of uremia may be induced by several causes. First, the metabolic products that accumulate in uremia may be toxic [55]. Second, alterations in plasma concentrations of catabolic hormones may also promote wasting. Eigler et al. showed that dogs infused with cortisone, epinephrine, and glucagon in quantities sufficient to raise plasma concentrations to levels found in acutely catabolic patients demonstrated sustained increased glucose production [29]. Since much of the glucose formed was probably derived from amino acids, particularly alanine and glutamine, it is likely that these endocrine disorders also promoted protein wasting. There is little information on the effects of these hormones in acute renal failure. Serum glucagon levels are increased in acute renal failure [14]. In chronic uremia there is evidence for increased sensitivity to the actions of glucagon [97]; however, Mondon and Reaven were unable to demonstrate enhanced sensitivity to glucagon in acutely uremic rats [79]. Although resistance to the actions of insulin are reported in chronic renal failure [26, 27], we are not aware of many data on insulin resistance in acute renal failure. Our experience in acutely uremic patients infused with hypertonic glucose suggests that glucose intolerance is common in this condition [31]. Parathyroid hormone, which may be increased in acute renal failure [71, 85], is another potentially catabolic agent [60].

Third, Hörl and Heidland have made the intriguing observation that proteolytic activity can be observed in the sera of some patients with acute renal failure who are very catabolic [48]. These observations suggest that in the sera of hypercatabolic, acutely uremic patients, there may be either increased quantities of proteases, which degrade proteins, a reduction in protease inhibitors, or changes in other factors that lead to enhanced protease activity. Enhanced activity of certain muscle proteases has been reported in patients with net protein catabolism [70]. To our knowledge, increased muscle or liver protease activity has not been described in uremic patients. In the acutely uremic rats who have increased muscle protein degradation, Flügel-Link et al. found that activity of the proteases cathepsin B_1 and cathepsin D, was not different from that of controls [33]. The role of protease activity in uremia would seem to be an important area for further investigation.

In addition to the potential catabolic effects of uremia per se, there are clearly other causes for wasting and malnutrition in acute renal failure. These include the following:

1. Many patients are unable to eat adequately because of anorexia or vomiting. These symptoms may be caused by acute uremia, underlying illnesses, or the anorectic effects of dialysis treatment. Other causes of poor food intake are medical or surgical disorders that impair gastrointestinal function and the frequent diagnostic studies that require the patient to fast for several hours.
2. The patient's underlying medical disorders are often a major cause of wasting. Chief among these catabolic conditions are infection, hypotension, surgical or nonsurgical trauma, and rhabdomyolysis.
3. Losses of nutrients in draining fistulas and during dialysis therapy may lead to wasting and malnutrition. Approximately 6 to 7 gm of free amino acids are removed during a 4-hour hemodialysis [40, 63, 74]. During intermittent peritoneal dialysis for approximately 24 to 32 hours, about 5 gm of amino acids are lost [13, 119]. With continuous ambulatory peritoneal dialysis (CAPD), about 1.5 to 3.5 gm of free amino acids are lost each day [41, 59]. Not much protein is removed during hemodialysis, but during acute intermittent peritoneal dialysis for about 36 hours, approximately 22 gm of total protein and 13 gm of albumin are lost [17]. During maintenance intermittent peritoneal dialysis for about 10 hours, about 13 gm of total protein and 8 to 9 gm of albumin are removed [17]. Many of these losses are from ascitic fluid washout. With CAPD, the 24-hour losses of total protein and albumin

are about 9 and 6 gm, respectively. In patients undergoing peritoneal dialysis who have acute peritonitis, protein losses can increase markedly. We have observed one such patient who lost 106 gm of protein during a 24-hour period. With antimicrobial treatment, protein losses may fall quickly but may not return to normal for many weeks.

Patients undergoing hemodialysis with glucose-free dialysate may lose 20 to 50 gm of glucose during a 4- to 6-hour procedure. Glucose losses depend in part on the dialyzer used and the blood glucose levels. There is net glucose absorption with peritoneal dialysis, because the dialysate contains glucose monohydrate, 1.5 to 4.25 gm/100 ml. Glucose absorption varies directly with the concentration of glucose in dialysate or the total quantity of glucose instilled. During CAPD, glucose absorption (y, gm/day) was equal to the quantity instilled each day (x, gm/day) as follows [43]: $y = 0.89x - 43$, $r = 0.91$, $p < 0.001$. In the experience of Grodstein et al., about 180 gm/day of glucose were absorbed during CAPD [43]. Water-soluble vitamins and probably other biologically active substances are also lost during both hemodialysis and peritoneal dialysis. Losses of the water-soluble vitamins during dialysis are readily replaced with oral or parenteral vitamin supplements.

4. Blood drawing, gastrointestinal bleeding, which may be occult, and blood sequestered in the hemodialyzer are other sources of protein depletion. A person with a hemoglobin of 12.0 gm/100 ml and a serum total protein of 7.0 gm/100 ml will lose approximately 16.5 gm of protein in each 100 ml of blood removed.

PAST EXPERIENCE WITH NUTRITIONAL THERAPY OF ACUTE RENAL FAILURE

Nutritional therapy has been advocated in acute renal failure for three major purposes: (1) To reduce uremic toxicity and metabolic derangements; (2) to maintain or improve overall nutritional and clinical status, particularly with regard to wound healing, immunologic function, and host resistance; and (3) to facilitate healing of the injured kidney.

In this section we will review the published literature on nutritional therapy in acute renal failure, particularly with regard to its effects on nutritional and metabolic status, metabolism of the kidney, recovery of renal function, and survival.

Experience with Nutritional Therapy for Patients with Acute Renal Failure

Prior to the mid-1960s, many clinicians advocated severe or total restriction of protein intake for patients with acute renal failure [16, 19, 21]. Small amounts of energy (e.g., 400 to 800 kcal/day) were given as candy, butterballs, or intravenous infusions of hypertonic glucose to reduce the rate of protein degradation. This therapy was based on Gamble's studies of lifeboat rations for healthy young men. Gamble's observations indicated that administration of 100 gm/day of sugar could substantially reduce net protein breakdown [38]; 200 gm/day of sugar could spare more protein, although the protein-sparing was not twice as great as with 100 gm/day of sugar. However, many physicians who applied these findings to acutely uremic patients may have worked under a misunderstanding: Gamble's studies were carried out in healthy volunteers who were clinically stable, whereas acutely uremic patients are often in a severely catabolic state and may have extra losses of nutrients from dialysis, wound drainage, and blood drawing.

Anabolic steroids were frequently employed because they could transiently decrease the UNA, the rate of rise of serum urea nitrogen (SUN) or nonprotein nitrogen, and the development of acidosis. In the 1960s, the Giordano-Giovanetti diet was developed for patients with chronic renal failure. This diet contained about 20 gm/day of protein, most of which was usually supplied by two eggs, which provided the recommended daily allowances for essential amino acids (again, for healthy young adults). Some clinicians advocated this diet for the acutely uremic patient who was able to eat because they believed that the diet could be utilized efficiently and would minimize the degree of protein wasting while it reduced the UNA and accumulation of nitrogenous metabolites [12].

These earlier forms of nutritional therapy were developed before dialysis treatment was readily available; usually, the primary goal of treatment was to reduce uremic toxicity, and the maintenance of good nutrition was a secondary goal. When dialysis became available, it was usually only employed for specific sequelae of renal failure, such as uremic symptoms, congestive heart failure, or hyperkalemia, and great efforts were often made to avoid the need for dialysis therapy. It is now generally accepted that early and frequent dialysis should be employed in patients with acute renal failure to prevent uremic signs and symptoms and decrease morbidity and mortality [103].*

With the advent of modern techniques for total parenteral nutrition and the more ready availability of dialysis, it was natural to apply the former treatment to patients with acute renal failure who were unable to eat even if it increased the need for dialysis therapy. Lee and coworkers, in 1967, described their experience in several patients with acute or chronic renal failure who were administered solutions containing casein hydrolysate, fructose, ethanol, and soya bean oil emulsion (Intralipid) by peripheral vein [66]. They reported that, despite the severity of the patients' illnesses, marked loss of weight did not occur and convalescence was shortened.

Dudrick et al. in 1969 and 1970, reported treating 10 acutely or chronically uremic patients with intravenous infusions of essential amino acids and hypertonic glucose into the subclavian vein [28, 114]. They described weight gain, improved wound healing, and stabilization or reduction in SUN levels. Decreased serum potassium and phosphorus and positive nitrogen balance were often observed. They also reported that anephric beagles who received intravenous infusions of essential amino acids and 57 percent glucose intravenously had a lower rise in SUN and a longer survival than anephric beagles who were given food or infusions of glucose (5 or 57 percent) alone [111].

Abel and coworkers published a series of studies in patients with acute renal failure who were treated with hypertonic glucose and eight essential amino acids, excluding histidine [1–5]. They reported that serum potassium, phosphorus, and magnesium fell, and SUN often stabilized or decreased. They carried out a prospective double-blind study in 53 patients with acute renal failure who were randomly assigned to receive infusions of either essential amino acids and hypertonic glucose or hypertonic glucose alone [4]. Total caloric intake averaged 1426 and 1641 kcal/day with the two solutions. Mean amino acid intake with the former preparation was about 16 gm/day. It was not stated whether patients ate food during the study. The patients receiving the essential amino acids and glucose had a higher incidence of recovery of renal function. However, overall mortality was not significantly improved in this group. The essential amino acid solution appeared to be particularly effective in patients with more severe renal failure, as indicated by the need for dialysis, and in those with serious complications, such as pneumonia and generalized sepsis. In the latter patients, hospital survival was significantly greater in those receiving essential amino acids and glucose than in those infused with glucose alone.

Baek and coworkers compared results in 63 patients treated with a fibrin hydrolysate and hypertonic glucose and 66 subjects who received varying quantities of glucose [9]. The rate of rise in

**Editor's Note:* It is not necessarily established that early prophylactic dialysis, especially in the surgical situation, reduces mortality. In many surgical situations (e.g., ruptured abdominal aortic aneurysm, massive trauma), patients may not tolerate early hemodialysis, and peritoneal dialysis may not be possible (e.g., when the retroperitoneum is not sealed). Thus, the use of a nutritional support regimen that delays the need for dialysis may be lifesaving.

SUN in the two groups was not different, but the incidence of hyperkalemia was less in the patients given the hydrolysate and glucose. Lower morbidity and mortality were reported in the patients who were given the hydrolysate. However, it is not clear whether the patients were randomly assigned to the two treatment regimens or even whether the two groups of patients were treated concurrently.

McMurray et al. and Milligan and associates examined the clinical course in patients with acute tubular necrosis who received either hypertonic glucose alone (200 to 400 kcal/day) or a mixture of essential and nonessential amino acids and hypertonic glucose that provided 12 gm of nitrogen/day and more than 2000 kcal/day [75, 77]. In patients with no complications, there was no difference in survival between the two treatment groups. However, in patients with three or more complications or with peritonitis, those who received 12 gm/day of amino acid nitrogen and hypertonic glucose had significantly greater survival as compared with the patients receiving low quantities of glucose alone. The study, however, was carried out retrospectively, and the patients who received amino acids and glucose were treated at a later time than were those who received glucose alone.

Blackburn, Etter, and MacKenzie reported experiments in 11 patients with mild acute renal failure who were given infusions providing 1.2% essential amino acids and 37% glucose, 2.0% essential and nonessential amino acids and 37% glucose, or 2.1% essential and nonessential amino acids and 52% glucose [15]. Infusion with more glucose was associated with a significant fall in SUN and creatinine, whereas there was a slight but not significantly greater decrease in SUN in patients receiving the essential amino acids as compared with those given both essential and nonessential amino acids. When nitrogen intake was increased to 4 to 5 gm/day, nitrogen balance improved and became almost neutral.

Abitbol and Holliday infused, in sequential order, glucose alone and glucose with essential amino acids to four anuric children who had the hemolytic-uremic syndrome, to one child with systemic lupus erythematosus and to one child with congenital nephrosis [6]. Nitrogen balance was negative with glucose alone and positive with glucose and essential amino acids; SUN rose more slowly with the latter solution. As energy intake increased from 20 to 70 kcal/kg/day, nitrogen balance became less negative. The children, who were malnourished at the onset of the study, were first given the glucose infusion and then the infusion of glucose and amino acids; the latter infusion was also higher in calories. These factors could account for the greater anabolic response to both the higher energy intake and the amino acid therapy.

Several studies have indicated that nitrogen requirements are high in acute renal failure and that nitrogen balance is difficult to attain with low-nitrogen diets. Leonard, Luke, and Siegel carried out a prospective study in patients with acute renal failure who were randomly assigned to receive infusions of 1.75% essential L-amino acids and 47% dextrose or 47% dextrose alone [67]. Patients who were able to eat or tolerate tube feeding were excluded from the study, and many had severe complicating illnesses. Most patients required dialysis frequently. The rate of rise in SUN was significantly less in the group receiving essential amino acids. However, mean nitrogen balance was approximately 10 gm/day negative in both groups, and there was no difference in the rate of survival or recovery of renal function in the two groups.

Spreiter, Myers, and Swenson carried out 32 studies in 14 patients with acute renal failure who were infused with various intakes of amino acids and hypertonic glucose [100]. Nitrogen balances became positive in only four subjects and at a time when the mean amino acid intake was 1.03 gm/kg/day, and glucose intake provided 50 kcal/kg/day. The study may have actually underestimated nutrient requirements, because patients often were not able to tolerate the fluid and nitrogen loads associated with the higher intakes until some days had passed and their clinical condition had improved. Thus, the patients may have received the higher nitrogen and energy intakes at a time when they were less ill and possibly more able to become anabolic.

Lopez-Martinez et al. studied the effects of parenteral nutrition for 12 days each in 35 septic patients with acute renal failure [69]. At the time of study, the patients were in the polyuric phase and were not very uremic; none had received dialysis therapy. Patients were given 4.4 gm/day of nitrogen from essential amino acids and 2000 kcal/day (group 1), or 15 gm/day of nitrogen from essential and nonessential amino acids and 3000 kcal/day, provided either by glucose (group 2) or by glucose and fat (group 3). Nitrogen balance, apparently estimated from the difference between nitrogen intake and UNA, was initially negative in all three groups and became more positive with time, particularly in groups 2 and 3. During the 12-day period of study, the grand mean of the nitrogen balance in groups 2 and 3 was each significantly more positive than in group 1.

Hasik et al. fed diets varying in protein content to nine patients with acute renal failure at a time when they were polyuric [45]. The authors concluded that these patients, who were probably not severely ill at the time of study, required 0.97 gm of protein/kg/day.

Since the patients in these last two studies were neither very uremic or ill, the results may be more applicable to the patient who is recovering from acute renal failure.

Feinstein et al. evaluated 30 patients with acute renal failure who were unable to eat adequately while they were randomly assigned to receive parenteral nutrition with glucose alone, glucose and 21 gm per day of the esential amino acids, or glucose and 21 gm per day of essential amino acids and 21 gm/day of nonessential amino acids [31]. Mean energy intake varied from 2,300 to 2,700 kcal/day and did not differ significantly among the groups. Patients were studied in a prospective, double-blind fashion; mean duration of study in the three groups was 9.0 ± [S. D.] 7.7 days. Many patients were in a markedly catabolic state, as determined from nitrogen balances, UNA, serum protein levels, and plasma amino acid concentrations. Mean nitrogen balance, estimated from the difference between nitrogen intake and UNA, which underestimates nitrogen losses, was − 10.4 ± 5.7 gm/day with glucose alone, −4.4 ± 7.3 gm/day with glucose and essential amino acids, and −8.5 ± 7.9 gm/day with glucose and essential and nonessential amino acids. Although nitrogen balance was not different with the three infusates, in a few patients who received essential or both essential and nonessential amino acids, the nitrogen balance was only slightly negative or, in one patient, positive. Serum potassium, phosphorus, and SUN often stabilized or decreased in all three treatment groups; these changes in serum levels were probably related to dialysis therapy, recovering renal function, or the natural history of the underlying metabolic disorders. There was no difference in the rapidity or incidence of recovery of renal function or in the rate of survival among the three treatment groups. In patients in whom renal failure could be attributed to hypotension, sepsis, or both, as compared with patients with renal failure from other causes, there was a significantly lower rate of recovery of renal function (17 percent) and survival (17 percent).*

Effect of Nutritional Therapy on Recovery of Renal Function

Several lines of evidence suggest that nutritional therapy might facilitate healing of the acutely failed kidney. The findings of metabolic studies of the proximal tubular cells of rats with acute tubular necrosis caused by injection of mercuric chloride indicate that there is increased synthesis of

**Editor's Note:* This study was well designed and much needed. It is particularly unfortunate that the number of patients was too small to draw conclusions concerning the effect of various amino acid composition on survival.

protein, nucleic acids, and phospholipids and accelerated growth that is apparent as early as the second day after injection [24, 25, 81, 108]. Toback has pointed out that this regrowth should increase the requirements for nutrients and that this greater demand occurs at a time when food intake is often depressed, and uremic toxicity is developing [106]. An increased need for nutrients by the injured kidney could be further accentuated by the low plasma amino acid concentrations that are present in many patients with acute renal failure [31]. Moreover, in rats with mercuric chloride-induced acute tubular necrosis, Toback et al. found that free leucine concentrations in regenerating renal cells were 17 percent below normal [107]. Protein synthesis may be reduced in cells deficient in a single amino acid, and deficiency of leucine, which has a special ability to stimulate protein synthesis, might particularly inhibit protein anabolism. Finally, Abel and coworkers found that in patients with acute renal failure who received intravenous glucose and essential amino acids as compared with glucose alone, there was a tendency for serum creatinine concentrations to decrease sooner and to lower levels [4].

Toback and coworkers carried out a series of studies on the effects of administering essential and nonessential amino acids and glucose in rats with acute tubular necrosis caused by intravenous injection of mercuric chloride [105, 107, 109]. Since cellular membranes are composed in large part of phospholipids and proteins, these investigators assessed new membrane formation in regenerating cells of renal cortical slices by the rate of incorporation of ^{14}C-choline into phospholipids. Choline is a precursor of phosphatidylcholine, which is the major phospholipid in membranes of renal cells [89]. During each of the first 4 days of acute renal failure, the rats who received intravenous infusions of essential and nonessential amino acids and glucose had higher rates of ^{14}C-choline incorporation into phospholipids than did rats receiving glucose alone.

Preincubation of cortical slices from the rats receiving amino acids without glucose also increased synthesis without changing the breakdown of phospholipids; this indicates that amino acids themselves may increase phospholipid synthesis in regenerating renal cells. The amino acids also increased the accumulation of ^{14}C-choline in renal cells and the V_{max} of the choline kinase and cholinephosphotransferase reactions, which catalyze the formation of phosphatidylcholine. Infusion of amino acids was also observed to raise the low leucine concentrations in renal cortical cells and to increase protein synthesis, as measured by incorporation of ^{14}C-leucine into protein [107]. Toback also observed that rats with mercuric chloride-induced acute tubular necrosis who received infusions of amino acids and glucose had a significantly lower serum creatinine level than those who received glucose alone or no infusion [105]. Thus, the rats with acute tubular necrosis that were given amino acids and glucose had greater rates of phospholipid and protein synthesis and decreased severity or enhanced recovery of renal function.

Oken and coworkers were unable to confirm beneficial effects of infusions of amino acids and glucose in rats with acute renal failure [82]. Rats were made acutely uremic by injection of mercuric chloride or glycerol. They were then infused with varying quantities of essential and nonessential amino acids and glucose, essential amino acids and glucose, or glucose alone. The uremic rats infused with large amounts of amino acids had very high SUN levels and much higher morbidity as compared with those given glucose alone or no infusion. The rats with glycerol-induced renal failure who received large quantities of amino acids were the only group receiving amino acids who had a significantly lower serum creatinine. However, this could have been due to the high mortality in this group; the rats that died might have had more severe renal failure and higher serum creatinine levels.

Lack of Conclusiveness in Current Reports

The authors believe that although the foregoing studies, when taken together, are suggestive, they do not demonstrate conclusively that treatment of acute renal failure with glucose and essential or essential and nonessential amino acids, as compared with glucose alone or no nutrition, will improve the rate of recovery of renal function, survival, or the nutritional status of the patient. Once the patient has entered the convalescent stage, the evidence is stronger that oral or parenteral nutrition with amino acids will improve nutritional status.

However, intuitively, it seems that nutritional therapy should benefit patients with acute renal failure, and there are probably several reasons why it has been so difficult to demonstrate a beneficial effect for intravenous nutrition. These may include the following:

1. The clinical course of patients with acute renal failure is so variable and often so complex that it may be necessary to study scores or possibly hundreds of patients in a randomized prospective study to define accurately the advantages of a specific nutritional therapy. For example, in most groups of patients with acute renal failure, some will die despite the most sophisticated medical treatment. Conversely, others will recover without special medical care. For another large segment of patients, survival may depend much more on the types of antibiotics, drainage procedures, or other medical interventions than on nutritional therapy. Thus, it might be anticipated that even if nutritional therapy is valuable, it may affect recovery of renal function or survival in only a small proportion of patients. Hence, to demonstrate its effectiveness in terms of recovery or survival, it may be necessary to study large numbers of patients. Alternatively, one may choose other outcome measurements that may vary more closely with adequacy of nutritional support (e.g., tissue amino acid concentrations, nitrogen balance, immune function, or wound healing). The limitation of the latter approach is that one must also demonstrate that improvement in such outcomes will, in fact, be associated with a more ultimate benefit, such as better rehabilitation or survival or lower hospital costs.

2. Since several studies now indicate that glucose and small quantities of amino acids will not correct the severe protein wasting incurred by many patients with acute renal failure, it may be necessary to infuse more amino acids to obtain a demonstrably better nutritional response.

3. Moreover, if the nutrient composition of the infusates is not optimal, this might adversely affect the clinical response of the patients. For example, there may be advantages to raising or lowering the proportions of certain amino acids in the parenteral solutions (see the following). Also, since the fluid load necessary to provide total parenteral nutrition may be hazardous to many acutely uremic patients, it would probably be beneficial to increase the nutrient concentrations and infuse smaller volumes.

4. It is very likely that the catabolic status of many acutely uremic patients is due to a variety of factors in addition to poor nutrition. Thus, to correct catabolism in some patients, it may be necessary to administer medicines that may alter or counteract specific catabolic or antianabolic processes (see Metabolic and Nutritional Status of the Patient with Acute Renal Failure and Newer Directions for Nutritional Therapy).

Nonetheless, it seems that patients who are very ill should fare better if they are nourished than if they are allowed to starve. The need for nutritional therapy may be particularly great for patients who are wasted, who cannot eat for extended periods, or who are in a very catabolic state. We therefore believe that until more definitive information is available, patients with acute renal failure, in general, should be administered sufficient oral or parenteral nutrition to attain the optimal nutritional status, provided the nutritional therapy does not jeopardize clinical status.

NUTRITIONAL TREATMENT FOR PATIENTS WITH ACUTE RENAL FAILURE

From the available data it is not possible to develop definitive protocols for nutritional treatment of patients with acute renal failure. The following methods are based on our analysis of the literature and personal experience.

Use of Urea Nitrogen Appearance

The quantity of nitrogen given to a patient with acute renal failure is often dictated by the patient's UNA, which is a simple, inexpensive, and accurate measure of net protein breakdown (synthesis minus degradation). The usefulness of the UNA is based on the fact that urea is the major nitrogenous product of protein and amino acid metabolism, and the UNA usually correlates highly with total nitrogen output. The UNA is calculated as follows:

UNA (gm/day) = urinary urea nitrogen (gm/day) + dialysate urea nitrogen (gm/day) + change in body urea nitrogen (gm/day) (1)

Change in body urea nitrogen (gm/day) = ($SUN_f - SUN_i$, gm/L/day) × BW_i (kg) × (0.60 L/kg) + ($BW_f - BW_i$, kg/day) × SUN_f (gm/L) × (1.0 L/kg) (2)

where i and f are the initial and final values for the period of measurement; SUN is serum urea nitrogen (grams per liter); BW is body weight (in kilograms); 0.60 is an estimate of the fraction of body weight that is body water; and 1.0 is the volume of distribution of urea in the weight gain or loss.

The estimated proportion of body weight that is water may have to be increased in patients who are edematous or lean and decreased in the obese or very young. Changes in body weight during the 1- to 3-day period of measurement of UNA are assumed to be due entirely to changes in body water. In patients undergoing hemodialysis or intermittent peritoneal dialysis, the urea concentration in dialysate is low and difficult to measure accurately, and UNA is usually calculated during the interdialytic interval. The term *urea nitrogen appearance* is used rather than *urea production* because some urea is degraded in the gastrointestinal tract. Virtually all the ammonia released from hydrolyzed urea seems to be converted back to urea [113], and this recycling will not affect the accuracy of the UNA as an indicator of net urea production or net protein breakdown. Also, it is not possible to measure the magnitude of urea recycling without isotopic studies.

In our experience, the relationship between UNA and total nitrogen output in chronically uremic patients not undergoing dialysis is as follows:

Total nitrogen output (gm/day) =
0.97 UNA (gm/day) + 1.93 (3)

If the patient is more or less in neutral nitrogen balance, the UNA also will correlate closely with nitrogen intake. Our data indicate that the relation between UNA and dietary nitrogen intake in clinically stable, nondialyzed chronically uremic patients is as follows:

Dietary nitrogen intake (gm/day) =
0.69 UNA (gm/day) + 3.3 (4)

Moreover, if both nitrogen intake and UNA are known, nitrogen balance can be estimated from the difference between nitrogen intake and nitrogen output estimated from the UNA. Pregnancy or large protein losses (e.g., nephrotic syndrome or peritoneal dialysis) can alter the relation between UNA and total nitrogen intake and output [18]. Similarly, acidosis in patients with sufficient kidney function to excrete large quantities of ammonia may change these relationships.

Sargent and Gotch have proposed an ingenious technique for assessing UNA in hemodialysis patients, which they refer to incorrectly as urea generation [94]. Their calculations are based on the SUN and body weight at the beginning of two consecutive hemodialyses and at the end of the first dialysis, the residual renal function, the dialyzer employed, the blood and dialysate flow rates, and the duration and other characteristics of the hemodialysis procedure. Although this technique is useful, it requires a somewhat complicated computer program and, in our preliminary experience, does not appear to be more accurate than the method described here.

Selection of Nitrogen Intake

In patients who have low rates of UNA (e.g., equal to or less than 4 to 5 gm per day) and who are not markedly wasted, it may be advantageous to prescribe a dietary intake or regimen of parenteral nutrition that is very low in nitrogen. This regimen usually will maintain neutral or only slightly negative nitrogen balance and will minimize the rate of accumulation of nitrogenous metabolites. Hence, dialysis therapy may be minimized or avoided. For patients with rates of UNA greater than 4 to 5 gm/day, we generally feed or infuse a greater amount of protein or amino acid nitrogen up to 1.0 to 2.0 gm/day greater than the UNA or 12 to 15 gm/day of nitrogen, whichever is less. With the lower nitrogen intakes, an additional 10 to 20 gm of amino acids may be given during each hemodialysis or peritoneal dialysis to replace amino acid and peptide losses. The larger nitrogen intakes may reduce the negative nitrogen balance of the patient. However, the UNA will almost invariably rise, and the large volume of fluid necessary to provide appropriate energy and amino acids will often increase the requirement for dialysis which may have to be carried out daily. Patients with greater residual renal function, higher fluid tolerance, and a more healthy cardiorespiratory system usually are more tolerant of the large nitrogen intakes. The more severely ill and oliguric patients may only be given 40–50 gm/day of protein or amino acids.

Enteral Therapy

In patients who are able to receive nourishment by eating, enteral tubes, or gastrostomy, these routes are generally preferable to intravenous administration; the latter is more hazardous, provides greater fluid loads, and is more costly. There are very few experimental data on enteral nutrition in patients with acute renal failure, and the treatment regimens are to a large extent based on experience derived from chronically uremic patients [56].

When the UNA is low (e.g., 4 to 5 gm/day or less), one may prescribe diets providing about 0.30 to 0.40 gm/kg/day of the nine essential amino acids (approximately 20 to 30 gm/day). An additional 0.04 to 0.14 gm/kg/day of protein of miscellaneous quality (about 3 to 10 gm/day) is contained in high-calorie, low-nitrogen foodstuffs, which provide most of the energy intake. In clinically stable, chronically uremic patients who are not receiving dialysis treatments and who have a low UNA, these diets should maintain neutral or near-neutral nitrogen balance. Where available, ketoacid or hydroxyacid analogues may be substituted for several essential amino acids. If the patient has a residual glomerular filtration rate of about 4 to 10 ml/min, it may be feasible to add more protein to these diets or even to give a diet providing 0.55 to 0.60 gm/kg/day of protein. About 20 to 24 gm/day of this protein should be of high biologic value.

If patients are clinically stable and undergo regular dialysis therapy, they should be prescribed the same protein intake that is recommended for patients undergoing maintenance dialysis [57]. Patients receiving hemodialysis should ingest about 1.0 to 1.2 gm/kg/day; those undergoing intermittent or continuous ambulatory peritoneal dialysis should receive about 1.2 to 1.3 gm/kg/day. Approximately 50 percent of this protein should be of high biologic value. The UNA can be monitored to ensure that nitrogen balance is not very negative. Hypercatabolic, severely ill patients may better tolerate 40–50 gm/day of protein or amino acids although nitrogen balance will be negative.

For patients who must be fed by an enteric tube or gastrostomy, there are many liquid protein or defined-formula (elemental) diets available. The composition and the clinical effects of these diets in nonuremic patients have been reviewed by Russell and by Young et al. [90, 118]. Experimental evidence indicates that when patients receive large quantities of amino acids (e.g., more than 30 to 40 gm/day), they should be given nonessential amino acids (see the following).

Total Parenteral Nutrition

Patients who are unable to receive enteral nutrition, who have a UNA of 4 to 5 gm/day or less, and are not very wasted are given 0.30 to 0.40 gm/kg/day of essential amino acids intravenously. With a higher UNA, both essential and nonessential amino acids are given; the amount infused is determined in the manner previously described. A typical formulation for total parenteral nutrition (TPN) in acutely uremic patients is shown in Table 18-1.

Composition of Amino Acid Preparations

Currently, most essential amino acid formulations are largely based on the recommended daily dietary intake for essential amino acids as proposed by Rose from his studies in healthy young adults [88]. Histidine is added because it is considered an essential amino acid in both normal men and chronically uremic patients [62]. Some workers have proposed adding tyrosine and arginine. Tyrosine can be derived in vivo only from phenylalanine or from catabolized peptides or proteins. Since the conversion of phenylalanine to tyrosine is impaired in uremia [52], and plasma, red cell, and muscle tyrosine is usually decreased in uremic patients [10, 32, 52, 84], several workers have suggested that tyrosine may be essential for uremic patients. Similarly, arginine is normally released by the kidney [104], and in renal failure, there may be a dietary requirement for this amino acid. However, there is as yet no convincing evidence that patients receiving low quantities of essential amino acids (e.g., 20 to 30 gm per day) benefit from the addition of either tyrosine or arginine to the diet.

Several lines of evidence suggest that the patient with renal failure might benefit from a different formulation of amino acids. First, in patients with acute or chronic renal failure, there is an abnormal pattern of plasma amino acids, and concentrations of both essential and nonessential amino acids are altered [31, 55]. In chronic renal failure, there tend to be low concentrations of plasma leucine, valine, and tyrosine and high levels of cystine, citrulline, N^{τ}-methylhistidine, and N^{π}-methylhistidine. In acute renal failure, alterations in plasma amino acid levels may be more pervasive [31]. Also, in chronically uremic patients, abnormal amino acid concentrations have been described in muscle by Bergström and coworkers [10], in blood cells by Ganda et al. [39], in leukocytes by Metcoff and associates [76], and in red cells by Flügel-Link, Jones, and Kopple [32]. Amino acid concentrations in these tissues have not been described in acute renal failure.

Furst, Alvesstrand, and Bergström fed nondialyzed chronically uremic patients low protein diets that were supplemented with a special formulation of essential amino acids and tyrosine [37]. In this preparation, the proportions of the essential amino acids were changed from the Rose formulation, so that threonine and valine were increased, tryptophan remained the same, and the other essential amino acids were reduced. Preliminary data suggest that plasma and muscle concentrations of essential amino acids became normal with this formulation. However, there are no data as to whether this preparation will improve the clinical status of patients with acute renal failure. A potential reason for increasing the content of branched-chain amino acids, particularly leucine, is that they may stimulate protein anabolism [36, 22].

Another question concerning amino acid formulation is whether nonessential amino acids should be included. When chronically uremic patients are given very low nitrogen intakes (i.e., 2.0 to 4.0 gm per day), it is unclear whether or not there is a need for nonessential amino acids. At higher nitrogen intakes, the argument for inclusion of nonessential amino acids in oral and parenteral preparations is much stronger. The evidence comes from several sources. First, in comparison with the daily dietary requirements for proteins or amino acids, the dietary need each day for essential amino acids is small. Rose recommended 12.7 gm/day as a safe intake for the eight essential amino acids, excluding histidine [88]. The difference between the dietary requirements for essential amino acid nitrogen and for total nitrogen is referred to as the need for nonspecific nitrogen. Thus, in a patient who receives 40 to 100 gm/day of amino acids, there may be no advantage to providing only those that are essential.

In addition, both animal and human studies have indicated that diets providing both essential and nonessential amino acids may be nutritionally superior to those that provide essential amino acids alone. Both the rat and the chick seem to grow better when a mixture of nonessential amino acids is the source of nonspecific nitrogen [86, 87, 101]. Moreover, normal humans who eat low-nitrogen diets may maintain more positive nitrogen balance when nonspecific nitrogen is provided as a combination of nonessential amino acids rather than as diammonium citrate, glycine, or a mixture of glycine and glutamic acid [7, 102]. Pennisi, Wang, and Kopple tube fed chronically uremic rats diets providing essential amino acids, essential and nonessential amino acids, or casein [83]. Growth was greater in the rats fed the latter two diets as compared with growth in rats fed only essential amino acids, even when comparisons were between isonitrogenous diets.

Nonessential amino acids are just as necessary for protein synthesis as essential amino acids, and a deficiency of a nonessential amino acid inside the cell could disrupt protein synthesis [112]. The metabolic costs of synthesizing the nonessential amino acids are not known. Also, since many amino acids share common transport mechanisms and compete for intracellular transport, a selective infusion of essential amino acids that might lead to high extracellular concentrations of some amino acids might impair intracellular movement of others. Conversely, a low extracellular concentration of an amino acid could lead to decreased intracellular movement of that amino acid and accelerated cellular transport of others.

Motil, Harmon, and Grupe's report on two children with acute renal failure is pertinent in this regard [80]. The children, who were very ill, had been infused with a relatively large per kilogram dose of eight essential amino acids without histidine. Analysis of their plasma indicated very low concentrations of histidine and the urea cycle amino acids ornithine, citrulline, and arginine. Plasma methionine and blood ammonia were increased, and a metabolic acidosis developed in the patients. When the children received an infusion of essential and nonessential amino acids, the amino acid pattern was more normal. We have also observed a striking elevation of plasma lysine, methionine, phenylalanine, and threonine in an older man with acute renal failure who received intravenously about 75 gm/day of eight essential amino acids without histidine. Concurrently with the infusion of these large quantities of essential amino acids, the patient became comatose and ultimately died. This patient had underlying illnesses that could account for his deterioration. Nonetheless, these findings suggest that large doses of only essential amino acids can disrupt amino acid metabolism and possibly cause clinical deterioration.

The foregoing considerations suggest that patients with acute renal failure who receive larger amounts of amino acids should be given histidine and a number of nonessential amino acids, which should probably include arginine, tyrosine, alanine, glycine, proline, and serine. The appropriate ratio of essential to nonessential amino acids is not known; in standard intravenous solutions, it is about 1:1, with histidine considered essential and arginine considered nonessential. For uremic patients, a more effective formulation might be 2:1 or 4:1 with a higher proportion of the essentials provided as branched-chain amino acids. In addition, supplementation with ketoacid or hydroxyacid salts of certain essential amino acids may be beneficial. These compounds can be converted to their respective essential amino acids by combining with amino groups. Thus, they may divert amino group metabolism away from urea formation. Ketoacids or hydroxyacids that are not converted to amino acids are primarily metabolized to carbohydrate or fat, or to carbon dioxide and water with liberation of energy. Further studies are needed to examine the potential value of such supplements.

When administering mixtures of essential and nonessential amino acids, it is probably preferable to use solutions of free L-amino acids rather than protein hydrolysates, because there may be compounds in the latter solutions that may not be well utilized and may accumulate in renal failure [53]. Also, a recent study has indicated that the latter preparation may contain hazardous concentrations of aluminum [54].

Energy, Vitamins, and Minerals

Since patients with acute renal failure are usually in negative nitrogen balance, large quantities of calories are probably indicated to reduce net protein breakdown. There is no easy way to estimate the energy expenditure or requirement in these patients, and we empirically administer 35 to 50 kcal/kg/day. If nitrogen balance, as determined by the difference between observed nitrogen intake and nitrogen output calculated from the UNA (see above), is negative, we try to provide an energy intake closer to 50 kcal/kg/day. Many researchers believe that there is little advantage to administering more than 4000 to 5000 kcal/day to patients in a catabolic state. In fact, in patients with higher energy intakes, the large quantity of carbon dioxide produced from the infused carbohydrate and fat can cause hypercapnia if pulmonary function is impaired [8].

Since most acutely uremic patients do not tolerate large water intakes, glucose is generally provided in a 70% solution; this preparation is usually mixed with equal volumes of an amino acid solution (Table 18-1). Patients receiving TPN for more than five to seven days should receive an infusion of 250 to 500 gm of lipid emulsions twice weekly to prevent essential fatty acid deficiency. Currently, both 10% and 20% lipid emulsions are available; they are essentially isotonic and provide 1.1 and 2.0 kcal/ml, respectively. In contrast, 70% dextrose D-glucose monohydrate) yields about 2.38 kcal/ml and is the parenteral solution that gives the greatest calories per milliliter. In catabolic states, glucose has been reported to promote a more positive nitrogen balance than do isocaloric quantities of lipids [68, 78]. Thus, in catabolic, acutely uremic patients, glucose has been used as the major source of calories, and lipids are used primarily to prevent essential fatty acid deficiency. However, recent studies suggest that lipids may be at least as effective as glucose in promoting net anabolism.

The vitamins and minerals employed with TPN are shown in Table 18-1. Vitamin requirements have not been well defined for patients with acute renal failure, and much of the recommended intake is based on information obtained from studies in chronically uremic patients or normal persons. Vitamin A is probably best avoided, because serum vitamin A levels are elevated in chronic renal failure. Even small doses of vitamin A have been reported to cause toxicity in chronically uremic patients [30]. Also, since most patients with acute renal failure receive TPN for only a few days to weeks, it is unlikely that deficiency of this fat-soluble vitamin will occur.

Although vitamin D is fat-soluable and vitamin D stores should not become depleted during a few days to weeks of TPN, the turnover of its most active form, 1,25-dihydroxycholecalciferol, is much faster. However, the requirement for this vitamin D analogue in acute renal failure has not yet been determined. Furthermore, at the present time, a parenteral preparation of 1,25-dihydroxycholecalciferol is not commercially available. Although vitamin K is a fat-soluble vitamin, deficiencies have been reported in postoperative nonuremic patients who were not eating and were receiving antibiotics [110]. Vitamin K supplements are therefore given routinely to patients receiving TPN. Pyridoxine hydrochloride, 10 mg per day, is recommended, because studies in patients undergoing maintenance hemodialysis indicate that this amount may be necessary to prevent or correct vitamin B_6 deficiency [61].

The recommended concentrations for minerals in TPN solutions (Table 18-1) must be tentative. If the serum concentration of an electrolyte is increased, it may be advisable to reduce the concentration or not to administer it at the onset of TPN. The patient must be monitored carefully, however, because hormonal and metabolic changes that often occur with initiation of TPN may cause serum electrolytes to fall rapidly; this is particularly likely for serum potassium and phosphorus. Conversely, a mineral deficit may indicate a need for greater-than-usual intake of that element. Again, metabolic changes can lead to a rapid rise in serum levels.

It must be emphasized that the nutrient content of the TPN solutions for acutely uremic patients must be carefully reevaluated each day and sometimes more frequently. This is particularly important because these patients may undergo rapid changes in their metabolic and clinical status. The actual techniques for TPN, complications of TPN, and methods for assessing nutritional and clinical status of patients receiving TPN have been described previously [58].

Peripheral and Supplemental Parenteral Nutrition

Peripheral parenteral nutrition has been advocated as an alternative to TPN. The solutions are infused into a peripheral vein, and the risks and expenses of inserting a central catheter are avoided. A limitation of peripheral parenteral nutrition is that osmolality of the infusate must be restricted to about 600 mOsm to prevent thrombophlebitis, and, even then, the needles or catheters must be changed frequently, usually every 18 to 48 hours. Isaacs et al. reported that the addition of heparin, 500 units/liter, and cortisol, 5 mg/liter, allowed solutions of 900 mOsm to be infused into a peripheral vein for an average of 114 hours before local inflammation required changing the infusion site [51]. In contrast to these infusates, a typical solution for TPN via a central vein has a tonicity of about 1800 mOsm. Thus, with peripheral parenteral nutrition, fewer nutrients can be infused per liter, and it has little or no role in the treatment of the hypercatabolic state, the wasted patient who needs added nutrients for repletion, the patient with oliguria or fluid intolerance, and the patient who will need parenteral nutrition for extended periods.

For patients with acute renal failure who are able to ingest some nutrients or tolerate some tube feedings, peripheral infusions may enable them to receive adequate nutrition without resorting to TPN. In such patients, it is often most practical to infuse 8.5 to 10% amino acids or 20% lipid emulsions into a peripheral vein and to administer as much as possible of other essential nutrients, including carbohydrates, through the enteral tract.

Peripheral vascular accesses that are used for hemodialysis can also be used for TPN [98, 120]. However, this technique probably increases the hazard of infection, and it should not be used in patients who will need a hemodialysis access for extended periods.

In patients who have marginally adequate intakes, supplemental amino acids and glucose may be given during hemodialysis treatment. Some nephrologists infuse 20 or 30 gm of the nine essential amino acids at the end of dialysis therapy [46]. However, since most patients who need nutritional supplements have decreased intake of energy and total nitrogen, we give 40 to 42 gm of essential and nonessential amino acids and 200 gm of D-glucose (150 gm of D-glucose if the dialysate contains glucose). This preparation is infused into the blood leaving the dialyzer at a constant rate throughout the dialysis procedure to minimize disruption of amino acid and glucose pools that occur with hemodialysis [116]. Patients who have low serum concentrations of phosphorus or potassium at the start of the dialysis treatment may need supplements of these minerals. With such infusions, plasma amino acids and glucose do not fall during dialysis, and over 85 percent of the infused amino acids is retained [116]. If the dialysate is glucose-free, the infusion is not stopped until the end of hemodialysis to prevent reactive hypoglycemia. Also, the patient should eat some carbohydrate 20 to 30 minutes before the end of the infusion. Otherwise, the infusion must be tapered, or a peripheral infusion of glucose must be started.

Newer Directions for Nutritional Therapy

Several pharmacologic techniques may have a role in facilitating anabolic processes or reducing catabolic rates in patients with renal failure. Preliminary results with each of these techniques in sick patients or experimental animals have been promising, although further studies are necessary to determine their potential role in patients with acute renal failure. These techniques involve the use of insulin, anabolic steroids, protease inhibitors, and adenine nucleotides.

Since insulin is the most potent known anabolic hormone, it is natural to question whether this compound could reduce protein wasting in sick patients. Two studies have now indicated that in nonuremic patients who have catabolic illnesses, insulin can reduce nitrogen output and negative nitrogen balance [47, 117]. Hence, there may be value in administering insulin routinely to acute renal failure patients with catabolic illness.

Anabolic steroids can also promote anabolism and have been used to treat acute or chronic renal failure patients with catabolic illness [34, 42, 44, 73, 115]. These compounds can decrease UNA and the rise in SUN, enhance positive nitrogen and potassium balance, retard the development of acidosis, and delay the need for dialysis therapy [34, 42, 73, 91]. In recent years, the use of anabolic steroids for treatment of renal failure patients with catabolic illness has been largely neglected because its effects last only several days to weeks, and dialysis therapy is readily available. However, dialysis treatment does not reduce catabolism and is often hazardous in severely ill patients. Since the period of critical illness in patients with acute renal failure is often only a few days to weeks, anabolic steroids might still be beneficial, even if they reduce net catabolism and UNA only transiently.

Anabolic steroids are not always effective, particularly in severe catabolic stress, and they can have masculinizing effects in women and children. These compounds may be ineffective unless the patient also receives nourishment. Many anabolic steroids can cause cholestatic jaundice, although this is not observed with testosterone or its esters (enanthate or propionate). Commonly used anabolic steroids include testosterone enanthate, testosterone proprionate, methandrostenolone, nandrolone decanoate, norandrolone phenproprionate, and norethandrolone.

Two therapeutic procedures that show exciting promise but have not yet been employed in patients are the use of protease inhibitors and adenine nucleotides. Hörl and Heidland described increased protease activity in ultrafiltrates of plasma from patients with acute renal failure with catabolic illness [48]. The protease inhibitor, alpha$_2$-macroglobulin, was undetectable in plasma from some of these patients. Addition of alpha$_2$-macroglobulin, in vitro, to plasma ultrafiltrates inhibited the proteolytic activity [49]. These findings suggest that in patients with acute renal failure who are under catabolic stress, enhanced activity of proteases in plasma and possibly other tissues may be a cause of accelerated protein wasting. If this is confirmed, such patients may eventually be treated with specific inhibitors of these proteases.

Siegel and coworkers studied the effects of infusion of magnesium chloride with either adenosine triphosphate, or diphosphate, or monophosphate into rats with acute renal failure secondary to ischemia [99]. The rats that received one of these adenine nucleotides with magnesium chloride had less impaired inulin clearance, renal blood flow, and osmolar clearance, a low fractional excretion of sodium, and less histologic evidence of renal injury as compared with rats

Table 18-1. *Typical Composition of TPN Infusate for Adults with Acute or Chronic Renal Failure*[a–c]

Volume	liters	1.0
Dextrose (D-glucose)	gm/L	350
Essential and nonessential free crystalline amino acids	gm/L	42.5–50
Energy (approx.)[d]	kcal/L	1339–1365
Electrolytes[e]		
Sodium[f]	mEq/L	50
Chloride[f]	mEq/L	25–35
Potassium	mEq/day	40
Acetate	mEq/L	35–40
Calcium	mEq/day	10
Phosphorus	mEq/day	20
Magnesium	mEq/day	8
Iron	mg/day	2
Vitamins		
Vitamin A[g]	USP units/day	
Vitamin K[h]	mg/week	4
Vitamin D[i]	USP units/day	See text
Vitamin E[j]	IU/day	10
Niacin	mg/day	20
Thiamin HCl (B_1)	mg/day	2
Riboflavin (B_2)	mg/day	2
Pantothenic acid	mg/day	10
Pyridoxine HCl (B_6)	mg/day	10
Ascorbic acid (C)	mg/day	100
Biotin	mg/day	200
Folic acid[h]	mg/day	1
Vitamin B_{12}[h]	μg/day	4

[a]For patients undergoing frequent hemodialysis or peritoneal dialysis, 1.5 to 2.0 L of the solution are administered each day; patients should receive 64 to 100 gm amino acids, and 70% dextrose is added as necessary to ensure that energy intake is at least 30–35 kcal/kg/day. Greater quantities of energy are often of value, but the fluid load may increase the need for dialysis. During dialysis treatment, amino acid and glucose losses can be replaced by increasing infusions (see text). For patients with chronic uremia (GFR < 10 ml/min) or acute renal failure who are not undergoing dialysis, 1 L of this solution is mixed with 400–600 ml of 70% dextrose in water to increase energy intake to about 2300–2800 kcal/day. Hypercatabolic uremic patients may need greater quantities of energy and amino acids. Infusion of 500 ml of lipid emulsion twice weekly can be used in place of some glucose and is particularly indicated in long-term TPN to prevent essential fatty acid deficiency.
[b]These nutrients are included in each bottle containing 500 ml of 8.5–10% crystalline amino acids and 500 ml of 70% dextrose. Exceptions are the vitamins and trace elements, which should be added to only one bottle per day.
[c]Composition and volume of infusate may have to be changed if patients are very uremic, acidotic, or volume overloaded; if serum electrolyte concentrations are not normal or relatively constant; or if dialysis therapy is not readily available.
[d]Approximate caloric value of dextrose monohydrate is 3.4 kcal/gm; amino acids, 3.5 kcal/gm.
[e]When adding electrolytes, the amounts intrinsically present in the amino acid solution should be taken into account.
[f]Refers to final concentration of electrolytes after any extra 70% dextrose has been added.
[g]Vitamin A is best avoided unless TPN is continued for more than several weeks.
[h]Should be given orally or parenterally and not in solution because of antagonisms.
[i]Currently, 1,25-dihydroxycholecalciferol is not commercially available for parenteral administration.
[j]May have to be increased with use of lipid emulsions.
Source: Adapted from J. D. Kopple. Nutrition and the Kidney. In R. E. Hodges, *Human Nutrition: A Comprehensive Treatise*. New York: Plenum, 1979. Vol. 4, pp. 409–457.

that either received no infusion or received adenosine triphosphate, magnesium chloride, or adenosine alone. Although the mechanism for these effects is unknown, it is tempting to speculate that adenine nucleotides and magnesium chloride may act by altering glomerulotubular or vascular dynamics or by improving energy metabolism in the injured and regenerating cells.

Nutritional Treatment for Patients with Chronic Renal Failure

Total parenteral nutrition regimens for patients with chronic renal failure are essentially similar to those for patients with acute renal failure. The major difference is that patients who are already undergoing regular dialysis therapy have greater nitrogen requirements because of the amino acid and protein losses during peritoneal dialysis. Hence, unless the frequency of dialysis treatments is reduced in these patients, they generally should not receive infusions containing small quantities of the essential amino acid preparations.

In general, patients undergoing maintenance hemodialysis three times per week should receive 1.0 to 1.2 gm/kg/day of essential and nonessential amino acids. Those undergoing regular intermittent peritoneal dialysis (10 hours/day, 4 days/week) or continuous ambulatory peritoneal dialysis should receive 1.2 to 1.3 gm/kg/day of these amino acids. With catabolic stress, the amino acid intake may be increased, as discussed for patients with acute renal failure, depending on the patient's fluid tolerance and the ease with which the patient can undergo frequent dialysis (e.g., four to five times per week). The considerations concerning the optimal formulation of the essential and nonessential amino acids are the same as for the patient with acute renal failure.

When administering parenteral nutrition to uremic patients, it is important to restrict fluid intake because of the oliguria. Therefore, 70% glucose solutions are generally used. When the solution is mixed with equal volumes of amino acids, one will attain a final glucose concentration of 35 gm/100 ml. A typical regimen for electrolyte and vitamin administration during TPN is shown in Table 18-1. Management of carbohydrate, fat, mineral, and vitamin intake is similar to that discussed for patients with acute renal failure.

Insulin resistance and glucose intolerance, which occur both in uremia and with catabolic illness, may lead to hyperglycemia, particularly because there is a high glucose intake with TPN. It is often necessary to add insulin to the infusate. The decreased plasma clearance of triglycerides in uremia may lead to hypertriglyceridemia, and uremic patients must be monitored closely when they receive fat emulsions. The techniques, complications, and methods for monitoring patients with TPN have been previously reviewed [58].

Although routine supplementation with intravenous or oral essential amino acids has been recommended for maintenance hemodialysis patients, recent reports indicate that supplemental essential amino acids or ketoacids are of little nutritional benefit when such patients eat a nutritious diet providing 1.0 to 1.2 gm of protein/kg/day. Patients undergoing maintenance hemodialysis who eat poorly may be given supplemental amino acids and glucose intravenously during hemodialysis treatment. The techniques for infusing amino acids and glucose during hemodialysis are the same as those described for patients with acute renal failure (see above).

REFERENCES

1. Abbot, W. M., Abel, R. M., and Fischer, J. E. Treatment of acute renal insufficiency after aortoiliac surgery. *Arch. Surg.* 103:590, 1971.
2. Abel, R. M., Abbott, W. M., Beck, C. H., Jr., Ryan, J. A., Jr., Fischer, J. E. Essential L-amino acids for hyperalimentation in patients with disordered nitrogen metabolism. *Am. J. Surg.* 128: 317, 1974.
3. Abel, R. M., Abbott, W. M., and Fischer, J. E. Intravenous essential L-amino acids and hypertonic dextrose in patients with acute renal failure. *Am. J. Surg.* 123:631, 1972.

4. Abel, R. M., Beck, C. H., Jr., Abbott, W. M., Ryan, J. A., Jr., Barnett, G. O., and Fischer, J. E. Improved survival and acute renal failure after treatment with intravenous essential L-amino acids and glucose. *N. Engl. J. Med.* 288:695, 1973.
5. Abel, R. M., Shih, V. E., Abbott, W. M., Beck, C. H., Jr., and Fischer, J. E. Amino acid metabolism in acute renal failure. *Ann. Surg.* 180:350, 1974.
6. Abitbol, C. L., and Holliday, M. A. Total parenteral nutrition in anuric children. *Clin. Nephrol.* 3:153, 1976.
7. Anderson, H. L., and Heindel, M. B. Effect on nitrogen balance of adult man of varying source of nitrogen and level of calorie intake. *J. Nutr.* 99:82, 1969.
8. Askanazi, J., Elwyn, D. H., Silverberg, B. S., Rosenbaum, S. H., and Kinney, J. M. Respiratory distress secondary to a high carbohydrate load: A case report. *Surgery* 87:596, 1980.
9. Baek, S. M., Makabali, G. G., Bryan-Brown, C. W., Kusek, J., and Shoemaker, W. The influence of parenteral nutrition on the course of acute renal failure. *Surg. Gynecol. Obstet.* 141:405, 1975.
10. Bergström, J., Fürst, P., Norrée, L.-O., and Vinnars, E. Intracellular free amino acids in muscle tissue of patients with chronic uremia: Effect of peritoneal dialysis and infusion of essential amino acids. *Clin. Sci. Mol. Med.* 54:51, 1978.
11. Bergström, J., and Hultman, E. Glycogen content of skeletal muscle in patients with renal failure. *Acta Med. Scand.* 186:177, 1969.
12. Berlyne, G. M., Bazzard, F. J., Booth, E. M., Janabi, K., and Shaw, A. B. The dietary treatment of acute renal failure. *Q. J. Med.* 141:59, 1967.
13. Berlyne, G. M., Lee, H. A., Giordano, C., DePascale, C., and Esposito, R. Amino acid loss in peritoneal dialysis. *Lancet* 1:1339, 1967.
14. Bilbrey, G. L., Faloona, G. R., White, M. G., Knochel, J. P., and Borroto, J. Hyperglucagonemia of renal failure. *J. Clin. Invest.* 53:841, 1974.
15. Blackburn, G. L., Etter, G., and MacKenzie, T. Criteria for choosing amino acid therapy in acute renal failure. *Am. J. Clin. Nutr.* 31:1841, 1978.
16. Blagg, C. R., Parsons, F. M., and Young, B. A. Effects of dietary glucose and protein in acute renal failure. *Lancet* 1:608, 1962.
17. Blumenkrantz, M. J., Gahl, G. M., Kopple, J. D., Anjana, V. K., Jones, M. R., Kessel, M., and Coburn, J. W. Protein loss during peritoneal dialysis. *Kidney Int.* 19:593, 1981.
18. Blumenkrantz, M. J., Kopple, J. D., Moran, J. K., Grodstein, G. P., and Coburn, J. W. Nitrogen and urea metabolism during continuous ambulatory peritoneal dialysis. *Kidney Int.* 20:78, 1981.
19. Borst, J. G. G. Protein catabolism in uremia. Effects of protein-free diet, infections, and blood-transfusions. *Lancet* 1:824, 1948.
20. Bozzetti, F., Terno, G., and Longoni, C. Parenteral hyperalimentation and wound healing. *Surg. Gynecol. Obstet.* 141:712, 1975.
21. Bull, G. M., Joekes, A. M., and Lowe, K. G. Conservative treatment of anuric uremia. *Lancet* 2:229, 1949.
22. Buse, M. G., and Reid, S. S. Leucine. A possible regulator of protein turnover in muscle *J. Clin. Invest.* 56:1250, 1975.
23. Cahill, G. F. Starvation in man. *N. Engl. J. Med.* 282:668, 1970.
24. Cuppage, F. E., Chiga, M., and Tate, A. Cell cycle studies in the regenerating rat nephron following injury with mercuric chloride. *Lab. Invest.* 26:122, 1972.
25. Cuppage, F. E., Cunningham, N., and Tate, A. Nucleic acid synthesis in the regenerating nephron following injury with mercuric chloride. *Lab. Invest.* 21:449, 1969.
26. DeFronzo, R. A. Pathogenesis of glucose intolerance in uremia. *Metabolism* 27:1866, 1978.
27. DeFronzo, R. A., Tobin, J. D., Rowe, J. W., and Andres, R. Glucose intolerance in uremia. Quantification of pancreatic beta cell sensitivity to glucose and tissue sensitivity to insulin. *J. Clin. Invest.* 62:425, 1978.
28. Dudrick, S. J., Steiger, E., and Long, J. M. Renal failure in surgical patients—treatment with intravenous essential amino acids and hypertonic glucose. *Surgery* 68:180, 1970.
29. Eigler, N., Saccà, L., and Sherwin, R. S. Synergistic interactions of physiologic increments of glucagon, epinephrine and cortisol in the dog. A model for stress-induced hyperglycemia. *J. Clin. Invest.* 63:114, 1979.
30. Farrington, K., Miller, P., Varghesez, Baillod, R. A., and Moorehead, J. F. Vitamin A toxicity and hypercalcaemia in chronic renal failure. *Br. Med. J.* 282:1999, 1981.
31. Feinstein, E. I., Blumenkrantz, M. J., Healy, H., Koffler, A., Silberman, H., Massry, S. G., and Kopple, J. D. Clinical and metabolic responses to parenteral nutrition in acute renal failure. A controlled double-blind study. *Medicine* (Baltimore) 60:124, 1981.
32. Flügel-Link, R. M., Jones, M. R., and Kopple, J. D. Red cell and plasma amino acid concentrations in renal failure (submitted).

33. Flügel-Link, R. M., Salusky, I. B., Jones, M. R., and Kopple, J. D. Enhanced muscle protein degradation and urea nitrogen appearance (UNA) in rats with acute renal failure (abstract). *Kidney Int.*, in press.
34. Freedman, P., and Spencer, A. G. Testosterone propionate in the treatment of renal failure. *Clin. Sci.* 16:11, 1957.
35. Fröhlich, J., Schölmerich, J., Hoppe-Seyler, G., Maier, K. P., Talke, H., Schollmeyer, P., and Gerok, W. The effect of acute uremia on gluconeogenesis in isolated perfused rat livers. *Eur. J. Clin. Invest.* 4:453, 1974.
36. Fulks, R. M., Li, J. B., and Goldberg, A. Effects of insulin, glucose, and amino acids on protein turnover in rat diaphragm. *J. Biol. Chem.* 250: 290, 1975.
37. Fürst, P., Alvesstrand, A., and Bergström, J. Effects of nutrition and catabolic stress on intracellular amino acid pools in uremia. *Am. J. Clin. Nutr.* 33:1387, 1980.
38. Gamble, J. L. Physiological information from studies on the life-raft ration. *Harvey Lect.* 42: 247, 1946–1947.
39. Ganda, O. P., Aoki, T. T., Soeldner, J. S., Morrison, R. S., and Cahill, G. F., Jr. Hormone-fuel concentrations in anephric subjects. Effect of hemodialysis with special reference to amino acids. *J. Clin. Invest.* 57:1403, 1976.
40. Giordano, C., DePascale, C., DeCristofaro, D., Capodicasa, G., Balestrieri, C., and Baczyk, K. Protein Malnutrition in the Treatment of Chronic Uremia. In G. M. Berlyne (Ed.), *Nutrition in Renal Disease.* Baltimore: Williams & Wilkins, 1968. Pp. 23–34.
41. Giordano, C., De Santo, N. G., Capodicasa, G., Di Leo, V. A., Di Serafino, A., Cirrillo, D., Esposito, R., Fiore, R., Damiano, M., Buonadonna, L., Cocco, F., and Di Iorio, B. Amino acid losses during CAPD. *Clin. Nephrol.* 14:230, 1980.
42. Gjorup, S., and Thaysen, J. H. The effect of anabolic steroid (Durabolin[R]) in the conservative management of acute renal failure. *Acta Med. Scand.* 167:227, 1960.
43. Grodstein, G. P., Blumenkrantz, M. J., Kopple, J. D., Moran, J. K., and Coburn, J. W. Glucose absorption during continuous ambulatory peritoneal dialysis. *Kidney Int.* 19:564, 1981.
44. Hampl, R., and Stárka, L. Practical aspects of screening of anabolic steroids in doping control with particular accent to nortestosterone radioimmunoassay using mixed antisera. *J. Steroid Biochem.* 11:933, 1979.
45. Hasik, J., Hryniewiecki, L., Baczyk, K., and Grala, T. An attempt to evaluate minimum requirements for protein in patients with acute renal failure. *Pol. Arch. Med. Wewn* 61:29, 1979.
46. Heidland, A., Kult, J. Long-term effects of essential amino acids supplementation in patients on regular dialysis treatment. *Clin. Nephrol.* 3:234, 1975.
47. Hinton, P., Allison, S. P., Littlejohn, S., and Lloyd, J. Insulin and glucose to reduce catabolic response to injury in burned patients. *Lancet* 1:767, 1971.
48. Hörl, W. H., and Heidland, A. Enhanced proteolytic activity—cause of protein catabolism in acute renal failure. *Am. J. Clin. Nutr.* 33:1423, 1980.
49. Hörl, W. H., Gantert, C., Auer, I. O., and Heidland, A. In vitro inhibition of protein catabolism by alpha-macroglobulin in plasma from a patient with post-traumatic acute renal failure. *Am. J. Nephrol.*, in press.
50. Hörl, W. H., and Heidland, A. Glycogen metabolism in muscle in uremia. *Am. J. Clin. Nutr.* 33: 1461, 1980.
51. Isaacs, J. W., Millikan, W. J., Stackhouse, J., Hersh, T., and Rudman, D. Parenteral nutrition of adults with a 900 milliosmolar solution via peripheral veins. *Am. J. Clin. Nutr.* 30:552, 1977.
52. Jones, M. R., Kopple, J. D., and Swendseid, M. E. Phenylalanine metabolism in uremic and normal man. *Kidney Int.* 14:169, 1978.
53. Jonxis, J. H. P., and Huisman, T. H. J. Excretion of amino acids in free and bound form during intravenous administration of protein hydrolysate. *Metabolism* 6:175, 1957.
54. Klein, G. L., Alfrey, A. C., Miller, N. L., Sherrard, J., Hazlet, T. K., Ament, M. E., and Coburn, J. W. Aluminum loading during total parenteral nutrition. *Am. J. Clin. Nutr.*, in press.
55. Kopple, J. D. Nitrogen Metabolism. In S. G. Massry and A. L. Sellers, (Eds.), *Clinical Aspects of Uremia and Dialysis.* Springfield, Ill.: Charles C Thomas, 1976. Pp. 241–273.
56. Kopple, J. D. Treatment with Low Protein and Amino Acid Diets in Chronic Renal Failure. In R. Borcelo, M. Bergeron, S. Carriere, J. H. Dirks, K. Drummond, R. D. Guttman, G. Lemieux, J. G. Mongeau, and J. F. Seely (Eds.), *Proceedings VIIIth International Congress of Nephrology.* Basel: S. Karger, 1978. Pp. 497–507.
57. Kopple, J. D. Nutritional therapy in kidney failure. *Nutr. Rev.* 39:193, 1981.
58. Kopple, J. D., and Blumenkrantz, M. J. Total Parenteral Nutrition and Parenteral Fluid Therapy. In M. H. Maxwell and C. R. Kleeman (Eds.), *Clinical Disorders of Fluid and Electrolyte Me-*

tabolism. New York: McGraw-Hill, 1980. Pp. 413–498.
59. Kopple, J. D., Blumenkrantz, M. J., Jones, M. R., Moran, J. K., and Coburn, J. W. Amino acid losses during continuous ambulatory peritoneal dialysis (CAPD). *Kidney Int.* 19:152A, 1981.
60. Kopple, J. D., Cianciaruso, B., and Massry, S. G. Does parathyroid hormone cause protein wasting? *Contrib. Nephrol.* 20:138, 1980.
61. Kopple, J. D., Mercurio, K., Blumenkrantz, M. J., Jones, M. R., Tallos, J., Roberts, C., Card, B., Saltzman, R., Casciato, D. A., and Swendseid, M. E. Daily requirement of pyridoxine supplements in chronic renal failure. *Kidney Int.* 19:694, 1981.
62. Kopple, J. D., and Swendseid, M. E. Evidence that histidine is an essential amino acid in normal and chronically uremic man. *J. Clin. Invest.* 55: 881, 1975.
63. Kopple, J. D., Swendseid, M. E., Shinaberger, J. H., and Umezawa, C. Y. The free and bound amino acids removed by hemodialysis. *Trans. Am. Soc. Artif. Intern. Organs* 14:309, 1973.
64. Lacy, W. W. Effect of acute uremia on amino acid uptake and urea production by perfused rat liver. *Am. J. Physiol.* 216:1300, 1969.
65. Law, D. K., Dudrick, S. J., and Abdou, N. I. Immunocompetence of patients with protein-calorie malnutrition. The effects of nutritional repletion. *Ann. Intern. Med.* 79:545, 1973.
66. Lee, H. A., Sharpstone, P., and Ames, A. C. Parenteral nutrition in renal failure. *Postgrad. Med. J.* 43:81, 1967.
67. Leonard, C. D., Luke, R. G., and Siegel, R. R. Parenteral essential amino acids in acute renal failure. *Urology* 6:154, 1975.
68. Long, J. M., Wilmore, D. W., Mason, A. D., Jr., and Pruitt, B. A. Fat-carbohydrate interaction: Effects on nitrogen-sparing in total intravenous feeding. *Surg. Forum* 25:61, 1974.
69. Lopez-Martinez, J., Caparros, T., Perez-Picouto, F., Lopez-Diez, F., and Cereijo, E. Nutritión parenteral en enfermos sépticos con fracaso renal agudo en fase poliúrica. *Rev. Clin. Esp.* 157:171, 1980.
70. Lundholm, K., Bylund, A.-C., Holm, J., and Schersten, T. Skeletal muscle metabolism in patients with malignant tumor. *Eur. J. Cancer* 12:465, 1976.
71. Massry, S. G., Arieff, A. I., Coburn, J. W., Palmieri, G., and Kleeman, C. R. Divalent ion metabolism in patients with acute renal failure: Studies on the mechanism of hypocalcemia. *Kidney Int.* 5:437, 1974.
72. McCormick, G. J., Shear, L., and Barry, K. G. Alteration of hepatic protein synthesis in acute uremia. *Proc. Soc. Exp. Biol. Med.* 122:99, 1966.
73. McCracken, B. H., and Parsons, F. M. Nilevar (17-ethyl-19-nor-testosterone) to suppress protein catabolism in acute renal failure. *Lancet* 2: 885, 1958.
74. McGale, E. H. F., Pickford, J. C., and Aber, G. M. Quantitative changes in plasma amino acids in patients with renal disease. *Clin. Chim. Acta* 38:395, 1972.
75. McMurray, S. D., Luft, F. C., Maxwell, D. R., Hamburger, R. J., Futty, D., Szwed, J., Lavelle, K. J., and Kleit, S. A. Prevailing patterns and predictor variables in patients with acute tubular necrosis. *Arch. Intern. Med.* 138:950, 1978.
76. Metcoff, J., Lindeman, R., Baxter, D., and Pederson, J. Cell metabolism in uremia. *Am. J. Clin. Nutr.* 30:1627, 1978.
77. Milligan, S. L., Luft, F. C., McMurray, S. D., and Kleit, S. A. Intra-abdominal infection and acute renal failure. *Arch. Surg.* 113:467, 1978.
78. Milne, C. A., MacLean, L. D., and Shizgal, H. M. Casein hydrolysate and intralipid vs casein hydrolysate and 25% glucose for hyperalimentation. *Surg. Forum* 25:52, 1974.
79. Mondon, C. E., and Reaven, G. M. Evaluation of enhanced glucagon sensitivity as the cause of glucose intolerance in acutely uremic rats. *Am. J. Clin. Nutr.* 33:1456, 1980.
80. Motil, K. J., Harmon, W. E., and Grupe, W. E. Complications of essential amino acid hyperalimentation in children with acute renal failure. *J.P.E.N.* 4:32, 1980.
81. Nicholls, D. M., and Ng, K. Regeneration of renal proximal tubules after mercuric chloride injury is accompanied by increased binding of aminoacyl-transfer ribonucleic acid. *Biochem. J.* 160:357, 1976.
82. Oken, D. E., Sprinkel, F. M., Kirschbaum, B. B., and Landwehr, D. M. Amino acid therapy in the treatment of experimental acute renal failure in the rat. *Kidney Int.* 17:14, 1980.
83. Pennisi, A. J., Wang, M., and Kopple, J. D. Effects of protein and amino acid diets in chronically uremic and control rats. *Kidney Int.* 13:472, 1978.
84. Pickford, J. C., McGale, E. H. F., and Aber, G. M. Studies on the metabolism of phenylalanine and tyrosine in patients with renal disease. *Clin. Chim. Acta* 48:77, 1973.
85. Pietrek, J., Kokot, F., and Kuska, J. Serum 25-hydroxyvitamin D and parathyroid hormone in patients with acute renal failure. *Kidney Int.* 13: 178, 1978.

86. Ranhotra, G. S., and Johnson, B. C. Effect of feeding different amino acid diets on growth rate and nitrogen retention of weanling rats. *Proc. Soc. Exp. Biol. Med.* 118:1197, 1965.
87. Rogers, Q. R., Chen, D. M., and Harper, A. E. The importance of dispensable amino acids for maximal growth in the rat. *Proc. Soc. Exp. Biol. Med.* 134:517, 1970.
88. Rose, W. C. The amino acid requirements of adult man. *Nutr. Abstr. Rev.* 27:631, 1957.
89. Rouser, G., Simon, G., and Kritchevsky, G. Species variations in phospholipid class distribution of organs: Kidney, liver and spleen. *Lipids* 4:599, 1969.
90. Russell, R. I. Progress report: Elemental diets. *Gut* 16:68, 1975.
91. Saarne, A., Bjerstaf, L., and Ekman, G. Studies on the nitrogen balance in the human during long-term treatment with different anabolic agents under strictly standardized conditions. *Acta Med. Scand.* 177:199, 1965.
92. Sapico, V. Enzyme alterations and subcellular translocation of inducible tyrosine aminotransferase in acute uremia. *Fed. Proc.* 32:506A, 1973.
93. Sapico, V., Shear, L., and Litwack, G. Translocation of inducible tyrosine aminotransferase to the mitochondrial fraction. *J. Biol. Chem.* 249: 2122, 1974.
94. Sargent, J. A., and Gotch, F. A. Mass balance: A quantitative guide to clinical nutritional therapy. *J. Am. Diet. Assoc.* 75:547, 1979.
95. Shear, L. Internal redistribution of tissue protein synthesis in uremia. *J. Clin. Invest.* 48:1252, 1969.
96. Shear, L., Sapico, V., and Litwack, G. Induction of hepatic enzymes and translocation of cytosol tyrosine amino transaminase (TAT) in uremic rats. *Clin. Res.* 21:707A, 1973.
97. Sherwin, R. S., Bastl, C., Finkelstein, F. O., Fisher, M., Black, H., Hendler, R., and Felig, P. Influence of uremia and hemodialysis on the turnover and metabolic effects of glucagon. *J. Clin. Invest.* 57:722, 1976.
98. Shils, M. E., Wright, W. L., Turnbull, A., and Brescia, F. A long-term parenteral nutrition through an external arteriovenous shunt. *N. Engl. J. Med.* 283:341, 1970.
99. Siegel, N. J., Glazier, W. B., Chaudry, I. H., Gaudio, K. M., Lytton, B., Baue, A. E., and Kashgarian, M. Enhanced recovery from acute renal failure by the postischemic infusion of adenine nucleotides and magnesium chloride in rats. *Kidney Int.* 17:338, 1980.
100. Spreiter, S. C., Myers, B. D., and Swenson, R. S. Protein-energy requirements in subjects with acute renal failure receiving intermittent hemodialysis. *Am. J. Clin. Nutr.* 33:1433, 1980.
101. Stucki, W. P., and Harper, A. E. Importance of dispensable amino acids for normal growth of chicks. *J. Nutr.* 74:377, 1961.
102. Swendseid, M. E., Harris, C. L., and Tuttle, S. G. The effect of sources of nonessential nitrogen on nitrogen balance in young adults. *J. Nutr.* 71:105, 1960.
103. Teschan, P. E., Baxter, C. R., O'Brien, T. F., Freyhof, J. N., and Hall, W. H. Prophylactic hemodialysis in the treatment of acute renal failure. *Ann. Intern. Med.* 53:992, 1960.
104. Tizianello, A., De Ferrazi, G., Garibotto, G., Gurreri, G., and Robaudo, C. Renal metabolism of amino acids and ammonia in subjects with normal renal function and in patients with chronic renal insufficiency. *J. Clin. Invest.* 65:1162, 1980.
105. Toback, F. G. Amino acid enhancement of renal regeneration after acute tubular necrosis. *Kidney Int.* 12:193, 1977.
106. Toback, F. G. Amino Acid Treatment of Acute Renal Failure. In B. M. Brenner and J. H. Stein (Eds.), *Acute Renal Failure.* London: Churchill Livingstone, 1980. Pp. 202–228.
107. Toback, F. G., Dodd, R. C., Maier, E. R., and Havener, L. J. Amino acid enhancement of renal protein synthesis during regeneration after acute tubular necrosis. *Clin. Res.* 27:432A, 1979.
108. Toback, F. G., Havener, L. H., Dodd, R. C., and Spargo, B. H. Phospholipid metabolism during renal regeneration after acute tubular necrosis. *Am. J. Physiol.* 232:E216, 1967.
109. Toback, F. G., Tegarden, D. E., and Havener, L. J. Amino acid-mediated stimulation of renal phospholipid biosynthesis after acute tubular necrosis. *Kidney Int.* 15:542, 1979.
110. Udall, J. A. Human sources and absorption of vitamin K in relation to anticoagulant stability. *J.A.M.A.* 194:127, 1965.
111. Van Buren, C. T., Dudrick, S. J., Dworkin, L., Baumbauer, E., and Long, J. M. Effects of intravenous essential L-amino acids and hypertonic dextrose on anephric beagles. *Surg. Forum* 23:83, 1972.
112. VanVenrooij, W. J. W., Henshaw, E. C., and Hirsch, C. A. Effects of deprival of glucose or individual amino acids on polyribosome distribution and rate of protein synthesis in cultured mammalian cells. *Biochim. Biophys. Acta* 259: 127, 1972.
113. Walser, M. Urea metabolism in chronic renal failure. *J. Clin. Invest.* 53:1385, 1974.

114. Wilmore, D. W., and Dudrick, S. J. Treatment of acute renal failure with intravenous essential L-amino acids. *Arch. Surg.* 99:669, 1969.
115. Wilson, J. D., and Griffin, J. E. The use and misuse of androgens. *Metabolism* 29:1278, 1980.
116. Wolfson, M., Jones, M. R., and Kopple, J. D. Amino acid losses during hemodialysis with infusion of amino acids and glucose. *Kidney Int.*, in press.
117. Woolfson, A. M. J., Healtley, R. V., and Allison, S. P. Insulin to inhibit protein catabolism after injury. *N. Engl. J. Med.* 300:14, 1979.
118. Young, E. A., Heuler, N., Russell, P., and Weser, E. Comparative nutritional analysis of chemically defined diets. *Gastroenterology* 69:1338, 1975.
119. Young, G. A., and Parsons, F. M. The effect of peritoneal dialysis upon the amino acids and other nitrogenous compounds in the blood and dialysates from patients with renal failure. *Clin. Sci.* 37:1, 1969.
120. Zincke, H., Hirsche, B. L., Amamoo, D. G., Woods, J. E., and Andersen, R. C. The use of bovine carotid grafts for hemodialysis and hyperalimentation, *Surg. Gynecol. Obstet.* 139:350, 1974.

Altered Gut Absorption in Disease

Roger J. May
Barbara J. Nath
Robert H. Schapiro

19

In the healthy person, the digestion and absorption of food is a marvelously integrated process. Although it contributes little to the process of digestion, the stomach does store and break down the food and release it in small increments into the duodenum. There the coordinated secretion of both pancreatic enzymes and bile promotes the major portion of intraluminal digestion. The fat-soluble substances are then incorporated with bile salts into mixed micelles and rendered suitable for intestinal absorption. Absorption itself depends on the presence of both adequate intestinal surface area and absorptive function, with certain functions being more effectively handled by some areas of the small intestine than others. For example, calcium and iron absorption occur primarily in the duodenum and proximal jejunum, whereas vitamin B_{12} and bile salt absorption occur almost exclusively in the ileum.

Specific diseases may interfere with this process in a variety of ways. The admixture of food with digestive enzymes may be disrupted (postgastrectomy state), or the production of the enzymes themselves may be inadequate (pancreatic insufficiency). The availability of bile salts to promote solubilization and absorption of fats may be limited because of (1) diminished production (liver disease), (2) denaturation by acid inactivation (pancreatic insufficiency), bacterial deconjugation (bacterial overgrowth syndrome), or (3) loss through interference with the enterohepatic circulation (ileal resection). Ultimately, absorption depends on the presence of an intact, healthy intestinal mucosa in contact with digested food. This may be affected by a variety of mechanisms in diseases that cause inflammation, stasis, or fistulization, or by resection of the small intestine (Crohn's disease, bowel resections). Depending on the area of the intestinal tract affected and the mechanisms of maldigestion or malabsorption, effects may differ markedly for different classes of nutrients.

Of course, in any disease involving the gut, anorexia and postprandial symptoms may limit caloric intake and magnify the effects of malabsorptive processes. Such disease-related restrictions of intake may be further exaggerated by dietary restrictions recommended by physicians themselves.

This chapter will deal with a variety of abdominal diseases commonly encountered in surgical practice. It is our intention to alert the reader to the spectrum of problems that might reasonably be anticipated in these conditions and to outline methods for their recognition and management.

MALABSORPTION IN LIVER DISEASE

Weight loss is a frequent finding in patients with chronic liver disease. In most cases, the major cause is inadequate caloric intake. Anorexia and nausea, frequent symptoms in liver disease, combine with the unpalatable restricted diets, which are often used in the management of such patients, to limit intake of both calories and vitamins. In alcoholic liver disease, the high caloric value of ethanol and the associated alcoholic gastritis further contribute to poor intake.

In some of these patients, however, actual malabsorption may be present and become clinically evident as diarrhea, steatorrhea, and malnutrition. In some instances, malabsorption is related to chronic ingestion of ethanol and is reversible with abstinence. In others, it is produced by the underlying liver disease and may be irreversible.

Alcohol-Related Effects

Chronic, heavy alcohol abuse may lead to disorders of both digestion and absorption. Tests of pancreatic secretory function in such patients may reveal normal or increased volumes of fluid output, but decreased enzyme and bicarbonate secretion. This abnormality is distinct from that observed with acute or chronic pancreatitis and is potentially reversible. The decreased secretion of enzymes is dependent on a coexistent low-protein diet and may be corrected by institution of a normal diet, even if alcohol intake is continued. Malabsorption is also a frequent finding in chronic alcoholic patients. During or immediately following binges, 50 to 80 percent of such patients have at least one abnormality of intestinal absorptive function. These abnormalities are also reversible, but only with both abstinence and the institution of a normal diet.

Ethanol itself does not appear to be directly toxic to the small bowel mucosa. With severe folate deficiency in the setting of chronic alcoholism, however, jejunal morphology may be markedly abnormal. Villous shortening, cuboidal epithelial morphology, and an increased infiltration of chronic inflammatory cells in the lamina propria may be present. With abstinence and adequate folate replacement, these morphologic changes revert to normal.

Experimental studies involving chronic alcoholic patients have documented jejunal malabsorption of fluid and Na^+ as well as numerous nutrients (D-xylose, folate, vitamin B_{12}, glucose, and thiamine). Chronic ethanol intake by itself inhibited jejunal absorption of fluid and Na^+ and caused variable absorption of vitamin B_{12}, but did not significantly affect the absorption of the other nutrients. Ethanol intake combined with folate deficiency produced more marked malabsorption of fluid and Na^+ and strikingly reduced the absorption of the other nutrients studied. As with the aforementioned morphologic changes, the absorption of all substrates reverted to normal with abstinence and institution of an adequate diet.

During prolonged binges, chronic alcoholic patients may develop frequent, watery stools. This clinical disorder presumably reflects the malabsorption of fluid, Na^+, and nutrients already described. Abnormal intestinal motility may also play a role. Fluoroscopic studies using barium have demonstrated a reduction of phasic contractions and an enhancement of propulsive, peristaltic contractions, resulting in more rapid intestinal transit.

When confronted with an afebrile chronic alcoholic patient with nonbloody diarrhea, the physician should have a high index of suspicion that the diarrhea is alcohol-related. The finding of a low serum folate level and hematologic evidence of folate deficiency should reinforce this impression. The feces should be free of blood, leukocytes, enteric pathogens, ova, and parasites, and the rectal mucosa should not be inflamed or friable on sigmoidoscopy. A diagnostic two-week trial of abstinence, adequate dietary intake, and folic acid supplementation is recommended. Resolution of the diarrhea during this trial confirms the diagnosis, whereas persistence of the diarrhea or steatorrhea, or both, indicates the need for investigations directed toward other causes.

Cirrhosis-Related Effects

Malabsorption in chronic liver disease seems to be limited to steatorrhea. An apparent reduction in D-xylose absorption probably results from abnormal distribution, metabolism, and excretion of the sugar rather than true intestinal malabsorption. Mild, irreversible steatorrhea appears to be a widespread complication of cirrhosis, regardless of the etiology of the liver disease. Approximately 50 percent of cirrhotic patients develop steatorrhea, but in most cases excretion does not exceed 10 gm fat per day and is probably of little clinical significance.

Despite the occasional association between Laennec's cirrhosis and chronic pancreatitis among alcoholic patients, pancreatic exocrine insufficiency does not appear to be a frequent cause of steatorrhea in patients with chronic liver disease. In several series, a poor correlation exists between the degree of pancreatic exocrine dysfunction, as measured by secretory testing, and the magnitude of the steatorrhea, suggesting the presence of additional factors.

Decreased hepatobiliary secretion of bile salts has been observed in most patients with cirrhosis complicated by steatorrhea. Following a test meal, the bile salt concentration in the aspirated intestinal contents from cirrhotics with steatorrhea is significantly lower than that found in cirrhotics without steatorrhea or in normal controls (Figure 19-1). In such patients, the intraluminal concentration of bile salts may approach or fall below the critical micellar concentration (1 to 2 mM). A reduction in micelle formation then results in decreased lipid incorporation into the micellar phase and, consequently, steatorrhea.

Decreased hepatobiliary secretion of bile salts may result from either a synthetic or a secretory defect. In patients with cirrhosis, the synthesis of bile acids, especially cholic acid, is diminished, and the size of the bile salt pool significantly reduced. Apparently, the reduction in bile salt synthesis in cirrhosis is a manifestation of a general reduction in hepatic synthesis and correlates roughly with the severity of the liver disease, as measured by ascites, hypoalbuminemia, and hypoprothrombinemia.

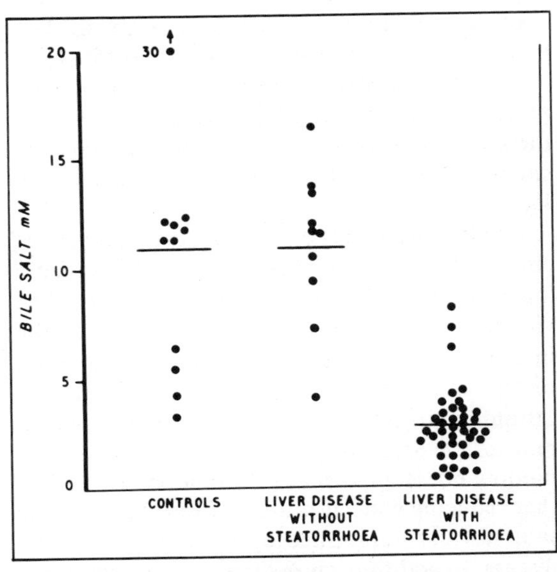

Figure 19-1. *Bile salt concentration of aspirated intestinal contents. (From B. W. D. Badley, et al. Diminished micellar phase lipid in patients with chronic nonalcoholic liver disease and steatorrhea.* Gastroenterology *58:781, 1970.)*

In chronic cholestatic liver disease, hepatobiliary secretion of bile salts may be impaired additionally by obstruction of the intra- and/or extrahepatic biliary tree. This phenomenon may explain the clinical observation that patients with advanced primary biliary cirrhosis may develop more severe steatorrhea, complicated by deficiencies of the fat-soluble vitamins.

In addition to potential defects in the incorporation of lipid into luminal micelles, cirrhotic patients may also suffer a defect in lipid absorption at the intestinal mucosal level. In one study done in cirrhotic patients, long-chain fatty acids in a micellar solution were perfused intraluminally and were found to be absorbed by the jejunum at a decreased rate compared with controls. This phenomenon may be due to chronic portal hypertension or mesenteric lymphatic congestion, or to an as yet uncharacterized abnormality of mucosal metabolism or transport. The incidence and clinical significance of the phenomenon remain unknown.

Finally, two drugs used in the management of chronic liver disease may, by themselves, cause malabsorption. Neomycin produces steatorrhea via three mechanisms: (1) direct toxicity to the intestinal mucosa; (2) intraluminal precipitation of bile salts and fatty acids; and (3) inhibition of intraluminal lipolysis. Cholestyramine, which reduces the pruritus of cholestasis by its bile acid-binding effect, predisposes to steatorrhea by further reducing concentrations of intraluminal bile salts already diminished by the underlying liver disease. In addition, cholestyramine directly binds the fat-soluble vitamins, especially vitamin D, and consequently increases their malabsorption.

In most cirrhotic patients, the mild steatorrhea of chronic liver disease is of little clinical significance. Weight loss in cirrhosis is more commonly caused by anorexia or other medical problems, such as malignancy or uncontrolled diabetes. When a question does exist concerning malabsorption, one should obtain a careful dietary history to quantitate caloric intake and a 72-hour stool collection for quantitative fecal fat determination to document the magnitude of steatorrhea. A fecal fat excretion of 15 gm per day or less is compatible with the underlying cirrhosis and is an unlikely cause of significant weight loss. Except in patients with primary biliary cirrhosis, the finding of a fecal fat excretion greater than 15 to 20 gm per day should suggest some cause of malabsorption other than cirrhosis and requires appropriate investigation.

Patients with chronic cholestatic liver disease, especially primary biliary cirrhosis, are at risk for developing clinical syndromes of fat-soluble vitamin deficiency, and appropriate vigilance should be maintained. Since these deficiencies develop secondary to malabsorption, optimal replacement therapy may be parenteral.

Vitamin A deficiency most commonly is first noted as a decrease in night vision and may be documented by a subnormal serum level of vitamin A. Adequate repletion by parenteral therapy (100,000 units IM each month) should be monitored by periodic measurement of the serum level. A persistent impairment of night vision has been reported in patients with primary biliary cirrhosis, despite adequate parenteral therapy with vitamin A; this impairment was associated with coincidental zinc deficiency and resolved once zinc supplements had been added to the vitamin A therapy.

Findings of ecchymoses and poorly controlled bleeding are usually secondary to clotting-factor deficiencies. In advanced cirrhosis, this may be due to impaired hepatic synthesis of these factors. In primary biliary cirrhosis, however, the clotting-factor deficiency is more likely to be produced by the malabsorption of vitamin K and may be corrected by adequate parenteral replacement with phytonadione. Ten milligrams should be given intramuscularly daily until the prothrombin time has been corrected and then monthly thereafter.

Patients with chronic liver disease, especially primary biliary cirrhosis, are at significant risk for the development of metabolic bone disease. The incidence of both osteoporosis and osteomalacia is increased and may be manifested as either asymptomatic radiographic osteopenia or symptomatic bone pain, compression fractures, and muscle weakness. In patients with primary biliary cirrhosis, the risk for the development of osteomalacia is sufficiently high to mandate a surveillance program accompanied by prophylactic therapy. Although a single determination of bone density is not a sensitive indicator of metabolic bone disease, annual or bi-annual assessment by bone densitometry may detect evidence of excessive bone loss. Periodic measurement should be made of serum calcium, phosphorous, magnesium, and 25-hydroxycholecalciferol (25-OHD_3) as well as urinary calcium excretion. The serum 25-OHD_3 should be maintained in the high-normal range with oral ergocalciferol (D_2) in a dose of at least 50,000 units per week. Since vitamin D absorption and enterohepatic circulation are closely dependent on adequate intestinal bile salt concentrations, larger doses of the vitamin may be necessary. Alternately one may use parenteral therapy with 100,000 units of vitamin D IM each month or oral 25-OHD_3 therapy (50 to 100 mcg per day). This latter preparation has the advantage of better absorption, but is more expensive and less readily available than D_2. In addition, an adequate calcium intake should be maintained (1.0 to 1.5 gm of elemental calcium per day) with periodic measurement of serum and urinary calcium to ensure a 24-hour urinary calcium excretion of 100 to 300 mg. Vitamin D toxicity or excessive calcium intake becomes evident as hypercalciuria (greater than 300 mg per day) or hypercalcemia.

A significant number of patients with metabolic bone disease in the setting of primary biliary cirrhosis have osteoporosis and do not benefit from the recommended measures for osteomalacia. For unclear reasons, these patients malabsorb calcium despite normal serum levels of 1,25-dihydroxycholecalciferol, and it is uncertain what therapy, if any, will prevent or arrest the development of their bone disease. Patients who do develop symptomatic bone disease should undergo an iliac crest bone biopsy to differentiate between osteoporosis and osteomalacia, since this distinction cannot be made radiographically. Thereafter, appropriate therapy should be individualized. Since bone densitometry, calcium determinations, and serum vitamin D levels are not infallible screening techniques, bone biopsy should be performed in the presence of symptoms suggestive of metabolic bone disease, even when these studies are normal.

MALABSORPTION IN PANCREATIC EXOCRINE INSUFFICIENCY

The exocrine pancreas plays a major role in digestion through the secretion of enzymes that catalyze the hydrolysis of fat, protein, and carbohydrate. Predictably, the development of pancreatic exocrine insufficiency may result in a clinical syndrome of marked malabsorption characterized by diarrhea and weight loss; quantitative fecal fat excretion may approach 50 to 80 gm/24 hours, and protein-calorie malnutrition may evolve despite increased dietary intake.

Pancreatic insufficiency may develop whenever the pancreas is unable to secrete quantities of enzymes sufficient to complete digestion. Insufficiency may result, therefore, from total or near-total surgical excision of the gland, obstruction of the pancreatic duct due to carcinoma or pancreatic stones, or inflammatory destruction of the gland by chronic pancreatitis. Although surgical drainage procedures may relieve ductal obstruction and pain in chronic pancreatitis, they do not, in general, improve exocrine secretory function.

Under physiologic conditions, the exocrine pancreas secretes a tenfold excess of digestive enzymes. Even with progressive loss of acinar tissue, steatorrhea and azotorrhea (protein malabsorption) require a 90 percent reduction in the secretion of lipase and trypsin, respectively. In chronic pancreatitis secondary to alcoholism, this process may require 10 to 20 years. During this period, the secretion of lipase may decrease more rapidly than that of trypsin, so that steatorrhea may precede azotorrhea. The digestion of carbohydrate is not so profoundly affected as that of fat and protein, presumably because of the modest activity of salivary amylase. Clinical evidence of fat-soluble vitamin deficiency is unusual, as absorption of these vitamins depends more on solubilization by bile salt micelles than on digestion by pancreatic enzymes. An increased intake of a balanced diet or the addition of oral vitamin supplements may allow adequate absorption despite steatorrhea.

Since malabsorption in pancreatic insufficiency is due to endogenous enzyme deficiency, medical therapy would appear to be straightforward, i.e., exogenous pancreatic enzymes administered in sufficient quantities should correct steatorrhea. In practice, however, this is not easily achieved. Clinical studies have identified three factors that affect the success of pancreatic enzyme replacement therapy: (1) choice of the enzyme preparation; (2) selection of an appropriate therapeutic schedule; and (3) improving delivery of enzymes into the duodenum.

Pancreatic enzyme therapy is available as three

Table 19-1. *Comparison of Enzyme Activities Present in Some Commercial Pancreatic Enzyme Preparations*

Preparation	Manufacturer	Type*	Enzyme Activity (U/Unit)				
			Lipase	Trypsin	Chymo-trypsin	Proteolytic Activity	Amylase
Ilozyme	Warren-Teed	T	3,600	3,444	2,807	6,640	329,600
Ku-Zyme HP	Kremers-Urban	C	2,330	3,082	2,458	6,090	594,048
Festal	Hoechst-Roussel	E	2,073	488	1,150	1,800	219,200
Cotazym	Organon	C	2,014	2,797	3,364	5,840	499,200
Viokase	Viobin	T	1,636	1,828	2,081	4,440	277,333
Gastroenterase	Wallace	E	553	778	995	1,420	108,600
Ro-Bile	Rowell	E	539	661	735	980	68,000
Entozyme	AH Robins	E	495	668	483	1,088	39,000
Enzapan	Norgine	E	297	381	425	2,200	29,100
Phazyme	Reed & Carnrick	E	210	620	405	870	15,800
Ku-Zyme	Kremers-Urban	C	170	25	47	110	37,700
Digolase	Boyle	C	44	143	117	195	16,850
Arco-Lase	Arco	T	29	106	113	240	19,000
Convertin	BF Ascher	E	28	458	387	690	40
Kanulase	Dorsey	T	11	590	568	990	517
Zypan	Standard Process	T	10	296	313	410	441

*T represents tablet; C, capsule; and E, enteric-coated tablet.
Source: D. Y. Graham, Enzyme replacement therapy of exocrine pancreatic insufficiency in man. *N. Engl. J. Med.* 296:1314, 1977. Reprinted by permission.

different types of preparations: (1) *pancreatin,* an alcohol extract of hog pancreas standardized for amylase and trypsin only; (2) *pancrelipase,* a lipase-enriched hog pancreatic preparation; and (3) *enteric-coated preparations,* pancreatic preparations covered with an acid-resistant polymer designed to dissolve only at the neutral pH of the duodenum. Careful in vitro testing has demonstrated wide variations in the lipase activity of commercial enzyme preparations. As shown in Table 19-1, lipase activity may range from 10 units per tablet to 3600 units per tablet, depending on the preparation. A recently released enteric-coated microsphere preparation contains approximately 2000 units per capsule. These activity values are significant, since a preparation's in vitro lipase activity correlates with its in vivo ability to reduce steatorrhea. Since enzyme preparations contain considerable amounts of the purines adenine and guanine, patients receiving conventional amounts of enzyme therapy may develop hyperuricosuria. It is unclear whether this phenomenon produces symptoms in patients with underlying hyperuricosuria or gout.

To correct steatorrhea in pancreatic insufficiency, enzyme therapy should optimally achieve a duodenal lipase concentration equivalent to 10 percent of postprandial pancreatic secretory capacity. It has been estimated that this may be achieved by delivering 8000 units of lipase per hour into the duodenum for four postprandial hours. This is equivalent to the ingestion of 8 tablets of high-potency pancreatin taken in a divided schedule during a meal. In the actual clinical situation, however, this regimen has corrected azotorrhea and has reduced, but not eliminated, steatorrhea. Administering the pancreatin on a regular schedule of two tablets every two hours while awake (32 tablets/day) was no more effective.

The failure of this regimen to correct steator-

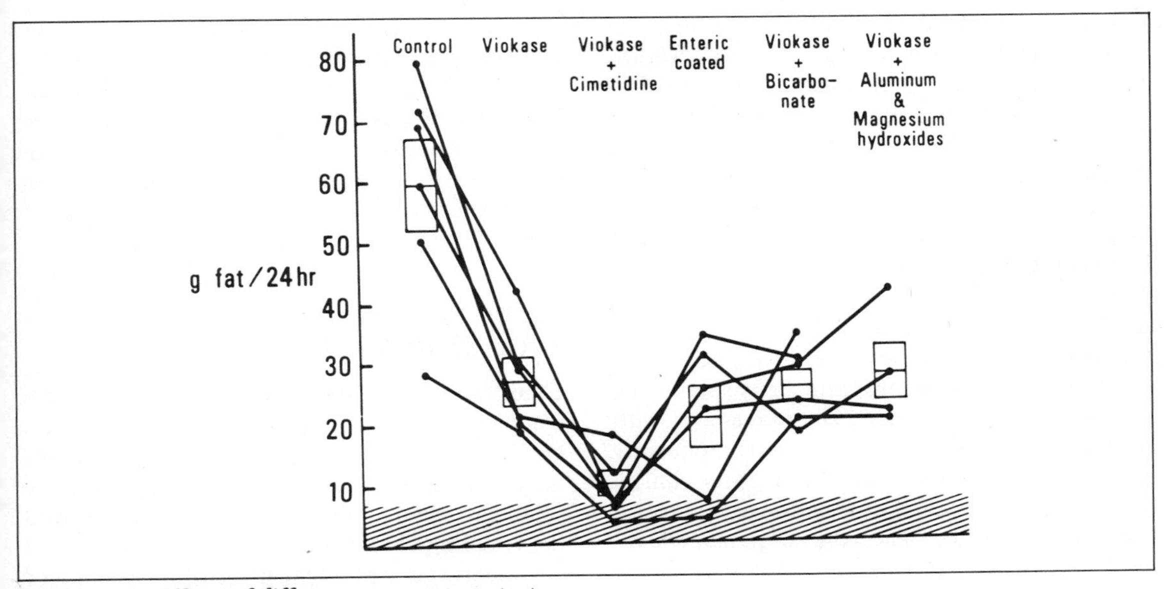

Figure 19-2. *Effects of different treatment on steatorrhea of pancreatic insufficiency in six patients. Normal values for fecal fat excretion (< 7 gm per 24 hours) are represented by hatched area. (From P. T. Regan, et al. Comparative effects of antacids, cimetidine, and enteric coating on the therapeutic response to oral enzymes in severe pancreatic insufficiency.* N. Engl. J. Med. *297:854, 1977. Reprinted by permission.)*

rhea is to a major extent related to gastric inactivation of the ingested enzymes. Following the ingestion of pancreatin, only 20 to 25 percent of the exogenous trypsin activity and 5 to 10 percent of the lipase activity are recovered from the duodenum. The fact that lipase is more acid-sensitive (inactivated at pH < 5) than trypsin may explain the relatively greater passage of exogenous trypsin into the duodenum and hence the more effective correction of azotorrhea. It has been further demonstrated in patients ingesting the same amount of pancreatin that the longer the gastric pH remained greater than 4, the greater the reduction in steatorrhea. Moreover, the higher the average duodenal pH, the greater the reduction in steatorrhea.

Since gastric acidity reduces the efficacy of pancreatic enzyme therapy, it would seem reasonable to augment such therapy with a regimen of acid neutralization. Indeed, as shown in Figure 19-2, the addition of cimetidine to pancreatin therapy does reduce steatorrhea more effectively than does pancreatin alone. In this one study, four of six patients who ingested 300 mg of cimetidine and 8 tablets of pancreatin (Viokase) experienced total correction of steatorrhea. The addition of bicarbonate (2.5 gm) or an aluminum-magnesium hydroxide antacid (30 ml) to pancreatin therapy was no more effective in reducing steatorrhea than pancreatin therapy alone. In addition to reducing gastric inactivation of lipase, cimetidine also reduces total gastric secretion and thus minimizes dilution of the ingested enzymes. Finally, in the more acidic, bicarbonate-depleted duodenum of the patient with pancreatic exocrine insufficiency, pH-induced precipitation of bile salts may cause significant reductions in micellar bile salts and, thus, micellar solubilized fatty acids. These reductions diminish intestinal absorption of hydrolyzed lipid and may only be corrected by the addition of cimetidine to standard pancreatin therapy.

Pancreatic preparations covered with an acid-resistant polymer are designed to survive passage through the stomach and then release their enzymes intact in the neutral pH of the duodenum. Early enteric-coated preparations were found to be less effective than conventional pancreatin in reducing steatorrhea. Since the stomach retards the emptying of all solids larger than several millimeters, these acid-resistant tablets were retained in the stomach until long after the meal had passed into the small intestine.

Recently, a new enteric-coated microsphere preparation has become available. When ingested, an outer capsule dissolves, releasing acid-resistant microspheres that are sufficiently small to be emptied from the stomach simultaneously with the meal. The enzyme content is then subsequently liberated in the duodenum. In an early clinical trial, microspheres and conventional pancreatin therapy reduced the steatorrhea of pancreatic insufficiency to the same extent, although microsphere therapy required fewer capsules and less total lipase activity per meal to achieve its effect.

The ideal of medical therapy is the total elimination of steatorrhea. In practical terms, the reduction of steatorrhea to less than 15 to 20 gm per day should allow weight gain, positive nitrogen balance, and the reduction or elimination of diarrhea. The patient should be instructed to adjust his meal schedule to four feedings per day with 20 to 25 gm of fat per meal. Each meal should be accompanied by 4 to 8 tablets of a high-potency pancreatin preparation in a divided schedule (2 tablets before, 4 tablets during, and 2 tablets after the meal). If diarrhea, weight loss, or gross steatorrhea persist on this regimen, cimetidine 300 mg, 30 minutes before meals, should be added. Alternatively, a trial of the new microsphere preparation might be undertaken. If necessary, further reduction of steatorrhea may be achieved by isocalorically substituting carbohydrate for fat in the diet. Total fat intake may then be supplemented by adding a preparation containing medium-chain triglyceride (MCT) to the diet as needed to maintain weight. Such preparations are composed of fatty acids of shorter chain-length (C-6 to C-10) than the usual dietary long-chain fatty acids, and are digested and absorbed more easily. Up to 30 percent of ingested MCT is absorbed intact. The remainder is hydrolyzed more readily by lipase and solubilized more easily by micelles. Consequently, MCT supplements may enhance dietary fat intake even when fat digestion and absorption are markedly abnormal, as in pancreatic insufficiency.

POSTGASTRECTOMY MALABSORPTION

Digestion in the upper gastrointestinal tract is a complex, multifactorial process. Acting as a reservoir, the normal stomach retains ingested solids until they have been dispersed into sufficiently small particles (2 mm) and then gradually empties the resulting chyme into the duodenum. The vagus innervates a pacemaker focus in the body of the stomach that initiates orderly peristaltic waves that effect this emptying of solids. Also under vagal innervation, "receptive" relaxation of the proximal stomach serves to accommodate increasing volumes of ingested and secreted fluid. Finally, optimal mixing of the chyme with biliary and pancreatic secretions in the duodenum enhances further digestion and ensures normal absorption of nutrients in the small intestine.

Gastric surgery may interfere with these events at any of several levels. Distal gastrectomy destroys the reservoir function of the stomach and promotes rapid emptying. With truncal vagotomy, gastric emptying of solids is occasionally slowed, and that of liquids increased. Alterations in gastroduodenal anatomy, such as occurs with Billroth II gastroenterostomy, produce asynchronous secretion of bile and pancreatic enzymes and poor mixing of these secretions with the chyme.

Alterations in these same events may also produce several postgastrectomy syndromes that do not produce malabsorption per se, but may affect food intake. Rapid gastric emptying may give rise to clinical symptoms of "dumping." Truncal vagotomy may be associated with rapid intestinal transit and watery diarrhea. Finally, altered anatomy, such as that seen with distal gastrectomy, may result in duodenogastric reflux and "reflux" (alkaline) gastritis.

Following gastric surgery, 20 to 40 percent of patients lose weight significantly below their preoperative baseline. This phenomenon seems to be a function of both decreased caloric intake and mild malabsorption. The vast majority have decreased caloric intake compared with their preoperative diet. Predictably, the incidence of steatorrhea varies with the amount of the stomach resected, occurring in 70 to 80 percent of patients following total gastrectomy, 50 to 60 percent following subtotal gastrectomy with Billroth II anastomosis (STG–BII), and 30 to 40 percent following truncal vagotomy and pyloroplasty (TV & P). In general, however, the coefficient of fat malabsorption in affected patients rarely exceeds 15 to 20 percent of the dietary intake; a greater degree of steatorrhea probably denotes significant coincidental disease, such as bacterial overgrowth or gluten-sensitive enteropathy.

Clinical studies of the metabolic effects of the newer gastric operations are more preliminary. Mean fecal fat excretion following selective vagotomy with pyloroplasty appears not to differ from that observed for TV & P. In contrast, the mean excretion following parietal cell vagotomy does not differ from that for unoperated patients with duodenal ulcer disease.

Following gastric surgery, gastric emptying of both liquids and solids is greatly altered. Studies employing nonabsorbable markers have shown that patients with subtotal gastrectomy with Billroth I anastamosis (STG-BI), STG-BII, and TV & P empty a liquid meal at approximately twice the rate of unoperated controls (Figure 19-3). Patients with TV & P tend to empty liquid even more rapidly than do patients with STG alone, probably owing to the loss of vagally mediated "receptive" relaxation of the stomach.

In all operated patients, duodenal concentrations of bile salts and pancreatic enzymes are reduced to a major degree because of dilution by rapidly emptied gastric contents. Total bile salt secretion in all operated groups appears normal, as does pancreatic exocrine output in the absence

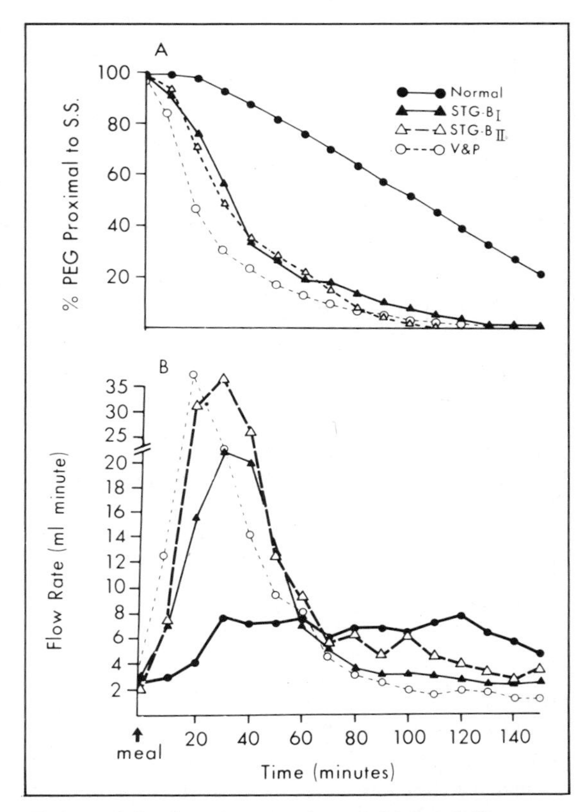

Figure 19-3. *Gastric emptying and jejunal flow rates after a 500-ml liquid meal of fat, protein, and hypertonic glucose in normal subjects and in those with various ulcer operations.* A *expresses the percentage of ingested meal marker (PEG) remaining proximal to the jejunum (SS) as time elapses after ingesting the meal.* B *illustrates the very high jejunal flow rates following the liquid meal. (From J. H. Meyer, Chronic morbidity after ulcer surgery. In M. H. Sleisenger and J. S. Fordtran (Eds.),* Gastrointestinal Disease *(2nd ed.) Philadelphia: Saunders, 1978. Pp. 947-969.*

of vagotomy. In patients with TV & P, however, pancreatic enzyme output in response to a test meal is only 40 percent of that of controls, despite a normal response to a maximal dose of cholecystokinin (CCK). Presumably, truncal vagotomy either reduces mucosal release of CCK or disrupts gastro- or enteropancreatic reflexes. Even with this reduction, pancreatic output should be ade-

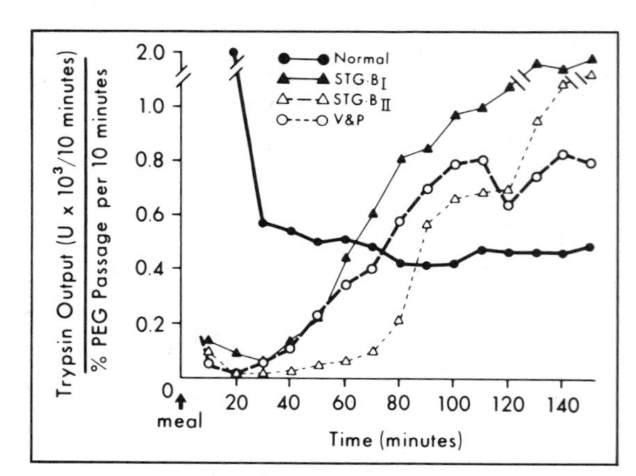

Figure 19-4. *Ratio of trypsin to the percentage of liquid meal marker (PEG) passing jejunal sampling site as a function of time after a test meal. (From I. MacGregor, et al. Gastric emptying of liquid meals and pancreatic and biliary secretion after subtotal gastrectomy or truncal vagotomy and pyloroplasty in man.* Gastroenterology *72:195, 1977.)*

quate in view of the normal, tenfold excess output of pancreatic enzymes. However, intraluminal dilution by gastric contents may reduce bile salt concentrations below the critical micelle concentration necessary for fat absorption.

Suboptimal concentrations of bile salts and pancreatic enzymes are further compromised by poor mixing of these agents with the meal owing to asynchrony between gastric emptying and digestive secretion. In all operated groups, rapid gastric emptying of a liquid meal results in passage of the meal downstream before large amounts of bile salts and pancreatic enzymes are secreted (Figure 19-4). Furthermore, in patients with STG-BII, the afferent loop may sequester a significant fraction of the digestive secretions until the meal has passed into the small intestine.

Although frequent, this form of postgastrectomy malabsorption is mild in severity. Only rarely does bacterial overgrowth play a significant role in postgastrectomy malabsorption. Achlorhydria, per se, does not seem to predispose to pathologic overgrowth; rather, altered intestinal motility appears to be a necessary prerequisite. Occasionally, in patients with STG-BII, an unusually long or partially obstructed afferent loop may provide an appropriate environment (pp. 602–606).

Infrequently, gastric surgery may unmask old disease rather than create new complications. Following gastric surgery, a patient with a previously subclinical small bowel disorder may develop clinically significant malabsorption owing to rapid emptying of gastric contents into the jejunum. In this manner, borderline lactase deficiency may manifest itself following partial gastrectomy as lactose intolerance, and the subclinical gluten-sensitive enteropathy, as symptomatic celiac sprue secondary to rapid gastric emptying of lactose and gluten, respectively.

Following gastric surgery, a patient whose weight falls significantly below his preoperative baseline should undergo an evaluation for malabsorption. The majority of these patients will have lost weight primarily as a result of inadequate caloric intake. Consequently, a careful dietary history should be obtained and, if possible, caloric intake quantitated during an inpatient work-up. A quantitative fecal fat determination should be performed while the patient is on a 100 gm fat diet. If fecal fat excretion is less than 15 gm per day, dietary counselling is indicated; this small magnitude of steatorrhea is consistent with that expected after gastric surgery, and weight loss is most likely a result of inadequate caloric intake. If fecal fat excretion is greater than 15 gm per day, further evaluation for underlying disease (e.g., bacterial overgrowth, pancreatic insufficiency, gluten-sensitive enteropathy) is indicated.

Metabolic Consequences of Gastrectomy

Anemia is the most common metabolic complication of gastric surgery. Following gastrectomy, the incidence of anemia increases with time; only 5 percent of patients with STG will be anemic or iron-deficient immediately postoperatively, but by 10 to 15 years, this number will have risen to 30 percent. Laboratory testing may reveal combined deficiency in 50 percent of patients with

STG, but it is unclear to what extent each factor-deficiency contributes to clinical anemia, if present. Iron deficiency is manifested earliest, folate deficiency later, and vitamin B_{12} deficiency quite late as body stores are depleted.

Postgastrectomy iron-deficiency anemia is a consequence of both gastrointestinal blood loss and iron malabsorption. Causes of blood loss in these patients include recurrent peptic disease as well as reflux gastritis. Although dietary iron intake is probably adequate, postoperative reduction in gastric acid secretion may interfere with iron absorption in four ways: (1) reduced peptic digestion and release of food-bound iron; (2) diminished conversion of ferric iron (Fe^{+3}) to the more soluble ferrous form (Fe^{+2}); (3) decreased formation of soluble iron-ligand complexes; and (4) loss of an unidentified iron-binding factor in gastric juice (not HCl), which enhances iron absorption. Since most iron absorption occurs in the duodenum and proximal jejunum, iron absorption may be particularly poor in patients with STG-BII.

The evaluation and management of iron-deficiency anemia in postgastrectomy patients is relatively straightforward. Stools should be screened for evidence of gastrointestinal bleeding; if such evidence is found, a thorough diagnostic search of both the upper and lower gastrointestinal tracts should be undertaken. Not infrequently, iron deficiency develops as a result of iron malabsorption alone without evidence of blood loss. In such instances, initial therapy should consist of oral ferrous sulfate, with or without sodium ascorbate to improve solubility. Simultaneous consumption of antacids may decrease iron solubility. Occasionally, iron absorption in the postgastrectomy patient may be so poor that parenteral iron therapy is indicated to replete and then maintain adequate body iron stores.

Anemia secondary to vitamin B_{12} deficiency is an uncommon complication of gastric surgical procedures less extensive than a total gastrectomy. As the parietal cells of the gastric body normally secrete 100 times the necessary amount of intrinsic factor (IF), distal gastrectomy does not significantly reduce the capacity to secrete IF, and consequently, early malabsorption of vitamin B_{12} is uncommon. Physiologic serum levels of gastrin, however, appear to exert a trophic effect on the parietal cells. Antrectomy and subsequent gastrin depletion may then predispose to late parietal cell atrophy, atrophic gastritis, and eventual IF deficiency.

Despite adequate dietary intake and normal secretion of IF, postgastrectomy patients may still malabsorb vitamin B_{12}. Because of rapid gastric emptying and suboptimal digestion, there may be diminished release of food-bound vitamin B_{12} and reduced efficiency of vitamin B_{12}- and IF-binding in the proximal jejunum. Crystalline vitamin B_{12} may be absorbed more efficiently than food-bound vitamin B_{12}, but it is unclear whether this phenomenon is of clinical importance.

If malabsorption of vitamin B_{12} is suspected, a Schilling test, stage I (without IF) should be performed. The potential contribution of bacterial overgrowth to vitamin B_{12} malabsorption can be documented by repeating the study with the addition of exogenous IF before and after antibiotic therapy. If vitamin B_{12} malabsorption is present, replacement therapy should consist of parenteral vitamin B_{12}, 100 mcg IM each month.

Folate deficiency with megaloblastic anemia is a rare complication of gastric surgery. In patients with poor gastric emptying of solids, especially those with phytobezoars, a low fiber diet may provide inadequate amounts of folate. As with vitamin B_{12}, diminished release of food-bound folate in the upper intestine may reduce the efficiency of folate absorption in the jejunum. If indicated, oral folate therapy (1 mg per day) should be instituted.

Metabolic bone disease is a common but late complication of gastric surgery. Changes in bone radiodensity are rarely seen before the sixth postoperative year. By 10 to 20 years, however, approximately a third of patients display bone-biopsy findings consistent with osteomalacia. The incidence of the lesion varies with the surgical procedure; it is rare after TV & P and much more frequent following STG-BII.

Osteomalacia following gastric surgery is caused by a deficiency of both calcium and vitamin D. Dietary avoidance of milk and milk products produced by postoperative lactose intolerance may limit intake. Although osteomalacia may exist in these patients independent of steatorrhea, the development of significant steatorrhea will, nevertheless, decrease absorption of both vitamin D and calcium and further predispose to the lesion. Furthermore, since the duodenum is the major site of calcium absorption, malabsorption of calcium is more common in patients with STG-BII than in patients with STG-BI or in unoperated controls.

Since osteomalacia is a common, late complication of gastric surgery, especially STG-BII, surveillance would seem prudent beginning 5 to 10 years postoperatively. Bone densitometry should be performed at one- to two-year intervals. If serial measurements demonstrate a decline in the bone density, an iliac crest bone biopsy should be performed to document osteomalacia. If present, osteomalacia should be managed with calcium and vitamin D supplements, as described elsewhere in this chapter.

MALABSORPTION DUE TO BACTERIAL OVERGROWTH

The size of the small intestinal bacterial population is controlled by gastric acidity, peristalsis, and mucosal antibacterial defenses. When altered intestinal motility or anatomy results in luminal stasis, or when access of bacteria to the small intestine is markedly increased, weight loss, steatorrhea, and B_{12} deficiency may develop. The combination of malabsorption and increased small bowel bacterial population is known as the bacterial overgrowth syndrome (also called the contaminated small bowel, blind loop, or small intestine stasis syndrome).

Mechanisms That Control Bacterial Growth

The upper gastrointestinal tract flora consists of less than 10^4 organisms per cc of intestinal fluid, composed predominantly of anaerobic streptococci, aerobic lactobacilli, dipththeroids, and fungi. A change in flora occurs in the distal ileum, with an increase in numbers of bacteria to 10^5 to 10^8 per cc, and the appearance of gram-negative coliforms and anaerobic Bacteroides species. Once the ileocaecal valve is crossed, there is a marked increase in number and variety of microorganisms, with anaerobes predominating. In bacterial overgrowth syndromes, the number of organisms in the proximal small bowel rises to 10^6 to 10^{11} per cc, usually accompanied by a predominance of enteric coliforms and strict anaerobes.

Most bacteria ingested with a meal are destroyed by gastric acid, the first barrier to bacterial overgrowth in the jejunum. In vitro studies indicate that the bactericidal activity of gastric juice is entirely pH (HCl)-dependent, with other constituents of gastric juice playing no role. In vivo, hypochlorhydria alone rarely results in clinically significant overgrowth, though there is a correlation between jejunal bacterial counts and reduced gastric acidity.

Studies performed in dogs subjected to varying degrees of vagal denervation and gastric resection (parietal cell vagotomy, selective vagotomy and pyloroplasty, truncal vagotomy and pyloroplasty, truncal vagotomy and antrectomy, and subtotal gastrectomy) demonstrated that elevated gastric pH alone did not alter jejunal flora. Significant bacterial overgrowth occurred, however, in all types of surgery except parietal cell vagotomy, suggesting that preservation of antroduodenal innervation may be a factor in limiting bacterial proliferation. Mild degrees of overgrowth did not necessarily result in malabsorption.

Intestinal motility is probably the most important factor in regulating intestinal bacterial counts. Nonsurgical conditions associated with abnormal motility, such as scleroderma, intestinal pseudo-obstruction, and diabetic autonomic neuropathy are often associated with intestinal stasis and malabsorption. Surgical manipulations that create excessively long or aperistaltic segments of intestine, as occasionally occurs in the afferent loop of a Billroth II anastamosis, may result in over-

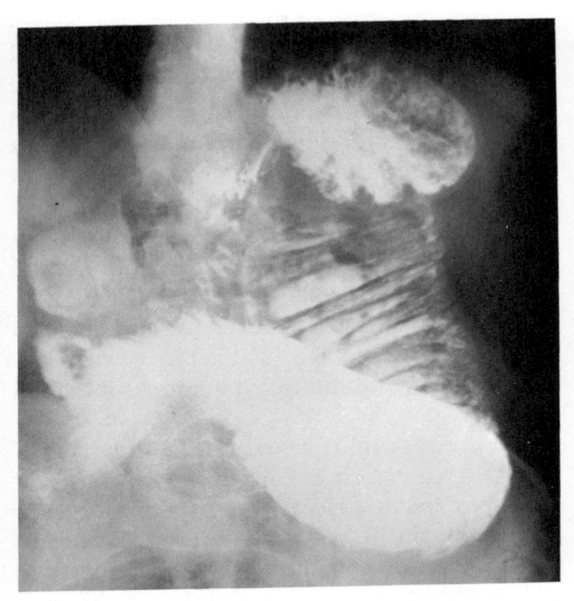

Figure 19-5. *Upper GI series in a patient with a Hofmeister gastrojejunostomy. The large, dilated afferent loop was best demonstrated by a combination of food followed by barium. (From J. R. Dreyfuss, On evaluating upper gastrointestinal symptoms by provocative study.* Radiol. Clin. North Am. *10:18, 1971.)*

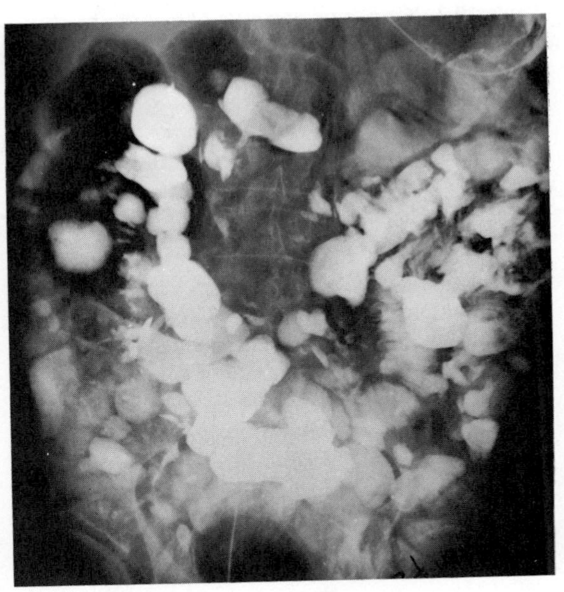

Figure 19-6. *Upper GI series demonstrating large duodenal and jejunal diverticula.*

growth (Figure 19-5). Gastric surgery that preserves intestinal continuity (Billroth I, vagotomy and pyloroplasty) is almost never associated with bacterial overgrowth. Decreased peristalsis may occur after circumferential muscle fibers are severed in the creation of a side-to-side anastamosis, and may be attended by the bacterial stasis syndrome.

A few patients with the Koch continent ileostomy have clinically significant bacterial overgrowth in the ileal reservoir. Similarly, multiple duodenal and jejunal diverticula (Figure 19-6) provide a reservoir for bacterial proliferation which then continuously bathes the more distal bowel with an excess of abnormal flora. Diverticula also alter motility and exaggerate these effects. Areas of small bowel stasis may also be created by strictures, adhesions, or tumors, causing varying degrees of overgrowth on this basis.

The ileocecal valve is an important boundary that keeps the predominantly anaerobic population of the colon separate from the small intestine. Surgical resection of this anatomic barrier may be associated with abnormal small intestinal flora and clinical evidence of bacterial contamination. Similarly, fistula formation (e.g., gastrocolic, jejunocolic, or cholecystocolic) may permit abnormal access of colonic bacteria to the upper gastrointestinal tract with consequent malabsorption, even when the amount of intestinal contents bypassing the absorbing areas is minimal.

Rare cases of partial biliary obstruction with cholangitis have been reported in which infected bile secreted into the intestine altered the jejunal flora and resulted in steatorrhea, B_{12} deficiency, and increased amounts of unconjugated bile acids. Conditions associated with bacterial overgrowth are listed in Table 19-2.

Pathophysiology

The effects of bacterial overgrowth range from no symptoms at all to profound malnutrition, with

Table 19-2. *Causes of Bacterial Overgrowth*

Postoperative anatomic changes	Afferent loop S/P Billroth II
	Gastroenterostomy
	End-to-side anastomosis
	Ileocecal valve resection
	Continent ileostomy
	Colectomy with postoperative ileus
	Jejunoileal bypass
Structural and motility disorders	Strictures: Crohn's disease, radiation enteritis
	Obstruction: adhesions, Crohn's disease, carcinoma
	Duodenal or jejunal diverticula
	Fistulas: gastrocolic, jejuno-colic, enteroenteric, cholecystocolic
	Cholangitis
	Intestinal pseudo-obstruction
	Scleroderma
	Diabetic autonomic neuropathy
Functional disorders	Malnutrition
	Tropical sprue
	Immune deficiency states
	Malabsorption in the elderly

weight loss and protein deficiency resembling kwashiorkor in severity. The more usual presenting symptoms are mild to moderate weight loss, B_{12}-related megaloblastic anemia, and diarrhea. Steatorrhea usually is in the vicinity of 20 to 40 gm per day, but may range as high as 70 gm per day.

Malabsorption in the bacterial overgrowth syndrome is primarily the result of abnormalities in bile acid metabolism and mucosal injury, with consequent disturbances of intraluminal digestion and mucosal function. Mucosal abnormalities tend to be patchy and are characterized by partial villous atrophy, increased numbers of mononuclear cells in the lamina propria, increased intracytoplasmic lysosomes, and mitochondrial swelling. The lesion is rarely as severe as that seen in celiac disease and is never associated with morphologic disruption of the brush border. Nevertheless, mucosal injury may cause occult blood and protein loss and malabsorption of sugars and amino acids owing to decreased amounts of brush border and intracellular enzymes. The agents causing mucosal injury are unknown, but most investigative speculation has centered around the effects of deconjugated bile acids. This mechanism may explain steatorrhea even with normal luminal concentrations of bile salts. Persistent malabsorption after elimination of abnormal bacteria is probably due to mucosal recovery lagging behind restitution of the normal intestinal flora.

Fatty acids and triglycerides, the products of lipolysis, are poorly soluble unless incorporated into micelles by the detergent action of conjugated bile salts. Excess bacteria, especially anaerobes, when present in adequate concentrations (10^6 organisms) in the small intestine, deconjugate bile salts, liberating free bile salts, which are ineffective in promoting micelle formation and are passively absorbed in the proximal small intestine. As mentioned, such free bile acids may also produce direct mucosal injury and impair uptake of fatty acids and triglycerides. Unconjugated bile acids and the hydroxy fatty acids produced by bacterial metabolism of unabsorbed fat are also colonic irritants, stimulating fluid and electrolyte secretion and producing a secretory diarrhea.

Although the mechanisms causing protein deficiency in bacterial overgrowth are not completely understood, there is evidence to support the role of decreased uptake and transport of amino acids and peptides due to decreased brush border peptidase activity. Bacterial catabolism of amino acid precursors, intraluminal metabolism of amino acids, and interference with amino acid absorption by deconjugated bile salts may also play a role. Endogenously shed proteins may be similarly affected.

Carbohydrate malabsorption is rarely a problem in adult patients with the contaminated small bowel syndrome, although it may be important in children. Mucosal injury may result in impaired disaccharidase activity and impaired mucosal monosaccharide absorption. The consequences of carbohydrate malabsorption—increased osmotic load and bacterial metabolism of unabsorbed carbohydrates—contribute to the diarrhea that is a common accompaniment to bacterial overgrowth.

Vitamin B_{12} deficiency occurs in the setting of bacterial overgrowth even though intraluminal vitamin B_{12} concentrations may be high. Vitamin B_{12}-intrinsic factor complexes are tightly bound to the cell surfaces of bacteria, especially anaerobes, where they are unavailable for absorption by the host. Ileal absorption per se is not impaired. Inactive metabolites of vitamin B_{12}, produced by the abnormal intestinal bacteria, compound the problem by blocking attachment of B_{12} to intrinsic factor and the B_{12}-IF complex to ileal receptor sites.

Folate absorption is normal, and serum folate levels may be elevated in some patients as a consequence of folate production by some bacterial species. In contrast to folate production, bacterial utilization of ingested nutrients may also be a factor in the malnutrition that may accompany the bacterial overgrowth syndrome.

In addition to these metabolic defects, a syndrome of episodic encephalopathy has been described in patients with short bowel syndrome and following jejunoileal bypass surgery. It is characterized by periods of disorientation, ataxia, slurred speech, and confusion that may last from two hours to several days. There are no obvious precipitants, but D-lactic acidosis has been documented in the serum of several patients during the periods of encephalopathy. Treatment with antibiotics usually cures the syndrome, even in those patients without documented D-lactic acidosis. Although tests to determine the presence of bacterial overgrowth were not reported, the encephalopathy appears to be related to products of bacterial metabolism, including D-lactate, since the salutory effects of the antibiotics presumably were due to eradication of abnormal gut flora.*

*Editor's Note: The encephalopathy following jejunoileal bypass conceivably could be related to changes in plasma amino acid patterns similar to those seen in liver disease.

Diagnosis

Diarrhea, steatorrhea, anemia, or weight loss complicating any of the surgical procedures or medical conditions already described should alert the physician to the possibility of bacterial overgrowth. If a qualitative stool exam using Sudan stain confirms the presence of neutral and split fats, a quantitative measurement should be made of 72-hour fecal fat excretion. The Schilling test with intrinsic factor will be low in bacterial overgrowth, owing to bacterial binding of B_{12} and intrinsic factor, even with normal serum B_{12} levels. The D-xylose test is usually low, probably owing to defects in mucosal uptake and to utilization of the sugar by bacteria.

Specific demonstration that bacterial overgrowth is the cause of these defects may be accomplished by intestinal intubation, with aspiration and culture of duodenal contents, and by breath tests. Demonstration of greater than 10^6 organisms per milliliter of intestinal fluid, composed of both anaerobes and aerobes, is considered positive. Because of the discomfort, inconvenience, and expense of this technique, it has been largely supplanted by breath tests. These tests assay breath excretion of either CO_2 or H_2, products of bacterial metabolism of administered substances. The bile acid breath test measures $^{14}CO_2$ in the breath, released when the amide bond linking ^{14}C-1-glycine with cholic acid is cleaved by bacteria. An early peak suggests the presence of abnormal concentrations of bacteria in the small intestine. The test does not, however, distinguish between patients with overgrowth and those in whom ileal disease or resection has led to bile salt losses into the colon and deconjugation of these bile salts by colonic bacteria. Occasional false-positive results occur in postcholecystectomy patients. In these patients, a reduced conjugated bile salt pool may magnify the apparent percentage of deconjugated bile acids. A false-negative rate of about 30 percent further limits the usefulness of this test.

The xylose breath test uses ^{14}C-D-xylose as the substrate. In normals, the small quantity of administered xylose should be entirely absorbed in

Table 19-3. *Causes of Diarrhea in Short Bowel Syndrome*

Causes	Site of Resection
Excess bile acids	Less than 100 cm of terminal ileum
Excess fatty acids	Greater than 100 cm of terminal ileum
Bacterial overgrowth	Ileocecal valve
Gastric hyper-secretion	Variable lengths of small bowel
Altered transit time	More rapid after distal than after proximal resections

the small intestine and excreted, largely unmetabolized, in the urine. When bacteria are present in the small intestine, they metabolize the xylose, and the CO_2 is absorbed and released in the breath. This test is of much shorter duration and greater specificity and sensitivity than the bile acid breath test.

The lactulose breath test measures hydrogen production after bacterial fermentation of this carbohydrate or its constituents. Radioisotopes are not required. False positives occur only in patients with rapid transit, in whom the early peak represents colonic bacterial metabolism. A 30 percent false-negative rate is in part related to the absence of hydrogen-producing organisms in some intestinal tracts. Although each breath test has a significant false-negative rate, together they correctly diagnose greater than 90 percent of patients with the contaminated small bowel syndrome.

Treatment

If an anatomic defect is responsible for bacterial overgrowth and is amenable to correction, surgery should be performed. In most cases, however, this option is not feasible, and medical management with antibiotics and nutritional supplements must be utilized. Bacterial overgrowth alone, without malabsorption, is not necessarily an indication for treatment.

The choice of antibiotics is largely empiric, since culture of small bowel contents yields a large variety of bacterial species and antibiotic sensitivities. Broad-spectrum antibiotics are most commonly used, preferably drugs with anaerobic activity. Tetracycline 250 mg PO q.i.d. is the usual first choice of antibiotic. Good results have also been achieved with chloramphenicol, ampicillin, metronidazole, erythromycin, and oral clindamycin. Remission is indicated by the normalization of fat absorption and of the Schilling test. This response usually occurs within seven to ten days and may persist for months, even when there has been a recurrence of bacterial overgrowth. Antibiotic therapy is usually given for 10 to 14 days. If a recurrence of malabsorption is documented, a second course of antibiotic therapy should be tried. For patients who require prolonged treatment, intermittent therapy (one week out of six) is a reasonable option. Alternation between two or three different antibiotics may also be helpful, especially during prolonged or intermittent therapy.

In some cases, nutritional manipulations alone may be adequate. Mild to moderate steatorrhea can be controlled on a limited (40 gm) fat diet or a diet rich in medium-chain triglycerides. Parenteral vitamin B_{12} and supplemental vitamins A, D, and K may also be valuable adjuncts to therapy.

MALABSORPTION DUE TO INFLAMMATORY BOWEL DISEASE

Malnutrition is a common complication of inflammatory bowel disease. Dietary intake is frequently subnormal due to stringent dietary restrictions, anorexia during flares in disease activity, and the association of eating with abdominal pain and diarrhea. In the presence of the catabolic state that accompanies disease activity, even normal caloric intake may be inadequate for nutritional needs. These factors may be operative in both ulcerative colitis and Crohn's disease. Malabsorption of fat, fat-soluble vitamins, B_{12}, and folate occurs only in patients with small intestinal involvement with Crohn's disease, but diarrhea and enteric losses of protein and minerals may complicate inflammatory bowel disease in any location. Certain vitamin deficiencies and absorptive defects may be compounded by side effects of drugs commonly used in treating inflammatory bowel disease: sulfasalazine, cholestyramine, and corticosteroids.

Disease Activity and Catabolic State

GROWTH RETARDATION

It has been estimated that about 25 percent of children and adolescents with inflammatory bowel disease suffer from growth retardation, inadequate weight gain, retarded bone development, and delayed puberty. Although some children with Crohn's disease have low serum levels of 25-OH-vitamin D, malabsorption of vitamin D and calcium are unusual, and vitamin supplementation does not reverse the growth retardation. Endocrine abnormalities have not been implicated. Thyroid function, adrenal function, somatomedin production, and the hypothalamic-pituitary axis all appear to be normal. Rather, growth retardation is due primarily to negative nitrogen and caloric balance. Severe reduction in caloric intake is the major factor, with enteric protein losses creating greater than normal nutritional requirements. Steroids often produce an acceleration in linear growth by suppressing inflammation, but prolonged administration of high-dose steroids may also contribute to growth retardation, especially when taken on a daily basis. Elective surgery for children with Crohn's disease is generally reserved for debilitated patients who have limited disease, and for whom growth is an urgent problem. Surgical resection may restore health in ulcerative colitis, but its efficacy in correcting growth deficiency in Crohn's disease of the small bowel is limited by the frequency of disease recurrence and by the absorptive problems stemming from the resection itself.

Dramatic restoration of normal growth and development has been achieved with aggressive oral alimentation, including nutritional supplements, elemental diets sometimes administered as a continuous intragastric infusion, supplemental oral vitamins and iron, and periodic intravenous administration of Intralipid. Such measures have been shown to produce a dramatic, albeit temporary, resumption of growth in children with severe growth failure due to inflammatory bowel disease. Parenteral hyperalimentation achieves the same ends more rapidly, but is usually reserved for patients who are entering the crucial period for growth, before epiphyseal closure occurs. In these patients, rapid reversal of growth retardation is important. The caloric intake required to achieve growth spurts in these patients is up to 90 percent greater than levels recommended for children without disease. Although protein consumption also increases concomitantly, the greater caloric intake is probably the most important factor in promoting normal growth. It may take three to four years of high calorie nutritional support before pre-illness height percentage levels are achieved.

WEIGHT LOSS

In adults with Crohn's disease, weight loss is also the consequence of protein-calorie malnutrition. As with children, inadequate caloric intake is one of the major contributing factors. Fat malabsorption may also be important in patients with bile salt deficiency due to extensive small bowel resection or severe ileal disease. Excessive protein loss is often a factor in weight loss, although its major effect is to lower serum protein levels.

Enteric protein losses may be as high as 15 times normal (normal protein losses are roughly the equivalent of 30 cc of plasma) and correlate with the length of bowel involved with disease. There is no correlation with other parameters of mucosal function, such as D-xylose absorption, amount of steatorrhea, or B_{12} metabolism. Excessive protein loss may result from lymphatic obstruction, mucosal ulceration and inflammation, and bacterial overgrowth.

Disaccharidase deficiency has been suspected in inflammatory bowel disease. Lactose intolerance was reported in 20 percent of patients with ulcerative colitis, but it is unclear how this figure differs from that found in the general population. Although suspected intolerance should be defined by lactose tolerance tests, it is inappropriate to prohibit milk products in all patients with inflammatory bowel disease.

Consequences of the Anatomic Site of Disease

Mucosal inflammation, surgical resection, fistulas, and stricture formation reduce the amount of functioning intestinal surface area. Mucosal inflammation interferes with absorption by reducing brush border enzymes and altering normal enterocyte metabolism. The effects of surgical resection depend on the length and segment of bowel removed. Jejunal resection may be better tolerated than ileal resection, since the ileum can more easily undergo adaptation. Hyperplasia of epithelial cells increases the amount of absorptive area and regenerates some lost brush border enzymes. Ileal resection, as well as extensive ileal disease, may especially compromise bile salt and B_{12} absorption, which are largely confined to this area of the bowel.

Fistula formation occurs in up to 30 percent of patients with Crohn's disease. Any fistula that bypasses a major segment of the small bowel, such as a gastrocolic fistula or jejunocolic fistula, usually results in diarrhea and weight loss. Enteroenteric fistulas between loops of ileum and right colon may have similar but less dramatic effects. Colonic bacterial colonization of the upper bowel occurs with gastrocolic or jejunocolic fistula and may produce a bacterial overgrowth syndrome (Figure 19-7). Diagnosis of enterocolic fistula is best made by barium enema rather than an upper GI series. When fistulization causes significant malabsorption, surgery should be performed to correct the anatomic defect.

Surgical resection of the ileocecal valve also predisposes to bacterial overgrowth by permitting the predominantly anaerobic bacterial population of the colon to submerge the less populous, mixed aerobic and anaerobic population of the distal ileum. Strictures due to ulceration and scarring in Crohn's disease cause stasis proximal to the stricture and alter intestinal motility both proximally and distally. Peristaltic clearing of bacteria is especially hampered if long segments of bowel are involved, and bacterial overgrowth is common in this setting.

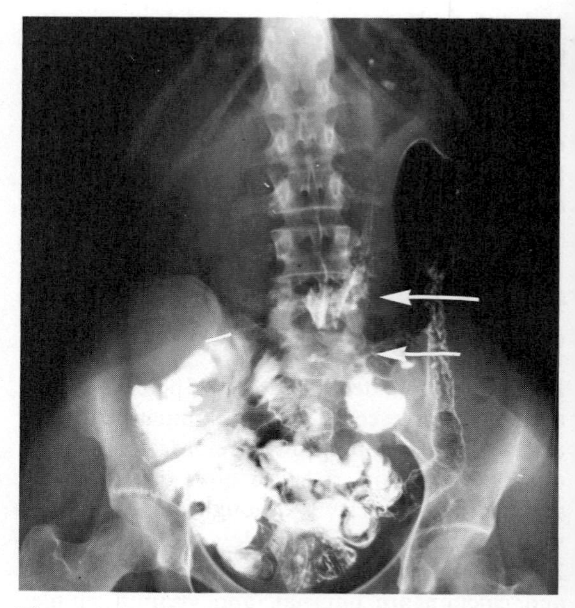

Figure 19-7. *This barium enema demonstrates a gastrocolic fistula in a patient with Crohn's disease with diarrhea and malabsorption. Upper arrow indicates the stomach, which contains barium refluxed through the fistula. Lower arrow indicates the fistulous tract originating in a segmental area of involvement in the mid-transverse colon. (Courtesy of Jack R. Dreyfuss, M.D.)*

Sequelae of Ileal Resection

The ileum is the site of bile salt reabsorption. When less than 100 cm of ileum has been resected, hepatic synthesis is adequate to replace the fraction of bile salts that escape reabsorption, and the size of the bile salt pool is preserved. Although steatorrhea usually does not result, a choleretic diarrhea does occur owing to the secretory effects of deconjugated bile salts on colonic mucosa. When more than 100 cm of ileum has been removed, bile salt losses usually become sufficient to diminish the size of the bile salt pool and impair intraluminal micelle formation. Both diarrhea and steatorrhea are common in this setting.

The treatment of diarrhea resulting from limited ileal resection is directed at binding bile salts in the intestinal lumen with cholestyramine resin in order to prevent their secondary effects on colonic mucosa. Limited amounts, 1 packet (4 gm cholestyramine) twice a day, or less, are usually sufficient to inhibit diarrhea. With more extensive ileal resection, the resultant steatorrhea is best treated by limitation of fat intake (40 gm a day fat diet) or the substitution of medium-chain triglycerides. The effect of cholestyramine is less predictable. Although preventing the secretory effects of unabsorbed bile salts on colonic mucosa, it may further decrease the availability of micelles and exacerbate steatorrhea.

Increased oxalate absorption and hyperoxaluria may occur in patients with extensive ileal disease or following ileal resection. Increased urinary levels of calcium oxalate predispose to calcium oxalate renal stone formation and recurrent nephrolithiasis. Following oral administration of an oxalate load, patients with ileal disease or resection have twice the urinary excretion of oxalate of normals. Oxalate is bound to calcium in the intestinal lumen. It is postulated that, in the presence of steatorrhea, luminal calcium is precipitated by excess fat in the stool, thereby making more free oxalate available for absorption. Normal excretion rates of oxalate in patients with ileostomies suggest that the colon is the site of absorption. In addition, experimental studies have demonstrated that the hydroxylated fatty acids and deconjugated bile salts that enter the colon in excessive amounts with ileal disease increase mucosal permeability and thereby facilitate oxalate absorption. Not all patients with steatorrhea are at risk for nephrolithiasis, however. Solubilizing substances, including citrate, magnesium, and sodium, are important in preventing renal stone formation. Patients with ileal disease, ileal resection, or jejunoileal bypass often have markedly decreased urinary excretion of citrate and magnesium, probably owing to malabsorption of these substances.

Treatment is directed toward decreasing urinary oxalate excretion or increasing urinary excretion of citrate and magnesium. A low oxalate diet may reduce hyperoxaluria, but since oxalate is ubiquitous in food, such a diet is often impractical. The best that can be done is to avoid high oxalate foods, such as tea, cocoa, chocolate, spinach, rhubarb, and beets. Supplemental oral calcium produces a fall in oxalate excretion, but patients need to be monitored for a corresponding increase in urinary calcium excretion. High doses of calcium are required, often in the range of 4 gm per day, before a decrease in urinary oxalate occurs. This treatment should be reserved for patients who have had recurrent calcium oxalate stones. Cholestyramine is effective in binding oxalate as well as bile salts, thereby reducing the amount of both available to the colon, but it may chelate vitamin K, folate, and other drugs. A low-fat diet limits the amount of intraluminal fatty acids in the colon. If hypocitraturia or hypomagnesemia is present, oral citrate or oral or parenteral magnesium should be administered.

Cholelithiasis occurs in 13 to 30 percent of patients with Crohn's disease, primarily those who have undergone extensive ileal resection. When diminished bile salt absorption exceeds the liver's synthetic capacity, hepatic bile salt secretion is diminished, and the biliary bile salt-cholesterol ratio is reduced. The bile may become supersaturated with cholesterol, which predisposes to cholelithiasis. A recent trial of ursodeoxycholic acid, which does not cause diarrhea and is absorbed passively in the proximal small intestine, was effective in unsaturating biliary bile in 6 patients with ileal resection. The drug, however, is still experimental, and long-term follow-up is not available.

VITAMIN DEFICIENCIES

Vitamin B_{12}

Vitamin B_{12} absorption occurs primarily in the ileum, and B_{12} malabsorption may be expected with resection of more than 100 cm of bowel. It is much less common with extensive ileal disease, presumably because mucosal involvement is variable enough to allow some absorption to occur. An abnormal Schilling test with added intrinsic factor defines B_{12} malabsorption due to ileal disease, assuming bacterial overgrowth is not present. Since body stores of vitamin B_{12} last 5 to 8 years, serum B_{12} levels are unreliable indicators of malabsorption. If malabsorption or deficiency is documented, monthly therapy with 100 μg of intramuscular vitamin B_{12} should be instituted. Improvement in an underlying inflammatory process in the ileum may correct B_{12} malabsorption.

Folate

Low serum folate levels occur in 60 percent of hospitalized patients with Crohn's disease, and low red cell folate levels in 25 to 35 percent. The incidence of megaloblastic anemia due to folate deficiency, however, is less than 20 percent. The overall incidence of folate deficiency and megaloblastic anemia in ambulatory patients with Crohn's disease is probably much lower.

Folate intake may be limited for a variety of reasons. Fruits and vegetables, rich dietary sources of folate, are often eliminated in a low-roughage diet. Anorexia commonly accompanies disease flares. A specific defect in mucosal folate transport has also been suggested. The drug, sulfasalazine, causes a 25 percent decrease in mean folate absorption in many patients. Since there appears to be an inverse correlation of folate deficiency with disease activity in hospitalized patients, an increased need for folate, perhaps related to cell turnover, probably also plays a role.

Patients with low fasting serum folate levels or with megaloblastic anemia due to folate deficiency should be treated with 5 mg of folate per day. Lesser doses are needed for maintenance. Patients receiving long-term sulfasalazine therapy should be screened for folate deficiency and appropriate folate replacement instituted if deficiency is present.

Vitamin A

Deficiency of vitamin A, a fat-soluble vitamin, may occur as a result of steatorrhea, although much less commonly than vitamin D deficiency. The major symptom is night blindness due to xerophthalmia. Rarely, keratomalacia may result in corneal destruction and blindness. In the gut, vitamin A deficiency leads to diminished mucus and glycocalyx production by goblet cells and epithelial cells, respectively. Diminished barrier function and increased absorption of potentially toxic macromolecules may be restored to normal by treatment with vitamin A (initially 100,000 units per day). Vitamin A levels should be checked even in the asymptomatic patient if significant steatorrhea is present.

Vitamin D

Deficiency of vitamin D usually parallels bile salt deficiency. The magnitude of vitamin D malabsorption tends to reflect the severity of steatorrhea and interference with the enterohepatic recycling of the fat-soluble forms of vitamin D. Reduced dietary intake of the vitamin plays only a minor role. Cholestyramine therapy may interfere with vitamin D absorption not only by worsening steatorrhea but also by binding vitamin D itself and reducing its enterohepatic circulation.

Osteomalacia and, less commonly, osteoporosis are consequences of vitamin D deficiency. A history of bone pain or the presence of osteopenia on X ray should prompt an evaluation of vitamin D and calcium status. Even in the absence of these clues, however, known severe ileal disease or extensive ileal resection should alert the physician to possible bone disease. Serum calcium, phosphorus, and alkaline phosphatase can be normal, even in the presence of significant bone disease. Twenty-four hour urine excretion of calcium may be low even in the asymptomatic patient and is, therefore, a helpful screening test. Bone densitometry is useful in demonstrating response to therapy, but is often normal even with significant disease. The most sensitive methods for detecting vitamin D deficiency are serum 25-OH vitamin D levels and bone biopsy. In patients with bone pain, demineralization noted on X ray examination, pathologic fractures, or abnormalities in serum calcium, phosphorus, or alkaline phosphatase, bone biopsy should be performed if the distinction between osteoporosis and osteomalacia cannot be made from the history or if the diagnosis is in doubt.

Replacement therapy with 50,000 units of oral ergocalciferol (D_2), once or twice a week, is usually adequate. Only rarely is parenteral vitamin D needed. Even patients with considerable steatorrhea respond to such large doses of oral vitamin D. Peak increases in 25-OH vitamin D_3 levels occur within one to three weeks, and levels should therefore be checked after three weeks of treatment. Oral 25-OHD_3 (calciferol) has the advantages of more rapid onset of action, shorter half-life, and better absorption in the presence of steatorrhea. Availability for routine use, however, is currently limited.

MINERAL DEFICIENCIES

Calcium

Abnormalities of calcium metabolism in patients with Crohn's disease most commonly result from hypomagnesemia, vitamin D deficiency, or steatorrhea-related formation of intraluminal calcium soaps. Sufficient calcium malabsorption to produce a negative calcium balance is infrequent in patients who have not undergone small bowel resection. When it does occur, it is usually in the presence of sizable enteric protein loss. In patients with hypocalcemia due to causes other than hypomagnesemia, supplementation with 1 to 1.5 gm of elemental calcium per day is adequate replacement. Serum calcium and 24-hour urine calcium should be measured six weeks after beginning supplements and then every six months once homeostasis has been achieved. Urine calcium levels between 100 and 300 mg per day should be sought. Vitamin D supplements should be included when 25-OH vitamin D levels are subnormal. If coexistent hypomagnesemia is present, this deficit should be corrected first, since magnesium is a required cofactor for parathormone action on bone. Normalization of magnesium levels may occasionally restore calcium levels to normal without supplemental calcium.

Magnesium

Hypomagnesemia in Crohn's disease is usually the consequence of diarrheal losses, whether the diarrhea is due to steatorrhea, fistula formation, or intestinal resection. Rarely, extensive Crohn's disease may result in magnesium malabsorption. Although magnesium is present primarily in the chlorophyll-containing foods that may be lacking in a low-residue diet, hypomagnesemia is rarely due to dietary deficiency alone. The mineralocorticoid effect of some corticosteroid medications promotes renal losses of magnesium, which may compound the effects of diarrheal losses.

Initial replacement therapy consists of intramuscular administration of 50 percent magnesium sulfate, 2 ml, three times a day, until the 24-hour urine magnesium has returned to normal (usually over 24 to 48 hours). Oral magnesium supplementation can be tried using magnesium chloride, 5 mEq/5 ml, 15 ml b.i.d. or t.i.d. This therapy may be accompanied by an unacceptable increase in diarrhea.

Zinc

Zinc absorption occurs primarily in the small intestine. In the rare zinc-deficient patient with Crohn's disease, zinc intake, as assessed by dietary history, is usually adequate. Malabsorption is assumed to be the major cause of deficiency. Total parenteral nutrition has been associated with zinc deficiency in the past, although most preparations now include zinc supplements.

Symptoms suggestive of zinc deficiency include acrodermatitis and taste impairment, especially of sweet substances. Zinc deficiency has been implicated in other complications of Crohn's disease, including anorexia, growth retardation, hypogonadism, impaired wound healing, and impaired cellular immunity, although the distinction between zinc deficiency and disease activity or other factors has not yet been determined. Serum zinc levels below 80 mcg/dl suggest zinc deficiency. Zinc may be orally supplemented with 220 mg of zinc sulfate PO t.i.d.

Iron

Iron deficiency in inflammatory bowel disease is usually the result of chronic blood loss from diseased areas of the small and large intestine. Bloody diarrhea is a common manifestation of disease activity in ulcerative colitis. In Crohn's disease, guaiac-positive stools are more commonly found in colonic disease, and the incidence of iron deficiency is therefore highest in this group, although blood loss can occur from any area involved with active disease. Major gastrointestinal hemorrhage due to Crohn's disease occurs in 6 to 12 percent of patients, primarily in the younger age group. Ferrous salts, 300 mg t.i.d., are usually adequate replacement.

MALABSORPTION IN THE SHORTENED BOWEL

The normal small intestine provides a surface area in excess of that needed for absorption, and so removal of limited segments is usually of no physiologic consequence. After resection of a major portion of small intestine, usually greater than 50 percent, clinical and metabolic effects become significant. The severity of these changes depends on the site of resection, the length and the function of remaining bowel, the presence or absence of the ileocecal valve, and the degree of intestinal adaptation after resection (Table 19-3).

Intestinal resections of the magnitude that result in short bowel syndrome are usually performed for small bowel infarction due to mesenteric vascular disease, volvulus, and strangulated internal or external hernias. Less commonly, they are done for Crohn's disease or trauma. At least two feet of jejunum or ileum are usually required to maintain adequate nutrition, although there are reports of long-term survival in patients with only six inches of remaining small intestine, in addition to the duodenum.

Pathophysiology

Resection of major segments of small intestine results in reduced surface area for nutrient absorption and shortens transit time. Luminal contents, therefore, may not mix adequately with pancreatic enzymes. If the nutrient stimulus to cholecystokinin (CCK) release is diminished because of decreased transit time, biliary and pancreatic secretions, which are in part controlled by CCK, may also be reduced. Although the duodenum and jejunum are the most active sites of iron, calcium, and magnesium absorption, the metabolic consequences of proximal resection are limited because of the ability of ileal epithelium to undergo hyperplasia. But since the ileum cannot take over the jejunum's function in the synthesis and release of secretin and CCK, decreased flow of pancreatic and biliary secretions may result in impaired lipolysis of dietary fat.

Loss of ileum has several specific metabolic consequences related to abnormalities in the transport of bile salts and vitamin B_{12}. These are discussed in detail in relation to intestinal resection for Crohn's disease (pp. 609–610). In brief, with shorter (less than 100 cm) ileal resections, unconjugated bile salts that have escaped reabsorption stimulate colonic secretion of water and sodium, causing a secretory diarrhea. Steatorrhea develops only with more extensive ileal resection, when so little surface area remains for bile salt reabsorption that enteric losses exceed the maximal rate of hepatic synthesis. Intraluminal bile salt concentrations are then inadequate for micelle formation. Fat malabsorption is accompanied by failure to absorb the fat-soluble vitamins, A, D, E, and K. Since vitamin D undergoes enterohepatic circulation independent of bile salts, deficiency of this vitamin is especially common after major ileal resection. Hydroxy-fatty acids, products of colonic bacterial metabolism of the unabsorbed fatty acids, impair colonic water reabsorption and contribute to the secretory diarrhea. Loss of the terminal ileum also results in vitamin B_{12} deficiency over several years as body stores are depleted. This process is accelerated if there is concomitant bacterial overgrowth, with intraluminal binding of B_{12} by bacteria.

The ileocecal valve functions as an anatomic barrier to colonic bacteria, helping to preserve the low bacterial count and the predominantly aerobic composition of ileal contents. Removal of the ileocecal valve can result in bacterial overgrowth, with its consequent steatorrhea and vitamin B_{12} malabsorption, even if much of the small bowel remains intact. Transit time is also prolonged by the intact valve, even with large segments of small bowel removed.

The colon functions as a reservoir for stool and the site of water and electrolyte reabsorption. Partial or total colectomy in the setting of small bowel resection may markedly exaggerate dehydration and electrolyte losses.

Gastric Hypersecretion

Gastric hypersecretion occurs in about 50 percent of patients after either proximal or distal small bowel resection. It begins within the first 24 hours following resection and diminishes after several weeks, although long-term changes in acid secretion have also been reported. The degree of hypersecretion is roughly proportional to the length of small intestine resected. The precise mechanism is obscure, although several possibilities have been suggested. High acid output may reflect diminished levels of secretin, CCK, VIP, serotonin, and GIP, all of which are products of small intestinal mucosa and inhibit gastric acid secretion. Elevated gastrin levels have also been documented, both in the fasting state and in response to a gastrointestinal test meal. Whether this increase in gastrin is due to altered gastrin catabolism or removal of inhibitory hormones is not clear. Since acid secretion in response to exogenous histamine or gastrin is unaffected by small intestinal resection, alterations in parietal cell function probably play no role. The primary stimulus appears to be the response to feeding.

This hypersecretory state may worsen steatorrhea and diarrhea, for reasons much the same as those that obtain in the Zollinger-Ellison syndrome. The lowered small intestinal pH inactivates pancreatic lipase. The excess amount of gastric juice results in an increased volume load. Peptic ulceration in the duodenum or small bowel is theoretically possible, but has rarely been documented.

Intestinal Adaptation

After small intestinal resection, absorption of a variety of nutrients improves over a period of several months following surgery, and this improvement is related to adaptive changes in the remaining small bowel. Data, derived primarily from animal studies, have shown that compensatory growth occurs in all layers of the bowel wall, with hyperplasia of villi predominating. Dilatation and lengthening of the intestine grossly correspond to increases in villous height and crypt depth. The number of cells per unit length of villus is unchanged, and the cell populations of villus and crypt are increased, suggesting that hyperplasia rather than hypertrophy is the mechanism whereby adaptation occurs. The total number of remaining villi may be increased or remain the same, and crypt number is constant. Hyperplastic changes in ileal mucosa begin as early as 48 hours after jejunectomy and reach a peak one to two weeks postoperatively. In humans, intestinal response is slower and may not reach its final state for as long as a year. Dilatation and lengthening of the intestine have been noted radiologically, although increases in villous height have not been documented. The degree of intestinal adaptation is greater after jejunal than after ileal resection. When combined with the specialized ileal absorptive functions, this may explain why proximal resections are usually better tolerated than distal ones. The rate of hyperplasia is maximal nearest the anastomosis.

Studies in laboratory animals after resections have demonstrated that, for a given length of intestine, there is enhanced uptake of monosaccharides, disaccharides, water, electrolytes, calcium, and amino acids, as well as bile acids and vitamin B_{12}. Accelerated jejunal absorption of bile acids occurs by passive diffusion, whereas higher rates of ileal absorption probably represent an accelerated rate of active transport. Enhanced carbohydrate and amino acid absorption appears to be related to the greater cell number rather than to improved absorption or increased disaccharidase or dipeptidase activity of each individual cell.

Although the overall intensity of adaptation in laboratory animals is directly proportional to the amount of intestine resected, in man, epithelial cell hyperplasia usually occurs only after extensive (75 to 80 percent) small bowel resection. Cellular hyperplasia has not been demonstrated with resections of 50 percent or less. Increased segmental absorption of glucose, water, and electrolytes following enterectomy does occur and corresponds to the improvement in weight and nutritional status that usually follows several months after surgery.

The factors responsible for these beneficial adaptive changes include luminal chyme, pancreatic and biliary secretions, and as yet unidentified humoral factors. Exogenous nutrients within the bowel lumen are required for cellular hyperplasia to occur, since no functional or morphologic adaptive changes occur in dogs or rats who receive only parenteral nutrition following intestinal resection. Epithelial hypoplasia occurs in the bypassed segment of bowel following jejunoileal bypass surgery and may be completely reversed by the instillation of intraluminal amino acids. This effect of chyme may account for the maximal stimulation of adaptation that occurs adjacent to the anastomosis. Since non-nutritive substances increase cell proliferation in bypassed loops of bowel, mechanical stimulation may also play a part.

Endogenous intraluminal substances are also important in promoting epithelial cell hyperplasia after intestinal resection. With proximal resection, the ileal mucosa is closer to the stomach and duodenum and, therefore, exposed to higher concentrations of gastric, duodenal, and pancreaticobiliary secretions. These have all been shown to increase villous size, with pancreaticobiliary secretions having the strongest influence. If the secretions are diverted from the proximal to the mid portion of the small intestine, distal hyperplasia results. Intestinal hypoplasia during parenteral alimentation is, therefore, probably the result of absence of luminal food and of the endogenous secretions stimulated by chyme.

The contribution of humoral factors to intestinal adaptation is supported by vascular parabiosis experiments in which villous hyperplasia occurs in the unoperated partners of animals subjected to enterectomy. Similarly, in Thiry-Vella fistulas of jejunum and ileum, hyperplasia occurs in all segments, although the greatest effects are in those segments in continuity.

Various enterotropic hormones have been suggested, including gastrin, glucagon, prolactin, mineralocorticoids, and pituitary hormones. Evidence for their specific contributions is equivocal.

Management

During the immediate postoperative period, problems with massive fluid and electrolyte shifts predominate. Most patients who have undergone a greater than 50 percent resection will require parenteral alimentation. Since the slow process of intestinal adaptation requires the stimulus of luminal nutrients, oral feedings should be initiated as soon as bowel motility resumes, usually during the second postoperative week. Depending on the extent of resection, complete oral nutrition may not be possible for several months. Initiation of oral feeding is best accomplished with diets that are lactose-free and low in long-chain triglycerides, yet include all essential nutrients. Medium-chain triglycerides, which do not require enzymatic digestion but are absorbed directly via the portal vein, may be added for their caloric effect. In severe cases, such elemental diets should usually be given in a diluted form and as a continuous

Table 19-4. *Suggested Vitamin and Mineral Supplements in Short Bowel Syndrome*

Supplement	Dosage
Fat-soluble vitamins	
Vitamin A	Oral: 25,000 units/tablets. 100,000–200,000 units/day in severe deficiency. Maintenance: 5,000–50,000 units/day. Monitor serum vitamin A levels.
Vitamin D	Oral: 50,000 units vitamin D_2 2–3×/week. 25-OH vitamin D 50–100 μg/day. Intramuscular: 100,000 units/month vitamin D_2. Dosage should be adjusted to maintain serum calcium in normal range and urine calcium excretion of 100–300 mg/24 hours.
Vitamin K	Oral: vitamin K_1 (Mephyton) 10 mg/day; or vitamin K_2 (Menadione) 4–12 mg/day. Intramuscular: vitamin K_1 10 mg/day. Intravenous: vitamin K_1 5–25 mg. Give slowly over 10–15 min.
Folic Acid	Initial therapy: 5 mg PO per day for 4–5 weeks. Maintenance: 100 μg/month IM.
Vitamin B_{12}	Initial therapy: cyanocobalamin 1000 μg/day IM for one week. Maintenance: 1000 μg/month IM.
Vitamin B complex	Multivitamin preparations containing thiamine 1.6 mg, riboflavin 1.8 mg, niacin 20 mg should be administered bid.
Calcium	Oral: 1–1.5 gm/day of elemental calcium as calcium gluconate 40 mg/500 mg tab.; or calcium carbonate as Titralac (400 mg Ca/5 ml) or OsCal (250 mg Ca/tablet; also contains 400 Units vitamin D_2/tablet). Intravenous: calcium gluconate injection, USP 10% solution, 10–30 ml administered slowly over 15–30 min, followed by IV drip of calcium gluconate (600–800 mg Ca/L) until serum calcium stabilizes with oral supplements.
Magnesium	Oral: magnesium chloride 500 mg (5 mEq/5 ml) 15 ml tid.; or magnesium gluconate tablets 500 mg (25 mg of magnesium) qid. Intramuscular: magnesium sulfate (20% solution) 10 ml bid. or tid.; or (50% solution) 2 ml bid. or tid. Intravenous: magnesium sulfate 0.5% solution. Maximum rate 1 mEq/min; maximum volume 1000 ml/24 hrs.
Iron	Oral: ferrous gluconate 300–600 mg tid.; or ferrous sulfate 320 mg tid. or qid. Intramuscular: Imferon. See drug package insert or PDR to calculate dosage based on hemoglobin. Intravenous: same as intramuscular.

infusion. Later, they may be tolerated at full osmolarity or in the form of multiple small meals.*

Diarrhea is common during this period and has several etiologies. The gastric hypersecretion that occurs within the first week presents a significant volume load to the gut. It can be effectively controlled by the administration of cimetidine and anticholinergics. Steatorrhea is an important cause of diarrhea, and stool fat losses should be quantitated early on. If significant, dietary intake should be limited to 30 gm or less of fat per day. For patients with an intact gallbladder to serve as a reservoir, low-fat diets may also decrease bile secretion and bile acid-mediated colonic irritation. When ileal resection of more than 100 cm has resulted in bile salt depletion, medium-chain

* *Editor's Note:* My own practice is to allow a mechanically soft diet with solid food. This is as well tolerated, or better, than various defined diets.

triglycerides may need to be substituted for long-chain fatty acids. When less than 100 cm of ileum has been removed, cholestyramine (4 to 8 gm per day) may be adequate to control diarrhea by binding excess bile salts. Since rapid transit may cause inadequate mixing of food with endogenous pancreatic enzymes, pancreatic supplements may help to limit the amount of steatorrhea. If the ileocecal valve has been resected, bacterial overgrowth should be sought by appropriate tests.

Although carbohydrate malabsorption is usually not a significant nutritional problem, after large jejunal resections, mucosal disaccharidase reduction may lead to diarrhea when lactose and other disaccharidases are ingested in any quantity.

Specific deficiencies of vitamins and minerals have been discussed in detail in the section on inflammatory bowel disease (pp. 610–612) and are only summarized here. Appropriate replacement therapy is listed in Table 19-4. The consequences of ileal resection include vitamin B_{12} and bile salt deficiency, and the latter in turn leads to steatorrhea, and vitamin D and calcium decreases. Ileal resection predisposes the patient to hyperoxaluria and urinary calculi as well as to cholelithiasis (pp. 608–609). Calcium and magnesium losses in the stool due to diarrhea further compound these metabolic abnormalities. Water-soluble vitamins, including folic acid and vitamin C, are absorbed along the entire length of jejunum and ileum and, therefore, are rarely deficient unless less than four feet of jejunum remains. As mentioned, parenteral vitamin B_{12} is usually required when more than 6 feet of terminal ileum has been removed. Duodenal resection often requires the administration of oral and sometimes parenteral iron supplements.

BIBLIOGRAPHY

Malabsorption in Liver Disease

Badley, B. W. D., Murphy, G. M., Bouchier, I. A. D., et al. Diminished micellar phase lipid in patients with chronic nonalcoholic liver disease and steatorrhea. *Gastroenterology* 58:781, 1970.

Halstead, C. H., Robles, E. A., and Mezey, E. Intestinal malabsorption in folate-deficient alcoholics. *Gastroenterology* 64:526, 1973.

Mezey, E. Liver disease and nutrition. *Gastroenterology* 74:770, 1978.

Mezey, E. Intestinal function in chronic alcoholism. *Ann. N.Y. Acad. Sci.* 252:215, 1975.

Pitchumoni, C. S., and Jerzy Glass, G. B. Alcohol injury to gastrointestinal mucosa. In G. B. Jerzy Glass (Ed.), *Progress in Gastroenterology,* New York: Grune and Stratton, 1977. Vol. III, pp. 717–758.

Pancreatic Insufficiency

DiMagno, E. P. Medical treatment of pancreatic insufficiency. *Mayo Clin. Proc.* 54:435, 1979.

DiMagno, E. P., Malagelada, J. R., Go, V. L. W., et al. Fate of orally ingested enzymes in pancreatic insufficiency. *N. Engl. J. Med.* 296:1318, 1977.

Graham, D. Y. Enzyme replacement therapy of exocrine pancreatic insufficiency in man. *N. Engl. J. Med.* 296:1314, 1977.

Graham, D. Y. An enteric-coated pancreatic enzyme preparation that works. *Dig. Dis. Sci.* 24:906, 1979.

Regan, P. T., Malagelada, J. R., DiMagno, E. P., et al. Comparative effects of antacids, cimetidine, and enteric coating on the therapeutic response to oral enzymes in severe pancreatic insufficiency. *N. Engl. J. Med.* 297:854, 1977.

Postgastrectomy Malabsorption

Eddy, R. L. Metabolic bone disease after gastrectomy. *Am. J. Med.* 50:442, 1971.

Fromm, D. Weight loss. In *Complications of Gastric Surgery.* New York: Wiley, 1977. Pp. 50–66.

MacGregor, I., Parent, J., and Meyer, J. H. Gastric emptying of liquid meals and pancreatic and biliary secretion after subtotal gastrectomy or truncal vagotomy and pyloroplasty in man. *Gastroenterology* 72:195, 1977.

Meyer, J. H. Chronic morbidity after ulcer surgery. In M. H. Sleissenger and J. S. Fordtran (Eds.), *Gastrointestinal Disease,* 2nd ed. Philadelphia: Saunders, 1978. Pp. 947–969.

Pryor, J. P., O'Shea, M. J., Brooks, P. L., et al. The long-term metabolic consequences of partial gastrectomy. *Am. J. Med.* 51:5, 1971.

Bacterial Overgrowth

Banwell, J. G., Kistler, L. A., Giannella, R. A., Weber, F. L., Lieber, A., and Powell, D. E. Small intestinal

bacterial overgrowth syndrome. *Gastroenterology* 80:834, 1981.
Gorbach, S. L. Intestinal microflora. *Gastroenterology* 60:1110, 1971.
Gracey, M. The contaminated small bowel syndrome: Pathogenesis, diagnosis, and treatment. *Am. J. Clin. Nutr.* 32:234, 1979.
Greenlee, H. G., Gelbart, S. M., DeOrio, A. J., Francescatti, D. S., Paez, J., and Reinhardt, G. F. The influence of gastric surgery on the intestinal flora. *Am. J. Clin. Nutr.* 30:1826, 1977.
Isaacs, P. E. T., and Kim, Y. S. The contaminated small bowel syndrome. *Am. J. Med.* 67:1049, 1979.
King, C. E., and Toskes, P. P. Small intestine bacterial overgrowth. *Gastroenterology* 76:1035, 1979.

Inflammatory Bowel Disease

Dobbins, J. W. Oxalate and intestinal disease. *J. Clin. Gastroenterol.* 1:165, 1979.
Gelts, D. G., Grand, R. J., Shen, G., Watkins, J. B., Werlin, S. L., and Boehme, C. Nutritional basis of growth failure in children and adolescents with Crohn's disease. *Gastroenterology* 76:720, 1979.
Gerson, C. D., Cohen, N., and Janowitz, H. D. Small intestinal absorptive function in regional enteritis. *Gastroenterology* 64:907, 1973.
Kirshner, B. S., Voinchet, O., and Rosenberg, I. H. Growth retardation in inflammatory bowel disease. *Gastroenterology* 75:504, 1978.
Krawitt, E. L., Beeken, W. L., and Janney, C. D. Calcium absorption in Crohn's disease. *Gastroenterology* 71:251, 1976.
Sitrin, M., Meredith, S., and Rosenberg, I. H. Vitamin D deficiency and bone disease in gastrointestinal disorders. *Arch. Intern. Med.* 138:886, 1978.

Short Bowel Syndrome

Dowling, R. H., Bell, G. D., and White, J. Lithogenic bile in patients with ileal dysfunction. *Gut* 13:415, 1972.
Tilson, M. D. Pathophysiology and treatment of short bowel syndrome. *Surg. Clin. North Am.* 60:1273, 1980.
Weser, E. The management of patients after small bowel resection. *Gastroenterology* 71:146, 1976.
Weser, E., Fletcher, J. T., and Urban, E. Short bowel syndrome. *Gastroenterology* 77:572, 1979.
Williamson, R. C. N. Intestinal adaptation. *N. Engl. J. Med.* 298:1393, 1444, 1978.

Nutrition and the Heart

Ronald M. Abel

20

When examining the possible effects of nutritional disorders on the heart, there are three important parts of this subject to be considered. One may consider the effects of changing nutritional status on the heart as an end organ, which must subsist on nutrient substrates supplied via its circulation similar to other organs of the body. Second, since the heart must function continually in order to maintain life, one may also ask what effects a certain degree of impairment of cardiac function would exert on the general nutritional status of the body. Finally, the clinical consequences of these areas of inquiry must be examined.

NUTRITION AND ATHEROGENESIS IN CORONARY HEART DISEASE

In developed nations, primarily in the Western World, the most widely publicized nutritional influence on heart disease is the effect of diet on the development of arteriosclerosis. Since the effects of diet and drug therapy on serum concentrations of cholesterol and other lipids is a vast subject in itself, we will not deal with the nutritional factors leading to this arterial disease in this chapter. The effects of coronary arteriosclerosis on cardiac structure and function are only *secondary* to the myocardial ischemia that results from inadequate delivery of oxygen-containing coronary blood flow through stenotic coronary arteries. The cardiomyopathy associated with coronary heart disease, so-called "ischemic cardiomyopathy," is not a primary cardiomyopathy in and of itself, but is rather an indirect effect of multiple areas of myocardial infarction with subsequent fibrosis. This myocardial disorder, once established, is probably unaffected by specific changes in diet.

THE HEART AS A "SPARED ORGAN"

Until recently, it was common knowledge in clinical cardiology that the heart was in some way "special" and did not suffer adversely from the untoward effects of starvation. Voit [95] is responsible for the initiation of this myth when, in 1866, he reported the results of an experiment involving only two cats, one of which was starved for 13 days and whose heart weighed only a bit less than the heart of the other cat, which was fed a normal diet. This uncontrolled and inadequately designed "scientific conclusion" was handed down from textbook to textbook of physiology, claiming that the heart is resistant to the effects of malnutrition. Using teleologic reasoning, this "wisdom of nature" principle that vital organs needed to be protected from the effects of starvation [37, 40] seemed quite reassuring to those who noted that the heart seemed to continue to pump adequately despite the ravages of end-stage undernutrition. Vasquez indicated that "inanition has no harmful effect on the heart" [96]. It was not until the inadvertent (and a few intentional) "prospective clinical studies" involving human starvation in the Nazi concentration camps during World War II that it became increasingly obvious that the heart, like other viscera, was subject to atrophy, fibrosis, and weakness associated with inadequate delivery of nutrient substrates. Since the publication of those reports and the addition of scientific inquiries (see the following) into the relationship between starvation and cardiac structure and function, it is now apparent that the heart may indeed be quite sensitive to nutritional inadequacies. In the discussions that follow, the effects of nutrient insufficiencies and excesses will be examined. The effects of undernutrition on clinical heart disease and schemes for correcting nutritional disorders in such patients will also be presented.

STARVATION AND THE HEART

Absolute starvation and even semi-starvation generally result in a clinical syndrome of protein-calorie undernutrition, whereas specific deprivation of protein intake, as would occur because of poverty, frequently results in a pure protein deficiency.

Until the last quarter century, the dictum that "death from starvation is death from pneumonia" dominated the interpretation of the autopsy examinations of patients dying from malnutrition. Since sepsis, primarily pulmonary, was identified in the vast majority of patients dying from starvation [35], there was no specific need to incriminate cardiac impairment as a direct cause of death in such patients. When analyzing data from individuals who died during the Warsaw Ghetto uprising, however, Follis reported cardiac atrophy in those who died during the starved state [38]. He observed that the average heart weight was only 220 to 275 grams and noted "brown atrophy" with loss of epicardial fat, particularly along the interventricular and atrioventricular grooves [69]. In a classic series of experiments on normal volunteers, Keys and coworkers [59] prospectively studied the precise effects of starvation and semi-starvation in man. He subjected individuals to hypocaloric diets, which resulted in the loss of approximately 25 percent of initial body weight within six months; the patients then received a suitable period of nutritional rehabilitation. They noted a decrease in heart size in all dimensions, and the hearts assumed more of a vertical position in the chest following weight loss. Arterial and venous pressure fell, and heart rate frequently diminished to extreme levels of bradycardia. The bradycardia associated with starvation was suggested (teleologically) to represent a valuable protective mechanisms, which paralleled the decrease in basal energy expenditure of starvation. An attempt to provide too rapid a nutritional repletion frequently resulted in early signs of congestive heart failure during the rehabilitative phase of these experiments [34].

Several investigators have confirmed that total protein-calorie deprivation may cause myocardial atrophy [11, 13, 41, 42, 43, 54, 78]. Gelfand et al. [42] discussed the development of "microcardia" resulting from malnutrition in a group of patients in whom tropical sprue played an important factor in the development, and later the maintenance, of malnutrition.

More recently, there has also been a growing and unfortunate experience with self-induced marasmus. Garnett et al. [41] reported the sudden and unexpected death in an otherwise healthy, but morbidly obese, young woman subjected to 30 weeks of therapeutic, total starvation to obtain rapid weight reduction. Cardiac death occurred as a result of refractory ventricular fibrillation. Normal serum potassium and calcium concentrations were present, although it is quite conceivable that total body electrolyte imbalances also existed. Autopsy examination revealed a dilated, atrophied heart weighing only 250 grams; ultrastructural examination confirmed the presence of atrophy and destruction of myofibrils.

A recent disastrous chapter in the history of weight reduction therapy was closed after the death of at least 58 young women ingesting so-called "liquid protein diets" in the United States during 1977 [32, 39]. In an attempt to control morbid obesity by limiting all nutrient intake to commercial products containing protein of dubious biologic value with no additional supplemental calories, these women developed sudden cardiac death without prior evidence of heart disease. Although these products were officially marketed to serve as "dietary supplements," they were clearly misused and abused by serving as the sole nutrient source and, hence, effecting a placebo-type of therapeutic benefit, which was not as easily obtained by the usual severe hypocaloric restrictions with ordinary foods. Although this type of therapy for morbid obesity had been used under carefully controlled clinical conditions with some success [17, 18], the uncontrolled and unregulated induction of acute starvation by these patients resulted in serious cardiac effects. Although many of the terminal arrhythmias (primarily ventricular tachycardia and fibrillation, which were unresponsive to ordinary therapeutic endeavors), could have been associated with electrolyte abnormalities, there were a number of deaths documented in which electrolyte patterns appeared normal [72]. The deaths almost certainly resulted from acute starvation and not from any toxic effects of the "liquid protein diets" on the myocardium itself. The autopsy material from this group of patients confirmed the presence of myocardial atrophy [82]. It has been suggested that the syndrome of QT prolongation may have resulted from a deficiency of certain trace elements not determined by routine clinical testing, but which may result following prolonged exposure to liquid protein diet [97].

We [3, 6] became interested in examining a laboratory model whose similarity to human protein-calorie malnutrition would permit precise measurements of cardiac structure and function on a controlled basis. In an attempt to prepare a suitable experimental animal model of protein-calorie malnutrition, several obstacles had to be overcome. It was clear that to obtain a detailed evaluation of starved myocardium, requiring hemodynamic, biochemical and morphologic assessments, we were required to perform terminal, invasive assessments of cardiac structure and function, thereby precluding the use of each animal as its own control. Accordingly, we took 25 pure-bred beagle dogs, heartworm-free, averaging one year of age, and following a suitable period of observation to ensure the absence of nutritional and other diseases, 17 of the animals were subjected to a hypocaloric, nitrogen-poor diet for an average of 50 days (range 35 to 60). The remaining 8 dogs served as controls and were fed an ordinary maintenance diet until the time of hemodynamic evaluation.

The dogs subjected to protein-calorie malnutrition were fed a diet prepared by mixing bovine liver extract, a multivitamin canine preparation, and an electrolyte mixture with agar so that the bulky diet produced satiety following feeding, yet the overall diet yielded no more than 8 to 9 grams of protein (1 to 1½ gm nitrogen) and approximately 50 to 60 kcal each 24 hours.

Following the loss of "adequate amounts" of weight to obtain protein-calorie malnutrition, six of the animals (designated "refed") were then given ordinary diets for an additional month, so that they regained all of the weight loss. Terminal biochemical, hemodynamic, and structural assessments were then obtained.

At the time of evaluation, all animals were anesthetized with morphine and alpha chloralose. The hemodynamic model used was the isovolumetric left heart preparation on total cardiopulmonary bypass (Figure 20-1). Briefly, using an extracorporeal circuit primed with freshly heparinized, homologous blood, variables of altering heart rate and aortic pressure were eliminated, and precise indices of left ventricular (LV) contractility were determined by measuring instan-

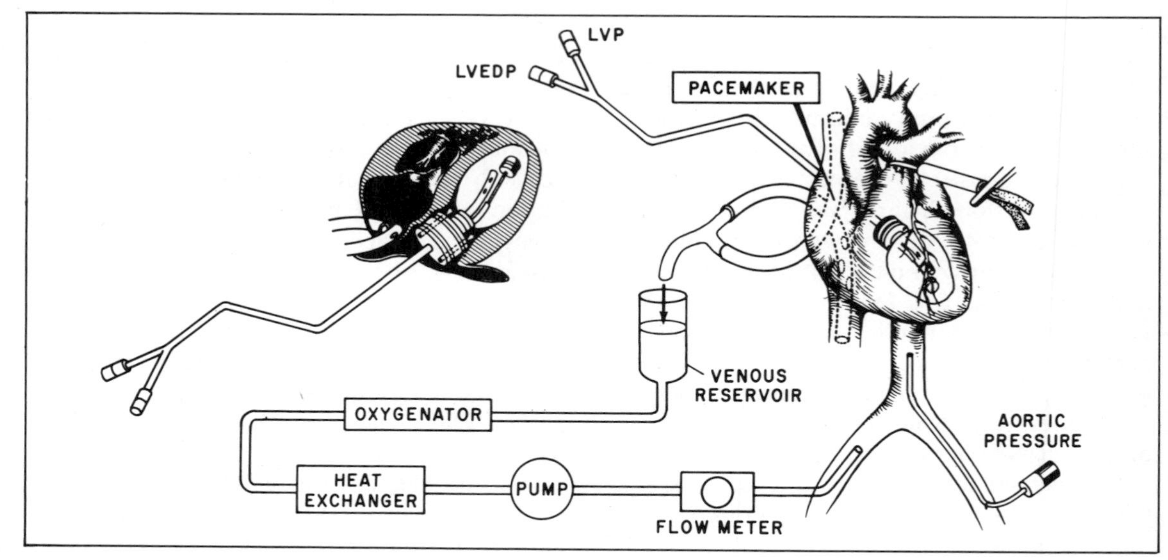

Figure 20-1. *Schematic representation of the preparation used to obtain isovolumetric LV contractions in controls and in dogs with protein-calorie malnutrition. (From Abel, R. M., et al. Adverse hemodynamic and ultrastructural changes in dog hearts subjected to protein-calorie malnutrition.* Am. Heart J. *97:733, 1979.)*

taneous changes in peak LV systolic pressure and the first derivative of LV pressure (LV dp/dt), to obtain the force-velocity and length-tension relations of the left ventricle. Furthermore, changes in LV compliance could be determined by examining the instantaneous relationship between the volume of saline placed in an intraventricular balloon and the LV end-diastolic pressure. Full-thickness biopsies of the right ventricle were examined for protein, water, glycogen, glucose, and amino acid content. Ultrastructural evaluation was performed by examining left and right ventricular myocardial specimens by routine light and electron microscopy.

The results indicated that the canine model, as described, was a reproducible and consistent one, with little individual variation from dog to dog (Table 20-1). The average weight loss in the protein-calorie malnutrition group was 42.1 ± 0.9 percent of initial body weight. The refed animals lost 40.7 ± 5.3 percent of initial body weight prior to refeeding and regained up to 106 percent initial body weight an average of 28.3 ± 2.8 days following refeeding with an ordinary diet [7].

There was a marked reduction in myocardial glycogen content in dogs subjected to protein-calorie malnutrition compared with controls (Table 20-1). Following refeeding, average myocardial glycogen concentrations were 126.4 ± 7.6 μmole/gm of dry tissue, which was not different from the control group, but significantly greater (Table 20-1) than those of malnourished animals ($p < 0.005$). There was a relative *increase* in protein concentration in malnourished hearts compared with those of controls, although this was apparent only when expressed in terms of dry weight, presumably owing to a decrease in nonprotein substrates, such as glycogen. The hearts were grossly edematous, as reflected by the increase in the wet/dry ratio (Table 20-1). Although the hearts were obviously atrophied as evidenced by a decrease in LV weight in malnourished dogs compared with controls, in the six refed animals, LV weight averaged 59.3 ± 4.6 gm, which was not significantly different from that in the control animals.

The hemodynamic changes (Table 20-2) included persistent and significant depression of LV function in dogs with protein-calorie malnu-

Table 20-1. *Total Body and Myocardial Composition Changes in Canine Protein-Calorie Malnutrition*

	Total Body				Left Ventricular Myocardium				
	Number of Experiments	Weight (kg) Initial	Weight (kg) Final	Weight Loss (%)	Weight (gm)	Glycogen (μmoles/gm dry wt.)	Protein (mg/gm dry wt.)	Glucose (μmoles/gm tissue)	Wet/Dry[a]
I Controls	8	11.8 ± 0.2[b]			66.5±1.3	135±6.9	581.2±30.8	5.13±0.87	4.75±0.13
II Protein-calorie malnutrition	11	11.7±0.3	6.8±0.2	42.1±0.9	47.5±1.4	58.6±10.5	714.7±17.5	4.38±0.95	5.72±0.21
Significance[c]		NS[d]			$p < 0.005$	$p < 0.005$	$p < 0.0025$	NS[d]	$p < 0.0025$

[a]Wet/Dry = wet weight divided by dry weight
[b]Mean standard error of the mean
[c]I vs II; Student's t-test for unpaired data
[d]NS = not significant
Source: R. M. Abel et al. Adverse hemodynamics and ultrastructural changes in dog hearts subjected to protein-calorie malnutrition. *Am. Heart J.* 97:733, 1979.

Table 20-2. *Hemodynamic Effects of Protein-Calorie Malnutrition at Increasing LV Intracavitary Volumes*

	Control (n = 8)			Protein-Calorie Malnutrition (n = 11)		
LV Volume (ml)	Peak LV Pressure (mm Hg)	LVEDP (mm Hg)	LV dp/dt max (mm Hg/sec)	Peak LV Pressure	LVEDP	LV dp/dt
3	99.1 ± 9.4*	0	2142 ± 359	80.8 ± 11.9 (NS)	3.5 ± 0.5 (NS)	1459 ± 225 (NS)
6	149.4 ± 9.0	1.6 ± 0.8	2687 ± 266	118.0 ± 11.2 ($p < 0.05$)	14.5 ± 7.2 (NS)	1986 ± 260 ($p < 0.05$)
9	168.7 ± 9.7	4.9 ± 1.7	3337 ± 318	148.5 ± 11.5 (NS)	25.4 ± 7.1 ($p < 0.01$)	2441 ± 308 ($p < 0.05$)
12	179.6 ± 4.7	10.6 ± 2.8	3492 ± 266	168.9 ± 11.8 (NS)	33.3 ± 4.5 ($p < 0.005$)	2733 ± 340 (NS)
15	191.0 ± 4.5	20.7 ± 3.5	3929 ± 594	176.8 ± 10.6 (NS)	39.0 ± 4.2 ($p < 0.0025$)	2980 ± 403 (NS)
18	188.7 ± 3.8	27.8 ± 3.8	3751 ± 392	174.5 ± 8.5 (NS)	42.3 ± 4.2 ($p < 0.01$)	2688 ± 295 ($p < 0.025$)
21	190.3 ± 4.4	35.0 ± 3.8	3338 ± 291	179.0 ± 7.5	46.9 ± 4.8	2699 ± 295 (NS)

NS = Not significant
*Standard error of the mean
Source: R. M. Abel et al. Adverse hemodynamic and ultrastructural changes in dog hearts subjected to protein-calorie malnutrition. *Am. Heart J.*, 97:733, 1979.

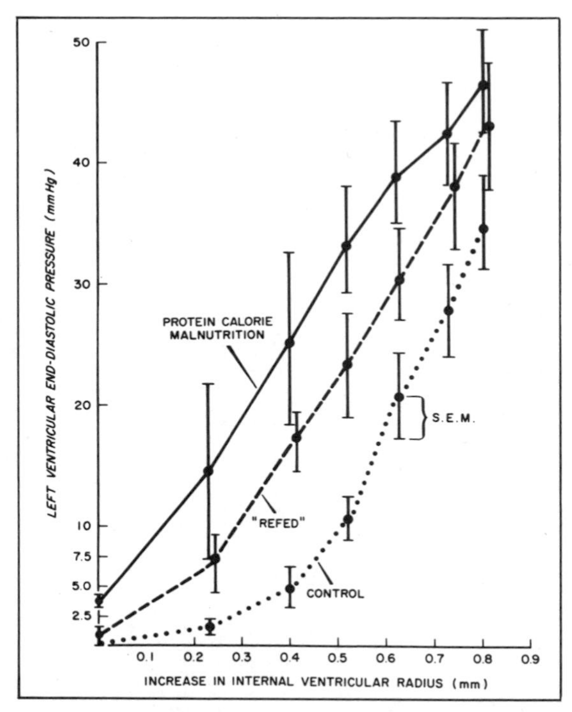

Figure 20-2. *Diastolic compliance relations in all animals. The significant increase in LV stiffness in protein-calorie malnutrition is incompletely reversed in the refed dogs.*

trition. This diminished inotropic state was reflected as a decrease in peak LV systolic pressure and a decreased LV dp/dt at similar LV volumes, compared with controls. A decrease in LV compliance (Figure 20-2) was observed in malnourished animals compared with controls; refed animals demonstrated some improvement in this decreased compliance, but did not return to control values.

Two basic histologic changes were observed in malnourished animals: myocardial atrophy and interstitial edema (Figure 20-3A, B). This impression was confirmed by direct measurement of mean myofiber diameter $24.1 \pm 0.5\ \mu$ compared with a diameter of $30.4 \pm 0.4\ \mu$ in control animals ($p < 0.001$).

We concluded that the short-term induction of protein-calorie malnutrition resulted not only in the "starvation edema" of generalized hypoproteinemia, but also in myocardial atrophy. The functional correlate of the myocardial edema was an increase in LV stiffness. The myocardial atrophy was presumably associated with the decrease in contractility. Following a short-term nutritional convalescence, refed animals demonstrated persistent abnormalities of LV function, including decreases in LV compliance and in maximum developed LV dp/dt.*

Whether adverse effects caused by undernutrition will prove to be entirely reversible following a more prolonged period of nutritional convalescence is unknown. It is also uncertain whether the results in these animal studies pertain to human disease states.

An additional hemodynamic observation was made during these studies [6, 7], when we chose to compare the force-velocity relationship of the left ventricle in protein-calorie malnutrition with that of normal animals (Figure 20-4). Since the calculation of LV wall force (tension) is dependent on the LV weight, peak systolic LV force is actually *greater* in the malnourished dogs for any given identical pressure because of the LaPlace equation [51], where $F = P \pi r^2$ and F = force, P = LV pressure, and R is the radius of the spheroid model utilized for the calculations and based upon the LV mass [26, 27, 65, 93].

Since peak LV wall tension is one of the major determinants of myocardial oxygen consumption [45], it is interesting to hypothesize that if such a mechanism is of clinical significance, relatively greater oxygen demands would exist in patients with ischemic heart disease who begin to suffer from concomitant malnutrition. That is, at a given availability of coronary blood flow through fixed coronary arterial stenoses, greater oxygen consumption would be anticipated from an atrophied left ventricle producing the same systolic pressure as in a normally nourished patient, assuming no other changes.

The mechanism by which the heart may undergo starvation-induced atrophy has been recently studied. Wildenthal and coworkers [101] noted significant increases in myocardial lysosomal en-

**Editor's Note:* These findings may explain the difficulty most clinicians have had in reversing cardiac cachexia with nutritional support.

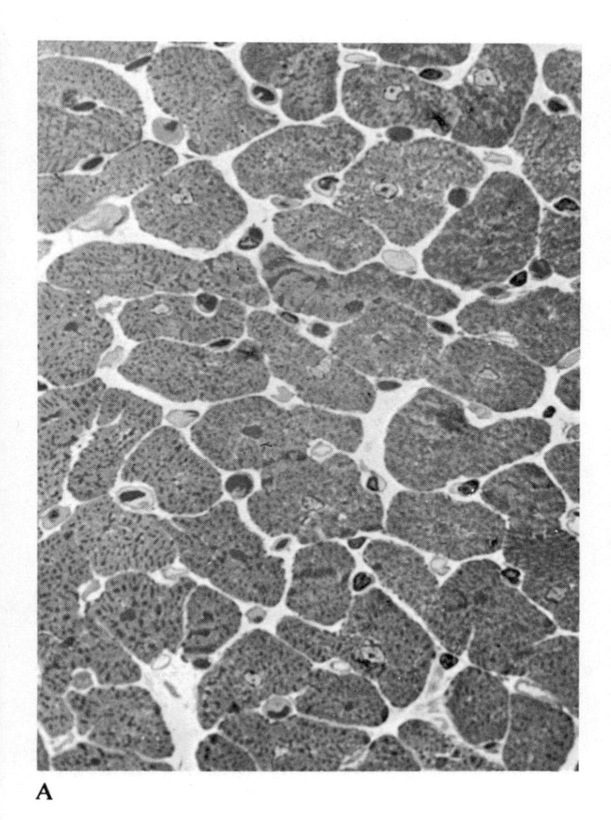

A

B

Figure 20-3. A, *Normal appearance of myofibers in control dogs (Epon-embedded section stained with Toluidine Blue, 385×).* B, *Biopsy of right ventricular myocardium in dog with protein-calorie malnutrition. In comparison to the control myocardium, there is marked interstitial edema and moderate cell atrophy (Epon-embedded section stained with Toluidine Blue, 385×). (From Abel, R. M. et al. Adverse hemodynamic and ultrastructural changes in dog hearts subjected to protein-calorie malnutrition.* Am. Heart J. *97:733, 1979.)*

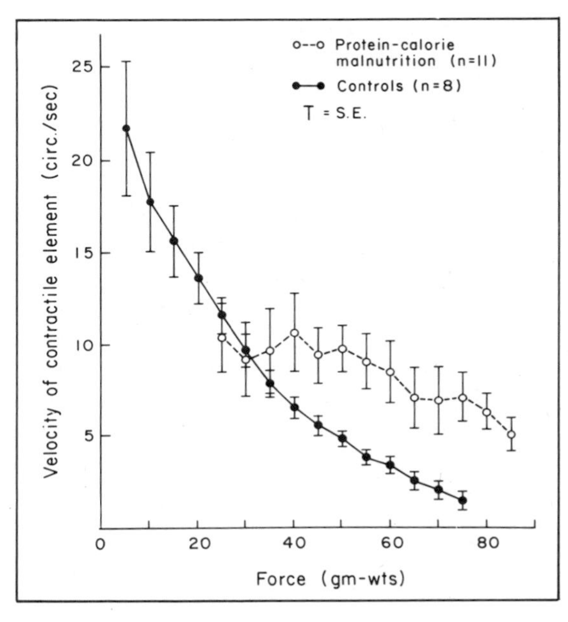

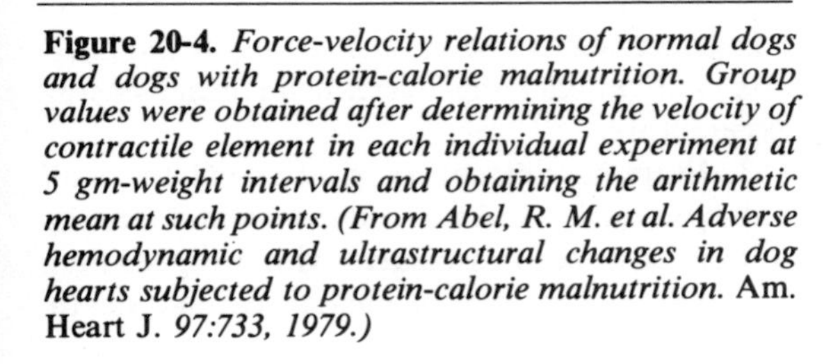

Figure 20-4. *Force-velocity relations of normal dogs and dogs with protein-calorie malnutrition. Group values were obtained after determining the velocity of contractile element in each individual experiment at 5 gm-weight intervals and obtaining the arithmetic mean at such points. (From Abel, R. M. et al. Adverse hemodynamic and ultrastructural changes in dog hearts subjected to protein-calorie malnutrition.* Am. Heart J. *97:733, 1979.)*

zymes, including the acid proteinase cathepsin D. Since no changes in cathepsin D were detected if experimental animals received protein-poor, but calorie-rich diets, it was concluded that caloric deficiency and not protein deficiency caused increases in lysosomal enzyme activity and, hence, myocardial atrophy. Cathepsin D activity is also known to be dependent on the ordinary adaptive mechanisms associated with the starved state. Increased free fatty acids and ketone bodies or a decrease in plasma insulin activity are associated with increases in cathepsin D activity and in the activity of other myocardial lysosomal enzymes [101]. It appears, therefore, that the starvation "signals" present in other organ systems are also present in the heart and provide the mechanism of organ atrophy during starvation.

PROTEIN DEFICIENCY ("KWASHIORKOR HEART DISEASE")

Kwashiorkor is a specific form of protein malnutrition initially described in African children whose diet consisted nearly entirely of protein-poor maize [57, 69, 102]. Although many of these patients also developed a form of nutritional cirrhosis characterized by fatty infiltration and periportal hepatic fibrosis, specific cardiac abnormalities appeared to coexist which were independent of the secondary effects of abnormal fluid and sodium retention of chronic liver disease.

Clinical cardiac features are characteristically those of biventricular failure, as evidenced by jugular venous distention and the development of a low cardiac output state with acrocyanosis and weak peripheral pulses [87]. Although heart size in starvation and semi-starvation generally decreases as a result of myocardial atrophy (see the foregoing) and decreased blood volume [21], kwashiorkor hearts generally tend to be enlarged and exhibit persistent tachycardia with low QRS voltage on the electrocardiogram. Following early stages of treatment, even greater increases in the cardiothoracic ratio are common, presumably secondary to ventricular dilatation in response to the increased fluid and electrolyte load associated with nutritional repletion [99]. Sudden cardiac death occurred in many of these children [85] and was thought to be due to fibrosis and degeneration of the cardiac conduction system. Additional pathologic findings of children dying of kwashiorkor included severe myofibrillar atrophy, patchy necrosis with round cell infiltration of the myocardium, and, in some areas, fatty infiltration [99].

Experimental models of a kwashiorkor-like protein deficiency heart disease have been produced in a variety of experimental animals. Experimental protein malnutrition in Rhesus monkeys [23] resulted in histologic changes similar to those described in kwashiorkor. The myocardial atrophy associated with primate protein deficiency was identified as a true atrophy, that is, a decrease in the size of all muscle fibers and not due to diminution in the *number* of fibers present [33]. The use of smaller, more hypermetabolic mammals for studies of protein deficiency states are fraught with the basic objections to any nutritional studies when using extremely small mammals. Nevertheless, Kyger and associates [63] observed that protein-deficient rats developed measurable decreases in myocardial contractility when compared with normally fed animals.

The effects of isolated protein deficiency or combined protein-calorie malnutrition on the heart may be summarized as follows:

1. The immediate clinical effects of starvation or semi-starvation in man are associated with a decrease in circulatory blood volume, and, therefore, a decrease in heart size, which may cause diminished myocardial performance by "moving to the left" in a classic ventricular function curve. That is, decreased circulatory volume leads to a decrease in ventricular preload and hence a decrease in LV output.
2. As the adaptive mechanisms of starvation take effect, a decrease in cardiac output and heart rate will parallel the decrease in basal energy expenditure.
3. Extreme degrees of protein-calorie malnutrition during unusual environmental circumstances have been associated with a higher than anticipated incidence of sudden cardiac death.

These deaths are associated with myocardial atrophy and myofibrillar degeneration, and although electrolyte imbalance has been implicated, the precise mechanism of the sudden cardiac death has not yet been identified.

4. Pure protein deficiency, as exemplified by kwashiorkor heart disease, appears to result in myocardial changes similar to those of starvation, although there appears to be a higher incidence of fatty infiltration with myocardial fibrosis.

5. Following nutritional resuscitation in both pure protein deficiency and protein-calorie malnutrition, the increase in cardiac size and cardiac dilatation, perhaps in association with depressed contractility due to myocardial atrophy, may result in a "flooding" of the circulatory system and exacerbate problems of congestive heart failure.

6. The reversibility of the pathologic and pathophysiologic effects of malnutrition on the heart has not been evaluated thoroughly. Preliminary evidence from our laboratory suggests that following short-term resuscitation of the malnourished experimental animal, there remains significant depression of ventricular performance compared with normals. These observations may parallel those reported by Keys and coworkers [59], who noted a prolonged period of disability following nutritional repletion from semi-starvation in normal volunteers. It is interesting to speculate that perhaps an additional adverse effect of even short-term fasting regimens for the management of morbid obesity may be the induction of long-term cardiac disability based on the failure of the heart to recover morphologically from a severe degree of myocardial atrophy and disintegration. Additional clinical and laboratory studies in these areas would be interesting.

CARDIAC CACHEXIA

Many patients suffering from states of chronic congestive heart failure as exemplified by rheumatic valvular heart disease develop weight loss, inanition, and a state of protein-calorie malnutrition. The mechanism of this "cardiac cachexia" is multifactorial in origin and may vary from patient to patient. The primary pathophysiologic mechanism appears to be secondary to increased central venous pressure with subsequent hepatic engorgement and hepatomegaly. The transmission of elevated hepatic venous pressure to the portal system can result in secondary portal hypertension with congestion of gastric mucosa. It has been suggested that this congestion and decreased motility result in postprandial distress and in the anorexia commonly associated with this state [58]. Additional factors including malaise, general weakness and the psychologic response to chronic illness resulting in a reactive depression may further diminish food intake. Furthermore, the relative unpalatability of a low-sodium diet to which most patients in chronic congestive heart failure must adhere may further cause patients to avoid eating. Another prevalent contributory factor is the anorexia and nausea of digitalis toxicity. Nephrotic syndrome, protein-losing gastroenteropathy, and fat malabsorption have also been reported to be secondary to the venous congestion of chronic congestive heart failure and may contribute to the decreased appetite seen in these patients.

This condition of decreased food intake associated with congestive heart failure can frequently lead to a hypermetabolic state which, in the presence of cellular hypoxia secondary to decreased cardiac output, can lead to accelerated cardiac atrophy, which in turn develops into a vicious cycle causing worsening of the congestive heart failure (see the foregoing) [19]. Severe cardiac cachexia has been reported to lead to potentially dangerous conditions [56, 60]. In patients with severe rheumatic valvular heart disease usually resulting in left and right ventricular hypertrophy, several individuals with severe malnutrition demonstrated unexpected cardiac atrophy, undoubtedly secondary to the effects of protein-calorie malnutrition. This inhibition of LV hypertrophy in response to spontaneous hypertension in rats fed a low-protein diet resulted in significant decrease in LV function [104]. Since the hypertrophic response is hemodynamically compensatory, a heart unable

Table 20-3. *Epidemiologic Data*

Group	No. of Patients	Age (Mean±SE)	Sex		Mortality		
			Male	Female	Lived	Died	Mortality (%)
1 Malnourished controls	24	59.5±2.7	8	16	21	3	12.5
2 Malnourished, hyperalimented	20	61.7±2.2	6	14	16	4	20
3 Nonmalnourished	22	54.8±2.3	13	9	22	0	0

Source: R. M. Abel et al. Malnutrition in cardiac surgical patients: Results of a prospective, randomized evaluation of early postoperative parenteral nutrition. *Arch. Surg.* 111:46, 1976. Copyright 1976, American Medical Association.

to achieve such increase in size would predictably function less well, particularly during periods of hemodynamic stress.

Therapy

Since the etiologic factors responsible for cardiac cachexia will persist for as long as congestive heart failure persists, the management of this form of malnutrition is difficult. A thorough nutritional assessment—including anthropomorphic, biochemical, and immunologic measurements—should be carried out in any patient in whom malnutrition is suspected. A history of weight loss and anorexia combined with the simple physical finding of decreased subcutaneous fat stores are generally sufficient to warrant a diagnosis of "cardiac cachexia." Active dietary counseling in an attempt to improve the palatability and balance of orally ingested diets may be beneficial; the addition of dietary supplements containing little, if any, sodium can also be helpful if tolerated. The difficulty lies in that these patients refuse to ingest large quantities of food because of early satiety and nausea following eating. In addition, because of chronic passive congestion to the splanchnic bed and viscera, absorption may not be optimal.

Patients who suffer from various degrees of cardiac cachexia and who are about to undergo open heart operations to palliate cardiac abnormalities constitute a special subgroup of patients. It has been a clinical impression that these patients, when subjected to open heart procedures, frequently develop prolonged requirements for artificial ventilation, difficulties with wound healing, decubitus ulcers, and other complications that might be worsened by the malnourished state. Because of the difficulties in reversing this state preoperatively, the complication rate in the malnourished patient following open heart surgery is high compared with that of nourished patients.

We [5] undertook a prospective, randomized study to determine whether immediate postoperative nutritional support would decrease the morbidity and mortality predicted from past anecdotal experiences in patients with cardiac cachexia undergoing open heart surgery. We selected patients above 18 years of age who had a recent history of weight loss exceeding 4.5 kg or an absolute weight loss of 15 percent below ideal, as predicted from life insurance charts. Malnourished patients were then divided into two groups, the first (group 1) serving as controls (Table 20-3) and the second (group 2) scheduled to receive immediate postoperative hyperalimentation. Patients in group 1 were matched as closely as possible for age, degree of preoperative cardiac disbility, and operative procedure. Group 2 patients received hyperalimentation with a special solution designed to deliver as high a concentration of nutrients in as small a fluid volume as feasible (Table 20-4).

Table 20-4. *Formulation of "Cardiac Hyperalimentation Solution" Used at the Massachusetts General Hospital, 1974*

Substance	Form Provided	Amount	Volume (ml)	Kcal
Protein equivalent	Freamine, 8.5%	28 gm	360	98
Dextrose	Dextrose, 70%	350 gm	500	1190
Potassium	Potassium acetate, 3 mEq/ml	30 mEq	10	
	Potassium phosphate, 2 mEq/ml	20 mEq	10	
Sodium		3.6 mEq		
Magnesium	Magnesium sulfate	4 mEq	5	
Chloride		17 mEq		
Ascorbic acid		500 mg	2	
Multivitamins	Berocca C MVI concentrate*		1.0	

*Used once weekly. Each 880 ml contains 4.5 gm nitrogen, approximately 1,300 kcal, and 2,280 mOsm/liter.
Source: R. M. Abel et al. Malnutrition in cardiac surgical patients: Results of a prospective, randomized evaluation of early postoperative parenteral nutrition. *Arch. Surg.* 111:45, 1976. Copyright 1976, American Medical Association.

Table 20-5. *Operative Procedures*

	Group			
Procedure	1	2	3	Total No.
Mitral valve replacement	13	10	5	28
Aortic valve replacement	5	3	5	13
Aortic and mitral valve replacements	3	1	3	7
Other valve procedures	1	4	3	8
Isolated aortocoronary bypass	0	0	4	4
Valve replacement plus aortocoronary bypass	2	1	2	5
Closure ductus arteriosus with aortic graft	0	1	0	1
Total	24	20	22	66

Source: R. M. Abel et al. Malnutrition in cardiac surgical patients: Results of a prospective, randomized evaluation of early postoperative parenteral nutrition. *Arch. Surg.* 111:45, 1976. Copyright 1976, American Medical Association.

Infusion rates of this solution were begun at 30 ml/hour and were increased by increments of 10 ml/hour/24 hours until the maximum fluid tolerance was achieved, generally between 50 to 60 ml/hour. Exogenous insulin was administered intravenously when indicated.

It was predicted that parenteral nutritional support in patients receiving hyperalimentation would be discontinued once oral intake exceeded 1,500 kcal/day, but following initiation of the study, it was clear that even by the time of hospital discharge, very few patients indeed would ingest this amount of food. Accordingly, hyperalimentation was then discontinued in patients by the fifth or sixth postoperative day, once an adequate fluid volume was obtained. The operative mortality in both malnourished groups was excessively high compared with that of the control patients. The operative procedures (Table 20-5) were roughly similar, although there was a higher incidence of coronary artery operations in patients who were not malnourished.

We were unable to observe any beneficial effects of routine postoperative hyperalimentation in group 2 patients; in fact, they sustained a slightly higher incidence of complications than all other groups (Table 20-6). We concluded that although patients judged to be malnourished *preoperatively* had less satisfactory results after cardiac surgery than a group of similar, but non-malnourished patients, we were unable to reverse the untoward effects of malnutrition by *postoperative* feeding. Blackburn and associates [19] reported in a small series of patients requiring triple cardiac valve replacement that an aggressive program of inpatient preoperative support might diminish the ill effects of cardiac cachexia. It is important to recall the kwashiorkor experience, however, in which too rapid a nutritional repletion in patients with already compromised cardiovascular systems could trigger the onset of frank pulmonary edema [53].

Although the cachexia associated with severe heart disease can participate in a vicious cycle leading to additional complications, particularly in the stressed surgical patient, there is new evidence that cardiac function itself may be impaired additionally by the cachectic state. Although preoperative nutritional repletion is justifiable and desirable and may even be feasible by certain techniques of nutritional support, particularly by the parenteral route, great caution must be exercised in attempting too rapid a reversal of the cachetic state for fear that congestive heart failure might worsen. Additionally, the potential hazards of infection in a persistent intravascular catheter in patients with valvular heart disease would raise the specter of infective endocarditis in any such patient who might develop a febrile course.

OBESITY

Since hypernutrition results in the most prevalent nutritional disorder in the United States, it would appear that if there were any etiologic mechanism by which obesity would directly produce cardiac failure, it would have become immediately apparent. There are many difficulties in identifying these factors, since many obese patients suffer from concomitant coronary heart disease, hypertension, and diabetes, all of which can directly result in significant LV dysfunction. In certain instances, however, in which no evidence of primary myocardial disease is demonstrable, a small subgroup of patients has been identified with significant cardiac impairment, as characterized by cardiomegaly with varying degrees of fatty infiltration of the myocardium [86]. It is also recognized that in certain instances of massive obesity, chronic hypoventilation, with the subsequent development of the so-called "Pickwickian syndrome," can occur in association with right ventricular hypertrophy and congestive heart failure. Further deterioration of this syndrome with the development of chronic cor pulmonale has been reported [25], but this is unusual in the absence of underlying primary pulmonary disease [64].

"High output" LV failure in the absence of hypertension and pulmonary disease was reported by Alexander [12] in 50 obese patients. At cardiac catheterization, excessive increases in LV work occurred with mild exercise, averaging 95 percent greater than predicted values. He proposed that myocardial hypertrophy and subsequent congestive heart failure may develop as a result of the increased cardiac work in obese patients, particularly during exercise.

The usual advice given to obese patients with heart disease is to effect significant weight reduction as soon as feasible. Reduction in total body adiposity may clearly result in a decrease in systemic hypertension and in the pulmonary insufficiency that may result from the mechanical difficulties in providing adequate alveolar ventilation in the morbidly obese. Furthermore, the hypermetabolic state, with subsequent high cardiac output failure, would conceivably be lessened as total adiposity is reduced. It should be remembered, however, that too rapid a weight loss, such as would be obtained by semi-starvation or by fad diets, may result in inadvertent rapid protein deficiency and the possibility of myocardial atrophy (see the foregoing).

Table 20-6. *Postoperative Complications*

Complication	Group				Total
	1 Malnourished Control	2 Malnourished Hyperalimented	1 and 2 All Malnourished	3 Nonmalnourished Control	
Excessive postoperative hemorrhage requiring re-exploration	1	1	2	2	4
Acute renal failure requiring dialysis	0	3	3	0	3
Pneumonia	2	6	8	1	9
Superficial wound infection	1	0	1	2	3
Mediastinitis	0	2	2	0	2
Respiratory failure requiring tracheostomy	3	4	7	0	7

Source: R. M. Abel et al. Malnutrition in cardiac surgical patients: Results of a prospective, randomized evaluation of early postoperative parenteral nutrition. *Arch. Surg.* 111:45, 1976. Copyright 1976, American Medical Association.

SPECIFIC NUTRIENT EXCESSES OR DEFICIENCIES

Tryptophan Metabolism

A peculiar distribution of valvular fibrosis has been associated with the carcinoid syndrome. In patients with advanced carcinoid syndrome with extensive hepatic metastases, cardiac lesions frequently occur on the tricuspid and pulmonic valve, presumably owing to the incomplete degradation of 5-hydroxytryptamine by the liver. The vasoconstrictive effects of 5-hydroxytryptamine (serotonin) are thought to cause ischemia of the endocardium with subsequent endomyocardial fibrosis [12, 44]. Since monoaminoxidases are present in sufficiently large quantities in the lung to degrade any unmetabolized serotonin after it passes through the right side of the heart, left-sided cardiac valvular lesions are exceedingly rare, even with massive pulmonary metastases.

Carcinoid-like endocardial lesions also occur in Uganda and other tropical countries in a syndrome of so-called endomyocardial fibrosis [29]. This lesion was first described in West African soldiers [16] and later defined by Davies and Williams [30, 31, 103]. The epidemiology of the disease appears to be related to increased consumption of bananas (plantains), a rich dietary source of serotonin. The excretion rate of 5-hydroxy indolacetic acid (5-HIAA) in patients consuming a high plantain diet is similar to the magnitude measured in patients with the carcinoid syndrome [28]. Endomyocardial fibrosis has been reproduced experimentally in guinea pigs by feeding them a diet rich in plantain [71]. McKinney [70] was able to reproduce these lesions by feeding a tryptophan-deficient diet (low-protein) supplemented by large quantities of serotonin, whereas similar animals given protein supplements in the form of casein failed to develop these lesions. Lesions have also been produced in the experimental animal fed a diet consisting of maize (Zea mays) [69]. These low-tryptophan diets were hypothesized to cause the endomyocardial fibrotic lesions on the basis of a relative serotonin excess similar to that seen in plantain feeding and the carcinoid syndrome. Spartz suggested that the production of these lesions experimentally required concomitant tryptophan deficiency and elevated serotonin intake coexisting with diminished hepatic function [88, 89]. The presumed mechanism, therefore, of the human condition seen in economically deprived regions in which protein-poor (and hence tryptophan-poor) diets coexist with high serotonin-containing foods (plantain, maize) and concomitant nutritional cirrhosis create the "perfect" experimental circumstances under which this rather unusual form of nutritional heart disease can occur. There is no evidence that a reversal of this dietary pattern can cause a clearing of the cardiac lesions, nor is it clear whether the endomyocardial fibrosis can respond to any specific therapy other than symptomatic.

Lipid Abnormalities, Vitamin E, and Selenium Deficiency

A syndrome of "nutritional muscular degeneration" of the myocardium and skeletal muscles was reported to occur in ruminants in certain parts of the world when they were fed diets containing large quantities of saturated fatty acids [74]. The mitrochondria of the muscle cells appear to be damaged by excessive quantities of these fatty acids in the absence of adequate antioxidants. Fatty infiltration with deposition in the myocardial interstitium follows the mitochondrial changes and, finally, round cell infiltration has been identified between the myofibers themselves. Similar lesions have been reported in the heart and other organs in the experimental animal fed rapeseed oil, a common ingredient in salad oils, margarines, and shortenings, which are used extensively in some human diets. Rapeseed oil, a major constituent of which is erucic acid (13-cis-docosenoic acid), also contains low concentrations of unsaturated fatty acids [14]. Transient myocardial lipidosis has been identified in a variety of small mammals [24, 84, 100], but never in man. It appears that an imbalance in the fatty acid composition of rapeseed oil may be the etiologic factor. Supplementing the diets in mice with betaine, a lipotrophic agent, minimized the toxic myocardial effects of rapeseed oil feedings [15].

Similar myocardial changes have been identified in the experimental animal fed vitamin E- or selenium-deficient diets, or both. For example, piglets born from vitamin E- and selenium-deficient sows develop myocardial changes, commonly known as "mulberry heart disease" [90]. Vitamin-E-deficient rabbits [22] develop an acute myocarditis that does not occur in rabbits fed alpha-tocopherol. Rats fed high concentrations of cod liver oil without additional tocopherol develop deposition of ceroid pigment in the myocardium and a high peroxide content in myocardial lipid extracts [91]. The pathogenesis of these cardiomyopathies is thought to be related to a lack of the selenoenzyme, glutathione peroxidase, and of vitamin E itself, which would ordinarily effect a protective lipoperoxidative influence [94].

It should be emphasized, however, that vitamin E/selenium deficiency or the myocardial damage of unsaturated fat ingestion have not been identified in man. Extensive reviews on the subject of possible vitamin E deficiency and cardiac disease have concluded that there is no basis for the claims that vitamin E deficiency is associated with human heart disease [55, 75]. Furthermore, the use of "megavitamin therapy" with massive doses of vitamin E, as advocated by some on the basis of anecdotal observations [84], has not been justified on the basis of carefully controlled scientific investigation [36, 66, 79].

Notwithstanding this lack of controlled studies, the sales of vitamin E supplements in "health food" stores reflect a substantial belief by the American public that large quantities of this agent may prevent or ameliorate the symptoms of coronary heart disease. The placebo effect of such therapy is thought to explain this continued interest. Prospective clinical studies will be necessary to put to rest the theories that vitamin E may be helpful for heart disease, as it has been suggested for the prevention of sexual inadequacy, chronic fatigue, and a host of other ailments [55], none of which have been proven.

Vitamin B_1 (Thiamine, Aneurin) Deficiency: Beriberi Heart Disease

The only known vitamin deficiency disease that affects the heart is due to chronic vitamin B_1 depletion, which was identified in the early twentieth century by Oriental physicians. This disease, as originally described, causes primarily right-sided cardiac symptoms and a "high-output" variety of cardiac failure characterized by a widened arterial pulse pressure, "pistol-shot" sounds over peripheral arteries, and tachycardia. This disease, frequently fulminant in nature, terminates in sudden cardiovascular collapse or the so-called *shoshin* beriberi, as described by the Japanese. Aalsmeer and Wenckebach [1] called the attention of the Occidental medical world to beriberi in 1928, following which this disease came to be recognized in the West.

Although isolated vitamin B_1 deficiency occurs endemically in the Orient because of the lack of whole-grain cereal ingestion, isolated B_1 deficiency failure rarely occurs in the west, since vitamin deficiency is frequently associated with global insufficiencies of many nutrient substances. For example, in a series of 120 patients identified with beriberi [98], the majority were also heavy consumers of alcohol and had a combination of what is now recognized as alcoholic cardiomyopathy and beriberi heart disease. When considering beriberi heart disease as the sole etiologic factor in the production of cardiac disability, Blankenhorn recommended the following criteria to warrant the diagnosis:

1. Enlarged heart with normal (sinoauricular) rhythm.
2. Dependent edema.
3. Elevated venous pressure.
4. Peripheral neuritis or pellagra.
5. Nonspecific changes in the electrocardiogram.
6. No other cause evident.
7. Gross deficiency of diet for three months or more.
8. Improvement or reduction of heart size after specific treatment.
9. Autopsy findings consistent with beriberi [20].

Although once treatment with adequate doses of thiamine is instituted, hemodynamic abnormalities generally rapidly return to normal [10, 80], failure to respond to adequate therapy in advanced stages may result from the myocardial fibrosis that is frequently noted in the terminal stages of the disease. A lack of response to treatment in patients with suspected beriberi heart disease and concomitant chronic alcoholism may suggest a primary influence of alcoholic cardiomyopathy rather than thiamine deficiency [11].

The ultimate hemodynamic mechanism of the cardiac disability is a decrease in total peripheral vascular resistance, which results in the secondary effects of increased heart rate, stroke index, blood volume, and a narrow arterial-venous oxygen difference [9]. Thiamine is required for normal oxidative metabolism both in man and in the experimental animal. Myocardium from thiamine-deficient dogs failed to utilize pyruvate and lactate normally [49]. Following four weeks of a thiamine-deficient diet fed to rats, myocardial concentrations of ATP decreased. Within three days following repletion of thiamine stores, cardiac pyruvate decarboxylase activity increases and cardiac pyruvate concentrations decrease as ATP levels revert toward normal [68]. There appears to be no difference in LV performance in thiamine-deficient rabbits compared with normals, however, suggesting that the primary defect in beriberi heart disease is indeed its peripheral action and diminution in vascular resistance [77].

The exact mechanism of the loss of peripheral vascular tone in beriberi heart disease is unknown. Although restitution of normal peripheral vascular resistance may occur following institution of thiamine therapy, persistent abnormalities of the circulation may exist due to irreversible, fibrotic changes in the myocardium, which result from the excessive demands placed on the heart during untreated stages of the disease.

The diagnosis of beriberi heart disease is infrequently made in the West because of a low index of suspicion. When presented with a patient demonstrating a high-output variety of cardiac failure, however, the disease must be included in the initial differential diagnosis. The use of pulmonary arterial-flow catheters to determine right-sided cardiac pressures and cardiac output is a mainstay of the bedside diagnosis of a high cardiac output state. In the absence of thyrotoxicosis, peripheral arteriovenous fistulas, or pregnancy, beriberi heart should be strongly suspected and, accordingly, patients should be treated empirically with 50 to 100 mg thiamine hydrochloride each day, administered by any route. Although it has been suggested that blood transketolase activity may be useful as a precise biochemical marker of thiamine deficiency [10], a more practical approach to the clinical problem has been the empiric administration of vitamins to all patients with suspected vitamin deficiency states. The epidemiologic relationship between alcohol abuse and suspected vitamin deficiency [57, 67] has encouraged the empiric use of thiamine to be administered to alcoholic patients even upon arrival to a hospital for a variety of emergency causes. The "cocktail" administered to alcoholic patients suffering from delirium tremens, bleeding esophageal varices, and a host of other syndromes associated with chronic alcoholism generally consists of a high concentration of calories as carbohydrate and a multivitamin preparation in which at least 50 mg of thiamine is administered daily. Since resting cardiac output is generally elevated in nutritional cirrhosis alone, the differentiation between the two diseases in their earlier stages may be difficult. It is possible that many patients with subclinical beriberi heart disease in the general population of chronic alcoholics suffering from malnutrition are never proved to have beriberi heart disease, since thiamine therapy, as indicated, often precludes confirmation of the diagnosis. Although the empiric use of *any* therapeutic regimen should generally be condemned, vitamin therapy to treat *potential* and probable vitamin deficiency states appears to be reasonable, since adverse side effects are extremely rare.

Although many food and vitamin cultists and faddists advocate vitamin therapy for heart disease, there is little evidence that human cardiac ailments can be produced by other isolated hypovitaminoses. Prolonged vitamin B_{12} deprivation in rats was reported to produce extensive myocardial fibrosis with distortion of mitochondria [76]. There have been no reports of abnormalities specifically attributed to vitamin B_{12} deficiency in humans, however, again reflecting the difficulty in indentifying a pure, isolated nutritional deficiency state naturally occurring in man.

ELECTROLYTE ABNORMALITIES

Magnesium Deficiency

Although there has been no documentation of human cardiac disease due to isolated magnesium deficiency, myocardial degeneration with subsequent fibrosis was described in rats reared on low magnesium diets [46]. Moore and coworkers [73] identified focal cardiac necrosis with calcification in calves fed similar diets, and calcification was also noted on the cristae of sarcomeres [52]. These interesting experimental observations may either be species-specific or have their relatively minor effects masked by global malnourished states.

Potassium Deficiency

Although acute changes in the serum concentration of potassium have obvious effects on myocardial contractility, unequivocal demonstration of chronic morphologic changes of a potassium deficient state have not been identified in man. Chronic potassium deficiency may result in marked depression of LV function [2, 48, 50, 81], and the altered mitochondria that have been identified in potassium-deficient experimental animals appear to result from a decreased uptake of calcium which may, in turn, cause negative inotropic effects [61]. Myocardial necrosis was also reported in rats fed a potassium-deficient diet [83]; Thomas and coworkers [92] concluded that the development of these myocardial lesions may also be dependent on concomitant deficiency of vitamin B_6.

Since chronic potassium deficiency in man is often associated with chronic malnutrition and dehydration, any potassium-specific effects are difficult to identify in man. The cardiac abnormalities identified in women ingesting "liquid protein diet" (see the foregoing) may have been related to chronic potassium deficiency, although this variable could not be separated from chronic protein-calorie malnutrition.

NUTRITIONAL SUPPORT IN PATIENTS WITH SEVERE CARDIAC DISEASE: CLINICAL EXPERIENCE

Although malnutrition and cardiac dysfunction may coexist, there is no reason that one clinical problem should necessarily interfere with or preclude therapy directed toward the other. That is, since there is no contraindication to nutritional support and all starving patients must be fed, a patient with severe cardiac illness resulting in congestive heart failure simply represents a "variation on the theme" of ordinary nutritional support. The difficulties with manipulating orally ingested diets in patients with cardiac cachexia represent only minor adjustments in patient management. The following discussion outlines these modifications of parenteral nutritional support.

Since most patients with "medical" problems related to congestive heart failure generally have intact gastrointestinal tracts, the vast experience with parenteral feedings in patients with severe cardiac illness has been immediately following cardiac surgery. A retrospective review [4] of patients undergoing a variety of cardiac surgical procedures revealed that approximately 3.1 percent of all patients required parenteral feeding in the postoperative period. The major indications for hyperalimentation in these patients were complications of a low cardiac output state and of the surgical procedure (e.g., acute renal failure was the major indication) (Table 20-7). Since only patients with complications received parenteral nutrition, survival in this subset was low (24 of 64 patients or 37.5 percent). Eight hundred forty-seven patient days of hyperalimentation were required to treat these patients for a mean of 13.2 days (range 3 to 47 days). Complications of hyperalimentation in this group were notably rare, consisting primarily of hyperglycemia due to poor glucose tolerance. There was no incidence of catheter-related sepsis in any of the patients, despite

Table 20-7. *Indications for Hyperalimentation in 64 Cardiac Surgical Patients*

Indications	No.
Acute renal failure	43
Malnutrition; poor wound healing	19
Inadequate oral intake secondary to central nervous system dysfunction	15
Significant prerenal azotemia with starvation	11
Inadequate gastrointestinal tract function (postoperative ileus, abdominal operation, etc.)	3
Total	92

Source: R. M. Abel et al. Hyperalimentation in cardiac surgery. *J. Thorac. Cardiovasc. Surg.* 67:296, 1974.

the fact that several of the patients had active, infective endocarditis at the time of therapy.

The major therapeutic changes encountered in the postoperative cardiac surgical patient requiring parenteral nutrition consist of modifications of the fluid and electrolyte pattern, modification of technique of catheter insertion and management, and determination of the therapeutic end-points of nutritional therapy.

Metabolic Considerations

Since the pathophysiologic mechanisms that result in congestive heart failure cause the renal tubule to conserve sodium (effects of secondary hyperaldosteronism and increased fluid volume), the general rule of thumb is not to administer any exogenous sodium unless extraordinary losses occur. For example, a patient with severe cardiac illness with a paralytic ileus requiring prolonged nasogastric drainage may conceivably require some sodium administration, but this is extremely rare. In the presence of palpable edema on physical examination or in the presence of pulmonary edema on chest roentgenogram, the total body sodium content is almost certainly elevated, and therefore appropriate therapy is directed toward eliminating water in excess of sodium. Since many of these patients are receiving concomitant diuretic therapy, this problem is easily managed by increasing the diuretic dose.

Problems with glucose intolerance occur more commonly in cardiac patients for many reasons. The overall incidence of diabetes mellitus is generally higher because of the older age population and because of the association between diabetes mellitus and coronary artery disease. Furthermore, low cardiac output states in chronic congestive failure result in a decrease in hepatic and peripheral skeletal muscle perfusion. Both of these may lead to decreased glucose utilization, which may not necessarily be due to an inadequacy of endogenous insulin stores. Furthermore, as already indicated (Table 20-4), the solutions given to patients with fluid retention should contain a higher concentration of nutrients than usual. The "ordinary" hyperalimentation solutions administered to general surgical patients usually consist of between 20 and 25 percent glucose, whereas solutions given to patients with heart disease should range between 35 and 50 percent glucose. Using low infusion rates initially, with progressive increases, will guard against rapid increases in blood glucose concentration. In our experience, however, approximately half of all patients with severe congestive heart failure receiving parenteral nutrition have required exogenous insulin therapy. As with all "ordinary" patients receiving total parenteral nutrition, we recommend that when insulin is required, it be added directly to the hyperalimentation solution itself, so that a constant carbohydrate-insulin ratio can be maintained. Furthermore, the absorption of insulin from subcutaneous sites, which tends to be quite irregular in patients with low cardiac output, will not further complicate nutritional therapy.

In the absence of concomitant renal failure, total body potassium stores are generally decreased in patients receiving continuous diuretic therapy. When patients begin to receive hyperalimentation solutions, the requirement for administered potassium is even greater than for "ordinary" patients, and therefore we recommend that between 50 and 60 mEq/L of potassium be administered, especially when diuretic therapy, with loop-active diuretics such as furosemide, is continued. Serum magnesium concentrations may also decline in association with diuretic therapy, and accordingly, magnesium stores need to be repleted as indicated in any "cardiac hyperalimentation solution" (see Table 20-4).

Fluid volume should be restricted to as small a quantity as feasible within the range of nutrient solubility and glucose tolerance. Since amino acid concentration is limited by the quantity available in commercial solutions, the major "savings" in free water administration occurs by concentrating the calorie source, in most instances by using dextrose 70 percent in water rather than lesser concentrations. Frequent monitoring of blood glucose concentrations is necessary in most patients because of the increased concentration of glucose in the solutions. We recommend that blood glucose concentrations be determined every six hours until a stable rate of infusion is achieved; it may then be monitored every 12 hours. With the onset of fever, use of glucocorticoid therapy, or other conditions that further decrease glucose tolerance, sharp attention must be paid to the possibilities of rapid rises in blood glucose, which may lead to hyperosmolar, nonketotic dehydration with coma. This complication is predictably poorly tolerated in patients with severe compromise of cardiac function, and accordingly, the best therapy is directed toward prevention.

Technical aspects of catheter insertion differ little from those for ordinary patients receiving central venous hyperalimentation, with the following exceptions, which result from increased right-sided cardiac pressure and bleeding difficulties: In patients with biventricular cardiac failure, since the right atrial (and hence central venous) pressure is generally elevated, it is unnecessary to place patients in the Trendelenberg position or to have them perform a Valsalva maneuver during catheter insertion or tubing changes. Furthermore, patients with severe congestive heart failure will not tolerate a flat, supine position for even a brief minute or two to insert the catheter. A semirecumbent position generally is satisfactory to permit catheter insertion without introducing air emboli. In patients who are being treated with heparin, it is recommended that the catheter be inserted at a time when the heparin activity is minimal (just prior to the next dose). If the heparin is being administered by constant intravenous drip, we recommend that the heparin be discontinued for several hours prior to catheter insertion. In patients receiving long-term oral anticoagulant therapy with sodium warfarin, it is probably the lesser of two hazards to proceed with venipuncture rather than to discontinue the anticoagulant therapy. In such instances it may be safer to elect the internal jugular site initially, since if unanticipated bleeding were to occur, direct pressure can more easily be placed on the neck than on the subclavian venipuncture site.

In patients with continued bacteremia, as in infective endocarditis, parenteral nutrition frequently is life-saving, especially in cases of concomitant hypermetabolism and malnutrition. The intravenous catheter used for parenteral nutrition should be changed every 72 to 96 hours to prevent secondary seeding of the intravascular catheter with bacteria.

These management guidelines represent only minor alterations in the ordinary care of patients receiving hyperalimentation solutions. The alternative to nutritional support in patients without functioning gastrointestinal tracts is the continued breakdown of lean body mass, with the consequences of malnutrition. It is clear, therefore, that the foregoing measures for providing safe parenteral nutrition are necessary for the patient's recovery from devastating complications.

Hemodynamic Effects of Intravenously Administered Nutrients

In the process of considering parenteral nutrition in patients with compromised cardiac function, it may be important to know whether the nutrient solutions themselves affect cardiac function. Ko and Paradise [62] reported positive inotropic effects of hypertonic dextrose in anesthesized rats. We [8] determined the cardiovascular effects of a commercially available infusion of carbohydrate-free amino acids in the canine isovolumetric heart preparation previously described. Within 5 min-

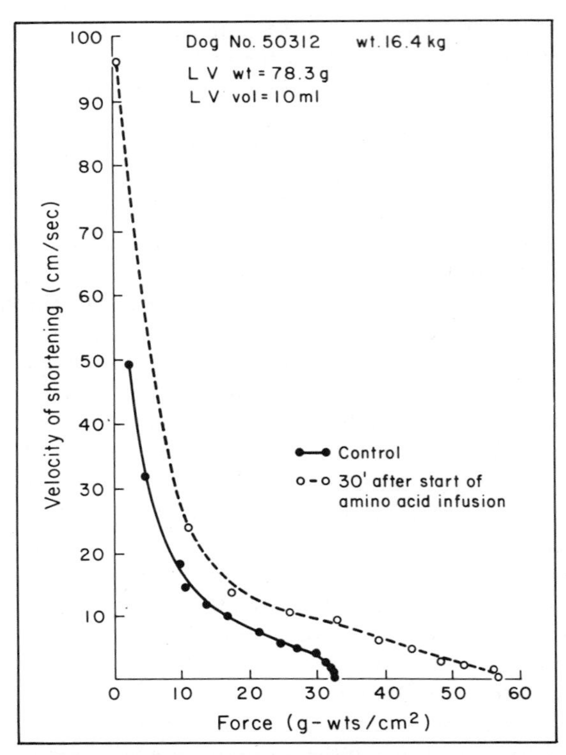

Figure 20-5. *Representative force-velocity curves from a typical experiment in which the effects of the amino acid infusions are to shift the curve upward and to the right, indicating improved myocardial performance. (From Abel, R. M., Subramanian, V. A., and Gay, W. A., Jr. Effects of an intravenous amino acid nutrient solution on left ventricular contractility in dogs.* J. Surg. Res. *23:204, 1977.)*

utes following initiation of a crystalline amino acid infusion (FreAmine), consistent improvements in LV function were noted in all animals as evidenced by an increased peak developed LV pressure and LV dp/dt max. Furthermore, the force-velocity relationships of the LV demonstrated consistent positive inotropic effects of this infusion (Figure 20-5). Although the mechanism of the positive inotropic action was not elucidated, we speculated that direct utilization of glucogenic amino acids, such as alanine, by the myocardium may be responsible for the observed beneficial effects.

We also reported that a 10 percent concentration of intravenous fat emulsion (Intralipid) produced consistently *negative* effects on canine myocardium in a similar preparation [47]. Furthermore, significant decreases in systemic vascular resistance repeatedly occurred following Intralipid infusion in the same preparation. On the basis of these studies, we concluded that rapid infusion of an intravenous fat emulsion should probably be avoided in patients with marginal cardiac reserve who cannot tolerate even brief episodes of hypotension. Whether these observations in the experimental animal relate to man remains to be determined, however.

Future Considerations

With an increasing life expectancy throughout the world, particularly in developed nations, a relatively greater percentage of patients with coexisting heart disease present with nutritional problems requiring aggressive nutritional support. Although the magnitude of this problem has not been determined, it is clear that under certain circumstances, such as cardiac cachexia in patients with rheumatic heart disease and complications following open heart surgery, nutritional support is vital. Interactions between the nutritional status of a patient vis à vis the requirements of his heart for adequate protein stores for myofibril synthesis and energy stores to "fuel the cardiac engine" are attractive areas for future investigation. One may tentatively conclude, however, that the heart certainly is not "spared" the ill effects of undernutrition and may, in fact, be a rather sensitive indicator of nutritional status.

REFERENCES

1. Aalsmeer, W. C., and Wenckeback, K. F. Herz and Kreislauf bei der ber-beri Krankheit. *Wien. Arch. Inn. Med.* 16:193, 1928.
2. Abbrecht, P. H. Cardiovascular effects of chronic potassium deficiency in dogs. *Am. J. Phys.* 223: 555, 1972.
3. Abel, R. M., Alonso, D. R., Grimes, J. B., and Gay, W. A., Jr. Biochemical, ultra-structural,

and hemodynamic changes in protein-calorie malnutrition in dogs. *Circulation* [Suppl. 3] 56: 55, 1977.
4. Abel, R. M., Fischer, J. E., Buckley, M. J., and Austen, W. G. Hyperalimentation in cardiac surgery. A review of sixty-four patients. *J. Thorac. Cardiovasc. Surg.* 67:294, 1974.
5. Abel, R. M., Fischer, J. E., Buckley, M. J., Barnett, G. O., and Austen, W. G. Malnutrition in cardiac surgical patients: Results of a prospective randomized evaluation of early postoperative parenteral nutrition. *Arch. Surg.* 111:45, 1976.
6. Abel, R. M., Grimes, J. B., Alonso, D., Alonso, M. L., and Gay, W. A., Jr. Adverse hemodynamic and ultrastructural changes in dog hearts subjected to protein-calorie malnutrition. *Am. Heart J.* 97:733, 1979.
7. Abel, R. M., Grimes, J. B., and Paul, J. Effects of refeeding on the hemodynamic consequences of protein-calorie malnutrition in dogs. Unpublished manuscript, 1979.
8. Abel, R. M., Subramanian, V. A., and Gay, W. A., Jr. Effects of an intravenous amino acid nutrient solution on left ventricular contractility in dogs. *J. Surg. Res.* 23:201, 1977.
9. Akbarian, M., and Dreyfus, P. M. Blood transketolase activity in beriberi heart disease. A useful diagnostic index. *J.A.M.A.* 203:77, 1968.
10. Akbarian, M., Yankopoulos, N. A., and Abelman, W. H. Hemodynamic studies in beriberi heart disease. *Am. J. Med.* 41:197, 1966.
11. Alexander, C. S. Nutritional heart disease. *Cardiovasc. Clin.* 41:221, 1972.
12. Alexander, J. K. Obesity and cardiac performance. *Am. J. Cardiol.* 14:860, 1964.
13. Alleyne, G. A. O. Cardiac function in severely malnourished Jamaican children. *Clin. Sci.* 30: 553, 1966.
14. Applequist, L. A., and Ohlson, R. *Rapeseed.* Amsterdam: Elsevier, 1972.
15. Ball, C. R., and Williams, W. L. Spontaneous and dietary-induced cardiovascular lesions in DBA mice. *Anat. Rec.* 152:199, 1976.
16. Bedford, D. E., and Konstam, G. L. S. Heart failure of unknown aetiology in Africans. *Br. Heart J.* 8:236, 1946.
17. Blackburn, G. L. Letter to editor. *N. Engl. J. Med.* 299:419, 1978.
18. Blackburn, G. L., Flatt, J. P., and Biestrian, B. R. Role of a Protein-Sparing Modified Fast in a Comprehensive Weight Reduction Program. In A. Howard (Ed.), *Recent Advances in Obesity Research.* London: Newman, 1975.
19. Blackburn, G. L., et al. Nutritional support in cardiac cachexia. *J. Thorac. Cardiovasc. Surg.* 73:489, 1977.
20. Blankenhorn, M. A. The diagnosis of beriberi heart disease. *Ann. Intern. Med.* 23:398, 1945.
21. Bloom, W. L., Gordon, A., and Smith, E. G., Jr. Changes in heart size and plasma volume during fasting. *Metabolism* 15:409, 1966.
22. Bragdon, J. H., and Levine, H. D. Myocarditis in vitamin E-deficient rabbits. *Am. J. Pathol.* 25: 246, 1949.
23. Chauhan, S., Nayak, N. C., and Ramalingaswami, V. The heart and skeletal muscle in experimental protein malnutrition in Rhesus monkey. *J. Pathol.* 90:301, 1965.
24. Charlton, K. M., et al. Cardiac lesions in cats fed rapeseed oils. *Can. J. Comp. Med.* 39:261, 1975.
25. Counihan, T. B. Heart failure due to extreme obesity. Case report. *Br. Heart J.* 18:425, 1956.
26. Covell, J. W., Furhrer, J. S., Boerth, R. C., and Ross, J., Jr. Production of isotonic contraction in the intact canine left ventricle. *J. Appl. Physiol.* 27:577, 1969.
27. Covell, J. W., Ross, J., Jr., Sonnenblick, E. H., and Braunwald, E. Comparison of the force-velocity relation and the ventricular function curve as measures of the contractile state of the intact heart. *Circ. Res.* 19:364, 1966.
28. Crawford, M. A. Excretion of 5-OH indolacetic acid in East Africans. *Lancet* 1:352, 1962.
29. Crawford, M. A. Endomyocardial fibrosis and carcinoidosis. A common denominator? *Am. Heart J.* 66:273, 1963.
30. Davies, J. N. P. Pathology of Central African natives. *East Afr. Med. J.* 25:454, 1948.
31. Davies, J. N. P., and Ball, J. D. The pathology of endomyocardial fibrosis in Uganda. *Br. Heart J.* 17:337, 1955.
32. Deaths associated with liquid protein diets. *Morbidity & Mortality Wkly. Rep.* (CDC) 26:383, 1977.
33. Deo, M. G., Sood, S. K., and Ramalingaswami, V Experimental protein deficiency: Pathological features in the Rhesus monkey. *Arch. Pathol. Lab. Med.* 80:14, 1965.
34. Dimondon, R., Henschel, A., and Keys, A. The electrocardiogram of man in semistarvation and subsequent rehabilitation. *Am. Heart J.* 35:584, 1948.
35. Dmochowski, J. R., and Moore, F. D. Choroba Glodowa. *N. Engl. J. Med.* 293:356, 1975.
36. Dongegan, C. K., et al. Negative results of tocopherol therapy in cardiovascular disease. *Am. J. Med. Sci.* 217:294, 1949.
37. Evans, C. L. *Starling's Principles of Human Physiology,* 9th ed. Philadelphia: Lea & Febiger, 1945. P. 1155.
38. Follis, R. H. *Deficiency Disease.* Springfield, IL: Thomas, 1958. P. 577.

39. Follow-up on deaths in persons on liquid protein diets. *Morbidity & Mortality Wkly. Rep.* (CDC) 26:443, 1977.
40. Foster, M. *A Textbook of Physiology*. New York: Macmillan, 1895. P. 1183.
41. Garnett, E. S., et al. Gross fragmentation of cardiac myofibrils after therapeutic starvation for obesity. *Lancet* 1:914, 1969.
42. Gelfand, M., Jones, J. J., and Thomas, G. E. Nutritional microcardia recovery of heart size and function with treatment. *Cent. Afr. J. Med.* 21: 107, 1975.
43. Gillanders, A. D. Nutritional heart disease. *Br. Heart J.* 13:177, 1951.
44. Gobel, A. J., Hay, D. R., and Sandler, M. 5-OH tryptamine metabolism in acquired heart disease associated with argentaffine carcinoma; preliminary communication. *Lancet* 2:1016, 1965.
45. Graham, T. P., Jr., et al. Control of myocardial oxygen consumption: Relative influence of contractile state and tension development. *J. Clin. Invest.* 47:375, 1968.
46. Greenberg, D. M., Anderson, C. E., and Tufts, E. V. Pathological changes in the tissues of rats reared on diets low in magnesium. *J. Biol. Chem.* 42:114, 1936.
47. Grimes, J. B., and Abel, R. M. Acute hemodynamic effects of intravenous fat emulsion in dogs. *J.P.E.N.* 3:40, 1979.
48. Gunning, J. F., Harrison, C. E., Jr., and Coleman, H. W., III. The effects of chronic potassium deficiency on myocardial contractility and oxygen consumption. *J. Mol. Cell Cardiol.* 4:139, 1972.
49. Hackel, D. B., Goodale, W. J., and Kleinerman, J. Effects of thiamine deficiency on myocardial metabolism in intact dogs. *Am. Heart J.* 46:883, 1953.
50. Harrison, C. E., Jr., et al. Myocardial and mitochondrial function in potassium depletion cardiomyopathy. *J. Mol. Cell Cardiol.* 4:633, 1972.
51. Hefner, L. L., et al. Relation between neural force and pressure in the left ventricle of the dog. *Circ. Res.* 11:654, 1962.
52. Heggtveit, H. A., Herman, L., and Mishra, R. K. Cardiac necrosis and calcification in experimental magnesium deficiency. A light and electron microscopic study. *Am. J. Pathol.* 45:757, 1964.
53. Heymsfield, S. B., et al. Cardiac abnormalities in cachetic patients before and during nutritional repletion. *Am. Heart J.* 95:584, 1978.
54. Higginson, J., Gillanders, A. D., and Murray, J. F. The heart in chronic malnutrition. *Br. Heart J.* 14:213, 1952.
55. Hodges, R. E. Vitamin E and coronary heart disease. *J. Am. Diet. Assoc.* 62:638, 1973.
56. Hottinger, V. A., Esell, O., and Uehlinger, E. *Hungerkronkeit, Hungerodem, Hungertuberkulose.* Basel: Benno, Schwabe, 1948. P. 181.
57. Jolliffe, N., and Goodhart, R. Beriberi in alcohol addicts. *J.A.M.A.* 111:380, 1938.
58. Jones, R. V. Fat malabsorption in congestive cardiac failure. *Br. Med. J.* 1:1276, 1961.
59. Keys, A., Henschel, A., and Taylor, H. L. The size and function of the human heart at rest in semi-starvation and in subsequent rehabilitation. *Am. J. Physiol.* 50:153, 1947.
60. Keys, A., et al. Laboratory of Physiological Hygiene. In A. Keys, J. Brosek, A. Henschel, and O. Mickelson (Eds.), *The Biology of Human Starvation.* Minneapolis: University of Minnesota, 1950. P. 494.
61. Kim, N. D., and Harrison, C. E. $45Ca^{2+}$ accumulation by mitochondria and sarcoplasmic reticulum in chronic potassium depletion cardiomyopathy. *Rec. Adv. Stud. Cardiac Struct. Metab.* 4:551, 1974.
62. Ko, K. K., and Paradise, R. R. The effects of substrates on contractility of rat atria depressed with halothane. *Anesthesiology* 31:532, 1969.
63. Kyger, E. R., et al. Adverse effect of protein malnutrition on myocardial function. *Surgery* 84: 147, 1978.
64. Levey, S. Obesity and heart failure. *Nutr. Rev.* 24:199, 1966.
65. Levine, H. J., and Britman, N. A. Force-velocity relations in the intact dog heart. *J. Clin. Invest.* 43:1383, 1964.
66. Levy, H., and Boas, E. P. Vitamin E in heart disease. *Ann. Intern. Med.* 28:1117, 1948.
67. Majoor, C. L. H. Alcoholism as a cause of beriberi heart disease. *J. R. Coll. Physicians Lond.* 12:143, 1978.
68. McCandless, D. W., et al. Cardiac metabolism in thiamine deficiency in rats. *Nutrition* 100:991, 1970.
69. McKinney, B. *Pathology of the Cardiomyopathies.* London: Butterworth, 1974. P. 360.
70. McKinney, B. Studies on the experimental production of endomyocardial fibrosis and cardiomegaly of unknown origin by dietary means. *Am. Heart J.* 90:206, 1975.
71. McKinney, B., and Crawford, M. A. Fibrosis in guinea pig hearts produced by plantain diet. *Lancet* 2:880, 1965.
72. Michiel, R. R., et al. Sudden death in a patient on a liquid protein diet. *N. Engl. J. Med.* 298:1005, 1978.
73. Moore, L. A., Hallman, E. T., and Sholl, E. B. Cardiovascular and other lesions in calves fed diets low in magnesium. *Arch. Path.* 26:820, 1938.
74. Oksanen, A., and Poukka, R. An electron micro-

scopial study of nutritional muscular degeneration (NMD) of myocardium and skeletal muscle in calves. *Acta Pathol. Microbiol. Scand.* 80:440, 1972.
75. Olson, R. E. Vitamin E and its relation to heart disease. *Circulation* 48:179, 1973.
76. Peterson, B. J., and Vahouny, G. V. Cardiac structure and function in vitamin B_{12} deprived rats. *J. Nutr.* 105:1567, 1975.
77. Phornphutkul, C., Gamble, W. J., and Monroe, R. E. Ventricular performance, coronary flow, and myocardial oxygen consumption in rats with advanced thiamine deficiency. *Am. J. Clin. Nutr.* 27:136, 1974.
78. Piza, J., et al. Myocardial lesions and heart failure in infantile malnutrition. *Am. J. Trop. Med. Hyg.* 20:343, 1971.
79. Rinzler, S. H., et al. Failure of alpha tocopherol to influence chest pain in patients with cardiac disease. *Circulation* 1:288, 1950.
80. Robin, E., and Goldschlager, N. Persistence of low cardiac output after relief of high output by thiamine in a case of alcoholic beri-beri and cardiac myopathy. *Am. Heart J.* 80:103, 1970.
81. Sack, D. W., Kim, N. D., and Harrison, C. E., Jr. Myocardial function and subcellular calcium metabolism in chronic potassium deficiency. *Rec. Adv. Stud. Cardiac Struct. Metab.* 5:203, 1975.
82. Saurs, H. E. Personal communication, 1978.
83. Schrader, G. A., Pricket, C. O., and Salmon, W. D. Symptomatology and pathology of potassium and magnesium deficiencies in the rat. *J. Nutr.* 14:85, 1937.
84. Shute, W. E., and Taub, H. G. A. *Vitamin E for Ailing and Healthy Hearts.* New York: Pyramid, 1972.
85. Sims, B. A. Conducting tissue of the heart in kwashiorkor. *Br. Heart J.* 34:828, 1972.
86. Smith, H. L., and Willins, F. A. Adiposity of the heart. *Arch. Med.* 51:911, 1933.
87. Smythe, P. M., Swanepoel, A., and Campbell, J. A. H. The heart in kwashiorkor. *Br. Med. J.* 1: 5271, 1962.
88. Spatz, M. Pathogenic studies of experimentally induced heart lesions and their relations to carcinoid syndrome. *Lab. Invest.* 13:288, 1964.
89. Spatz, M. Tryptophan metabolism and cardiac disease. *Ann. NY Acad. Sci.* 156:152, 1969.
90. Sweeny, P. R., and Brown, R. G. Ultrastructural changes in muscular distrophy: I. Cardiac tissue of piglets deprived of vitamin E and selenium. *Am. J. Pathol.* 68:479, 1972.
91. Sylven, C., and Glavind, J. Peroxide formulation, vitamin E and myocardial damage in the rat. *Int. J. Vitam. Nutr. Res.* 47:9, 1977.
92. Thomas, R. M., Mylon, E., and Winternitz, M. C. Myocardial lesions resulting from dietary deficiency. *Yale J. Biol. Med.* 12:345, 1940.
93. Taylor, R. R., et al. Quantitative analysis of left ventricular function in the intact sedated dog. *Circ. Res.* 21:99, 1967.
94. Van Vleet, J. F., Ferrans, V. J., and Ruth, G. R. Ultrastructural alterations in nutritional cardiomyopathy of selenium-vitamin E deficient swine: I. Fiber lesions. *Lab. Invest.* 37:188, 1977.
95. Voit, C. Uber die Verschiedenheiten der Erweiss-Ersetzung bein hungern. *Z. Biol.* 2:309, 1866.
96. Vasquez, H. *Diseases of the Heart.* (Translated and edited by G. F. Laidlow.) Philadelphia: Saunders, 1924. P. 743.
97. Warren, S. E., and Vieweg, W. V. R. Letter to editor. *N. Engl. J. Med.* 299:419, 1978.
98. Weiss, S., and Wilkins, R. W. The nature of the cardiovascular disturbances in nutritional deficiency states (beriberi). *Ann. Intern. Med.* 11: 104, 1937.
99. Wharton, B. A., et al. The myocardium in Kwashiorkor. *Q. J. Med.* 38:107, 1969.
100. Wildenthal, R. Hormonal and nutritional substrate control of cardiac lysosomal enzyme activities. *Circ. Res.* 39:441, 1976.
101. Wildenthal, R., et al. Dietary control of cardiac lysosomal enzyme activities. *Rec. Adv. Stud. Cardiac Struct. Metab.* 8:519, 1975.
102. William, C. D. Kwashiorkor: Nutritional disease of children associated with maize diet. *Lancet* 2:1151, 1935.
103. Williams, A. W., Ball, J. D., and Davies, J. N. P. Endomyocardial fibrosis in Africa: Its diagnosis distribution and nature. *Trans. R. Soc. Trop. Med. Hyg.* 48:290, 1954.
104. Yokota, Y., et al. Effects of low protein diet on cardiac function and ultrastructure of spontaneously hypertensive rats loaded with sodium chloride. *Rec. Adv. Stud. Cardiac Struct. Metab.* 12:157, 1978.

Specific Modes of Therapy

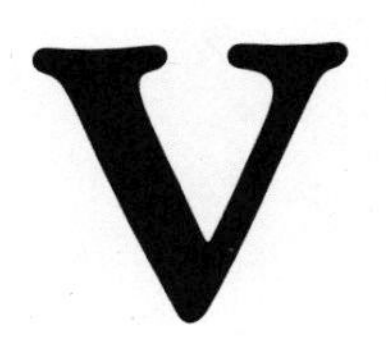

Energy Supply in Total Parenteral Nutrition

Khursheed N. Jeejeebhoy
Errol B. Marliss

21

Nutrients are ingested or infused to provide the basic needs for growth, maintenance, and repair of normal body constituents. In addition, ingested nutrients are used as supply fuels, which are oxidized to provide energy for the aforementioned processes and for such vital functions as heat production, respiration, locomotion, and circulation. The living organism is constantly consuming fuel and generating energy to remain alive. In the absence of nutrients, the organism draws primarily upon disposable stores, which, in the human, are glycogen and fat, but it also consumes essential tissues by utilizing structural protein for energy. This latter source is undesirable because if excessive or prolonged consumption occurs, it ultimately results in death. Hence the provision of energy sources is essential to the proper functioning of the patient, so that such protein "autophagy" does not occur and essential tissues are preserved and provided with sufficient energy to function normally. However, it is equally axiomatic that protein equilibrium and net synthesis require that exogenous protein be provided.

SOURCES OF ENERGY

The human body can utilize many sources of energy, each through its own set of metabolic pathways. However, in the administration of total parenteral nutrition, certain constraints make only a few sources suitable for the provision of energy on a large scale.

Constraints

Calorie Density

The ability to provide a high calorie-to-fluid volume ratio is critical so that the patient can receive sufficient calories without having to be infused with excessive volumes of fluid.

Complete Utilization and Negligible Excretion

As a corollary to the first constraint it is clear that even if a calorie-dense solution can be infused, the loss of a substantial part of such an infusion into the urine or by accumulation in the body fluids will effectively prevent the patient from utilizing the infused nutrient.

FREEDOM FROM TOXICITY IN THE DOSES REQUIRED TO MEET ENERGY NEEDS

The nutrient or its metabolic products should not adversely affect the vascular system, the central nervous system, or indeed the function of any organ.

COST

This is an important factor in the provision of nutrients, since their use on a large scale in parenteral nutrition programs is so costly that strict controls are required. The cost/benefit ratio of any nutrient must be subject to precise monitoring.

OSMOLALITY

The osmolar concentration of the solution influences its effect on veins. Hypertonic solutions are injurious to veins and certainly cannot be given into peripheral veins. Hence, any regimen involving the use of peripheral veins cannot employ markedly hypertonic solutions. This has been offset by the use of central venous infusions; however, even with this route there is a significant incidence of caval injury and thrombosis, which may be reduced by the use of infusions having a lower tonicity.

When all these criteria are met, it is clear that at present only two sources of energy are suitable. They are glucose and triglyceride-containing lipid emulsions. These two, and others, will be discussed in this chapter.

Glucose

Ordinarily this physiologic carbohydrate fuel is readily and completely utilized, and has no known toxic effects in this situation. When endogenous insulin secretion is known or highly suspected to be insufficient, the utilization of glucose can be enhanced by infused insulin so that hyperglycemia and glycosuria can be controlled and prevented. The high osmotic pressure of a solution that is sufficiently calorie-dense to meet energy requirements is a disadvantage. It is also poorly utilized in the face of insulin resistance and does not supply essential fatty acids. Furthermore, recent studies have indicated that a significant amount of infused glucose may be synthesized into fatty acids prior to becoming available for oxidation. This process increases carbon dioxide output. Since fatty acid synthesis is an energy-requiring process, there is a decrease in the net energy available for other purposes. These aspects will be discussed later in the text. Recent evidence has shown that in injured septic patients, glucose infusion increases oxygen consumption and catecholamine excretion.

Fat

Fat emulsions are made up of three groups of constituents: triglyceride, an emulsifying agent, and an added agent to give an acceptable osmolar concentration. The initial experience with lipid emulsions in the United States was disastrous and resulted in the publication of literature suggesting that lipid caused a host of side effects including liver function abnormalities, pulmonary insufficiency, fever, jaundice, shock, and adverse effects on immunity. However, this applied to only a specific product, Lipomul (Upjohn Co., Kalamazoo, Mich.). Concurrently in Sweden, using painstaking research methods, Wretlind and his colleagues developed and perfected a lipid emulsion, Intralipid (Vitrum, Stockholm, Sweden), which is made up of soya bean triglyceride, purified egg phospholipid as emulsifier, and glycerol to determine the osmolality. This emulsion could be used in dogs to provide total caloric replacement without reaction over a 4-week period [16], had a particle size and clearance comparable to those of chylomicrons [18], demonstrated elimination characteristics comparable to those of chylomicrons [17], and showed negligible uptake by the reticuloendothelial system. Furthermore, it is hydrolyzed by lipoprotein lipase in the same way as chylomicrons [8]. More recently Ota et al. [37] have shown that this lipid actually enhances the reactivity of lymphocytes to antigens and does not depress immunity.

At the time of this writing, another emulsion has become available. It is made from safflower oil and is called Liposyn (Abbott, Chicago, Ill.). It has the same clearance and utilization characteristics as Intralipid and appears to be similarly free of toxicity. However, long-term experience with this lipid emulsion is still awaited.

Amino Acids

After amino acids are transaminated or deaminated, the resulting carbon skeletons are oxidized either directly via subsequent conversion to pyruvate or entry into the tricarboxylic acid cycle, or indirectly by prior conversion to glucose (gluconeogenesis). However, this is a costly way of providing energy. Furthermore, infusion of amino acids in quantities to provide sufficient energy will result in the production of urea in amounts large enough to induce an osmotic diuresis, and azotemia, which varies according to the adequacy of renal function.

Alcohols, Polyols, and Other Mono- and Disaccharides

Ethanol can be used as a source of calories, but its utilization is limited by central nervous system effects, altered redox state, and risk of hepatic damage. Sorbitol has been advocated as a source of calories, but studies have shown that between 20 and 40 percent of the infused sorbitol is excreted renally [24]. Furthermore, in a controlled study in which the thrombogenic effect on peripheral veins of 10 percent sorbitol was compared with that of 10 percent glucose, sorbitol was not found to be superior to glucose [24]. Xylitol is another polyol used as a source of energy, but it causes oxaluria and oxalosis of the kidney. Maltose, the disaccharide of glucose, has half the osmolality of glucose, but its metabolic availability when it is given intravenously is controversial. Fructose has been advocated because its intracellular transport is not insulin-dependent. However, in large does it depletes hepatic ATP, raises lactate (and hence uric acid) levels, and has been claimed to result in relatively higher plasma triglyceride levels than glucose. Although the latter may not be the case, it does not have sufficient merit to be used in preference to glucose, with the addition of insulin if necessary.

METABOLIC FATE AND INTERRELATIONSHIPS OF ENERGY SOURCES

A scheme of these relationships is given in Figure 21-1. The three major nutrients—carbohydrate, fat, and protein—are interrelated metabolically in three ways. *First,* all these nutrients can provide substrates for oxidation in the Krebs cycle (Figure 21-1, *1*). *Second,* biosynthesis of one of these nutrients can occur from others in specified ways. In this regard, α-keto acids can be synthesized into nonessential amino acids (Figure 21-1, *2*) by transamination, with glutamic acid as the nitrogen donor. In muscle, alanine is synthesized from pyruvate (Figure 21-1, *3*), with the amino group being derived by transamination from other amino acids originating from muscle protein catabolism, especially the branched-chain amino acids—valine, leucine, and isoleucine. Recently it has been shown that by providing the keto or hydroxy analogue of certain essential amino acids exogenously, one can cause biosynthesis of essential amino acids to occur, thus showing that it is the carbon skeleton of these amino acids that is essential. Fatty acid synthesis occurs in the liver from acetyl-CoA (Figure 21-1, *4A*) derived from pyruvate, a product of carbohydrate metabolism. This pathway is a major source of fatty acids in patients infused with large amounts of carbohydrate. Likewise, the glycerol for triglyceride synthesis (Figure 21-1, *4B*) can be derived from dihydroxyacetone phosphate, a metabolite of glucose. Glucose, on the other hand, can be synthesized via the gluconeogenic pathway (Figure 21-1, *5*) from substrates derived from amino acid metabolism. Although it is currently popular to consider "the" gluconeogenic amino acid to be alanine, Figure 21-1 shows that its carbon skeleton is derived from pyruvate, which in turn is derived

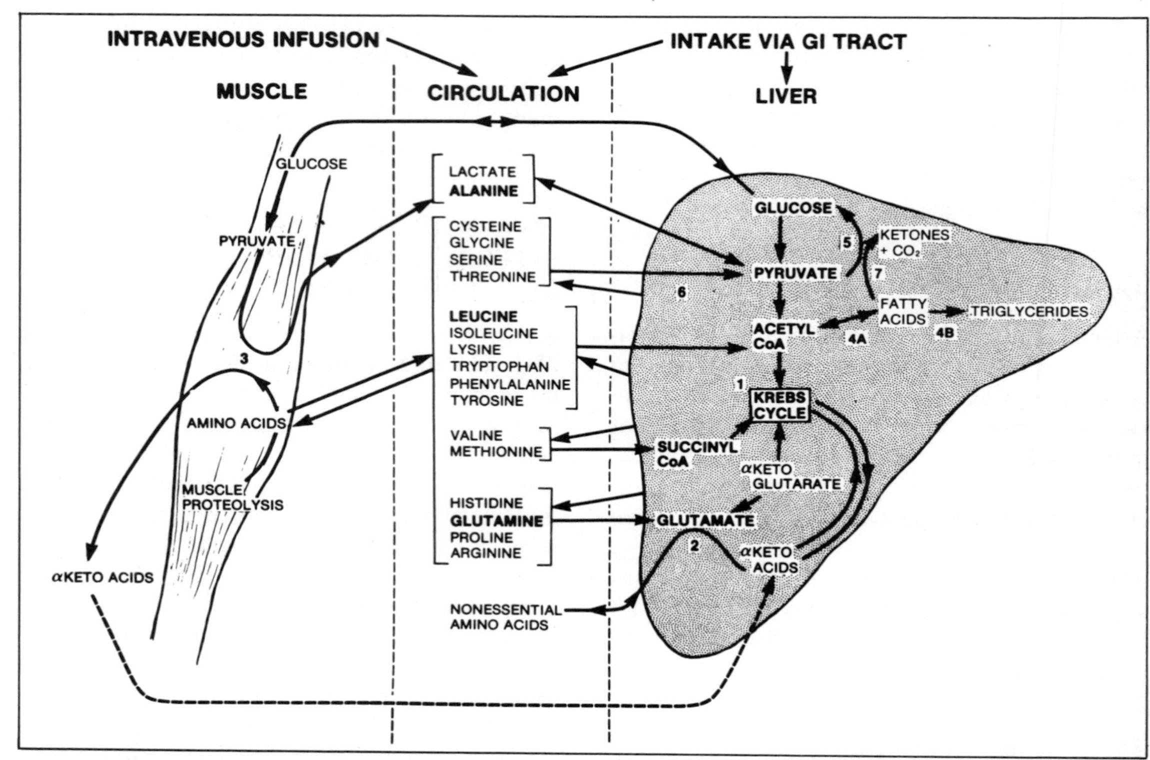

Figure 21-1. *Scheme of interrelationships of energy sources and their metabolites. For discussion, see text.*

primarily from glucose. Hence the "alanine-glucose cycle" does not lead to net glucose synthesis from amino acid precursors unless the pyruvate is derived from other amino acids (Figure 21-1, *6*) [38]. In this respect alanine and lactate are analogous as gluconeogenic precursors, since no *net* new glucose is produced from lactate derived from glucose and recycled (via the Cori cycle) back to glucose in the liver. Experimental studies have shown that in fasted animals, pyruvate derived from amino acids in muscle is quantitatively of minor importance as a source of pyruvate for gluconeogenesis [38]. Thus alanine can equally be regarded as no more than an amino group carrier to rid muscle of otherwise potentially toxic ammonia, which the liver synthesizes into urea for subsequent excretion. *Third,* while the naturally occurring fatty acids themselves cannot be converted to glucose, it should be recognized that the energy-requiring gluconeogenic pathway is "fueled" by fatty acid oxidation (Figure 21-1, *7*). Hence, energy from oxidation of one substrate supports the biosynthesis of others.

In the case of fatty acid oxidation by the liver, the "byproducts" are the ketone bodies, acetoacetate and 3-hydroxybutyrate. Thus, in states in which fat-derived fuels are the primary energy source, elevation in ketone body levels is expected. This occurs whether fatty acids are derived from endogenous lipid stores or from infusion of triglyceride emulsions. When gluconeogenesis is accelerated as a primary event (as in certain forms of trauma), again this link between gluconeogenesis and fatty acid oxidation results in accelerated ketogenesis. A fundamental principle of control of all the foregoing processes is that the pathways do not usually operate in both directions simultaneously. Thus, in states of isocaloric provision of glucose exogeneously, that glucose will be oxidized and used as substrate for fatty acid synthesis, and gluconeogenesis and fatty acid oxidation will be shut off. In the opposite direction, with fat as the principal energy source, gluconeogenesis to provide the necessary fuel for obligate glycolytic tissues (erythrocytes, CNS, skin, etc.) will be active. But when both glucose and lipid are available, the net adjustment of these pathways is determined by the proportion of each provided.*

These interrelationships are important in recognizing that there is nothing exclusive about any one substrate, and that infusion of any one energy source will influence the utilization of other sources. A discussion of the hormonal mediation of these responses follows.

Utilization of Energy Sources in Pathologic States

Malnutrition

In malnutrition and fasting, there is mobilization of fatty acid from adipose tissue stores to provide energy for peripheral tissues, including muscle. In addition, there is an obligatory release of amino acids from muscle protein and this leads to wasting. The carbon skeletons of the released amino acids are used for gluconeogenesis to provide fuel for the central nervous system and other glucose-utilizing tissues. In prolonged fasting, ketogenesis becomes well established, and ketones are used as fuels by the central nervous system, displacing glucose in part. Additionally, associated with increased ketonemia and a rise in plasma free fatty acid levels, the mobilization of amino acids from muscle is reduced. Hence in malnutrition and starvation, endogenous lipids are selectively utilized as fuel and protein loss is curtailed, but does persist [7]. If carbohydrates are administered in this state, their utilization for energy and insulin levels will increase in proportion to the amount given in relation to total needs. Such energy supply will also serve to decrease gluconeogenesis from protein and, hence, protein loss. This protein-sparing effect of carbohydrate has been known for a century, but popularized in the past several decades [12]. In otherwise normal individuals, exogenous fat given with amino acids as energy will also spare protein, though without elevating insulin levels.

Trauma

In trauma the metabolic rate is increased and energy expenditure rises. Kinney et al. [27] have estimated that this increase may be 25 percent above normal for multiple fractures and as much as 40 to 100 percent with burns. Wilmore [45] considers that this increase in metabolic rate is due to the elevation of catecholamines together with other hormonal stimuli, such as increased growth hormone and glucagon levels [2]. In addition, Greenberg et al. (unpublished observations) and Batstone et al. [5] have obtained evidence suggesting that corticosteroids are also an important factor in the catabolic reaction observed with surgery and burns, respectively. However, Wolfe et al. [48] have found no relationship between altered glucose metabolism and any alteration in the hormonal milieu.

Associated with a rise in metabolic rate in the injured patient, there is increased gluconeogenesis, increased nitrogen loss, and insulin resistance. Despite this increased flow of glucose it is not used as the primary metabolic fuel [48] because the respiratory quotient in these patients is only 0.70 to 0.75, indicating that fat oxidation still provides the primary energy substrate [27, 45]. Furthermore in burned patients, during glucose infusion with or without insulin, the proportion of glucose oxidized fell as uptake increased, showing that the availability of this substrate as the primary source of energy is limited and is not enhanced by insulin [48]. In these patients it is of interest that the high rate of gluconeogenesis cannot be cur-

**Editor's Note:* While this may occur normally, in deranged metabolic situations, such as sepsis, such controls may not operate as well.

tailed by glucose infusions alone [15]. Furthermore, in trauma the muscle appears to completely oxidize only 50 percent of the glucose extracted from the circulation, the remainder being released, only after partial oxidation, as lactate [9, 45]. The increase in muscle lactate output and the consequent increase in blood lactate are associated with increased gluconeogenesis. Clowes et al. [9] have indicated that in the traumatized subject, muscle also does not use fatty acids effectively and thus increases the need to oxidize amino acids as a source of fuel. The nitrogen released by oxidation of endogenous amino acids from muscle flows out as alanine, resulting in a further increase in the availability of substrate for gluconeogenesis. The enhanced rate of gluconeogenesis derives its energy needs from fatty acid oxidation. Hence, fatty acid utilization is enhanced, and the respiratory quotient falls to 0.70 to 0.75. Viewed in another way, it can be shown that in such patients, despite the increased nitrogen wasting, 80 percent of the total metabolic energy is derived from fat [27, 45].

In contrast to the findings of Clowes et al. [9] and a corresponding conclusion drawn from selected literature by Ryan [40] that fatty acid mobilization and ketogenesis are impaired in trauma, are the findings of Greenberg (unpublished observations) in patients undergoing major surgery and of Batstone et al. [5] and Carlson [8] in patients with burns. In these studies, fatty acid mobilization and ketogenesis did occur during the early phase of injury, but the levels fell after the first few days. Experimentally, Barton et al. [4] showed that ketone body production after early injury was normal, but peripheral utilization was increased. Hence, the availability of fat substrates in injury is still controversial and requires direct measurement by isotopic and regional metabolic studies.

Infection

The effects of injury and infection on nutrient utilization have often been considered together. More recently, attempts have been made to distinguish the effects of infection from those of injury per se. Infections are associated with an increased metabolic rate; for example, peritonitis may be associated with a 50 percent increase in metabolic rate [27], and Clowes et al. [9] have shown an average increase in metabolic rate of about 30 percent in patients having infection uncomplicated by trauma or shock. In contrast, the presence of septic shock is associated with a fall in metabolic rate owing to poor perfusion and, possibly, the effect of endotoxin on the oxidative mechanism of the cell [9]. The uptake of glucose by muscle is increased by infection, but lactate output rises to a degree that suggests that only 25 percent of the glucose is being fully oxidized. This finding, together with the observation that free fatty acid utilization is only one-seventh that of the fasting patient despite only a 50 percent reduction in free fatty acid levels, suggests that the muscle must obtain a significant part of its energy from amino acid oxidation. This assumption is supported by the higher nitrogen loss seen in these patients and the greater release of alanine from muscle, which may amount to three times the output in controls [9]. Gluconeogenesis is increased, as expected from the hormonal milieu (inappropriately low insulin and high glucagon, corticosteroids, catecholamines, and growth hormone), and the increase in lactate and alanine output by muscle makes substrates available for gluconeogenesis by the liver. However, with septic shock and endotoxemia, gluconeogenesis falls, lactate and alanine levels rise, and blood glucose levels approach normal [9, 45]. In extreme septic shock, hypoglycemia may occur.

Therefore, it appears that with infection muscle continues to rely on endogenous protein as a source of energy, despite the availability of glucose and fatty acids. Hence, in such patients the traditional sources of nonprotein energy may not be of any value, and in fact it is not clear whether anything other than amino acids can provide metabolic fuel for muscle under these circumstances.

Lipoprotein Abnormalities

In type I and type V hyperlipoproteinemia, the utilization of circulating triglycerides is impaired because of reduced or absent lipoprotein lipase activity, preventing the hydrolysis of the circulating triglyceride into fatty acids. In type IV hyperlipoproteinemia, increased carbohydrate intake is associated with a rise in circulating triglyceride levels, presumably from increased hepatic VLDL-triglyceride synthesis from the glucose provided.

Liver and Renal Diseases

In liver disease, especially cirrhosis and chronic liver failure, there is insulin resistance and carbohydrate intolerance. In consequence, hyperglycemia and hyperinsulinemia occur with carbohydrate infusions. In contrast, there is no evidence for the impaired utilization of lipids.

In chronic renal disease there are impaired carbohydrate and fat tolerances, both of which are corrected by dialysis. Furthermore, it has been shown that infused lipid emulsions do not adversely affect the dialysis membrane in its ability to clear the blood of such waste products as urea and electrolytes.

Diabetes Mellitus

Since insulin is a primary regulator of the responses to altered nutritional states and has been described as a factor in several of the aforementioned abnormal states, predicted responses of diabetics to parenteral nutrition and to these pathologic states are correspondingly exaggerated. Absolute insulin deficiency, in insulin-dependent (juvenile-onset type) diabetics, has been described as a "superfasted state," in which all early fasting metabolic adjustments are amplified (fat mobilization, gluconeogenesis, protein mobilization) and exacerbated by the inability to generate a "fed-state" response to exogenous nutrients. Thus, utilization of both exogenous and endogenously overproduced nutrients is impaired. The administration of either glucose or lipid, or mixes of both, to such diabetics would thus produce catastrophic effects unless appropriate amounts of insulin (determined by the nutrient composition and its rate of delivery) are concurrently provided. This is easily done by merely adding insulin to infusates, titrating the amount against glycemia, glucosuria, and ketone levels. When this is done, there is no contraindication to the use of any nutrient mix considered appropriate to the state being treated.

In the non-insulin-dependent (maturity-onset-type) diabetic, the metabolic state is the integrated result of the magnitude of insulin deficiency and insulin resistance present. The majority of such patients are obese, and their insulin levels may range from low compared with normal weight or obese nondiabetics, all the way to high compared with normal weight or even with obese nondiabetics. The requirement for parenteral nutrition in such individuals is most often associated with stress states, in which insulin secretory capacity is further suppressed. These states often convert such diabetics into "apparent" insulin-dependent diabetics, now termed "insulin-requiring." Without insulin treatment, marked hyperglycemia and its consequences—or even ketoacidosis—may appear. Therefore, in any case of isocaloric or hypercaloric parenteral nutrition in such individuals, insulin therapy should be introduced at the outset and continued throughout treatment, again with careful monitoring. Without it, the risk of hyperosmolar, hyperglycemic states is significant.

Often in the course of acute illness in previously undiagnosed diabetics, hyperglycemia develops, precipitated by suppression of insulin secretion and elevation of antiinsulin hormone levels. If unrecognized, marked hyperglycemia may rapidly evolve, with all its untoward consequences. Therefore all candidates for TPN must be tested for diabetes at the outset and at intervals during treatment. Especially vulnerable are individuals with renal failure and those receiving high-dose corticosteroids, or any drug known to be capable of impairing insulin secretion (e.g., diazoxide, phenytoin) or previously described as being associated with hyperglycemia (e.g., some diuretics, l-asparaginase, azathioprine, lithium, pentamidine).

On the other hand, our observations have shown that providing 50 percent of the total caloric input as lipid emulsion frequently abolishes or greatly reduces the degree of hyperglycemia and thus obviates the need to add exogenous insulin. The introduction of fat does not adversely alter nitrogen balance when compared with an all-glucose infusion [23]. Hence, mixed lipid-glucose infusions are recommended for these patients.

PROTEIN-SPARING ACTION OF ENERGY SUBSTRATES

Concept of Protein-Sparing and Factors Modifying the Protein-Sparing Effect of Energy Sources

In 1946 Gamble [12], in his now classic "life raft" studies, showed that the infusion of glucose reduced by 50 percent the nitrogen loss (as urea) from protein catabolism. This effect was referred to as the protein-sparing effect of glucose. Later Cahill et al. [7] showed that in prolonged fasting, a rise in circulating nonprotein fuels, such as fatty acids and ketones, was associated with a fall in urinary nitrogen, one interpretation of which is that fuels derived from fat can inhibit the breakdown of muscle protein.

These effects demonstrate that availability of nonprotein energy, both as glucose and as fat, can inhibit the breakdown of endogenous protein in the absence of exogenous protein. Since the early 1900s, it has been known that with a fixed protein intake, nitrogen balance improves with the addition of energy as either carbohydrate or fat [33]. More recently, Blackburn et al. [6] and others, including ourselves [33], have shown that infusing amino acids alone results in a reduced net negative balance of nitrogen, indicating that exogenous amino acids are also protein-sparing. The key finding in all these studies has been the inability to attain positive nitrogen balance when one energy substrate was used alone or when amino acids were combined with hypocaloric (i.e., less than metabolic needs) amounts of carbohydrate or fat.

By contrast, amino acids combined with carbohydrate in quantities exceeding the energy requirements of the patient have resulted in a positive nitrogen balance. Similarly, the use of fat also has been associated with a positive nitrogen balance [23]. Hence, protein anabolism can only be attained by combining amino acids with an energy source in amounts sufficient to meet or exceed the requirements of the patient.

In addition to a positive nitrogen balance, it can be shown that such a combination indeed results in an increase in total body nitrogen when the gamma emission of neutron bombardment is measured and in total body potassium using whole body counting of ^{40}K (Figure 21-2) [32]. It is the universal experience that such patients gain body weight and tissue by a variety of measures.

Role of Carbohydrate versus Fat in Nitrogen Sparing. The Modifying Effects of Malnutrition, Infection, and Trauma

It appears that in both malnutrition and trauma the major part of the oxidized fuel is fat [9, 27, 45]. Furthermore, even when glucose is infused as the sole exogenous energy substrate, Holroyde et al. [20] have shown that 30 to 50 percent of the carbon dioxide excreted comes from sources other than glucose, indicating that glucose fails to provide all the carbon required for oxidation in the situations examined. Fat might be expected to be the natural substrate for the provision of the nonprotein energy in these situations. In contrast to this simple theory, however, the results of experimental studies comparing the relative efficacy of carbohydrate and fat in promoting positive nitrogen balance are controversial. The weight of evidence now supports the equivalence of fat and carbohydrate in many clinical situations. However, studies by Long et al. [31] and McDougall et al. [34] on critically ill burned patients suggested that despite excellent utilization of exogenously infused lipid, this substrate did not reduce nitrogen loss. In contrast, the infusion of glucose did significantly reduce nitrogen excretion. The maximum reduction in nitrogen excretion was found

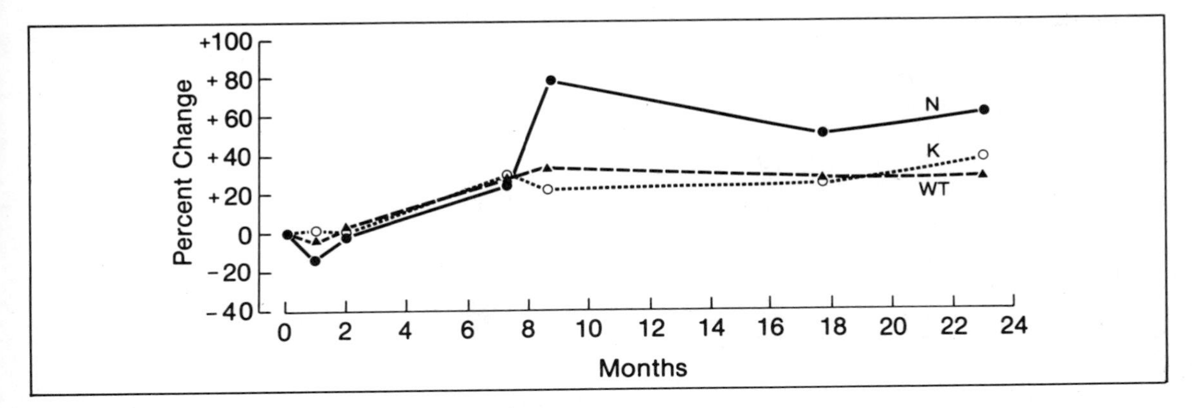

Figure 21-2. *Course with time of one patient's changes in body weight, total body potassium (naturally occurring ^{40}K determined in whole-body counter) and total body nitrogen (as determined by neutron capture gamma analysis).*

to occur when the infusion rate of glucose was equal to the metabolic requirements for energy. These studies were widely interpreted as suggesting that lipid had no role in promoting nitrogen retention during parenteral nutrition.

On the other hand, another controlled crossover trial of glucose and lipid sources [23] of nonprotein energy in patients with malnutrition and a variety of gastrointestinal disorders, including those with infection and inflammation such as Crohn's disease, pancreatitis, and peritonitis, showed that lipids and carbohydrates were comparable in promoting nitrogen retention. In this study a mixture of 5 percent amino acid and 5 percent dextrose solution, delivering 1 gm/kg of ideal body weight, was infused throughout the study. On an average these patients therefore received a constant intake of 60 gm of amino acids and 60 gm of dextrose. In addition, the patients were randomized to receive either glucose or lipid at 40 kcals/kg of ideal body weight. After a week of this regimen, the additional nonprotein energy source was switched, making each patient his or her control for comparing the two substrates. By randomizing the order, the effect of any change due to improvement in the clinical state was minimized. It will be seen from Figures 21-3 to 21-5 that the glucose infusion resulted in higher levels of pyruvate and lactate, both glucose-derived substrates, and that the circulating concentrations of free fatty acids and ketones were suppressed. Plasma glucose levels were not different, but they had higher insulin and lower glucagon levels. In contrast, during lipid infusion there were lower pyruvate and lactate levels with higher concentrations of fat-derived substances, namely free fatty acids and ketones, with lower insulin and higher glucagon levels. Despite these very different substrate-hormone profiles, the nitrogen balance was comparable after the initial three days of study on each substrate. During the initial three days of infusion, there was slightly higher nitrogen retention with glucose. However, after the initial three days nitrogen retention was comparable. In addition, it was noted that during lipid infusion, a higher free fatty acid level was associated with a lower nitrogen excretion, showing the nitrogen-sparing effect of exogenous fatty acids and indicating that during exogenous fat infusions, additions of agents such as heparin improve nitrogen retention.

Wilmore [45] has reconciled differences between studies from his center and those of Jeejeebhoy et al. [23] by suggesting that in hypermetabolic patients the neurohormonal drive may reduce the ability to adapt to fat utilization. Other investigators have also noted that fat and carbohydrate are comparable in promoting nitrogen

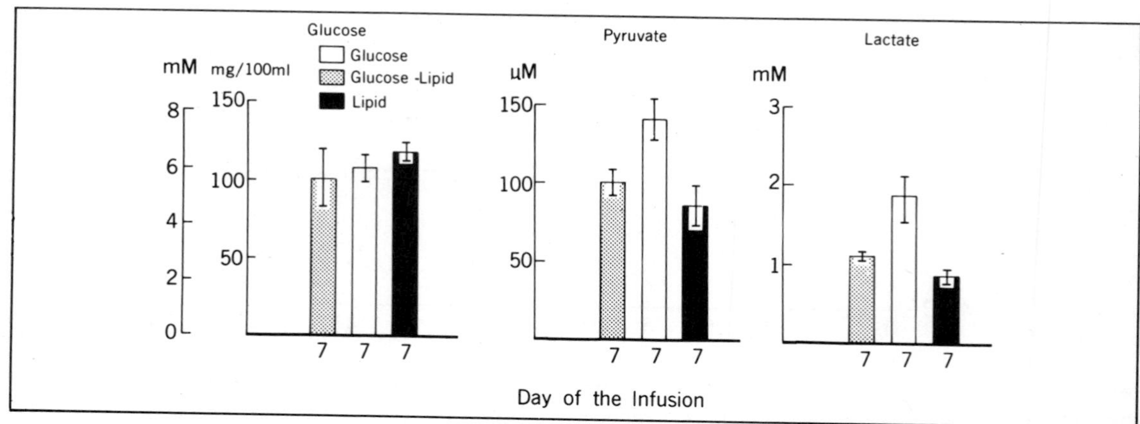

Figure 21-3. *Serum concentrations of glucose, pyruvate, and lactate during 24-hour infusions of total parenteral nutrition containing 1 gm of amino acids per kg of ideal body weight. The form of nonprotein calories, prescribed to maintain normal body weight, was randomly given in turn for 1 week at a time as 100% glucose; 50% glucose, 50% lipid (Intralipid); or 17% glucose, 83% lipid (Intralipid).*

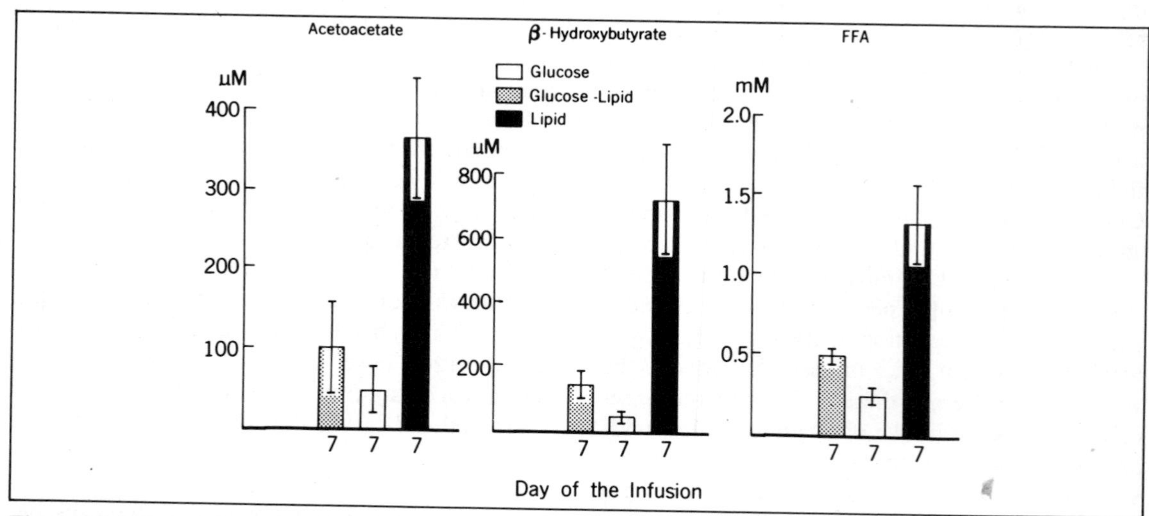

Figure 21-4. *Serum concentrations of acetoacetate, β-hydroxybutyrate, and plasma free fatty acids under the conditions noted in Figure 21-3.*

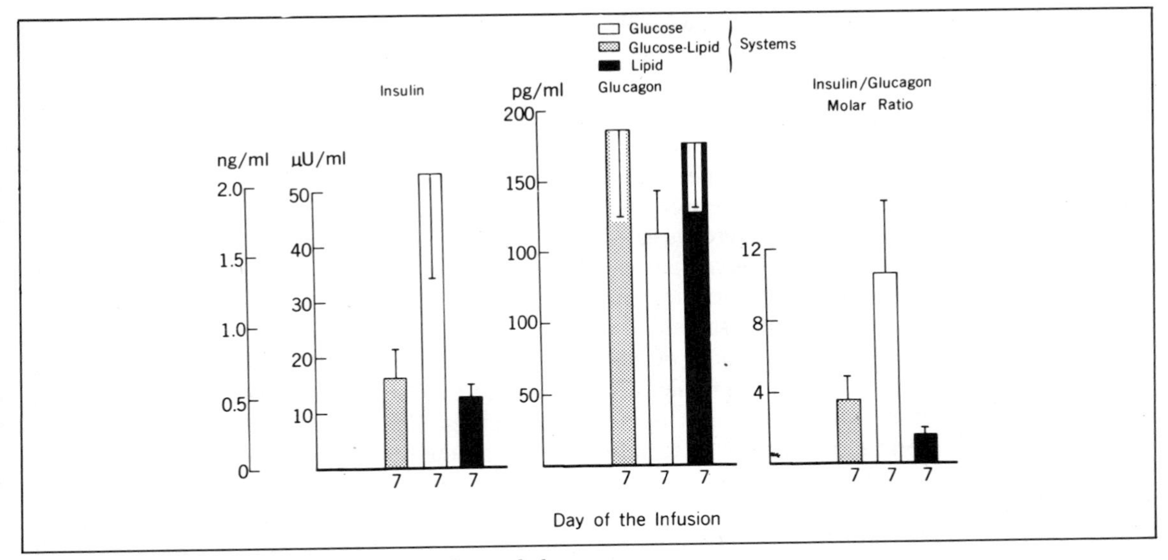

Figure 21-5. *Plasma immunoreactive insulin and glucagon and their molar ratio, under the conditions noted in Figure 21-3.*

balance in patients in a variety of conditions similar to those studied by us [3, 13, 49]. Recently, Wannemacher et al. [43] have shown that in monkeys infected with *pneumococci,* exogenous glucose and lipid had equal protein-sparing actions and both were clearly superior to that of amino acids alone. Long et al. [30] have shown in rats that glucose and lipid are comparable in normal animals and in those with 20 percent burns, but that glucose was superior in animals with 40 percent burns. In these studies it was shown that the protein-sparing actions of both glucose and lipid were reduced with increasing trauma, so that energy substrates alone did not appear to be sufficient to blunt the catabolic action of trauma or sepsis. Similarly, the more recent data of Long et al. [30] suggest that glucose and lipid are comparable in promoting nitrogen retention in all situations except severely catabolic states, as exemplified by 40 percent burns. Recent data on whole body composition by MacFie et al. [32] indicate that total body nitrogen increases only when lipid is added to the TPN regimen.

TECHNIQUES OF INFUSING LIPID AS AN ENERGY SOURCE

Metabolic Considerations

Over the years numerous studies have shown that nutrients are most effectively utilized when given simultaneously. Hence it is appropriate that intravenous fat be infused concurrently with the other nutrients. Also by infusing nutrients gradually, the circulating substrate profile remains at near steady-state levels, and rapid and marked increases in triglyceride or fatty acid levels are thereby avoided.

Despite the dogmatic pronouncements about the danger of mixing fat with glucose and amino acids because of the risk of breaking the emulsion, experimental and practical experience has shown otherwise. When lipid has been infused concurrently with a glucose-amino acid solution through a Y connector in the manner to be described later in this chapter, no untoward effects have been reported from an experience with infusion of 36,000 units over 10 years at the Toronto General Hospital. Furthermore, published metabolic studies indicate excellent utilization of fat when it is given this way. There is therefore no evidence to support the alleged requirement for separately infusing fat and dextrose-amino acid mixtures.

The next metabolic consideration is the most appropriate ratio of fat to carbohydrate. It is clear from what has been noted earlier that nitrogen balance is comparable in many studies irrespective of the nature of the nonprotein energy source, the only exception being patients with severe burns—who do not constitute the majority given parenteral nutrition. This being the case, a decision regarding the type of infusion will be based mainly on other criteria. These are the: (1) route of administration, (2) substrate-hormone profile, (3) need for specific factors only available in lipid, (4) effect of infusion on fluid and electrolyte balance, (5) effect on ventilatory load, and (6) maintenance of normal biochemical parameters. These criteria will be discussed when we present the advantages and disadvantages of fat as a caloric source compared with glucose.

Peripheral Infusion Technique

Solutions Used

Amino Acids; Dextrose; Electrolytes; Vitamins; Trace Elements in a Mix. A five percent amino acid solution with 12.5 percent dextrose is made by mixing equal volumes of commercially available 10 percent amino acids with 25 percent dextrose. In most adults, about 1,500 ml/24 hours is sufficient to meet amino acid requirements. Electrolytes are added to this infusion to provide about 115 to 120 mEq Na, 80 to 100 mEq K, 20 mEq Ca, 25 to 30 mEq Mg, and 500 to 600 mg P/24 hours. Vitamins are added as indicated in previously published papers [22]. Trace elements are likewise introduced as required. When 20 percent lipid becomes available, 500 ml distilled water will have to be added to 1,500 ml of the aforementioned mix to make up 2,000 ml, reducing the osmolality.

Lipid Emulsion. Concurrently with the amino acid-dextrose mix just described, 1,500 ml of a 10 percent lipid emulsion is infused. When 20 percent lipid becomes available, more calories can be given in the same volume at a lower osmolality by infusing 1,000 ml of this lipid and diluting the amino acid-dextrose with 500 ml of distilled water.

Method of Infusion

The success of the peripheral venous infusion depends on strict adherence to the method to be described. The amino acid-dextrose mixture must be infused concurrently and at the same rate as the lipid through a Y connector to avoid thrombophlebitis. The entire success of the method depends on the lipid mixing and diluting the amino acid-dextrose mixture to a near-isotonic state. It is desirable to use a two-channel Holter pump (model No. 921, Extracorporeal Medical Specialities, King of Prussia, PA) so as to ensure uniform infusion of the viscous lipid and the dextrose-amino acid mixture.

Nutrient Prescription. This infusion provides 75 gm of amino acids, 650 kcals of dextrose, and 1,650 kcals of lipid, giving a total caloric input of about 2,300 kcals in 3,000 ml of fluid. From these figures it is apparent that sufficient calories and protein can be given by this system to induce anabolism. Thereby, such a peripheral system can provide sufficient calories to restore tissue proteins. If more fluids can be given, as in patients with fistulas, the caloric input can be increased further. Also, when 20 percent lipid becomes available, the lipid input can be increased.

Equipment Required. (Figure 21-6)

19-gauge butterfly needle or 18-gauge Angiocath Teflon intravenous catheter placement unit (Deseret Co., Sandy, Utah)
500 ml normal saline (initially)
Straight IV tubing
Intralipid tubing (if Intralipid is to be given)
Alcohol swabs
Povidone iodine 10 percent solution (PI)

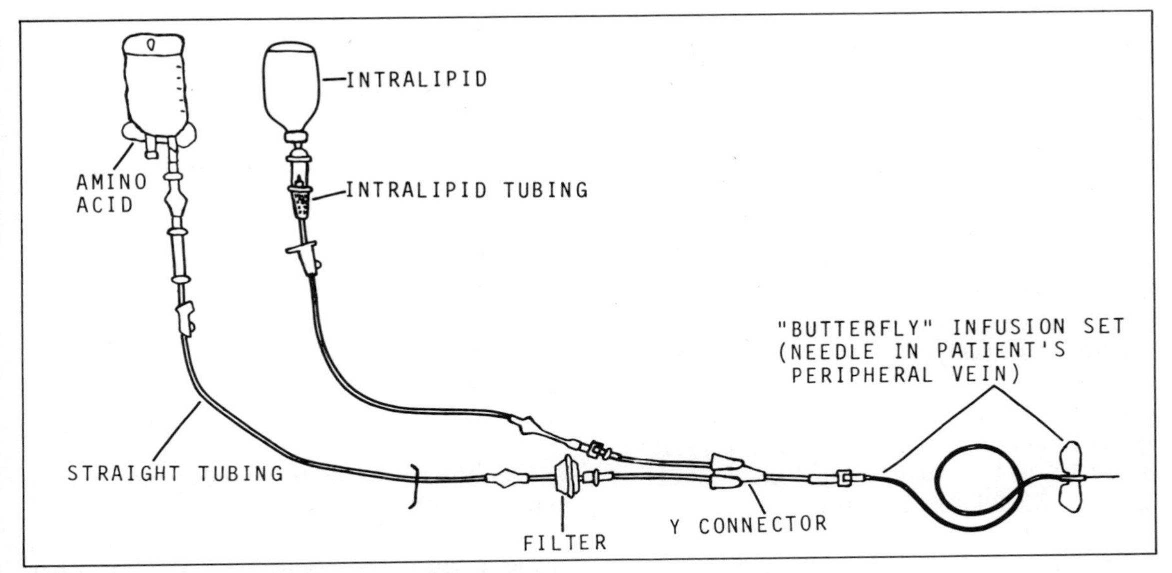

Figure 21-6. *Scheme of peripheral venous infusion for total parenteral nutrition.*

Tourniquet
Y connector (to allow mixing of lipid with the other solutions as close to point of IV entry as possible)
Filter

Procedure. (Note: The IV nurse or doctor should insert the butterfly needle or catheter.)

1. Explain to the patient what is to be done and why.
2. Bring all the necessary equipment to the bedside and connect and flush the IV tubing with saline.
3. Place the tourniquet on the arm; clean the skin with alcohol and apply Povidone. Insert the butterfly needle or catheter. Release the tourniquet and connect the tubing.
4. Open the control clamp on the IV to run quickly at first, then regulate.
5. Tape the butterfly needle or catheter securely.
6. When the saline flush is running properly, the nutrient mixture can be started (Figure 21-6).

Central Venous Infusion Techniques

The central venous catheter is inserted and cared for in the usual way [39]. To infuse lipids, the central route is used with minor modifications as follows.

Solutions Used

Amino Acids; Dextrose; Electrolytes; Vitamins; Trace Elements in a Mix. The solutions used consist of 5 percent amino acids and 25 percent dextrose made up by mixing commercially available 10 percent amino acid with 50 percent dextrose in equal volumes. In an average adult 1.5 to 2 liters of this solution are infused with lipid per 24 hours. Electrolytes, vitamins, and trace elements are added to the solution as indicated under the peripheral infusion system. Details of these additives have been published elsewhere and can be reviewed by the interested reader.

Lipid Infusion. The aforementioned mixture is infused with 1,000 or 1,500 ml of 10 percent lipid concurrently by means of a Y connector, as described previously. When 20 percent lipid becomes available, a smaller volume can be used.

METHOD OF INFUSION

The two solutions are infused concurrently by means of a standard drip system. No pumps are necessary. The dextrose concentration in the final infusate using this technique is diluted by the lipid emulsion to about 16 percent, reducing the danger of hypoglycemia in the event that the drip is discontinued abruptly.

Nutrient Prescription. This system provides 100 gm of amino acids, 1,250 to 1,700 kcals of glucose, and 1,100 to 1,650 kcals of lipid, giving a total of 2,350 to 3,350 kcals/24 hours.

Technique. The hub of the central venous line is attached to a connecting length of intravenous tubing (e.g., Extension Set 30″, by Abbott Hospital Supplies, Abbott Laboratories, North Chicago, Ill.), which is then connected to the Y connector (Figure 21-7). The remaining connections are as given under peripheral infusion (see Figure 21-6).

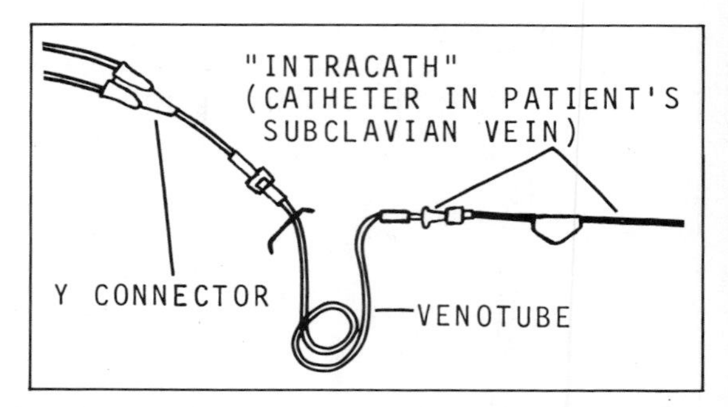

Figure 21-7. *Scheme of proximal modifications of Figure 21-6 for central vein infusion for total parenteral nutrition.*

ADVANTAGES AND DISADVANTAGES OF FAT AS A CALORIE SOURCE COMPARED WITH GLUCOSE

Substrate-Hormone Profile

It will be seen from Figures 21-3 to 21-5 that the substrate hormone profile depends on the nature of the nonprotein calories infused. It is quite clear that the substrate-hormone profile is closest to the postprandial state when half the calories are given as glucose and half as lipid (glucose-lipid). The insulin levels are largely within the postprandial range. Hence this ratio of calories provides the system most comparable to that observed in the postabsorptive state. The modest insulin response required to utilize the substrate infused makes it attractive when there is insulin resistance and in non-insulin-dependent diabetics. Using this ratio of calories, or when more fat is infused as in a peripheral system, we have rarely had to give insulin to our patients, thus improving the simplicity of the method and reducing the need for frequent monitoring. Correspondingly, the reduced glucose concentration required when lipid is given as a caloric source has simplified the technique for ambulatory patients who are receiving parenteral nutrition at home. The lower circulating levels with a glucose-lipid infusion reduce the need to use pumps, or to carefully taper the infusion in order to avoid hypoglycemia upon its termination. Toleration of abrupt stoppage or change of infusion is useful in case of mishap or sudden alteration in circumstances, and allows ambulatory patients to take the infusion in units that can be easily discontinued, thus allowing flexibility of the system to suit the social needs of the patient.

It has been claimed that lipid infusions may cause a cardiac arrhythmia because of high free fatty acid levels. It should be noted, however, that with a 1:1 lipid-to-glucose calorie ratio, the free fatty acid levels are comparable to those seen with an oral diet. Furthermore, the opposite problem of high lactate levels is also avoided in patients with conditions sometimes associated with lactic acidosis.

Fluid and Sodium Balance

It has been shown by Spark et al. [42] and by others that high insulin levels and carbohydrate feeding result in marked sodium retention, an undesirable development in patients prone to pulmonary complications and those with heart failure. This theoretic possibility has been confirmed by Hill [19], and Yeung et al. [50] who showed by careful body composition studies that during glucose-based hyperalimentation, a major part of the increase in body weight was due to water. In our own unpublished studies using a glucose-lipid based system, such water retention does not occur.*

Respiratory Quotient and Carbon Dioxide Load

When carbohydrate alone is infused, the respiratory quotient (RQ = CO_2 excreted / O_2 consumed) rises to 1.0, or higher if fat synthesis occurs. With a mixed intake of lipid and carbohydrate, the RQ is between 0.80 and 0.85. Hence, there is at least a 15 to 20 percent lower CO_2 load to be excreted when lipid is infused. Recently, using an all-glucose system, Askanazi et al. [1] showed that glucose infusion increases the CO_2 load and especially increases oxygen consumption and the ventilatory effort in hypermetabolic patients. The same group has also noted difficulty in weaning patients off respirators because of this high CO_2 load and could only do so by reducing caloric intake. Respiratory failure with high glucose loads has now been described [10]. Clearly, if fat is used as a source of calories, the CO_2 load could be reduced without reducing caloric intake.

Potential Complications of Lipid Infusion—Fact and Fiction

In older literature, the use of earlier lipid preparations (such as Lipomul), which proved to be toxic by reason of the particular lipid or emulsifier used, has led to the accumulation of references that are often quoted to indicate the hazards of lipid infusions. It is important to emphasize that modern lipid sources, available in North America, do not show these effects.

**Editor's Note:* Part of the problem with increased fluid retention may be due to excessive volumes infused.

Utilization of Fat in Trauma

It is often claimed that fat is not utilized in the traumatized patient. This appears not to be the case. Wilmore et al. [46] showed increased clearance of infused fat in catabolic patients, as did Hallberg [17].†

Utilization of Fat in Sepsis

Fat clearance is shown to be reduced in septic animals, and hence it was concluded that fat is not utilized in septic patients. However, a controlled study by Wannemacher et al. [43] showed that while triglyceride levels were higher in infected animals infused with lipid, there was no difference in nitrogen retention or recovery from the infection when compared with glucose-infused animals. It should be noted also that hyperglycemia is also common during sepsis and that in end-stage sepsis all substrates are poorly utilized.‡

Effect of Fat Emulsions on the Reticuloendothelial (RE) System

It is commonly believed that fat emulsions are taken up by the RE system, reducing the ability to combat infection. However, with Intralipid, Gigon et al. [14] and Scholler [41] found no accumulation in the RE system. Furthermore Huth et al. [21] showed that while Lipomul-like emulsions using cottonseed oil reduced tolerance to endotoxin, the same phenomenon was not observed with soya bean oil emulsions such as Intralipid.

Effect on the Coagulation System

Disseminated intravascular coagulation has been reported after use of cottonseed oil emulsions, but no such effect and, indeed, no abnormality of

†*Editor's Note:* Clearance may not be synonymous with utilization.

‡*Editor's Note:* While in end-stages of sepsis utilization of all substrates is depressed, a number of studies, including those cited earlier, suggest that in "ordinary" but severe sepsis glucose may be better utilized than fat.

coagulation in vivo has been reported during infusion of soya bean oil emulsions.

Effect on Liver and Renal Disease

Liver disease is commonly believed to be a contraindication to lipid. However, on theoretical and practical grounds, this cannot be justified. The lipid emulsions are hydrolyzed by lipoprotein lipase mainly situated outside the liver, and the fatty acids thus released are taken up largely by muscle and adipocytes. In contrast, excess carbohydrate has to be converted to fatty acids in the liver [47] and then excreted as lipoproteins. Hence carbohydrates place a greater load on the liver than do fats. This is attested to by the observation that a high-carbohydrate infusion reproducibly induces a fatty liver [25, 26, 35], whereas high-fat infusions rarely do so. Furthermore, Jeejeebhoy et al. [25, 26] have shown that isocaloric replacement of carbohydrate with lipid to the extent of 30 to 50 percent of total calories reproducibly clears the liver of the fat observed when an all-glucose system has been infused.

In practice, Zohrab et al. [51] found that when lipid was given in a TPN mixture up to 2 gm/kg ideal body weight/day in patients with jaundice and abnormal liver function tests, no adverse effect was seen, and in fact the liver function abnormalities improved during infusion. Similar results have been reported by Lee [28], Michel et al. [36], and Zumtobel and Zehle [52].*

In renal disease, both glucose and lipid utilization are reduced [11, 44], but this abnormality is corrected by dialysis; furthermore, lipids do not influence the clearance of electrolytes and dialyzable nitrogenous products during hemodialysis [29].

Partial Parenteral Nutrition

In a number of gastrointestinal conditions the patient may be able to tolerate only a limited amount of normal or elemental diet. Under these circumstances, balance of the nutrient requirements (after taking into account any energy reserves as fat) can be easily made up through peripheral parenteral nutrition, using the technique described earlier. This is especially useful in selected patients with esophageal and gastric obstruction, intractable diarrhea, anorectal disease, and partial bowel obstruction, as a temporary measure pending definitive treatment. By means of this method, optimal nutrition can be provided by all available routes and by simple techniques.

In conclusion, there is increasing evidence for the role of lipid as an energy source during parenteral nutrition, and earlier and less fortunate experience should not influence further exploration of the use of modern and nontoxic fat emulsion in parenteral nutrition.

**Editor's Note:* The concern is not so much liver disease but liver failure. In the latter case, it is not clear that fatty acids are cleared by the liver. It is known that manufacture of the ketone bodies is decreased in liver failure.

REFERENCES

1. Askanazi, J., Carpentier, Y. A., Elwyn, D. H., Nordenstrom, J., Jeevananda, M., Rosenbaum, S. H., Gump, F. E., and Kinney, J. M. Influence of total parenteral nutrition on fuel utilization in injury and sepsis. *Ann. Surg.* 191:40, 1980.
2. Aulick, H. L., Wilmore, D. W., and Mason, A. D. Mechanism of glucagon calorigenesis. *Fed. Proc.* 35:401, 1976.
3. Bark, S., Holm, I., Hakansson, I., et al. Nitrogen-sparing effect of fat emulsion compared with glucose in the postoperative period. *Acta Chir. Scand.* 142:423, 1976.
4. Barton, R. N. Ketone Body Metabolism After Trauma. In R. Porter and J. Knight (Eds.), *Energy Metabolism in Trauma* (Ciba Foundation Symposium). London: Churchill Livingstone, 1970. Pp. 173–182.
5. Batstone, G. F., Alberti, K. G. M. M., Hinks, L., et al. Metabolic studies in subjects following thermal injury: Intermediary metabolites, hormones, and tissue oxygenation. *Burns* 2:207, 1976.
6. Blackburn, G. L., Flatt, J. P. Clowes, G. H. A., et al. Peripheral intravenous feeding with isotonic amino acid solutions. *Am. J. Surg.* 125:447, 1973.
7. Cahill, G. F., Jr. Starvation in man. *N. Engl. J. Med.* 282:668, 1970.
8. Carlson, L. A. Mobilization and Utilization of Lipids After Trauma: Relation to Caloric Homeostasis. In R. Porter and J. Knight (Eds.), *Energy Metabolism in Trauma* (Ciba Foundation Symposium). London: Churchill Livingstone, 1970. Pp. 155–171.

9. Clowes, G. H. A., O'Donnell, T. F., Blackburn, G. L., et al. Energy metabolism and proteolysis in traumatized and septic man. *Surg. Clin. North Am.* 56:1169, 1976.
10. Covelli, H. D., Black, W. J., Olsen, M. S., Beekman, J. F. Respiratory failure precipitated by high carbohydrate loads. *Ann. Intern. Med.* 95:579, 1981.
11. Cramp, D. G., Moorhead, J. F., and Wills, M. R. Disorders of blood lipids in renal disease. *Lancet* 1:672, 1975.
12. Gamble, J. L. Physiological information gained from studies on the life raft ration. *Harvey Lectures,* 1946/47. Series 42, p. 247.
13. Gazzaniga, A. B., Bartlett, R. H., and Shobe, J. B. Nitrogen balance in patients receiving either fat or carbohydrate for total intravenous nutrition. *Ann. Surg.* 182:163, 1975.
14. Gigon, J. P., Enderlein, F., and Scheidegger, S. Uber das Schicksal infundierter Fettemulsionen in der menschlichen Lunge. *Schweiz. Med. Wschr.* 96:71, 1966.
15. Gump, F. E., Long, C. L., Illian, P., et al. Studies of glucose intolerance in septic, injured patients. *J. Trauma* 14:378, 1974.
16. Hakansson, I. Experience in long-term studies on nine intravenous fat emulsions in dogs. *Nutr. Diet.* 10:54, 1968.
17. Hallberg, D. Elimination of exogenous lipids from the blood stream. An experimental methodological and clinical study in dog and man. *Acta Physiol. Scand.* (Suppl. 259) 65:1, 1965.
18. Hallberg, D., and Wersall, J. Electron-microscopic investigation of chylomicrons and fat emulsions for intravenous use. *Acta Chir. Scand.* (Suppl.) 325:23, 1964.
19. Hill, G. L., McCarthy, I. D., Collins, J. P., et al. A new method for the rapid measurement of body composition in critically ill surgical patients. *Br. J. Surg.* 65:732, 1978.
20. Holroyde, C. P., Myers, R. N., Smink, R. D., et al. Metabolic response to total parenteral nutrition in cancer patients. *Cancer Res.* 37:3109, 1977.
21. Huth, K. W., Schoenborn, W., and Borner, J. Zur Pathogenese der Unvertraglichkeitserscheinungen bei parenteraler Fettzufuhr. *Med. Ernah.* 8:146, 1967.
22. Jeejeebhoy, K. N. Total parenteral nutrition (TPN) —a review. *Ann. Roy. Coll. Phys. Surg.* (Canada) 9:287, 1976.
23. Jeejeebhoy, K. N., Anderson, G. H., Nakhooda, A. F., et al. Metabolic studies in total parenteral nutrition with lipid in man: Comparison with glucose. *J. Clin. Invest.* 57:125, 1976.
24. Jeejeebhoy, K. N., Anderson, G. H., Sanderson, I., et al., Total Parenteral Nutrition. In J. G. G. Ledinghan (Ed.), *Advanced Medicine Symposium 10.* London: Pitman Medical, 1974. Pp. 132–150.
25. Jeejeebhoy, K. N., Langer, B., Tsallas, G., et al. Total parenteral nutrition at home: Studies in patients surviving 4 months to 5 years. *Gastroenterology* 71:943, 1976.
26. Jeejeebhoy, K. N., Zohrab, W. J., Langer, B., et al. Total parenteral nutrition at home for 23 months without complication and with good rehabilitation. A study of technical and metabolic features. *Gastroenterology* 65:811, 1973.
27. Kinney, J. M., Long, C. L., and Duke, J. H. Carbohydrate and Nitrogen Metabolism After Injury. In R. Porter and J. Knight (Eds.), *Energy Metabolism in Trauma. Ciba Foundation Symposium.* London: Churchill Livingstone, 1970. Pp. 103–126.
28. Lee, H. A. The Rationale for Using a Fat Emulsion (Intralipid) as Part Energy Substrate During Intravenous Nutrition. In J. M. Greeps, P. B. Soeters, R. I. C. Wesdorp, C. W. R. Phaf, and J. E. Fischer (Eds.), *Current Concepts in Parenteral Nutrition.* Hague: Martinus Nijhof, 1977. Pp. 261–271.
29. Lee, H. A., Sharpstone, P., and Ames, A. C. Parenteral nutrition in renal failure. *Postgrad. Med. J.* 43:81, 1967.
30. Long, J. M., III, Souba, W. W., and Dudrick, S. J. Effect of calorie intake and stress on nitrogen excretion. *J.P.E.N.* 2:Abst. 84, July 1978.
31. Long, J. M., Wilmore, D. W., Mason, A. D., Jr., et al. Fat carbohydrate interaction: Nitrogen-sparing effect of varying caloric sources for total intravenous feeding. *Surg. Forum* 25:61, 1974.
32. MacFie, J., Smith, R. C., and Hill, G. L. Glucose or fat as a non-protein energy source? A controlled clinical trial. *Gastroenterology* 80:103, 1981.
33. Marliss, E. B. An Overview of Amino Acid Metabolism. The Determinants of Protein Homeostasis in Parenteral Nutrition. In *Symposium on Clinical Nutrition Update: Amino Acids.* Chicago: AMA, 1977. Pp. 34–45.
34. McDougal, W. S., Wilmore, D. W., and Pruitt, B. A., Jr. Effect of intravenous near isosmotic nutrient infusions on nitrogen balance in critically ill injured patients. *Surg. Gynecol. Obstet.* 145:408, 1977.
35. Messing, B., Bitoun, A., Galian (1) A., et al. La steatose hepatique au cours de la nutrition parenterale depend-elle de l'apport calorique glucidique? *Gastroenterol. Clin. Biol.* 1:1015, 1977.
36. Michel, H., Raynaud, A., Crastes de Paulet, Mme., et al. Tolerance du cirrhotique aux lipides intra-veineux. *Congres International de Nutrition*

Parenterale. Montpellier, France, Sept. 12-14, 1974.

37. Ota, D. M., Copeland, E. M., Corriere, J. N., et al. The effects of a 10% soya-bean oil emulsion on lymphocyte transformation. *J.P.E.N.* 2:112, 1978.
38. Ruderman, N. B. Glucose Metabolism. A. Control of Glucose Production: Hepatic Glycogenolysis and Gluconeogenesis. In R. Assan, J. R. Girard, and E. B. Marliss (Eds.), *Diabetes Mellitus: A Pathophysiologic Approach to Clinical Practice.* New York: Wiley, in press.
39. Ryan, J. A., Jr. Complications of Total Parenteral Nutrition. In J. E. Fischer (Ed.), *Total Parenteral Nutrition.* Boston: Little, Brown & Co., 1976. Pp. 55–100.
40. Ryan, N. T. Metabolic adaptations for energy production during trauma and sepsis. *Surg. Clin. North Am.* 56:1073, 1976.
41. Scholler, K. L. Transport and Speicherung von Fettemulsion-teilchen. *Z. prakt. Anasth. Wiederbel.* 3:193, 1968.
42. Spark, R. F., Arky, R. A., Boulter, P. R., et al. Renin, aldosterone and glucagon in the natriuresis of fasting. *N. Engl. J. Med.* 292:1335, 1975.
43. Wannemacher, R. W., Kaminski, M. V., Neufeld, H. A., et al. Protein-sparing therapy during pneumococcal infection in rhesus monkey. *J.P.E.N.* 2:507, 1978.
44. Westervelt, F. B., and Schreiner, G. E. The carbohydrate intolerance of uremic patients. *Ann. Intern. Med.* 57:266, 1962.
45. Wilmore, D. W. Alterations in Intermediary Metabolism. In T. King and K. Reemtsmak (Series Eds.), *The Metabolic Management of the Critically Ill. Reviewing Surgical Topics.* New York: Plenum, 1977. Pp. 129–170.
46. Wilmore, D. W., Moylan, J. A., Helmkamp, G. M., et al. Clinical evaluation of a 10% intravenous fat emulsion for parenteral nutrition in thermally injured patients. *Ann. Surg.* 78:503, 1973.
47. Wolfe, R. R. Personal communication.
48. Wolfe, R. R., Durkot, M. J., Allsop, J. R., et al. Glucose metabolism in severely burned patients. *Metabolism* 28:1031, 1979.
49. Woolfson, A. M. J., Heatley, R. V., and Allison, S. P. Insulin to inhibit protein catabolism after injury. *N. Engl. J. Med.* 300:14, 1979.
50. Yeung, C. K., Smith, R. C., and Hill, G. L. Effect of an elemental diet on body composition: A comparison with intravenous nutrition. *Gastroenterology* 77:652, 1979.
51. Zohrab, W. J., McHattie, J. D., and Jeejeebhoy, K. N. Total parenteral nutrition with lipid. *Gastroenterology* 64:583, 1973.
52. Zumtobel, V., and Zehle, A. Postoperative parenterale Ernahrung mit Fettemulsionen bei Patienten mit Leberschaden. *Langenback's Arch. klin. Chir. Suppl. Chir. Forum,* 1972. P. 179.

Central Hyperalimentation

Josef E. Fischer
Herbert R. Freund

22

HISTORY OF PARENTERAL NUTRITION

The history of intravenous nutrition is short—a brief, recent chapter in the long history of intravenous therapy. Shortly after William Harvey's discovery of the blood circulation in 1628, Sir Christopher Wren gave the first intravenous morphine injection to a dog. The practical application of intravenous nutrition has its roots in the work of Pasteur and of Lister, and continues to rely on the modern development of chemistry and biochemistry. In 1913, Henriques and Anderson, realizing the allergic reaction that follows infusion of foreign protein, hydrolyzed casein and used the mixture to intravenously feed a goat, claiming nitrogen equilibrium. Dr. Robert Elman, in 1936, reported the first successful administration of protein hydrolysate in humans [36].

The first apparently successful case of parenteral nutrition in an infant was reported in 1944 from the Johns Hopkins University, where Helfrick and Abelson supported an infant with intractable diarrhea by the intravenous administration of fat (coconut milk) and protein [62]. A landmark in the development of intravenous nutrition was the work of W. C. Rose and colleagues, determining the requirements of essential amino acids in man [94, 95]. Additional experimental and clinical observations suggested that protein deficiency profoundly affects the outcome of surgery.

The classic works of Cuthbertson [26], Habif and associates, and the many important contributions from Dr. Jonathan Rhoad's laboratory stressed the nutritional importance of post-injury catabolism. Efforts to obtain nitrogen equilibrium at this time by intravenous nutrition were only occasionally successful because of many limitations. The volume of fluid infused, often 7.0 liters per day, could not be managed by the weak diuretics then available. Large infusion volumes were required by the low caloric density of nutrients, 4 calories per gram of glucose or per gram of protein hydrolysate. Alcohol, with a caloric density of 7 calories per gram, was not available. Finally, nutrients had to be infused in tolerable concentrations. A 5% dextrose solution, approximately isotonic, offers only 150 gm or 510 calories/3 liters, which was the daily volume infused; a 10% solution of glucose, marginally tolerated by peripheral veins, yields only 340 calories/liter.

Clearly, fat emulsions or hypertonic dextrose solutions were necessary. Emmett and Holt, in the 1930s, introduced the use of fat emulsions. However, clinical trials with these solutions revealed serious, and at times fatal, side effects. By the middle 1950s, Intralipid, a soybean oil emulsion, became available in Europe, and systematic intravenous nutrition of patients began with intravenous fat, small amounts of glucose, and protein given via peripheral veins [33]. In the United States, however, no fat emulsions were available, and the use of 10% glucose required the infusion of 5 liters supplying the patients with 2000 calories a day, to which were added 80 to 100 gm of protein hydrolysate.

Dudrick, in 1966, working in Rhoad's laboratory, realized that to achieve positive nitrogen balance, a calorie to nitrogen ratio of approximately 150 to 250:1 was necessary. In order to administer such a concentrated solution of glucose and amino acids, central venous access was essential. The groundwork for the central venous access was laid by a French surgeon, Aubiniac, working in Vietnam, who perfected subclavian venipuncture as a means of achieving rapid transfusion in battle casualties. Dudrick placed catheters centrally in young beagle puppies and demonstrated that normal growth and development could be achieved by the use of total parenteral nutrition alone [33]. The first human patient, a baby with almost no gastrointestinal tract, was successfully treated and parenteral nutrition in the United States was launched [34].

After Dudrick's first publication, advances rapidly followed. Protein hydrolysate solutions were largely replaced by solutions of crystalline amino acids in more nutritionally efficient proportions and thus better utilized. Fat emulsions were reintroduced in the United States, and the technical aspects of catheter insertion and maintenance were improved. The differentiation of parenteral nutrition has begun. For example, patients with renal disease and hepatic disease currently receive amino acid solutions specially formulated for their disease states. The pediatric patient has differing nutritional requirements as does, in all probability, the regrowing, profoundly depleted adult patient. Patients with burns, cardiac failure, massive trauma, injury, and sepsis probably constitute special situations for which special solutions or special regimens should be designed and administered.

BASIC INGREDIENTS AND CONSIDERATIONS IN CENTRAL HYPERALIMENTATION

Protein

The nutritional requirement for protein, supplied parenterally as amino acids, is increased in many disease states. In traumatized or septic patients, increased caloric needs are met in part by breakdown of lean body mass. It is said, although supporting data are difficult to find, that death ensues when patients lose 40 percent of their lean body mass. Wasting of the intercostal muscles and the diaphragm, together with low resistance to infection, sets the stage for pneumonia. Whether the protein requirements of healthy individuals are sufficient for patients who are sick, severely catabolic, depleted, or septic is not yet clear.

In a series of investigations over two decades, Rose and his coworkers defined the nutritionally essential amino acids, the carbon skeletons of which could not be synthesized by man [94, 95]. These essential amino acids include phenylalanine, methionine, lysine, threonine, tryptophan, and the three branched-chain amino acids—valine, leucine, and isoleucine. Other amino acids such as arginine and, particularly, histidine may not be synthesized rapidly enough in infants and in renal failure [14]. The essential amino acids, however, may be synthesized by transamination if the carbon skeleton is provided as the alpha-keto carboxylic acid, as recently demonstrated by Walser et al. [115, 116].

The requirement for protein, however, cannot be viewed as separate from the requirement for calories. Nitrogen retention and equilibrium can be achieved by providing up to 1.7 gm/kg of synthetic L-amino acids alone, without the provision of any carbohydrate calories [10, 60], although urea accumulates rapidly. When glucose in the amount of 55 calories/kg is provided, only 0.5 gm/kg of crystalline amino acids is required for nitrogen equilibrium [10]. The metabolic fate of protein or amino acids also depends on the type and the number of calories simultaneously provided. If carbohydrate alone is also provided, most of the administered protein is incorporated into muscle protein under the influence of insulin. If both fat and carbohydrate are provided, amino acids are distributed both to the periphery and to the liver, and liver weight and nitrogen content increase [84].

Administered or ingested protein does not form the only available supply of amino acids, however, as there is rapid turnover of body protein (up to 300 gm of free amino acids per day) [84]. Many of these amino acids are reincorporated into protein, provided adequate amounts of energy are available. When adequate amounts of energy fuels are not administered, catabolism apparently proceeds unchanged while synthesis of protein decreases, as is the case in trauma or in the presence of severe infection. This is not surprising, as protein synthesis is an energy-consuming process. Thus, administration of adequate calories is important not only for the maintenance of lean body mass, but also to maximize the efficiency of utilization of administered protein and the reincorporation of endogenously available amino acids into protein.

The branched-chain amino acids (valine, leucine, and isoleucine) are unique among the amino acids in that they directly provide a source of energy for skeletal muscle, which may become important when intracellular utilization of glucose is blocked, as is the case in sepsis or massive injury. The branched-chain amino acids are not only utilized by the muscle as energy substrate, but serve also as a source for nitrogen and perhaps also carbon skeleton for the production of alanine in gluconeogenesis. In addition, branched-chain amino acids may take part in regulating the rate of muscle protein breakdown and synthesis [87]. The beneficial effects and applications of the branched-chain amino acids in trauma, sepsis, and liver failure will be discussed later in this chapter, as well as elsewhere in this volume.

Carbohydrate

Glucose is the most widely available and widely used energy fuel. Six carbon fragments are broken down into three carbon fragments, which then enter the Cori cycle, providing a major portion of the body's energy requirements. Although other carbohydrates, such as fructose, xylitol, and sorbitol, have been utilized clinically as alternative energy sources, they all are converted to glucose prior to utilization. Thus, the argument that other carbohydrates may be more suitable in the post-traumatic state when glucose intolerance is apparent does not withstand close scrutiny. It makes little sense to administer other carbohydrates, which require energy for transformation into glucose prior to utilization, instead of glucose itself with adequate amounts of insulin to promote its utilization. In addition, there are other disadvantages:

Fructose is largely converted into glucose. Production of lactate and pyruvate is increased, and fructose, especially in infants and in severely ill and septic patients, has a tendency to provoke fatal lactic acidosis. Fructose is approximately three times as expensive as glucose.

Xylitol, another widely regarded substitute for glucose, is hepatotoxic. The patient with trauma and sepsis already risks hepatic decompensation and does not need the added insult of xylitol.

Glucose in blood or urine is easy to assay in all hospitals. This is not the case for other carbohydrates. Fructose and other substances may be detected as reducing substances in the urine, but not by the glucose oxidase method (Dextrostix) so widely used for determining urinary reducing substances (mainly glucose). Glucose oxidase techniques (Dextrostix) will detect neither xylitol nor sorbitol. Thus, excessive blood and urine concentration of these substances are not as easily detected as are excessive concentrations of glucose.

Fat

With the exception of linoleic acid and some of the polyunsaturated fatty acids that the body apparently cannot synthetize except from other unsaturated fatty acids, the presence of fat in the diet may not be essential. Excessive carbohydrate and protein may ultimately end up as adipose tissue. There are, however, several theoretic advantages for utilizing fat in any intravenous regimen:

1. Fat is part of the normal diet, and there may be beneficial effects of dietary fat of which we are unaware.
2. In its anhydrous form, fat yields 9 calories/gm when totally oxidized, as opposed to only 3.3 to 4 calories/gm of glucose when totally oxidized.
3. Protein is distributed both to the liver and to the periphery in the presence of fat and carbohydrate, but it is not clear whether protein is distributed as much to the liver in the absence of fat [84].

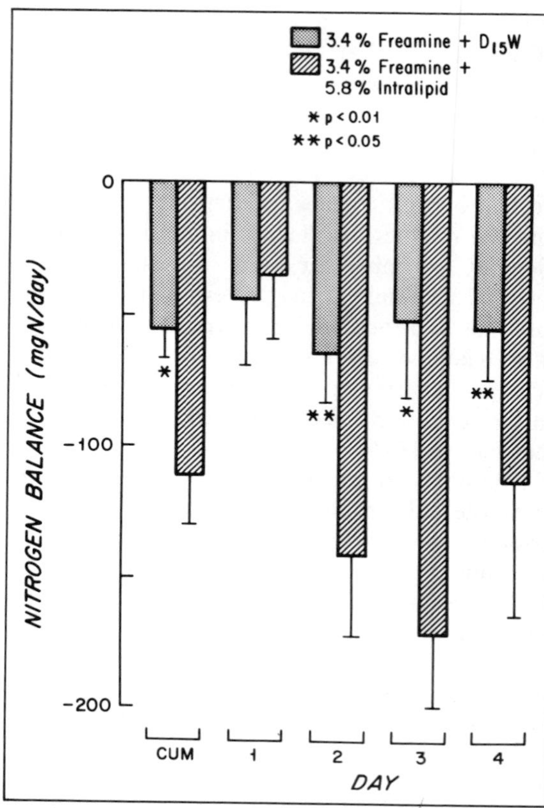

Figure 22-1. *Comparison of daily and mean nitrogen balance in rats treated with amino acids and isocaloric hypertonic dextrose or fat. Note that on each day, with the exception of the first, there is an advantage to those animals treated with hypertonic dextrose. This is seen only in the presence of amino acids. The two are equivalent with respect to nitrogen balance in the absence of amino acids. (From H. Freund et al., Is intravenous fat nitrogen sparing in the injured rat?* Am. J. Surg. *140:377, 1980.)*

Considerable confusion exists as to the fate of administered fat and its effect on lean body mass catabolism. Intralipid, the soybean oil and egg phosphatide emulsion now available, contains a certain amount of glycerol as a stabilizing agent in the emulsion, and this is easily available as three carbon fragments to be rapidly synthesized to glucose [16]. A certain amount of carbohydrate is therefore available within the lipid emulsion itself. Nor is it clear whether fat is protein-sparing under all circumstances. Jeejeebhoy et al. [66] compared a regimen containing amino acids and glucose with one containing amino acids, 17 percent glucose, and 83 percent fat. He found that nitrogen balance with both systems was positive and similar, and he concluded that exogenously infused lipid is a suitable source of nonprotein calories. Long et al. [70] detected no nitrogen-sparing effect of Intralipid in their study of 5 patients after injury or surgery. In our own studies in traumatized rats, Intralipid and glucose, when infused without any added protein, exhibited an identical nitrogen-conserving quality. However, when amino acids are added, glucose exhibits a decisively better nitrogen-conserving quality than isocaloric amounts of Intralipid (Figure 22-1) [51]. Similarly, Souba et al. [104] infused different combinations of carbohydrate and fat and found nitrogen excretion in normal and mildly stressed rats to be inversely related to both carbohydrate and fat. However, in severely stressed rats, the effect of fat on nitrogen excretion was abolished, leading to the conclusion that under significant stress, fat is unable to spare protein [104]. Thus the controversy over the efficacy of fat as a caloric source in stress continues.

Despite the lack of ability to define indications for use of fat emulsions in routine intravenous nutrition, essential fatty acid deficiency may be prevented by the administration of 4 to 10 percent of the caloric requirement as fat emulsion [80]. Essential fatty acid deficiency has become increasingly recognized, both biochemically and clinically, in patients receiving total parenteral nutrition. Recently Goodgame et al. [58] presented evidence that essential fatty acid deficiency begins early in the course of parenteral nutrition, confirming earlier work by Wene et al. [117]. Levels of linoleic and eicosatrienoic acid were abnormal after one week. Arachidonic acid levels were abnormal after two weeks, and all patients had triene-tetraene ratios greater than 0.4 after four weeks of fat-free parenteral nutrition. These biochemical abnormalities respond rapidly to the intravenous administration of fat emulsions. We observed similar results in a group of patients with fatty acid deficiency [47]. Although it has not been clearly established that essential fatty acid deficiency is injurious, except perhaps to red cell membranes and (to a questionable degree) to wound healing, we recently presented evidence that essential fatty acid deficiency may result in prostaglandin deficiency (Figure 22-2). As prostaglandins are mediators in a variety of physiologic and pathologic processes, essential fatty acid and prostaglandin deficiency may result in derangements of multiple functions regulated by prostaglandins. A significant fall in intraocular pressure during fat-free parenteral nutrition may be useful for the diagnosis of essential fatty acid-prostaglandin deficiency (Figure 22-3) [47]. To prevent essential fatty acid deficiency, 500 ml of 10% fat emulsion, every other day or twice weekly, should be administered. This should be started early in the course of parenteral nutrition, as essential fatty acid and prostaglandin deficiency occurs early, particularly in depleted patients. Equally efficacious in prevention of essential fatty acid deficiency is the oral ingestion of any unsaturated oil, such as sunflower, safflower, or corn oil margarine, approximately 25 to 50 ml/day, into any orifice of the gastrointestinal tract. When used as a caloric source, fat emulsions may be infused via central vein, but can also be infused via peripheral vein as they are iso-osmotic. When given through a peripheral vein, the fat emulsion can be infused together with a protein or amino acid solution and a 5 to 10% glucose solution in what is known as the "lipid system." In this form

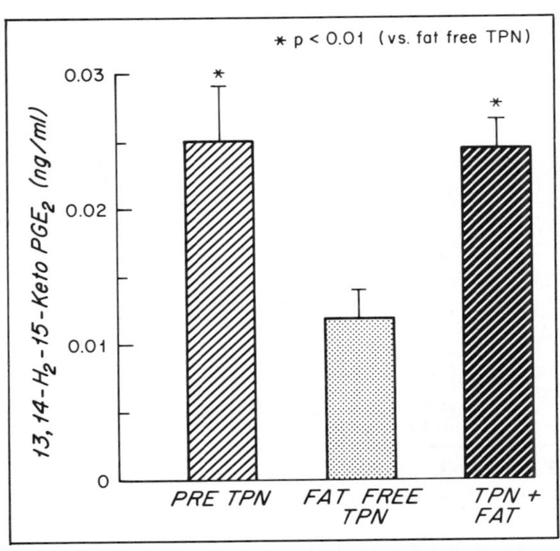

Figure 22-2. *Measurements of prostaglandins in patients undergoing fat-free total parenteral nutrition. Prostaglandin deficiency appears within 10 days of the initiation of fat-free parenteral nutrition. Normal levels of prostaglandins are restored after the administration of intravenous fat or after the patients eat fat. (From H. Freund et al. Essential fatty acid deficiency in total parenteral nutrition: detection by changes in intraocular pressure.* Ann. Surg. *190:139, 1979.)*

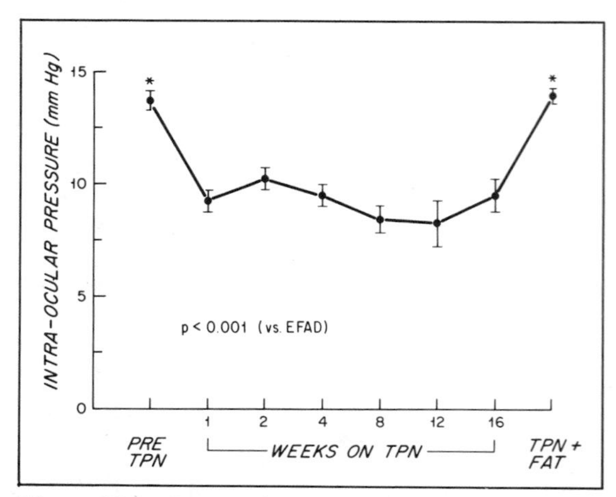

Figure 22-3. *Intraocular pressure as measured in patients on fat-free total parenteral nutrition. Note that within one week after the initiation of total parenteral nutrition without a source of fat, intraocular pressure falls, presumably secondary to prostaglandin deficiency. (From H. Freund et al. Essential fatty acid deficiency in total parenteral nutrition: detection by changes in intraocular pressure.* Ann. Surg. *190:139, 1979.)*

of therapy, the insertion site of the fat into the protein-dextrose mixture should be as close to the vein as possible in order to avoid lengthy contact of the two solutions in the tubing. The safe amount of fat is 2 gm/kg/day, higher in infants.

Vitamins

Vitamins are an essential part of our diet, performing as cofactors in a variety of metabolic processes. There is comparatively little information concerning the need for vitamins in different disease states, and little information is available to indicate requirements during total parenteral nutrition (TPN). Requirements of the relatively nontoxic B and C vitamins increase in disease and injury [11], and large excesses may be given with impunity.

Some doubt that the fat-soluble vitamins need to be given at all. Diseases of excess of vitamins A, D, and E do exist and have been observed in patients receiving parenteral nutrition. Thus, it seems wise to limit these vitamins, which in general are stored in adequate amounts or to barely above minimal requirements, until further data are forthcoming. Our practice is to include vitamins B and C in every bottle of hyperalimentation mixture, whereas fat-soluble vitamins are added only once a week in the form of MVI concentrate, 2.5 ml per bottle. Folic acid mixtures, B_{12}, and vitamin K are oxidized in glucose amino acid mixtures and must be given intramuscularly or orally. Recently Lowry et al. [71] conducted a study of vitamin requirements in patients receiving total parenteral nutrition and came up with similar conclusions, namely administration of vitamin B and C daily and the administration of 2 ampules of MVI per week (see Chapter 8, Vitamins).

Trace Metals

Trace metals are another dietary component we take for granted. Whereas there has been a significant amount of work concerning zinc and its possible importance in nutrition, very little is known about copper, chromium, selenium, iodine, manganese, and many other trace elements. Much of our knowledge concerning trace metal requirements derives from the study of patients receiving long-term parenteral nutrition, usually at home, in whom deficiency states have developed. As is the case with many other micronutrients, stores may be dangerously low and difficult to measure in such patients. As trace metals are toxic when given in excess, their administration should be conservative [17]. Furthermore, some imbalances, such as a zinc:copper imbalance, might be harmful. See also Chapter 9, "Trace Metals."

Zinc Deficiency

A shortage of zinc is generally associated with abnormalities in wound healing, dermatitis, alopecia, and disturbances in taste. In infants, zinc deficiency may lead to thymic atrophy, immune incompetence, and irritability. Plasma zinc is probably not a reasonable estimate of total

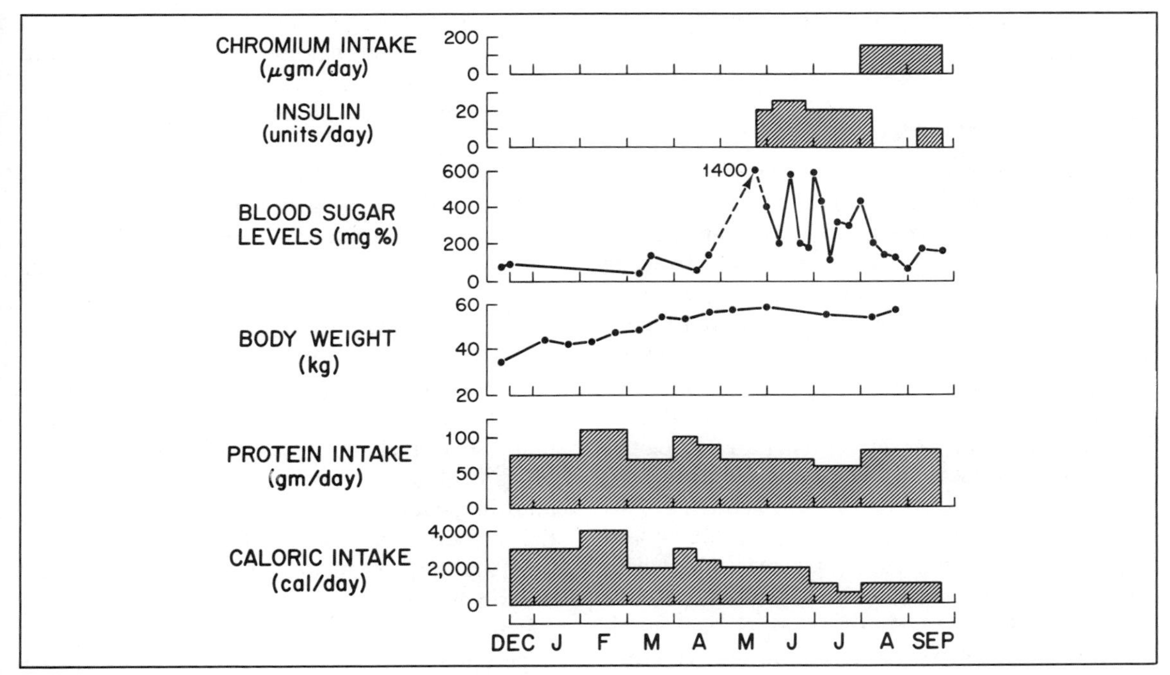

Figure 22-4. *Demonstrated chromium deficiency in a patient on long-term parenteral nutrition and sepsis. This patient was relatively stable with respect to blood sugar for approximately five months. At the end of the fifth month, she demonstrated a marked elevation in blood sugar with great difficulty in controlling her blood sugar. She also developed a peripheral neuropathy and an encephalopathy, which initially was interpreted as being hepatic or perhaps septic encephalopathy. Chromium deficiency was documented. After restoration of normal chromium intake, her need for insulin and her blood sugar returned to normal. Encephalopathy and neuropathy cleared. (From H. Freund et al. Chromium deficiency during total parenteral nutrition.* J.A.M.A. *241:496, 1979. Copyright 1979, American Medical Association.)*

body zinc. As with many of the other trace metal deficiencies, zinc deficiency is not often seen in patients on short-term parenteral nutrition. It is also becoming clear that the zinc to copper ratio may be more important than the absolute amount of zinc itself. Zinc deficiency is associated with a characteristic rash in the perioral area and in the flexion creases, as well as darkening of the skin in flexion creases [68]. Zinc deficiency is closely related to muscle protein catabolism, as urinary zinc loss is associated with aminoaciduria, but significant amounts of zinc may be lost in the stool as well, particularly in patients with diarrhea [119]. With the increase in the severity of the injury and increased muscle catabolism, there is also an increase in zinc requirements. We usually prescribe a supplement of 3 to 6 mg zinc/day, starting with the initiation of parenteral nutrition.

Copper

Copper has recently been associated with megaloblastic anemia, especially in long-term hyperalimented patients [85, 113]. The anemia commonly associated with parenteral nutrition is not due to copper deficiency, at least in our experience. If copper supplementation is required, 0.5 to 1 mg as the sulfate may be used per liter of hypertonic dextrose in amino acids without exceeding the solubility limit. The requirement for copper in stable patients is probably 0.5 to 2 mg/day.

Chromium Deficiency

Chromium deficiency has been associated with the development of a diabetic state and peripheral neuropathy, corrected by the administration of chromium [67]. This again seems only to occur in long-term patients with minimal or no oral intake. Recently, we observed the development of severe glucose intolerance and metabolic encephalopathy in a patient after 6 months of total parenteral nutrition. The administration of 150 μg chromium per day initially and 15 μg per day later reversed all symptoms (Figure 22-4) [45].

Recently, selenium deficiency was diagnosed by measuring erythrocyte, plasma, and whole blood selenium levels in New Zealand patients receiving TPN [12]. However, no clinical manifestations of deficiency were reported. It seems reasonable to assume that there are other essential trace elements of which we are not yet aware (see Chap. 9, Trace Metals).

INDICATIONS FOR PARENTERAL NUTRITION

Disease States in Which Parenteral Nutrition Is Considered Primary Therapy (Affects Outcome)—Efficacy Demonstrated

Gastrointestinal Fistulas

The role of hyperalimentation in the management of gastrointestinal fistulas is to promote fistula closure by providing maximal bowel rest and adequate nutritional support. Using total parenteral nutrition, favorable effects on fistula closure rates and increased survival have been demonstrated in many institutions. In 1960, mortality rates ranged from 47 to 62 percent and were directly related to fistula output, sepsis, malnutrition, and electrolyte imbalance [35]. No patient judged to have severe malnutrition survived [35]. Sheldon et al. recognized the importance of nutrition in these patients and noted that when more than 3000 calories/day were provided (largely by nonintravenous techniques), mortality dropped to 14 percent [100]. With the advent of parenteral nutrition and improvement in techniques and solutions, mortality rates for gastrointestinal fistula dropped to 6 to 21 percent, and closure rates of 70 percent or more were reported [5, 40, 73, 102]. Recently, Soeters and Fischer [102] reported a series of 404 gastrointestinal fistulas and compared the results in patients before and after 1970. Comparing the pre- and posthyperalimentation era, although spontaneous closure rates were increased, mortality was unchanged suggesting that the improvement in survival of patients with gastrointestinal cutaneous fistulas is more likely due to the introduction of antibiotics, respiratory support, and improvement in anesthesia and patient monitoring. Similar conclusions were reached by Reber et al. [91]. The widespread addition of hyperalimentation to the treatment of gastrointestinal cutaneous fistulas has improved spontaneous closure and is a valuable part of the present regimen for treating gastrointestinal fistulas. The decrease in mortality, however, cannot be attributed to parenteral nutrition [102]. The main cause of death is no longer malnutrition, but sepsis.

Short Bowel Syndrome

In patients who have undergone massive resection of their small bowel for mesenteric thrombosis, mesenteric emboli, or volvulus, or in patients with regional enteritis who have undergone multiple extensive resective procedures, there may be little alternative to long-term permanent parenteral nutrition. In these patients, the surface area of small bowel available for absorption is too small, and parenteral nutrition must be carried out at home. Some patients who have had resections ultimately regain enough bowel function to permit resumption of oral nutrition, particularly if an ileocecal valve is present [99]. However, immediately following operation their management should involve parenteral nutrition for at least two months, followed by gradual reintroduction of orally ingested food. As oral intake is resumed, absorption improves over several months. In patients with a very short gut—as little as 6 to 12 inches of jejunum anastomosed to the left colon—hyperalimentation is required for at least one to two years, until the gut has hypertrophied and complete nutritional support by oral feeding is possible. We have not found the predigested enteral diets of much value in this group of patients because the high osmolarity of these solutions often provokes severe diarrhea.

Renal Failure

The mortality in post-traumatic acute renal failure has remained unchanged at 55 to 65 percent since the Korean war. If all the problems with renal failure could be solved by aggressive dialysis, nearly 100 percent survival would result, assuming that other problems are dealt with. Nonetheless, despite the recent advances in intensive care, antibiotic treatment, and dialysis, mortality has not decreased in twenty years. Patients with acute tubular necrosis are hypercatabolic for reasons as yet unknown. In Europe, where extensive dialysis facilities were lacking, dietary therapy of chronic renal failure was undertaken with excellent results. Diets containing quantities of protein usually considered insufficient enabled patients with chronic renal insufficiency to live in nitrogen equilibrium by re-utilizing their own urea nitrogen [53, 54]. Intravenous modification of this Giordano-Giovannetti diet was first used by Dudrick and his coworkers [37]. After favorable initial experience with this solution at the Massachusetts General Hospital [1], a randomized double-blind prospective study was carried out in a homogeneous group of patients with acute tubular necrosis. Patients receiving eight essential L-amino acids, in hypertonic dextrose with vitamins, were compared with patients given hypertonic dextrose solution with vitamins alone. Dialysis requirements remained the same in the two groups, but those treated with essential amino acids and hypertonic dextrose appeared to recover from renal failure approximately 48 hours earlier, and the mortality rate decreased from 56 percent in the control group to 25 percent in the group treated with essential amino acids in hypertonic dextrose, a statistically significant difference [2]. Since that time it has been our practice to treat all patients with acute tubular necrosis with essential amino acids and hypertonic dextrose, a solution that is now commercially available as Nephramine. This solution will be discussed in detail subsequently.

Major Burns

There is no metabolic insult greater than a major burn. Basal metabolic requirements in excess of 200 percent of normal are seen; urinary excretion of nitrogen may approach 30 gm/24 hours; and even 9,000 to 10,000 calories a day may be insufficient to avoid major weight loss in these patients [118].

In these patients, the rapid breakdown of lean body mass for gluconeogenesis may result in wasting of the respiratory muscles, so that breathing and coughing are impaired, and weaning from the respirator is impossible. Moreover, the acute malnutrition developing in burn patients secondary to catabolism results in deranged immune competence, reduced phagocytic activity, and increased susceptibility to infection. In the past, it has been difficult to prove that patients with major burns treated with aggressive nutritional supplementation show a higher survival rate [118]. More recently, however, a prospective randomized study has convincingly demonstrated that increasing the percentage of calories derived from protein is associated with increased survival, secondary to improved host resistance [8].

However, catheter sepsis in patients with burns is more common and appears to be somewhat different from that in other groups, which usually is related not to hematogenous seeding, but to breaks in approved catheter technique. In patients with burns, hematogenous seeding seems much more common because bacteremias are frequent, high grade, and of long duration. Septic venous thrombosis was first described as another lethal hazard of TPN in burn patients [108]. Therefore, the protocol for parenteral nutrition in burn patients is different. Central venous catheters should be kept in place for no longer than 48 to 72 hours, used for all infusions, and the catheter site rotated on a regular basis between the two internal jugulars and the two subclavians, or if the need arises, between the two femoral veins.

Parenteral nutrition must be used in conjunction with oral intake, as it is impossible to satisfy the metabolic demands by parenteral route alone. Despite anorexia and early malfunction of the gastrointestinal tract, more than 5000 calories per day may be achieved by tube feedings or by voluntary oral intake, or by both, after a few days when the ileus has subsided [118].

Diseases in Which Efficacy Has Not Been Satisfactorily Demonstrated: Primary Therapy

Inflammatory Bowel Disease

In inflammatory bowel disease, hyperalimentation permits bleeding, edema, and acute inflammation to subside while providing optimal nutrition and bowel rest. The results of a number of prospective, but not randomized, studies permit several generalizations concerning the treatment of inflammatory bowel disease by hyperalimentation [42, 92, 93].

1. The most favorable situation is in the patient with regional enteritis (Crohn's disease) confined to the small bowel. A remission rate of approximately 75 percent can be achieved for as long as 10 years, although the mean duration of remission is approximately one year. The period of treatment is usually 3 to 6 weeks, depending on the severity of the disease and the nutritional state of the patient.
2. Steroids may be decreased under the cover of parenteral nutrition to approximately 5 to 10 mg of predisone per day. We have tended to maintain patients on this dosage. The few patients in whom steroid therapy was stopped tended to relapse quite early.
3. The presence of granulomatous disease involving the colon is associated with a lower remission rate.
4. Parenteral nutrition does not affect the course of ulcerative colitis. In a prospective but not randomized study, patients undergoing total proctocolectomy for ulcerative colitis had earlier discharge from the hospital, fewer postoperative complications, and perhaps less ileostomy dysfunction when treated with total parenteral nutrition preoperatively [92]. In the acutely ill and catabolic patient with fulminant ulcerative colitis, preoperative nutritional support enables the patient to tolerate total one-stage proctocolectomy with fewer complications and a much smoother postoperative course than experienced by patients undergoing a two-stage procedure without preoperative nutrition. We prefer the one-stage operation over two operations, since at times, after rectal resection the second-stage procedure has been required on an emergency basis within one week of colectomy because of continuing hemorrhage.

Anorexia Nervosa

It is our impression that in this group of very difficult patients, breaking the cycle of "voluntary" anorexia, weakness, and malnutrition is of utmost importance. We have been impressed by the fact that patients who receive hyperalimentation while undergoing psychiatric treatment for anorexia nervosa do respond better to psychotherapy.

Support Provided by Parenteral Nutrition—No Effect on Primary Disease—Efficacy Demonstrated

Radiation Enteritis

Large doses of radiation in the intra-abdominal or pelvic cavity interfere with growth and replacement of the brush border of the gut, resulting in diarrhea and malabsorption in the acute stage, and later, in some degree of fibrosis and stenosis of the small bowel. Predigested elemental diets are not successfully utilized. It is reasonable to assume that bowel rest with adequate nutrition by vein will ultimately result in healing of the bowel and resumption of oral intake. However, there is no evidence to suggest that healing and resumption of gastrointestinal absorption will result in chronic cases of radiation enteritis, in which fibrosis is present, under the influence of parenteral nutrition. In these cases, the patient is maintained on total parenteral nutrition at home, as will subsequently be discussed.

Acute Gastrointestinal Toxicity Due to Chemotherapeutic Agents

Toxicity from chemotherapeutic agents affecting the brush border of the gastrointestinal tract and the absorbing cells is becoming more common with the development and dissemination of cancer chemotherapy. Fortunately, this is usually a self-limiting complication, as healing takes place after cessation of toxic drugs. Parenteral nutrition in these patients furnishes adequate protein and calories for healing of the gastrointestinal tract and for maintaining the patient in good nutritional status while he is unable to take any oral diet.

Disease States in Which the Value of Hyperalimentation As Support Is Not Completely Established or Is Still Questionable

Hyperalimentation Prior to Major Surgery

This is perhaps the area in which the largest potential indication for parenteral nutrition exists. Patients facing major surgery for a variety of reasons, including neoplasms, often have lost a significant amount of weight. Although the body's economy usually favors the wound and enables healing at the expense of other tissues, it is not clear that this also occurs in depleted cancer patients. Holter and Fischer [63] carried out a preliminary prospective study in which patients with neoplasms who had lost more than 10 lbs body weight were randomized for either perioperative hyperalimentation, beginning 72 hours before surgery and continued postoperatively until 1500 calories were taken by mouth or by standard intravenous therapy. These two groups were matched for age and operation with a group of patients whose weight loss was minimal or nonexistent (making a total of three groups). Although only 84 patients were studied, there appears to be a lower incidence of major complications (13% vs 19%), better weight gain, and increased albumin levels in the group receiving perioperative hyperalimentation. If trends continue, these findings will be statistically significant in a study of 300 patients (100 in a group).

Recently, a similar prospective study of patients undergoing surgery for esophageal carcinoma demonstrated that patients who receive hyperalimentation 5 to 7 days preoperatively and 6 to 7 days postoperatively can revert to a positive nitrogen balance during their entire perioperative course [81]. Patients who did not receive parenteral nutrition were in continuous negative nitrogen balance through the entire period. Patients who received perioperative parenteral nutrition exhibited a more "complete and uncomplicated wound healing" (whatever that means!) when compared to those who did not receive parenteral nutrition. Another experimental and clinical study indicates that immediate postoperative infusion with both amino acids and carbohydrates leads to a metabolic pattern of rapid healing and homeostatic stability [82]. A series of recent retrospective studies by Mullen and coworkers have utilized measurements of various biochemical and anthropometric parameters to define a population at risk for surgery. The PNI or prognostic nutritional index relies mostly on protein parameters such as plasma albumin and transferrin, as well as skin tests. In retrospect, those patients having severe derangements (deficiencies) in these parameters manifest higher risk for operation.

What must be and has not been demonstrated is: (1) Can one identify a population at risk? (2) Once one identifies the population at risk, can the risk be altered by short-term parenteral nutritional support pre- and postoperatively? While Mullen's retrospective studies claim such a group can be identified, the largest prospective study reaches the opposite conclusion [98a]. In a recent study in a fairly large number of patients with esophageal and gastric carcinoma, preoperative preparation and postoperative support with TPN decreased the mortality, but this improved result was not limited to patients who were malnourished [80a]. Thus, neither question has been answered in a satisfactory manner. In both dogs and patients undergoing surgery, adequate enteral feeding resulted in marked positive nitrogen balance within minutes of surgery. In dogs, this early postoperative hyperalimentation resulted also in increased albumin and globulin production as early as 24 hours after surgery, a 6.2 times increase in DNA synthesis in the bowel wound, and a 3 to 4 times increase in bursting pressure of the abdominal wall and bowel 96 hours postoperatively [82]. In a recently published experimental study, dietary protein restriction did not affect growth characteristics or composition of a rat tumor, but retarded growth and increased the loss of carcass protein of the host, findings supporting efforts for nutritional support for the tumor-bearing host [72]. From these observations, it would seem as if preoperative and postoperative nutritional support may offer important clinical benefits, which must yet be established on a firmer footing.

Patients Undergoing Cardiac Surgery

Patients with end-stage rheumatic heart disease often manifest cardiac cachexia, in which low cardiac output and presumably inadequate provision of nutrients to the periphery result in decreased lean body mass, overall weakness, and debility. The operative mortality in these patients is high [3]. Since Starling commented in 1912 that the heart was not affected by malnutrition, very little attention has been given to the effect of nutrition on the heart. This dictum has gone unchallenged until recently when Abel et al. [4] and Kyger et al. [69] demonstrated the adverse effects of protein-calorie malnutrition or protein deficiency on cardiac performance. Peak left ventricular pressure, left ventricular dp/dt, and stroke volume were depressed. Histologic findings of note were interstitial edema and myocardial atrophy. When animals with impaired cardiac performance secondary to protein depletion were replenished with intravenous infusion of crystalline amino acids and glucose, an improvement in force-velocity, length-tension, and left ventricular diastolic compliance relationship was noted. In a clinical prospective randomized study, Abel et al. [3] compared malnourished and well-nourished patients undergoing open heart surgery for valve replacement. Malnutrition proved to be a significant risk factor. Malnourished patients required longer respiratory support and had more postoperative complications and a longer hospital stay. In this study, however, no apparent benefit was demonstrated from a 5-day course of hyperalimentation beginning immediately postoperatively. It is now appreciated that 5 days of postoperative hyperalimentation is not likely to restore nutritional adequacy. Perioperative nutrition may require 7 to 10 days of preoperative nutrition (or longer) and nutritional support through the postoperative period as long as needed.

Pancreatitis

Pancreatitis is a disease of varying etiology, resulting in profound hemodynamic, metabolic, pulmonary, and renal alterations. Simultaneously, gastrointestinal tract function is disturbed. The combination of alcoholism (a principal etiologic factor in pancreatitis), chronic malnutrition, and gastrointestinal dysfunction in the form of malabsorption or prolonged paralytic ileus, or both, further complicates the nutritional status of these patients. Patients surviving an acute severe episode of pancreatitis may die of inadequate nutritional support. This deterioration will, of course, be enhanced by any surgical intervention in these patients, and unfortunately patients with severe pancreatitis tend to be subjected to repeated surgical interventions. The overall mortality in severe pancreatitis varies between 20 and 48 percent. Feller et al. [39] reported an unrandomized series of patients with severe pancreatitis in whom they believed that mortality was reduced to 14 percent by nutritional support with hyperalimentation. However, the interpretation of this study was hampered by the absence of a control group. In a more recent retrospective study of 46 admissions for severe pancreatitis, Goodgame and Fischer [57] reported an overall mortality rate of 20 percent, with hyperalimentation having no effect on early mortality. However, patients who were unable to eat for more than one month fared no worse in terms of survival than did those whose disease resolved in less than 30 days, indicating the success of nutritional support, keeping those patients alive for 50 to 90 days before they were able to take oral feedings. The operative mortality was 22 percent, lower than the 26 to 56 percent commonly reported. Catheter sepsis rate in this group of patients was 17 percent, much higher than the 3 percent in the general hospital population and, for some reason, very high in the first week. It thus appears that in the treatment of severe acute pancreatitis, hyperalimentation should be regarded as useful for maintaining nutritional integrity in the face of a severe illness and a malfunctioning gastrointestinal tract. At present, however, there is no evidence that parenteral nutrition alters the early course of acute pancreatitis.

Patients Requiring Prolonged Respiratory Support for Respiratory Insufficiency

As prolonged respiratory support becomes more common and sophisticated, the need for nutritional support becomes mandatory. It may well be that many patients are unable to be weaned from the respirator because they have catabolized their muscle mass, including diaphragm and respiratory muscles, for energy needs and gluconeogenesis. Nutritional support to prevent this breakdown is essential. Once the respiratory muscles have been cannibalized, it is not clear whether they can be replenished. Other factors not yet investigated are the nutritional requirements of the lungs themselves, particularly during respiratory failure and artificial support. Nor is it known what types of foodstuff the lung requires. We know, for example, that the lung manufactures surfactant, which contains much fat. It is not known, however, whether fat would be beneficial to pulmonary function or healing, or both. If so, this might prove to be important both in adult respiratory distress and in respiratory distress syndromes of the newborn. No controlled studies in these areas have been reported, as these patients are difficult to study and compare owing to the multiple factors and systems involved in their catabolic state and the respiratory failure. Recently, in a preliminary study, it was demonstrated that malnourished patients were unable to be weaned from controlled ventilation despite the fact that all criteria for discontinuation from controlled ventilation were met. Only 10 days later, when nutritional status improved, was weaning possible [90].

Applications for Which Hyperalimentation Is Still Considered Experimental

Malignancy

In neoplastic disease, a group of cells escapes from normal metabolic control and declares nutritional independence. When a tumor is present, surgical or other wounds are no longer the only beneficiaries of amino acids and other factors mobilized for healing. Nutritional support in excess of normal needs will perhaps circumvent the tumor and allow normal wound healing to take place. Between the nutritional demands of their tumors and the anorexia that often accompanies neoplastic disease, many cancer patients die of starvation. If this cycle can be broken, patients might respond better to cancer therapy. Recently much work has been published indicating that malnutrition contributes to the anergy (lack of response to a battery of skin delayed recall antigens) and depressed host immunocompetence [28, 121] common in advanced malignancies, thus making infection more likely. For all the aforementioned reasons, nutritional support in the cancer patient seems of utmost importance.

On the other hand, a note of caution is appropriate; nutrition to the patient will also nourish the cancer. When adequate nutrition was provided to animals with cancer, increased tumor growth paralleled increased body weight [20, 107]. Lowry et al. [72] demonstrated that dietary protein restriction did not affect tumor growth, but retarded body growth and caused lysis of carcass protein of the rat host. Daly et al. [27], by supplying adequate intravenous nutrition, were able to restore body weight and host immune competence in malnourished tumor-bearing rats without stimulating tumor growth. Although contradictory, these findings support efforts attempting nutritional repletion of the tumor-bearing host. One can identify several groups of patients with malignancy who might potentially benefit from parenteral nutrition:

1. Patients who have lost weight and undergo radical surgical procedures. In a group of 84 patients with gastrointestinal malignant disease, Holter and Fischer [63] found that significant weight loss was associated with an increased incidence of postoperative complications and mortality. Perioperative hyperalimentation resulted in a trend toward weight gain, increased albumin levels, and decreased incidence of major complications, which was not statistically significant in the number of patients tested.
2. Patients who have lost immunologic competence secondary to malnutrition and in whom return of immunologic competence might better enable them to withstand their tumors. However, there is no evidence at present that the return of immunologic competence to such patients will signify anything other than the restoration of reasonable nutrition [23, 30]. It has definitely not been established that the patient will be able to deal better with his tumor.
3. Patients who, because of malnutrition, have been denied chemotherapy and radiation therapy for widespread neoplastic disease. It is in this group that most of the present work has been done. Parenteral nutrition can be safely given to patients with low white cell counts and who are at risk for sepsis [24]. Moreover, there is at least a small group of patients to whom chemotherapy and radiotherapy would have been previously denied who become candidates for such therapy and, presumably, may benefit from treatment [30]. However, in most patients, neither parenteral nutrition nor any other form of nutritional supplementation can reverse the course of the disease. Whether these patients would benefit from earlier or altered nutritional supplementation is not clear.

Patients in a State of Immune Incompetence

Fatal septic complications continue to be of major importance in surgical patients, despite the improvement in surgical techniques, asepsis, and the use of antibiotics. The state of host resistance until recently, however, has not been considered in the risk assessment of the surgical patient. In a study of 55 severely injured and septic patients, McLean et al. [74] assessed cell-mediated immunity by testing skin reactivity to mumps, PPD, *Trichophyton, Candida,* and Varidase antigens, response to DNCB sensitization, and by testing lymphocyte activity to mitogen and to allergenic leukocytes. They found the mortality to be 100 percent in the totally anergic group and 7 percent in patients with normal response. In a prospective study of 50 preoperative patients, 62 percent of the patients with impaired cellular immune response had infectious complications, most of them septicemia, whereas in the group of patients with normal response, only a 5 percent incidence of wound infections with no other major infection occurred [86]. These results were confirmed in a larger group of 520 preoperative, postoperative, post-traumatic, or nonoperative patients [79]. Sequential testing in individual patients was of even greater prognostic value. In patients who remained normally reactive or became normal, sepsis rate was 10.1 percent and mortality rate 8.4 percent. However, a sepsis rate of 57.6 percent and a mortality rate of 78 percent occurred in patients developing abnormal responses or those whose responses did not improve. Meakins et al. documented abnormalities of neutrophil chemotaxis and T-lymphocyte rosetting in a group of anergic patients, abnormalities that may account for the increased infection and mortality rates in these patients [79]. When cutaneous responses became normal, chemotaxis returned to nearly normal. Furthermore, there was a significant correlation between absence of neutrophil chemotaxis, phagocytosis, and bactericidal killing to explain the inability of the anergic patient to respond to infection. More recently, the emergence of a plasma inhibitor in anergy leading to decreased neutrophil chemotaxis and the increased risk for sepsis was described [25]. Others suggested that immunocompetence is compromised by inhibitory monocytes and suppressor T-lymphocytes appearing following trauma. Trauma, shock, malnutrition, infection, and old age were shown to be associated with anergy [9, 13, 15]. More recently, however, it has become clear that the conditions under which skin tests are applied largely determine response and that anergy is a relatively nonspecific finding [109a]. In a recent review, Meakins and coworkers concluded that while anergy was sometimes predictive of prognosis in a statistical sense, i.e., in a large population, it was of little value in a given patient [79a].

Protein-calorie malnutrition is known to alter immune response and host resistance to infection [28, 121]. An excellent correlation was found to exist between malnutrition, as measured by body cell mass determination, and the presence of anergy [105]. However, abnormal body composition consistent with poor nutritional state was noted in both anergic and nonanergic patients, indicating that other factors are operative as well. With the identification of patients who are at risk for developing sepsis, the question of reversing the anergic state is of prime importance. Attention has been focused on nutritional status and nutritional support of the anergic patient. Restoration of body cell mass by nutritional support is associated with the returning of cutaneous responses to normal and thus supports the use of total parenteral nutrition in anergic patients [23, 30]. Alexander reported improvement of neutrophil bactericidal function in burn patients receiving oral rather than parenteral hyperalimentation, with a concomitant reduction of sepsis [7] and, in a landmark study, a decreased mortality rate in burned children prospectively randomized by burn size and differing only in increased protein as a percentage of calories in the group demonstrating significantly increased survival [8]. Daly et al. showed in rats that proper nutritional repletion with protein and nonprotein calories will return immunocompetence [28]. However, Sheldon et al. showed that the return of immunocompetence in rats receiving hyperalimentation does not change their poor response to a septic challenge [89]. Thus, although multiple factors contribute to anergy or depressed host resistance, the only readily reversible factor is malnutrition. Enteral or parenteral nutrition constitutes the best single method so far to treat the anergic patient. Anergy is often (but not always) a reversible state, and aggressive early use of total parenteral nutrition in these patients might prove lifesaving.

Home Hyperalimentation

Owing to the widening experience in hyperalimentation and the development of new pumps and more chemically inert venous catheters, safe home hyperalimentation has become a reality. Indications for this procedure are the prolonged inability to maintain adequate nutrition orally, as in patients with severe Crohn's disease of the bowel, who have had repeated resections or in whom there is insufficient functional length of bowel remaining, or in patients who have suffered massive venous or arterial thrombosis of the gastrointestinal tract. Other, more rare indications are chronic radiation enteritis with fibrosis, extensive diverticulosis of the small bowel, unresponsive sprue, and isolated carcinomatosis of the abdominal cavity in patients who are being treated with chemotherapy or irradiation.

The two basic techniques for home parenteral nutrition vary in their source of nonprotein calories. In the United States, an indwelling central venous catheter and a glucose amino acid infusion are commonly used. In Canada, as well as in France, patients have been treated by the combination of glucose-amino acid and lipid. Our group has used the Broviac-Scribner and, more recently, the Hickman catheter which utilizes a silicon-rubber catheter with a Teflon sleeve and a long subcutaneous tunnel, which emerges on the upper abdomen and can be easily reached by the patient for dressing change and connection to the infusion set. Generally, the patient receives 2000 to 3000 ml of hyperalimentation fluid overnight, and this fluid contains approximately 80 to 120 gm of amino acids and 2000 to 3000 calories. Many patients are able to supplement the intravenous intake with limited oral intake, thus supplying themselves with some vitamins, trace elements, and fatty acids.

Patients can also be given continuous infusion over 24 hours by means of a life-vest-like arrangement and a portable battery driven pump. Our own preference is for an overnight infusion, utilizing an infusion pump that allows the patient to sleep without interruption, adequately protected by a variety of alarms. The infusion is begun at approximately 200 ml per hour, with or without preliminary priming. This infusion rate proceeds overnight for 8 to 12 hours, depending on the patient's need, and is then tapered in 2 to 3 hours, again depending on the patient. In this way the patient is nourished during sleep and is free to work and conduct a normal life during the day with his catheter plugged. Training the patients for home parenteral nutrition involves a complicated system of educating and teaching the patient, his family, the community physician, and the pharmacist supplying the solutions to the patient. This training is one of the functions of the hyperalimentation unit (see Practical Aspects of Parenteral Nutrition). From our experience and the experience of many other groups in the United States, Canada, and France, home hyperalimentation seems to be a feasible solution for many patients who would otherwise have repeated and prolonged hospitalizations.

Another important factor in home hyperalimentation is that under these circumstances it is much less expensive than hyperalimentation in the hospital itself. In our exprience, the annual expenses per patient per year come to about $35,000 to $60,000, whereas the expense of hyperalimentation in the hospital is $500/day (including hospital bed).

SPECIALIZED HYPERALIMENTATION SOLUTIONS FOR SPECIFIC DISEASE STATES

Whereas ten years ago the only protein solution available was in the form of protein hydrolysate (usually casein or fibrin), recently crystalline synthetic amino acid solutions have been introduced. Nitrogen equilibrium is achieved with 0.5 gm of protein equivalent/kg when crystalline amino acids are used compared to 0.8 gm/kg of protein hydrolysate [10]. One important advantage of synthetic amino acid solutions is that special solutions may be tailor-made for specific disease states which present difficulties in nitrogen utilization or erquirements, or both, for special amino acids. Currently available crystalline amino acid solutions usually contain the 8 essential amino acids and a variable number of nonessential amino acids. They come in different concentrations and are mixed with different volumes of 50 to 70% dextrose, depending on the formula required for certain patients. To the mixture of glucose and crystalline amino acids, we add electrolytes, both water and fat soluble vitamins, trace elements, and HCl or acetate for acid-base balance, as indicated. Fixed electrolyte formulas make the preparation of solutions simpler, safer, and more efficient. One liter of hyperalimentation solution usually contains 35 to 42.5 gm amino acids, 250 gm dextrose, electrolytes, vitamins, and trace elements. A patient would usually need 2 to 5 liters/day, offering 2000 to 5000 calories/day and 85 to 200 grams of amino acids/day.

Cardiac Failure and Respiratory Insufficiency

The limiting factors of nutritional support in both respiratory insufficiency and cardiac failure are fluid intolerance and salt restriction. In severe cases of cardiac cachexia requiring hyperalimentation before surgery, the maximum fluid intake would be limited to 1,000 to 1,500 ml per day with one gram of sodium. In patients with severe depletion, cardiac insufficiency severely limits the ability of the patient to tolerate large initial volumes of solution. The fluid limitation in severe respiratory insufficiency might be similar. In order to reduce fluid intake while maintaining adequate caloric and protein intake, a solution containing 4.25 percent crystalline amino acids and 35 to 40 percent dextrose may be used, enabling the administration of 3000 calories/day in a total volume of 2 liters. However, with increasing glucose concentration, the danger of metabolic and septic complications increases, particularly in the severely injured or septic patient. It should be remembered in patients in respiratory failure that respiratory work consumes energy and nitrogen, that most of these patients are severely catabolic, and that it is of utmost importance to give adequate amounts of calories and nitrogen in order to help them both to wean from the respirator and to overcome their basic catabolic insult. One should remember that in a few patients with respiratory insufficiency and sepsis, increasing carbohydrate may result in excessive production of CO_2. It is sometimes necessary to give both highly concentrated nutritional solutions and additional diuretics in order to supply large amounts of calories and protein without fluid accumulation. An unanswered question is whether adequate nutrition might result in more rapid healing of damaged lungs.

Renal Failure

The mortality of surgical patients with acute renal failure has remained exceedingly high since the Korean war, about 56 to 67 percent. For unclear reasons, renal failure produces a hypercatabolic state. Dietary therapy of chronic renal failure has been undertaken in a number of countries lacking expensive dialysis equipment. A modification for intravenous use of the Giordano-Giovannetti diet was first reported by Dudrick and his coworkers with encouraging results [32]. Giordano [53] and Giovannetti [54] had shown that in patients with chronic renal failure, positive nitrogen balance, lowering of BUN, and improved patient well-being could be achieved by providing essential amino acids and limiting the amount of nonessential amino acids. Under such circumstances, urea is split by the gut bacteria to ammonia, which is reabsorbed and made available for synthesis by eventual transamination into nonessential amino acids. Adequate protein synthesis thus can take place at a lower nitrogen intake than had been previously suspected. After an initial anecdotal experience at the Massachusetts General Hospital [1], a randomized double-blind prospective study was undertaken to ascertain whether the provision of essential amino acids and hypertonic dextrose in patients with acute tubular necrosis would influence outcome and rate of dialysis. It was expected that the frequency of dialysis would decrease. However, the need for dialysis was unchanged, whereas renal failure appeared to abate 48 hours earlier in patients treated with essential amino acids and hypertonic dextrose as opposed to hypertonic dextrose alone. Moreover, the mortality rate decreased from 56 to 25 percent [2]. Since the patients in both groups were comparable, the only apparent explanation for the different mortality in the two groups was the provision of amino acids in the treated group. Since that time, all patients with acute tubular necrosis are treated by parenteral nutrition with essential amino acids and hypertonic dextrose, now commercially available as Nephramine (McGaw Laboratories: 12.7 gm of eight L-essential amino acids, 350 gm of dextrose, insulin, and vitamins, in a total of 750 ml). The total glucose concentration thus reaches 47 percent, and the osmolarity of the solution is 2100 mOsm per liter. The high concentrations of glucose in a small volume enables even an oliguric patient to receive a substantial amount of calories. In the presence of the usual gastrointestinal tract losses in surgical patients, an intake of 2000 to 2500 calories daily is easily achieved.

Optimal formulation of solutions for use in renal failure remains controversial. Although others have argued for a more complete formulation earlier in the course of the disease, we continue to emphasize large doses of essential amino acids, which appear to increase nonspecific host resistance while elevating BUN slowly [46, 109]. The same amino acid formula is also available as an elemental diet (Amin-aid, McGaw Laboratories), which may be substituted for the intravenous form in patients whose gastrointestinal tract is functioning.

Since urinary glucose is notoriously unreliable in renal failure, the blood glucose should be checked at least twice daily when therapy is started. Insulin is added to the bottle as necessary, according to blood sugar levels. Hypokalemia, hypomagnesemia, and hypophosphatemia occur regularly, sometimes as soon as eight hours after the initiation of renal failure fluid infusion. Electrolytes should be checked at least every day at the outset, and subsequently every other day. Once renal failure becomes established and the need for dialysis becomes chronic, all essential and nonessential amino acids should be administered to prevent protein depletion, as there is an additional loss of 250 mg of amino acid nitrogen per hour of dialysis. At this stage, our patients undergo dialysis three times a week, and we infuse a regular amino acid formulation, mixed in a 35 to 40% dextrose solution so as to minimize the infused fluid load.

Liver Disease and Hepatic Encephalopathy

Cirrhosis and its complications form the sixth most common cause of death in the United States. The patient with hepatic insufficiency poses a classic dilemma in nutrition. Although adequate amounts of calories and protein are required, it is specifically the protein to which such patients are intolerant. In the cities of the United States, the most common cause of liver disease is alcoholism. We are often confronted with a patient suffering from chronic malnutrition in whom a major catastrophe such as gastrointestinal bleeding has occurred, necessitating surgical intervention with further aggravation of the catabolic state. Added to this is the almost inevitable hepatic deterioration that follows any major stress in the patient with liver disease. Although nutritional support is sorely needed, these patients often do not tolerate protein or standard amino acid formulations, which result in hepatic encephalopathy and coma.

Recently an experimental solution has been developed which appears to be well tolerated by patients with hepatic insufficiency and encephalopathy [43]. The solution is partially the result of Baldessarini and Fischer's studies in brain neurotransmitter changes in hepatic coma, which suggested that a CNS accumulation of serotonin, an inhibitory neurotransmitter [12], a depletion of the central nervous system norepinephrine [29], and an accumulation of octopamine [41, 97] might be causally related to hepatic encephalopathy. These abnormalities have, in turn, been related to abnormal peripheral metabolism of amino acids, with a resultant abnormal plasma amino acid profile: increased aromatic amino acids, phenylalanine, tyrosine, methionine, free but not necessarily total tryptophan, and decreased branched-chain amino acids. This pattern results in abnormal brain concentrations of monoamine precursors, resulting in neurotransmitter derangements. The purpose of such infusional therapy is to normalize plasma amino acid patterns and to improve encephalopathy. This solution with reduced aromatic amino acids and increased amounts of branched-chain amino acids was devised and tested in animals [6, 96, 101] and subsequently in humans [43, 44]. Administered with a 25% dextrose solution, it successfully corrected neurologic derangements occurring after portacaval shunt in dogs, with the animals remaining neurologically normal despite the administration of up to 4 gm protein equivalent/kg/day [6, 101]. Patients with chronic liver failure and acute decompensation tolerated the infusion of 60 to 120 gm of amino acids per day and awoke from coma [43]. Our subsequent experience with 70 patients (unpublished data) confirms the initial impression of excellent tolerance of large amounts of amino acids with a simultaneous correction of plasma amino acid profile, reversal of encephalopathy, and, in some, improvement in hepatic function. Three randomized, prospective, multicenter trials have confirmed the efficacy of branched-chain amino acid enriched solutions given with hypertonic dextrose: not only were such solutions well tolerated in patients with hepatic insufficiency requiring nutritional support, but they also improved hepatic encephalopathy [97a, 20a, 109a]. In two trials in which fat was the primary caloric source, efficacy has not been demonstrated. For further information, please see the chapter on hepatic failure (Chap. 17). Recently, the same amino acid formulation has also become available as an enteral feeding formula. Early experience with this oral formula showed similarly favorable results [50], and a randomized prospective trial has shown efficacy [63a].

Hyperalimentation in Trauma, Injury, and Sepsis

The metabolic consequences of infection have been the subject of increased interest in recent years. Characteristically, sepsis is a major catabolic insult leading to increased muscle breakdown and nitrogen loss. This progressive proteolysis is accompanied by modified carbohydrate and fat energy metabolism. Insulin resistance, developing in sepsis, decreases the ability to oxidize glucose in the periphery, probably secondary to decreased intracellular penetration of glucose, and results in a diabetic-type glucose tolerance curve. However, plasma insulin levels are sufficiently elevated and fat tissue sufficiently sensitive to insulin to cause an antilipolytic effect, which may lead to further energy deficit. The availability of fuels in sepsis is therefore limited, and the body turns to muscle breakdown and amino acid oxidation to supply energy needs. In a clinical study of 40 septic patients, most of them suffering severe abdominal sepsis, a characteristic plasma amino acid pattern was present—increased aromatic amino acids, taurine, cystine, and methionine. Alanine, aspartic acid, glutamic acid, and proline were increased to a lesser extent, while the branched-chain amino acids (valine, leucine, and isoleucine) were within normal limits (Figure 22-5) [49]. This amino acid pattern suggests extensive muscle protein degradation to satisfy energy needs. Muscle breakdown results in release into the circulation of large amounts of almost all amino acids, with the exception of the branched-chain amino acids, which are the only amino acids the muscle itself is able to oxidize and utilize to supply its own energy requirements, and alanine and glutamine. Furthermore, the oxidation of branched-chain amino acids supplies the nitrogen and perhaps also the carbon skeleton for alanine synthesis in muscle, the latter circulating to the liver for use in gluconeogenesis [37, 66]. The utilization of the branched-chain amino acids for muscle energy requirements and of alanine for gluconeogenesis may in part explain the normal plasma levels of the branched chain amino acids and the only mildly elevated levels of alanine. The remaining amino acids released into the circulation after muscle breakdown, namely the aromatic and sulphur-containing amino acids, must

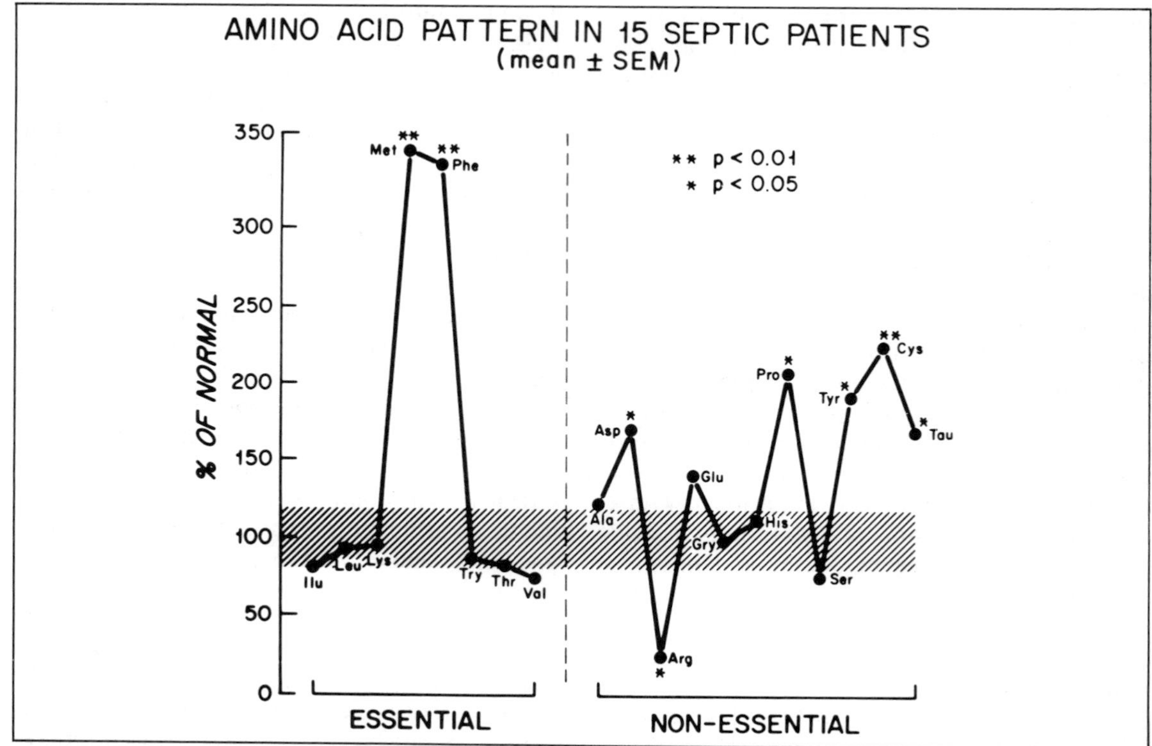

Figure 22-5. *Plasma amino acid pattern in 15 patients with sepsis. The pattern is similar to that seen in liver disease in that aromatic amino acids are elevated including phenylalanine and tyrosine. Branched chain amino acids tend to be low normal. The sulfur-containing amino acids, cysteine, taurine, and methionine are increased to a considerably greater extent with respect to cysteine and taurine than are seen in liver disease. (From H. R. Freund, J. A. Ryan, Jr., and J. E. Fischer, Amino acid derangements in patients with sepsis: treatment with branched chain amino acid rich infusions.* Ann. Surg. *188:423, 1978.)*

be metabolized by the liver. However, protein synthesis in the liver, except for acute-phase plasma proteins, is reduced, as is (in all probability) overall hepatic catabolism of aromatic amino acids, because of hepatic dysfunction occurring early in sepsis [61, 110, 111], and the aromatic and sulphur-containing amino acids accumulate. Because of the disturbed amino acid pattern and apparent central role of the branched-chain amino acids in muscle catabolism, in a group of 10 septic patients we attempted to restore the plasma amino acid pattern to normal and to supply additional amounts of branched-chain amino acids by the technique of hyperalimentation using a 24% glucose solution, insulin, and an amino acid mixture rich in branched-chain amino acid, but poor in tryptophan, methionine, and phenylalanine [49]. In these patients, normalization of the plasma amino acid pattern was achieved, probably owing to decreased efflux of amino acids from the skeletal muscle, as suggested by the in vitro experiments by Odessey et al. [87, 88]. By supplying an easily utilizable energy source for the muscle in the form of the branched-chain amino acids, further skeletal muscle breakdown was prevented (Figure 22-6).

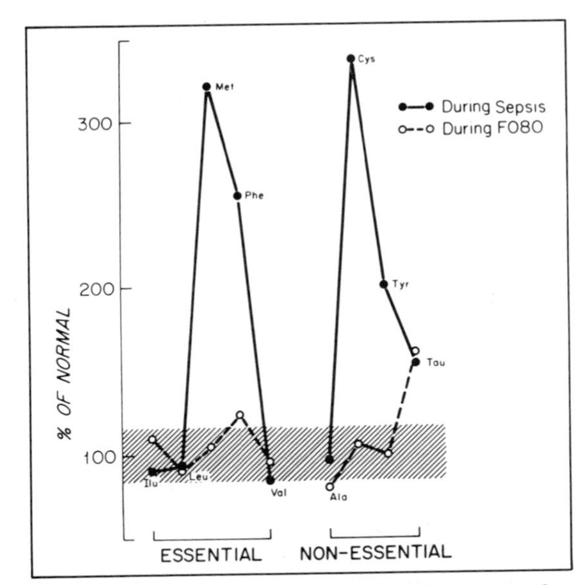

Figure 22-6. *The results of administration of a branched-chain enriched amino acid solution, F080, during septic encephalopathy. In 10 individual patients with the plasma amino acid pattern shown, administration of F080 in amounts of 80 to 100 gm amino acids/24 hr resulted in awakening from encephalopathy coincident with normalization of the plasma amino acid pattern. Some hepatic decompensation was present in these patients.*

The metabolic response to injury similarly results in a rapid breakdown of muscle protein as substrate for energy production and gluconeogenesis and mobilization of body fat, with the resulting negative nitrogen balance and weight loss. Skeletal muscle is a major site of protein loss after injury. Muscle protein breakdown, in addition to being economically wasteful if allowed to proceed for prolonged periods, also leads to relative deficiency of those essential amino acids, such as leucine, isoleucine, and valine, which are extensively oxidized by the muscle as energy source and substrate for gluconeogenesis. This relative deficiency might have deleterious effects on availability of these and other essential amino acids for protein synthesis.

The branched-chain amino acids (valine, leucine, and isoleucine) are the only essential amino acids that are principally oxidized by the skeletal muscle [18, 19, 75, 87, 88, 122]. Oxidation of the branched-chain amino acids supplies energy to the muscle and nitrogen for the glucose alanine cycle and muscle glutamine synthesis [37, 38, 56, 76, 88, 114]. In addition to being easily available energy substrate for the skeletal muscle, the branched-chain amino acids, according to recent in vitro experiments, also may have regulatory functions [19, 52, 87]. Recently, in a series of animal experiments and clinical studies, we were able to show that:

1. Early nutritional support in the post-injury state can result in nitrogen equilibrium or even mild positive nitrogen balance. Thus, the obligatory catabolic phase, as viewed by Moore, can be minimized or even abolished by the provision of enough protein and calories [48].
2. The infusion of only the three branched-chain amino acids in the immediate postoperative period is as effective in achieving nitrogen equilibrium as other more balanced amino acid solutions (Figure 22-7).
3. The nitrogen-conserving quality of amino acid solutions in the post-injury period might be improved by increasing the amounts of branched-chain amino acids.
4. A balanced amino acid solution containing adequate amounts of essential and nonessential amino acids, together with a high (45 to 50%) concentration of branched-chain amino acid, may be a more appropriate amino acid formulation in the post-injury patient.

It would thus appear that such a combination of amino acids with hypertonic glucose and insulin can result in early reversal of nitrogen balance or even immediate post-injury positive nitrogen balance and improvement in protein and energy metabolism during sepsis. In a series of preliminary as yet unpublished studies, we have observed that a high branched-chain acid mixture is superior to standard amino acid mix-

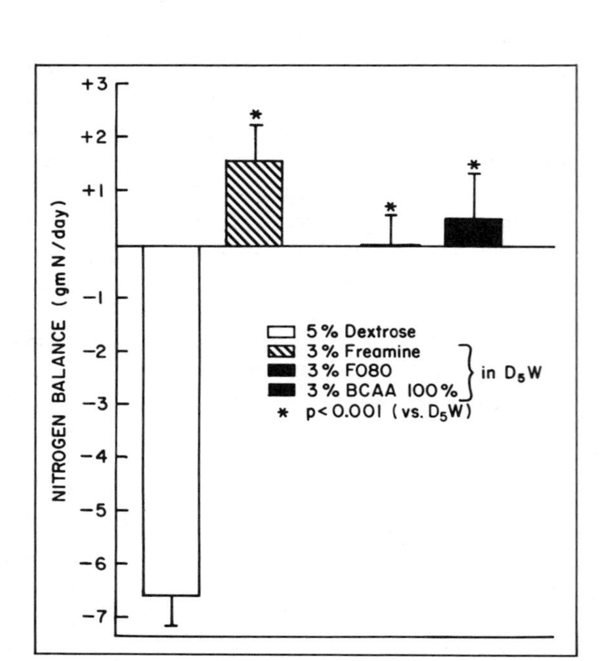

Figure 22-7. *Mean daily nitrogen balance in a group of 35 patients treated with either 5% dextrose or 3% amino acid solution, including Freamine, F080, or the branched-chain amino acids alone, following surgery of moderate severity. Of interest is the ability of the branched-chain amino acids alone, with hypocaloric dextrose to maintain nitrogen equilibrium. (From H. Freund et al. Infusion of the branched chain amino acids in postoperative patients: anticatabolic properties.* Ann. Surg. *190:18, 1979.)*

tures in critically ill septic patients with respect to improved nitrogen balance and decreased muscle breakdown, as manifested by decreased excretion of 3-methylhistidine.

COMPLICATIONS

Complications of parenteral nutrition may be classified under three headings: technical, metabolic, and septic.

Technical

Technical complications are the most common complications of hyperalimentation and are related to the act of placing the catheter through a large-bore needle into a region crowded with many vital structures and to the mere presence of the catheter, a foreign body, in a large vein. Complications are much more common in the subclavian approach than in the jugular vein approach and include:

1. Pneumothorax with higher incidence in cachectic patients.
2. Arterial laceration.
3. Hemothorax, the result of leakage of blood from the subclavian vein, especially in a thin patient, even in a nontraumatic insertion.
4. Mediastinal hematoma, which in patients with insufficient clotting factors may result in mediastinal decompression and even death.
5. Nerve injury to the brachial plexus or one of its branches, or, in the case of a jugular vein cannulation, phrenic nerve, vagus nerve, or recurrent laryngeal nerve injury.
6. Hydrothorax, which may result from the perforation of the catheter through the subclavian vein leading to the administration of solution into the pleural cavity.
7. "Sympathetic effusions" that are generally the result of the mediastinal hematoma. They may occur on both sides and are generally associated with symptoms of fever, tachycardia, tachypnea, and anterior chest pain.
8. In the left jugular vein cannulation, the thoracic duct may be injured, an occurrence that is rare, but is reported in patients with lymphatic obstruction due to cancer of the stomach and in patients with hepatic cirrhosis.
9. Air embolism is an unusual but dramatic complication that may occur during the process of insertion when the syringe is removed in order to thread the catheter, during tubing changes by the nursing staff, if the intravenous line inadvertently becomes detached from the catheter, or after the intravenous catheter has been pulled out and before the tract can seal properly. Air embolism usually occurs in a patient who is hypovolemic, upright, and breathing deeply, so that there is negative intrathoracic pressure. Air embolism can be prevented if the patient per-

forms a Valsalva maneuver in the Trendelenburg position when the catheter is being inserted or when the tubing is being changed. Whenever the catheter is removed, ointment and a small air-occlusive dressing should be placed over the insertion site for 24 hours.

10. Catheter embolism is another rare complication that is usually due to faulty technique, namely, the pulling of the catheter back through the sharp needle, shearing off the catheter tip with subsequent migration into the venous tree and lungs.

Other rare complications are erosion of the catheter tip into a bronchus as well as spontaneous later perforation and penetration through the right atrium or other venous structures. Therapy in these cases consists of identifying the problem and treating it appropriately. It is important to remember that the catheter tip should be located in the superior vena cava and not in the right atrium.

Late complications, particularly large vein thrombosis, are far more common than is recognized or reported. In a study of 34 autopsies among 200 patients who had received hyperalimentation, thrombosis was observed in approximately 20 percent. Many of these patients had catheters in place for only 2 to 3 days, and thrombosis was undoubtedly secondary to an agonal low flow state. However, if patients are examined closely for signs of swelling at the base of the neck, a slight increase in the diameter of the arm, an increase in the venous pressure of the associated arm, and a venous prominence along the chest wall and neck, subclavian or internal jugular thrombosis may be suspected and confirmed by venography. This complication undoubtedly is partially related to the polyvinyl chloride present in the catheter, which is a more reactive substance than that of silastic or Teflon-coated catheters. When thrombosis of a great vein is suspected, we usually remove the catheter as soon as possible, if necessary introduce a new catheter on the opposite side, and treat the patient with heparin; streptokinase treatment is also useful. Recanalization occurs in most patients within a few weeks. Septic thrombosis is another rare complication, albeit a life-threatening one. As subclavian septic thrombosis does not lend itself easily to excision, we treat these patients by anticoagulation and massive antibiotics. However, it should be remembered that prevention of this complication is much easier than its treatment.

Metabolic Management

Metabolic management may be grouped into prevention of deficiency states resulting from the omission of certain nutrients generally available in the diet and disorders of glucose metabolism, which are specific for parenteral nutrition.

Electrolyte Deficiency or Imbalance

With the introduction of more standardized hyperalimentation solutions, electrolyte imbalances or deficiencies became quite uncommon. In patients receiving four liters of hypertonic glucose and amino acids per day, at least 100 mEq of sodium, 160 to 200 mEq of potassium (with normal renal function), 90 to 100 mEq of phosphorus, and 28 to 32 mEq of magnesium are required. Once the requirements for phosphate and magnesium have been met, calcium generally is not a problem in patients treated over the short term because of the large calcium stores. However, it is customary to supply 9 to 18 mEq of calcium per day, despite the fact that this may be insufficient.

Zinc Deficiency

As with other trace metals, the requirement for zinc has been inadequtely investigated. Plasma zinc is probably not an accurate estimate of total body zinc. Zinc deficiency, like deficiencies of other trace metals, is rarely seen in patients receiving short-term parenteral nutrition (less than 3 or 4 weeks). Furthermore, zinc requirements cannot be considered in isolation, but must be related to other trace metals, mainly copper. As zinc is discussed in our treatment of trace metals earlier in this chapter, we will mention only requirements to avoid deficiency. We supplement patients with 3 to 6 mg of zinc per day, beginning with the initiation of parenteral nutrition. Supplementation should be increased in very depleted patients whose stores are probably low and in patients with excessive gastrointestinal losses or cirrhosis [119].

Copper Deficiency

Deficiency of copper has mainly been observed in patients receiving hyperalimentation at home. The anemia of copper deficiency may be mistaken for folic acid and vitamin B_{12} deficiency. If copper supplementation is required, up to 2 mg per day of the sulfate salt may be used without exceeding the solubility limit and meeting the daily required dose.

Chromium Deficiency

Chromium deficiency has been associated with the development of a diabetic state and peripheral neuropathy. Again this seems to occur only in long-term patients with minimal or no oral intake. Recently we have observed the development of severe glucose intolerance and metabolic encephalopathy in a patient after 6 months of total parenteral nutrition. The administration of 15 micrograms per day of chromium chloride should be adequate to meet daily requirements. (See more extensive discussion of trace elements earlier in this chapter and in Chapter 9.)

Essential Fatty Acid Deficiency

Essential fatty acid deficiency has become increasingly recognized, both biochemically and clinically, in patients receiving total parenteral nutrition. Recently, Goodgame et al. [58] and Wene et al. [117] presented evidence that essential fatty acid deficiency begins early in the course of parenteral nutrition. The characteristic biochemical changes of essential fatty acid deficiency are lower levels of linoleic and arachidonic acid, high levels of 5, 8, 11 eicosatrienoic acid, and an increase in the triene to tetraene ratio. These biochemical abnormalities respond to the intravenous administration of fat emulsions. Although it has not been clearly established that essential fatty acid deficiency is injurious, except perhaps to red cell membranes and, to a questionable extent, to wound healing, there seems to be no reason to allow it to occur, particularly as 500 ml of 10% fat emulsion every other day or twice weekly will essentially remove concern about this complication. Clinically, the principal lesion is a characteristic dry flaky skin rash, with small reddish papules and loss of hair to variable degrees. We have recently demonstrated that essential fatty acid deficiency results also in prostaglandin deficiency and results in changes in intraocular pressure, which we regard as probably one of many derangements or deleterious effects of prostaglandin deficiency [47]. To prevent essential fatty acid deficiency, 4 to 10 percent of the total caloric intake should be given either as a fat emulsion or by the administration of any unsaturated oil such as corn, sunflower, safflower, or margarine, approximately 25 to 50 ml a day, into any orifice of the gastrointestinal tract. This also has the advantage of being less expensive. We usually start fat administration with the initiation of hyperalimentation. Recently, some have argued for the infusion of an optimal amount of fat as being beneficial to the viscera, particularly the liver. The figure of 25 percent of total calories as fat seems most appropriate [83].

Glucose Metabolism

Hypoglycemia

The most common cause of hypoglycemia is a slowing of the infusion because of mechanical problems. This often occurs when the rate of infusion has been increased to meet the infusion schedule and then stopped suddenly. Insulin is then secreted in increased amounts, and when suddenly glucose is no longer provided, hypoglycemia results. Excessive insulin administration, of course, may be responsible for symptomatic hypoglycemia. Another curious form of hypoglycemia is secondary to the endogenous overproduction of insulin, which may occur in patients receiving rapid infusions of glucose. These patients may be symptomatic with blood sugar levels of 30 mg/100 ml at a time when infusion rates as rapid as 185 to 200 ml/hr of 25% glucose are being administered. Slowing the infusion will abolish symptomatic hypoglycemia in these patients.

Hyperglycemia

The most dangerous metabolic complication in hyperalimentation is hyperglycemia. The most common cause of hyperglycemia is too rapid initiation of the infusion. It is our practice to start the infusion at the rate of 60 ml/hr and increase infusion rate by 20 ml/hr every 24 to 48 hours, depending on age and tolerance. The elderly patient may not tolerate this rate of infusion and may require additional insulin, but young patients without pancreatic disorders generally secrete enough insulin to tolerate infusion of this magnitude. Patients may spill glucose in the urine during the first 24 to 48 hours while they are increasing their endogenous insulin production, but exogenous insulin should not be administered unless blood sugar is elevated. Similarly, patients may become glucose-intolerant after surgery and slowly regain tolerance again. In a study performed by Ryan et al. [98], patients at risk of hyperglycemia included patients with pancreatitis, patients who have undergone pancreatic resection, and patients with liver disease. When a patient who was previously stable and glucose-tolerant develops hyperglycemia, emerging sepsis should be suspected. Hyperglycemia may antedate clinical sepsis by 18 to 24 hours.

Diabetes

Considered by some to be a relative contraindication to parenteral nutrition, diabetes has not been a problem in our experience, as in most patients amino acid release of insulin simplifies control of blood glucose. The most dangerous state of hyperglycemia is hyperosmotic hyperglycemic nonketotic coma, which may arise and develop with surprising suddenness. Fever, obtundation, osmotic diuresis, and blood sugar levels of 700 to 1400 mg/100 ml are present. This complication must be diagnosed early and treated with large amounts of insulin (up to 200 units of insulin intravenously over a 24-hour period) and the infusion of large amounts of hypo-osmotic solutions, usually 0.45% saline. After the hyperosmolar hyperglycemia nonketotic coma has been successfully treated, hyperalimentation may be reinstituted cautiously, with the expectation that the patient will tolerate it well provided the predisposing cause of hyperglycemia has been removed. It should be remembered that hyperglycemic hyperosmolar nonketotic coma still carries a mortality rate of over 50 percent, and it is easier to prevent than to treat.

Liver Function Derangement

Patients receiving hyperalimentation solutions frequently manifest derangement in liver disease tests, particularly elevations of SGOT, SGPT, and alkaline phosphatase levels and, rarely, hyperbilirubinemia. These abnormalities of SGOT, SGPT, and alkaline phosphatase levels usually resolve promptly when hyperalimentation is discontinued [31]. To date, all components of parenteral nutrition solutions have been accused of being responsible for the hepatic dysfunction. Glucose has been implicated as causing fatty changes in the liver resulting in liver function derangements, particularly in the pediatric age group [21], whereas others have claimed that fat emulsions reverse fatty infiltration of the liver in patients receiving only hypertonic glucose-amino acid infusions [78]. Recently, amino acid solutions have been implicated as causing liver function derangements due to a tryptophan breakdown product in the solution [59]. In a study of 35 patients receiving peripheral solutions containing 5% dextrose and 3% amino acid formulations differing in their branched-chain amino acid concentrations, we found derangements in liver function tests in the form of elevations in SGOT levels in the patients receiving 5% dextrose with Freamine and 5% dextrose with F080 (a solution rich in branched-chain amino acids reported beneficial in the treatment of liver patients). Only the two groups receiving 5% dextrose only and 5% dextrose with three branched-chain amino acids did not develop any liver function derangements. We conclude that even infusing only 5% dextrose with 3% amino acid formulations can cause liver function derangements, and that the culprit may be one of the infused amino acids, the branched-chain amino acids excluded [48].

Infection Control

Sepsis is the most frequent and potentially the most serious complication in patients receiving total parenteral nutrition. Catheter sepsis in a patient receiving intravenous hyperalimentation is defined as an episode of clinical sepsis for which no other anatomic septic focus can be identified and which resolves upon removal of the hyperalimentation catheter. Confirmatory evidence includes positive blood and catheter tip cultures. In 2078 patients collected from 31 hospitals that used a reasonable protocol for administering hyperalimentation, the total incidence of septicemia was 7 percent [98]. Fungemias counted for 54 percent of the septicemias, but the rate of disseminated candidiasis was low. In 200 patients studied at the Massachusetts General Hospital, 355 catheters were used and catheter sepsis was associated with 11 percent of the patients and 7 percent of catheters [98]. Only eight of the catheters (2.3%) were associated with fungemias. One patient died of catheter-related sepsis. In a more recent prospective study done by Colley et al. [22], at the Massachusetts General Hospital, 179 patients receiving hyperalimentation through 224 catheters were studied. Among this group, five cases of catheter sepsis were identified (2.8%), while an additional three patients were suspected to suffer from catheter sepsis but without clear-cut evidence, to a total of 4.5 percent catheter sepsis. This relatively low sepsis rate occurring in hyperalimentation patients is a surprise, considering the depleted patient's disposition to infection. The patient's primary illness often impairs his resistance to infection. Most hyperalimentation patients are malnourished and debilitated, often suffering from such diseases as diabetes, azotemia, cancer, liver insufficiency, burns, gastrointestinal fistulas, abscesses, and gastrointestinal dysfunction. A great number of them are receiving antibiotics, steroids, radiation therapy, or chemotherapy, all of which are known to cause interference with host defense mechanisms. The catheter itself, a foreign body, must be passed through the skin into the bloodstream and remain there for extended periods as another obvious nidus of bloodstream infection. The solution itself may promote growth of organisms and might have been contaminated during preparation or later through repeated breaks in the sterility of the infusion apparatus at different points. However, all these factors seem to play only a minor role in hyperalimentation catheter sepsis. In our experience, the seeding of the hyperalimentation catheter from other sources is rare. Although bacteremia occurs and seeding of catheters seems common in patients with burns, owing to the presence of frequent and high-grade bacteremia, seeding of the fibrin sleeves around catheters in regular TPN patients is uncommon. In our experience and that of others, skin microorganisms, mainly *Staphylococcus,* are the organisms generally seen in catheter sepsis [22, 98], presumably originating at the catheter's site of entry and advancing along the catheter. If the site of entry is not properly cared for, microorganisms grow in whatever medium is supplied, including tissue juices mixed with glucose or collected under the dressing around the catheter.

One of the purposes of the hyperalimentation unit is the prevention of sepsis (see Practical

Aspects of Parenteral Nutrition). Once sepsis occurs, another objective of the unit is to investigate its epidemiology in order to try to avoid further infections. Among factors predisposing to catheter sepsis are poor nursing techniques, shortage of nursing staff, and improper attention to protocol, particularly when dealing with IV tubing changes, dressing changes, and catheter insertion. Another factor is the time of the year. Infection rate in the summer is increased, probably owing to the high temperature and the accumulated perspiration under the dressings.

Another factor that previously was thought to predispose to catheter sepsis is the duration of catheterization. However, in a study by Ryan et al., although the septic catheters were in place 4 days longer, (16.5 days versus 12.5 days), compared to the nonseptic catheters, sepsis was no more frequent when catheters remained in place for months [98]. The peak incidence in this study of the appearance of sepsis was approximately 2 weeks following insertion. Once the patient has reached equilibrium with the foreign body, the incidence decreases markedly and is not reduced by changing catheters after a given period of time.

In a more recent prospective study by Colley et al. [22], 7 of 8 catheter infections occurred within 20 days after their insertion. After 21 days, only one catheter in 65 (1.5%) was infected, whereas before the twentieth day, 7 of 159 were infected (4.4%). As mentioned earlier, skin microorganisms are the most common in catheter sepsis, *Staphylococcus epidermidis* being the most common in recent years. Other much less frequent offenders include coliform bacilli, klebsiella, enterococcus, pseudomonas, and the most serious, *Candida albicans*. In a study by Ryan of 200 patients on total parenteral nutrition and 355 catheters, there was a catheter infection rate of 7 percent, including 8 cases of fungal infection, most of them *Candida albicans*, and 13 cases of bacterial infection, 9 of them staphylococcal [98]. Whereas it is usually relatively easy to recognize bacterial infections, fungal infections are difficult to diagnose. Many patients receiving total parenteral nutrition may have positive cultures for fungi in the sputum, the urine, and wounds, i.e., colonization. It is essential, however, to differentiate between the patient who is colonized and the one with significant invasive candidiasis. Glew and coworkers [55] suggested that such a judgment is possible when *Candida* precipitins are determined by the use of crossed immunoelectrophoresis, in which antibodies to the cell or to the cellular protein in the fungus may be differentiated.

The presence of antibodies to the cell wall and not to the protein suggests that deep invasion has not taken place, whereas antibodies to the fungal protein indicate deep invasion necessitating treatment. If a fungus grows in blood cultures or antibodies to cell protein are present, the catheter must be removed. Fungemia usually disappears when the catheter is removed. However, once infusion of high-glucose solutions is resumed, blood cultures for fungi may again become positive. Consequently, the only method of supporting the patient nutritionally if oral or tube feedings are not feasible is the administration of dilute solutions of glucose and amino acids, with or without fat emulsions, through peripheral veins while fungemia is being treated. Some of our more recent studies have demonstrated a disturbing tendency for fat emulsions to support candida growth, at least in vitro.

Managing the Patient with Suspected Catheter Sepsis

If a patient who had previously been afebrile suddenly spikes a fever when receiving hyperalimentation, the hyperalimentation bottle should be taken down, the tubing and filter changed and a new bottle hung, and the bottle and the tubing should be cultured. Rarely, pyrogens or bacterial contamination of the bottle will be responsible for the fever. Blood cultures should be drawn, and a thorough search made for possible sources of fever. Among the more obvious sources of fever are pneumonia, intra-abdominal abscess, urinary tract infection, and wound infection. The practice of promptly removing the catheter, if no source is found, results in the removal of three or four "innocent" catheters for every catheter responsible for a septicemia. In a recent study by Colley et al. [22], 52 catheters were pulled for suspicion of sepsis. Of these 52 catheters, only five (9%) were responsible for catheter sepsis. In another 10 patients, fevers were designated by Colley et al. as noninfected catheter fever. These patients developed fever while receiving hyperalimentation, but no apparent cause for the fever was found. Cultures of blood and catheter tip drainage yielded negative results. However, the fever returned to normal within two or three days after the catheter was removed. The explanation for this kind of fever is probably the chemical irritation by the foreign material in these catheters, mostly PVC, interacting with the intima of the vein and causing a chemical type phlebothrombosis or thrombophlebitis. Even pooling these 10 cases and the five cases of proven sepsis, 70 percent of catheters are unnecessarily removed.

It is not necessary to treat patients with bacteremia secondary to suspected line sepsis with antibiotics unless fever persists after the line is pulled. In most instances, the infection clears once the infected catheter is removed. Serial blood specimens for culture should then be drawn to rule out persistence of bacterial or fungal infection. If results of blood culture continue to be positive, this is an indication for long-term use of antibiotics. It has been our practice to wait approximately 24 hours before replacing the hyperalimentation line. Certainly the new catheter should not be inserted before the old one is removed, since seeding may occur. In a few patients in whom the line was promptly reinserted on the opposite side shortly after removal of the other line, without giving infection an opportunity to clear, infection immediately recurred, with the same organism growing on the new line.

As stated earlier, patients with established fungemia require complete cessation of high-glucose infusions. The treatment of established fungemia involves the administration of amphotericin B or a similar agent for 6 weeks. This decision should not be undertaken lightly, since amphotericin B is a highly toxic drug. Exceptional in this respect are leukemic patients, in whom we tend to start amphotericin therapy on clinical grounds, that is, when the suspicion of sepsis occurs although results of repeated blood cultures are negative. Another problem with fungal infection is that the microorganism may lie dormant. A common place for a fungus to multiply while the patient is asymptomatic is in the retinal vessels or the superior mesenteric artery, where a mycotin aneurysm may result. When discussing catheter sepsis in hyperalimentation, it is clear that the easiest way to treat catheter sepsis is to prevent it, and this by the combined effort of all participants in the unit. Preparation of sterile solutions in the pharmacy, daily aseptic changes of intravenous tubing and filters, strict adherence to aseptic techniques while inserting the catheter, maintenance of clean catheter entry sites by dressing changes every other day, and the use of povidone-iodine ointment at the insertion site will decrease the incidence of infection, both bacterial and fungal. Likewise, maintaining the catheter for hyperalimentation only, avoiding the administration of other solutions such as blood, plasma, or antibiotics; blood sample drawing; or CVP measurements will also prevent line sepsis.

Practical Aspects of Parenteral Nutrition

Organization of the Parenteral Nutrition Unit and Team

The goal of a parenteral nutrition unit and team should be to provide safe nutritional support to all patients throughout the institution. The two approaches to the organization of the nutritional support unit in a general hospital setting are as follows:

The Team as a Primary Physician. The patient is under the direct care of the hyperalimentation team for the administration of parenteral nutrition, with other aspects of the illness being cared for by consultants. Geographic segregation is sometimes used in this approach. This in turn means that all lines are put in by one or a few individuals and that dressing changes are performed by a single or only several nurses.

The Team as a Consultant. The patient is cared for by his primary physician, with the hyperalimentation team serving as a consultant for nutrition. The team is responsible for maintaining quality control throughout the hospital. Under this system there is no geographic segregation, nor is it the responsibility of only one person to put in the hyperalimentation lines. Dressings are changed and the patient cared for by the regular hospital staff, while a central controlling individual or group of individuals oversees the administration and quality control of parenteral nutrition. This group of individuals, usually termed the "hyperalimentation team," serves as liaison among physician, nurse, pharmacist, dietitian, and patient receiving hyperalimentation therapy.

There are several advantages to the first approach. It may be argued that parenteral nutrition is safer, the chances of error minimized, and the administration of parenteral nutrition more efficient. There are also distinct disadvantages. Hospital personnel have less exposure to an important and widely used treatment modality, and parenteral nutrition may be less readily utilized. Physicians may resent the transfer of a patient from service to service for the purpose of treatment with parenteral nutrition. Finally, and perhaps most important, the primary disease for which the patient is being hospitalized may not be treated with as much interest by a physician acting only as a consultant.

At the Massachusetts General Hospital and later at the University of Cincinnati Medical Center, we have chosen the second approach. By exposing more of the hospital personnel to this technique, the use of parenteral nutrition has increased over the years. We have collaborated extensively with the respiratory unit, infectious disease unit, renal group, gastrointestinal group, and many others, all of whom have made invaluable contributions to our work. Although the implementation of safe conduction and quality control of parenteral nutrition is more difficult when dealing with many separate patient care areas, the achievement of hospital-wide sepsis rates of 2.3 percent is a clear indication that quality control is possible. This, of course, requires a dedicated staff, trained nurses, constant vigilance, and cooperation of all parties involved.

The hyperalimentation unit is usually located in an office that is staffed by a secretary and a research assistant. Each morning the secretary obtains from the pharmacy staff the names and locations of patients who are receiving parenteral nutrition. For each patient, a punch card and eventually an entry on a computer program is prepared. On this card or the computer program, the principal diagnosis, indication for TPN, solution used, complications, blood chemistry, nitrogen balance, skin testing, and the like are entered. These cards serve as a constantly updated file for all patients and various disease states and as a source of prospective and retrospective analysis of patients treated with parenteral nutrition. Research assistants are involved in data collection, and multiple clinical studies are usually ongoing.

The pharmacy is responsible for the manufacture and quality control of the solutions supplied to patients under orders of the various physicians in the hospital. It is customary for the hyperalimentation unit to have one to three physicians intimately involved in the management of the hyperalimentation patients throughout the hospital. These physicians are available for consultation, if required, for placing lines, and for follow-up of all the patients. In addition, they are involved in clinical and animal research pertaining to basic nutritional and metabolic problems. A large number of other physicians from other units and services of the hospital are generally involved in collaborative projects; these physicians may be attached to the renal unit, the gastrointestinal unit, the infectious disease and epidemiology service, or the clinical biochemistry and pathology laboratories.

The backbone of the hyperalimentation unit consists of the hyperalimentation nurse clinicians. Their primary task is educating the nursing staff and evaluating and maintaining the quality control of the nursing staff and care of patients. In addition, at least once every 48 hours, these nurses see every single patient who is receiving hyperalimentation. In general, before parenteral nutrition is initiated, they reassure, teach, and explain to patients what hyperalimentation is, as well as the benefits and complications, especially preparing patients for the catheter insertion procedure. Usually one of the nurses is present for the insertion of the parenteral nutrition catheter. Once a week, members of the hyperalimentation unit, consisting of one or more physicians, nurse clinicians, a research nurse, a pharmacist, and a dietician, meet to discuss morbidity, administrative problems, to follow the various clinical studies that are in progress, or to discuss basic problems of nutrition and new developments reported in the literature or at recent meetings.

Protocol

One of the main purposes of a parenteral nutrition unit is to make the administration of parenteral nutrition as easy, convenient, and safe as possible for both physician and patient. This is done in the following way. Parenteral hyperalimentation carts, which are stocked with all the materials needed for the proper insertion of catheters, are placed at strategic locations throughout the hospital. In addition to the prepackaged subclavian placement sets, which contain anything and everything needed for a safe subclavian vein cannulation, they contain acetone, alcohol, iodine, all the intravenous solutions, elastoplast and dressing kits, tincture of benzoin, printed order sheets, and even preprinted chest roentgenogram requisitions for the placement of a line. Each patient care area, in addition to stocking the subclavian placement sets, also stocks a number of dressing change kits, so that proper dressing changes can be carried out easily and with the proper equipment. The hyperalimentation unit prepares and circulates guidelines for the care of the patient receiving hyperalimentation. These guidelines usually contain an introductory part dealing with solutions available, indications for hyperalimentation, technique of catheter insertion, maintenance of catheters, a review of complications, and an extensive nursing care manual describing how to assist with the insertion of a hyperalimentation line, dressing change procedures, bottle, intravenous set and filter changes, and what to do when and how.

We prefer to have the total care of the patient carried out by the ordinary floor nursing staff. The ward nurses are instructed by the hyperalimentation nurses to take care of regulation of drips, dressing changes, and overall care of the patient. It is bad for morale to remove a given aspect of patient care from the hands of the primary nurses under the guise that it is too complicated. The result will be poor overall patient care, which might prevent the use of hyperalimentation in some patients. Since physicians are considerably harder to regulate, we have adopted the stance that as much of the patient care as possible should be carried out by the nurse.

The responsibility of the physician includes making the decision to initiate parenteral nutrition, starting the hyperalimentation line if he or she feels comfortable in doing so, and giving daily orders for hyperalimentation solutions. Writing the orders for parenteral nutritional solutions has been simplified by the use of preprinted standardized order forms on which all the physician has to do is check the appropriate type of formulation and the rate of infusion he wishes to administer to his patient (Figure 22-8). A protocol is also included for each solution. In this way, ordering is simplified and the physician is relieved of tiresome daily calculations of electrolytes and other ingredients of the hyperalimentation solution. This also increases efficiency in an institution in which more than 100 bottles of hyperalimentation solution may be manufactured daily. A copy of the orders is delivered to the pharmacy, where all the solutions are manufactured under laminar flow hood with utmost

CGH-122a
12/78

University of Cincinnati Medical Center
Cincinnati General Hospital

PHYSICIAN'S ORDER FORM
Parenteral Nutrition - Central Formulation

DATE ______________ TIME ______________ **ORDERS MUST BE IN THE PHARMACY BEFORE 9:30 A.M.**

FOR THIS ENTRY SEND YELLOW COPY TO PHARMACY

SOLUTIONS FROM PHARMACY
CHECK **ONE** FORMULA FOR EACH BOTTLE

BOTTLE	STANDARD	ADDED Na	ADDED INSULIN	ADDED Na & INSULIN	ADDED K	ADDED K & Na	ADDED K & INSULIN	ADDED K, Na & INSULIN
#1								
#2								
#3								
#4								
#5								

ADDITIVES:

INDICATE **TOTAL** AMOUNT OF EACH ADDITIVE DESIRED PER BOTTLE (INCLUDE THE BASIC AMOUNT IN EACH BOTTLE PLUS THE ADDITIONAL DESIRED TO EQUAL THE **TOTAL.**)

RATE ______________ ML/HR ______________ M.D.

DATE ______________ TIME ______________ **ORDERS MUST BE IN THE PHARMACY BEFORE 9:30 A.M.**

FOR THIS ENTRY SEND PINK COPY TO PHARMACY

SOLUTIONS FROM PHARMACY
CHECK **ONE** FORMULA FOR EACH BOTTLE

BOTTLE	STANDARD	ADDED Na	ADDED INSULIN	ADDED Na & INSULIN	ADDED K	ADDED K & Na	ADDED K & INSULIN	ADDED K, Na & INSULIN
#1								
#2								
#3								
#4								
#5								

ADDITIVES:

INDICATE **TOTAL** AMOUNT OF EACH ADDITIVE DESIRED PER BOTTLE (INCLUDE THE BASIC AMOUNT IN EACH BOTTLE PLUS THE ADDITIONAL DESIRED TO EQUAL THE **TOTAL.**)

RATE ______________ ML/HR ______________ M.D.

DATE ______________ TIME ______________ **ORDERS MUST BE IN THE PHARMACY BEFORE 9:30 A.M.**

FOR THIS ENTRY SEND GOLDENROD COPY TO PHARMACY

SOLUTIONS FROM PHARMACY
CHECK **ONE** FORMULA FOR EACH BOTTLE

BOTTLE	STANDARD	ADDED Na	ADDED INSULIN	ADDED Na & INSULIN	ADDED K	ADDED K & Na	ADDED K & INSULIN	ADDED K, Na & INSULIN
#1								
#2								
#3								
#4								
#5								

ADDITIVES:

INDICATE **TOTAL** AMOUNT OF EACH ADDITIVE DESIRED PER BOTTLE (INCLUDE THE BASIC AMOUNT IN EACH BOTTLE PLUS THE ADDITIONAL DESIRED TO EQUAL THE **TOTAL.**)

RATE ______________ ML/HR ______________ M.D.

Figure 22-8. *Physician's order form for central formulation used at the University of Cincinnati Medical Center. Numerous carbon copies are available, which are collected by the pharmacy each day. The variety of solutions minimizes the chance of error and enables one to handle almost any metabolic situation.*

attention to sterility. At two o'clock in the afternoon, all the solutions are delivered to the floors where the patients are located, and the hyperalimentation day starts. The nurses on the floor change the bottle that is hanging, even if it still contains solution, and change the IV tubing and the filter connected to the IV tubing, and the patient starts his new hyperalimentation day with a fresh solution, a fresh IV set, and a fresh filter.

The infusion is initiated at a rate of 60 ml/hr. The rate is increased by 20 ml/hr every 1 to 2 days, depending mainly on age (volume tolerance) and glucose tolerance. The full daily requirement is reached within a few days and maintained. When a patient is to be operated on, his infusion rate is tapered to 80 ml/hr, kept at this rate during surgery and the first postoperative day, then gradually increased according to need and tolerance.

Infusion rate regulation can be done either manually or by a pump or controller. Manual control requires enough nurses to check the rate every 30 minutes. If enough nurses are available, we find this half-hourly check preferable. If not, an infusion rate controller may be used. However, it should be remembered that this controller also should be checked periodically in order to avoid unwanted rate changes or occlusion of the line.

The patient's urine is examined routinely every 6 hours for sugar and acetone. Twice weekly blood is drawn to be tested for urea, creatinine, sugar, electrolytes, liver function, calcium, phosphorus, magnesium, ammonia, hemoglobin, hematocrit, white blood count, prothrombin time, or any appropriate special test. We avoid any additional blood drawing if possible. The dressing over the insertion site of the subclavian or jugular catheter is changed three times a week by floor nurses who have been instructed and certified by the hyperalimentation nurses. We use povidone-iodine ointment on the entrance site and an air-occlusive dressing. The hyperalimentation nurses are responsible not only for the teaching of routines, dressing change procedures, and helping with insertion of the catheter, but also for the teaching of basic principles of hyperalimentation and nutrition. This is done by lectures, seminars, or workshops. In addition, the hyperalimentation nurses are responsible for quality control, done by daily visits to the floors and the checking of the patient's chemistries, blood cultures, vital signs, dressings, and infusion rates. The nurses report to the head nurse on the floor if they find something that should be corrected and to the hyperalimentation physician or physicians, who then take further steps if needed. We have recently added both a clinical pharmacist and a dietitian to the hyperalimentation team. The former plays an important role in patient monitoring as well as in improving liaison with the pharmacy.

The addition of a dietitian to the hyperalimentation team reflects our belief that when the gut is available and functional it should be utilized. Her role is the education of the hospital staff and the standardization of enteral feeding throughout the hospital.

Finally, and here it is clearly last but not least, the research nurse plays a critical role in helping to plan the numerous studies, coordinating them, supervising, and finally, when completed, helping to analyze and collate the results.

Catheter Insertion

Perhaps the single most important act in parenteral nutrition is catheter insertion. One purpose of the hyperalimentation team is to provide such a service if needed, although in some institutions many of the house staff and the attending physicians prefer to place their own catheters. Sterile line insertion is facilitated by prepackaging of insertion and dressing kits and by placing hyperalimentation carts throughout the hospital. Insertion of the catheter is carried out in the patient's bed, generally with the assistance of one of the hyperalimentation nurses. We prefer to insert subclavian catheters because the dressing is easier and the patients generally are more comfortable. However, we realize there may be fewer complications with the insertion of an internal jugular vein catheter. Placement of the subclavian or internal jugular catheter for hyperalimentation

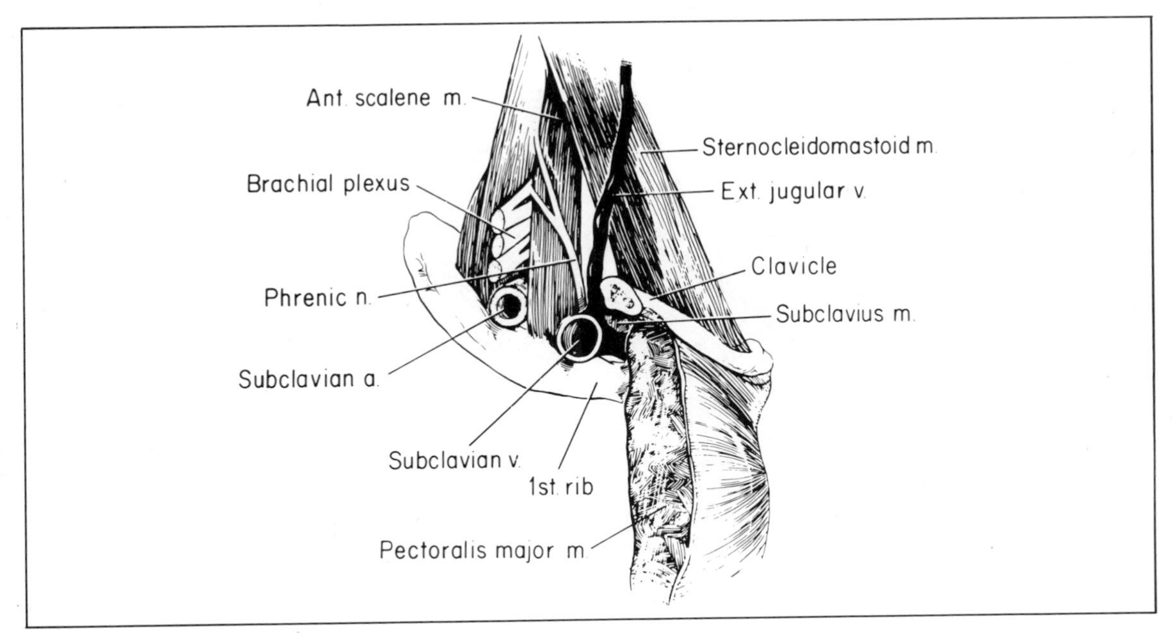

Figure 22-9. *A section of the thoracic inlet through the area of the subclavian vein. Note that the subclavian vein is the most anterior structure in a thoracic inlet.*

is never an emergency procedure. It should be carried out carefully and with the patient well hydrated and with adequate nursing help. The patient should be given a sedative before the procedure; we prefer Valium and Demerol by vein. Before starting the procedure, both the physician and the nurse take time to explain to the patient what the procedure is all about, why we are doing it, what the patient should expect out of it, and what the complications are. We find this quite valuable as the patient is less frightened and will not flinch at an inappropriate time.

Positioning is important. The patient is placed in Trendelenburg position to aid in the filling of the subclavian veins. Arms are relaxed at the sides. A roll between the shoulder blades throws the clavicles backward and makes it easier to approach the subclavian vein. The landmark for the insertion of the subclavian catheter is generally 1 cm inferior and 1 cm medial to the midpoint (bend) in the clavicle. After preparation with acetone as a defattening agent, iodine or povidone-iodine, and alcohol, with alcohol being left on the skin for approximately two minutes, the area is carefully draped. The operator should be gloved and gowned and all those in the room should be masked. Using a 3-ml syringe with 2% lidocaine (Xylocaine) and a 22-gauge needle, a wheal should be raised and Xylocaine infiltrated in the expected path of the needle, particularly around the periosteum of the clavicle. Using the same syringe and 22-gauge needle, the vein is located. Locating the vein with a 22-gauge needle avoids excessive exploration with the bigger 14-gauge needle used for insertion of the catheter. When the vein is located with a small needle, another syringe with a 14-gauge needle is used to enter the vein. The catheter is threaded and the needle removed.

Several important technical points should be noted. First, the subclavian vein is the most anterior structure in the thoracic inlet (Figure 22-9). It runs behind the proximal third of the clavicle and is separated from the subclavian artery by the scalenus anterior muscle. The brachial plexus and the apex of the lung are posterior to the subclavian artery. Thus, if the

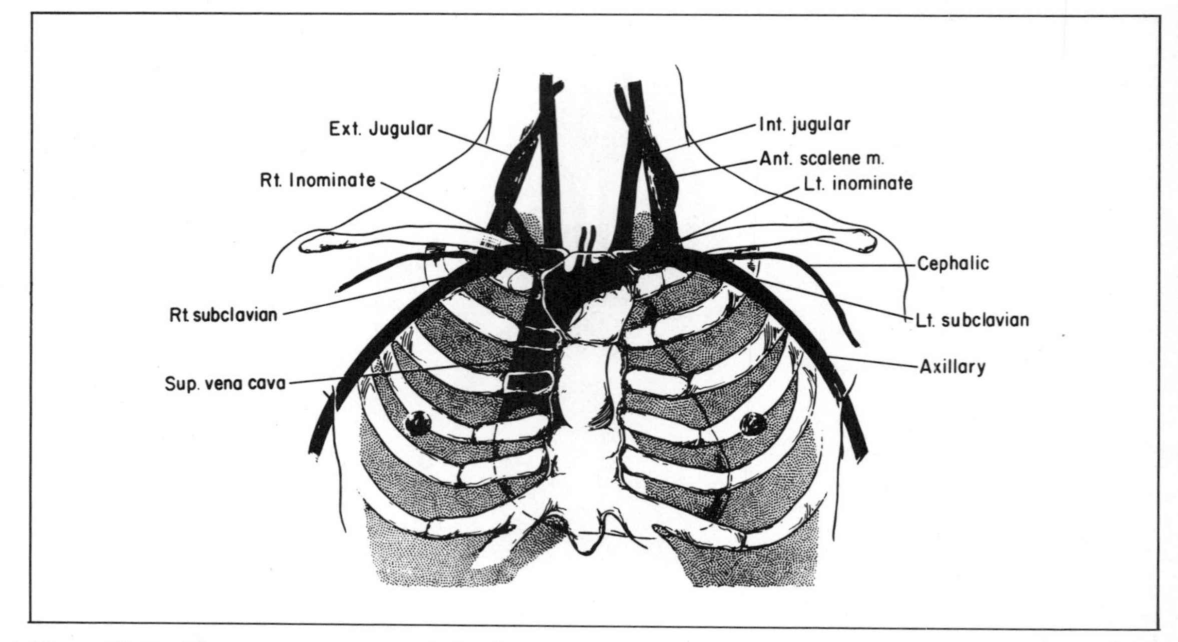

Figure 22-10. *The venous anatomy of the thoracic inlet. Note the transverse lie of the subclavian veins. The horizontal course of the subclavian vein is larger on the left than on the right. It is also easier for a right-handed person to cannulate the left subclavian vein.*

needle is kept no more than 10 degrees from the horizontal, potentially vulnerable structures will not be hit, even if the subclavian vein is not found. The second important point is that the direction of the left subclavian is more horizontal, whereas the right subclavian describes an arch, with a shorter horizontal traverse. By starting 1 cm below and 1 cm medial to the bend in the clavicle, the operator may expect that if the point of the needle is aimed toward a spot one fingerbreadth above the sternal notch, the vein will be found (Figure 22-10). A continuous aspirating motion on the syringe, usually a 2- to 3-ml syringe so that it can be placed horizontally without difficulty, is helpful. Usually a "pop" is felt as the needle enters the subclavian, and dark venous blood is obtained. At this point, the patient should be asked to perform a Valsalva maneuver; the hub of the needle is tilted cephalad and the catheter inserted as quickly as possible while the patient is still holding his breath. If the catheter does not thread and is not easily withdrawn, both the needle and the catheter should be withdrawn together to prevent the catheter from shearing off within the vein. Once the catheter is in place, it is secured with one 3:0 or 4:0 silk stitch at the site of entrance, and no other suture is necessary. Povidone-iodine ointment is put on the insertion site and an appropriate dressing is applied.

An infusion of isotonic solution, usually 5% dextrose, is begun through the newly placed line. Before leaving the patient, we usually lower the bottle and observe for blood return through the catheter to ascertain that the catheter is in the vein. After every central catheter placement, a chest roentgenogram is performed to confirm the location of the tip of the catheter and check for pneumothorax. Once the catheter tip is confirmed radiographically to be lying in the superior vena cava, infusion of 20% dextrose or the appropriate hyperalimentation solution is started.

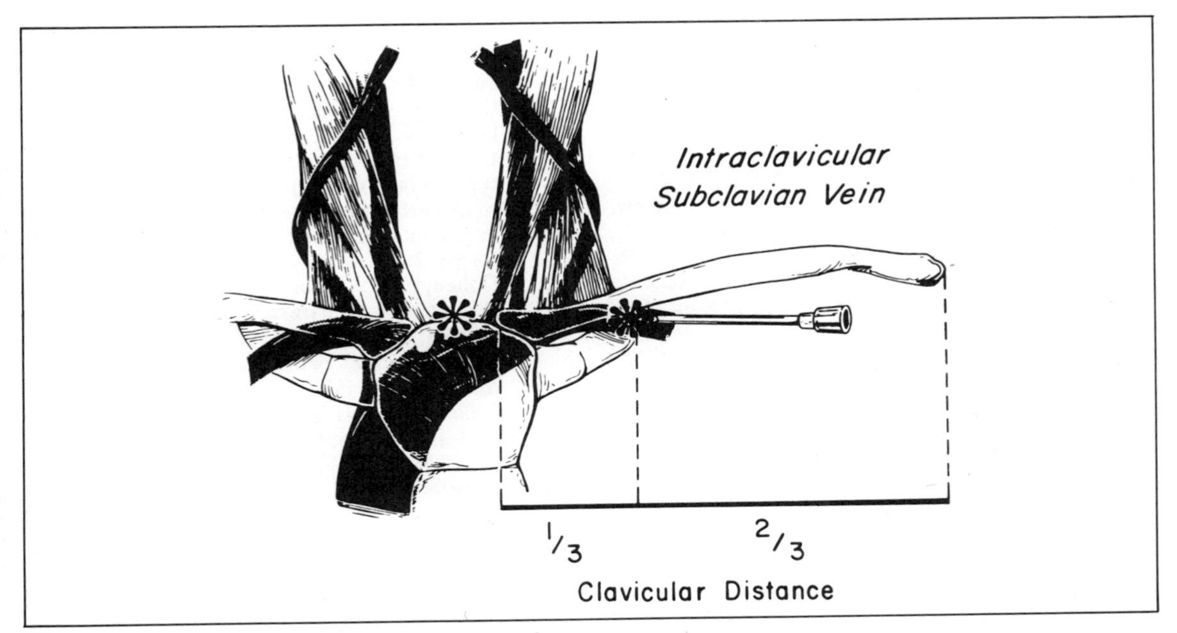

Figure 22-11. *The position of the needle in cannulating the subclavian vein. Note that one approaches the subclavian vein through the medial third of the thoracic inlet, aiming for that portion of the subclavian vein behind the clavicle.*

In placing an internal jugular catheter, the operator uses a point 5 cm above the clavicle at the posterior edge of the posterior belly of the sternocleidomastoid muscle. The internal jugular vein may be approached by aiming the needle toward the suprasternal notch with a lifting motion immediately under and in the plane of the fascia of the sternocleidomastoid (Figure 22-11). Insertion at a 30-degree angle is carried out. The internal jugular vein may also be entered by the anterior approach, in which the carotid artery is displaced to one side, the anterior edge of the sternocleidomastoid to the other side, and the needle introduced in the horizontal plane at a 30-degree angle toward the internal jugular vein. The internal jugular vein again may be identified first with a 22-gauge needle, which is also used for creating the skin wheal and locally anesthetizing the tract for the 14-gauge needle. Again, no hypertonic infusion should be undertaken until the location of the tip of the catheter in the superior vena cava is radiologically confirmed.

REFERENCES

1. Abel, R. M., Abbott, W. M., and Fischer, J. E. Intravenous essential L-amino acids and hypertonic dextrose in patients with acute renal failure: Effects on serum potassium phosphate and magnesium. *Am. J. Surg.* 123:632, 1972.
2. Abel, R. M., Beck, C. H., Jr., Abbott, W. M., Ryan, J. A., Barnett, G. O., and Fischer, J. E. Improved survival from acute renal failure following treatment with intravenous essential L-amino acids and glucose. *N. Engl. J. Med.* 288:695, 1973.
3. Abel, R. M., Fischer, J. E., Buckley, M. J., Barnett, G. O., and Austin, G. W. Malnutrition in cardiac surgical patients. *Arch. Surg.* 111:45, 1976.
4. Abel, R. M., Subramanian, V. A., and Gay, W. A. Effect of an intravenous amino acid nutrient solution on left ventricular contractility in dogs. *J. Surg. Res.* 23:201, 1977.
5. Aguirre, A., Fischer, J. E., and Welch, C. E. The role of surgery and hyperalimentation in

therapy of gastrointestinal-cutaneous fistulae. *Ann. Surg.* 180:393, 1974.

6. Aguirre, A., et al. Plasma amino acids in dogs with two experimental forms of liver damage. *J. Surg. Res.* 16:339, 1974.
7. Alexander, J. W. Emerging concepts in control of clinical infection. *Surgery* 75:934, 1974.
8. Alexander, J. W., MacMillan, B. G., Stinett, J. D., Ogle, C., Bozian, R. C., Fischer, J. E., Oakes, J. B., Morris, M. J., and Krummel, R. Beneficial effects of aggressive protein feeding in severely burned children. *Ann. Surg.* 192: 505, 1980.
9. Alexander, J. W., Ogle, C. K., Stinett, J. D., and MacMillan, B. G. A sequential prospective analysis of immunologic abnormalities and infection following severe thermal injury. *Ann. Surg.* 188:809, 1978.
10. Anderson, G. H., Patel, D. G., and Jeejeebhoy, K. N. Design and evaluation by nitrogen balance and blood aminograms of an amino acid mixture for total parenteral nutrition of adults with gastrointestinal disease. *J. Clin. Invest.* 53:904, 1974.
11. Baker, E. M. Vitamin C requirements in stress. *J. Clin. Nutr.* 20:583, 1967.
12. Baldessarini, R. J., and Fischer, J. E. Serotonin metabolism in rat brain after surgical diversion of the portal venous circulation. *Nature* 245:25, 1973.
13. Bauer, A. R., et al. The depression of T-lymphocytes after trauma. *Am. J. Surg.* 136:674, 1978.
14. Bergstrom, J., et al. Intravenous nutrition with amino acid solutions in patients with chronic uremia. *Acta Med. Scand.* 191:368, 1972.
15. Bjornson, A. B., Altemeier, W. A., and Bjornson, H. S. Host defense against opportunist micro-organisms following trauma. *Ann. Surg.* 188:102, 1978.
16. Brennan, M. F., et al. Glycerol: Major contributor to the short term protein sparing effect of fat emulsions in normal man. *Ann. Surg.* 182:386, 1975.
17. Brocks, A., Reid, H., and Glazer, G. Acute intravenous zinc poisoning. *Br. Med. J.* 1:1330, 1978.
18. Buse, M. G., and Buse, J. Effect of free fatty acids and insulin on protein synthesis and amino acid metabolism of isolated rat diaphragms. *Diabetes* 16:753, 1967.
19. Buse, M. G., and Reid, S. S. Leucine, a possible regulator of protein turnover in muscle. *J. Clin. Invest.* 58:1250, 1975.
20. Cameron, I. L., and Pavlat, W. A. Stimulation of growth of a transplantable hepatoma in rats by parenteral nutrition. *J. Natl. Cancer Inst.* 56:597, 1976.

20a. Cerra, F., Cheung, N. K., Fischer, J. E., Kaplowitz, N., Schiff, E., Dienstag, J. L., Mabry, C. D., Leevy, C. M., and Kiernan, T. A multicenter controlled study of branched chain enriched amino acid infusion (Hepatamine-F080) in patients with hepatic encephalopathy. *Hepatology* 2:683, 1982. (Abstract).

21. Cohen, I. T., Dahms, B., and Hays, D. M. Peripheral total parenteral nutrition employing a lipid emulsion (Intralipid): Complications encountered in pediatric patients. *J. Pediatr. Surg.* 12:837, 1977.
22. Colley, R., et al. Does fever mean infection in central total parenteral nutrition. *J.P.E.N.* 3: 32, 1979.
23. Copeland, E. M., MacFadyen, B. V., Jr., and Dudrick, S. J. Effect of intravenous hyperalimentation on established delayed hypersensitivity in the cancer patient. *Ann. Surg.* 184:60, 1976.
24. Copeland, E. M., MacFadyen, B. V., Jr., McGown, C., and Dudrick, S. J. The use of hyperalimentation in patients with potential sepsis. *Surg. Gynecol. Obstet.* 138:377, 1974.
25. Criston, N. V., and Meakins, J. L. Neutrophil function in surgical patients: Two inhibitors of granulocyte chemotaxis associated with sepsis. *J. Surg. Res.* 26:355, 1974.
26. Cuthbertson, D. P. Post traumatic metabolism: A multi-disciplinary challenge. *Surg. Clin. North Am.* 58:1045, 1978.
27. Daly, J., Copeland, E. M., and Dudrick, S. J. Effect of intravenous nutrition on tumor growth and host immunocompetence in malnourished animals. *Surgery* 84:655, 1978.
28. Daly, J., Dudrick, S. J., and Copeland, E. M. Effects of protein depletion and repletion on cell-mediated immunity in experimental animals. *Ann. Surg.* 188:791, 1978.
29. Dodsworth, H. M., et al. Depletion of brain norepinephrine in acute hepatic coma. *Surgery* 75:811, 1974.
30. Dudrick, S. J., Copeland, E. M., and MacFadyen, B. V., Jr. The Nutritional Care of the Cancer Patient. In J. M. Greep, P. B. Soeters, R. I. C. Wesdorp, C. W. R. Phaf, and J. E. Fischer (Eds.), *Current Concepts in Parenteral Nutrition.* The Hague: Martinus Nijoff, 1977. P. 187 ff.
31. Dudrick, S. J., MacFadyen, B. V., Jr., VanBuren, C. T., Ruberg, R. L., and Maynard,

A. T. Parenteral hyperalimentation: Metabolic problems and solutions. *Ann. Surg.* 176: 259, 1972.
32. Dudrick, S. J., Steiger, E., and Long, J. M. Renal failure in surgical patients: Treatment with intravenous essential amino acids and hypertonic dextrose. *Surgery* 68:180, 1970.
33. Dudrick, S. J., Vars, H. M., Rawnsley, H. M., and Rhoads, J. E. Total intravenous feeding and growth in puppies. *Fed. Proc.* 25:481, 1966.
34. Dudrick, S. J., Wilmore, D. W., Vars, H. M., and Rhoads, J. E. Can intravenous feeding as a sole means of nutrition support growth in the child and restore weight loss in an adult? An affirmative answer. *Ann. Surg.* 169:974, 1969.
35. Edmunds, L. H., Jr., William, G. M., and Welsh, E. E. External gastrointestinal fistulas arising from the gastrointestinal tract. *Ann. Surg.* 152:445, 1960.
36. Elman, R., and Weiner, D. O. Intravenous alimentation with special reference to protein (amino acid) metabolism. *J.A.M.A.* 122:796, 1939.
37. Felig, P. The glucose alanine cycle. *Metabolism* 22:179, 1973.
38. Felig, P., et al. Alanine: Key role in gluconeogenesis. *Science* 167:1003, 1970.
39. Feller, J. H., et al. Changing methods in the treatment of severe pancreatitis. *Am. J. Surg.* 127:196, 1974.
40. Fischer, J. E. Management of high intestinal fistulas. *Adv. Surg.* 9:139, 1975.
41. Fischer, J. E., and Baldessarini, J. E. False neurotransmitters and hepatic failure. *Lancet* 2:75, 1971.
42. Fischer, J. E., Foster, G. S., Abel, R. M., Abbott, W. M., and Ryan, J. A. Hyperalimentation as primary therapy for inflammatory bowel disease. *Am. J. Surg.* 125:165, 1973.
43. Fischer, J. E., Rosen, H. M., Ebeid, A. M., James, J. H., Keane, J. M., and Soeters, P. B. The effect of normalization of plasma amino acids on hepatic encephalopathy in man. *Surgery* 80:77, 1976.
44. Fischer, J. E., Yoshimura, N., James, J. H., Cummings, M. G., Abel, R. M., and Deindoerfer, F. Plasma amino acids in patients with hepatic encephalopathy: Effects of amino acid infusions. *Am. J. Surg.* 127:40, 1974.
45. Freund, H., Atamian, S., and Fischer, J. E. Chromium deficiency during total parenteral nutrition. *J.A.M.A.* 241:496, 1979.
46. Freund, H., Atamian, S., and Fischer, J. E. Comparative study of parenteral nutrition in renal failure using essential and non-essential amino acid-containing solutions. *Surg. Gynecol. Obstet.* 151:652, 1980.
47. Freund, H., Floman, N., Schwartz, B., and Fischer, J. E. Essential fatty acid deficiency in total parenteral nutrition: Detection by changes in intraocular pressure. *Ann. Surg.* 190:139, 1979.
48. Freund, H., Hoover, H. C., Jr., Atamian, S., and Fischer, J. E. Infusion of the branched-chain amino acids in postoperative patients: Anticatabolic properties. *Ann. Surg.* 190:18, 1979.
49. Freund, H., Ryan, J. A., and Fischer, J. E. Amino acid derangements in sepsis. Treatment with branched-chain amino acid rich infusions. *Ann. Surg.* 188:423, 1978.
50. Freund, H., Yoshimura, N., and Fischer, J. E. Long term therapy of chronic hepatic encephalopathy with a branched-chain amino acid enriched elemental diet. *J.A.M.A.* 242:347, 1979.
51. Freund, H., Yoshimura, N., and Fischer, J. E. Is intravenous fat nitrogen sparing in the injured rat? *Am. J. Surg.* 140:377, 1980.
52. Fulks, R. M., Li, J. B., and Goldberg, A. L. Effects of insulin, glucose and amino acids on protein turnover in rat diaphragm. *J. Biol. Chem.* 250:280, 1975.
53. Giordano, C. Use of exogenous and endogenous urea for protein synthesis in normal and uremic subjects. *J. Lab. Clin. Med.* 62:231, 1963.
54. Giovannetti, S., and Maggiore, Q. A low-nitrogen diet with protein of high biological value for severe chronic uraemia. *Lancet* 1: 1000, 1964.
55. Glew, R. H., et al. Serologic tests in the diagnosis of systemic Candidiasis. *Am. J. Med.* 64: 586, 1978.
56. Goldberg, A. L., Odessey, R. Oxidation of amino acids by diaphragms from fed and fasted rats. *Am. J. Physiol.* 223:1384, 1972.
57. Goodgame, J. T., and Fischer, J. E. Parenteral nutrition in the treatment of acute pancreatitis. *Ann. Surg.* 186:651, 1977.
58. Goodgame, J. T., Lowry, S. F., and Brennan, M. F. Essential fatty acid deficiency in total parenteral nutrition: Time course of development and suggestions for therapy. *Surgery* 84: 271, 1978.
59. Grant, J. P., et al. Serum hepatic enzyme and bilirubin elevations during parenteral nutrition. *Surg. Gynecol. Obstet.* 145:573, 1977.

60. Greenberg, G. R., et al. Protein sparing therapy in postoperative patients. *N. Engl. J. Med.* 294: 1411, 1976.
61. Heinburger, S. L., et al. Correction of hepatocellular dysfunction during endotoxemia. *J. Surg. Res.* 24:442, 1978.
62. Helfrick, S. W., and Abelson, N. M. Intravenous feeding of complete diet in a child. *J. Pediatr.* 25:400, 1946.
63. Holter, A. R., and Fischer, J. E. The effects of perioperative hyperalimentation on complications in patients with carcinoma and weight loss. *J. Surg. Res.* 23:31, 1977.
63a. Horst, D., Grace, N., Conn, H. O., Schiff, E., Schencker, S., Viteri, A., Law, D., and Atterburg, C. E. A double-blind randomized comparison of dietary protein and an oral branched-chain amino acid (BCAA) encephalopathy (PSE). *Hepatology* 1:518, 1981. (Abstract).
64. Howard, J. M. Studies of the absorption of glucose following injury. *Ann. Surg.* 141:321, 1955.
65. Iber, F. L., et al. The plasma amino acids in patients with liver failure. *J. Lab. Clin. Med.* 50:417, 1957.
66. Jeejeebhoy, K. N., Anderson, G. H., Nakhooda, A. F., Greenberg, G. R., Sanderson, I., and Marliss, E. B. Metabolic studies in total parenteral nutrition with lipid in man. *J. Clin. Invest.* 57:125, 1976.
67. Jeejeebhoy, K. N., Langer, B., Tsallas, G., Chu, R. C., Kuksis, A., and Anderson, G. H. Total parenteral nutrition at home: Studies in patients surviving four months to five years. *Gastroenterology* 71:943, 1976.
68. Kay, R. G., et al. A syndrome of acute zinc deficiency during total parenteral hyperalimentation in man. *Ann. Surg.* 183:331, 1976.
69. Kyger, E. R., et al. Adverse effects of protein malnutrition on myocardial function. *Surgery* 84:147, 1978.
70. Long, J. M., et al. Effect of carbohydrate and fat intake on nitrogen excretion during total intravenous feeding. *Ann. Surg.* 185:417, 1977.
71. Lowry, S. F., Goodgame, J. T., Maher, M. M., and Brennan, M. F. Parenteral vitamin requirements during intravenous feeding. *Am. J. Clin. Nutr.* 31:2149, 1978.
72. Lowry, S. F., Goodgame, J. T., Norton, J. A., Jones, D. C., and Brennan, M. F. Effect of chronic protein malnutrition on host-tumor composition and growth. *J. Surg. Res.* 26:79, 1979.
73. MacFadyen, B. V., Jr., and Dudrick, S. J. Management of gastrointestinal fistulae with parenteral hyperalimentation. *Surgery* 74:100, 1973.
74. MacLean, L. D., et al. Host resistance in sepsis and trauma. *Ann. Surg.* 183:207, 1975.
75. Manchester, K. L. Oxidation of amino acid by isolated rat diaphragm and the influence of insulin. *Biochem. Biophys. Acta* 100:295, 1965.
76. Marliss, E. B., et al. Muscle and splanchnic glutamine and glutamate metabolism in postabsorptive and starved man. *J. Clin. Invest.* 50:814, 1971.
77. Mattson, W. J., et al. Alterations of individual free amino acids in brain during acute hepatic coma. *Surg. Gynecol. Obstet.* 130:263, 1970.
78. McDonald, A. T. J., Phillips, M. J., and Jeejeebhoy, K. N. Reversal of fatty liver by Intralipid in patients on total parenteral alimentation. *Gastroenterology* 64:885, 1973.
79. Meakins, J. L., et al. Delayed hypersensitivity indicator of acquired failure of host defense in sepsis and trauma. *Ann. Surg.* 186:241, 1977.
79a. Meakins, J. L., Christou, N. V., Forse, A., and Shizgal, H. M. Malnutrition and Anergy in the Surgical Setting. In J. E. Fischer (Ed.), *Relevance of Nutrition to Sepsis: Report of the Third Ross Conference on Medical Research.* Columbus, Ohio: Ross Laboratories, 1982. Pp. 285–296.
80. Meng, H. C. Fat Emulsions in Parenteral Nutrition. In J. E. Fischer (Ed.), *Total Parenteral Nutrition.* Boston: Little, Brown, 1976. Pp. 305–334.
80a. Miller, J. M., Brenner, U., Dienst, C., and Pichlmaier, H. L. Preoperative parenteral feeding in patients with gastrointestinal carcinoma. *Lancet* 1:68, 1982.
81. Moghissi, K., et al. Parenteral nutrition in carcinoma of the esophagus treated by surgery: Nitrogen balance and clinical studies. *Br. J. Surg.* 64:125, 1977.
82. Moss, G., et al. Postoperative metabolic patterns following immediate total nutritional support: Hormone levels, DNA synthesis, nitrogen balance, and accelerated wound healing. *J. Surg. Res.* 21:383, 1976.
83. Mullen, J. L., Buzby, G. P., Walman, M. T., Gertner, M. H., Hobbs, C. L., and Rosato, E. F. Prediction of operative morbidity and mortality by preoperative nutritional assessment. *Surg. Forum* 30:80, 1979.
84. Munro, H. N. A General Survey of Pathological Changes. In H. N. Munro and J. B. Allison (Eds.), *Mammalian Protein Metabolism.* Philadelphia: Saunders, 1959. Vol. II, Pp. 267–319.

85. Palmisano, D. J. Nutrient deficiencies after intensive parenteral alimentation. *N. Engl. J. Med.* 291:799, 1974.
86. Pietsch, J. B., Meakins, J. L., and MacLean, L. D. The delayed hypersensitivity response: Application in clinical surgery. *Surgery* 82:349, 1977.
87. Odessey, R., and Goldberg, A. L. Oxidation of Leucine by rat skeletal muscle. *Am. J. Physiol.* 223:1376, 1972.
88. Odessey, R., Khairallah, E. A., and Goldberg, A. L. Origin and possible significance of alanine production by skeletal muscle. *J. Biol. Chem.* 249:7623, 1974.
89. Petersen, S. R., Sheldon, G. F., and Carpenter, B. A. Failure of hyperalimentation to enhance survival in malnourished rats with E. coli-hemoglobin adjuvant peritonitis. *Surg. Forum* 30:60, 1979.
90. Raciti, A., et al. Effects of nutrition on weaning from controlled ventilation in patients with chronic obstructive pulmonary disease and sepsis. *J.P.E.N.* 3:27, 1979.
91. Reber, H. A., Roberts, C., Way, L. W., et al. Management of external gastrointestinal fistulas. *Ann. Surg.* 188:460, 1978.
92. Reilly, J. Inflammatory Bowel Disease. In J. E. Fischer (Ed.), *Total Parenteral Nutrition.* Boston: Little, Brown, 1976. P. 187.
93. Reilly, J., et al. Hyperalimentation in inflammatory bowel disease. *Am. J. Surg.* 131:192, 1976.
94. Rose, W. C., Coon, M. J., and Lambert, G. F. The amino acid requirements of man: The role of the caloric intake. *J. Biol. Chem.* 210:331, 1954.
95. Rose, W. C., and Wixom, R. L. The amino acid requirements in man: XVI. The role of the nitrogen intake. *J. Biol. Chem.* 217:997, 1955.
96. Rosen, H. M., et al. Influences of exogenous intake and nitrogen balance on plasma and brain aromatic amino acid concentrations. *Metabolism* 27:383, 1978.
97. Rossi-Fanelli, F., et al. Octopamine plasma levels and hepatic encephalopathy. *Clin. Chim. Acta* 67:261, 1976.
97a. Rossi-Fanelli, F., Riggio, O., Cangiano, C., Cascino, A., Stortoni, M., Merli, M., and Capocaccia, L. Intravenous branched chain amino acid (BCAA) infusions vs. lactulose (L) in the treatment of hepatic encephalopathy (HE): A controlled study. *Gastroenterology* 82:1226, 1982. (Abstract).
98. Ryan, J. A., et al. Catheter complications in total parenteral nutrition: A prospective study of 200 consecutive patients. *N. Engl. J. Med.* 290:757, 1974.
98a. Ryan, J. A., Jr., and Taft, D. A preoperative nutritional assessment does not predict morbidity and mortality in abdominal operations. *Surg. Forum* 31:96, 1980.
99. Scheflan, M., et al. Intestinal adaptation after extensive resection of the small intestine and prolonged administration of parenteral nutrition. *Surg. Gynecol. Obstet.* 143:757, 1976.
100. Sheldon, G. F., et al. Management of gastrointestinal fistulas. *Surg. Gynecol. Obstet.* 113:490, 1971.
101. Smith, A. R., et al. Alterations in plasma and CSF amino acids, amines, and metabolites in hepatic coma. *Ann. Surg.* 187:343, 1978.
102. Soeters, P. B., Ebeid, A. M., and Fischer, J. E. Review of 404 patients with gastrointestinal fistulas: Impact of parenteral nutrition. *Ann. Surg.* 190:189, 1979.
103. Soeters, P. B., and Fischer, J. E. Insulin, glucagon, amino acid imbalance and hepatic failure. *Lancet* 2:880, 1976.
104. Souba, W. W., Long, J. M., and Dudrick, S. J. Energy intake and stress as determinants of nitrogen excretion in rats. *Surg. Forum* 29:76, 1978.
105. Spanier, A. H., et al. The relationship between immune competence and nutrition. *Surg. Forum* 27:332, 1976.
106. Steiger, E., Daly, J. M., Allen, T. R., Dudrick, S. J., and Vars, H. M. Postoperative intravenous nutrition: Effects on body weight, protein regeneration, wound healing and liver morphology. *Surgery* 73:686, 1973.
107. Steiger, E., Oram-Smith, J., Miller, E., Kno, L., and Voss, H. M. Effects of nutrition on tumor growth and tolerance to chemotherapy. *J. Surg. Res.* 18:455, 1975.
108. Stein, J. M., and Pruitt, B. A. Suppurative thrombophlebitis, a lethal iatrogenic disease. *N. Engl. J. Med.* 282:1452, 1970.
109. Stinnett, J. D., Wunder, J. A., and Alexander, J. W. Alterations on complement metabolism during protein malnutrition and restoration by selected amino acids. *Fed. Proc.* 39:888, 1980. (Abstract).
109a. Strauss, E., Santos, W. R., Carrtapalti DaSilva, E., Laret, C. M., Capacci, M. L., and Bernadini, A. P. A randomized controlled clinical trial for the evaluation of the efficacy of balanced amino acid solution compared to neomycin in hepatic encephalopathy. Submitted for publication.
109b. Twomey, P., Ziegler, D., and Rombeau, J.

Utility of skin testing in nutritional assessment: A critical review. *J. Parent. Nutr.* 6:50, 1982.

110. Vaidyanath, N., Birkhahn, R., Border, J. R., Oswald, G., Trietley, G., Yuan, T. F., Moritz, E., and McMenamy, R. H. Plasma concentrations and tissue uptake of free amino acids in dogs in sepsis and starvation: Effects of glucose infusion—some effects of low alimentation. *Metabolism* 27:641, 1978.
111. Vaidyanath, N., Oswald, G., Trietley, G., Weissenhoffer, W., Moritz, E., McMenamy, R. H., Birkhahn, R., Yuan, T. F., and Border, J. R. Turnover of amino acids in sepsis and starvation: Effect of glucose infusion. *J. Trauma* 16: 125, 1976.
112. Van Rij, A. M., et al. Selenium in total parenteral nutrition. *J.P.E.N.* 3:25, 1979.
113. Vilter, R. W., et al. Manifestations of copper deficiency in a patient with systemic sclerosis on intravenous hyperalimentation. *N. Engl. J. Med.* 291:188, 1974.
114. Wahren, J., Felig, P., and Hagenfeldt, L. Effect of protein ingestion on splanchnic and leg metabolism in normal men and in patients with diabetes mellitus. *J. Clin. Invest.* 57:987, 1976.
115. Walser, M., Sapir, D. G., and Maddrey, W. C. The Use of Alpha-Keto Analogues of Essential Amino Acids. In J. E. Fischer (Ed.), *Total Parenteral Nutrition.* Boston: Little, Brown, 1976. Pp. 413–430.
116. Walser, M., et al. The effect of keto analogues of essential amino acids in severe chronic uremia. *J. Clin. Invest.* 52:678, 1973.
117. Wene, J. D., Connor, W. E., and denBesten, L. The development of essential fatty acid deficiency in healthy men fed fat-free diets intravenously and orally. *J. Clin. Invest.* 56:127, 1975.
118. Wilmore, D. W., and Pruitt, B. A., Jr. Parenteral Nutrition in Burn Patients. In J. E. Fischer (Ed.), *Total Parenteral Nutrition.* Boston: Little, Brown, 1976. Pp. 231–252.
119. Wolman, S. L., et al. Zinc in total parenteral nutrition: Needs and metabolic effects. *Gastroenterology* 74:1113, 1978.
120. Wretlind, A. Complete intravenous nutrition. Theoretical and experimental background. *Nutr. Metab.* 14:Suppl:1, 1972.
121. Wunder, J. A., Stinnett, J. D., and Alexander, J. W. The effects of malnutrition on variables of host defense in the guinea pig. *Surgery* 84: 542, 1978.
122. Young, V. The Role of Skeletal and Cardiac Muscle in the Regulation of Protein Metabolism. In H. N. Munro (Ed.), *Mammalian Protein Metabolism.* New York: Academic Press, 1969. Vol. IV, pp. 585–674.

Physiologic Approach to Peripheral Parenteral Nutrition

Joel B. Freeman
Robert J. Fairfull-Smith

23

Since the advent of total parenteral nutrition (TPN), nutritional support has become an area of special interest for many investigators. Practically all major centers now have the capability of sustaining metabolic and nutritional needs for long periods in patients who cannot consume adequate nutrition orally. As knowledge and experience accumulate, more biochemical and physiologic problems present themselves. These complex metabolic interrelationships are dealt with in other parts of this book. The purpose of this chapter is to discuss the problem of peripheral parenteral nutrition (PPN). PPN implies the administration of sterile water, electrolytes, nitrogen, and calories by peripheral vein.

In 1947, Robert Elman published his text, *Parenteral Alimentation in Surgery*. Historically, it is apparent that many routes other than the subclavian have been used for alimentation. These include peripheral veins, the subcutaneous space and the rectum. Clearly, the problem of surgical malnutrition was appreciated by Elman and his contemporaries. They founded the basis for modern nutritional support systems. The lack of advancement between 1945 and 1968 is best expressed on page 29 of Elman's book, where it is stated, "When the patient possesses few veins, the occurrence of phlebitis may make it difficult or impossible to continue." That Elman understood the importance of simultaneously infusing glucose and protein is demonstrated by his many allusions to combinations of 10% glucose with amino acids. Indeed, classic experiments that determined the now well-known requirement of 150 nonprotein calories for each gram of nitrogen were performed in malnourished but relatively stable patients and animals. Many nitrogen balance data showed that when 10 gm nitrogen were administered, as protein hydrolysates, daily, nitrogen balance during the infusion of amino acids *alone* was superior to that obtained during the infusion of nonprotein solutions. Finally, data were presented to show that the addition of small amounts of glucose (100 gm/day) to the amino acid solutions improved nitrogen balance. As one reviews the innumerable amino acid infusion studies, both with and without caloric sources, dating from 1970 to the present, one feels that many of the experiments performed by Elman and his contemporaries have been repeated!

EFFECTS OF CRYSTALLOID INFUSIONS

Routine pre- and postoperative care with 5% glucose, in water or salt, delivers 50 gm glucose/liter. At a rate of 125 ml/hr, the patient will receive 3 liters or 600 calories daily. The average postoperative patient at rest requires about 35 calories/kg of ideal body weight (approximately 2500 calories per day). Three liters of 5% glucose provides one-quarter of these energy requirements and no protein. Salt solutions provide no calories. Hence, it is axiomatic that patients receiving such solutions by peripheral vein are being starved. In well-nourished patients, this is tolerated for short periods. Parenthetically, the role of starvation in postoperative fatigue, even after elective surgery, is an intriguing consideration.

The diagnosis of malnutrition is most easily made by a common-sense approach, which includes a good history and an accurate visual assessment of the patient. The following factors are strong indicators of existing malnutrition: (1) a history of prolonged inadequate intake, (2) a protracted illness, (3) a 10 percent weight loss, and (4) serum albumin under 3.5 gm.

Administration of 100 to 150 gm glucose daily (3 liters of 5% dextrose) only partially meets total energy requirements, leaving a deficit of 1900 (2500 − 600) calories. These extra calories are needed to meet energy demands, such as muscular function, cardiac contractility, and the synthesis of new protein. In this hypocaloric situation, extra calories are derived from protein. Amino acids from the protein pool are constantly being rechanneled through various cycles for synthesis of new protein. However, amino acids can also be used as substrates for gluconeogenesis. This means that the amino acid is deaminated, and the remaining carbon skeleton is used to produce glucose. Conversion of body protein to glucose is expensive and wasteful. The body is able to produce approximately 3.5 gm glucose for each gram of nitrogen. However, considerable energy investment is required to form the protein originally. All of this energy plus the metabolic energy required to convert protein to glucose is lost during gluconeogenesis. Furthermore, the human body contains only 15 percent of ideal weight as protein, meaning that the average 70-kg patient has only 10.5 kg protein. In contrast to amino acids, glucose is used primarily for energy production. Therefore, further increments of exogenous glucose, without simultaneous protein administration, do not result in protein *synthesis.* However, glucose, administered to patients postoperatively, reduces nitrogen losses because energy requirements are partially met, thereby reducing the amount of gluconeogenesis required. Small additional benefits would result if 10% rather than 5% glucose was given, but this would not improve protein synthesis and, furthermore, would increase phlebitis. Complete nutritional support requires the simultaneous administration of both nitrogen and calories in the familiar ratio of 150 nonprotein calories/gm nitrogen. Long-term administration of calories and nitrogen in this ratio requires administration through the subclavian vein. Despite our many advances with respect to technique and infection control, subclavian venipuncture is still potentially hazardous, especially for routine postoperative care. The essential role of PPN is to provide some nutritional support for patients in whom the indications for TPN by subclavian vein are not absolute.

PERIPHERAL AMINO ACID INFUSIONS

During TPN, 25% glucose is infused simultaneously with amino acids. Hence, all energy requirements are met by glucose, while protein requirements are met by the infused amino acids. The need for gluconeogenesis is obviated. The same holds true if part of the calories are infused as fat rather than glucose. When all calories are infused as 25% glucose, serum insulin levels are elevated threefold. From a teleologic point of view, the body has evolved to preserve fat when calories are plentiful. Metabolically, this is facilitated by high insulin levels, which inhibit lipoprotein lipase, the enzyme responsible for breakdown of body fat. Insulin also promotes synthesis of triglycerides from glucose. Conversely, when glucose is not plentiful, as in starvation, glycogen reserves are used for energy. These reserves can maintain a patient for 12 to 20 hours. In order to maintain blood glucose levels, the body switches to amino acid catabolism (gluconeogenesis). Large quantities of nitrogen appear in the urine. Nitrogen input is absent, resulting in a markedly negative balance [7]. With time, urinary nitrogen excretion falls owing to an acceleration of fat hydrolysis, which provides free fatty acids and glycerol as fuel, hence sparing protein. However, complete adaptation to fat utilization takes 5 to 10 days. During this period, body protein stores are severely depleted.

When amino acids are infused without glucose, insulin levels are low. According to the original theory of Blackburn and Flatt, these low insulin levels would have a permissive effect on fat mobilization, providing the body with a large endogenous supply of fuel [16]. Simultaneously, the infused amino acids would be available for synthesis of new protein. Initial studies showed that nitrogen balance during infusion of amino acids alone was markedly superior to that obtained during infusion of glucose alone [4]. The addition of glucose to the amino acids resulted in a greater nitrogen deficit, suggesting that glucose, by raising serum insulin, was detrimental to the regimen. Unfortunately, the amino acid and amino acid plus glucose infusion periods were not isonitrogenous. Furthermore, these data were questioned because many investigators could not believe that insulin was anything other than a favorable anabolic hormone.

Between 1974 and 1978, many investigators compared the effects of amino acids to glucose. All were able to demonstrate the superiority of amino acids over glucose alone [14, 18, 29, 30, 48]. Our data, obtained both from normal volunteers and postoperative patients, showed an improvement of nitrogen balance from approximately −12 gm/day during glucose infusion to −1 gm/day during infusion of 5% amino acids [17–20]. When 5% amino acids (150 gm protein a day) were used, nitrogen balance was superior to that obtained during infusion of 3% amino acids (90 gm/day) [18]. When 50 gm glucose was added to each of the 3 liters of amino acid solutions infused daily, a 5% amino acid–5% glucose solution resulted. This was similar to solutions used during the 1940s, the only difference being the greater extent of metabolic measurements. All investigators examined free fatty acid levels, ketone bodies, and insulin. Infusion of amino acids alone resulted in a tenfold increase of free fatty acid levels and a twofold increase of ketone bodies. This strongly suggested lipolysis. Simultaneously, there was a significant fall in insulin levels, with the aforementioned marked improvement in nitrogen balance. In question was the validity of the assumption that the low insulin levels were causally related to the improved nitrogen balance. Hence, other experiments were carried out, wherein amino acids were infused with and without glucose, both study periods being isonitrogenous. The addition of glucose resulted in a slightly improved, but statistically insignificant, nitrogen balance from approximately −1 gm/day to nitrogen equilibrium [20]. During amino acid plus glucose infusion, insulin levels rose to control levels. This suggested that the improvement of nitrogen balance was independent of serum insulin. During infusion of amino acids with glucose, free fatty acid and ketone body levels fell, but not to control levels. This was interpreted to mean that part of the patient's calories were being provided endogenously (from fat), while the remainder came from exogenous glucose [14, 24]. Other studies confirmed these results, although several demonstrated statistically significant improvements in nitrogen balance when glucose was added [14, 24, 29, 30, 52]. Numerically, however, all studies were similar. They also showed that doubling the amount of glucose (from 50 to 100 gm/liter of amino acids) produced a 10% glucose solution, which further improved nitrogen balance. This is not surprising. Indeed, if glucose concentrations were progressively increased, we would soon have a standard hyperalimentation solution! However, peripheral vein tolerance to hyperosmotic solutions prevents the administration of glucose concentrations greater than 10%. Greenberg substituted fat isocalorically for glucose during PPN and showed that regardless of the caloric source, nitrogen balance was always superior to that achieved by calorie-free amino acid infusions [14]. Other evidence also exists showing that glucose, or any nonprotein caloric source, will maximize utilization of amino acids during PPN. In 1939, Elman showed that the addition of small amounts of glucose reduced urinary nitrogen losses during amino acid infusions. These early studies accounted for the development of the popular 5% dextrose–5% protein hydrolysate solution. During infusion of amino acids alone, breakdown of endogenous as well as some of the exogenously administered amino acids continues. Hence, urinary nitrogen losses are large, even though nitrogen balance is improved when compared to infusion of glucose alone. Tweedle et al. showed that utilization of infused amino acids for protein synthesis was favored by providing exogenous glucose [48]. Howard produced similar results [30]. Some of Howard's patients were obese and some were lean, again confirming our studies done in lean and obese surgical patients [18, 20]. Elwyn and his colleagues gave amino acids with and without glucose in a crossover design and again demonstrated the beneficial effects of adding glucose to the amino acid solution [14].

That most studies have been carried out using nitrogen balance is certainly open to criticism. Nitrogen balance techniques have many sources of error, particularly in the study of patients in differing nutritional states. Our studies partially resolved these problems because they were carried out for relatively long (10- to 14-day) metabolic periods, in a metabolic ward, and after assuring constant nitrogen excretion prior to beginning the experiment. The fact that at least 10 papers on protein sparing have demonstrated improved nitrogen balance attests to the efficacy of protein sparing. In addition, other investigators have carried out more sophisticated studies. Skillman et al. measured the albumin synthesis rate in postoperative patients. Albumin synthesis was 66 percent greater in patients receiving 3.5% amino acids than in those receiving glucose alone [45]. Spanier et al. measured body composition preoperatively and 5 days postoperatively in patients receiving either 5% glucose or 5% protein intravenously. Patients receiving glucose had a significant loss of both body fat and body cell mass, whereas patients receiving amino acids either maintained or had a slight increase in body cell mass [46]. Yoshida measured albumin synthesis rates in rats who were first protein depleted and then treated with intraperitoneal amino acids for 5 weeks. Incorporation of ^{15}N into albumin was higher in rats fed with amino acids than in those on a protein-free diet [42, 53]. Elwyn et al. used oxygen consumption and carbon dioxide production to assess energy utilization. Their well-designed crossover study showed that protein sparing with small amounts of glucose reduced nitrogen excretion and resting metabolic expenditure below levels resulting from amino acids alone [13, 14]. O'Keefe and Sender used ^{14}C-leucine to measure protein turnover postoperatively [42]. They showed that protein *synthesis* rather than *breakdown* was inhibited and suggested a need for stimulating protein synthesis in postoperative patients. From this, one could infer that provision of nitrogen as amino acids to improve synthesis might be as important as provision of energy to prevent breakdown. Greenberg et al. studied postoperative patients who received amino acids alone, with glucose, or with isocaloric amounts of lipid [26]. They also found improved nitrogen balance with intravenous amino acids, but with no distinguishable benefits from carbohydrate versus lipid calories. Fat mobilization from endogenous fat stores adjusts to meet caloric deficits [20]. Patients mobilize more fat in inverse proportion to the numbers of calories supplied. The fact that Greenberg's study showed no beneficial effect from glucose added to the amino acids is probably accounted for by the lack of crossover design.

In summary, during starvation or surgical

stress, all body glucose is utilized within 24 hours. This necessitates gluconeogenesis from protein. As a result, insulin levels are low. This has a permissive effect on the mobilization of body fat producing free fatty acids and ketone bodies for fuel. Normally, high ketone body levels stimulate insulin (except in diabetes), which in turn prevents excessive fat breakdown. The process is similar during semi-starvation, as when a patient receives 5% glucose. The administered glucose spares some protein, but gluconeogenesis must continue, since the patient needs 2500 calories daily while receiving only 600 (3 liters of 5% glucose = 150 gm × 4 calories/gm = 600 calories). The need for proteolysis to produce glucose is high in the early stages of starvation, but it is gradually reduced over the ensuing 5 to 10 days as the patient becomes adapted to fat utilization.

Amino acids with small amounts of exogenous lipid or carbohydrate calories improve nitrogen balance and protein synthesis. The real question is which patients need amino acids, particularly when periods of starvation are short or the patient's nutritional status is relatively good. The answer to this obviously rests with the clinical judgment of the physician, who must individualize in attempting to determine who should receive simple glucose regimens, PPN, or TPN. The well-nourished patient seems to tolerate starvation well, but protein is still required because protein breakdown is continual. Since the period of starvation is short (as with cholecystectomy), recovery should be rapid when oral intake resumes. However, even well-nourished patients require 7 to 10 days to re-establish nitrogen equilibrium after elective surgery. Malnourished patients, particularly those with reduced fat stores from pre-hospital morbidity (as in carcinoma of the esophagus) or patients with burns, fever, sepsis, or massive trauma, require 35 to 50 calories/kg combined with 1 to 1.5 gm protein/kg body weight from the outset. Malnutrition is common in hospitalized patients and is compounded by surgical trauma or by the use of postoperative 5% glucose without adequate protein, or by both. Hence, patients are not prepared for complications that may ensue. The extremely malnourished patient or the patient with a catastrophic complication clearly requires TPN. We recommend PPN for patients who do not have absolute indications for subclavian catheter insertion and TPN. In such patients, protein sparing is acceptable nutritional support and can be beneficial for the safe peripheral infusion of nitrogen to correct mild to moderate malnutrition. Protein sparing should be used for short (7- to 10-day) periods until enteral nutrition can be resumed or until the patient clearly requires TPN. Protein sparing is not intended as a global substitute for 5% glucose in routine postoperative care. Nitrogen balance during amino acid infusions is clearly superior to that obtained with 5% glucose. The 5% amino acid solution is superior to the 3% solution. During amino acid infusion, body fat is mobilized, and the resulting ketosis is well tolerated. The addition of glucose partially inhibits lipolysis and improves rather than worsens nitrogen balance. Insulin is not the mediating hormone for the improved nitrogen balance observed during protein sparing, and elevated insulin levels are not detrimental to nitrogen retention. All available evidence indicates that insulin is an anabolic hormone. Sophisticated body composition and labeling studies have shown that amino acid infusions are beneficial.

GLYCEROL AS A PROTEIN-SPARING AGENT

Amino acids are an expensive component of TPN solutions, as is pharmacy mixing time. When one orders protein sparing, these cost factors should be remembered, particularly if the amino acids are diluted with water or glucose, or both. Pharmacy mixing time for PPN solutions is nearly identical to that required for regular parenteral nutrition.

Glycerol is a glucose precursor, accounting for 7 percent of synthesized glucose in the postoperative state and rising to 20 percent in the fasted state. Glycerol infusion results in increased glucose production [41]. Glycerol infusion has a minimal effect on circulating levels of insulin and glucagon. Any short-term protein-sparing effects of lipid emulsions are due to the glycerol component alone [5]. Glycerol can be heat-autoclaved with amino acids to make a pre-mixed solution suitable for PPN. In contrast, glucose must be added to amino acids after sterilization. This results in increased pharmacy mixing time.

Culebras et al. infused 3.4% amino acids with and without 75 gm glycerol [10]. They demonstrated significant improvement in nitrogen balance during the amino acid plus glycerol period. Smith and Stoski, in our hospital, studied 40 patients undergoing major abdominal surgery, randomly assigned to receive 3% amino acids, with or without 3% glycerol, at 40 ml/kg/day. All patients were within 20 percent of ideal body weight and had no serious renal, hepatic, or metabolic disease. The solution was infused for 5 days, beginning the morning after surgery. The study was double-blind. No adverse reactions were encountered. Mean cumulative nitrogen balances for the 5-day study period were +12.2 gm for the amino acid plus glycerol group versus −2.8 gm for the amino acid alone group ($p < 0.05$). In contrast to other studies, insulin levels rose in patients who received amino acids plus glycerol. This again proves that protein sparing and nitrogen balance are not dependent on insulin levels. The incidence of thrombophlebitis was not increased by the addition of glycerol to the amino acid solution.

In summary, an amino acid–glycerol–electrolyte mixture is a stable solution which, in contrast to amino acids with glucose, can be heat-sterilized. Therefore, the solution is readily available for immediate use without pharmacy mixing and is clearly superior to amino acids alone for PPN.

INTRAVENOUS FAT

One of the great advantages of protein-sparing is that carbohydrate intolerance, seen during regular TPN, is eliminated. However, it is not necessary to use hypocaloric regimens simply to avoid carbohydrate intolerance. There are now two fat emulsions available. Intralipid is soybean oil mixed with egg yolk phospholipid to form an emulsion suitable for intravenous use. Because the solution is hypotonic, lysis of red cells would occur, and therefore glycerol (25 gm/500 ml 10% Intralipid) is added to make the solution isotonic. The adjusted pH is 7.5, and a 500-ml bottle contains 50 gm fat (450 calories) plus 25 gm glycerol (100 calories), with an osmolarity of 280 mOsm/liter. Liposyn, a more recently introduced safflower oil emulsion, has a similar but not identical composition.

Intravenous fat can be used during parenteral nutrition as (1) prevention and treatment of essential fatty acid deficiency, (2) peripheral parenteral nutrition, and (3) a partial substitute for glucose during subclavian hyperalimentation. In essence, the latter two are similar. During TPN with 25% glucose, the glucose concentration may be reduced by giving lipid through a Y-connected intravenous tubing. For example, a patient with glucose intolerance could have the 25% glucose–5% amino acid solution reduced to 10% glucose–5% amino acids, which provides only 100 gm glucose (400 calories) per liter. If the patient received 2.5 liters daily, only 250 gm glucose (1000 calories) would be administered. The simultaneous infusion of 1.5 liters of lipid would provide an additional 1650 calories. Because Intralipid is an emulsion, it must be administered by Y-connector close to the vein. Any solutions added to the Intralipid could destroy the emulsion, resulting in toxicity. In the foregoing example, the patient would receive 4 liters of water daily, which might exceed pulmonary tolerance. Clearly, to substitute lipid for glucose calories during TPN requires scrupulous management of water balance and carbohydrate tolerance. For example, the glucose could be increased to 15 or even 20%, while the Intralipid is reduced from three to two bottles daily. Alternatively, diuretics could be used.

The use of Intralipid in PPN is similar. Five percent amino acids in 5 or 10% glucose are infused by peripheral vein. A 5% amino acid–5% glucose solution contains 50 gm protein and 50 gm glucose per liter. If the patient received 1.5

liters daily, 75 gm each of protein and glucose would be infused. The 300 calories derived from glucose are inadequate unless supplemented by 500 ml of 10% Intralipid, by Y-connector, every 8 hours. This provides an additional 1650 calories. In our experience, this peripheral Intralipid system has limited usefulness because of the paucity of peripheral veins frequently encountered in those patients who most require the nutrition. Unless a skilled intravenous team is available, subcutaneous infiltrations occur frequently, especially at night. Each time this occurs, nutritional deficits accrue. Over the course of a week, calorie and nitrogen deficits become significant. Whenever nutritional support is critical, the subclavian route is recommended. In sick patients, the same criticisms apply equally to protein sparing.

There are other disadvantages of the Intralipid system. Lipid costs $25 per 500 ml (550 calories) compared to $3 for 500 ml of 50% glucose (1000 calories). The lipid system requires a Y-tubing, which is somewhat cumbersome and more expensive, although this is certainly not an insurmountable problem. Early studies suggested that nitrogen retention during fat infusion was inferior to that observed with carbohydrate infusion. However, more recent, well-designed crossover studies suggest that this difference may not be as great as was originally believed [23, 38, 47]. Substituting fat for glucose calories does not eliminate the risk of systemic bacterial and mycotic infections. In fact, Intralipid supports luxuriant growth of a broader variety of microorganisms than do other major parenteral products [11]. Intralipid should remain refrigerated until immediately prior to use and should not hang longer than twelve hours. This prevents bacterial growth.

Intralipid is an efficient caloric source. It results in positive nitrogen balance and weight gain when given with other appropriate nutrients. Free fatty acid levels rise and the respiratory quotient falls. Further evidence that the fat is utilized is provided by infusing ^{14}C-labeled fat, which results in the elimination of ^{14}C carbon dioxide from the lungs. The fat particles are approximately equal in size to chylomicrons and are metabolized in much the same way as orally ingested fat. The accepted range of tolerance is 2 to 4 gm fat/kg body weight daily. Fat may be utilized and cleared even more rapidly in septic patients [2]. Some investigators add 500 units of heparin, which may improve fat clearance by accelerating the hydrolysis of triglycerides [5]. On the other hand, heparin may raise serum free fatty acids to toxic levels [8]. Few would recommend the use of lipid emulsions without glucose. Glucose prevents gluconeogenesis of the administered protein and provides fuel both for the brain and to prime the Krebs cycle. It thus improves the metabolism of free fatty acids derived from Intralipid and reduces fatty acid accumulation in the liver. Millipore filters cannot be used because of the size of the fat particles. Early in our experience, test doses were given for the first hour, and serum was analyzed to ensure adequate clearance. These tests are seldom carried out now, but may be important in critically ill patients or when liver function is impaired.

The peripheral lipid system eliminates problems of glucose tolerance. By the central route, home parenteral nutrition with lipid becomes more feasible because the patient can receive the fluids over a shorter time period without glycosuria. Peripheral nutrition avoids subclavian catheterization, which is advantageous in septic patients or when facilities for inserting and maintaining the catheter are not available. Hyperosmolarity does not occur with the lipid system. Intralipid 20% is useful when fluids need to be restricted. This recently introduced product provides 3000 calories in 1500 ml. Fluid restriction normally is not a consideration if the subclavian vein is available and if the patient tolerates concentrated glucose.

ESSENTIAL FATTY ACID DEFICIENCY (EFAD)

During TPN with 25% glucose, the high insulin levels inhibit mobilization of body fat. Twelve percent of body fat is linoleic acid—the primary essential fatty acid. Hence during TPN with 25%

glucose–5% amino acids, the patient receives a fat-free solution and cannot mobilize his own adipose tissue. A 500-ml bottle of 10% Intralipid contains 50 gm fat, of which 55% (27 gm) is linoleic acid. Ten percent Liposyn (the safflower oil emulsion) contains 78% (39 gm) linoleic acid per 500 ml. To prevent EFAD, approximately 4% of total calories must be given as linoleic acid. These requirements will be met if the patient receives 1 liter of 10% Intralipid (54 gm linoleic acid) weekly. Patients who receive Intralipid as a continual calorie source, either by subclavian or peripheral vein, do not develop EFAD. Malnourished adult patients and infants who have reduced fat stores may develop overt EFA deficiency sooner and will require one or more units of lipid emulsion daily for 7 to 10 days.

TOXICITY OF LIPID EMULSIONS

The safety record of the soybean lipid emulsion is good. The following comments probably apply equally to the recently introduced safflower lipid emulsion. Fever, chills, nausea, and vomiting, frequently alluded to, are not common in our experience. This is always difficult to sort out because there are many other possible causes for such symptoms in sick patients. Hematologic complications observed with cottonseed emulsions used in the 1950s are no longer problematic. Lipid emulsions support the growth of bacteria and fungi [11]. Furthermore, Intralipid is cleared by the reticuloendothelial system and has been shown to inhibit chemotaxis of neutrophils [15, 51]. Therefore, Intralipid may enhance the risk of bacterial infection in certain patients. If a lipid–amino acid–glucose mixture is given by subclavian vein, is the infection rate less than when the same solution is given peripherally? Such comparative studies have not been done, but one could predict that infection rates would be lower with the peripheral system because the catheter is changed frequently.

Jaundice, coagulation defects, and the overloading syndrome seen with the cottonseed emulsion are not problematic with the safflower or soybean emulsions. The fat particles are phagocytosed by the reticuloendothelial system, particularly the Kupffer cells in the liver. This appears to be innocuous and resolves when lipid infusions are discontinued. The newer 20% safflower emulsion has a higher osmolarity (330 mOsm/liter) and a slightly larger particle size (0.16 microns), but contains twice as many calories in the same volume. Recent reports suggest that this product may have great potential, particularly for patients in whom water restriction is important [12, 52]. Intralipid does not potentiate fistula output in patients with pancreatic fistulas [28]. However, it should be used cautiously in patients with pancreatitis and hypertriglyceridemia.

Patients with lipid disorders should have lipid administered cautiously, since they may have difficulty clearing the triglycerides. Cholesterol is elevated in most patients, but returns to normal when the infusion is stopped. Much of the recent literature centers around clearance tests for intravenous fat and the fate of the fat particles taken up by the reticuloendothelial system. Critically ill patients oxidize fat in preference to carbohydrate [2]. Lindholm et al. confirmed that critically ill patients were able to clear triglycerides from the circulation [36]. Adding heparin to lipid emulsions may improve triglyceride clearance, but may also raise fatty acids to toxic levels. The latter should be avoided in patients with disturbances of cardiac conduction.

Pediatric patients can also clear lipid emulsions, even when critically ill [1]. However, lipid emulsions may spuriously elevate serum bilirubin levels in newborns [44].

Levene et al. reported 8 pre-term infants who died after Intralipid infusions. All had fat accumulation in the lungs. They suggested that such fat accumulation might be an unrecognized cause of ventilation/perfusion defects [35]. Fat pigment accumulates in the Kupffer cells, but not in the hepatocytes of patients and dogs treated for long periods with Intralipid. The recommended dose of 2 to 4 gm fat/kg/day should not be exceeded. There are 50 gm of fat in each 500-ml bottle of 10% lipid emulsion. Fat accumulation in the reticuloendothelial system and a potential susceptibility to infection have already been alluded to. Exceeding the recommended dose may further enhance this susceptibility. Much of the lipid emulsion is taken up by the liver and spleen prior to hydrolysis. This implies a necessity for cautious administration in patients with liver disease. However, many investigators have used lipid emulsions for nutritional support of critically ill patients with liver disease without noting side effects. This may be related in part to the preference for fat as an energy source during sepsis [2]. Also, recent evidence suggests that some of the lipid emulsion is metabolized by muscle. Nevertheless, failure of lipid clearance owing either to liver disease or to exceeding the recommended doses should be borne in mind, particularly for patients with severe cachexia, sepsis, or organ failure. Experimental studies have shown that drugs, such as tetracycline, that block the reticuloendothelial system, may impair fat clearance. Pediatric patients are particularly susceptible to the fat overload syndrome characterized by hepatosplenomegaly, coma, a deterioration in clinical status, and foamy fat vacuoles in the reticuloendothelial system and peripheral leukocytes [3, 21].

Lipid emulsions contain triglycerides, phospholipids derived from egg lecithin, and small amounts of cholesterol. Triglycerides are apparently phagocytosed by the cells of the reticuloendothelial system and subsequently hydrolyzed by lipoprotein lipase to free fatty acids and glycerol. Since many factors affect this clearance process, it is not surprising to observe variation in the reports of serum lipid abnormalities during lipid infusions. Triglycerides are moderately elevated when the 4.5% amino acid–10% glucose–10% lipid system is used [32]. Short-term infusion studies with lipid emulsions, particularly in the absence of glucose, show greater rises in triglycerides. Patients with lipid disorders may respond similarly. Even if triglyceride levels do rise during parenteral nutrition, MacFadyen et al. showed that levels tend to decrease with time. This is, in part, attributable to enzymatic adaptation wherein lipid is more efficiently cleared, and also to the simultaneous administration of carbohydrate, which appears to optimize fat utilization [39]. It is interesting to note that triglyceride levels increase to similar levels during fat-free parenteral nutrition with 25% dextrose–4.5% amino acids.

In contrast to triglycerides, cholesterol and phospholipid concentrations are markedly elevated in the serum of pediatric and adult patients receiving lipid emulsions. The rises in serum cholesterol and phospholipid concentrations are significantly greater during the lipid–carbohydrate–amino acid type of parenteral nutrition than with the fat-free, 25% glucose–amino acid system [32]. Serum cholesterol, in one report, rose from 133.5 to 422.6 mg/100 ml, although these changes were temporary and returned to normal two weeks after infusion was discontinued. Koga confirmed this and also corroborated MacFadyen's impression that the rise in lipid levels, followed by a plateau over long periods of infusion, implied an adaptive enhancement for lipid metabolism during lipid infusion [34]. Soybean oil contains small amounts of unesterified cholesterol and phospholipids, but large amounts of triglycerides. Yet, serum cholesterol and phospholipid levels are increased markedly during lipid infusion, especially in comparison to the small elevations of triglycerides. Simultaneously, an abnormal lipoprotein called lipoprotein X appears in the plasma [27, 40]. The clinical significance of this abnormal pattern is not yet known, but it closely resembles the lipid profile found in patients with obstructive jaundice. These abnormalities have been observed in infants, adults, and experimental animals. Griffin et al. reported that most of the hyperphospholipidemia is attributable to the Intralipid itself. At least 50 percent of the cholesterol increment is from endogenous sources, presumably representing leeching of cholesterol from tissues into plasma in order to clear the elevated lecithin-derived phospholipids. The abnormal lipoprotein X is apparently associated with this clearing mechanism and disappears, along with the other lipid abnormalities, when Intralipid infusion is discontinued [27]. In summary, these data suggest that clearance mechanisms for phospholipids contained in lipid emulsions are exceeded during lipid infusion, resulting in a serum lipid pattern resembling that observed in patients with cholestasis.

TPN with 25% glucose–5% amino acids is associated with cholestasis, and many investigators have observed an increased incidence of acalculous cholecystitis. This is more common in children than in adults. The etiology is believed to be a lack of pancreatic and intestinal stimulation. It is of interest that the addition of lipid to the TPN regimen does little to alter this potential complication. Gimmon showed that a carbohydrate–lipid–amino acid mixture induced increased bile lithogenicity in rats when given either intravenously or through a gastrostomy [25]. Van Der Linden and Nakayama administered 1000 ml of 10% Intralipid to 8 patients prior to cholecystectomy. Compared to 8 controls, who received normal saline, the patients who received Intralipid had crystals in their hepatic bile and increased bile lithogenicity [49].

Utilization of fat for energy is initiated by lipoprotein lipase, which hydrolyzes triglycerides into glycerol and fatty acids. Free fatty acids are progressively broken down by two carbon fragments, each of which combines with coenzyme A to form acetyl coenzyme A, which in turn combines with oxaloacetic acid and is converted to energy, carbon dioxide, and water. Insulin and glucose levels are low during starvation and protein sparing. This reduces the amount of oxaloacetic acid. Hence, ketone bodies are formed from the acetyl CoA. Conversely, when glucose is added to amino acid mixtures, energy provisions increase while insulin levels rise. Urinary nitrogen excretion in well-nourished patients given 5% glucose is 10 to 12 gm daily. If Ringer's lactate is substituted for 5% glucose, urinary nitrogen rises by 15 to 20%. Malnourished patients adapt to their state of starvation by reducing protein breakdown through the use of fatty acids and ketone bodies as energy sources. The same adaptation process occurs during fat infusion. Hence, short-term lipid studies in well-nourished patients inevitably show little improvement in nitrogen balance, particularly with hypocaloric peripheral regimens. Conversely, substituting lipid for carbohydrate calories over the long term and/or in malnourished patients yields improved nitrogen balance data simply because the body has adapted, or is rapidly learning to adapt, to fat metabolism. With this background, one can appreciate that PPN given prophylactically need include only amino acids, possibly with small amounts of glucose. If the patient's clinical condition fails to improve and provided peripheral vein access remains constant, lipid can be added to the regimen with expected improvements in nitrogen retention.

Two important variables should be remembered when attempting to interpret data from studies that compare caloric sources. First, there are 25 gm glycerol/500 ml Intralipid, which is metabolized as carbohydrate. Hence, lipid infusion studies are not carbohydrate-free. Second, nitrogen excretion varies in direct proportion to the patient's nutritional state and to the number of nonprotein calories administered. Therefore, a patient on protein sparing (3 liters of 5% amino acids daily) receives 150 gm protein (24 gm nitrogen) and will have nitrogen balance data influenced by both nitrogen intake and basal nitrogen excretion. If the patient is well-nourished and therefore losing 10 to 12 gm urinary nitrogen a day, net nitrogen balance will differ from that of an 80-year-old malnourished, starvation-adapted female with bowel obstruction, who might lose only 6 gm nitrogen daily. Nitrogen excretion is higher in obese patients and in males versus females. The amount of nitrogen excreted in the first few days after commencement of hypocaloric or acaloric protein sparing is considerably higher, primarily because much of the infused nitrogen is being used for gluconeogenesis. Many of our patients lost 24 gm nitrogen daily for the first 2 to 4 days of protein sparing [19]. This emphasizes the importance of knowing individual daily, as well as mean, nitrogen excretions for the total metabolic period when interpreting data. It is also important to know whether a washout phenomenon occurs when the study is completed. This would be characteristic of short-term (3 to 4 days) studies, wherein large amounts of nitrogen may be lost in the urine when the study is ended and therefore not measured. Seven- to ten-day study periods, as carried out in our patients, usually yield stable urinary nitrogen excretions. We did not find large amounts of excessive nitrogen lost in the urine following completion of the study.

THE NEED FOR NONPROTEIN CALORIES DURING PERIPHERAL PARENTERAL NUTRITION

The preceding evidence clearly establishes the efficacy of peripheral amino acid infusions for certain patients. One hundred and fifty grams of glucose added daily to these amino acids is not harmful, except with regard to its potentiation of phlebitis. Wolfe et al. showed that the provision of various caloric sources, from hypocaloric to eucaloric levels, continued to maximize utilization of infused amino acids [52]. Interestingly, low-dose glucose tended to lower serum amino acid levels while simultaneously improving nitrogen balance. This suggested increased utilization of amino acids. When glycerol or lipid was added to the amino acid solutions, nitrogen balance improved, but not to the extent observed during infusion of amino acids with glucose. Regardless of which caloric source was used, when intake was eucaloric, nitrogen utilization was maximized. From this, we can conclude that the use of 5% glucose as a caloric source during protein sparing is simple and efficient. When more calories are necessary, the addition of lipid increases caloric load while minimally affecting peripheral veins. Nitrogen balance improves because of the added calories. There would be little justification for using lipid without glucose in PPN [52]. In this situation, any potential benefits of lipid on protein sparing are due to glycerol. Brennan et al. and Wolfe et al. were able to separate the protein-sparing effects of lipid-derived fatty acids from those due to glycerol to confirm this [52, 53]. Each bottle of lipid contains 25 gm glycerol, added for tonicity. Also, glycerol is released from the triglycerides in the lipid emulsion during hydrolysis.

If lipid is added to a peripheral amino acid–glucose regimen and if peripheral veins remain accessible, long-term nutritional studies comparing this to standard TPN show equally good results [23, 32]. Paradis and Freund each showed that the isocaloric substitution of fat for carbohydrate, while amino acid infusion remained constant, actually increased nitrogen negativity [22, 43]. The reason for this discrepancy lies in the choice of the subject or experimental animal. Formerly, it was believed that in the presence of trauma or sepsis, more nitrogen would be spared with 25% glucose than with fat. This conflicts with metabolic studies from Kenney's lab, which show a preference for fat utilization in critically ill patients [2]. Similarly, Burke has shown that septic patients may not utilize administered glucose even though serum glucose levels are within normal limits [6]. Also, 25% glucose is difficult to administer to septic patients if glucose tolerance is poor. Water and carbon dioxide production are additional complications of 25% glucose infusions, particularly important in patients who require ventilatory support. Paradis and Freund did not include combinations of glucose and fat, which maintained caloric input while lowering glucose concentration. MacFie et al. studied patients who received 50 calories/kg/day as either 25% glucose or 10% glucose and enough Intralipid calories to make the two groups isocaloric. Amino acid infusions were identical. They showed that the combination of fat and glucose was more effective than hypertonic glucose alone for energy purposes [38].

Fewer comparative studies are available in the pediatric literature. This is because of the overwhelming success of the peripheral–lipid–glucose system in pediatric patients, in whom lower volume and caloric requirements make it possible to easily deliver the necessary numbers of calories and protein by peripheral vein [9].

To date, fat emulsions have been used primarily as sources of essential fatty acids and to supplement peripheral parenteral nutrition regimens. Their use as a major source of calories remained limited because of cost. There is a recent trend toward aligning intravenous nutrition to that of the normal diet. Every available study indicates that combinations of glucose and fat for parenteral nutrition are superior to those using fat or carbohydrate alone [2, 33, 38].

MANAGEMENT OF PERIPHERAL CATHETERS

Peripheral catheters should be treated like subclavian catheters with respect to sterility, dressing care, and protocols to monitor serum metabolic parameters. Infusions can be continued for long periods if the butterfly needle is carefully taped. Examining the catheter by removing the tape may, of itself, cause infiltration. The tape should be applied to the wings of the butterfly and should not elevate the needle tip. The needle tip can be continuously viewed if a semiporous membrane (Op-Site) is applied. We have used this material both peripherally and on subclavian catheters for 18 months with good success. It is permeable to air, thus preventing skin maceration, and permits the dressing to remain intact for a week or longer. It is translucent, permitting frequent inspection of the catheter without disturbance. Its firm, adherent qualities minimize catheter movement. As long as the needle tip is visible, infiltration or phlebitis will be diagnosed early. The catheter can then be removed and inserted elsewhere, and the initial site re-used later. Conversely, when severe local reactions occur, as on the dorsum of a hand, that area will be unavailable for 7 to 14 days.

Isaacs found that cortisol was the most effective agent for delaying the onset of phlebitis at the infusion site [31]. It acts locally and does not require metabolic alteration for conversion into its active component. Five hundred units of heparin may also be added to each liter of solution. The pH of the infused solution may be important, and many have proposed adding bicarbonate to bring the pH of the amino acid–dextrose solution closer to 7. Interestingly, studies comparing heparin, cortisol, and bicarbonate in various combinations have not been done. Antibiotic ointment on the catheter site may prevent phlebitis, as has been shown for centrally inserted catheters. Substituting Silastic or Teflon for polyvinyl catheters may also delay the onset of phlebitis [37]. Metal butterfly needles are the least reactive, but their stiffness predisposes to local infiltration. Polyvinyl catheters are too irritating and seldom last longer than 48 to 72 hours.

PPN AND TPN COMPARED

PPN is sometimes conceived as distinct from central parenteral nutrition. This is not true, as can be seen by comparing the various regimens. Consider a simple protein-sparing solution. If a patient is given 3 liters of 5% amino acids daily, he receives 150 gm protein (24 gm nitrogen) and no calories. If 50 gm glucose are added to each of the amino acid bottles, the patient receives 3 liters of a 5% amino acid–5% glucose solution or 24 gm nitrogen and 150 gm glucose (600 calories) daily. In the peripheral Intralipid system, the patient receives 1.5 liters of 10% lipid through a Y-connector. To prevent water overloading, the glucose–amino acid volume must be reduced from 3 to 1.5 liters. The patient now receives 300 glucose calories, 1650 calories from the Intralipid, and 75 grams of protein. Calories are increased at the expense of reducing protein intake. During TPN with 5% amino acids and 25% glucose, the patient still receives 150 gm protein, but now with 3000 glucose calories.

PPN avoids subclavian catheterization and provides better infection control. Nursing care is probably less complicated, although many experienced nurses would debate this point. The use of a subclavian catheter for long-term intravenous infusion is simpler, provided one has the expertise to insert and care for the catheter. Finally, PPN avoids hyperosmolarity.

On the debit side, PPN requires higher volumes of fluid or lesser amounts of protein and calories. Problems with access to veins or infiltration of catheters result in further periods of inadequate calorie and nitrogen administration. Peripheral vein access can be particularly difficult in critically ill patients. The Y-tubing, used with the lipid system, makes administration more complicated and expensive.

Even with TPN, the patient seldom receives more than basal caloric and nitrogen requirements, particularly in the presence of sepsis or severe malnutrition. Hence, permitting patients to starve for 5 to 7 days by giving 5% glucose seems unwise in principle and destined to increase the nutritional debt.

Sedentary adult patients require 35 calories and 0.5 to 1.0 gm protein/kg in a ratio of 150 nonprotein calories/gm nitrogen infused. Well-nourished adults having transitory medical or surgical problems that interrupt regular enteral feeding seem to tolerate the malnutrition induced by peripheral hypocaloric glucose feeding. In situations of pre-existing malnutrition or unpredictable periods of starvation combined with surgical stress, prophylactic parenteral nutrition seems indicated. To carry out the latter by TPN via subclavian vein is efficient, but not without risk. The simplest method of supportive PPN is to infuse amino acids as a 3% or 5% solution by peripheral vein. This significantly improves nitrogen balance and protein synthesis. Increasing the caloric value by adding 50 gm glucose per liter will further improve nitrogen balance, although with a greater incidence of phlebitis. With either regimen, some of the infused amino acids will be used in part to meet energy needs through gluconeogenesis. Hence, with protein sparing, nutritional deficits continue to accrue unless more calories are given. To achieve this, the use of a 10% lipid emulsion seems eminently justified, particularly when facilities for inserting and caring for subclavian catheters are not readily available. TPN, providing 3000 to 4000 calories per day either as glucose or glucose combined with fat, remains the ultimate treatment of severely malnourished patients. Essential to this discussion is the understanding that protein stores in the body are limited. Most is stored as muscle, and the remainder consists of amino acids used in important metabolic pathways. Protein is not stored as fuel in the body. Catabolism of body protein through gluconeogenesis, under conditions of starvation or administration of protein with inadequate calories, uses protein for fuel rather than for its more important structural or visceral functions. Early nutritional support in patients whose hospital course and period of starvation are unpredictable, using isotonic amino acids with or without glucose, will minimize calorie and protein deficits. These deficits can be difficult and time-consuming to correct even with TPN. Conversely, most patients tolerate elective surgery extremely well, and when the patient's course in hospital is uncomplicated, protein sparing should not replace routine 5% glucose infusions.

REFERENCES

1. Andrew, G. Lipid metabolism in the neonate. *J. Pediatr.* 88:273, 1976.
2. Askanazi, J., Carpentier, Y. A., and Elwyn, D. H. Influence of total parenteral nutrition on fuel utilization in energy sepsis. *Ann. Surg.* 191:40, 1980.
3. Bellin, R. P., Bivins, A., Jona, J. Z., and Young, V. L. Fat overload with a 10% soybean oil emulsion. *Arch. Surg.* 111:1391, 1976.
4. Blackburn, G. L., Flatt, J. P., Clowes, G. H. A., Jr., et al. Protein-sparing therapy during periods of starvation with sepsis or trauma. *Ann. Surg.* 177:588, 1973.
5. Brennan, M. F., Fitzpatrick, G. F., Cohen, K. H., and Moore, F. D. Glycerol: major contributor to short-term protein-sparing effects of fat emulsions. *Ann. Surg.* 182:386, 1975.
6. Burke, J. F., Wolfe, R. R., Mullany, C. J., Mathews, D. E., and Bier, D. M. Glucose requirements following burn injury: Parameters of optimal glucose infusion and possible hepatic and respiratory abnormalities following excessive glucose intake. *Ann. Surg.* 190:274, 1979.

7. Cahill, G. F. Starvation in man. *N. Engl. J. Med.* 282:668, 1970.
8. Cohen, I. T., Dahms, B., and Hays, D. M. Peripheral total parenteral nutrition in pediatric patients. *J. Pediatr. Surg.* 12:837, 1977.
9. Coran, A. G. The long-term total intravenous feeding of infants using peripheral veins. *J. Pediatr. Surg.* 8:801, 1973.
10. Culebras, J. M. Nitrogen sparing in normal man: Effect of glycerol and amino acids given peripherally. *Surg. Forum* 27:37, 1976.
11. Deitel, M., Kaminsky, B. M., and Fukasa, M. Growth of common bacteria and Candida in 10% soybean oil emulsion. *Can. J. Surg.* 10:531, 1975.
12. Desai, N. S., Piecoro, J. J., and Cunningham, M. D. Comparison of safflower oil 20% and 10% emulsion as a potential calorie source in total parenteral nutrition in infants. *Clin. Res.* 28: 871A, 1980.
13. Elwyn, D. H. Nutritional requirements of adult surgical patients. *Crit. Care Med.* 8:9, 1980.
14. Elwyn, D. H., Gump, G. E., Iles, M., et al. Protein and energy sparing of glucose added in hypocaloric amounts to peripheral infusions of amino acids. *Metabolism* 27:325, 1978.
15. Fischer, J. W., Hunter, K. W., and Wilson, S. R. Intralipid and reticuloendothelial clearance. *Lancet* 2:1300, 1980.
16. Flatt, J. P., and Blackburn, G. L. The metabolic fuel regulatory system: Implications for protein-sparing therapies during caloric deprivation and disease. *Am. J. Clin. Nutr.* 27:175, 1974.
17. Freeman, J. B. Peripheral parenteral nutrition. In *Symposium on the Nutritional Requirements of Surgical Patients. Can. J. Surg.* 21:489, 1978.
18. Freeman, J. B., Stegink, L. D., Meyer, P. D., Thompson, R. G., and DenBesten, L. Metabolic effects of amino acids vs. dextrose infusion in surgical patients. *Arch. Surg.* 110:916, 1975.
19. Freeman, J. B., Stegink, L. D., Wittine, M. F., et al. The current status of protein sparing. *Surg. Gynecol. Obstet.* 144:843, 1977.
20. Freeman, J. B., Stegink, L. D., Wittine, M. F., et al. Lack of correlation between nitrogen balance and serum insulin levels during protein sparing with and without dextrose. *Gastroenterology* 73:31, 1977.
21. Freund, V., Krausz, Y., Levij, I. S., and Eliakim, M. Iatrogenic lipidosis following prolonged TPN. *Am. J. Clin. Nutr.* 28:1156, 1975.
22. Freund, H., Yoshimura, N., and Fischer, J. E. Does intravenous fat spare nitrogen in the injured rat? *Am. J. Surg.* 140:377, 1980.
23. Gazzaniga, A. B., Barlett, R. H., and Shobe, G. B. Nitrogen balance in patients receiving either fat or carbohydrate for total intravenous nutrition. *Ann. Surg.* 182:163, 1975.
24. Gazzaniga, A. B., Day, A. T., Bartlett, R. H., et al. Endogenous calorie sources and nitrogen balance. *Arch. Surg.* 111:1357, 1976.
25. Gimmon, Z., Kelley, R. E., Simko, V., Fischer, J. E. TPN solution induces increase in lithogenicity of bile in the rat. *Gastroenterology* 79: 1021, Part 2, 1980 (Abstract).
26. Greenberg, G. R., Marliss, E. B., Anderson, G. H., et al. Protein sparing therapy in postoperative patients: Effects of added hypocaloric glucose or lipid. *N. Engl. J. Med.* 294:1411, 1976.
27. Griffin, E., Breckenridge, W. C., Kuksis, A., et al. Apperance and characterization of lipoprotein X during continuous Intralipid infusion in the neonate. *J. Clin. Invest.* 64:1703, 1979.
28. Grundfest, S., Steiger, E., Selinkoff, P., and Fletcher, J. A study of the effect of intravenous fat emulsion in patients with pancreatic fistulas. *J.P.E.N.* 3:26, 1979.
29. Hoover, H. C., Grant, J. P., Gorschboth, C., et al. Nitrogen-sparing intravenous fluids in postoperative patients. *N. Engl. J. Med.* 293:172, 1975.
30. Howard, L., Dobs, A., Chodos, R., Chu, R., and Loludice, T. A comparison of administering protein alone and protein plus glucose on nitrogen balance. *Am. J. Clin. Nutr.* 31:226, 1978.
31. Isaacs, J. W., Millikan, W. J., Stackhouse, J., et al. Parenteral nutrition of adults with a 900 milliosmolar solution viȧ peripheral veins. *Am. J. Clin. Nutr.* 30:552, 1977.
32. Jeejeebhoy, K. N., Anderson, G. H., Nakhooda, A. F., et al. Metabolic studies in total parenteral nutrition with lipid in man. *J. Clin. Invest.* 57:125, 1976.
33. Kirkpatrick, J. R., Dahn, M., and Lewis, L. Selective versus standard hyperalimentation. A randomized prospective study. *Am. J. Surg.* 141:116, 1981.
34. Koga, Y., Ikida, K., and Inokuchi, K. Effect of complete parenteral nutrition including fat emulsion on plasma lipid. *Surgery* 76:278, 1974.
35. Levene, M. I., Wigglesworth, J. S., and Desai, R. Pulmonary fat accumulation after Intralipid infusion in a pre-term infant. *Lancet* 2:815, 1980.
36. Lindholm, M., Rossner, S., and Eklund, J. Intralipid clearance from the circulation in intensive care patients. *J.P.E.N.* 3:26, 1979.
37. MacDonald, A. S., Master, S. K. P., and Moffitt, E. A. A comparative study of peripherally inserted silicone catheters for parenteral nutrition. *Can. Anaesth. Soc. J.* 24:263, 1977.
38. MacFie, J., Smith, R. C., and Hill, G. L. Glucose or fat as a nonprotein energy source? *Gastroenterology* 80:103, 1981.
39. MacFadyen, E. V., Dudrick, S. J., Tagudar, E. P., et al. Triglyceride and free fatty acid clearance in patients receiving complete parenteral nutrition

using a 10% soybean oil emulsion. *Surg. Gynecol. Obstet.* 137:813, 1973.
40. Miyahara, T., Jujiwara, H., Yae, Y., et al. Abnormal lipoprotein in plasma of patients receiving 10% soybean emulsion. *Surgery* 85:566, 1979.
41. Nikkila, E. A., and Ojala, K. Gluconeogenesis from glycerol in fasting rats. *Life Sci.* 3:243, 1964.
42. O'Keefe, S. J., and Sender, P. M. Catabolic loss of body nitrogen in response to surgery. *Lancet* 2:1035, 1974.
43. Paradis, C., Spanier, A. H., Calder, M., and Shizgal, H. N. Total parenteral nutrition with lipid. *Am. J. Surg.* 135:164, 1978.
44. Shennan, A. T. The effect of intralipid on estimation of serum bilirubin in the newborn. *J. Pediatr.* 88:285, 1976.
45. Skillman, J. J., Rosenoer, V. M., Smith, P. C., et al. Improved albumin synthesis in postoperative patients by amino acid infusion. *N. Engl. J. Med.* 295:1037, 1976.
46. Spanier, A. H., Carmody, P., Milne, C. A., et al. Preservation of body cell mass following major abdominal surgery. *Surg. Forum* 26:3, 1975.
47. Stein, T. P., Buzby, G. P., Leskiw, M. J., et al. Protein and fat metabolism in rats during repletion with total parenteral nutrition. *J. Nutr.* 111: 154, 1981.
48. Tweedle, D. E. F., Fitzpatrick, G. F., Brennan, M. F., Culebras, J. M., Wolfe, B. M., et al. Intravenous amino acids as the sole nutritional substrate. *Ann. Surg.* 186:60, 1977.
49. Van Der Linden, W., and Nakayama, F. Effect of intravenous fat emulsion on hepatic bile. *Acta Chir. Scand.* 142:401, 1976.
50. Wilkinson, S. A., Radmacker, P., and Adamkin, D. H. Comparison of 10% and 20% safflower oil. *Clin. Res.* 28:845, 1980.
51. Wilson, S. R., Hunter, K. W., and Mease, A. D. Diminished bacterial defenses with intralipid. *Lancet* 2:819, 1980.
52. Wolfe, B. M., Culebras, M. D., Sim, A. J. W., Ball, M. R., and Moore, F. D. Substrate interaction in intravenous feeding: Comparative effects of carbohydrate and fat on amino acid utilization in fasting man. *Ann. Surg.* 186:518, 1977.
53. Yoshida, H., Abei, T., and Abe, T. Trial on the evaluation of the effectiveness of parenterally administered amino acids. *Acta Chir. Scand.* [Suppl.] 466:24, 1976.

Enteral Alimentation

Laura E. Matarese

24

If the gastrointestinal tract is functional and accessible, it is always the preferred route for nutritional support for several reasons. First, absorption of nutrients by the portal system with subsequent delivery to the liver may better support visceral, particularly hepatic, protein synthesis and regulation of metabolic processes. Second, certain processes that occur in the wall of the gut, such as transamination, are bypassed during parenteral feedings. In addition, alimentation via the parenteral route results in increased splanchnic blood flow, with increased cardiac output, which requires increased energy expenditure for processing these substances [35]. Also, isocaloric, isonitrogenous solutions given via the gastrointestinal route have been shown to have the advantage—in both weight gain and nitrogen retention—over those solutions given intravenously [3, 52, 69]. Recent studies from our own laboratory, however, have revealed no difference when catheter sepsis was carefully controlled, suggesting that the differences previously observed may have been due to catheter sepsis.

Enteral alimentation is not without potential complications, and requires proper administration and monitoring. However, it can usually be administered without employing a surgical technique; it is simpler to use and readily available in most institutions; and it is much less expensive than parenteral methods.

NUTRIENT COMPONENTS

The ingredients and nutritional values of enteral formulas vary greatly. The quality and quantity of protein, carbohydrate, and fat supplied in a specific formula is a major consideration in formula selection. In addition, the vitamin and mineral content may vary.

Protein

Although it is conventional to speak of protein requirements, the true requirement is not for protein as such, but rather for specific amino acids and for nonessential amino acid nitrogen. These are derived from any or all of the following: (1) intact protein in the form of eggs, milk, or pureed meat; (2) protein isolates from milk (casein), soybean, or egg white; (3) hydrolyzed protein from casein, fish, meat, soy, and whey, with added amino acids; (4) short-chain peptides; or (5) free amino acids.

Protein digestion in the normal intestinal tract proceeds fairly rapidly in the first 100 cm of the jejunum [99]. Relatively few studies, however, have been performed to determine protein digestion and absorption in various disease states. With severe pancreatic insufficiency or malabsorption secondary to a short or damaged small bowel, it has been proposed that single amino acids are better absorbed from either hydrolyzed protein or free amino acids than from intact protein. There are increasing data, however, indicating that the absorption of certain di- and tripeptides may be more rapid and uniform than that of individual free amino acids [1, 2, 5, 6, 24, 36, 64, 71]. However, the differences thus far appear largely academic except in special situations.

Recent studies on the effects of dietary manipulation and various pathologic conditions on peptide transport indicate that, in general, absorption of amino acids is more severely affected than that of peptides. A peptide diet would be more advantageous than a diet with free amino acids for the treatment of patients with celiac sprue, tropical sprue, and short bowel syndrome, all of which have reduced rates of amino acid absorption [2, 64, 88, 90, 95]. Similarly, in the malnutrition that follows jejunocolostomy for obesity, jejunal absorption of the free amino acid, leucine, is reduced, but absorption of the dipeptide, gly-leu, is unaffected [36]. Patients with hereditary defects in transport of either basic amino acids and cystine (cystinuria) or neutral amino acids (Hartnup disease) have little or no impairment of intestinal absorption of amino acids from dipeptide solutions [5, 50, 72, 96, 102].

Patients with pancreatic insufficiency may have serious impairment of protein digestion and increased loss of protein in the feces [28]. Since the brush border membrane of the intestinal mucosa can efficiently hydrolyze peptides with three to six amino acid units, the administration of oligopeptides to these patients would supply a useful nitrogen source and circumvent the problem of impaired protein digestion. Although no human data on peptide absorption in pancreatic insufficiency are yet available, rats with exocrine pancreatic insufficiency utilize a diet containing 85 percent of its nitrogen source in one form of oligopeptides better than a diet with its entire nitrogen source as free amino acids [56]. Finally, the use of a peptide formula as opposed to a free amino acid solution affords a nitrogen source with less osmotically active, more palatable characteristics [97].

In addition to evaluating the amount and source of protein in an enteral formula, the number of kilocalories supplied must also be considered. The amount of nitrogen retained is proportional to the amount of energy supplied [112]. Protein supplied without sufficient nonprotein kilocalories fails to result in positive nitrogen balance because the protein is used as an energy substrate. The kilocalorie/nitrogen ratio (K/N) for a normal, active 70 kg man is approximately 300:1 [74]. However, in illness or injury, patients require a lower K/N ratio, in part because both energy and protein needs are elevated. Formulas with K/N ratios above 200:1 may provide inadequate protein for the stressed patient, whereas formulas with K/N ratios below 100:1 may provide excessive protein, which is used as an energy source with possible rise of blood urea nitrogen and ammonia. Blackburn and Bistrian state that protein requirements for anabolism can be met when the ratio of nonprotein kilocalories to nitrogen is approximately 150:1 [9]. Kinney adopted a range of 120:1 to 180:1 for the K/N ratio when total kilocalories (protein and nonprotein) are used [63]. Peters and Fischer showed a parenteral ratio of 160:1 to be most efficacious [81].

To ensure that protein requirements are met, the quality, as well as the quantity, of protein should be considered. The quality is determined primarily by the amounts of essential amino acids found in the protein. In order for anabolism to occur, all amino acids, both essential and nonessential, must be present simultaneously in appropriate amounts.

Carbohydrates

Carbohydrates comprise the major source of kilocalories (40 percent to 90 percent) in most formulas. Thus, consideration of the nature of the carbohydrate becomes important, since it affects the tolerance of the feeding. Similarly, carbohydrates exert the greatest effect on osmolality. When simple sugars, such as glucose or sucrose, are used as a carbohydrate source, the osmolality is higher than in a formula with more complex carbohydrates. These hyperosmolar solutions often result in problems of abdominal discomfort, diarrhea, and dumping. However, this can be avoided by the use of less osmotically active starches, dextrins, and glucose oligosaccharides. Oligosaccharides are polymers of monosaccharides that contain two to six molecules of simple sugars; these are hydrolyzed by enzymes in the intestinal mucosa without the need for pancreatic amylase. Thus, these formulas can be useful for patients with severe pancreatic exocrine insufficiency. Since oligosaccharides and complex carbohydrates are not sweet, they can be used for patients who have an aversion to sweet-tasting foods.

The absorptive and digestive capacity of the mucosa should be considered when choosing a carbohydrate source, since most carbohydrates are hydrolyzed and absorbed primarily at the intestinal brush border. In disaccharidase deficiency, undigested sugar remains in the intestinal lumen where it exerts an osmotic force in the colon, drawing fluids into the lumen. Bacterial action on the sugar causes the production of acid and gas; osmotic diarrhea ensues. The resulting diarrhea may increase malabsorption of other nutrients. Other common side effects include: borborygmi, cramping, and distention.

Almost any step from the hydrolysis of starch to utilization of the monosaccharides in the tissue has the potential for a defect. However, deficiency in amylase has not been evident, even in cases of severe pancreatic insufficiency [42]. The inability to absorb one or another of the monosaccharides exists in some individuals. The most prevalent instance of carbohydrate intolerance is for lactose. Lactase is required to split the disaccharide, lactose, into its component monosaccharides, glucose and galactose, which are absorbed in the small intestine [98]. This intolerance is known to cause diarrhea and other gastrointestinal disturbances [47, 60]. Lactose intolerance occurs when an insufficient amount of the enzyme, lactase, is present in the brush border of intestinal villi [27, 70]. If the quantity of lactose presented to the intestinal cells is greater than the hydrolytic capacity of the available lactase, owing either to a low lactase level or to the ingestion of an unusually large quantity of lactose, the unhydrolyzed lactose passes into the large intestine, drawing water from the tissues into the intestines, resulting in rapid movement of the intestinal contents along the gut [66, 75]. As with other disaccharidase deficiencies, fermentation of the sugar by bacteria forms irritating, volatile acids. Flatulence, cramps, belching, and watery, explosive diarrhea may result [22, 66].

Certain disease states of the intestine, such as tropical sprue, celiac sprue, regional enteritis, protein calorie malnutrition, and gastrointestinal infections such as cholera and giardiasis can result in insufficient levels of lactase. Some drugs, including neomycin, kanamycin, and colchicine, also produce lactase deficiency [8]. Gastric surgery and short bowel syndrome can also cause a relative deficiency [76].

The two other types of lactose intolerance are genetic, or primary, and acquired, or secondary. Individuals who tolerate lactose in infancy, but later develop intolerance, are examples of primary lactase deficiency. When lactose intolerance is the secondary result of disease, normal tolerance often returns as the ailment is treated and cured. In genetic, or primary, intolerance, lactose must be eliminated from the diet [76].

In general, limitations on the use of carbohydrates are few. But they must be recognized and dealt with, as the results of intolerance can be serious and debilitating in some instances.

Sucrose is widely used in the average diet to enhance flavor. However, sucrose used as the sole source of carbohydrate in an enteral feeding can result in a high osmolality.

Lactose, although not as sweet as sucrose, contributes to the palatability of a formula, but the incidence of intolerance makes it questionable for inclusion in some therapeutic regimens. Most patients, however, do not exhibit symptoms of intolerance if lactose levels are kept low or if the feeding is administered slowly.

Starches are not easily suspended in liquid. Therefore, their value for use in enteral formulas is questionable. Corn syrup solids, or glucose oligosaccharides, are partial hydrolysates of starch, are easily digested, dissolve in water, and, like starch, are not nearly as osmotic as simple sugars. Owing to their bland taste, they have little, if any, effect on the flavor of an enteral feeding.

Fat

Dietary fat provides a highly concentrated form of energy. In addition, fat acts as carrier for the fat-soluble vitamins and also supplies essential fatty acids. Because it is insoluble, fat does not contribute to the osmolality of a formula and often enhances the flavor. The amount of fat available in commercial formulas varies considerably.

Fat may contribute from less than 1 percent to as much as 47 percent of kilocalories in these preparations. Most commercial formulas contain long-chain triglycerides (LCT), such as corn oil, soy oil, or safflower oil, as the fat source. Some products contain medium-chain triglycerides (MCT) and combine these, in varying amounts, with a long-chain triglyceride such as soy or corn oil. The rationale for such mixtures is not apparent. Thus, more data are needed to determine whether there is any advantage to the use of various combinations and proportions of long-chain triglycerides and medium-chain triglycerides in individuals with normal bowel function.

Digestion and absorption of fat depends on the presence of pancreatic lipase and bile salts. The triglycerides of all long chain fats are absorbed rapidly, and no one oil has any advantage over others in patients with normal digestion and absorption. When significant maldigestion or malabsorption is present, a formula that is low in fat or contains MCT oil may be advantageous. Unlike long-chain triglycerides, medium-chain triglycerides do not depend on pancreatic lipase or bile salts for effective absorption. Medium-chain triglycerides pass through the intestinal epithelium directly into the portal system rather than through lymphatic circulation [58].

Ingestion and absorption of large amounts of medium-chain triglycerides without adequate carbohydrate may be associated with increased ketone body production and acidosis [104, 119]. Medium-chain triglycerides should be used with caution in patients with hepatic cirrhosis or portacaval shunts who have a tendency to hepatic encephalopathy, since elevated levels of shorter-chain fatty acids may be associated with reversible coma in these patients. Short-chain fatty acids have been used in these patients without any ill effects.

There is no need to prescribe formulas containing medium-chain triglycerides unless the patient has maldigestion and/or malabsorption of fat. The amount of dietary linoleic acid found to prevent both biochemical and clinical evidence of deficiency in animal and man is 1 to 2 percent of dietary kilocalories [74]. The American Academy of Pediatrics has recommended that 3 percent of kilocalories be supplied as essential fatty acids in infant formulas [4]. For those individuals whose fat intake is below 25 percent of total kilocalories, 3 percent of energy as linoleic acid should be a satisfactory minimum intake. However, for those consuming 35 percent of dietary energy as fat, 8 to 10 percent of total kilocalories should be essential fatty acids [74].

Vitamins and Minerals

In addition to protein, carbohydrate, and fat, vitamins and minerals are required by the body. Generally, only small quantities of these substances are needed, although the requirements for certain vitamins may be increased in some states of illness or injury.

Most commercial formulas are designed to meet the Recommended Dietary Allowances (RDA) for vitamins in approximately 2 liters of formula. Certain vitamins may be increased in commercial formulas when compared with the RDA. The vitamin E content of these products sometimes exceeds the RDA, since more is required when the amount of polyunsaturated fatty acids (PUFA) is high [74]. This relationship is probably of little concern, since the primary dietary sources of PUFA—vegetable oils—are also the richer sources of vitamin E.

Commercial formulas may also be fortified with additional ascorbic acid, since requirements increase during stress and illness [57]. The B-complex vitamins—folacin, thiamine, riboflavin, pyridoxine, niacin, biotin, pantothenic acid, vitamin B_{12}, and possibly choline—serve a variety of complex metabolic functions. When the metabolic rate or cell turnover is high, as in patients with infections or malignant tumors, the demand for the B-complex vitamins rises [41, 51]. The requirements for thiamine and niacin are related to the caloric intake [41, 54, 74], and the requirements for riboflavin and pyridoxine are related to protein intake [55, 74, 89]. Therefore, these vitamins should be increased in proportion to an increase in the caloric or protein density of a formula. Vitamin K may have to be administered if it is not included in the formula.

Specific RDAs are not available for some minerals, because the exact amount that the body requires is not known. Instead, ranges of safe daily intake are suggested.

Calcium and phosphorus should be provided in a ratio of 1:1, according to current recommendations [29, 74]. Higher phosphate levels decrease the absorption of dietary calcium, because phosphate forms an insoluble complex with calcium [29].

Since most synthetically produced commercial formulas are lacking in a full complement of trace elements, it is advisable to allow the patient to progress to natural table food as soon as possible and whenever possible.

Water

If it were possible to say that one nutrient is more essential than another, most would agree that it is water. Yet, it is often not considered when providing enteral nutritional support. The human body can survive for weeks, months, and even years without certain vitamins and minerals, but will survive only a few days without water.

Approximately 6 percent of the water in the adult body and 15 percent of that in the infant's body turns over each day. Water leaves the body through several pathways—urinary losses, respiratory losses through the lungs, evaporative losses through the skin, and enteric losses through the feces. The body obtains water from several sources—as preformed water in liquids and foods and as a product of oxidation. The major source, approximately 900 to 1500 ml per day, is the fluid consumed as beverages.

Fluid requirements vary with age. Adults require approximately 35 ml/kg. Children and infants require 50 to 60 ml/kg and 150 ml/kg, respectively. Requirements are increased above normal when extrarenal fluid losses are high, as occurs with fever, severe diarrhea, vomiting, excessive sweating, and fistula drainage. With increased losses and the administration of a hyperosmolar formula, dehydration can develop.

Provision of adequate water to satisfy a patient's thirst will usually meet fluid requirements.

However, certain patients are unable to communicate their thirst or to consume liquids orally to satisfy thirst. Thus, a precise intake and output record for each patient is necessary to determine and meet fluid requirements. Clinical signs and laboratory determinations of dehydration should also be closely monitored. Development of dehydration and hypernatremia can and should be prevented in all patients.

The actual water content of enteral formulas varies considerably from approximately 70 percent to 95 percent. Most of the formulas ensure an adequate intake of water. However, additional water should be provided if necessary to meet fluid requirements.

Residue

A normal healthy adult excretes 75 to 170 gm of feces daily. About 70 percent of the feces is water, and the remainder is a variety of organic and inorganic material [87]. The exact composition of the stool varies with the type of diet consumed. Diets that are low in residue result in decreased stool mass. In addition, stool passage is less frequent and transit time is increased [7].

Low-residue feedings are often indicated before certain diagnostic procedures. Gutwein et al. used a defined formula liquid diet rather than a traditional clear liquid diet in preparation for a barium enema [48]. This may be beneficial for the malnourished patient who must undergo numerous tests. However, for those patients who must be maintained on long-term enteral feedings, a formula that approximates the residue of a normal diet should be considered.

Osmolality

Osmolality is a measure of the concentration of particles (solutes) in a feeding that affects the osmotic balance between the gut and the vascular system. It is expressed in mOsm/kg H_2O. Osmolality is a similar but not identical concept to osmolarity, which is the standard measure of concentration used with intravenous solutions. This is expressed in mOsm/L. Osmolarity refers to the number of particles of a solution (solvent plus solute). Osmolarity is thus influenced by the volumes of all the solutes contained in the solution, and by the temperature, whereas osmolality is not. Although there are only small clinical differences between the terms osmolality and osmolarity, osmolality is generally considered the correct and preferred term when referring to enteral products.

The osmolality of a solution is based on the number of dissolved particles in the solution—the greater the number of particles, the higher the osmolality. At a given concentration, the smaller the particle size, the greater the number of particles present and the higher the osmolality. A high-molecular-weight carbohydrate is a large particle; a low-molecular-weight carbohydrate is a smaller particle. Since the size of the particle is inversely proportional to the osmolality of the solution, a solution of high-molecular-weight carbohydrates has a lower osmolality than an isocaloric solution of low-molecular-weight carbohydrates.

Whole proteins are high-molecular-weight molecules that have little or no osmotic effect. However, smaller peptides of lower molecular weight exert a greater osmotic effect. Individual amino acids, which are smaller particles than peptides, have an even greater osmotic effect, similar to that of low-molecular-weight carbohydrates.

Since fats are not water-soluble and do not form a solution in water, they have no osmotic effect.

Salts such as sodium chloride or potassium chloride, which dissociate in solution, are small particles that have a great effect on the osmolality of a solution.

Thus, enteral feedings that have high concentrations of simple carbohydrates, amino acids, and electrolytes have the greatest effect on the osmolality, and consequently, on tolerance. The food in a normal diet has a higher average osmolality than most commercial formulas.

The osmolality of normal body fluids is approximately 300 mOsm/kg. The body attempts to keep the osmolality of the contents of the stomach and intestine at this level. When a concentrated solution of high osmolality is ingested, large amounts of water enter the stomach and intestines by osmosis from the fluid surrounding the organs in an attempt to dilute and equalize the concentration of the solution. The amount of water drawn in is proportional to the osmolality; the higher the osmolality of the solution, the larger the amount of water required to reduce the osmolality of the solution. A large amount of water rushing into the gastrointestinal tract causes a feeling of fullness, increased activity of the intestinal tract, and in some cases nausea. The feeding solution may move through the tract too rapidly for the water to be reabsorbed, resulting in diarrhea.

Isotonicity in terms of osmolality is defined as 300 mOsm/kg H_2O. In general, the closer an enteral feeding is to isotonic, the lower the potential for complications such as diarrhea, dumping, nausea, and vomiting. However, an isotonic formula is not a guarantee that all patients will tolerate a feeding without complications. Administration techniques are often more critical in preventing complications than is the osmolality of the feeding. Tolerance of higher osmolalities can be built up gradually. Thus, the concentration of a feeding may have to be manipulated until tolerance is established. Finally, small (30 to 50 mOsm) differences in osmolality of different formulas are usually not clinically insignificant.

Renal Solute Load

Renal solute load is a measure of the concentration in a feeding solution of the particles that the kidney must work to excrete. The higher the renal solute load, the greater the stress on kidney function.

The main contributors to renal solute load are protein, yielding urea as its end product, and the electrolytes—sodium, potassium, and chloride.

Ziegler and Fomon have devised a simple method for estimating renal solute load [120]. In general, each milliequivalent of sodium, potassium, and chloride yields one milliosmole (mOsm), and 1 gm of protein yields 4 mOsm in young children and an estimated load of 5.7 mOsm in adults.

Kidneys of normal healthy adults can usually concentrate urine to approximately 1200 mOsm/liter. However, the ill patient may have impaired urinary concentrating ability. Large quantities of water may be required for solute excretion. For the volume-sensitive patient, however, the renal solute load can be controlled by regulating the amount of electrolytes and protein in an enteral formula.

FORMULAS FOR ORAL AND TUBE FEEDINGS

There is no standardization of terminology of enteral nutrition products. Consequently, this has resulted in much confusion. Essentially, there are only two categories of commercial products: nutritionally complete and nutritionally incomplete. They have two fundamental uses: total nutritional support and supplemental feedings.

Nutritionally Complete Formulas

Enteral formulas that supply protein, carbohydrate, fat, vitamins and minerals in sufficient quantities to maintain the nutritional status of a normal, healthy individual receiving no other source of nourishment are considered nutritionally complete. In the strictest sense of the definition, all such products are "defined formula diets." "Defined formula" implies that they have been formulated to provide specific amounts of nutrients in a certain volume. "Diets" implies food substances habitually consumed in the course of normal living or adopted for a particular state of health or disease.

The formulas in this category vary greatly in composition and cost. These products form a progression, spanning the gap between parenteral nutrition and normal food, and differ from one another in clinical application, depending on the individual patient's ability to digest and absorb nutrients. Most nutritionally complete formulas provide 1 kilocalorie per milliliter. There are some available with a higher caloric density. Protein, fat, vitamin, and mineral concentrations vary considerably. Thus, different amounts of different products may be required to meet a patient's needs.

Blenderized Formulas

Blenderized formulas consist of whole foods that have been blenderized to liquid form (Table 24-1). Although they are available commercially, some institutions prepare their own in the dietary kitchen. These formulas are usually administered as tube feedings for patients whose gastrointestinal tracts are completely functional, but who cannot or will not take food by mouth.

The blenderized formulas have the advantage of being composed of regular table food and therefore contain all the nutrients contained in natural food. The protein sources, usually egg, meat, and milk, provide protein of the highest biologic value. Since these formulas are composed of natural foods, they can claim the highest fiber content of all commercial products.

There are also some disadvantages to the blenderized formulas. With continually rising food and labor costs, these formulas are relatively expensive to prepare. Owing to the viscosity of the feeding, a large-bore feeding tube is required for administration. Depending on the institution, there may or may not be a recipe for a standardized tube feeding. As a result, assurance of quality and consistency becomes questionable. In addition, contamination of the formula during preparation is not uncommon, with resultant nausea, vomiting, and diarrhea. Finally, many of these formulas contain lactose, which may be contraindicated in a percentage of the population.

Milk-based and Lactose-free Formulas

Milk-based and lactose-free formulas are commercially prepared formulas designed to meet the nutritional requirements of adults (Tables 24-2 and 24-3). In general, they require a functioning gastrointestinal tract for digestion and absorption of nutrients. They are indicated to supply both total nutrition for patients who cannot swallow or chew, or lack appetite, and supplemental nutrition for patients whose intake of normal food is not adequate to meet their individual requirements. These formulas can be given orally or via tube, depending on the patient's condition. They vary in protein, carbohydrate, and fat source, as well as lactose content, vitamin and mineral concentration, osmolality, renal solute load, residue, viscosity, and palatability. Milk-based and lactose-free formulas are often considered to be feedings for general use since they are so versatile.

There are several advantages to these formulas. Most are palatable and inexpensive to use. Their formulation is standardized, thus the composition is consistent and they are sterile prior to opening. They are generally less viscous and have an even, free-flowing consistency. As a result, smaller-bore feeding tubes may be utilized.

There are also disadvantages. First, these formulas generally require full digestive and absorptive abilities, and are therefore not applicable in all clinical situations. Second, the fact that these formulas are standardized makes them unacceptable for patients who are unable to tolerate any of the components of the formula.

Chemically Defined, Elemental, or Defined-Formula Diets

There is much confusion over the use of the terms chemically defined diets, elemental diets, and defined-formula diets. According to O'Hara, Kennedy, and Lizewski, chemically defined diets contain amino acids, simple sugars, essential fatty acids, vitamins, and minerals [77]. The components of these diets are clearly defined, chemically discrete components [114]. "Elemental" refers to the simplest constituent part; existing as an uncombined chemical element. However, since these diets usually are neither chemically defined nor "elemental," they are

Table 24-1. *Blenderized Formula*

	Compleat-B (Doyle)	Vitaneed (Organon)
Kcal/ml	1	1
Protein, gm/L; (source)	40.0 (beef, nonfat milk)	35 (beef, Ca caseinate)
Fat, gm/L; (source)	40.0 (corn oil, beef fat)	40 (soy oil)
Carbohydrate, gm/L (source)	120.0 (hydrolyzed cereal, maltodextrin, sucrose)	130 (corn syrup solids, maltodextrin)
Lactose, gm/L	24.4	0
Minerals/L		
Calcium, mg	625.0	575.0
Phosphorus, mg	1250.0	525.0
Magnesium, mg	250.0	250.0
Iron, mg	11.3	12.0
Sodium, mEq	51.6	23.9
Potassium, mEq	33.6	31.9
Chloride, mEq	22.9	21.0
Iodine, mcg	93.8	150.0
Zinc, mg	9.4	10.0
Copper, mg	1.3	1.5
Manganese, mg	2.5	
Volume required to meet 100% RDA, ml	1,600	1,470
Kcal/gm N_2	131/1	157/1
mOsm/kg H_2O	390	400
Preparation	Ready to use	Ready to use
Comments	Commercially prepared blenderized tube feeding, requires digestion and absorption	Commercially prepared blenderized tube feeding, requires digestion and absorption

Table 24-2. *Milk-Based Formula*

	C.I.B. (Carnation)	Forta Pudding (Ross)	Meritene Liquid (Doyle)
Kcal/ml	1	1.6	1
Protein, gm/L; (source)	58 (milk, soy protein, sodium caseinate)	45 (nonfat milk)	60 (nonfat milk, Na caseinate)
Fat, gm/L; (source)	31 (milk fat)	65 (soy oil)	33 (corn oil, mono-diglycerides)
Carbohydrate, gm/L (source)	135 (lactose, sucrose, corn syrup solids)	227 (modified starch)	115 (lactose, corn syrup solids, sucrose)
Lactose, gm/L	100	60	56.7
Minerals/L			
Calcium, mg	1371.0	1333	1250.0
Phosphorus, mg	1105.0	1333	1250.0
Magnesium, mg	458.5	447	333.3
Iron, mg	18.0	2	15.0
Sodium, mEq	42.0	64	39.8
Potassium, mEq	71.9	51	42.7
Chloride, mEq		39	47.0
Iodine, mcg	146.9	400	125.0
Zinc, mg	15.5	20	12.5
Copper, mg	2.27	2.2	1.7
Manganese, mg		4.4	3.3
Volume required to meet 100% RDA, ml	1373	880	1200
Kcal/gm N_2	88/1	197/1	79/1
mOsm/kg H_2O			550–610
Preparation	Powder	Ready to use	Ready to use
Comments	Palatable, easily available, inexpensive, requires digestion and absorption	Supplemental, requires digestion and absorption	Supplemental, high protein, requires digestion and absorption

Meritene + Milk (Doyle)	Sustacal Pudding (Mead Johnson)	Sustacal + Milk (Mead Johnson)	Sustagen + Water (Mead Johnson)
1	1.9	1	1.8
69 (nonfat milk, whole milk)	45 (nonfat milk)	60 (nonfat milk, whole milk)	109 (nonfat milk, whole milk, Ca caseinate)
34.5 (milk fat)	63 (soy oil)	24 (milk fat)	16 (milk fat)
119 (corn syrup solids)	213 (sucrose, modified starch)	134 (sucrose, corn syrup solids)	312 (corn syrup solids, glucose)
103.7	646	86	105
2307.0	1467	1611	3333
1922.5	1467	1333	2500
384.5	400	375	416
17.3	18	17	19
41.8	35	40	54
75.6	50	65	93
61.8	40	40	15
144.8	150	140	156
14.4	15	14	21
1.9	2	2.0	2
3.8	0.5	3.0	5.2
1040	1000	720	960
71/1	240/1	80/1	78/1
690		760	1334
Powder	Ready to use	Powder	Powder
Supplemental, high protein, requires digestion and absorption	Supplemental, requires digestion and absorption	Supplemental, tube feeding, requires digestion and absorption	Supplemental, high calorie, high protein, requires digestion and absorption

Table 24-3. *Lactose-Free Formula*

	Citrotein (Doyle)	Ensure (Ross)	Ensure Plus (Ross)
Kilocalories/ml	0.7	1	1.5
Protein, gm/L (source)	43 (egg albumin)	37 (sodium + calcium caseinates, soy protein isolates)	55 (sodium + calcium caseinates, soy protein isolates)
Fat, gm/L (source)	2 (partially hydrogenated soy oil)	37 (corn oil)	53 (corn oil)
Carbohydrate, gm/L (source)	129 (maltodextrin, sucrose)	145 (corn syrup, sucrose)	200 (corn syrup, sucrose)
Lactose, gm/L	0	0	0
Minerals/L			
Calcium, mg	1111	500	634
Phosphorus, mg	1111	500	634
Magnesium, mg	444	200	317
Iron, mg	40	9	14
Sodium, mEq	31	32	46
Potassium, mEq	19	32	49
Chloride, mEq	28	30	45
Iodine, mcg	166	75	105
Zinc, mg	16	15	23
Copper, mg	2.2	1.0	1.6
Manganese, mg	55	2.0	2.1
Volume required to meet 100% RDA, ml	NA	1900	2000
Kcal/gm N_2	71/1	153/1	146/1
mOsm/kg H_2O	496	450	600
Preparation	Powder	Ready to use	Ready to use
Comments	Protein, vitamin, mineral supplement	Supplemental, requires digestion and absorption	Supplemental, requires digestion and absorption

Isocal (Mead Johnson)	Isocal HCN (Mead Johnson)	Isomil (Ross)	Magnacal (Organon)
1	2	0.7	2
34 (sodium caseinate, soy protein)	75 (calcium + sodium caseinate)	20 (soy protein isolate, L-methionine)	70 (calcium + sodium caseinates)
44 (soy oil, MCT)	91 (soybean oil, MCT)	36 (coconut oil, soy oil)	80 (soy oil)
132 (glucose oligosaccharides)	225 (corn syrup)	68 (corn syrup, sucrose)	250 (maltodextrin, sucrose)
0	0	0	0
600	670	700	1000
500	670	500	1000
200	270	50	400
9	12	12	18
22	35	13	43
32	36	18	32
28	34	10	27
75	100	150	150
10	20	5	30
1.0	2	0.5	2.0
2.5	3.3	0.2	5
2000	1000	NA	1000
167/1	145/1	194/1	154/1
300	740	250	590
Ready to use	Ready to use		Ready to use
Tube feeding, requires digestion and absorption, isotonic	High calorie, high protein, supplemental, tube feeding, requires digestion and absorption	Infant formula	High calorie, high protein, supplemental, tube feeding, requires digestion and absorption

Table 24-3. (Continued)

	Mull-soy (Syntex)	NeoMull-soy (Syntex)	Osmolite (Ross)
Kilocalories/ml	0.7	0.7	1
Protein, gm/L (source)	30 (soy flour)	19 (soy protein isolates, L-methionine)	37 (sodium + calcium caseinates, soy protein isolates)
Fat, gm/L (source)	37 (soy oil)	36 (soy oil)	38.5 (corn oil, soy oil, MCT)
Carbohydrate, gm/L (source)	55 (sucrose, invert sucrose)	65 (sucrose)	145 (glucose oligosaccharides)
Lactose, gm/L	0	0	0
Minerals/L			
Calcium, mg	1268	845	500
Phosphorus, mg	846	634	500
Magnesium, mg	79	79	200
Iron, mg	11	11	9
Sodium, mEq	11	17	23.5
Potassium, mEq	13	23	27
Chloride, mEq	16	11	23
Iodine, mcg	159	159	75
Zinc, mg	8.5	3.2	15
Copper, mg	1	0.4	1.0
Manganese, mg	1.5	2.7	2.0
Volume required to meet 100% RDA, ml	NA	NA	1900
Kcal/gm N_2	121/1	205/1	153/1
mOsm/kg H_2O	252	275	300
Preparation			Ready to use
Comments	Infant formula	Infant formula	Tube feeding, requires digestion and absorption, isotonic

Precision HN (Doyle)	Precision Isotonic (Doyle)	Precision LR (Doyle)	Portagen (Mead Johnson)
1	1	1	1
44 (egg albumin)	30 (egg albumin)	26 (egg albumin)	35 (sodium caseinate)
0.5 (soy oil)	31 (soybean oil)	1 (soy oil)	48 (MCT oil, corn oil, lecithin)
218 (maltodextrin, sucrose)	150 (glucose oligosaccharides, sucrose)	250 (maltodextrin, sucrose)	115 (corn syrup solids, sucrose)
0	0	0	<0.3
335	667	530	938
335	667	530	604
135	267	211	208
6	12	10	19
41	35	30	20
22	27	22	32
32	30	30	24
50	100	80	73
5.0	10	8	9
0.7	1.3	1.5	1.6
1.3	2.7	2.5	3
2850	1560	1710	1000
117/1	183/1	215/1	154/1
557	300	525	354
Powder	Powder	Powder	Powder
Supplemental, tube feeding, high biologic value protein, absorbed in upper gut	Supplemental, tube feeding, high biologic value protein, isotonic, absorbed in upper gut	Supplemental, tube feeding, high biologic value protein, absorbed in upper gut	Supplemental, tube feeding, requires digestion and absorption

Table 24-3. (Continued)

	Prosobee (Mead Johnson)	Renu (Organon)	Sustacal HC (Mead Johnson)
Kilocalories/ml	0.7	1	1.5
Protein, gm/L (source)	25 (soy protein isolate, L-methionine)	35 (sodium + calcium caseinates, soy protein isolates)	61 (calcium + sodium caseinate)
Fat, gm/L (source)	33 (soy oil)	40 (soy oil)	58 (partially hydrogenated soybean oil)
Carbohydrate, gm/L (source)	67 (corn syrup solids)	150 (maltodextrin, sucrose)	190 (corn syrup solids, sucrose)
Lactose, gm/L	0	0	0
Minerals/L			
Calcium, mg	790	500	840
Phosphorus, mg	530	500	840
Magnesium, mg	74	200	340
Iron, mg	12.5	9	15
Sodium, mEq	18	22	36
Potassium, mEq	19	32	38
Chloride, mEq	12	24	36
Iodine, mcg	48	75	130
Zinc, mg	5	15	13
Copper, mg	0.6	1	2
Manganese, mg	1.1	2.5	2
Volume required to meet 100% RDA, ml	NA	2000	1000
Kcal/gm N_2	150/1	153/1	134/1
mOsm/kg H_2O	160	300	650
Preparation	Ready to use or concentrated liquid	Ready to use	Ready to use
Comments	Infant formula, milk-free formula with soy isolate	Tube feeding, requires digestion and absorption	Supplemental, requires digestion and absorption

Sustacal Liquid (Mead Johnson)	Travasorb (Travenol)	Travasorb MCT (Travenol)
1	1	1
60 (sodium + calcium caseinates, soy protein isolates)	35 (sodium caseinate, soy protein isolate	49 (lactalbumin, potassium caseinate)
23 (soy oil)	35 (corn oil)	33 (MCT, sunflower oil)
138 (sucrose, corn syrup solids)	136 (sucrose, corn syrup solids)	123 (corn syrup solids)
0	0	0
1000	500	500
920	500	500
380	200	200
17	9	9
40	30	15.2
53	31	44.5
44	28	34.2
140	75	75
14	15	15
1.9	1	1
3.0	2	2
1100	2000	1000
80/1	153/1	102/1
625	488	312
Ready to use	Ready to use	Powder
High protein, supplemental, requires digestion and absorption	Supplemental, requires digestion and absorption	Supplemental, tube feeding, requires digestion and absorption

often referred to as "defined-formula diets" (Table 24-4) [93].

The impetus for the development of the defined-formula diet came from the space program in an effort to provide astronauts with complete nutrition while generating minimal fecal output [43, 115]. Nutrients were supplied in the simplest or most "elemental" forms. Protein was supplied as free amino acids; carbohydrates were provided as glucose oligosaccharides; a minimum of fat was supplied as long-chain fatty acids to prevent essential fatty acid deficiency.

Although these diets had been developed for the space program, their value in the treatment of patients with reduced digestive and absorptive capability soon became apparent. Several changes in the properties of these diets occurred, until the defined-formula diet evolved and became available for medical use.

The defined-formula diets are nutritionally complete. When adequate amounts of these diets are given, the requirements for kilocalories, essential amino acid and nonessential amino acid nitrogen, carbohydrate, fat, vitamins, and minerals can be met for most individuals.

Although defined-formula diets have been designed to be used as meal replacements, they can be used as supplements. Patients with some absorptive capacity are sometimes maintained on a combination of parenteral and defined-formula enteral nutrition.

Another property of the defined-formula diet is the minimal digestion required for their absorption and utilization. They are almost totally absorbed in the duodenum and proximal jejunum, leaving only the endogenous residue to enter the large bowel [23, 44, 73, 85, 105, 116]. They provide nutrients in a readily assimilable form, requiring little digestion. However, the effects of defined formula diets on pancreatic-biliary-intestinal secretions remain controversial. Decreases in enzymes associated with protein digestion, both in the pancreas and in the intestinal mucosa, have been reported [13, 14, 16, 80]. However, Ragins et al. observed an increased output of volume, protein, and bicarbonate secretion from chronic pancreatic fistulas after bolus injections of a defined-formula diet into the stomachs of dogs with duodenal fistulas and cannulated pancreatic ducts [83]. Yet, the same diet injected through a Thiry-Vella loop did not stimulate pancreatic secretion. Cassim and Allardyce found that the infusion of a defined-formula diet into the proximal jejunum of dogs resulted in a pancreatic secretory response, but the fluid was enzyme-poor and HCO_3 rich [20]. Thus two factors seem to be important: (1) feeding past the stomach and (2) minimizing acid secretion.

Glucose-based defined-formula diets have been reported to cause a reduction of gastrointestinal bacterial flora. Thus, these diets have been used for preoperative colonic preparation, since they permit a reduction in the fecal flora, provide nutritional support, and prevent the development of antibiotic-resistant organisms [26, 38, 40, 59]. However, early studies showing both a qualitative and a quantitative decrease in three types of intestinal microflora—bacteroid organisms, coliforms, and enterococci—have not been duplicated by later investigations [117]. Bounous and Devroede found no significant difference in total anaerobes, aerobes, and coliforms, but a significant decrease in the number of enterococci in the stool of patients receiving a defined-formula diet [15].

A reduction in the excretion rate of fecal bile acid during the administration of a defined-formula diet has been reported [26]. Thus it may be useful in diarrheal states induced by excessive fecal excretion of bile acids, as occurs following ileal resection or vagotomy.

A significant reduction in gastric acid secretion has been shown to occur in both man and dogs receiving defined-formula diets [17, 84]. This is due to a reduction in the cephalic phase of gastric secretion and a reduction in the physical stimulatory effects of the predigested formula. In addition, bolus feeding of two defined-formula diets resulted in delayed gastric emptying [17].

There are several disadvantages and potential hazards associated with the use of defined-formula diets. These products are relatively un-

Table 24-4. *Defined-Formula Diets*

	Criticare HN (Mead Johnson)	Flexical (Mead Johnson)	Nutramigen (Mead Johnson)
Kcal/ml	1	1	0.7
Protein, gm/L (source)	38 (hydrolyzed casein, 70% free amino acids, 30% peptides)	23 (casein hydrolysate, crystalline amino acids)	22 (casein hydrolysate)
Fat, gm/L (source)	3 (safflower oil)	34 (soy oil, MCT)	26 (corn oil)
Carbohydrate, gm/L (source)	220 (maltodextrin, modified corn starch)	152 (glucose oligosaccharides, modified tapioca starch)	88 (sucrose, modified tapioca starch)
Lactose, gm/L	0	0	0
Minerals/L			
Calcium, mg	530	600	630
Phosphorus, mg	530	500	470
Magnesium, mg	210	200	70
Iron, mg	9.5	9	10
Sodium, mEq	27	15	10
Potassium, mEq	34	32	20
Chloride, mEq	30	28	10
Iodine, mcg	79	75	50
Zinc, mg	10	10	4
Copper, mg	10	1.0	0.6
Manganese, mg	2.6	2.5	1
Volume required to meet 100% RDA, ml	2000	2000	
Kcal/gm N_2	148/1	270/1	174/1
mOsm/kg H_2O	650	550	443
Preparation	Ready to use	Powder	Powder or liquid
Comments	Tube feeding, uses peptide carrier system + free amino acids, absorbed in upper gut	Supplemental, tube feeding, absorbed in upper gut	Hypoallergenic formula with protein in hydrolyzed form

Table 24-4. (Continued)

	Pregestimil (Mead Johnson)	Travasorb HN (Travenol)	Travasorb STD (Travenol)
Kcal/ml	0.7	1	1
Protein, gm/L (source)	19 (casein hydrolysate, amino acids)	45 (hydrolyzed lactalbumin, 25% 5–10 peptide links, 25% 2–3 peptide links, 50% free amino acids)	30 (hydrolyzed lactalbumin, 25% 5–10 peptide links, 25% 2–3 peptide links, 50% free amino acids)
Fat, gm/L (source)	27 (corn oil, MCT)	13 (MCT, sunflower oil)	13 (MCT, sunflower oil)
Carbohydrate, gm/L (source)	91 (corn syrup solids, tapioca starch)	175 (glucose oligosaccharides)	190 (glucose oligosaccharides)
Lactose, gm/L	0	0	0
Minerals/L			
Calcium, mg	626	500	500
Phosphorus, mg	417	500	500
Magnesium, mg	73	200	200
Iron, mg	13	9	9
Sodium, mEq	13	40	40
Potassium, mEq	19	30	30
Chloride, mEq	16	38	38
Iodine, mcg	47	75	75
Zinc, mg	4	7.5	7.5
Copper, mg	0.6	1	1
Manganese, mg	0.2	1.3	1.3
Volume required to meet 100% RDA, ml		2000	2000
Kcal/gm N_2	205/1	114/1	183/1
mOsm/kg H_2O	348	560	550
Preparation	Powder	Powder	Powder
Comments	Infant formula for use in severe digestive and absorptive disorders	Supplemental, tube feeding, uses peptide carrier system + free amino acids, absorbed in upper gut.	Supplemental, tube feeding, uses peptide carrier system + free amino acids, absorbed in upper gut.

Vital (Ross)	Vivonex (Eaton)	Vivonex HN (Eaton)
1	1	1
42 (whey, soy + meat protein hydrolysate, free essential amino acids)	21 (L-amino acids)	42 (L-amino acids)
11 (safflower oil, MCT)	1.4 (safflower oil)	0.9 (safflower oil)
185 (glucose oligo- + polysaccharides, sucrose)	226 (glucose oligosaccharides)	210 (glucose oligosaccharides)
0.825	0	0
666	555	333
666	555	333
266	222	133
12	10	6.0
17	20.4	23
30	30	30
19	20.4	23
100	83	50
10	8	5
1.3	1.1	0.7
1.3	1.6	1
1500	1800	3000
124/1	272/1	124/1
460	550	810
Powder	Powder	Powder
Supplemental, tube feeding, uses peptide carrier system + free amino acids, absorbed in upper gut.	Supplemental, tube feeding, absorbed in upper gut	Supplemental, tube feeding, absorbed in upper gut, high protein

palatable. Even with the use of flavor packets, most patients are reluctant to sustain an adequate oral intake.

These diets may also result in gastrointestinal side effects. The high percentage of simple sugars may result in osmotic diarrhea. Nausea may occur if the diet is ingested too rapidly. Gastric retention may also result, especially if the diet is administered by an intragastric feeding tube.

The hyperosmolar nature and high carbohydrate content of these formulas introduces the potential for hypertonic dehydration, hyperosmolar nonketotic coma, and osmotic diuresis.

Finally, these diets are significantly more expensive than diets composed of intact nutrients.

Nutritionally Incomplete

Modular Enteral Feedings

Modular enteral feedings supply one single nutrient or combinations of nutrients in insufficient quantities to maintain the nutritional status of a normal, healthy individual receiving no other source of nourishment (Table 24-5). Such products are considered to be nutritionally incomplete and are referred to as "feeding modules." They can be used as supplemental feedings or as total nutrition when combined in appropriate amounts.

Only a few currently available products consist of a single nutrient, and they are feeding modules in the strictest sense of the definition. They are usually used to supplement the caloric content of an enteral feeding or regular table food, but can be used with other feeding modules.

Most nutritionally incomplete foods are combinations of two macronutrients (e.g., protein and carbohydrate; fat and carbohydrate). Some contain micronutrients (vitamins and/or minerals) and are also used as supplements, but can be combined with feeding modules or other enteral formulas to produce a nutritionally complete feeding.

INDICATIONS

In general, patients with functioning gastrointestinal tracts who cannot take food by mouth and/or cannot meet nutritional requirements are candidates for special oral and tube feedings.

Gastrointestinal Disease

Enteral nutritional support has been used in a variety of gastrointestinal diseases. Defined-formula diets have been used in the treatment of fistulas of the gastrointestinal tract [11, 18, 85, 105], and are sometimes used in conjunction with parenteral nutrition. Although defined-formula diets may not be effective in all cases, patients with low-intestinal fistulas and gastroduodenal fistulas with distal feeding respond best to these diets. Patients with high gastroduodenal fistulas can be fed below the fistula by means of an enteric feeding tube or a jejunostomy. Intragastric feedings may be given to patients who have low small-bowel fistulas with at least 100 cm of functioning proximal small bowel. The successful application of defined-formula diets in the management of gastrointestinal, rectourethral, and gastrointestinal-cutaneous fistulas have also been reported [30, 46, 82, 100, 118].

Since defined-formula diets require little or no digestion in the upper alimentary tract and no micelle formation, they may be advantageous in the management of patients with maldigestion or malabsorption. Thus, a few patients with short bowel syndrome may benefit from administration of these diets [34, 103, 106]. However, these diets should be introduced slowly and at a low concentration in order to prevent excessive diarrhea. In our own experience, these patients have not tolerated these diets.

Defined-formula diets have also been used in the treatment of patients with ulcerative colitis and Crohn's disease [19, 86, 107]. The low-residue nature of these diets allows bowel rest while providing nutrients necessary for recovery.

The use of defined-formula diets in the treatment of pancreatitis is based on the belief that these diets stimulate less pancreatic secretion. As discussed previously, this is not well established.

Enteral alimentation may be employed in patients with chronic partial obstruction. The feeding may be given below the site of obstruction (e.g., via a gastrostomy in patients with esophageal obstruction or jejunostomy).

Metabolic Abnormalities

Special enteral formulas have also been used in the treatment of patients with significant specific metabolic abnormalities (Table 24-6). Formulas containing essential amino acids have been given to patients with renal disease to improve nutritional status.

An enteral formula has been developed to supplement the diet of patients with serious hepatic insufficiency secondary to cirrhosis. Its amino acid composition has a relatively high branch-chain amino acid content and a relatively low aromatic amino acid content. It is specially formulated for the patient with hepatic insufficiency who cannot utilize large quantities of aromatic amino acids. It should be supplemented with vitamins and electrolytes as required by the patient's metabolic state.

Inborn Error of Metabolism

Several formulas have been developed for the treatment of various inborn errors of metabolism (Table 24-6). Infants with branched-chain keto-aciduria (maple syrup urine disease) require special dietary manipulation. The branch-chain amino acids undergo transamination and form their corresponding keto acids. In this inborn error of metabolism, these keto acids cannot undergo oxidative decarboxylation. This results in elevated blood levels of amino acids and keto acids. A special diet powder has been formulated with an amino acid mixture free of branched-chain amino acids. The powder contains fat, carbohydrate, vitamins, and minerals essential for infants.

Children with phenylketonuria (PKU) lack the enzyme phenylalanine hydroxylase which results in phenylalanine being metabolized via other metabolic pathways and not to tyrosine. The only mode of treatment, at present, is dietary. There are currently two commercial formulas available for the nutritional support of these children. One is a low-phenylalanine formula, which is a casein hydrolysate supplemented with methionine, tryptophan, tyrosine, corn oil, sugar, vitamins, and minerals. A powder has also been developed which supplies all essential amino acids (except phenylalanine), vitamins, and minerals. The use of this product allows the inclusion of a greater variety of other foods that contain phenylalanine.

A powder low in tyrosine and phenylalanine has been designed for patients with hereditary tyrosinemia. For infants with homocystinuria who lack the enzyme cystathionine synthase and cannot convert methionine to cystathionine, there is a soy protein powder containing no added methionine.

Hypermetabolic States

Special enteral formulas have also been prepared to meet excessive protein and caloric requirements. Larkin and Moylan prevented weight loss and nitrogen deficits in severely burned patients with complete enteral nutritional support [67]. Likewise, patients suffering from multiple trauma and fractures can be supported with various enteral formulas. Septic patients, in whom parenteral alimentation may be contraindicated, have been maintained on enteral formulas [10, 92, 111].

Neoplasia

Anorexia, weight loss, and chronic malnutrition are hallmark symptoms of neoplasia. The etiology of the malnutrition is multifactorial, resulting from the disease process, treatment, emotional stress, and psychosocial factors. Enteral formulas may be used as supplements or total nutritional support in an attempt to prevent the wasting and chronic malnutrition observed in this group of patients.

Nonallergenic Food Sources

Several commercially available formulas are suitable substitutes for cow's milk in individuals

Table 24-5. *Modular Feedings*

	Amount needed to give 1000 Kcal	Protein, gm/1000 K	Fat, gm/1000 K	Carbo-hydrate, gm/1000 K	Minerals/1000 K		mOsm/kg H_2O	Prepara-tion	Comments
					Sodium, mEq	Potassium, mEq			
Aminess Tablets (Cutter)	333 Tablets	230	7	16.7	0	0		Tablets	Supplemental, essential amino acids plus histidine in tablet form
Cal-Power (General Mills)	550 gm liquid	0.6	0	272	2.39	0.70		Liquid	Carbohydrate source
Casec (Mead Johnson)	270 gm dry weight	237.6	5.4	0	6	2.10		Powder	Protein source
Controlyte (Doyle)	198 gm dry weight	Trace	48.0	143	0.85	0.20	590	Powder	Caloric source, low protein, low electrolytes, lactose free
dp Hi p.e.r. Protein (General Mills)	258 gm dry weight	206	10	21	22.4	9.90		Powder	Protein source, low electrolytes
EMF Liquid (Control Drugs)	481 ml liquid	243	0	6.97	51	4.91		Liquid	Protein source
EMf Soup (Control Drugs)	280 gm dry weight	195	8.3	36	357	34		Powder	Protein and caloric source
Gevral (Lederle)	285 gm dry weight	171	6	67	19	3.65		Powder	Protein and caloric source
Hi Density Nutrition (Control Drugs)	270 gm dry weight	183	5.2	52.4	Negligible	39		Powder	Protein and caloric source
Hy-Cal (Beecham-Massengill)	407 ml liquid	0.1	0.1	244	2.41	0.07		Liquid	Carbohydrate source
Lipomul-Oral (Upjohn)	167 ml liquid	0.1	111	1.1	2.9	0.09		Liquid	Fat source, lactose free
Liprotein (Upjohn)	184 gm dry weight	83	64	22	8.0	43		Powder	Protein, fat source
Lonalac (Mead Johnson)	196 gm dry weight	53	55	74	1.7	48		Powder	Protein source, low sodium, contains lactose
Lytren (Mead Johnson)	3333 ml standard dilution	0	0	253	100	83	290	Liquid	Electrolyte and carbohydrate source
MCT Oil (Mead Johnson)	120.5 gm liquid	0	120.5	0	0	0	Negligible	Liquid	Medium Chain Triglycerides
Microlipid (Organon)	222 ml liquid	0	111	0	0	0	80	Liquid	Fat source, lactose free

Moducal (Mead Johnson)	500 ml liquid	0	0	250	0.5	6.5	250	Liquid	Carbohydrate source
Pedialyte (Ross)	500 ml liquid	0	0	250	150	100		Liquid	Electrolyte and carbohydrate source
Polycose (Ross)	263 gm dry weight	0	0	250	12	2.5	250	Powder or liquid	Glucose oligosaccharides
Probana (Mead Johnson)	1500 ml standard dilution	60	32	118	41	47		Powder or liquid	High protein formula with banana powder for celiac conditions and diarrhea, contains lactose
Pro Mix (Beatrice Scientific)	284 gm dry weight	227	0	22.7	18.5	116.5		Powder	Protein source
Sumacal (Organon)	1000 ml liquid	0	0	250	4.34	3	680	Liquid	Carbohydrate source
Sumacal Plus (Organon)	400 ml liquid	0	0	312.5	4.6	4.2	890	Liquid	Carbohydrate source

Table 24-6. *Special Formulations*

	Amin-Aid (McGaw)	CHO-Free (Syntex)	Hepatic Aid (McGaw)
Kcal/ml	1.9	0.4	1.6
Protein, gm/L (source)	19 (crystalline essential amino acids)	19 (L-methionine, soy protein isolate)	43 (↑ branched chain, ↓ aromatic amino acids)
Fat, gm/L (source)	66 (partially hydrogenated soybean oil)	36 (soy oil)	36 (soybean oil, lecithin, mono + di-glycerides)
Carbohydrate, gm/L (source)	330 (maltodextrin, sucrose)	(none)	287 (maltodextrin, sucrose)
Lactose, gm/L	0	0	0
Minerals/L			
Calcium, mg		899	negligible
Phosphorus, mg		687	negligible
Magnesium, mg		79	negligible
Iron, mg		11	negligible
Sodium, mEq	<15	16	negligible
Potassium, mEq		23	negligible
Chloride, mEq		12	negligible
Iodine, mcg		159	negligible
Zinc, mg		5	negligible
Copper, mg		0.42	negligible
Manganese, mg		3	negligible
Volume required to meet 100% RDA, ml	NA	NA	NA
Kcal/gm N_2	600/1	106/1	207/1
mOsm/kg H_2O	900	125	900
Preparation	Powder	Powder	Powder
Comments	Supplemental, tube feeding, low electrolytes, indicated for renal disease	Supplemental, tube feeding, carbohydrate free	Supplemental, tube feeding, low electrolytes, indicated for liver disease

Lofenalac (Mead Johnson)	MSUD Diet Powder (Mead Johnson)	Phenyl-Free (Mead Johnson)	Product 3200 AB (Mead Johnson)
0.7	0.7	0.8	0.7
22 (casein hydrolysate, amino acids)	11.5	42 (casein hydrolysate, amino acids)	22 (casein hydrolysate)
26.5 (corn oil)	29	14 (corn oil)	26
86 (corn syrup solids, tapioca starch)	90	135 (corn syrup solids, tapioca starch)	87
0		0	
625	694	1250	631
468	379	937	474
73	74	145	74
12.5	13	25	13
13	14	22.5	14
17	12	37.5	17.5
13	15	29	13
46.8	47	94	47
4	4.2	8	4.2
0.625	0.63	1.25	0.63
1	1	2	1
NA	NA	NA	NA
259/1	355/1	94/1	173/1
356			
Powder	Powder	Powder	Powder
Low phenylalanine formula for use in PKU	Diet powder free of branched-chain amino acids for use in Maple Syrup Urine Disease	Supplemental, phenylalanine free for use in PKU	Low tyrosine, low phenylalanine formula for use in tyrosinemia

Table 24-6 (Continued)

	Product 3200 K (Mead Johnson)	Product 3232 A (Mead Johnson)
Kcal/ml	0.7	0.7
Protein, gm/L (source)	20.5 (soy protein isolate)	22 (casein hydrolysate)
Fat, gm/L (source)	36	28 (MCT oil)
Carbohydrate, gm/L (source)	66	87 (tapioca starch)
Lactose, gm/L		
Minerals/L		
Calcium, mg	631	632
Phosphorus, mg	421	473
Magnesium, mg	63	74
Iron, mg	13	13
Sodium, mEq	11	14
Potassium, mEq	15	17.5
Chloride, mEq	12	13
Iodine, mcg	47	47
Zinc, mg	5.2	4.2
Copper, mg	0.63	0.63
Manganese, mg	1	1
Volume required to meet 100% RDA, ml	NA	NA
Kcal/gm N_2	188/1	174/1
mOsm/kg H_2O		
Preparation	Powder	Powder
Comments	Soy protein isolate infant formula without added methionine for use in homocystinuria	Protein hydrolysate base for use with added carbohydrate in diagnosing carbohydrate disorders

with galactosemia, lactase deficiency, or allergy to milk protein (see Table 24-3). They are given to infants, children, and adults in amounts that supply adequate fluid and nutrients.

Mechanical Obstruction

No longer do patients suffering from dysphagia or obstructions of the head and neck region have to be subjected to chronic weight loss and poor nutrition. With the advent of soft, flexible small-bore tubes, enteral formulas may be administered to prevent chronic malnutrition and support healing.

Preoperative Bowel Preparation

With the availability of low-residue, clear liquid enteral formulas, there is no reason to subject patients, especially the critically ill, to days of clear liquid fluids for preoperative bowel preparation. These special formulas may be used alone or to supplement the clear liquid diet [40, 59]. Likewise, enteral feedings may be utilized for preoperative nutritional replenishment in order to maximize benefits and minimize risks of an operation.

Early Postoperative Feeding

Defined-formula diets have been administered postoperatively to provide the patient with nutritional support as well as fluid. Since the stomach is the principal site of postoperative ileus, feedings may be administered via needle-catheter jejunostomies [53] (see Chap. 25).

Anorexia

Anorectic patients can be supported nutritionally with enteral formulas, either orally or via a feeding tube. Thus, nutritional status can be preserved until appetite returns.

CONTRAINDICATIONS

There are several contraindications to the use of special enteral feedings. If adequate oral intake can be maintained, there is no need to prescribe special formulas. The acutely ill with some degree of ileus may not tolerate enteral feedings. If the ileus is adynamic or cannot be bypassed, enteral alimentation should not be attempted. In some cases, intestinal obstruction, which cannot be bypassed, will eliminate the enteral alternative. Enteral alimentation is contraindicated for those with intractable vomiting and enterocutaneous fistulas. In these instances, the parenteral route may be more feasible until the patient's condition stabilizes.

FORMULA SELECTION

As new enteral products become available, the selection of an appropriate formula becomes more complicated.

Selection is based on several factors. The first step in formula selection is assessment of nutritional status to determine nutrient needs. Patients in hypermetabolic states, such as those associated with burns and trauma, may require a feeding that has a high caloric density. Likewise, patients who cannot tolerate large volumes of fluid may benefit from feedings with high caloric density.

Digestive capability and absorptive capacity must also be assessed. Patients with impaired digestive capabilities (e.g., pancreatitis, bile duct obstruction) or absorptive capacity (e.g., massive bowel resection, Crohn's disease) may require feedings in a simple, readily available form (i.e., hydrolyzed protein, peptide formulas or free amino acids, simple sugars, low fat content). However, if the gastrointestinal tract is fully functional, these formulas are not indicated. Rather, a more complete formula, with intact protein, complex carbohydrate, and a higher percentage of fat would be more approriate.

The feeding route must also be considered. Feedings delivered directly into the small intestine may necessitate the use of formulas as near isotonic as possible.

Finally, other medical conditions, such as food allergies or lactose intolerance, which may preclude the use of some formulas, should also be considered. Certain medications may cause such side effects as nausea, diarrhea, cramping, and distention, any of which may contraindicate enteral tube feedings if the medication cannot be withdrawn. In this instance, parenteral alimentation may be warranted.

TECHNIQUES OF ADMINISTRATION

In order to ensure the safe delivery of enteral formulas, several principles should be noted.

The volume and concentration of the formulas delivered should be individually tailored to the patient, based on current medical condition, formula selection, prior intake, and feeding site. Severely malnourished patients who have been without oral intake for several weeks, or have consumed minimal amounts of food, require a period of adaptation to feeding before full strength and volume can be tolerated.

These diets should be introduced at isotonic concentrations. Generally, tube feedings should be started at 50 ml/hr. If the patient tolerates the feeding this rate can be advanced. If the patient is being fed intragastricly, the concentration is advanced first and then the volume. With feedings into the small bowel, the volume should be increased first by 25 ml/hr every 8 to 12 hours as tolerated, and then the concentration can be increased. Rate and concentration should not be altered simultaneously. If the feeding is not tolerated, reduce the rate or concentration to the levels tolerated by the patient. Gradually advance again, giving the patient time to adjust to each increase.

There are several methods of delivery. The feeding may be administered by bolus delivery, which involves the rapid administration of the formula by syringe. Generally, the patient is fed a volume of 300 to 400 ml of feeding four to six times daily. Feedings given by this method allow the sudden delivery of a large, hyperosmolar bolus of formula, which is poorly tolerated and can result in nausea, diarrhea, vomiting, distention, cramps, or aspiration.

Enteral feedings also may be delivered by intermittent infusion. With this method, the prescribed volume of formula is administered over a 20- to 30-minute period. Some of the problems associated with bolus delivery are eliminated, but tolerance may still be poor in some patients.

Continuous administration is the preferred method of delivery. Feedings may be delivered by continuous drip over a 16- to 24-hour period. The use of a pump or controller is more desirable than gravity drip because constant drip can be maintained and accidental bolus delivery is less likely to occur. Drop rates should be checked every hour for accuracy.

COMPLICATIONS

The complications of parenteral alimentation are well known. The problems associated with enteral alimentation have been less well described. However, it should be recognized that enteral alimentation is not totally innocuous.

Tube Misplacement and Perforation

Tube misplacement, a serious complication of enteral alimentation, can be avoided if care is taken during intubation. Placement of a feeding tube into the trachea and administration of an enteral feeding can be lethal. Placement of a tube into the stomach or small bowel should always be confirmed, by x-ray examination if the tube is radiopaque or by injecting air and listening with a stethescope over the epigastric area. Passage of feeding tubes into the pleural space of newborns has been reported [62]. Retroperitoneal perforation of the second portion of the duodenum [94, 101], intraperitoneal perforation of the third portion of the duodenum [12, 94] or jejunum [21], and perforation of the second portion of the duodenum into the right pelvis [37] have been reported with the use of polyvinyl chloride tubes. These tubes become rigid during prolonged use and pose a potential hazard [49]. The advent of soft, pliable small-bore tubes decreases the potential for this complication.

Aspiration

Aspiration is the most dangerous potential hazard of enteral alimentation. This commonly occurs in weak, debilitated and comatose patients, especially if the cardia is intubated and free reflux into the esophagus occurs. Olivares et al. studied 720 autopsy cases of neurologic patients. They found that lethal aspiration had occurred in an average of 9.5 percent of the cases studied and that gastric tubes increase the risk of aspiration sixfold [78]. Transpyloric feeding tubes may decrease the potential for aspiration, since two sphincters, the pylorus and lower esophageal, can theoretically prevent or lessen the potential for aspiration. Elevation of the head of the bed to an angle greater than 30 degrees and avoidance of night feedings may reduce the risk of aspiration. Checking for gastric distention and gastric residuals is also advisable. It has been suggested that the rate of the feeding should be adjusted when residuals are more than 150 ml [45]. In our institution, if the residual is greater than 100 ml, the feeding is turned off and the physician notified.

Fluid and Electrolyte Imbalance

Dehydration, hypernatremia, and azotemia associated with hyperosmolar, high-protein enteral feedings appear to be less well-recognized than when due to other causes. The occurrence of hypernatremia and hyperchloremia as manifestations of dehydration in the unconscious or debilitated patient who cannot communicate or alleviate thirst has been reported [109]. Normally the sensation of thirst serves as an adequate guide for water intake; but when the sensation cannot be experienced, as in the unconscious patient, or cannot be alleviated, as in the debilitated patient, serious discrepancies in fluid and electrolyte balance may ensue. In 1954, Engel and Jaeger first described dehydration, hypernatremia, hyperchloremia, and azotemia as a complication of nasogastric tube feeding [32]. This has been described as the "tube feeding syndrome" [109]. It can result from excessive protein intake accompanied by inadequate fluid intake.

Investigation of this syndrome has been reported in some detail [25, 32, 39, 108, 109, 113]. Most patients with hypernatremia due to the administration of hyperosmolar tube feedings experience this complication primarily as a result of a water deficit rather than an excess of sodium [31, 32, 65, 68]. However, an increase in total body sodium could occur as a result of a moderate or high sodium content of the feeding and a low urinary excretion of sodium. Next to the intake of large amounts of protein without adequate water, a moderate-to-high intake of sodium may constitute the most important factor resulting in the "tube feeding syndrome." Finally, administration of hyperosmolar solutions may result in osmotic diarrhea, leading to additional fluid losses, hypernatremia, dehydration, fever, coma, and death. These complications may be avoided by administering free water and monitoring serum electrolytes, osmolality, BUN, and intake and output.

Diarrhea and Constipation

Diarrhea is one of the most commonly mentioned complications of tube feedings. It can result when one or a combination of factors is present, including administration of hyperosmolar solutions, bacterial contaminations, lactose intolerance, low serum albumin, and concurrent drug therapy.

Administration of a hyperosmolar solution into the lumen of the gut often results in bloating, hypermotility, and osmotic diarrhea. Initial dilution of hyperosmolar solutions to a hypotonic or isotonic concentration, with a gradual increase in concentration as tolerated, helps to eliminate this problem. In addition, delivery by continuous drip rather than by bolus allows the gut to adapt to the constant osmolar load.

Bacterial contamination of the feeding formula is preventable by ensuring cleanliness during preparation, storage, and administration of the feeding solution. Schreiner et al. demonstrated a high rate of bacterial contamination of infant formulas administered by continuous drip, probably introduced during the mixing and hanging of the formula [91]. Changing the feeding container and tubing every 12 to 24 hours also reduces the risk of excessive bacterial growth. At this time there are limited data on the length of time a feeding should be hung. Hanging times of 8 to 24 hours have been suggested [33, 91, 110]. At our institution, feedings are warmed to room temperature after being refrigerated and hung for a maximum of 6 hours. Special blenderized feedings prepared in the dietary kitchen are hung for a maximum of 4 hours.

Lactose intolerance may be caused by a primary lactase deficiency or may be a temporary consequence of malnutrition or disease. Undigested lactose creates a hyperosmolar load in the gut that precipitates the dumping syndrome and osmotic diarrhea. Treatment requires the use of lactose-free feedings.

Serum albumin aids in maintaining colloidal osmotic pressure, which in turn increases the absorptive capacity of villous capillaries. Low serum albumin levels, therefore, may result in decreased absorptive power in the villi, leading to malabsorption and diarrhea. This is often the case with patients who require enteral alimentation by tube. These patients may have lowered serum albumin as a result of chronic malnutrition or as a consequence of the disease state. Parenteral administration of albumin may aid in correcting the problem, provided feedings are given concurrently so that albumin is not utilized as an energy source [61].

Drug therapy may also be responsible for inducing diarrhea. If treatment with the drug(s) cannot be discontinued, diarrhea can be expected to continue. However. the use of antidiarrheal agents (Kaopectate, Lomotil, Paregoric, or decolorized tincture of opium) may be effective. These can be administered through the feeding tube or directly to the feeding if necessary.

Constipation may result from long-term enteral feedings. Since most commercially available feedings are designed to be low in fiber, chronic constipation may ensue. Thus, the addition of fiber to the feeding or the administration of medications or enemas, or both may be indicated.

Gastrointestinal Disturbances

Other gastrointestinal symptoms may result from administration of enteral feedings. These include abdominal cramps, distention, nausea, and vomiting. These problems are generally avoided when appropriate feedings are administered by continuous drip as opposed to bolus delivery. Abdominal cramping can be relieved by administering the feeding at room temperature and at a slower rate if necessary. If the rate of the feeding falls behind, no attempt should be made to "catch up." If the patient experiences nausea, the feeding should be stopped and the gastric residuals checked. Nausea may be relieved by stopping the feeding for approximately 1 hour or slowing the rate. If gastric distention is the cause of the nausea, ambulation may be advantageous [45]. If the patient begins to vomit, the feeding should be turned off immediately to prevent aspiration.

Irritation-Inflammation

Irritation and inflammation of the nose, esophagus, or sphincters may result from the prolonged use of stiff feeding tubes. Proper intubation and taping of the tubes help to alleviate this problem. In addition, use of small-bore soft tubes decreases the incidence of irritation and inflammation.

Vitamin K Deficiency

Patients receiving prolonged enteral alimentation may develop extended prothrombin times. This may be avoided by administering vitamin K on a weekly basis or as required.

Subjective Complications

Special care should be taken to satisfy the psychologic and social needs of the patient undergoing enteral alimentation. The person being enterally alimented is denied the social, cultural, and religious aspects of eating. Padilla et al. reported that the most common and most distressful experiences of nasogastric tube feeding were: sensory irritations and sensory deprivation [79].

The patient often feels as if he or she has lost all control. Even the manner in which they are to be nourished is decided for them. Thus patient involvement is extremely important. Encouraging the patient to assist in the feeding allows the person a measure of control over something that deals with the very crux of his or her existence—nutrition.

Finally, the patient may feel self-conscious about his or her appearance to others when a tube is passed transnasally. Encourage ambulation. Physical and occupational therapy may further assist the patient in maintaining social normalcy.

MONITORING

Patients receiving enteral nutritional support should be monitored, just as patients receiving parenteral nutrition are, twice weekly initially and once or twice weekly thereafter. Values for sodium, potassium, chloride, BUN, osmolality, calcium, phosphorus, magnesium, total protein, albumin, transferrin, bilirubin, ammonia, blood sugar, and prothrombin time should be determined regularly.

Daily weights should be obtained on all patients receiving tube feedings unless contraindicated (e.g., in patients with fractures of the pelvis). The patient's weight provides a means of assessing whether kilocalorie and fluid requirements are being met or exceeded. Careful monitoring of intake and output is essential in assessing fluid balance and the amount of nutrition supplied by the tube feeding.

The patient should also be observed for gastrointestinal symptoms of intolerance: diarrhea, nausea, vomiting, cramping, and distention.

Finally, an assessment of nutritional status should be made in order to evaluate the efficacy of the enteral formula.

REFERENCES

1. Adibi, S. A. Intestinal transport of dipeptides in man: Relative importance of hydrolysis and intact absorption. *J. Clin. Invest.* 50:2266, 1971.
2. Adibi, S. A., Fogel, M. R., and Agrawal, R. M. Comparison of free amino acid and dipeptide absorption in the jejunum of sprue patients. *Gastroenterology* 67:586, 1974.
3. Allardyce, D. B., and Groves, A. C. A comparison of nutritional gains resulting from intravenous and enteral feedings. *Surg. Gynecol. Obstet.* 139:180, 1974.
4. American Academy of Pediatrics, Committee on Nutrition. Commentary on breast-feeding and infant formulas, including standards for formulas. *Pediatrics* 57:278, 1976.
5. Asatoor, A. M., Cheng, B., Edwards, D. G., et al. Intestinal absorption of two dipeptides in Hartnup disease. *Gut* 11:380, 1970.
6. Asatoor, A. M., Harrison, B. D., Milne, M. D., and Prosser, D. I. Intestinal absorption of an arginine-containing peptide in cystinuria. *Gut* 13:95, 1972.
7. Attebery, H. R., Sutter, V. L., and Finegold, S. M. Effect of a partially chemically defined diet on normal human fecal flora. *Am. J. Clin. Nutr.* 25:1391, 1972.
8. Beline, M. S., and Bayless, T. M. Intolerance of small amounts of lactose by individuals with low lactase levels. *Gastroenterology* 65:735, 1973.
9. Blackburn, G. L., and Bistrian, B. R. Curative Nutrition: Protein-Calorie Management. In H. A. Schneider, C. E. Anderson, and D. B. Coursin (Eds.), *Nutritional Support of Medical Practice.* Hagerstown, MD: Harper & Row, 1977.
10. Blackburn, G. L., and Bistrian, B. R. Nutritional care of the injured and/or septic patients. *Surg. Clin. North Am.* 56:1195, 1976.
11. Bode, H. H. Healing of faecal fistula initiated by synthetic low residue diet. *Lancet* 2:954, 1970.
12. Boros, S. F., and Reynolds, J. W. Duodenal perforation: A complication of neonatal nasojejunal feeding. *J. Pediatr.* 85:107, 1974.
13. Bounous, G., Deuroede, G., Hugon, J., and Charvel, C. Effects of an elemental diet on the pancreatic proteases in the intestine of the mouse. *Gastroenterology* 64:577, 1973.
14. Bounous, G., Gentile, J. M., and Hugon, J. Elemental diet in the management of the intestinal lesion produced by 5-fluorouracil in the rat. *Can. J. Surg.* 14:298, 1971.
15. Bounous, G., and Devroede, G. J. Effects of an elemental diet on human fecal flora. *Gastroenterology* 66:210, 1974.
16. Brown, R. A., Thompson, A., McArdle, A., and Gurd, F. N. Alteration of exocrine pancreatic storage enzymes by feeding an elemental diet: A biochemical and ultrastructural study. *Surg. Forum* 21:391, 1970.
17. Bury, K. D., and Jambunatham, G. Effects of elemental diets on gastric emptying and gastric secretion in man. *Am. J. Surg.* 127:59, 1974.
18. Bury, K. D., Stephen, R. V., and Randall, H. T. Use of a chemically defined liquid elemental diet for nutritional management of fistulas of the alimentary tract. *Am. J. Surg.* 121:174, 1971.
19. Bury, K. D., Turnier, E., and Randall, H. T. Nutritional management of granulomatous colitis with perineal ulceration. *Can. J. Surg.* 15:1, 1972.

20. Cassin, M. M., and Allardyce, D. B. Pancreatic secretion in response to jejunal feeding of elemental diet. *Ann. Surg.* 180:228, 1974.
21. Chen, J. W., and Wong, P. W. K. Intestinal complications of nasojejunal feeding in low-birthweight infants. *J. Pediatr.* 85:109, 1974.
22. Condon, J. R., Westerholm, P., and Tanner, N. C. Lactose malabsorption and postgastrectomy milk intolerance, dumping and diarrhea. *Gut* 10:311, 1969.
23. Couch, R. B., Watkins, D. M., Smith, R. R., et al. Clinical trials of water-soluble chemically defined diets. *Fed. Proc.* 19:13, 1960.
24. Craft, I. L., Geddes, D., Hyde, C. W., Wise, I. J., and Matthews, D. M. Absorption and malabsorption of glycine peptides in man. *Gut* 9:425, 1968.
25. Cramer, L. M., Haverback, C. Z., and Smith, R. R. Hypertonic dehydration complicating high protein nasogastric tube feeding. *Med. Ann. D.C.* 27:331, 385, 1958.
26. Crowther, J. S., Drasar, B. S., Goddard, P., et al. The effect of a chemically defined diet on the faecal flora and faecal steroid concentration. *Gut* 14:790, 1973.
27. Dahlquist, A., Hammond, J. B., Crane, R. K., et al. Intestinal lactase deficiency and lactose intolerance in adults. *Gastroenterology* 45:488, 1963.
28. Davenport, H. W. Intestinal Digestion and Absorption of Protein. In *Physiology of the Digestive Tract,* 4th ed. Chicago: Year Book, 1977.
29. DeLuca, H. F. The Vitamins: Section B. Vitamin D. In R. S. Goodhart and M. E. Shils (Eds.), *Modern Nutrition in Health and Disease,* 6th ed. Philadelphia: Lea & Febiger, 1980.
30. Duke, J. H., Jr., Kinney, J. M., Broell, J. R., and Long, C. L. Metabolic evaluation of high calorie alimentation in surgical patients. *Surg. Forum* 81:74, 1970.
31. Editorial: Hypernatremia in tube fed patients. *Br. Med. J.* 1:1179, 1963.
32. Engle, F. L., and Jaeger, C. Dehydration with hypernatremia, hyperchloremia and azotemia complicating nasogastric tube feeding. *Am. J. Med.* 17:196, 1954.
33. Fason Fitzpatrick, M. Controlling bacterial growth in tube feedings. *Am. J. Nursing* 67: 1246, 1967.
34. Feldman, E. J., Peters, T. J., McNaughton, J., and Dowling, R. H. Adaptation after small bowel resection: Comparison of oral versus intravenous nutrition. *Gastroenterology* 66:691, 1974.
35. Fischer, J. E. Parenteral and enteral nutrition. *Disease-a-Month* 24:68, 1978.
36. Fagel, M. R., Ravitch, M. M., and Adibi, S. A. Absorptive and digestive function of the jejunum after jejunoileal bypass for treatment of human obesity. *Gastroenterology* 71:729, 1976.
37. Fogel, R. S., Smith, W. L., and Gresham, E. L. Perforation of feeding tube into right renal pelvis. *J. Pediatr.* 93:122, 1978.
38. Freeman, J. B., Egan, M. C., and Millis, B. J. The elemental diet. *Surg. Gynecol. Obstet.* 142: 925, 1976.
39. Gault, M. H., Dixon, M. E., Doyle, M., and Cohen, W. M. Hypernatremia, azotemia and dehydration due to high-protein tube feeding. *Ann. Intern. Med.* 68:778, 1968.
40. Glotzer, D. J., Boyle, P. L., and Silen, W. Preoperative preparation of the colon with an elemental diet. *Surgery* 74:703, 1973.
41. Goldsmith, G. A. Curative Nutrition: Vitamins. In H. A. Schneider, C. E. Anderson, and D. B. Coursin (Eds.), *Nutritional Support of Medical Practice.* Hagerstown, MD: Harper and Row, 1972.
42. Gray, G. M. Intestinal digestion and maldigestion of dietary carbohydrates. *Annu. Rev. Med.* 22:391, 1971.
43. Greenstein, J. P., Birnbaum, S. M., Winitz, M., and Otey, M. C. Quantitative nutritional studies with water-soluble chemically defined diets: IV. *Arch. Biochem. Biophys.* 72:396, 1957.
44. Greenstein, J. P., Birnbaum, S. M., Winitz, M., and Otey, M. C. Quantitative nutritional studies with water-soluble chemically defined diets: I. Growth, reproduction and lactation in rats. *Arch. Biochem. Biophys.* 72:396, 1957.
45. Griggs, B. A., and Hoppe, M. C. Update: Nasogastric tube feeding. *Am. J. Nurs.* March, 481, 1979.
46. Grundy, D. J. Small bowel fistula treated with low-residue diet. *Br. Med. J.* 2:531, 1971.
47. Gudmand-Hoyer, E., Dahlquist, A., and Jarnun, S. The clinical significance of lactose malabsorption. *Am. J. Gastroenterol.* 53:460, 1970.
48. Gutwein, I., Baer, J., and Holt, P. R. Formula diet preparation for barium enema: Impact on health care and costs. *Arch. Intern. Med.* 141: 993, 1981.
49. Hayhurst, E. G., and Wyman, M. Morbidity associated with prolonged use of polyvinyl feeding tubes. *Am. J. Dis. Child.* 129:72, 1975.
50. Hellier, M. D., Holdsworth, C. D., Perrett, D., et al. Intestinal dipeptide transport in normal and cystinuric subjects. *Clin. Sci.* 43:659, 1972.
51. Herbert, V., Colman, N., and Jacob, E. The Vitamins: Section J. Folic Acid and Vitamin B_{12}. In R. S. Goodhart and M. E. Shils (Eds.):

Modern Nutrition in Health and Disease, 6th ed. Philadelphia: Lea & Febiger, 1980.
52. Hindmarsh, J. T., and Clark, R. G. The effects of intravenous and intra-duodenal feeding on nitrogen balance after surgery. *Br. J. Surg.* 60: 589, 1973.
53. Hoover, H. C., Jr., Ryan, J. A., Anderson, E. F., and Fischer, J. E. Nutritional benefits of immediate postoperative jejunal feeding of an elemental diet. *Am. J. Surg.* 139:153, 1980.
54. Horwit, M. D. The Vitamins: Section E. Niacin. In R. S. Goodhart and M. E. Shils (Eds.), *Modern Nutrition in Health and Disease,* 6th ed. Philadelphia: Lea & Febiger, 1980.
55. Horwit, M. K. The Vitamins: Section F. Riboflavin. In R. S. Goodhart and M. E. Shils (Eds.), *Modern Nutrition in Health and Disease,* 6th ed. Philadelphia: Lea & Febiger, 1980.
56. Imond, A. R., and Stradley, R. P. Utilization of enzymatically hydrolysed soybean protein and crystalline amino acid diets by rats with exocrine pancreatic insufficiency. *J. Nutr.* 104:793, 1974.
57. Irwin, M. I., and Hutchins, B. K. A conspectus of research on vitamin C requirements of man. *J. Nutr.* 106:823, 1976.
58. Isselbacher, K. J. Biochemical aspects of fat absorption. *Gastroenterology* 50:78, 1966.
59. Johnston, W. C. Oral elemental diet: A new bowel preparation. *Arch. Surg.* 108:32, 1974.
60. Jussila, J., Launrala, K., and Gorbatow, O. Lactase deficiency and a lactose-free diet in patients with "unspecific abdominal complaints." *Acta Med. Scand.* 186:217, 1969.
61. Kaminisk, M. V. Enteral hyperalimentation. *Surg. Gynecol. Obstet.* 143:12, 1976.
62. Kassner, E. G., Baumstack, A., Balsan, D., and Haller, J. O. Passage of feeding catheters into the pleural space: A radiographic sign of trauma to the pharynx and esophagus in the newborn. *Am. J. Roentgenol.* 128:19, 1977.
63. Kinney, J. M. Energy Requirements of the Surgical Patient. In W. F. Ballinger, J. A. Collins, W. R. Drucker, S. J. Dudrick, and R. Zeppa (Eds.), *Manual of Surgical Nutrition.* Philadelphia: Saunders, 1975.
64. Klipstein, F. A., and Corcino, J. J. Malabsorption of essential amino acids in tropical sprue. *Gastroenterology* 68:239, 1975.
65. Knowles, H. C., Jr. Symposium on water and electrolytes. Hypernatremia. *Metabolism* 5:508, 1956.
66. Kretchmer, N. Lactose and lactase. *Sci. Amer.* 227:71, 1972.
67. Larkin, J. M., and Moylan, J. A. Complete enteral support of thermally injured patients. *Am. J. Surg.* 131:722, 1976.
68. Leaf, A. The clinical and physiologic significance of the serum sodium concentration. *N. Engl. J. Med.* 267:24, 77, 1962.
69. Lickley, H. L. A., Track, N. S., Vranic, M., and Bury, K. D. Metabolic responses to enteral and parenteral nutrition. *Am. J. Surg.* 135:172, 1978.
70. McMichael, H. B., Webb, J., and Dawson, A. M. Jejunal disaccharidases and some observations on the cause of lactase deficiency. *Br. Med. J.* 2:1037, 1966.
71. Mathews, D. Intestinal absorption of peptides. *Physiol. Rev.* 55:537, 1975.
72. Milne, M. D., and Asatoor, A. M. Peptide Absorption in Disorders of Amino and Transport. In D. M. Mathews and J. W. Payne (Eds.), *Peptide Transport in Protein Nutrition.* New York: North Holland/American Elsevier, 1975. P. 167.
73. Morgan, A., Filler, R. M., and Moore, F. D. Surgical nutrition. *Med. Clin. North Am.* 54: 1367, 1970.
74. National Academy of Sciences. Recommended Dietary Allowances, 9th ed. Washington, D.C.: Nat. Res. Council, 1980.
75. National Dairy Council. Lactose intolerance. *Dairy Council Digest.* 42:31, 1971.
76. Necomer, A. D. Disaccharide deficiencies. *Mayo Clinic Proc.* 48:648, 1973.
77. O'Hara, J. G., Kennedy, S., and Lizewski, W. Effects of long-term elemental nasogastric feeding on elderly debilitated patients. *Can. Med. Assoc. J.* 108:977, 1973.
78. Olivares, L., Segovia, A., and Revuetta, R. Tube feeding and lethal aspiration in neurological patients: A review of 720 autopsy cases. *Stroke* 5:654, 1974.
79. Padilla, G. V., Grant, M., Wong, H., Hansen, B. W., Hansen, R. L., Bergstrom, N., and Kubo, W. R. Subjective distresses of nasogastric tube feeding. *J. Par. Ent. Nutr.* 3:53, 1979.
80. Perrault, J., Devroede, G., and Bounous, G. Effects of an elemental diet in healthy volunteers. *Gastroenterology* 64:569, 1973.
81. Peters, C., and Fischer, J. E. Studies on calorie to nitrogen ratio for total parenteral nutrition. *Surg. Gynecol. Obstet.* 151:1, 1980.
82. Porter, J. M., Snowe, R. F., and Silver, D. Tuberculous enteritis with perforation and abscess formation in childhood. *Surgery* 71:254, 1972.
83. Ragins, H., Levenson, S. M., Signer, R., Stamford, W., and Seifler, E. Intrajejunal administration of an elemental diet at neutral pH avoids pancreatic stimulation. *Am. J. Surg.* 126:606, 1973.
84. Rivilis, J., McArdle, H. W., Wlodek, G., and

Gurd, F. N. Effects of an elemental diet on gastric and secretion. *Ann. Surg.* 179:226, 1974.
85. Rocchio, M. A., Chung-Ja, C., Haas, K. F., and Randall, H. T. Use of chemically defined diets in the management of patients with high output gastrointestinal cutaneous fistulas. *Am. J. Surg.* 127:148, 1974.
86. Rocchio, M. A., Chung-Ja, C., Haas, K. F., and Randall, H. T. Use of a chemically defined diet in the management of patients with inflammatory bowel disease. *Am. J. Surg.* 127:469, 1974.
87. Rothman, M. M., and Katz, A. B. Analysis of feces. In H. L. Bockus (Ed.), *Gastroenterology,* 2nd ed. Philadelphia: Saunders, 1964. Vol. 2.
88. Sadikal, F. Dipeptidase deficiency and malabsorption of glycylglycine in small intestinal disease. *Gut* 12:276, 1971.
89. Sauberlick, H. E., and Canham, J. E. The Vitamins: Section I. Vitamin B_6. In R. S. Goodhart and M. E. Shils (Eds.), *Modern Nutrition in Health and Disease,* 6th ed. Philadelphia: Lea & Febiger, 1980.
90. Schedl, H. P., Pierce, C. E., Rider, A., et al. Absorption of L-methionine from the human small intestine. *J. Clin. Invest.* 47:417, 1968.
91. Schreiner, R. L., Eitzen, H., Gfell, M. A., Kress, S., Gresham, E. L., French, M., and Moye, L. Environmental contamination of continuous drip feedings. *Pediatrics* 63:232, 1979.
92. Scrimshaw, N. S. Effect of infection on nutrient requirements. *Am. J. Clin. Nutr.* 30:1536, 1977.
93. Shils, M. E., Block, A. S., and Chernoff, R. Liquid formulas for oral and tube feeding. Memorial Sloan-Kettering Cancer Center, 1979.
94. Siegle, R. L., Rabinowitz, J. G., and Sarasuhn, C. Intestinal perforation secondary to nasojejunal feeding tubes. *Am. J. Roentgenol.* 126: 1229, 1976.
95. Silk, D. B. A., Kumar, P. J., Perrett, D., et al. Amino acid and peptide absorption in patients with coeliac disease and dermatitis herpetiformis. *Gut* 15:1, 1974.
96. Silk, D. B. A., Perrett, D., and Clark, M. L. Jejunal and ileal absorption of dibasic amino acids and an arginine-containing dipeptide in cystinuria. *Gastroenterology* 68:1426, 1975.
97. Silk, D. B. A., Chung, Y. C., Kim, Y. S., et al. Comparison of oral feeding of peptide and amino acid meals to normal human subjects. *Gastroenterology* 70:937, 1976.
98. Simoons, F. J. Primary adult lactose intolerance and the milking habit. A problem in biological and cultural interrelations. *Digestive Diseases* 14:819, 1969.
99. Sleisenger, M. H., and Brundberg, L. L. Malabsorption. In L. H. Smith (Ed.), *Major Problems in Internal Medicine.* Philadelphia: Saunders, 1977. P. 39.
100. Smith, A. M., and Veenema, R. J. Management of rectal injury and rectourethral fistulas following radical retropubic prostatectomy. *J. Urol.* 103:778, 1972.
101. Sun, S. C., Samuels, S., Lea, J., and Marquis, J. R. Duodenal perforation: A rare complication of neonatal nasojejunal feeding. *Pediatrics* 55:371, 1975.
102. Tarlow, M. J., Seakins, J. W. T., Lloyd, J. K., et al. Absorption of amino acids and peptides in a child with a variant of Hartnup disease and coexistent coeliac disease. *Arch. Dis. Child.* 47:798, 1972.
103. Thompson, W. R., Stephens, R. V., Randall, H. T., and Bowen, J. R. Use of the "space diet" in the management of a patient with extreme short bowel syndrome. *Am. J. Surg.* 117:449, 1969.
104. Uzawa, H., Schlierf, G., Chirman, S., et al. Hyperglyceridemia resulting from intake of medium chain triglycerides. *Am. J. Clin. Nutr.* 15:365, 1964.
105. Voitk, A., Echave, V., Brown, R., McArdle, A. H., and Gurd, F. N. Elemental diet in the treatment of fistulas of the alimentary tract. *Surg. Gynecol. Obstet.* 137:68, 1973.
106. Voitk, A., Echave, V., Brown, R., and Gurd, F. N. Use of elemental diet during the adaptive stage of short gut syndrome. *Gastroenterology* 65:419, 1973.
107. Voitk, A., Echave, V., Feller, J. H., Brown, R. A., and Gurd, F. N. Experience with elemental diets in the Rx of inflammatory bowel disease. *Arch. Surg.* 107:329, 1973.
108. Walike, J. W. Tube feeding syndrome in head and neck surgery. *Arch. Otolaryngol.* 89:117, 1969.
109. Welt, L. G., Seldin, D. W., Nelson, W. P., German, W. J., and Peters, J. P. Role of the central nervous system in metabolism of electrolytes and water. *Arch. Intern. Med.* 30:355, 1952
110. White, W. T., Acuff, T. E., Sykes, T. R., and Dobbie, R. P. Bacterial contamination of enteral nutrient solution: A preliminary report. *J. Par. Ent. Nutr.* 3:459, 1979.
111. Wilmore, D. W. Alimentation in injured and septic patients. *Heart Lung* 5:791, 1976.
112. Wilmore, D. W. Energy and Nitrogen Metabolism in Disease. In *Current Approaches to Nutritional Therapy of the Hospitalized Patient.* Abbott-Ross Research Conference, Amerlia Island, FL, 1975.
113. Wilson, W. S., and Meinert, J. K. Extracellular hyperosmolarity secondary to high-protein naso-

gastric tube feeding. *Ann. Intern. Med.* 47:585, 1957.

114. Winitz, M., Seedman, D. A., and Graff, J. Studies in metabolic nutrition employing chemically defined diets: I. Extended feeding of normal human adult males. *Am. J. Clin. Nutr.* 23:525, 1970.
115. Winitz, M., Graff, J., Gallacher, M., Narhin, A., and Seedman, D. A. Evaluation of chemical diets as nutrition for man-in-space. *Nature* 205: 741, 1965.
116. Winitz, M., Birnbaum, S. M., Sugimura, T., and Otley, M. C. Quantitative Nutritional and In Vivo Metabolic Studies with Water-Soluble Chemically Defined Diets. In *Amino Acids, Proteins and Cancer Biochemistry*. Greenstein Memorial Symposium, 1960.
117. Winitz, M., Adams, R. F., Seedman, D. A., et al. Studies in metabolic nutrition employing chemically defined diets: II. Effects on gut microflora populations. *Am. J. Clin. Nutr.* 23: 546, 1970.
118. Wolfe, B. M., Keltner, R. M., and William, V. L. Intestinal fistula output in regular, elemental and intravenous alimentation. *Am. J. Surg.* 124:803, 1972.
119. Yeh, Y., and Zee, P. Relation of ketosis to metabolic changes induced by acute medium-chain triglyceride feeding in rats. *J. Nutr.* 106:58, 1976.
120. Ziegler, E. F., and Foman, S. J. Fluid intake, renal solute load and water balance in infancy. *J. Pediatr.* 78:561, 1971.

Jejunal Feeding

John A. Ryan, Jr.

25

In 1858 Wilhelm Busch of Bonn, Germany, treated a woman who had been gored in the abdomen by a raging bull. The injury severed her upper jejunum and resulted in a jejunal fistula and subsequent malnutrition. Her condition was considered to be too grave for operation. Busch fed a diet of eggs, flour, meat, and meat broth into the jejunal opening. The patient thrived on this treatment, and over a period of five months gained 19 pounds. This was the first recorded case in which a feeding had been given directly into the jejunum [16].

This case permitted all the elements of jejunal feeding to be observed: (1) jejunal access, (2) indication, (3) diet, (4) method, and (5) result. In this chapter the historical development of these same five elements will be traced from Busch's initial effort to current experience. They will be considered separately, although they have points of overlap. The importance of jejunal feedings and jejunostomy has varied with changes in abdominal operations, knowledge of gastrointestinal physiology, emphasis on nutrition, and availability of alternative methods of furnishing fluid and nutrition in the postoperative patient. The purpose of this chapter is to define the current role of jejunal feeding and describe techniques and methods which are safe and effective.

JEJUNAL ACCESS

Jejunostomy

Busch's report became famous throughout Europe, but 20 years passed before a surgeon's knife rather than a bull's horn created the next jejunostomy. In 1878 Surmay, in Le Havre, France, performed a jejunostomy in a patient with obstructing gastric carcinoma by drawing the jejunum through the wound, suturing it to the skin, and making a small opening through which a tube could be introduced for feeding (Figure 25-1). His first patient died 30 hours after the operation [99, 100]. Independently, in 1885 three English surgeons—Robertson, Gould, and Golding-Bird—performed jejunostomies with similar techniques on three patients with far-advanced gastric cancer [38, 53, 81]. All three patients died early postoperatively. One of the

Special thanks to K. Peter Kretschmer, M.D., for translation of the German references.

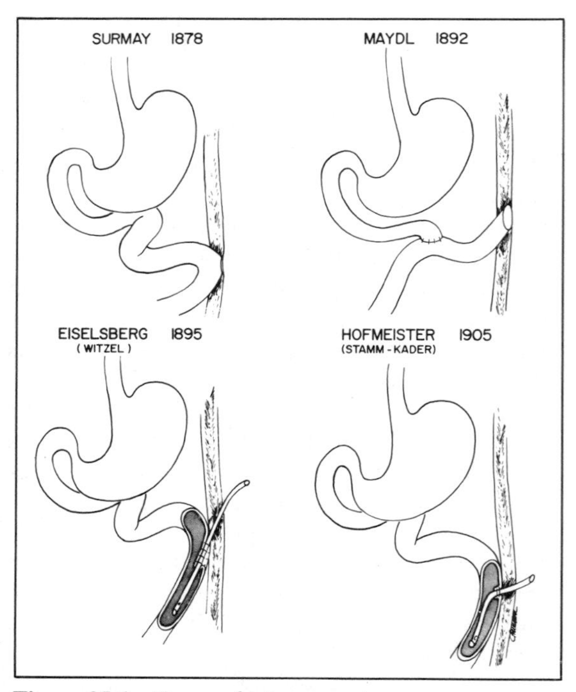

Figure 25-1. *Types of jejunostomies.*

patients died because of a complication of the jejunostomy, the infusion of diet into the peritoneal cavity causing peritonitis. The skin level jejunostomy underwent several modifications, but the techniques were rarely successful because of loss of intestinal contents and reflux of diet [82]. Despite a high mortality, significant complications, and poor function, these early reports sparked interest in jejunostomy as palliation in gastric malignant disease.

The first continent jejunostomy was described by Maydl, in Vienna, in 1892 [59] (Figure 25-1). This Roux-en-Y jejunojejunostomy afforded permanence, continence, ability to use solid foods, and lack of dependency on an indwelling tube. Its influence lasted until modern times, despite its technical complexities [15].

Eiselsberg, the Professor of Surgery at Utrecht, described a technique for jejunostomy in 1895 in which a 12- or 16-mm rubber tube was placed through a serosal lined tunnel, and the jejunum was sutured to the abdominal wound [30] (Figure 25-1). The technique was modeled after the Witzel gastrostomy [114] and has since been called the Witzel jejunostomy. Because of the simplicity and excellent function of this method, it was adopted widely and is still the most popular type of jejunostomy [55]. Unless the tube was large, the jejunostomy rarely leaked intestinal contents. Originally Eiselsberg planned reoperation with jejunal closure if jejunal feedings became unnecessary [30]; later he realized that the fistula would close spontaneously [54].

In 1905 Hofmeister described a technique for jejunostomy in which a double purse-string suture created a serosal tunnel for the tube at right angles to the jejunal entry point [42] (Figure 25-1). This technique was based on gastrostomy techniques of Stamm [90] and Kader [47]. This type of jejunostomy is still in common use and is referred to as the Stamm jejunostomy.

Despite the early development of surgical techniques and isolated reports of benefit in the early 1900s, jejunostomy was not widely used because of early deaths and numerous complications. In 1933 Barber reported that only 20 Witzel jejunostomies had been done at Bellevue Hospital in the preceding 13 years. Nine patients died less than two weeks postoperatively, and diarrhea, leakage around the jejunostomy tube, obstruction by the tube, and difficulty in maintaining the tube's position occurred frequently [12] (Figure 25-2).

Operative Access Without Jejunostomy

Because of the fear of complications of tube jejunostomy, some surgeons obtained jejunal access by tubes passed through the nose and positioned into the jejunum intraoperatively. The first was Andresen, who in 1918 passed a nasojejunal tube through a gastrojejunostomy for feeding in a patient with peptic ulcer disease [8]. This concept was popularized in 1937 by W. Osler Abbott and A. J. Rawson, a gastroenterologist and a mechanical engineer who

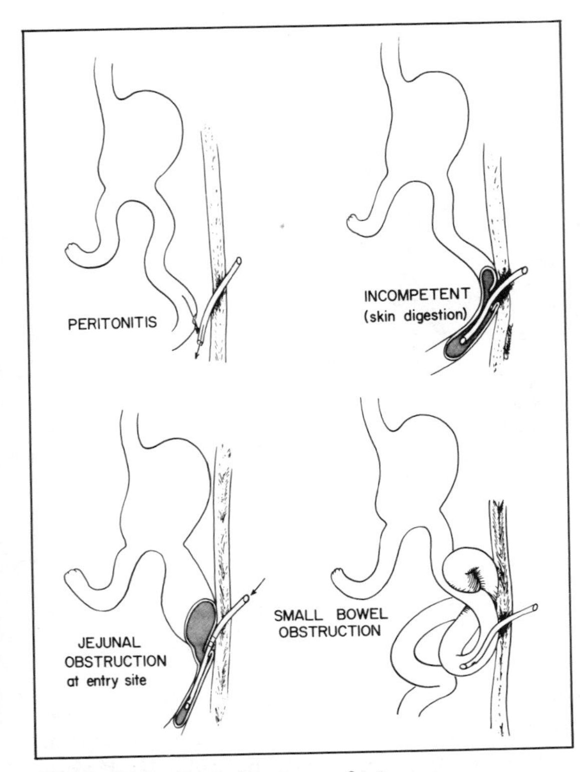

Figure 25-2. *Complications of jejunostomy.*

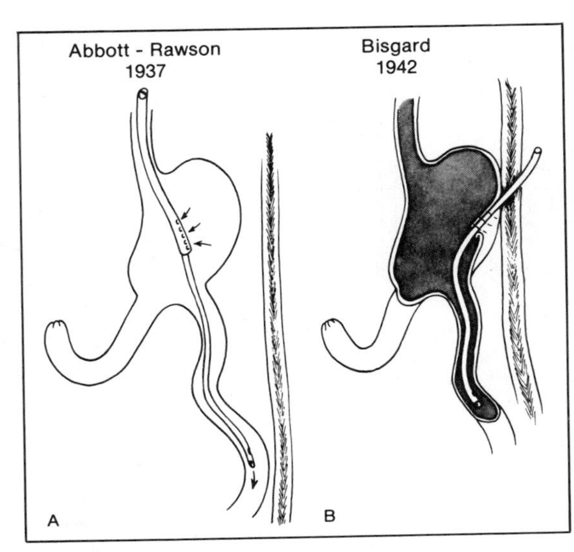

Figure 25-3. *A. Nasal jejunal tube. B. Gastrojejunal tube.*

worked with Isadore Ravdin, Chief of Surgery at the University of Pennsylvania [1–3, 77, 91]. Their Abbott-Rawson double-lumen tube for gastric decompression and jejunal feeding was used extensively in cases of gastrojejunostomy and gastrectomy [78–80] (Figure 25-3). Surgeons at Bellevue, who had used jejunostomy sparingly in the 1920s and 1930s [12], adopted postoperative nasojejunal feeding widely in the 1940s [22, 68]. Bisgard passed a tube through a gastrostomy incision and threaded it through a gastrojejunal anastomosis in order to have access to the jejunum for feeding [13] (Figure 25-3). His idea was later adapted with double-lumen tubes for gastric decompression and jejunal feeding. Recently Moss suggested a triple-lumen tube for postoperative esophagogastric decompression and duodenal or jejunal feeding, which is a further adaptation of these ideas [66].

The main drawback of nasojejunal feeding in the postoperative patient is that the tubes necessarily are large-bore in order to also allow gastric decompression. Large tubes are complicated by rhinitis, pharyngitis, otitis media, poor cough, pulmonary atelectasis, increased upper respiratory secretions, and gastroesophageal reflux leading to esophagitis, stricture, and aspiration pneumonia. Since the nasojejunal tube is uncomfortable, it is usually removed as soon as gastric decompression is unnecessary, and thus long-term access to the jejunum, which might otherwise be desirable, is lost.

Nonoperative Jejunal Access

A small-gauge nasojejunal catheter is satisfactory for jejunal feeding, and can be placed without the necessity for operation. In 1910 Einhorn described the first example of tube feeding below the level of the stomach [28]. In 1918 he fed a patient with a postoperative duodenal fistula by a nasojejunal catheter, with eventual healing of the fistula [29]. Morawitz and Henning [65], in 1929, and Abbott [3], in 1940, re-emphasized naso-

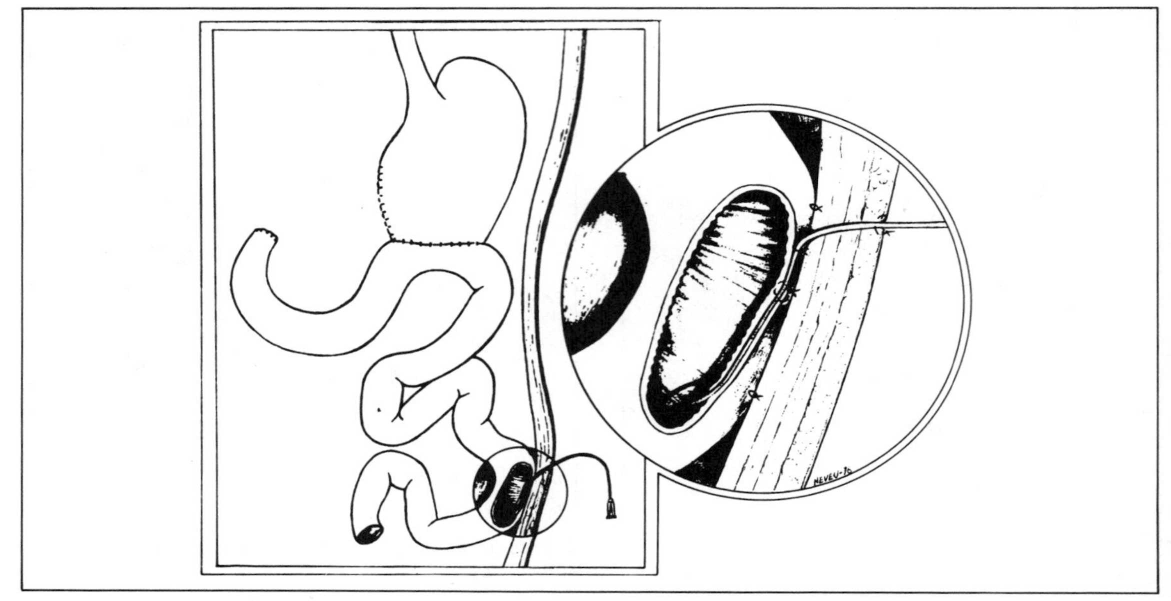

Figure 25-4. *Needle catheter jejunostomy. (From J. A. Ryan, C. P. Page, and L. Babcock, Early post-operative jejunal feeding of elemental diet in gastro-intestinal surgery.* Am. Surg. *47:393, 1981.)*

jejunal access for feeding of medical or surgical patients. In 1951 Fallis and Barron described a mercury-weighted, fine polyethylene catheter which, after nasal introduction, would pass by gravity and peristalsis into the jejunum [34]. Currently, similar tubes of polyethylene [25] and silicone elastomer [49] are commercially available.

Mercury-weighted tubes occasionally do not pass to the desired level of the jejunum. The main indication for this type of jejunal access is gastrointestinal obstruction, fistula, or pancreatic inflammation, and thus the proper position of the tip of the tube below the diseased area is of utmost importance. When the tip of the catheter fails to proceed to the jejunum by peristalsis, other methods are available for proper positioning: (1) An angiographic flexible guidewire may be passed, during fluoroscopy, to the desired level of the jejunum, and a fine polyethylene catheter threaded over the guidewire. The guidewire is removed, a blunt needle is inserted, and the catheter is suitable for a fine liquid diet. (2) An extra-long fine polyethylene or Teflon catheter may be inserted through the biopsy channel of a flexible fiberoptic endoscope, which has been passed to the desired level of the jejunum. The endoscope is withdrawn over this long catheter.

Needle Catheter Jejunostomy

A modified Witzel jejunostomy technique, which is extremely simple and safe, has recently been advocated and called a needle catheter jejunostomy. In 1951 Usher first used polyethylene rather than rubber for a jejunostomy catheter [103]. In 1954 McDonald used a trocar needle to place a polyethylene catheter into the jejunum [63]. Delaney adapted this technique, using a 14-gauge needle to create a seromuscular tunnel for a 16-gauge polyethylene catheter [23]. Experience with this needle catheter jejunostomy has confirmed its safety and ease [6, 7, 24, 45, 71–73, 85].

A 16-gauge, 24-inch polyethylene catheter is placed in the mobile portion of the jejunum distal to the ligament of Treitz or to a gastrojejunal anastomosis. The 14-gauge, 2¾-inch needle is removed from the catheter and inserted through a 4-0 silk purse-string suture into the seromuscular layer of the antimesenteric border of the jejunum. A lengthy tunnel is created by telescoping the intestines over the needle. The needle is turned into the lumen, and 12 inches of catheter are inserted into the jejunum. The plastic hub of the catheter is amputated, and the needle is withdrawn. A separate seromuscular suture anchors the catheter to the jejunal wall.

A similar 14-gauge needle is placed percutaneously through the abdominal wall at a point where the jejunum lies naturally, usually in the left upper quadrant, and the catheter is passed out of the abdomen through it. The jejunum is anchored to the abdominal wall with two 4-0 silk sutures, and the catheter is sutured to the skin. An 18-gauge blunt needle adapts the catheter to standard connecting tubing (Figure 25-4).

Because of the small size of the catheter, encroachment on the lumen and reflux through the entry point do not occur, and rapid sealing of the hole when the catheter is withdrawn is assured. Because of the mobility of the small intestines, the jejunum should be tacked to the abdominal wall to safeguard against dislodgment of the tube from the jejunal lumen and delivery of diet into the peritoneal cavity.

Page reported three minor complications in 156 consecutive needle catheter jejunostomies. No incidents of intra-abdominal leakage, perforation of the jejunum, incompetency, jejunal obstruction, small bowel obstruction, or persistent jejunal fistula occurred [72, 73] (see Figure 25-2). Ascites or far-advanced peritonitis may be a contraindication to jejunostomy because tube enterostomies heal poorly in these conditions.

INDICATIONS

Busch's historic jejunal feeding was done as a preoperative nutritional preparation. This was remarkable because even today surgeons rarely think of restoring nutrition before operation. In 1858 no surgeon would have done a laparotomy to establish a jejunostomy to replete a patient for a subsequent abdominal procedure. A half century passed before this concept was introduced.

Palliation

The original jejunostomies were done as palliation for gastric cancer. In 1885 Gould reported an operative mortality rate for gastrectomy of 77 percent, and for gastroenterostomy, 73 percent [53]. In 1895 Eiselsberg reported his personal mortality rate of 50 percent for gastrectomy and 25 percent for gastroenterostomy [30]. Thus, a simple jejunostomy had real appeal for a surgeon facing an advanced gastric malignancy, despite a respectable mortality rate of its own. Jejunostomy was employed in the worst operative risks, patients in whom gastrectomy or gastroenterostomy were not feasible. In 152 cases of gastric cancer seen between 1896 and 1903 by Eiselsberg, the following operations were done: gastrectomy, 33; gastroenterostomy, 77; and jejunostomy, 42 [54]. As recently as 1952 Brintall reported 34 Maydl jejunostomies performed over a four-year period for palliation of unresectable tumors of the pharynx, esophagus, or stomach [15].

Small Bowel Obstruction

In the early part of this century jejunostomy was advocated in acute obstruction of the small intestine. Death was thought to be due to the absorption of toxins. Jejunostomy under local anesthesia through a small incision was used to decompress the obstructed bowel and remove the toxins [39, 57, 58, 76, 88, 105]. When the "toxin theory" was exposed as an imposter of electrolyte imbalance, dehydration, malnutrition, and intestinal infarction, jejunostomy gave way to operations that relieved obstruction rather than just decompressing them. Baker, however, popularized long intestinal tube jejunostomy for decompression coincident with relieving obstruction of the small bowel. The tube was used as a stent to prevent early and late reobstruction postoperatively [10, 11].

Peptic Ulcer Disease

In 1886 Rydygier established gastrojejunostomy as the principal operation for peptic ulcer disease. It remained so for the next forty years despite isolated reports of marginal ulcer. In 1895 Eiselsberg reported a 60-year-old woman with an obstructing pyloric mass and a second lesion in the cardia that was interpreted as unresectable cancer and for which a palliative jejunostomy was performed. With jejunal feeding, the tumor disappeared, the woman gained 21 kg, and she was able to return to a normal diet. Eiselsberg deduced that the condition was not malignant and reasoned that simple jejunostomy had afforded absolute rest to the stomach, allowing healing [30]. Eiselsberg in Vienna and Mayo-Robson in London advocated jejunostomy as the treatment of benign inflammatory conditions of the stomach in order to avoid the dreaded jejunal ulcer seen with gastrojejunostomy [32, 61]. Many surgeons used jejunostomy as the sole treatment of peptic ulcer disease when the inflammation was too severe for excision or gastrojejunostomy or when the patient was too ill or malnourished for an intestinal anastomosis [20, 26, 41, 56, 60, 64, 106, 115].

In 1897 Schlatter reported the first total gastrectomy and noted maintenance of nutrition. This report influenced surgeons to accept jejunal feeding as a feasible way to maintain patients long-term [67]. Early reports of long-term jejunostomy feedings in benign conditions confirmed its efficacy [30, 31]. By 1930 gastrectomy became the operation of choice for severe peptic ulcer disease, eclipsing the interest in therapeutic jejunostomy. But even as late as 1933, Mensing in Wisconsin reported 54 cases of benign peptic ulcer treated with simple jejunostomy with a recurrence rate of four ulcers in two years [64].

Preliminary Measure

The idea of preliminary jejunostomy was first recommended in 1901 by Stieda in Konigsberg in order to improve the physical and nutritional condition of patients with obstructing cancers of the stomach or benign pyloric scarring, so that radical gastrectomy or gastrojejunostomy could be done safely later. Stieda recognized that early postoperative deaths after gastric operations labeled as "collapse" occurred because severely depleted patients were prepared for operation by decreasing fluid intake, underwent laparatomy without the benefit of fluid, and were maintained in the postoperative period with a starvation regimen until healing occurred. He made strong recommendations for subcutaneous infusions of fluid and rectal enemas of fluid and nutrients. In severely debilitated patients with gastric disease, he advocated nothing more than jejunostomy, so that fluids and nutrients could be given to prepare a patient for later resection or anastomosis [96].

Preliminary jejunostomy proved to have little value in gastric cancer because the patient usually died before nutrition could be restored, but since jejunostomy often reduced inflammation while restoring nutrition in benign ulcer disease, a planned preliminary jejunostomy with later resection was adopted in isolated cases [54, 61]. In 1933 Hillman reported a case of recurrent ulcer with gastro-jejunal-colic involvement, which was treated initially with jejunostomy. Nine weeks later the inflammation had subsided to the point that simple gastrectomy was possible [41].

Today, with the availability of total parenteral nutrition, preliminary jejunostomy is rarely employed. However, if a surgeon unexpectedly finds severe inflammation, which makes a gastric procedure hazardous, particularly in a catabolic patient, preliminary jejunostomy may be considered.

Complementary Measure

The complementary jejunostomy (simultaneous, prophylactic, or adjunctive) was first suggested in 1902 by Gibson, when he performed a jejunostomy during a gastric resection for antral cancer. The patient died on the fourth postoperative day, and this may explain the reason that no further report of complementary jejunostomy occurred until Heyd added a jejunostomy in order to safeguard the suture integrity of a gastrojejunostomy in 1926 [39].

In 1929 Kirschner, Professor of Surgery at Tubingen, reported 60 prophylactic jejunostomies with gastric resection for cancer and ulcer. He recognized the nutritional and fluid deprivation of patients coming to gastrectomy and the stress and starvation that the operation and postoperative recovery added. He realized that administration of fluids and nutrients by rectum or subcutaneous infusions were insufficient. The decreased oral intake because of fear of suture line dehiscence and gastric atony could be overcome by jejunostomy performed coincident with gastric resection, allowing unlimited fluid and nutrition postoperatively. He stated that with jejunal feeding there was increased resistance of his patients to death by collapse or infection [50].

These ideas met receptive minds on both sides of the Atlantic at a time when increasing numbers of gastrectomies were being performed. Intravenous therapy was still in its infancy, and surgeons recognized that postoperative Murphy drip enemas and subpectoral infusions did not meet the needs of their patients [79, 106]. Ravdin showed that hypoproteinemia adversely affected anastomotic function [77], and Studley correlated increased weight loss with increased mortality after gastric resection [98]. Jejunostomy or nasojejunal access was recommended as a routine complement to gastric procedures by many authorities in the 1930s and 1940s [5, 19, 20, 22, 68, 78, 80, 94, 95, 106, 115].

Complementary jejunal access was also recommended in the operative correction of duodenal atresia, duodenal obstruction, and other anomalies of the upper gastrointestinal tract in neonates. The ability to give prolonged postoperative jejunal feeding through nasojejunal tubes, gastrojejunal tubes, and jejunostomy decreased the mortality rate in these infants [6, 7, 27, 40, 112].

Supplementary Measure

With the increased incidence of gastric operations, supplementary (secondary) jejunostomy

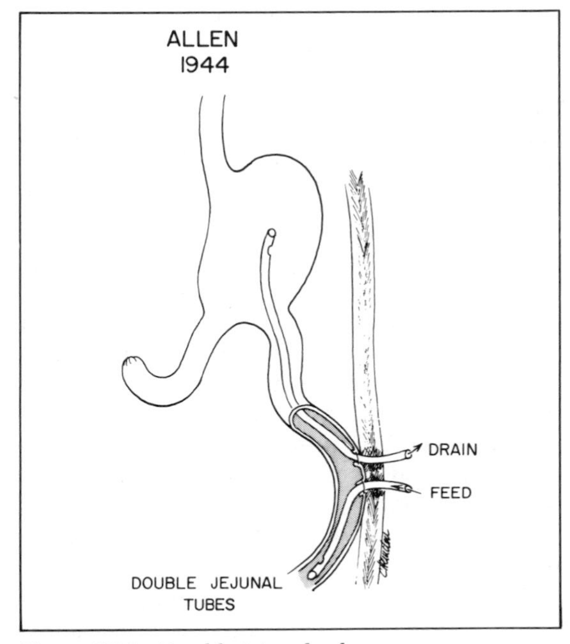

Figure 25-5. *Double jejunal tubes.*

became necessary for the relief of postoperative complications such as duodenal [48] or biliary fistula [94] and stomal obstruction [106, 110]. In 1941 Allen and Welch reported 15 cases of stomal obstruction occurring in 282 gastric resections in the previous 5 years at the Massachusetts General Hospital and recommended jejunostomy if the original anastomosis was not working one week postoperatively [4]. Their philosophy changed 3 years later when they shifted to complementary jejunostomy with gastrectomies [5] (Figure 25-5).

Current Indications

The relative indications for jejunal feeding by the mid-twentieth century were documented by Boles and Zollinger at Ohio State, who reported a 4-year experience with 103 jejunostomies performed for upper gastrointestinal diseases: primary or palliative, 7; preliminary, 7; complementary, 85; and supplementary, 4 [14].

Today many of the standard indications for

jejunostomy are not applicable. Malignant obstruction is not well palliated because the obstruction is not relieved and longevity is not increased. The mortality and morbidity of palliative gastrectomy and gastrojejunostomy are low enough to give these operations precedence over simple jejunostomy in incurable cases [70].

Jejunostomy for peptic ulcer disease, either as primary or preliminary therapy, makes little sense today because, except in rare cases, the most severe ulcers can be treated safely with vagotomy and drainage procedures. The need for preliminary jejunostomy for nutritional preparation has been eliminated by the availability of total parenteral nutrition, which puts the upper gastrointestinal tract at rest, restores nutrition, and is easier on the patient than a laparotomy for jejunal access, even if done under local anesthesia.

The use of supplementary jejunostomy for gastric stomal dysfunction also has been eclipsed by total parenteral nutrition. A surgeon should not forget, however, that if a reoperation is necessary for persistent stomal dysfunction, postoperative abscess, upper gastrointestinal tract fistula, or postoperative pancreatitis, a jejunostomy should be considered in addition to the corrective procedure. In certain instances nasojejunal access by gravity, fluoroscopic guidewire, or endoscopic placement can be established.

Complementary jejunostomy during operations on the upper gastrointestinal tract remains the most common indication for jejunal access. Paralleling a decrease in gastric operations has been an increase in operations on the pancreas, esophagus, and hepatobiliary tree. Resections for pancreatic neoplasms and chronic inflammation, a variety of operations for ductal drainage in chronic pancreatitis, and aggressive operative approaches to acute pancreatitis [51, 107, 111] are now commonplace [35]. Esophageal resection for cancer or advanced stricture with reconstructions using intestinal interpositions are frequently done. Pancreatic and esophageal diseases cause striking malnutrition and require major operative procedures with extensive dis-

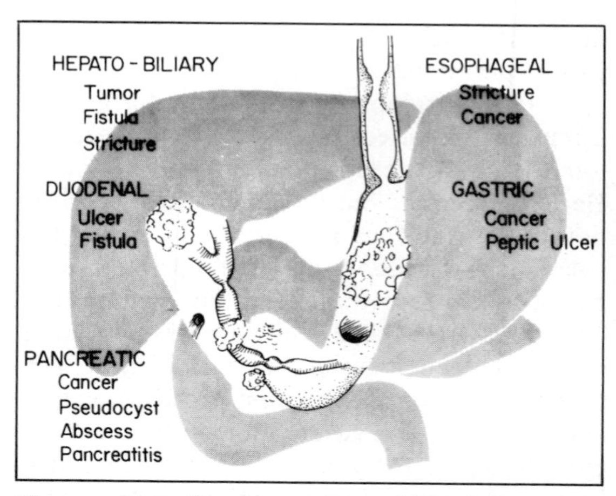

Figure 25-6. *Diagnoses for which jejunostomy should be considered as part of operative therapy.*

section, blood loss, and threat of infection, all associated with increased catabolic response. In addition, the postoperative course is often prolonged and complicated before return to a normal oral diet. Hepatic resections for tumor and trauma and reconstructive biliary operations usually do not have the preoperative malnutrition associated with esophageal and pancreatic diseases, but their postoperative courses are often more complicated and catabolic.

Patients who face major operations of the esophagus, stomach, pancreas, duodenum, and hepatobiliary systems, especially when malnourished preoperatively, may be candidates for jejunostomy established at the time of corrective operation (Figure 25-6). Gastrostomy is preferable to jejunostomy when either is feasible because of greater tolerance to diets and to methods of feeding. Gastrostomy for feeding purposes, however, is not as realiable as jejunostomy in upper abdominal operations because of the possibility of stomal dysfunction, fistula, or continued inflammation at the operative site.

DIET

One of the important limitations of jejunal feeding has been the lack of an ideal diet. Theoretically, the ideal diet would have the following characteristics: (1) nutritionally complete, (2) easily digested and absorbed, (3) low residue, (4) low fat, (5) low lactose, (6) low osmolarity, (7) drips by gravity through fine catheters, (8) stable, (9) easy to prepare, and (10) inexpensive. The definition of these ideal characteristics and the search for such a diet has gone on since Busch made his first observations. Just as William Beaumont in 1833 observed gastric digestion in the gunshot gastric fistula of Alexis St. Martin, so Busch observed the jejunal response to various foods in his patient with the bull-gored jejunal fistula. Proteins and carbohydrates were well tolerated despite the lack of gastric, biliary, and pancreatic digestion, but melted butter, a source of fat, caused reversed peristalsis, cramps, and diarrhea.

Jejunal Foods

Unfortunately, subsequent surgeons did not adopt Busch's conclusions or his reliance on observation of jejunal response to determine the ideal diet. They used normal dietary principles and foods for jejunal feeding. One of the reasons for the popularity of the Maydl jejunostomy was that solid, good-tasting foods could be fed at regular mealtimes. Even with the Witzel tube, regular feedings often simulated meals, sometimes with a disregard for a balanced diet or jejunal tolerance. In 1926 Heyd fed the diet listed in Table 25-1 through a No. 28 French Witzel jejunostomy [39]. The patient received orange juice, Cream of Wheat, eggs, and milk for breakfast, soup for lunch, a before-dinner syringeful of whiskey or wine, cereal for dinner, and chocolate milk before bedtime. Little attention was given to the electrolyte or vitamin content of these diets, and deficiencies were occasionally discovered [33].

Table 25-1. *Heyd's Jejunal Food Schedule*

Time	Feeding
7 AM, Arising	Water, one glass, 6 oz.
20 minutes later	Orange juice, 6 oz. Cream of Wheat, etc.
9 AM	Two eggs, soft boiled, egg-nog Glass of milk and lactose
11 AM	Soup Butter
1 PM	Cocoa
2 PM	Water, one glass
4 PM	Rice, cream Sugar, milk
6 PM	Whiskey, 1 oz., or wine Water, one glass
7 PM	Cereal
9 PM	Milk and lactose
10 to 11 PM	Chocolate Water, one glass

Scott-Ivy Pabulum

In 1931 at Northwestern Medical School H. G. Scott, a physiologist, and Andrew C. Ivy, a pharmacologist, described a diet for jejunal feeding which was widely adopted as the Scott-Ivy Pabulum [87] (Table 25-2) [115]. This diet was a nutritionally complete, thick liquid prepared by the mixture of multiple ingredients specifically for jejunal feeding. Attention was paid to vitamins and minerals. Its drawbacks were a high content of milk carbohydrate (lactose), fat, and osmotically active sucrose. It contained 13 constituents and was complex to prepare. Its semisolid nature required mechanical pumping through large tubes to avoid clogging.

Hollander Formula

In 1945 Franklin Hollander, a scientist in the Gastroenterology Research Laboratory of Mt. Sinai Hospital, reported a new diet, which he believed had important advantages in jejunal feeding [43, 44]. The Hollander formula was not based on milk and was low in fat and osmolarity. Its protein was an enzymatic digest of casein and pancreas, and its carbohydrate was an enzymatic digest of cereal starch. It was liquid and could

Table 25-2. *Scott-Ivy Pabulum*

Vitamine Feeding—added to the regular feedings once daily						
	Measure	Weight in Grams	Carbo-hydrate	Protein	Fat	Calories
Orange juice	1/2 cup	100	10.0	1.0		
Egg	One			6.0	6.0	
Viosterol	3 drops					
Haliver oil	5 drops					
Harris yeast tablet	One					
			10	7	6	120

Jejunal Feeding						
	Measure	Weight in Grams	Carbo-hydrate	Protein	Fat	Calories
Milk	1-1/2 qt.	1,500	75.0	45.0	52.5	
Cream	1 pt.	500	20.0	15.0	100.0	
Sugar	3/4 cup	150	150.0			
Flour	1 cup	120	90.0	13.0	1.5	
Peptone	1/2 cup	80		80.0		
Ringers	1,000 ml.)					
Water	1,000 ml.)*					
			335	153	154	3,340

Dissolve sugar in water. Add peptone. After both sugar and peptone have been thoroughly dissolved in the water, heat for several minutes. Mix flour with part of the milk to a smooth paste. Mix peptone solution with flour and milk. Bring mixture to a boil quickly over a hot flame but do not allow to boil. Stir vigorously, keeping a sub-boiling point until it thickens to the consistency of a thick cream soup or thin flour paste mixture. Strain, cool. Keep in refrigerator.

*Or 2,000 ml water, and 2 tablespoonsful salt.
Source: Modified from J. A. Wolfer, Jejunostomy with jejunal alimentation. *Ann. Surg.* 101:708, 1935.

pass through small tubes. Its main drawbacks were difficulty in preparation, because of its 12 constituents, and expense, because of the protein and carbohydrate sources. Variations of this diet were used for postoperative nasojejunal feeding by the groups at the University of Pennsylvania and at Bellevue [22, 68, 80] (Table 25-3) [43].

Homogenized Milk

Because of the complexity in preparation, the use of the Scott-Ivy and Hollander formulas waned when Case, a surgical research fellow working with Zollinger at Ohio State in 1949, popularized the use of homogenized milk as an inexpensive, readily available, and easy to use jejunal diet [17]. Whereas whole milk with large fat globules caused cramps and diarrhea, homogenized milk with smaller, finely emulsified particles of fat was better tolerated. With the addition of vitamins, milk was considered a complete diet. For long-term jejunal feedings the diet was fortified with protein and starch hydrolysates.

Table 25-3. *Hollander Formula*

Items	Amount	
	Per Liter	Per 2400 Calories
Water	760 ml	1,824 ml
Amigen	85 gm	204 gm
Dexin	150 gm	360 gm
Cream (18.5%; density 1.01 at 19° C.)	85 ml	204 ml
Salt mixture[a]	10 gm	24 gm
Vitamins (minimum amounts)		
Halibut liver oil[b]	0.33 ml	0.8 ml
Blexin[b]	5.8 ml	14.0 ml
Ascorbic acid	63 mg	150 mg

[a]The salt mixture is prepared in the following proportions:

NaCl	100 gm	4.8 gm
KCl	100 gm	4.8 gm
$MgSO_4 .7 H_2O$	46 gm	2.2 gm
Ca gluconate. H_2O	100 gm	4.8 gm
Na_2HPO_4 dried	160 gm	7.0 gm (ca)

[b]International Vitamin Corp.
As prepared in our diet kitchen, the material is made up in larger quantities than this and distributed among a number of bottles, each containing about 900 ml of the mixture.
Source: F. Hollander, S. Rosenak, and R. Colp, A synthetic predigested aliment for jejunostomy feeding. *Surgery* 17:754, 1945.

Because of its simplicity, the homogenized milk diet and other diets with a milk base were widely used in the 1950s with mixed results. Lactose was the main carbohydrate source. Although at that time physicians did not know about lactase deficiency and lactose intolerance, individual patients' gastrointestinal tracts were not immune to this ignorance. The homogenized milk diet had a 15 percent incidence of cramps, bloating, and diarrhea [14].

Elemental Diet

In the 1970s the pharmaceutical laboratories made several complete liquid diets commercially available. One category of diets was low in osmolarity, but was made of complex proteins, carbohydrates, and a moderate amount of fat. These diets were marketed for oral and nasogastric administration to patients with normal gastrointestinal tracts. The other group of diets was high in osmolarity and had predigested proteins and carbohydrates. These elemental diets were recommended for patients with diseases of the gastrointestinal tract.

One of the elemental diets (Vivonex) underwent thorough investigation at the National Institutes of Health in 1965 as a diet useful for space travel [113]. The first use in patients was reported by Stephens and Randall in 1969 [93]. Vivonex HN* (Table 25-4) has been widely used for jejunal feeding. It is nutritionally complete, easily digested and absorbed, low in fat, lactose-free, easily dripped by gravity through small tubes, easy to prepare, and stable. Its drawbacks are its expense and high osmolarity secondary to the glucose oligosaccharides and individual amino acids. Despite these drawbacks, jejunal use of the diet has proved nutritionally beneficial in a wide variety of patients. The diet has particular advantages as a jejunal feeding after pancreatic operations because it is less stimulating to pancreatic secretions than other diets [18, 62, 75, 104].

*Eaton Laboratories, Norwich Pharmaceutical

Table 25-4. *Vivonex HN (Per Liter)**

Calories	1,000
Carbohydrates	
Glucose oligosaccharides	210 gm
Lactose	0
Protein	
L-amino acids (nitrogen)	42 gm (6.67 gm)
Fats	
Safflower oil (linoleic acid)	.44 gm
Osmolarity	844 mOsm

*Contains minerals, vitamins, and trace elements in normal dietary levels.

The search for the ideal diet continues. The high osmolarity and expense of Vivonex HN (its major drawbacks) could be eliminated by substituting a more complex protein or protein hydrolysates for the amino acids. Protein digestion is not usually a limiting factor in diet tolerance, and amino acids can be absorbed just as rapidly as peptides as in free form. The insertion and maintenance of a jejunostomy must be free of complications in order to justify its routine use. The needle catheter jejunostomy satisfies this criterion. The ideal jejunal diet should be able to be delivered through a fine catheter such as a needle catheter jejunostomy.

METHOD

The method of jejunal feeding has influenced its effectiveness and use. In 1885 Golding-Bird noted that a pint of jejunal formula caused severe attacks of indigestion, but that 10 ounces were well tolerated [38]. Despite this, Maydl in 1892 gave two massive feedings per day 5 or 6 hours apart [59]. In 1908 Eiselsberg documented the case of a 41-year-old woman who was fed for 6 years through a jejunal tube because of severe gastritis. She gained weight on a diet of milk, meat broth, gruel, and eggs that was given in 8 separate portions from 6:00 AM until 10:00 PM [31]. Most patients were fed by small bolus injections every 1 to 2 hours through a syringe [8].

Continual Drip

In 1922 Kelling reported the first jejunal feeding by gravity drip [48]. His patient was a 59-year-old woman who developed a lateral duodenal fistula after a Billroth I gastrectomy for cancer. A supplementary jejunostomy was performed, and 200 ml of a mixture of flour, eggs, and meat broth was dripped by gravity over 2 hours. The feeding was given several times each day and eventually increased to 500 ml over 2 hours. This method simulated the normal physiology of gastric emptying into the small intestine. In this country, gravity drip was first reported in 1932 by Stewart at the Massachusetts General Hospital [94]. A patient with a biliary fistula was fed the Scott-Ivy Pabulum and the fistula losses through a jejunostomy, receiving at one point 4000 calories and 10 liters of fluid per day.

In 1935 Wolfer at Northwestern University reported the first large clinical experience with the Scott-Ivy Pabulum as a jejunal feeding and suggested an infusion by continual gravity drip at a rate of 100 ml/hr for an entire 24-hour period [115]. The Hollander formula was also given by continual infusion [43, 44]. The homogenized milk diet was initially given by gravity drip, but after a period of adaptation, small bolus feedings of 200 ml were given approximately every 2 hours [14, 17].

When continual drip installation was adopted, mechanical pumps became important to ensure even delivery, to prevent sudden accidental infusions of large volume, and to prevent clogging of the tubes by the viscous diets. Several centers reported the use of "home engineered pumps" [21, 64, 92, 115]. Today a wide variety of pumps and controllers are available commercially.

The jejunum responds to a bolus of a hyperosmolar diet by the secretion of enough fluid to obtain isotonicity. Decreased plasma volume and increased levels of bradykinin and serotonin result and cause vascular and gastrointestinal side effects similar to the weakness, sweating, lightheadedness, hyperperistalsis, cramps, and diarrhea commonly seen in postgastrectomy patients with dumping syndrome. If hypertonic diets are delivered to the jejunum by gravity drip

Table 25-5. *Postoperative* Small Bowel Function*

	Author	Method	Observation
Motility	Hoyer [46]	Barium studies of stomach and small bowel, oral administration	Small bowel motility continues virtually without interruption; traditional "postoperative ileus" is limited to stomach for 24–48 hours and to colon for 3–5 days
	Wells [108, 109]	Auscultation Balloon kymography Barium studies administered orally or through nasojejunal tubes	
	Nachlas [69]	Barium studies administered orally or through nasojejunal tubes	
Absorption	Tinckler [101]	Tritiated water given through nasojejunal tubes	Normal absorption of water measured by venous samples
	Argyropoulous [9]	Xylose given orally in patients lying on right side after vagotomy and pyloroplasty	Normal absorption of xyloses measured by urine samples
	Tomkins [102]	Ringer's lactate delivered to jejunum through gastrojejunostomy tube	Normal functional extracellular fluid volume and Na^+ balance measured by ^{35}Sulfurisotope dilution method
	Glucksman [37]	Glucose, ^{22}NaCl, polyethyleneglycol (PEG) introduced into duodenum	Normal glucose and Na^+ absorption measured by venous samples and double-lumen duodenal tube
	Shoemaker [89]	Glucose, NaCl, PEG, inulin infused directly into jejunum by triple lumen nasojejunal tube	Normal absorption of water and Na^+ measured by triple-lumen technique

*Studies on patients within 24 hours of operation.
Source: J. A. Ryan, C. P. Page, and L. Babcock, Early postoperative jejunal feeding of elemental diet in gastrointestinal surgery. *Am. Surg.* 47:393, 1981.

or pump control at a rate of 1 to 2 ml/min (1,440 to 2,880 ml/day), the jejunum can achieve isotonicity of its contents by secretion without marked side effects. Full-strength Vivonex HN has 844 mOsm/liter. Its tolerance in the jejunum is dependent on a slow even rate of delivery and a gradual increase from dilute to full-strength concentration.

Patients' gastrointestinal tracts have varied tolerance to hyperosmotic diets, and a degree of adaptation occurs with time. Once the gastrointestinal tract becomes accustomed to the inflow of jejunal feedings, more leeway is possible with the rate, concentration, and constituents of the jejunal diet.

Early Postoperative Feeding

Today most jejunostomies are performed in conjunction with major abdominal operations. The question of how soon after the operation jejunal feedings can begin is important. Despite scientific and clinical experience to the contrary, surgeons generally believe that postoperative ileus after laparotomy or general anesthesia prevents small bowel use. However, ileus is limited to the stomach for 1 to 2 days and to the colon for 3 to 5 days postoperatively. Small bowel motility and absorption are present immediately [85] (Table 25-5). Vast clinical experience has confirmed that the small bowel can be used for

Table 25-6. *Early Postoperative Jejunal Feeding of Elemental Diet*[a] *(Guidelines for 70 Kg Adult)*

Postop Day	Strength	Rate (ml/hr)	24-hour Volume (ml)	24-hour Calories
1	1/3	50	1,200	400
2[b]	1/3	100	2,400	800
3	1/3	125	3,000	1000
4	1/2	125	3,000	1500
5	2/3	125	3,000	2000
6	3/4	125	3,000	2250
7	1	125 (Reduce rate when patient eating)	3,000	3000

[a]Vivonex HN—Add 1 ampule of vitamins and 40 mEq KCl each day when concentration is less than full strength (1 cal/ml).
[b]Intravenous needle discontinued.

both fluid and nutrition as early as the first postoperative day if gastric decompression is also used [7, 8, 13, 14, 17, 22, 24, 27, 43, 45, 52, 63, 68, 78, 80, 85, 86, 94, 97, 115].

How early postoperatively the jejunal feeding is begun determines how soon anabolic recovery begins, but more important than a few extra days of nutritional advantage is the assurance of jejunal access should prolonged nutritional support become necessary.* Intrinsic small bowel disease, extensive adhesions, partial small bowel obstruction, and peritonitis prevent early postoperative feeding.

Our guidelines for early postoperative jejunal feeding of elemental diet are listed in Table 25-6. The physician orders the elemental diet daily, specifying concentration and rate. The pharmacy prepares a 24-hour supply of elemental diet, packaging it in four disposable plastic containers, each appropriate for 6 hours of feeding. Electrolytes can be added to the diet as needed. Food coloring prevents any confusion with intravenous fluid. The nursing staff administers the elemental diet through a drip chamber and tubing normally used for intravenous fluids. Pumps or controllers are optional (Figure 25-7 A, B). The patient is monitored for input and output, gastrointestinal tolerance, glucose tolerance, electrolyte balance, calorie count, and daily weight.

Nutritional support services organized institutionally for the administration of total parenteral nutrition should also concern themselves with enteral feedings. A team of physicians, dietitians, pharmacists, and nurses who establish protocols, select diets and equipment, control costs, and keep abreast of developments in the field, can greatly benefit patients receiving tube feedings.

*One noteworthy example of early jejunal feeding was reported by the Russian army surgeon Panikov in World War II. During explorations of abdominal battle wounds he introduced a trocar into the jejunum and fed a mixture of milk, butter, eggs, sugar, salt, and distilled alcohol. He claimed great benefit including early wound healing that allowed soldiers to return to battle [74].

RESULTS

The early reports of jejunal feeding were case examples that explained indications, techniques, complications, and subjective evaluations of nutritional worth. The first prospective survey of the nutritional value of jejunal feedings came in the 1940s, when early postoperative feeding through nasojejunal tubes resulted in positive

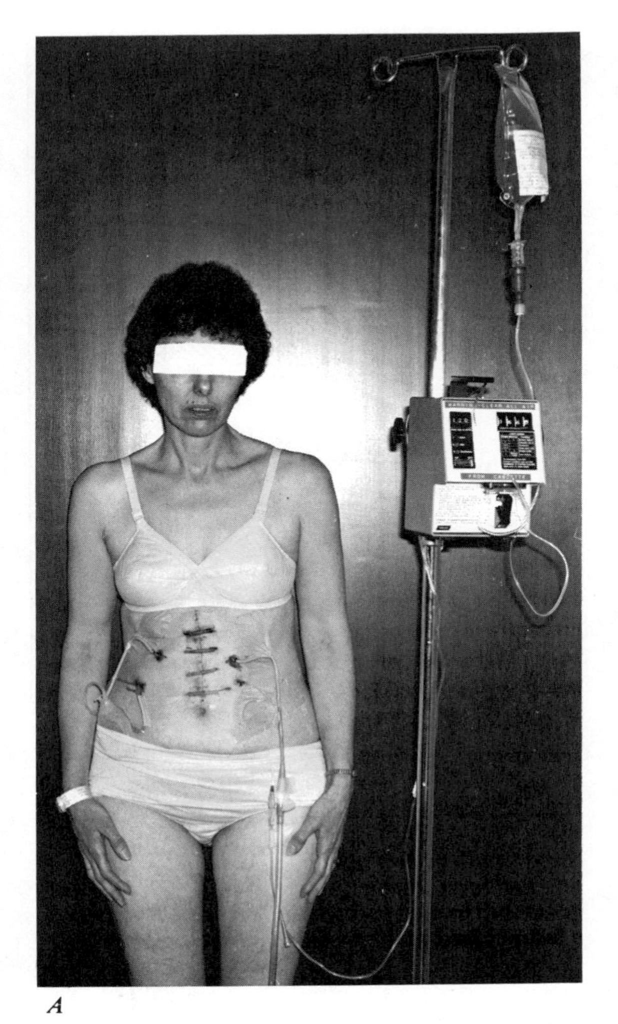

A

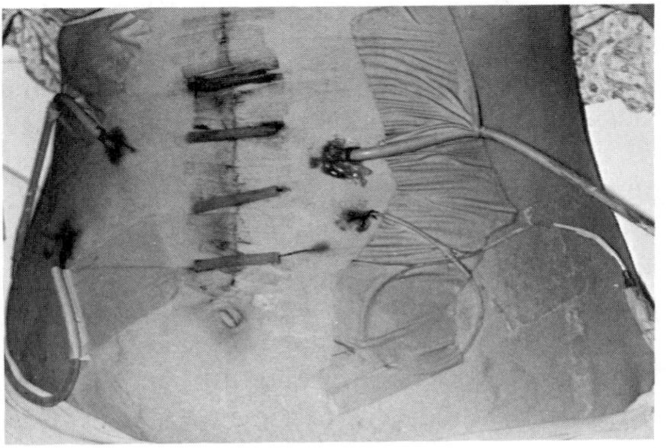

B

nitrogen balance in small series of patients undergoing gastrectomy [22, 68, 80].

The nutritional benefits of early postoperative feeding of elemental diet through a needle catheter jejunostomy have been reported more recently. In a randomized series of patients undergoing colectomy, the group with jejunal feeding received a daily total mean for the first 10 postoperative days of 2283 calories and 14.1 gm nitrogen compared to 800 calories and 3.4 gm nitrogen for the group receiving standard intravenous therapy. The patients with jejunal feeding lost 2.4 percent of their body weight in one month compared to 6.1 percent weight lost for the control patients. Jejunal feeding did not suppress appetite [85].

Twenty consecutive patients undergoing major upper gastrointestinal operations received a daily mean of 1468 calories and 9.7 gm nitrogen jejunally for the first 10 postoperative days. Mean total intake, including oral food, was 1890 calories and 11.7 gm nitrogen per day for the first 10 postoperative days. Mean postoperative weight loss at 2 and 4 weeks was 2.8 percent and 3.5 percent of preoperative weight [85]. Ten patients received jejunal elemental diet for longer than one month because of postoperative complications or adjunctive therapy for cancer. The mean weight loss in this group was 2.8 percent. Figure 25-8 is an example [85].

Positive nitrogen balance was achieved and weight was preserved by the use of early postoperative jejunal feeding of elemental diet in a randomized series of patients undergoing a variety of extensive esophageal, gastroduodenal, hepatobiliary, and pancreatic procedures. Mean cumulative 10-day nitrogen balance in 26 patients in the group receiving jejunal feedings was positive 13.4 gm. Mean weight loss was less than one

Figure 25-7. *A. A 42-year-old woman receiving elemental diet by continual pump administration through a needle catheter jejunostomy after cholecystectomy, common duct exploration, and lesser sac drainage for necrotizing pancreatitis. B. A close-up view. Note gastrostomy tube, biliary tube, and pancreatic drain.*

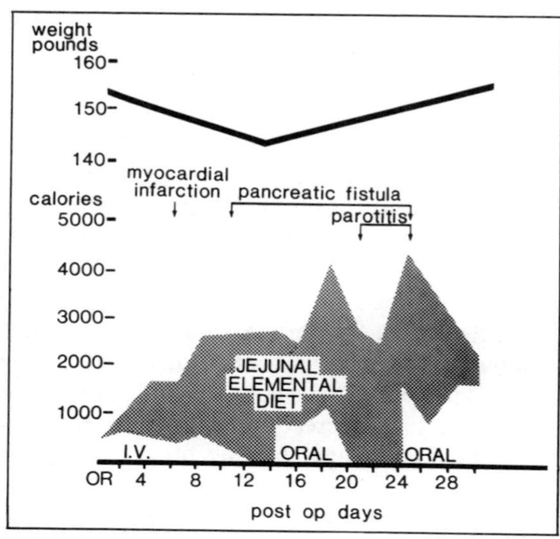

Figure 25-8. *Record of a 58-year-old man who received early feeding through a needle catheter jejunostomy after a Whipple procedure for carcinoma. Note caloric intake and weight preservation despite complications. (From J. A. Ryan, C. P. Page, and L. Babcock, Early postoperative jejunal feeding of elemental diet in gastrointestinal surgery.* Am. Surg. *47:393, 1981.)*

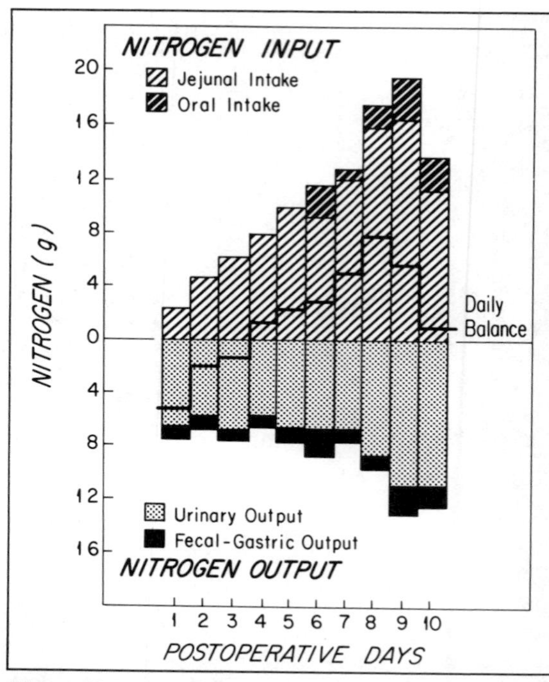

Figure 25-9. *Record of a 53-year-old woman who received early jejunal feeding after a 75 percent distal pancreatectomy, cholecystectomy, and transduodenal sphincteroplasty. She achieved positive nitrogen balance on the fourth postoperative day and had a 10-day cumulative nitrogen balance of positive 17 gm.*

pound. Mean cumulative 10-day nitrogen balance for 22 control patients treated with standard intravenous therapy was negative 45 gm. Mean weight loss was 8 pounds. Study patients required intravenous needles for only 2 days compared to 8 days for the controls [45]. Figure 25-9 gives an example of nitrogen balance in a patient receiving early postoperative jejunal feeding after pancreatic resection.

Besides the nutritional advantages, early postoperative jejunal feeding fulfills fluid requirements. It permits early discontinuance of intravenous catheters with avoidance of patient discomfort, catheter sepsis, sepsis related to contamination of intravenous infusions, catheter thrombophlebitis, and suppurative thrombophlebitis. The necessity of restarting intravenous catheters is also eliminated, decreasing the workload of the intravenous nursing teams.

With a jejunal catheter in place the necessity for nutrition via central venous catheters with their mechanical, thrombotic, septic, and metabolic hazards can often be avoided [83, 84]. Enteral feeding is less expensive than parenteral nutrition. Page has demonstrated the cost effectiveness of routine needle catheter jejunostomy in complex upper abdominal operations. Without access to the jejunum, a certain percentage of these patients would require total parenteral nutrition postoperatively. The savings in these patients because of jejunal feedings justify routine postoperative jejunal feeding in this type of case [73]. In addition, enteral feedings in comparison to total parenteral nutrition are more physiologic, require less laboratory monitoring, are more easily adapted to home use, and provide greater versatility because the catheter does not occlude with intermittent use. Enteral support is feasible in institutions of any size.

Whether the prevention of weight loss and negative nitrogen balance is an important goal that surgeons should strive for in the early postoperative period is unknown. Supplemental nutrients add little to wound healing in most patients. The rehabilitation of patients undergoing major abdominal operations depends to a large extent on physical activity, exercise tolerance, and motivation. Whether additional nutritional support reduces postoperative weakness, improves exercise tolerance, and prompts an early return to full function has not been established. The main benefit of complementary jejunostomy and early postoperative jejunal feeding occurs in malnourished patients who undergo major operative insults and who have prolonged postoperative recoveries due to complications.

The techniques of jejunostomy were well established by the turn of the century, when tubes were placed for palliation of far-advanced gastric cancer, and normal foods were given at varying intervals. The situation was stable until 1930 except for the occasional use of jejunostomy as the primary treatment of peptic ulcer disease. For most gastric procedures performed from 1900 until 1930, postoperative treatment consisted of nutrient and saline enemas and subcutaneous infusion of fluid. Standard intravenous therapy, as we know it today, did not begin in earnest until the late 1930s, and because of pyrogens, fear of fluid overload, and unavailability, it did not become routine until the late 1940s and 1950s.

Between 1930 and 1950, jejunal feedings had their greatest use. Gastrectomy was applied widely for cancer and ulcer in patients who often were dehydrated and malnourished. The importance of hypoproteinemia and malnutrition on postoperative morbidity and mortality was established, and the inability of subcutaneous infusion and nutrient enemas to counteract malnutrition was recognized. Jejunostomy or nasojejunal tubes were recommended for routine use after gastric operations. During this period the major advances in jejunal diets and methods of feeding were accomplished. Attention was paid to ensuring adequate amounts of nutrients, minerals, and vitamins, and to finding diets that were easily tolerated by the jejunum. Important in these developments was the collaboration of surgeons with physiologists, gastroenterologists, pharmacologists, and members of industry.

After 1950 the influence of routine postoperative jejunal feedings waned. Intravenous fluid therapy became widely available, safe, and familiar to the surgical profession. The practice of gastric resection decreased because of the decreasing incidence of gastric cancer and the use of vagotomy and drainage for ulcer. Earlier referral for operation resulted in patients with less debility and malnutrition. By 1970, with the widespread endorsement of total parenteral nutrition, fewer jejunostomies were perceived as necessary.

During the same period, however, an increased number of operations on the pancreas, esophagus, and hepatobiliary tree brought a new group of poorly nourished patients to face major operative procedures and catabolic postoperative courses. A resurgence of interest in nutrition, in part a byproduct of the developments in total parenteral nutrition, created a renaissance of intestinal application for nourishing postoperative patients. The complex dietary preparations of the 1930s and 1940s were replaced by commercial diets that were easy to prepare and use.

This chapter has concluded that needle catheter jejunostomy, established during major upper abdominal operations as a route for elemental diet by continual drip, can fulfill protein, caloric, and fluid requirements early postoperatively so as to achieve positive nitrogen balance and avoid weight loss and dehydration while securing an avenue for long-term feeding. The technique is simple and safe and is recommended to surgeons in their operative procedures in the upper abdomen.

REFERENCES

1. Abbott, W. O., and Rawson, A. J. A tube for use in the postoperative care of gastroenterostomy cases. *J.A.M.A.* 108:1874, 1937.
2. Abbott, W. O., and Rawson, A. J. Tube for use in postoperative care of gastroenterostomy patients—a correction. *J.A.M.A.* 112:2414, 1939.
3. Abbott, W. O. Fluid and nutritional maintenance by the use of an intestinal tube. *Ann. Surg.* 112:584, 1940.
4. Allen, A. W., and Welch, C. E. Jejunostomy for the relief of malfunctioning gastroenterostomy stoma. *Surgery* 9:163, 1941.
5. Allen, A. W., and Donaldson, G. Jejunostomy for decompression of the postoperative stomach. *Surgery* 15:565, 1944.
6. Andrassy, R. J., Page, C. P., Feldtman, R. W., Haff, R. C., Ryan, J. A., and Ratner, J. A. Continual catheter administration of an elemental diet in infants and children. *Surgery* 82:205, 1977.
7. Andrassy, R. J., Mahour, G. H., Harrison, M. R., Muenchow, S. K., Mishalany, H. G., and Woolley, M. M. The role and safety of early postoperative feeding in the pediatric surgical patient. *J. Pediatr. Surg.* 14:381, 1979.
8. Andresen, A. F. R. Immediate jejunal feeding after gastroenterostomy. *Ann. Surg.* 67:565, 1918.
9. Argyropoulous, G. D., and White, M. E. E. Gastrointestinal functioning following vagotomy and pyloroplasty. *Arch. Surg.* 93:578, 1966.
10. Baker, J. W. A long jejunostomy tube for decompressing intestinal obstruction. *Surg. Gynecol. Obstet.* 109:519, 1959.
11. Baker, J. W., and Ritter, K. J. Complete surgical decompression for late obstruction of the small intestine, with reference to a method. *Ann. Surg.* 157:759, 1963.
12. Barber, W. H. Jejunostomy. *Ann. Surg.* 97:553, 1933.
13. Bisgard, J. D. Gastrostomy—jejunal intubation. *Surg. Gynecol. Obstet.* 74:239, 1942.
14. Boles, T., and Zollinger, R. M. Critical evaluation of jejunostomy. *Arch. Surg.* 65:358, 1952.
15. Brintall, E. S., Daum, K., and Womack, N. A. Maydl jejunostomy. *Arch. Surg.* 65:367, 1952.
16. Busch, W. Beitrag zur Physiology der Verdauungsorgane. *Virchow's Arch.* 14:140, 1858.
17. Case, C. T., Zollinger, R. M., McMullen, C. H., and Brown, J. B. Observations in jejunal alimentation. *Surgery* 26:364, 1949.
18. Cassim, M. M., and Allardyce, D. B. Pancreatic secretion in response to jejunal feeding of elemental diet. *Ann. Surg.* 170:228, 1974.
19. Clute, H. M., and Bell, L. M. Jejunostomy for postoperative feeding. *Ann. Surg.* 114:462, 1941.
20. Colp, R., and Druckerman, L. J. The indication for jejunal alimentation in the surgery of peptic ulcer. *Ann. Surg.* 117:387, 1943.
21. Cornell, A., and Hollander, F. An improved continuous drip apparatus with special reference to the use of alumina gels in the therapy of peptic ulcer. *Rev. Gastroenterol.* 9:354, 1942.
22. CoTui, Wright, A. M., Mulholland, J. H., Carabba, V., Barcham, I., and Vinci, V. J. Studies on surgical convalescence. *Surgery* 120: 99, 1944.
23. Delany, H. M., Carnevale, N. J., and Garvey, J. W. Jejunostomy by a needle catheter technique. *Surgery* 73:786, 1973.
24. Delany, H. M., Carnevale, N., Garvey, J. W., and Moss, C. M. Postoperative nutritional support using needle catheter jejunostomy. *Ann. Surg.* 186:165, 1977.
25. Dobbie, R. P., and Hoffmeister, J. A. Continuous pump-tube enteric hyperalimentation. *Surg. Gynecol. Obstet.* 143:273, 1976.
26. Downes, W. A. Jejunostomy: Its value in the treatment of certain ulcers of the stomach and as a palliative measure in inoperable carcinoma of the stomach. *Surg. Clin. North Am.* 1:1619, 1921.
27. Ehrenpreis, T., and Sandblom, P. Duodenal atresia and stenosis. *Acta Paediat.* (Stockholm) 38:109, 1949.
28. Einhorn, M. Duodenal alimentation. *Med. Rec.* 78:92, 1910.
29. Einhorn, M. A case of perforation of the duodenum treated successfully by duodenal (jejunal) alimentation. *Med. Rec.* 94:927, 1918.
30. Eiselsberg, A. F. Ueber Ausschaltung inoperabler Pylorus-Stricturen nebst Bemerkungen uber die Jejunostomie. *Arch. Klin. Chir.* 50:919, 1895.
31. Eiselsberg, A. A case of linitis plastica of the stomach (Brinton) cured by jejunostomy. *Surg. Gynecol. Obstet.* 7:254, 1908.
32. Eiselsberg, A. Zur Ausschaltung des Magens-durch die Jejunostomie. *Arch. Klin. Chir.* 112: 1026, 1919.
33. Eusterman, G. B. Deficiency disease developing during the course of jejunal feeding. *Proc. Staff Meet. Mayo Clin.* 4:285, 1929.
34. Fallis, L. S., and Barron, J. Gastric and jejunal alimentation with fine polyethylene tubes. *AMA Arch. Surg.* 65:373, 1952.
35. Freeman, J. B., Egan, M. C., and Millis, B. J. The elemental diet. *Surg. Gynecol. Obstet.* 142: 925, 1976.

36. Gibson, C. L. The creation of an artificial valvula-fistula (b) as an adjunct to certain operations on the stomach. *M.&S.J.* 147:341, 1902.
37. Glucksman, D. L., Kalser, M. H., and Warren, W. D. Small intestine absorption in the immediate postoperative period. *Surgery* 60:1020, 1966.
38. Golding-Bird, C. H. Jejunostomy. *Br. Med. J.* 2:1063, 1885.
39. Heyd, C. G. Jejunostomy. *Am. J. Surg.* 1:188, 1926.
40. Hicken, F., Coray, Q. B., Snow, S., and Jackson, E. G. Complete duodenal obstruction in the newborn. *Am. J. Surg.* 111:461, 1946.
41. Hillman, O. S. Jejunostomy in the treatment of massive gastric ulcer. *Br. Med. J.* 1:221, 1933.
42. Hofmeister, F. *Verhandl. D. Naturf. Aerzte* 77:95, 1905.
43. Hollander, F., Rosenak, S., and Colp, R. A synthetic predigested aliment for jejunostomy feeding. *Surgery* 17:754, 1945.
44. Hollander, F., and Sober, H. A. A modified synthetic predigested aliment for protracted jejunostomy feeding. *Surgery* 25:500, 1949.
45. Hoover, H. C., Ryan, J. A., Anderson, E. J., and Fischer, J. E. Nutritional benefits of immediate postoperative jejunal feeding of elemental diet. *Am. J. Surg.* 139:153, 1980.
46. Hoyer, A. Abdominal distention and intestinal activity following laparotomy. *Acta. Radiol.* [Suppl.] 83:1, 1950.
47. Kader, B. Zur Technik der Gastrostomie. *Zentralbl. Chir.* 23:665, 1896.
48. Kelling, G. Zur Verschluss der Duodenal fistel nach Magenresektion. *Zentralbl. Chir.* 49:779, 1922.
49. Keoshian, L. A., and Nelsen, T. S. A new design for a feeding tube. *Plast. Reconstr. Surg.* 44:508, 1969.
50. Kirschner, M. Die Prophylaktische Jejunostomie bei Magenoperation. *Arch. Klin. Chir.* 157:561, 1929.
51. Lawson, D. W., Daggett, W. M., Civetta, J. M., et al. Surgical treatment of acute necrotizing pancreatitis. *Ann. Surg.* 172:605, 1970.
52. Lee, M. Intra-alimentary drip feeding following partial gastrectomy. *Postgrad. Med. J.* 33:78, 1957.
53. Lee, R. J., and Gould, P. Cancer of the pyloris and duodenum; jejunostomy; death. *Lancet* 2: 1092, 1885.
54. Lempp, H. Ueber den Werth der Jejunostomie. *Arch. Klin. Chir.* 76:323, 1905.
55. Liffmann, K. E., and Randall, H. T. A modified technique for creating a jejunostomy. *Surg. Gynecol. Obstet.* 134:663, 1972.
56. Lilienthal, H. Inoperable indurated ulcer of lesser curvature of stomach: Jejunostomy. *Ann. Surg.* 61:496, 1915.
57. Linton, R. R. Enterostomy. *Am. J. Surg.* 25:55, 1934.
58. Long, J. W. Enterostomy, a perfected technique. *J.A.M.A.* 68:833, 1917.
59. Maydl, K. Ueber eine neue Methode zur Ausfuhrung der Jejunostomie und Gastroenterostomie. *Wiener Med. Wochen Schr.* 42:740, 1892.
60. Mayo, W. J. Jejunostomy. *Am. J. Med. Sci.* 143:469, 1912.
61. Mayo-Robson, A. W. Jejunal and gastrojejunal ulcers. *Br. Med. J.* 1:1, 1912.
62. McArdle, A. H., Echave, W., Brown, R. A., and Thompson, A. G. Effect of elemental diet on pancreatic secretion. *Am. J. Surg.* 128:690, 1974.
63. McDonald, H. A. Intrajejunal drip in gastric surgery. *Lancet* 1:1007, 1954.
64. Mensing, E. H. Jejunal feeding in the treatment of "stubborn" duodenal ulcers; and other indications for jejunostomy. *Wis. Med. J.* 32:168, 1933.
65. Morawitz, P., and Henning, N. Uber Jejunale Ernahrung. *Klin. Woch.* April 9, 1929. Pp. 681–683.
66. Moss, G., Bievenbaum, A., Bova, F., and Slavin, J. A. Postoperative metabolic patterns following immediate total nutritional support; hormone levels, DNA synthesis, nitrogen balance, and accelerated wound healing. *J. Surg. Res.* 21:383, 1976.
67. Moynihan, B. G. A. The operation of jejunostomy, with a report of two cases. *Br. Med. J.* 1:1599, 1902.
68. Mulholland, J. H., CoTui, Wright, A. M., and Vinci, V. J. Nitrogen metabolism, calorie intake and weight loss in postoperative convalescence. A study of eight patients undergoing partial gastrectomy for duodenal ulcer. *Ann. Surg.* 117:512, 1943.
69. Nachlas, M. M., Younis, M. T., Roda, C. P., and Wityk, J. J. Gastrointestinal motility studies as a guide to postoperative management. *Ann. Surg.* 175:510, 1972.
70. Pack, G. T., and McNeer, G. Palliative operations for gastric cancer. *Rev. Gastroenterol.* 16:291, 1949.
71. Page, C. P., Ryan, J. A., and Haff, R. C. Continual catheter administration of an elemental diet. *Surg. Gynecol. Obstet.* 142:184, 1976.
72. Page, C. P., Carlton, P. K., Andrassy, R. J., Feldtman, R. W., and Ryan, J. A. Safety of

operative needle-catheter gastrointestinal intubation for the administration of elemental diet. Presented August 28, 1978, International Society of Parenteral Nutrition, Rio De Janeiro. *J. Par. Ent. Nutr.* 2:194, 1978.
73. Page, C. P., Carlton, P. K., Andrassy, R. J., Feldtman, R. W., and Shield, C. F. Safe, cost effective postoperative nutrition: Defined formula diet via needle-catheter jejunostomy. Presented at Southwestern Surgical Congress, April 26, 1979, Las Vegas. *Am. J. Surg.* 138:939, 1979.
74. Panikov, P. A. Spasokukotski's method of feeding abdominal wounds. *Am. Rev. Soviet Med.* 1:32, 1943.
75. Ragins, H., Levenson, S. M., Singer, R., et al. Intrajejunal administration of an elemental diet at neutral pH avoids pancreatic stimulation. *Am. J. Surg.* 126:606, 1973.
76. Ravdin, I. S. Anatomical exposure for jejunostomy. *Surg. Gynecol. Obstet.* 40:426, 1925.
77. Ravdin, I. S., Stengel, A., Jr., and Prushankin, M. Control of hypoproteinimia in surgical patients. *J.A.M.A.* 114:107, 1940.
78. Ravdin, I. S., Royster, H. P., Riegel, C., and Rhoads, J. E. Surgical care of patients with gastric cancer before and after operation. *Arch. Surg.* 46:871, 1943.
79. Rhoades, J. E. Riegel, D., Koop, C. E., and Ravdin, I. S. The problem of nutrition in patients with gastric lesions requiring surgery. *West. J. Surg. Obstet. Gynecol.* 51:229, 1943.
80. Riegel, C., Koop, C. E., Drew, J., Stevens, L. W., and Rhoads, J. E. The nutritional requirements for nitrogen balance in surgical patients during early postoperative period. *J. Clin. Invest.* 26:18, 1947.
81. Robertson, G. J. A case of fibrous stricture of the pylorus, enterostomy, death. *Br. Med. J.* 1:376, 1885.
82. Rosenak, S., and Hollander, F. Surgical jejunostomy for alimentation. A historical review. *Clinics* 3:638, 1944.
83. Ryan, J. A., Abel, R. M., Abbott, W. M., et al. Catheter complications in total parenteral nutrition: A prospective study of 200 consecutive patients. *N. Engl. J. Med.* 280:757, 1974.
84. Ryan, J. A. Complications of total parenteral nutrition. In J. E. Fischer (Ed.), *Total Parenteral Nutrition.* Boston: Little, Brown, 1976.
85. Ryan, J. A., Page, C. P., and Babcock, L. Early postoperative jejunal feeding of elemental diet in gastrointestinal surgery. *Am. Surg.* 47:393, 1981.
86. Sagar, R., Harland, P., and Shields, R. Early postoperative feeding with elemental diet. *Br. Med. J.* 1:293, 1979.
87. Scott, H. G., and Ivy, A. C. Jejunal alimentation; an experimental study in dogs. *Ann. Surg.* 93:1197, 1931.
88. Senn, N. *Intestinal Surgery.* Chicago: W. T. Keener, 1889.
89. Shoemaker, C. P., and Wright, H. K. Rate of water and sodium absorption from jejunum after abdominal surgery in man. *Am. J. Surg.* 119:62, 1970.
90. Stamm, M. Gastrostomy by a new method. *Med. News* 65:324, 1894.
91. Stengel, A., Jr., and Ravdin, I. S. Maintenance of nutrition in surgical patients with a description of orojejunal method of feeding. *Surgery* 61:511, 1939.
92. Stengel, A., and Vars, H. M. An apparatus for continuous intravenous injection in unanesthetized animals. *J. Lab. Clin. Med.* 24:525, 1935.
93. Stephens, R. V., and Randall, H. T. Use of concentrated, balanced liquid elemental diet for nutritional management of catabolic states. *Ann. Surg.* 170:642, 1969.
94. Steward, J. D. Gravity feeding by jejunostomy. *Ann. Surg.* 96:225, 1932.
95. Steward, J. D., Hale, H. W., and Schaer, S. M. Management of protein deficiency in surgical patients. *J.A.M.A.* 136:1017, 1948.
96. Stieda, A. Uber die Vorbereitung und Nachbehandlung bei Magenoperation. *Arch. Klin. Chir.* 63:715, 1901.
97. Stone, H. H. Transanastomotic jejunal feeding of newborn infants. *Am. J. Surg.* 123:63, 1972.
98. Studley, H. O. Percentage of weight loss, a basic indicator of surgical risk. *J.A.M.A.* 106:458, 1936.
99. Surmay, M. De l'enterostomie. *Bull. Gen. Ther.* 94:445, 1878.
100. Surmay, M. Observation d'enterostomie. *Bull. Gen. Ther.* 95:198, 1878.
101. Tinckler, L. F., and Kulke, W. Postoperative absorption of water from the small intestines. *Gut* 4:8, 1963.
102. Tomkins, R. K., Kraft, A. R., and Zollinger, R. M. Alternate method of surgical fluid administration. *J. Surg. Res.* 8:397, 1968.
103. Usher, R. C. Use of the polyethylene catheter for jejunostomy feeding. *Am. J. Surg.* 82:408, 1951.
104. Voitk, M. D., Brown, R. A., Echave, V., McArdle, A. H., Gurd, F. M., and Thompson, A. G. Use of an elemental diet in the treatment of complicated pancreatitis. *Am. J. Surg.* 125:223, 1973.
105. Walker, I. J. Jejunostomy. *Bost. Med. Surg. J.* 186:108, 1922.
106. Walters, W., and Hartman, H. R. Preoperative

and postoperative care of patients with lesions of the stomach and of the duodenum. *Arch. Surg.* 40:1063, 1940.

107. Warshaw, A. L., Imbembo, A. L., Civetta, J. M., and Daggett, W. M. Surgical intervention in acute necrotizing pancreatitis. *Am. J. Surg.* 127:484, 1974.
108. Wells, C. A., Rawlinson, K., Tinckler, L., Jones, H., and Saunders, J. Ileus and postoperative intestinal motility. *Lancet* 2:136, 1961.
109. Wells, C., Rawlinson, K., Tinckler, L., Jones, H., and Saunders, J. Postoperative gastrointestinal motility. *Lancet* 1:4, 1964.
110. Wesson, H. R. Postoperative gastric retention treated by jejunostomy for feeding. *Proc. Staff Meet. Mayo Clin.* 12:747, 1937.
111. White, T. T., and Heimbach, D. M. Sequestrectomy and hyperalimentation in the treatment of hemorrhagic pancreatitis. *Am. J. Surg.* 132: 270, 1976.
112. Wilkinson, A. W., Hughes, E. A., and Stevens, I. H. Neonatal duodenal obstruction; the influence of treatment on the metabolic effects of operation. *Br. J. Surg.* 52:410, 1965.
113. Winitz, M., Graff, J., Gallager, N., et al. Evaluation of chemical diets as nutrition for man in space. *Nature* 205:741, 1965.
114. Witzel, O. I. Zur Technik der Magenfistelanlegung. *Zentralbl. Chir.* 18:601, 1891.
115. Wolfer, J. A. Jejunostomy with jejunal alimentation. *Ann. Surg.* 101:708, 1935.

A Critical Evaluation of the Results of Total Parenteral Nutrition in Various Disease States: Cost and Benefit

J. Thomas Goodgame, Jr.

26

It is both fitting and paradoxical to conclude a book on surgical nutrition with an evaluation of the applicability of the major technical advance in this field. It has been made abundantly clear that techniques for maintaining nutritional integrity are now available regardless of the severity of the illness or the organ system failure that may supervene. As the technical questions are answered (how to?), operational questions take their place (whether to?). The contributions of others (outlined in preceding chapters) have demonstrated the feasibility of parenteral nutrition in major burns, neoplasia, inflammatory disease, sepsis, and trauma with minimal added morbidity. The relative benefit of the necessary expenditures of money, personnel, and time has not been as clearly demonstrated. At this time, some critical assessment of the efficacy of total parenteral nutrition (TPN) seems appropriate to define its role as "optimal care" and to define areas in which resources may be pointed in other directions without detriment to patients. Other areas of medical technical advances have had to wrestle with these considerations (e.g., hemodialysis, extensive surgery for aggressive neoplasia, antibiotics given prophylactically), and there has often been no clear-cut answer to the dilemma of when the use of the technique was justified.

The cost of parenteral nutrition is much more easily quantified than its benefits. The real cost of parenteral nutrition is approximately 150 to 300 dollars a day. This includes solutions, specialized nursing, physician's fees, intravenous and pharmaceutical supplies, and pump rentals. This excludes the cost of the hospital room, "standard" laboratory and x-ray examinations, and "standard" nursing and physician intervention. The complications of the procedure are, in most centers, minimal, but must be included in any assessment of the cost of the technique. One to four percent of the catheter insertions result in some misadventure: pneumothorax, hydrothorax, thrombosis of the subclavian or internal jugular vein, air embolism, and so on. The true incidence of great vein thrombosis is not known, but it is likely to be higher than the 4% incidence mentioned, possibly between 5–10%. Whether subclavian thrombosis is decreased in man by use of silastic catheters, as suggested by animal experiments, is not clear. Three to seven percent of the catheters inserted have to be removed for septic complications [52]. It is hard to quantify these events as to their effect on cost, but the number of patients involved makes the contribution to overall expense slight. Home hyperalimentation has been estimated to cost approximately 20,000 to 36,000 dollars per year or about one-third the cost of a similar period of in-hospital care [16].

Quantification of the benefits of parenteral nutrition involves at least two definitional questions. First, in order to benefit the patient, does parenteral nutrition have to improve the outcome of the illness or does it simply have to maintain or restore nutritional integrity? It is appropriate here to specifically assert that nutritional health is, in general, to be preferred to the state of malnutrition (though the differentiation is often difficult), and TPN is unquestionably able to maintain some semblance of nutritional integrity.

For purposes of argument, TPN will be assumed to be superb therapy for borderline or abnormal nutrition. It is not ideal, to be sure, but that is not the issue. Our task is to examine the data for alteration in disease outcome by parenteral nutrition. Our contention would be that as a therapeutic or support modality, TPN should alter the course of an illness in some quantifiable way apart from restoration of parameters of nutritional integrity before it can be considered unequivocally beneficial in the management scheme of individual patients. Obviously, subjective clinical criteria, such as feelings of well-being, are important considerations, but contributions in terms of mortality, morbidity, complications, and length of hospital stay should assume primary importance in our assessment. Second, when one speaks of benefits to the patient, it must be specified to what modality of treatment TPN is being compared. In many conditions, the options for nutritional management are at least three other than TPN: starvation, semi-starvation with standard IV fluids ± suboptimal IV nutritional supplements, and enteral support with dietary supplements or tube feedings. Much of the clinical data generated by the extensive experience with TPN has been compared to the first of these modalities (if any controls have been attempted at all). Too often, however, enthusiastic accolades about the contributions of TPN to patient care in a particular disease entity emerge without identifiable control groups with which to evaluate end results. The following represents an attempt at critical analysis of the existing clinical data regarding the contribution of parenteral nutrition in particular pathologic situations in humans.

PEDIATRIC PROBLEMS

Because of the rapid growth rate, low nutritional reserve, and fear of irreversible neurologic damage secondary to malnutrition, pediatricians have enthusiastically adopted parenteral nutrition in critically ill infants [66].

The major problems in the pediatric age group that have been treated with total parenteral nutrition in a primary or adjunctive setting are very-low-birth-weight infants, respiratory distress syndrome, intractable diarrhea in infancy, and major surgery of the gastrointestinal (GI) tract in infants.

Very-Low-Birth-Weight Infants

Heird and Winters [33] published an uncontrolled series of 14 consecutive low-birth-weight infants (mean, 863 gm, range 720 to 1,150 gm) fed intravenously for an average of 18 days (range 5 to 24 days). In 8 of these infants, an intake of 100 calories/kg/day was possible for 15.5 days. Of the 14 in which the protocol was begun, 8 survived (5 died of respiratory insufficiency and 1 of sepsis). After follow-up of 18 to 39 months, 3 are normal neurologically, 2 are definitely abnormal, and 2 are "suspect." When compared to historical controls (Table 26-1) from 2 years prior to the use of parenteral nutrition, the efficacy of TPN in producing growth and positive nitrogen balance is unequivocal. The contribution to the outcome in these patients is less convincing.

Table 26-1. *Comparison of Standard Nutritional Management and TPN in Infants of Less than 1200 gm*

	Standard Management		TPN
Number of infants	23		14
Birth weight (gm)	943		863
Average daily weight gain (gm)	20.0		21.1
Time to regain body weight	18.2d	$p < .01$	8.9d
Time to achieve discharge weight	76.4d		79.8d
Age of nonsurvivors	7.3d		27.3d
Mortality rate	56.5%	$p < .01$	42.9%

Source: W. C. Heird and R. W. Winters, Total parenteral nutrition: The state of the art. *J. Pediatr.* 86:2, 1975.

Table 26-2. *Influence of Nutritional Support on Late Growth and Development of Survivors of Infant Respiratory Distress Syndrome*

	No TPN	Percentile	TPN	Percentile
Six months				
Height Index	1.06 ± 0.29	50–75	1.09 ± 0.26	50–75
Weight Index	1.01 ± 0.38	50–75	1.02 ± 0.32	50–70
One year				
Height Index	1.00 ± 0.23	50	1.00 ± 0.18	50
Weight Index	0.99 ± 0.42	50	0.88 ± 0.23	25–50

Source: T. Gunn, G. Reaman, E. W. Outerbridge, and E. Colle. Peripheral total parenteral nutrition for premature infants with the respiratory distress syndrome: A controlled study. *J. Pediatr.* 92:608, 1978.

Respiratory Distress Syndrome

Gunn et al. [30], examined 40 premature infants with respiratory distress syndrome and randomly assigned them to TPN (about 80 calories/kg/day) or no TPN (about 56 calories/kg/day) groups. The clinical characteristics (sex, birth weight, number of infants less than 1,500 gm, and gestational age) were similar in 2 groups. The mortality in the TPN group (3 of 20) was not significantly different from that of the no TPN group (6 of 20). However, the increased number of deaths in the no TPN group were due to an increased number of deaths in infants weighing less than 1,500 gm. Five of 8 died in the no TPN group and 2 of 7 died in the TPN group. All of these deaths occurred in the first 10 days of life. Table 26-2 evaluates the somatic growth of the survivors of the 2 groups at 6 and 12 months. No differences are detectable. There were 2 survivors with severe neurologic deficits, both in the TPN group.

The survival rate in the less than 1,500 gm group (37%) without TPN is consistent with other series [19] and strikingly inferior to the 71 percent survival in the TPN group, suggesting a trend to beneficial outcome using TPN. This is obviously an area for further controlled studies.

Intractable Diarrhea in Infancy

There are no randomized controlled studies in this area, but two small series [36, 40] with 12 of

12 survivors in an illness that historically has a 40 percent mortality [5] serve to justify parenteral nutritional support as an integral part of the therapy of this condition. No statement concerning efficacy can be made.

Surgery of the Gastrointestinal Tract in Infants

Data as to the efficacy of TPN in altering the outcome of patients with surgery of the gastrointestinal tract are primarily testimonial. There are no controlled studies. Heird and Winters [33] noted, after a detailed study of 21 patients for at least 12 months postoperatively, that 15 of the 21 patients who had required TPN for support had normal GI function. Two of the patients had special diet requirements, and the remaining four had died. They assess this result as a "dramatic positive outcome in a group of patients who, prior to the advent of TPN, would have had a very high mortality rate."

ADULT PROBLEMS

Gastrointestinal Fistulas

Since the classic work of Edmunds, Williams, and Welch [13] in isolating and identifying the causes of morbidity and mortality in gastrointestinal fistulas, therapy has improved to the extent that the usual outcome is favorable. Of the three major causes of death in the 1960 series, only sepsis remained as a common lethal complication in the more recent reports. Many of the authors of contemporary reviews of the therapy of GI fistulas enthusiastically endorse TPN as a bulwark of therapy and a factor that has revolutionized the care of these patients. In reality, two recent extensive reviews credit the progress in the 1960s (non-TPN nutritional support, control of sepsis, more careful monitoring, volume and electrolyte repletion, better respiratory support) with the major role in decreasing mortality from approximately 50 percent to less than 30 percent in more recent series. The effect of parenteral nutrition itself is once again less obvious. For example, it is generally stated that the management of fistulas with TPN produces several beneficial consequences:

1. Decrease in GI secretions. Although data in dogs seem clear [31], the effect of TPN on human GI tract secretions is less obvious. Some observers relate up to an 85 percent decrease in intestinal secretory activity [45], but others report that reduction in fistula output after initiation of TPN occurred in less than 50 percent of cases [3, 57].
2. Correction of protein depletion. It is difficult to attribute correction of albumin and total protein values to TPN in these patients when most series specifically stress the importance of intravenous replacement of whole blood and albumin as a part of the initial resuscitative and maintenance programs. In fact, Aguirre et al. [3] report that 14 of 38 patients with fistulas who were managed with TPN remained hypoproteinemic despite their parenteral nutrition and albumin infusions. Because of albumin's long half-life, it is unusual for serum albumin to increase rapidly with hyperalimentation. Further, recent studies from this laboratory [39a] cast doubts on whether albumin concentrations are accurate reflections of synthesis, since dilution is an uncorrected factor. Plasma levels of short turnover proteins may reflect better maintenance of hepatic protein synthesis, at least, with nutritional support.
3. Decrease in mortality. As with many of the other parameters by which success in such a complicated problem as intestinal fistulas is measured, mortality is a multifactorial problem. Sepsis, it is agreed, is the major cause of death in these patients now that malnutrition has largely been eliminated [3, 57]. The contribution of parenteral nutrition to the elimination or reduction of the incidence of sepsis is speculative. Two groups have spoken to the specific point of whether TPN itself has altered mortality figures in this group of patients. Fischer [16, 57] reports that prior to the utilization of TPN at the Massachusetts General Hospital (between 1960 and

Table 26-3. *Influence of TPN on Mortality and Closure of Gastrointestinal Fistulas*

Series	No. of Cases	TPN	Spontaneous Closure (%)	Total Closure	Mortality (%)
Edmunds et al. 1960 [13]	157	no			44
Sheldon et al. 1971 [56]	51	yes	15	82%	16
Voitk et al. 1973 [61]	29	no	75	75%	28 (16% if deaths from metastatic cancer are excluded)
MacFadyen et al. 1973 [45]	62	yes	71	92%	6
Bury 1974 [8]	80	no	70	79%	17
Aguirre et al. 1974 [3]	38	yes	29	79%	21
Fischer 1974 [16]	119	no	10		15
Reber et al. 1978 [49]	72 (1968–1971)	yes 35% no 65%	26	58/72	22
	114 (1972–1977)	yes 71% no 29%	35	89/114	22
Soeters et al. 1979 [57]	404 (1945–1975) 128 (1970–1975)	yes 57% no 43%	31	86/128	21

1970), 119 patients with GI fistulas were treated, with an overall mortality of 15 percent. Between 1970 and 1975, 138 patients with GI fistulas were treated with TPN as an important part of their management regimen, with an overall mortality of 21 percent. Reber et al. [49] reported their experience with patients of different time periods whose principal statistical difference was the presence or absence of TPN in the regimen. They found no difference in the fistula-related mortality (11%) or total mortality (22%) in the two groups. Tabulation of mortality figures in several large series, with and without parenteral nutrition, is given in Table 26-3.

4. Increase in spontaneous closure rates. As mentioned in previous discussion, the heterogeneity of the populations reported and the underlying etiologies of their fistulas make conclusions about the impact of TPN practically impossible. As seen in Table 26-3, spontaneous closure rates vary in the TPN series from 15 to 70 percent, with similar figures present in the series that had relied on GI feedings to maintain nutritional stability. Reber et al. [49] were able to see a difference in spontaneous closure rates in their populations managed with TPN (26 of 71, 37%) and without TPN (9 of 41, 22%) from 1972 to 1977. Soeters and Fischer [57], reported an increase in spontaneous closure rate from 10 to 31 percent. It appears that the etiology of the fistula, control of sepsis, location of the fistula, and anatomic considerations far outweigh the mechanism of nutritional support in determining spontaneous closure. There is no evidence to support the claim that parenteral nutrition is more efficacious than other methods of nutritional support in promoting spontaneous closures of intestinal fistulas [45, 56, 61]. However, nutritional support, in and of itself, is associated with an increased rate of spontaneous fistula closure.

Short Bowel Syndrome

It is obvious to all observers that TPN has dramatically altered the end result of the loss of massive amounts of small bowel. Prior to clinical use of

TPN, survival was judged to be dependent on the length and location of the remaining small bowel [32]. With the advent of prolonged parenteral nutrition, many patients have survived total or near-total resection of the small bowel for many years [54]. Eventual weaning from TPN to a form of oral nutrition still remains a problem, depending on the age of the patient, the length of bowel left [53], and the time elapsed from insult, but a few centers are committed to essentially life-long maintenance of nutritional integrity via TPN and an "artificial gut" [7, 53]. The ethical issues here are similar to those cited for long term hemodialysis and are beyond the scope of this review.

Inflammatory Bowel Disease

The answers to two major questions would summarize the contributions of parenteral nutrition to the care of patients with inflammatory bowel disease. Unfortunately, randomized controlled studies directed at these questions have not as yet been done and seem unlikely to be done, considering the nature of patients referred for TPN, and the tentative answers are based on retrospective reviews from various institutions. First, is TPN a useful adjunct to the therapy of inflammatory bowel disease? The consensus in the literature is a resounding *yes*. Fazio et al. [14] retrospectively analyzed their experience in inflammatory bowel disease with 58 patients in whom TPN was used as support and found that they fell into three groups. Thirty-six of the 58 proceeded with their surgical procedure as planned at the time of their admission to the hospital, but 30 of these 36 were believed to have had their course improved (definition unclear) by TPN. Six of the 36 were thought to have had courses unaltered by TPN. A second group of 9 of the 58 total patients had their operative procedures simplified after a course of TPN. The third group of 13 of 58 patients avoided their planned operation on the basis of clinical improvement during TPN. Unfortunately, evaluation of these data is made difficult by the lack of a concurrent control group. Data from other centers [60] suggest that a greater than 70 percent remission rate results from standard medical therapy. There is a similar 70 percent remission rate when elemental diets are used during acute exacerbations of inflammatory bowel disease [8, 62]. Reilly et al. [50] have carefully examined their experience with TPN in inflammatory bowel disease:

1. In the patients with regional enteritis or granulomatous colitis, surgery was avoided in 14 of 23 patients (once again, the 70 percent number appears).
2. In the patients with ulcerative colitis in whom standard medical therapy was unable to control the disease, addition of TPN did not add to the ability to avoid surgery.
3. In the same ulcerative colitis group, when compared to a group not undergoing hyperalimentation, but having similar surgical procedures, there was no difference in morbidity or mortality. There was a trend to decreased length of hospital stay, and some patients were converted from two-stage to one-stage procedures.

The second question is: What role does TPN have as "primary therapy" for inflammatory bowel disease? Fazio et al. [14] looked at 23 patients in whom they considered TPN as primary therapy (although it is unclear whether steroids or ACTH were also used). In 15 of the 23 or 65 percent (70% is again the magic number!), remission was obtained, whereas 8 of 23 went on to operation. Fleming et al. [20] examined 7 patients with extensive Crohn's disease managed primarily with home TPN and concluded that no complications, except malnutrition, were prevented or reversed by this regimen. The patients did increase their total body weight, serum albumin, and hemoglobin concentrations during TPN. It seems clear that TPN can ameliorate protein-calorie malnutrition in these patients, but any other asserted benefits remain unproven.*

Pancreatitis

The rationale for utilization of TPN in acute pancreatitis rests on two premises. First, maintenance of nutritional integrity in the absence of a completely functional GI tract and in the presence of severe illness is beneficial, particularly if the course is prolonged. Second, TPN may represent active intervention in the pathophysiology leading to the acute exacerbation (reversal of malnutrition, prevention of organ system failure, decreasing pancreatic exocrine secretion). Once again, no randomized prospective studies exist here. Retrospective clinical studies of Feller et al. [15], utilizing a primarily medical approach to severe pancreatitis with aggressive correction of nutritional depletion with TPN and enteral feedings, demonstrated a mortality rate of 14 percent, an improvement over previous experience in that institution, thought to be primarily due to attention to nutritional details. Lawson et al. [42] used a primarily operative approach to severe pancreatitis in a group that had a 100 percent mortality in their previous experience. The operations had included placement of jejunostomy catheters and preceded the availability of TPN. With subsequent aggressive enteral nutritional replacement, 11 of 15 or 74 percent of these critically ill patients survived. We reviewed a similar group of medically and surgically managed patients from the same institution who had been parenterally nourished during the acute phase of their illness, with an overall 80 percent survival [25]. In a subset of these patients, with nonfunctioning GI tracts for greater than one month, 12 of 15 or 80 percent survived. The similarity of these survival numbers has lead us to the tentative conclusion that the first premise, maintenance of nutritional integrity is important, is true. Table 26-4 tries to examine the second premise and reveals that TPN seems to have little if any effect on the incidence or outcome of the complications of acute pancreatitis, such as renal or respiratory failure. It should be remembered, however, that TPN was begun after 4 to 5 days, and the die was cast. Thus, we concluded that at least when begun 4–5 days after onset of disease, TPN is simply sophisticated nutritional support rather than active intervention directed against the poorly understood pathophysiology. Any method of enteral or parenteral feeding in this disease seems to offer equivalent benefits.

Anorexia Nervosa and Delayed Gastric Emptying

Two other areas in which TPN has been advocated as an adjunctive measure are anorexia nervosa and stomal obstruction following gastric resection. In anorexia nervosa, the malnutrition can be effectively controlled by TPN, but the centrally placed catheter offers a portal of entry for manipulative behavior. There is no evidence that enteral administration of diets via nasal or oral tubes is any less effective than parenteral feedings in this condition.

In delayed gastric emptying, a problem seen in less than 3 percent of gastric resections, functional rather than anatomic abnormalities predominate [9]. Whether nutritional support with TPN will alter the management and outcome of these patients is still unstudied. However, in the last 7 to 10 years a subtle difference in strategy has appeared. Jordan and Walker [39], in 1972, reviewed 21 patients with postgastrectomy emptying problems. On the basis of their review, they recommended operative intervention within 3 weeks, with placement of gastrostomy and jejunostomy tubes, as a minimal approach.

**Editor's Note:* A good deal of the problem in ascertaining whether TPN is efficacious in the tr[illegible]tment of inflammatory bowel disease relates to the control group. Most patients referred for TPN represent the failures of medical therapy. Logically, the control group would use medical therapy—no TPN. In most cases, this therapy is the one that has failed. The dilemma is obvious.

Table 26-4. *Complications of Acute Pancreatitis in Selected Published Series*

Author	Total Number of Patients and Selection Factor	TPN	Overall Mortality	Renal Failure		Respiratory Failure		Surgical Mortality
				Incidence	Mortality	Incidence	Mortality	
Goodgame [25]	46 (severe pancreatitis)	Yes	9/46 (20%)	7/46 (15%)	4/7 (57%)	13/46 (28%)	8/13 (62%)	8/36 (22%)
Gordon [27]	41 (unselected)	No	6/41 (15%)	6/41 (15%)	3/6 (50%)			
Interiano [37]	50 (unselected)	No	5/50 (10%)			9/50 (18%)	5/9 (55%)	
Gleidman [24]	26 (malignant pancreatitis)	No	9/26 (35%)					9/16 (56%)
Feller [15]	83 (severe pancreatitis)	Yes	12/83 (14%)			18/83 (22%)	8/18 (44%)	
Frey [22]	306 (unselected)	No	78/306 (25%)	19/306 (6%)	18/19 (95%)			36/211 (17%)
Ranson [48]	31 (severe pancreatitis)	?	15/31 (48%)	10/31 (32%)	6/10 (60%)	12/31 (39%)	9/12 (75%)	10/21 (48%)
Lawson [42]	15 (severe pancreatitis)	No	4/15 (26%)					4/16 (26%)

Cohen and Ottinger [9], reviewing 46 similar patients in a time period ending in 1974, found that only 10 percent had mechanical or anatomic factors responsible for the gastric obstruction. They recommended an aggressive diagnostic evaluation to rule out this possibility, to be followed by an extended period of nutritional support with TPN, reserving reoperation for mechanical obstruction of the gastric or efferent stoma or "the requirement for a feeding jejunostomy." No comparison of the two approaches has yet appeared in the literature.

Renal Failure

The treatment of acute renal failure with intravenous L-amino acids and hypertonic glucose (renal failure fluid—RFF) remains as the indication for which there is the most clinical support. The classic study of Abel et al. [1], which examined the effect of RFF versus hypertonic glucose alone in a randomized prospective double-blind clinical trial, demonstrated that the recovery from acute renal failure could be improved by utilization of the experimental mixture. Twenty-one of 28 patients receiving RFF recovered from their renal failure, whereas only 11 of 25 given glucose alone recovered ($p = 0.02$). Complications during the period of acute renal failure (pneumonia, generalized sepsis, and GI hemorrhage) were handled significantly better by the RFF group with respect to survival than by the control population. Baek et al. [6] examined 129 consecutive patients with acute renal failure admitted to an ICU. Sixty-six were given hypertonic glucose alone (greater than 100 gm per day) and 63 were given hypertonic glucose plus fibrin hydrolysate. The division of patients was done in a non-random fashion. The mortality in the glucose-alone group was 70 percent, but in the TPN group the mortality was 46 percent. TPN seemed to improve the survival rate in subgroups with septic and cardiovascular complications and in both the dialyzed and nondialyzed subgroups of these patients. For the continuing controversy as to whether essential amino acids alone or a low dose of essential and nonessential amino acids is more appropriate, see the chapter on renal failure (Chap. 18). The important message is that nutritional support is beneficial.

In summary, there is good clinical evidence that parenteral nutrition can promote recovery from an episode of acute renal failure. Survival from the complications of renal failure also seems to be improved by TPN. It is unclear whether in-hospital survival of chronic failure is affected by TPN [43].

Hepatic Failure

The magnitude of the problem of alcoholism and resultant hepatic dysfunction, combined with the frequency of hepatic failure in patients with multi-system illnesses, make nutritional support in hepatic failure a major clinical concern. Provision of adequate nitrogen for protein conservation and synthesis without aggravating encephalopathy has been a dilemma most recently attacked by Fischer and his coworkers. For this purpose they used a parenteral nutrition formula with diminished concentrations of aromatic amino acids (phenylalanine, tyrosine, tryptophan) and increased concentrations of the branched-chain amino acids (valine, leucine, and isoleucine) [18]. This approach has proved successful in supporting a small number of patients with concomitant infusion of large amounts of intravenous nitrogen and improvement in mental status [17]. Whether this approach will succeed in improving hepatic function and augmenting survival in these patients has yet to be demonstrated; more recent studies [21] suggest improved survival in alcoholic hepatitis, similar to what has been reported as a result of an aggressive nutritional support [47]. A randomized prospective study is in progress.*

*Editor's Note: As of February 1982, three multicenter trials in Italy, Brazil, and the United States have demonstrated the efficacy of BCAA enriched amino acid solutions in nutritional support and treatment of patients with hepatic encephalopathy. In these studies, glucose was used as a caloric source. In two other studies in France, with fat as a caloric source, efficacy was not demonstrated. All studies but one are unpublished at this time (F. Rossi-Fanelli et al. Branched chain amino acids vs. lactulose in the treatment of hepatic coma: A controlled study. *Dig. Dis. Sci.* 27:929, 1982).

Cancer

The combination of aggressive chemotherapeutic, surgical, and radiation attempts at cancer therapy and the increasing experience with parenteral nutrition have led to the use of TPN as an adjunct in the treatment of many tumors. Initial experiences were reported to have resulted in few complications, no evidence of increased tumor growth, diminution in weight loss, and increased feelings of well-being among the patients so treated [10, 55]. Many additional uncontrolled experiences have accumulated substantiating these observations. It seems clear that TPN can prevent malnutrition and correct existing nutritional deficits in this as in all other groups of patients examined. The critical questions remain:

1. Does correction of nutritional deficits affect the course of antitumor therapy?
2. Does maintenance of nutritional integrity improve the survival of these patients or reduce the complications of their therapy?

Copeland et al. [11] reported a group of 39 nutritionally depleted patients with malignant disease, 95 percent of whom were able to complete a planned course of radiation therapy, despite their poor-risk status, when supported by total parenteral nutrition. Lanzotti et al. [41] retrospectively analyzed 30 patients with non-oat cell bronchogenic carcinoma undergoing aggressive chemotherapy with five drugs. Ten patients had received TPN during their course and 20 had not. They found that 5 of 10 of the TPN group were responders to the chemotherapeutic regimen, whereas 6 of 20 of the non-TPN group had a response. When the groups were further subdivided to exclude those patients who had lost less than 6 percent of their usual body weight (that is, to look at only those people who were nutritionally depleted when they began therapy), a statistical difference emerged. Fifty percent of the TPN group had responded, whereas none of the non-TPN group had demonstrated a clinical response. It is of interest that no difference in GI or hematologic toxicity could be detected between the two groups.

Table 26-5. *Response of Tumor to Experimental Regimen*

	TPN	No TPN
Partial response	4 (31%)	1 (7%)
Stable disease	8 (62%)	8 (62%)
Progressive disease	1 (7%)	4 (31%)

Source: B. F. Issell et al. Protection against chemotherapy toxicity by IV hyperalimentation. *Cancer Treat. Rep.* 62: 1139, 1978.

Issell et al. [38] have published the only randomized prospective study comparing TPN with no TPN in a chemotherapeutic adjuvant setting. Twenty-six patients with extensive squamous cell carcinoma of the lung were treated with chemotherapy and immunotherapy. Thirteen received TPN during their first course of therapy and 13 did not. Statistically significant less myelosuppression, as measured by the lowest recorded neutrophil and total leukocyte counts, was seen in the TPN group. Table 26-5 illustrates the relationship of chemotherapeutic response to TPN administration. There was no significant difference seen in tumor response between the two groups.

The National Cancer Institute has an ongoing randomized prospective study comparing TPN with standard enteral nutritional support in children undergoing aggressive chemotherapy for metastatic Ewing's sarcoma, osteogenic sarcoma, neuroblastoma, and rhabdomyosarcoma. Though the numbers are still small and the study is ongoing, no differences between the groups in response or survival have been noted. As expected, while the control group lost 3.25 kg during the course of therapy (6% of original weight), the TPN group gained 4.5 kg. Table 26-6 summarizes our clinical data in this group of patients as of November, 1978.

It is worthwhile to mention that careful metabolic studies by Holroyde et al. have demon-

Table 26-6. *Total Parenteral Nutrition as an Adjunct to Aggressive Chemotherapy—NCI 11/28/78*

	Total Patients	Survival	NED	Mean Survival Time (wks)	Died in Chemotherapy
TPN	9	5	1/5	43 (2–91)	1/4
Control	10	6	6/6	40 (3–95)	4/5

strated that TPN in patients with cancer results in respiratory quotients greater than 1.0 (implying fat synthesis rather than CO_2 production from the administered carbohydrate). They also observed moderate lactic acidemia in 25 percent of the patients studied. We have reported profound lactic acidosis in one patient with a bulky tumor who was given hypertonic glucose as a therapeutic adjunct.

On the basis of data at hand, prophylactic TPN does not seem warranted prior to or during cancer therapy. Treatment of existing or developing nutritional depletion prior to or during aggressive radiation or chemotherapy may improve the chances of completing the planned course of therapy without altering the end result.

PREOPERATIVE PREPARATION

Studley noted, in 1936, that patients who exhibited loss of 20 percent of usual body weight prior to gastric surgery experienced a 33 percent mortality, whereas those who had lost no weight had only 3.5 percent operative mortality [59]. This correlation between malnutrition and surgical complications has been extended with the findings that 16 to 50 percent of the patients admitted to a VA Hospital for elective surgery were malnourished as defined by low serum albumin, low transferrin level, and/or cutaneous anergy [46]. These malnourished patients then had the preponderance of postoperative complications seen in this study.

Several studies have looked at the ability of short-term preoperative or postoperative TPN to improve the clinical course of malnourished patients.

Abel et al. [2] compared, in a randomized prospective fashion, the clinical course of malnourished cardiac patients, 20 treated with postoperative TPN and 24 treated without TPN. The mortality in the TPN group was 20 percent and in the control group 12.5 percent (no significant difference). Postoperative parenteral nutrition had no effect on such parameters as time of required ventilatory assistance, return to full consciousness, renal failure, pneumonia, total hospital stay, or cost of hospitalization. Holter and Fischer [35] examined the effect of 48 to 72 hours of preoperative TPN, followed by postoperative TPN, on the course of malnourished patients undergoing GI surgery for malignant disease, and compared them to two control groups, one that did not lose weight and another with similar weight loss randomized not to receive TPN. The group with weight loss and no TPN had a significant morbidity and mortality as compared with the no-weight-loss group. The group with weight loss and TPN had an identical mortality, but morbidity which was intermediate. At the time of the report the authors extrapolated that if the beneficial trend were to become statistically significant, an additional 200 patients would have to be added to the study. The study is now in progress.

Although there is no current evidence that short-term pre- or postoperative TPN will influence the outcome of major surgery in nutritionally depleted patients, there are merely suggestions of an effect for which studies are now in progress.*

**Editor's Note:* Since preparation of this chapter, a recently published study documents decreased mortality in patients undergoing preoperative parenteral nutrition prior to major

POST-TRAUMATIC CATABOLIC STATES (BURNS, MAJOR TRAUMA, AND SEPSIS)

There are no studies of comparative modalities of nutritional support or of nutritional support versus starvation in regard to the end results of this critically ill group of patients. It is widely accepted that because some GI dysfunction usually accompanies these conditions, early hyperalimentation may alleviate some of the obligate loss of body mass and, inferentially, make survival more likely. There is clear evidence of elevated caloric needs with resting metabolic expenditures as high as 125 to 200 percent of normal [29]. This increased caloric expenditure is accompanied by profound changes in hormonal and metabolic substrate levels, including hyperglycemia, increased hepatic gluconeogenesis, increased glucose turnover [23, 28], decreased insulin-to-glucagon molar ratio [51, 64], and alterations of serum and muscle amino acid composition different from those seen in starvation alone [65]. Major trauma leads to loss of body nitrogen and muscle mass [44]. There is good evidence that positive nitrogen and caloric balance can usually be restored with increased intake, either intravenously or enterally [12, 63]. Additional sparing of protein can be induced by exogenous insulin [67].

Recently, Alexander and coworkers [4] have reported evidence that increasing the percentage of calories given as protein in the diet in a randomized stratified study of burned children resulted in increased survival, which was accompanied by increased measurable parameters of nonspecific host resistance. The study, however, was done orally, with most of the protein and calories administered orally or by tube feeding and only occasionally by vein.

Definitive answers of relative efficacy in this group of patients in regard to parenteral nutrition must await a clear categorization of this heterogeneous group regarding severity of insult, nutritional status, hormonal picture, and metabolic profile. However, at present, there is no evidence that early parenteral nutrition alters the clinical course other than to reduce weight loss.

Freund, Fischer, and coworkers [21] have argued for a specially designed solution, for treatment of patients with sepsis. This proposed solution, currently under investigation, would contain a higher ratio of the branched-chain amino acids, with the hypothesis that under stress and sepsis improved outcome will result, increased branched chain amino acids resulting in decreased protein breakdown. In addition the branched-chain amino acids may be utilized as an energy source. Other perhaps beneficial effects of the branched-chain amino acids include preventing or improving septic metabolic encephalopathy [21].

Although TPN represents a powerful tool for maintaining and restoring nutritional integrity in the acutely and chronically ill patient, the enthusiasm for its impact on particular pathologic processes is largely unproven. TPN can preserve body weight in almost all patient groups studied, although this may be largely fat rather than lean body mass. There is evidence for improved outcome with TPN in premature infants with respiratory distress syndrome, children with intractable diarrhea, patients with short bowel syndrome, and those with acute renal failure.

Other studies utilizing nutrition also demonstrate improved outcome in a few cases, largely in burns [4] and alcoholic hepatitis [47], but most of these patients have been fed orally. There may be a difference between the efficacy of the oral and intravenous routes. All agree that the malnourished patient does not fare as well as the well-nourished patient in any therapeutic setting. However, the question that remains is whether a malnourished patient can be converted to a well-nourished patient with improved outcome in a relatively short period by intravenous techniques.

This work certainly does not represent an inclusive list of the indications for parenteral nutrition, but it does demonstrate the limited

---

operations for gastrointestinal carcinoma (J. M. Muller, C. Dienst, U. Brenner, and M. Pichlmaier, Preoperative parenteral feeding in patients with gastrointestinal carcinoma. *Lancet* 1:68, 1982).

amount of controlled experience with TPN in other disease entities. The energy that has been fruitfully directed toward developing the methodology and techniques that make TPN possible must now be directed toward more completely defining its optimal role in patient care.

REFERENCES

1. Abel, R. M., Beck, C. H., Jr., Abbott, W. M., Ryan, J. A., Barrett, G. O., and Fischer, J. E. Improved survival from acute renal failure following treatment with intravenous essential L-amino acids and glucose. *N. Engl. J. Med.* 288: 695, 1973.
2. Abel, R. M., Fischer, J. E., Buckley, M. J., Barrett, G. O., and Austen, W. G. Malnutrition in cardiac patients: Results of a prospective randomized evaluation of early postoperative TPN. *Acta Chir. Scand.* [Suppl.] 466:77, 1977.
3. Aguirre, A., Fischer, J. E., and Welch, C. E. The role of surgery and hyperalimentation in therapy of gastrointestinal-cutaneous fistulae. *Ann. Surg.* 180:393, 1974.
4. Alexander, J. W., MacMillan, B. G., Stinnett, J. D., Ogle, C. K., Bozian, R. C., Fischer, J. E., Oakes, J. B., Morris, M. J., and Krummel, R. Beneficial effects of aggressive protein feeding in severely burned children. *Ann. Surg.* 192:505, 1980.
5. Avery, G. B., Villavicencio, O., Lilly, J. R., and Randolph, J. G. Intractable diarrhea in early infancy. *Pediatrics* 41:712, 1960.
6. Baek, S., Makabali, G. G., Bryan-Brown, C. W., Kusek, J., and Shoemaker, W. C. The influence of parenteral nutrition on the course of acute renal failure. *Surg. Gynecol. Obstet.* 141:405, 1975.
7. Broviac, J. W., and Scribner, B. H. Prolonged parenteral nutrition in the home. *Surg. Gynecol. Obstet.* 139:24, 1974.
8. Bury, K. D. Elemental Diets. In J. E. Fischer (Ed.), *Total Parenteral Nutrition.* Boston: Little, Brown, 1976. Pp. 395–412.
9. Cohen, A. M., and Ottinger, L. W. Delayed gastric emptying after gastric surgery. *Ann. Surg.* 184:689, 1976.
10. Copeland, E. M., Daly, J. M., and Dudrick, S. J. Nutrition as an adjunct to cancer treatment in the adult. *Cancer Res.* 37:2451, 1977.
11. Copeland, E. M., Sonehon, E. A., MacFadyen, B. V., Rapp, M. A., and Dudrick, S. J. Intravenous hyperalimentation as an adjunct to radiation therapy. *Cancer* 39:609, 1977.
12. Davies, J. W. L. The Nutrition of Patients with Burns. In J. R. Richards and J. M. Kinney (Eds.), *Nutritional Aspects of Care in the Critically Ill.* Edinburgh: Churchill Livingstone, 1977. Pp. 595–624.
13. Edmunds, L. H., Jr., Williams, G. M., and Welch, C. E. External fistulas arising from gastro-intestinal tract. *Ann. Surg.* 152:445, 1960.
14. Fazio, V. W., Kodner, I., Jagelman, D. G., Turnball, R. B., and Weakley, F. L. Inflammatory disease of the bowel: Parenteral nutrition as primary or adjunctive treatment. *Dis. Colon Rectum* 19:574, 1976.
15. Feller, J. H., Brown, R. A., Tonssaint, G. P. M., and Thompson, A. G. Changing methods in the treatment of severe pancreatitis. *Am. J. Surg.* 127:196, 1974.
16. Fischer, J. E. Hyperalimentation. In C. Rob (Ed.), *Advances in Surgery.* Chicago: Year Book, 1977. Vol. II, pp. 1–69.
17. Fischer, J. E., Rosen, H. M., Ebeid, A. M., James, J. H., Keane, J. M., and Soeters, P. B. The effects of normalization of plasma amino acids on hepatic encephalopathy in man. *Surgery* 80:77, 1976.
18. Fischer, J. E., Yoshimura, N., James, J. H., Cummings, M. G., Abel, R. M., and Diendorfer, F. Plasma amino acids in patients with hepatic encephalopathy: Effects of amino acid infusion. *Am. J. Surg.* 127:40, 1974.
19. Fitzhardinge, P. M., Pape, K., Aistikaitis, M., Boyle, M., Ashby, S., Rowley, A., Netley, C., and Swyer, P. R. Mechanical ventilation of infants of less than 1501 gm birth weight: Health, growth and neurologic sequelae. *J. Pediatr.* 88: 17, 1971.
20. Fleming, C. R., McGill, O. B., and Berkner, S. Home parenteral nutrition as primary therapy in patients with extensive Crohn's disease of the small bowel and malnutrition. *Gastroenterolcgy* 73:1077, 1977.
21. Freund, H., Dienstag, J., Lehrich, J., et al. Infusion of branched-chain amino acids in patients with hepatic encephalopathy. *Ann. Surg.* 192: 209, 1982.
22. Frey, C. The operative treatment of pancreatitis. *Arch. Surg.* 98:406, 1969.
23. Giddings, A. E. B. The control of plasma glucose in the surgical patient. *Br. J. Surg.* 61:787, 1974.
24. Gleidman, M. L., Balooke, H. G., and Rosen, R. G. Acute pancreatitis. *Curr. Probl. Surg.* August, 1970.
25. Goodgame, J. T., Jr., and Fischer, J. E. Parenteral nutrition in the treatment of acute pancreatitis: Effect on complications and mortality. *Ann. Surg.* 186:651, 1977.
26. Goodgame, J. T., Jr., Pizzo, P., and Brennan,

M. F. Iatrogenic lactic acidosis, association with hypertonic glucose administration in a patient with cancer. *Cancer* 42:800, 1978.

27. Gordon, D., and Calne, R. Y. Renal failure in acute pancreatitis. *Br. Med. J.* 3:801, 1972.
28. Gump, F. E., Long, C., Killian, P., and Kinney, J. M. Studies of glucose intolerance in septic injured patients. *J. Trauma* 14:378, 1974.
29. Gump, F. E., Martin, P., and Kinney, J. M. Oxygen consumption and caloric expenditure in surgical patients. *Surg. Gynecol. Obstet.* 137: 499, 1973.
30. Gunn, T., Reaman, G., Outerbridge, E. W., and Colle, E. Peripheral total parenteral nutrition for premature infants with the respiratory distress syndrome: A controlled study. *J. Pediatr.* 92:608, 1978.
31. Hamilton, R. F., Davis, W. C., Stephenson, D. V., and Magee, D. F. Effects of parenteral hyperalimentation on upper gastrointestinal tract secretions. *Arch. Surg.* 102:348, 1971.
32. Harrison, R. J., and Booth, C. C. Massive resection of the small intestine after occlusion of the superior mesenteric artery. *Gut* 1:237, 1960.
33. Heird, W. C., and Winters, R. W. Total parenteral nutrition: The state of the art. *J. Pediatr.* 86:2, 1975.
34. Holroyde, C. P., Myers, R. N., Smink, R. D., Putnam, R. C., Paul, P., and Reichard, G. A. Metabolic response to total parenteral nutrition in cancer patients. *Cancer Res.* 37:3109, 1979.
35. Holter, A. R., Rosen, H. M., and Fischer, J. E. The effect of TPN on major surgery in patients with malignant disease: A prospective study. *Acta Chir. Scand.* [Suppl.] 466:86, 1977.
36. Hyman, C. J., Reiter, J., Rodman, J., and Drash, A. L. Parenteral and oral alimentation in the treatment of the nonspecific protracted diarrheal syndrome of infancy. *J. Pediatr.* 78:17, 1971.
37. Interiano, B., Stuard, I. D., and Hyde, R. W. Acute respiratory distress syndrome in pancreatitis. *Ann. Intern. Med.* 77:923, 1972.
38. Issell, B. F., Valdivieso, M., Zaren, H. A., Dudrick, S. J., Freireich, E. J., Copeland, E. W., and Bodey, G. P. Protection against chemotherapy toxicity by IV hyperalimentation. *Cancer Treat. Rep.* 62:1139, 1973.
39. Jordan, G. L., and Walker, L. L. Severe problems with gastric emptying after gastric surgery. *Ann. Surg.* 177:660, 1973.

39a. Karlberg, I., Kern, K., and Fischer, J. E. Albumin turnover in sarcoma-bearing rats in relation to cancer anorexia. *Am. J. Surg.* in press, 1982.

40. Keating, J. P., and Ternberg, J. L. Amino Acid-hypertonic glucose treatment for intractable diarrhea in infants. *Am. J. Dis. Child.* 122:226, 1971.
41. Lanzotti, V. J., Copeland, E. M., George, S. L., Dudrick, S. J., and Samuels, M. L. Cancer chemotherapeutic response and intravenous hyperalimentation. *Cancer Chemother. Rep.* 59: 437, 1975.
42. Lawson, D. W., Daggett, W. M., and Civetta, J. M., et al. Surgical treatment of acute necrotizing pancreatitis. *Ann. Surg.* 172:605, 1970.
43. Leonard, C. D., Luke, R. G., and Seigel, R. R. Parenteral essential amino acids in acute renal failure. *Urology* 6:154, 1975.
44. Long, C. L., Spencer, J. L., Kinney, J. M., and Geiger, J. W. Carbohydrate metabolism in man. *J. Appl. Physiol.* 31:102, 1971.
45. MacFadyen, B. V., Dudrick, S. J., and Ruberg, R. L. Management of gastrointestinal fistulas with parenteral hyperalimentation. *Surgery* 74: 100, 1973.
46. Mullen, J. L., Gertner, M. H., Buzby, G. P., Goodhart, G. L., and Rosato, E. F. Implications of malnutrition in the surgical patient. *Arch. Surg.* 114:121, 1979.
47. Nasrallah, S. M., and Galambos, J. T. Amino acid therapy in alcoholic hepatitis. *Lancet* 2: 1276, 1980.
48. Ranson, J. H. C., Rifkind, K. M., and Rosen, D. F., et al. Prognostic signs and the role of operative management in acute pancreatitis. *Surg. Gynecol. Obstet.* 139:69, 1974.
49. Reber, H. A., Roberts, C., Way, L. W., and Dunphy, J. E. Management of external gastrointestinal fistulas. *Ann. Surg.* 188:460, 1978.
50. Reilly, J., Ryan, J. A., Strole, W., and Fischer, J. E. Hyperalimentation in inflammatory bowel disease. *Am. J. Surg.* 131:192, 1976.
51. Rocha, D. M., Sauternsanio, F., Fallona, G. R., and Unger, R. H. Abnormal pancreatic alpha-cell function in bacterial infections. *N. Engl. J. Med.* 288:700, 1973.
52. Ryan, J. A., Jr., Abel, R. M., Abbott, W. M., Hopkins, C. C., Chasney, T. M., Colley, R., Phillips, K., and Fischer, J. E. Catheter complications in total parenteral nutrition: A prospective study of 200 consecutive patients. *N. Engl. J. Med.* 290:757, 1974.
53. Scheflan, M., Gall, S. J., Perrotto, J., and Fischer, J. E. Intestinal adaptation after intensive resection of the small intestine and prolonged administration of parenteral nutrition. *Surg. Gynecol. Obstet.* 143:757, 1976.
54. Schribner, B. H., Cole, J. J., Christopher, T. G., Vizzo, J. E., Atkins, R. C., and Blagg, C. R.

Long-term total parenteral nutrition. *J.A.M.A.* 212:457, 1970.
55. Schwartz, G. F., Green, H. L., Bendon, M. L., et al. Combined parenteral hyperalimentation and chemotherapy in the treatment of dessemi-nated solid tumors. *Am. J. Surg.* 121:169, 1971.
56. Sheldon, G. F., Gardiner, B. N., Way, L. W., and Dunphy, H. M. Management of gastrointestinal fistulas. *Surg. Gynecol. Obstet.* 133:385, 1971.
57. Soeters, P. B., Ebeid, A. M., Fischer, J. E. Review of 404 patients with gastrointestinal fistulas: Impact of parenteral nutrition. *Ann. Surg.* 190:189, 1979.
58. Solassol, C., Joyeux, H., Etco, L., Pujol, H., and Romieu, C. New techniques for long-term intravenous feeding. *Ann. Surg.* 179:519, 1974.
59. Studley, H. O. Percentage of weight loss: A basic indication of surgical risk in patients with chronic peptic ulcer. *J.A.M.A.* 106:458, 1936.
60. Truelove, S. C., and Jewell, D. P. Intensive intravenous regimen for severe attacks of ulcerative colitis. *Lancet* 1:1067, 1974.
61. Voitk, A. J., Eschave, V., Brown, R. A., McArdle, A. H., and Gurd, F. N. Elemental diet in the treatment of fistulas of the alimentary tract. *Surg. Gynecol. Obstet.* 137:68, 1973.
62. Voitk, A. J., Eschave, V., Feller, J. H., et al. Experience with elemental diets in the treatment of inflammatory bowel disease. Is this primary therapy? *Arch. Surg.* 107:329, 1973.
63. Wilmore, D. W. Nutrition and metabolism following thermal injury. *Clin. Plast. Surg.* 1:603, 1974.
64. Wilmore, D. W., Moylan, J. A., Pruitt, B. A., Lindsey, C. A., Faloona, G. R., and Unger, R. H. Hyperglucagonaemia after burns. *Lancet* 1:73, 1974.
65. Wilson, R. E., Christensen, C., and LeBlanc, L. P. Oxygen consumption in critically ill surgical patients. *Ann. Surg.* 176:801, 1972.
66. Winick, M. Malnutrition and brain development. *J. Pediatr.* 74:667, 1969.
67. Woolfson, A. M. J., Heatley, R. V., and Allison, S. P. Insulin to inhibit protein catabolism after injury. *N. Engl. J. Med.* 300:14, 1979.

Index

Index